NATURAL COMPOUNDS
in CANCER THERAPY

NATURAL COMPOUNDS
in CANCER THERAPY

JOHN BOIK

Editor: Silvine Farnell
Cover design: Michelle Lundquist

Publisher's Cataloging-in-Publication (Provided by Quality Books, Inc.)

Boik, John.
     Natural compounds in cancer therapy / [John Boik].--
1st ed.
     p. cm.
     Includes biographical references and index.
     ISBN 0-9648280-1-4

     1. Cancer--Alternative treatment. 2. Herbs--
Therapeutic use. 3. Alternative medicine. I. Title.

     RC271.A62B65 2001   616.99'406
                                    QBI00-971

Library of Congress Control Number: 2001117271

Disclaimer
Medical knowledge is constantly expanding. As new experimental and clinical experiences are gained, modifications to research and treatment protocols are required. The author and publisher of this book have consulted sources believed to be reliable in their effort to provide information that is complete and true to the body of knowledge available at the time of publication. However, due to the possibility of human error or changes in medical knowledge, neither the author, publisher, nor any other party involved with the publication or preparation of this book warrants that the information contained herein is fully accurate or complete, and these parties are not responsible for any omissions or errors, or for the results obtained from using this information. Readers are advised to confirm all such information with appropriate written sources and experts in the field. Neither the publisher nor author advocate the use of any particular therapy but believe this information should be made available to the public. There is always some risk involved in therapy, and the publisher and author are not responsible for any adverse effects, lack of efficacy, or consequences that may result from using the material presented in this book.

Copies can be ordered directly from:
     Oregon Medical Press, LLC
     315 10th Avenue North
     Princeton, Minnesota 55371, USA
     Phone: (763) 389-0768
     Fax: (612) 395-5239
     Sales: 800-610-0768
     e-mail: sales@ompress.com
     web: secure online ordering at www.ompress.com

Web Site
Please visit the Oregon Medical Press web site at www.ompress.com. Our intent is to use this web site as a vehicle for collecting and disseminating information from practitioners, researchers, patients, and product suppliers who have an interest in the material contained in this book. **In addition, the web site contains errata as well as research updates to the material in this book.** If you do not have access to the web, errata and research updates are available from the Oregon Medical Press office for a $5.00 postage and handling fee.

CONTENTS

As a practicing cancer physician, I find my patients often come to their appointments with a sheaf of papers downloaded from the Internet, seeking guidance. John Boik's previous book, *Cancer and Natural Medicine*, is dog-eared because it has been a constant source of information in my own practice. I am delighted to add his new book, *Natural Compounds in Cancer Therapy*, to my shelf; it deserves to be included in the personal reference library of every researcher and cancer doctor. But most of all, it is my hope this book will be read by every cancer patient interested in including natural compounds in his or her treatment.

Cancer patients and cancer physicians are two sides of a single coin: we share similar hopes and dilemmas. Patients hope to be cured of cancer without paying an unbearable price; doctors hope to cure the cancer without harming the patient. Understandably, cancer patients want to survive not only the disease but also the treatment, without loss of function or quality of life. The dilemma, of course, is that when you blast cancer with the big guns of modern Western medicine, little may be left standing after the smoke clears.

Faced with dismaying treatment options, it is no wonder that horrified patients turn to alternative therapies. Unfortunately, in seeking to educate themselves, they find information that is unscientific, disorganized, or biased by media or commercial hype. That is why everyone should welcome this book; it is honest, scientific, it organizes the available information, and it fills a huge need—for patients, doctors, researchers, and everyone concerned with better treatments for cancer.

As its starting point, this groundbreaking book adopts the scientific approach. Scientists and physicians demand proof that alternative treatments work, and the book adheres to the scientific accountability necessary to satisfy these demands. This approach is also important for patients because it helps them see cancer as a multifaceted process, not a sole event. Boik shows us why each part of the process is a potential target for treatment, and why all parts will be inhibited most effectively when combinations of compounds are used. In other words, instead of looking for a single magic bullet to cure cancer, we would do well to consider that a holster full of carefully chosen ones might produce the greatest good. Overall, this book is unique in integrating basic information on molecular biology with clinical targets for cancer therapy, and will be of use to anyone wanting to understand either.

In addition to the scientific information it provides, the book makes a crucial contribution by drawing a clear, organized picture of what we know so far about natural compounds. Today, doctors and patients alike have to sort through an overwhelming bombardment of information on both natural and traditional cancer therapies. Boik gives us an extremely valuable overview of what is known and what remains to be learned. The use of natural compounds in cancer therapy is a field still in its infancy, as he states, but publication of this book is a huge step forward.

For the patient, this book addresses the hype in the lay media about the merits of natural compounds and counters it with solid, scientific information. It emphasizes the scientific rationale for a multipronged approach and provides an organized starting point for a team effort by patients and their doctors.

For the physician, Boik delivers a better scientific understanding of the activities of natural compounds and the scientific basis for using them in applied cancer therapy. Physicians desperately need this information for two reasons. First, traditional Western medicine in the past has discounted the role of natural compounds in cancer therapy because the scientific approach was lacking. Second, the modern physician needs to serve patients who are sorting through more information than ever before. With this book, the value of using natural compounds in cancer therapy will gain new respect because it makes the scientific framework accessible to the physician for the first time.

For the researcher, this book organizes the details of the work done so far, which for the most part is at the level of in-vitro (test tube) and animal studies. But it also provides the big picture, indicating how the results of these studies can guide human investigations—the next logical and necessary step toward developing effective natural compounds for cancer treatment. It will help researchers set the direction for this undertaking.

Natural Compounds in Cancer Therapy fills the gap between patient expectations and the reality of scientific information available in the field. It is a bridge between the skepticism of physicians and the hope of patients. John Boik provides physicians, patients, and researchers with a map of where we are, where we need to go, and how we will get there.

I hope that one day we will not need to label medicine as alternative or traditional, complementary or integrative, Eastern or Western, but simply "Good Medicine."

Good medicine will be defined as medicine that prevents illness, cures disease, avoids injury to the body, and brings comfort to the soul of the patient. We will help cancer patients by curing them sometimes, treating them meanwhile, comforting them ever, hoping with them always.

Israel Barken, M.D.
Urologic Oncologist

Chairman and Medical Director
Prostate Cancer Research and Education Foundation
San Diego, California

This book discusses numerous natural compounds that show promise in the treatment of cancer. It examines fully what research has told us about them, and it proposes ways of using them that could significantly increase their value in cancer treatment beyond what has previously been demonstrated. To understand the meaning of this new approach, one needs to see it in the context of the big picture of cancer research.

We stand at a turning point in the field of cancer chemotherapy. The last 50 years have been dominated by drugs that are not highly specific to cancer cells. Being nonspecific, these drugs also destroy normal cells, and in the process can cause significant and sometimes deadly adverse effects. Before long, a new generation of more powerful but less toxic drugs promises to be available. These new drugs will target events and processes that are more specific to cancer cells, and thus they will not be as harmful to normal cells. This revolution in therapy is already evident in the laboratory, and within the next 10 years or so it will become evident in the clinic. The ability to design and test this new generation of drugs comes from the many scientific discoveries made over the last 20 years that allow us to peer into the workings of a cancer cell at the molecular level. By seeing more clearly how cancer cells work, we are now better able to design drugs to halt their proliferation and spread. This new approach of targeting the mechanisms by which cancer cells prosper has been called, appropriately, a mechanism-based approach.

These developments paint a very encouraging picture for the eventual success of modern medicine in its battle to defeat cancer. But with such promising drugs on the horizon, the reader may ask, "Why does it make sense to turn to the study of natural compounds?"

WHY NATURAL COMPOUNDS?

There are three main reasons why natural compounds are worth studying. First, natural compounds that show anticancer potential fit into the mechanism-based approach as perfectly as a hand fits into a glove. All the natural compounds discussed in this book have been reported to inhibit cancer. Although most of the information available comes from preclinical (test tube and animal) studies, as is the case with most new mechanism-based drugs, some human studies have also been conducted. There is solid evidence that these compounds inhibit cancer by interfering with one or more of the mechanisms that researchers now feel are central to

cancer progression. In fact, some of the natural compounds discussed here have been used as probes in studies that unraveled the mechanisms of cancer progression.

This is not to imply that these natural compounds have been clinically proven to inhibit cancer. Multiple human trials will be needed for that. What matters is that the preclinical information presented here, as well as data from the human trials, is promising. And the most crucial point, central to this book, is that the beneficial effects of these compounds are likely to be much more apparent when they are used in large combinations, permitting additive and synergistic interactions to occur.

Second, although the future does look bright for eventual success in the fight against cancer, we are not there yet. Much more work remains to be done. As a science, the field of natural compound research can contribute to a greater understanding of cancer and a faster development of successful therapies.

Third, we must study natural compounds because they are already being used in cancer treatment (and in the treatment of other diseases). For better or for worse, hundreds of thousands if not millions of patients around the world are experimenting with natural compounds in their efforts to heal themselves of cancer. Researchers estimate that anywhere from 10 to 80 percent of U.S., European, Australian, and Mexican cancer patients use some form of complementary medicine as part of their overall therapy.[1-12, a] For many of these patients, the use of natural compounds is an essential part of the complementary approach. For example, two studies in the United States have reported that roughly 40 to 60 percent of cancer patients who use some form of complementary medicine include the use of herbs, vitamins, antioxidant, or all three.[12, 13] Most of these patients are using natural compounds without the guidance of their oncologist or any real guidance from scientific studies. Because the popularity of using natural compounds in cancer treatment appears to be growing rather than declining, we are compelled to study natural compounds so that we can properly guide the public.

---

[a] *Superscript numbers throughout the book refer to the numbered references at the end of each chapter. Hence, some numbers will occasionally be repeated or appear out of sequence.*

OBSTACLES TO RESEARCH ON NATURAL COMPOUNDS

Certainly, natural compounds have received some research attention, as is evidenced by the many studies in this book. But this is still a small number of studies compared to what is needed. There appear to be two main reasons why research is still lacking.

First, structure patents, granted for new and unique chemical structures, are impossible to obtain for the natural compounds discussed here, since their structures are already common knowledge. For this reason, these compounds are not generally thought of as profitable. Use patents, granted for a new and unique use of a compound, are somewhat easier to obtain for natural compounds, but these patents are less valuable than structure patents.

The ability to obtain a patent, especially a structure patent, is a very important aspect of drug development. A massive number of studies are required to test a drug and get it approved for market, and the cost of these studies can be many millions, possibly hundreds of millions of dollars. Pharmaceutical companies recoup this investment by either licensing their patent to other manufacturers or by acting as the sole manufacturer themselves. Since a large portion of the total research money available comes from pharmaceutical companies, the natural compounds discussed in this book have not received the full attention they deserve.[a]

Second, adequate attention is not given to the natural compounds I discuss because none are likely to become the "silver bullet" miracle cancer cure for which everyone has been searching. In fact, when used alone, the inhibitory effects of most of these compounds would be considered modest at best. Their true potential will be realized only when they are used in synergistic combinations, and here they may shine.

SYNERGISTIC INTERACTIONS

Until now, the search for miracle cures has meant that compounds not likely to be silver bullets are often viewed as unworthy of further investigation. It is my belief, however, that this search for the silver bullet is actually one reason we have not yet found many suitable cancer treatments. The new mechanism-based approach informs us that many different events contribute to the eventual success of a cancer. Any single drug can at best target a small number of these events, leaving the rest to occur uninterrupted. Moreover, we know that cancer cells have some ability to adapt to therapy. We can imagine that a cancer cell can adapt better to one or a few interrupted events than to many. Hence, my central thesis is that the most successful cancer therapies will be those that target all the primary events involved in cancer cell survival. The second part to this thesis is that to accomplish this task, multiple compounds used in combination will be necessary. Natural compounds are ideally suited for this type of application; they are active at reasonable concentrations, and yet their mild nature allows a variety of large combinations to be used safely.

There are several reasons why the concept of using large synergistic combinations of compounds has not been embraced by Western medical science. First, although small combinations of chemotherapy drugs are routinely used in research and clinical practice, the size of these combinations is normally limited to about three to five agents.[b] Larger combinations are not tested because as the size of the combination increases, so does the expense, technical difficulty, and potential for adverse effects. For example, the statistical analysis of interactions becomes very difficult with combinations larger than about five compounds. Nonetheless, this book considers combinations containing perhaps 15 to 18 compounds. Although this may seem excessive to some readers, we must keep in mind that these are relatively nontoxic compounds and that combinations of this size or slightly smaller have been routinely used in herbal medicine traditions from around the world. Thus humans have been following this general practice with some success for many hundreds, if not thousands of years. With a focused effort, we should be able to overcome any technical difficulties that the study of large combinations of natural compounds may present.

Another reason this concept of large combinations has not been embraced is because many agents must be available for testing. Some pharmaceutical firms, especially smaller firms, have only a few cancer drugs under development. These firms have little incentive to spend money showing their product works best when combined with products from competitors.

One last reason is that since the first half of the 1900s, regulatory agencies and medical researchers have preferred to work with pure, well-defined substances. In contrast, most of the compounds discussed here are

---

[a] *For those readers who have the ability and interest to help fund anticancer research on natural compounds, please see Appendix M.*

[b] *Note that the combinations of chemotherapy drugs in current use tend to contain agents that primarily focus on a single cellular target: the interruption of DNA activity. Thus such combinations do not address the full spectrum of events important in cancer progression and do not meet the criteria suggested here for optimal design of combinations.*

commonly used in the form of concentrated plant extracts. These extracts are complex mixtures, and combinations of these extracts are even more complex. It is only very recently that the U.S. Food and Drug Administration (FDA) has considered granting Investigational New Drug (IND) status to complex plant extracts. (IND status is needed for human studies.) Humans have been using complex mixtures much longer than isolated compounds, and the new openness of regulatory agencies is both promising and welcome.

In spite of any difficulties involved in testing large combinations, this work needs to be done. For one thing, large combinations hold more promise than single agents or small combinations. In addition, large combinations of natural compounds are already being used (perhaps haphazardly) by many thousands of cancer patients. An even larger number of patients use them for treatment of other diseases. Thus, however complex their study, we have a responsibility to apply ourselves to the task.

PURPOSES OF THIS BOOK

The first purpose of this book is to inform the reader what has been accomplished in the field. This necessarily entails a description of how natural compounds fit into the mechanism-based approach. It also requires discussions on dose calculations, toxicology, and other aspects of clinical use. Some of the information on dose and toxicology has not been previously published and was developed exclusively for this book.

I have tried not only to synthesize the total body of information into a coherent whole but also to construct a framework the reader can use to understand new information on these compounds as data become available. Moreover, as more studies are conducted, the usefulness of additional natural compounds will undoubtedly come to light, and some compounds discussed here may no longer seem as valuable. It is hoped that the structure provided here will assist evaluation of these new compounds.

The second purpose is to propose a thesis as to how natural compounds (or other drugs) might best be used in cancer treatment. This thesis has two parts: 1) the most successful cancer treatments will be those that address all the primary events in cancer progression; 2) large combinations will be needed to accomplish this task. Clearly, this book does not prove the thesis; but it does take the first step by arguing that the thesis is plausible and deserves full investigation. As part of these arguments, original research conducted by my colleagues and myself is presented in Chapter 13, which illustrates the potential benefits of large combinations.

The third purpose is to help guide future research in natural compounds. By presenting the available information as a whole, I hope to make the gaps where information is lacking more obvious, and to steer future research toward the study of combinations. Also, by presenting information on doses and other clinical aspects, I hope to guide the development of future study designs. As a simple example, I encourage future animal studies to use orally administered compounds at doses relevant to human use, a practice, unfortunately, often not followed.

I want to be clear I am not suggesting that patients self-medicate, nor am I suggesting natural compounds be used in lieu of beneficial conventional treatments when they are available. In fact, in some instances the best use of natural compounds will probably be as adjuncts to conventional treatments, and I have accordingly devoted an entire chapter to this topic. Thus my final purpose is to educate patients to help them work more effectively with their practitioners, who in turn should find much supportive information here for developing their own recommendations. Because this book is based primarily on preclinical information, the suggestions herein are not intended as ready-made treatment plans. Obviously, much work remains to determine the safety and efficacy of the compounds discussed. In those cases where patients and their doctors feel that certain combinations of natural compounds may be useful, I trust they will use them wisely, with caution, and after consulting other resources.

In writing this book, I am attempting to reach the patient, the doctor, and the researcher—three quite different audiences. With the patient in mind, I have placed the most technical material in the appendices. A less technical book at such an early stage of development in the field would not have been as appropriate because a simplified guide would not be as effective in advancing research on natural compounds as I hope this book will be.

ORGANIZATION

The book is divided into three parts, with Chapter 1 serving as an introduction to Parts I and II. Chapter 1 provides an overview of the anticancer strategies promoted in this book, discusses in more detail the need for using combinations of compounds, briefly introduces the compounds discussed in later chapters, and provides some practical information for understanding the concentrations and doses reported here.

Part I (Chapters 2 to 6) discusses the various events involved in cancer progression at the cellular level, including genetic changes, proliferation, cell death, and the communication that occurs between cancer cells and other cells. Each chapter briefly discusses the natural compounds likely to affect these events. The purpose of these discussions is both to show how natural compounds can affect cancer through multiple means and to set the stage for the more clinical discussions of each compound in Part III.

In Part II (Chapters 7 to 12) the focus shifts from cancer at the level of the cell to cancer at the level of the organism. Here we discuss the interactions that occur between groups of cancer cells (i.e., tumors) and the body, including angiogenesis, invasion, metastasis, and interactions with the immune system. Again, each chapter includes a brief discussion of the natural compounds likely to affect these events.

Parts I and II contain the most challenging scientific material, and the reader may find it useful to read these chapters sequentially, since all terms are explained as they are introduced. To further assist the reader, an acronym list is included and the index is extensive.

In Part III, the focus shifts to the individual compounds, the evidence for their efficacy, and the clinical considerations involved in using them. The introduction to Part III (Chapter 13) discusses synergism and presents research by my group and others supporting the thesis that synergism is a hopeful approach. Chapter 13 briefly explains my approach in estimating doses and evaluating toxicology and also contains information on how combinations can be designed. Chapter 13, along with Chapters 1 and 2, should be considered essential reading, because they introduce the material that forms the basis of the book.

Chapters 14 to 22 are organized according to the type of compound in question. For example, polysaccharides are discussed in Chapter 16 and lipids are discussed in Chapter 17. This type of organization is used in many textbooks of pharmacognosy, the study of crude drugs of natural origin; it is convenient here since many of the compounds within a given chemical family have similarities in clinical application. The discussion on each compound includes a review of test tube, animal, and human anticancer studies; an analysis of their implications; and estimates of a required dose. The last chapter, Chapter 23, focuses specifically on potential interactions between natural compounds and chemotherapy and radiotherapy.

The technical material in the appendices includes chemical structure diagrams for each compound and a table of molecular weights (Appendix A); a discussion on pharmacokinetic and pharmacodynamic modeling, along with a discussion on the methods used to scale animal doses to their human equivalents (Appendix B);

and supplementary information for various chapters (Appendices C to H, and K). Appendix I discusses two models I developed to estimate the oral clearance of natural compounds based on their chemical structure (oral clearance is a value used in estimating doses). It then discusses predictions of toxicity made for natural compounds using the TOPKAT model, which also bases estimates on chemical structure. Lastly, it presents the methods used to estimate an equivalent oral dose based on an intraperitoneal or subcutaneous dose. Appendix J contains a technical discussion of the pharmacokinetics of most of the natural compounds and explains the dose calculations made for each. Appendix L gives information on the computer programs used to develop some of my data, as well as the companies that make the programs. Lastly, Appendix M informs readers of the fund my colleagues and I have set up at M. D. Anderson Cancer Center at the University of Texas in Houston that will receive tax-deductible donations to conduct the kind of research on natural compounds this book calls for.

This book is a continuation of my first book, *Cancer and Natural Medicine*.[14] There are, however, some significant differences between the two. Whereas the first book discussed nearly two hundred natural compounds that may be useful, this book narrows that list to about three dozen judged to have the greatest potential or to be of the greatest interest. Furthermore, the discussions on clinical considerations here are more advanced. The reader is referred to my first book for information on theories of Traditional Chinese Medicine (TCM) in cancer treatment, Eastern and Western psychological therapies in cancer treatment, and additional natural compounds that may be useful in cancer treatment, including many Chinese herbs.

POTENTIAL CRITICISMS

This book discusses some controversial issues, and it will not be without its critics. One likely criticism is the lack of clinical evidence to prove or come close to proving that natural compounds are indeed beneficial in the treatment of human cancers. Certainly, randomized, double-blind, placebo-controlled studies, the gold standard in proving efficacy, have not been conducted for most of these natural compounds, much less for combinations of them. It is not my intent to declare that natural compounds will cure cancer but to provide a snapshot of a promising field in its infancy and to suggest ways in which the field might best mature.

Another criticism likely to arise is that the dose estimates in Part III are so rough they have little value. It is true they must be refined. For many compounds, only limited information is available on which to base dose estimates, and as I state in numerous places, most estimates provide only rough, ballpark values. They should not be taken as fact by patients or doctors. They do, however, represent the best estimates available so far. Again, this is a field in its infancy. I believe these values are worthwhile, in that they provide researchers with rough estimates for designing future studies and challenge them to develop more accurate estimates. Also, with judicious consideration, prudent caution, and consultation of other resources, doctors and patients working together may find some of these estimates helpful in guiding treatment.

ACKNOWLEDGMENTS

There are many people I would like to thank for their gracious help in putting this book together. I regret I am unable to mention every doctor, researcher, chemist, and pharmacologist who was kind enough to answer my many questions. I thank Hauser Inc. and M. D. Anderson Cancer Center at the University of Texas in Houston, who funded the research on synergism carried out by my colleagues and myself; Bill Keeney and David Bailey, of Hauser Inc., for their backing and assistance; Robert Newman, of M. D. Anderson Cancer Center, for his wisdom and support; Israel Barken, M.D., for his kind contribution of the foreword; my steadfast editor, Silvine Farnell, whose impassioned insistence on clear writing forced me to blossom as an author; Sarah Whalen, who edited and fine-tuned the final draft of the manuscript; Susan Fogo, who created the first draft for many of the illustrations; and Michelle Lundquist, for her design of a beautiful book cover.

I would also like to thank the many companies and individuals who offered software assistance, without which I could not have written this book. My thanks to Pharsight Inc., for use of their pharmacokinetic, pharmacodynamic, and noncompartmental analysis program WinNonlin®; MathSoft Inc., for use of their mathematics, scientific graphing, and data analysis programs Mathcad and Axum; ChemSW Inc., for use of their computational chemistry program Molecular Modeling Pro™; Daniel Svozil and Hans Lohninger, for use of their molecular descriptor program Topix; BioComp Systems Inc., for use of their neural network program NeuroGenetic Optimizer; and Douglas A. Smith of Oxford Molecular Group for providing toxicity assessments of natural compounds using the TOPKAT model. Additional information on these companies can be found in Appendix L.

Finally, I thank my family for their loving kindness, faith, and enduring support.

John Boik
January 2001

REFERENCES

[1] Kennedy BJ. Use of questionable methods and physician education. J Cancer Educ 1993; 8(2):129–31.

[2] Hauser SP. Unproven methods in cancer treatment. Curr Opin Oncol 1993; 5(4):646–54.

[3] Lerner IJ, Kennedy BJ. The prevalence of questionable methods of cancer treatment in the United States. CA 1992; 42:181–191, 192.

[4] McGinnis LS. Alternative therapies, 1990: An overview. Cancer 1991; 67(6 Suppl):1788–92.

[5] Downer SM, Cody MM, McCluskey P, Wilson PD, et al. Pursuit and practice of complementary therapies by cancer patients receiving conventional treatment. BMJ 1994; 9309(6947):86–9.

[6] Van der Zouwe N, Van Dam FS, Aaronson NK, Hanewald GJ. Alternative treatments in cancer; extent and background of utilization. Ned Tijdschr Geneeskd 1994; 138(6):300–6.

[7] Pawlicki M, Rachtan J, Rolski J, Sliz E. Results of delayed treatment of patients with malignant tumors of the lymphatic system. Pol Tyg Lek 1991; 46(48–49):922–3.

[8] Morant R, Jungi WF, Koehli C, Senn HJ. Why do cancer patients use alternative medicine? Schweiz Med Wochenschr 1991; 121(27–28):1029–34.

[9] Munstedt K, Kirsch K, Milch W, et al. Unconventional cancer therapy—survey of patients with gynaecological malignancy. Arch Gynecol Obstet 1996; 258(2):81–8.

[10] Risberg T, Lund E, Wist E, et al. The use of non-proven therapy among patients treated in Norwegian oncological departments. A cross-sectional national multicentre study. Eur J Cancer 1995 Oct; 31A(11):1785–9.

[11] Schraub S. Unproven methods in cancer: A worldwide problem. Support Care Cancer 2000 Jan; 8(1):10–5.

[12] Richardson MA, Sanders T, Palmer JL, et al. Complementary/alternative medicine use in a comprehensive cancer center and the implications for oncology. J Clin Oncol 2000 Jul; 18(13):2505–2514.

[13] Sparber A, Jonas W, White J, et al. Cancer clinical trials and subject use of natural herbal products. Cancer Invest 2000; 18(5):436–9.

[14] Boik J. Cancer and natural medicine: A textbook of basic science and clinical research. Princeton, MN: Oregon Medical Press, 1996.

BACKGROUND FOR PARTS I AND II

Part I of this book discusses cancer at the cellular level, and Part II discusses cancer at the level of the organism. The latter refers to interactions between groups of cancer cells (tumors) and the body. As we will see, a conglomeration of interrelated events occur within an individual cancer cell, as well as between tumors and the body, which allows a cancer to proliferate and spread. For convenience, I refer to these as procancer events. For example, one procancer event is the production of enzymes by tumors that allows them to invade local tissues. The mechanism-based approach to cancer treatment used throughout this book views each of these procancer events as a potential target for cancer inhibition. Although a very large number of procancer events occur during a tumor's life, to simplify and focus this approach, I group them into seven primary clusters of events. The inhibition of these seven event clusters thus becomes the goal of the mechanism-based approach outlined here.

This chapter defines the seven event clusters and identifies each with a strategy for cancer inhibition. In addition, we look more closely at why combinations of compounds will be most effective at inhibiting these seven clusters and why the synergism that occurs within combinations is needed for natural compounds to be effective. We will also look at how combinations of compounds might be designed, then introduce the natural compounds to be discussed. Finally, some practical information is provided to help the reader understand the concentrations reported and the relationship between animal doses and their human equivalents.

It seems useful to start with the basics of what occurs in cancer; thus we begin with a look at how normal cells behave and how a normal cell becomes a cancer cell during carcinogenesis.

DEVELOPMENT OF CANCER AND CHARACTERISTICS OF CANCER CELLS

Imagine a healthy tissue containing thousands of cells. Each cell serves the greater good, which is the continuation of a person's life. Each cell is programmed so that when the cell is old or no longer needed, it dies a peaceful and timely death. This death is called apoptosis. All cells are in communication, which allows for the smooth repair and replacement of tissues and other aspects of cell behavior. Communication takes place either indi-

rectly, via exchange of messenger compounds such as hormones and growth factors, or directly, via cell-to-cell contact. Contact allows cells to respond to the "feel" of neighboring cells, via cell adhesion molecules, and to exchange messenger molecules through cell-to-cell portals called gap junctions. With the help of proper communication, appropriate cells proliferate when new cells are needed, and when enough new cells have been produced, cell division stops.

Cancer cells are the descendants of a normal cell in which something has gone wrong. In this normal cell, some kind of internal or external stress causes a mix-up in its genetic code (its DNA). This event is said to "initiate" the cell to a precancerous state. After its DNA has been damaged, the cell withdraws from close communication with its neighboring cells. Interrupted cell-to-cell communication is a common result of DNA damage or other forms of cellular damage. Separated from the regulatory controls of its community, it is now at the mercy of its environment. Let us say that the environment around this cell contains a promoting agent, which is a compound that stimulates cell proliferation. In response to the promoting agent, this precancerous cell divides to produce daughter cells, and these daughter cells divide to produce more daughter cells, and so on. All are proliferating only in response to the promoting agent. The promoting agent may be a chemical foreign to the body, or it could come from a natural process such as inflammation. One day, the worst occurs. The genetic instabilities passed down through the generations finally result in one cell that becomes capable of self-stimulation, and on this day an autonomous cancer cell is born. This cell no longer requires the promoting agent to stimulate its proliferation. The role of the promoting agent is made obsolete by the cell's ability to make proteins such as growth factors that stimulate proliferation.

This original cancer cell divides to produce daughter cells, these cells also divide, and soon there is a population of cancer cells. As they divide, they develop malignant characteristics, such as the ability to invade and metastasize. They also develop other characteristics that help assure survival, for example, the ability to evade the immune system, to mutate when faced with adverse conditions, and to induce the growth of new blood vessels through the process called angiogenesis. The development of these characteristics marks the third stage in carcinogenesis, the first two stages being initiation and promotion, respectively. In this book, I use the term *progression* to refer to both the third stage of carcinogenesis proper and to the entire postpromotion period of the cancer's life. This correctly implies that progression is an ongoing, evolving process.

Compared to normal cells, cancer cells have lost touch with their neighboring cells, their community purpose, and even largely with one another. They are a race of self-serving, easily adaptable cells, whose proliferation continues with the slightest provocation. They use more than their fair share of resources, live longer than their fair share of time, and produce more than their share of offspring. In short, they exhibit the two deadly characteristics of cancer: uncontrolled proliferation and uncontrolled spread.

SEVEN STRATEGIES FOR CANCER INHIBITION

To be clear, not all cancers develop exactly as in the scenario above. This scenario is common, however, and within it lies the foundation for all our discussions on cancer inhibition. From it, we can identify seven clusters of procancer events:

1. *Induction of genetic instability.* Each cancer cell carries within itself genetic instability, and this instability increases the chances the cell will be able to mutate as needed to adapt to its environment.

2. *Abnormal expression of genes.* In essence, the function of genes is to make proteins—a process called gene expression. When they are expressed, some genes produce proteins that inhibit cancer progression, and others produce proteins that facilitate it. In cancer cells, abnormal expression of genes occurs, resulting in too few proteins that inhibit cancer and too many that facilitate it.

3. *Abnormal signal transduction.* Signal transduction is the movement of a signal from outside the cell toward the cell's nucleus, where it can stimulate proliferation or other activities. One important source of external signals comes from growth factors. Growth factors are soluble molecules that bind to specific receptors on the cell's surface and stimulate the cell's activities. A second source of external signals comes from cell adhesion molecules (CAMs). Cells interact with their environment through CAMs located on their surface. Cell adhesion molecules are proteins that act like fingers to regulate the degree of contact with other cells and tissues and inform cells of their surroundings. Other factors are also involved in signal generation and signal transduction. For example, cancer cells can produce their own growth factors, thereby allowing self-stimulation; they can produce

extra receptors for growth factors; and they can produce free radicals, which can make growth factor receptors more responsive to stimulation.

4. *Abnormal cell-to-cell communication.* By decreasing their contact with normal cells, cancer cells are freed to act independently. As mentioned previously, cell-to-cell communication occurs via portals between adjacent cells (gap junctions) and through cell adhesion molecules. Normal cell-to-cell communication through gap junctions maintains homeostasis and discourages cancerlike behavior. Normal CAM activity keeps cells in place and prevents signal transduction that may be initiated by abnormal CAM activity.

5. *Induction of angiogenesis.* Angiogenesis is the growth of new blood vessels toward and within tumors (or other tissues). Solid tumors require angiogenesis in order to grow. Tumors need blood vessels to supply oxygen and nutrients, and the blood vessels created by angiogenesis provide the channel by which tumor cells metastasize to distant locations.

6. *Invasion and metastasis.* Tumors can spread both locally, via invasion of adjacent tissues, and distantly, via metastasis through the blood and lymph circulation. The spread of cancer, along with uncontrolled proliferation, is a central hallmark of malignancy.

7. *Immune evasion.* Cancer cells shield themselves from immune attack, thereby evading destruction; they can hide from immune cells by employing various camouflaging techniques or can produce immunosuppressive compounds that impair the ability of immune cells to function.

These seven event clusters provide the targets for the anticancer strategies laid out in this book. Each of the seven clusters of procancer events is illustrated in Figure 1.1.

Since each of these seven clusters is a target for therapy, we can identify seven strategies for cancer inhibition. Keep in mind that natural compounds can be used to carry out each of these seven strategies and that the best results will be seen when all seven are used together. The seven strategies are as follows:

1. *Reduce genetic instability.* Genetic instability is aggravated by oxidative stress (stress caused by free radicals). Cancer cells exist in an oxidative environment, and although such an environment kills some cells, many continue to survive. As oxidative stress increases, the declining population of surviving cells exhibits greater instability and higher mutation rates, in theory eventually producing more

aggressive and successful cancers. Thus one way of reducing genetic instability is by reducing oxidative stress. Other possible means of reducing genetic instability are discussed in Chapter 2.

2. *Inhibit abnormal expression of genes.* One way that gene expression can be normalized is through modifying the activity of transcription factors. Transcription factors are proteins that act as switches in the nucleus to turn on gene expression. Genes that inhibit cancer progression are commonly underexpressed in cancer cells, and genes that facilitate cancer are commonly overexpressed. Therefore, cancer can be inhibited by normalizing the activity of those transcription factors that control the expression of these genes. The use of natural compounds to affect transcription factors is discussed in Chapter 5.

3. *Inhibit abnormal signal transduction.* The movement of a signal from outside the cell toward the nucleus relies on several proteins (including kinase enzymes and ras proteins, discussed later), and so signal transduction can be inhibited by blocking the actions of these proteins; using natural compounds for this purpose is discussed in Chapter 4. Signal transduction is a normal process needed by healthy cells, but in cancer cells the volume of signal transduction is excessive, and the signals that flow favor proliferation and spread. Thus the intent is not to eliminate signal transduction but to bring it down to normal levels.

4. *Encourage normal cell-to-cell communication.* Normal cell-to-cell communication can be fostered by improving gap junction communication and by normalizing CAM activity. Natural compounds that encourage normal cell-to-cell communication are discussed in Chapter 6.

5. *Inhibit tumor angiogenesis.* Like signal transduction, angiogenesis is a normal process; it is needed during wound healing and in other situations. Angiogenesis in tumors, however, unlike that in normal conditions, is uncontrolled and ongoing. Our intent then is not to eliminate angiogenesis but to normalize its occurrence by normalizing the factors that control it. Angiogenesis is most successful if certain chemicals called angiogenic factors are present, as well as

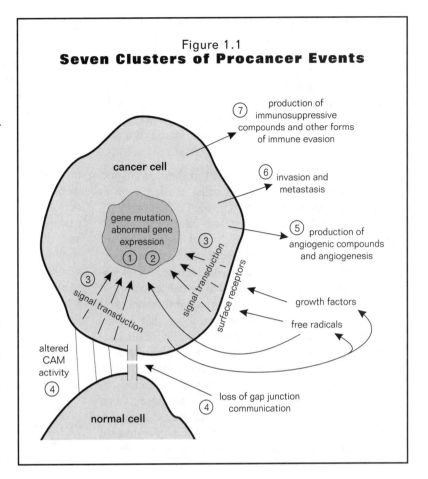

Figure 1.1
Seven Clusters of Procancer Events

certain environmental conditions, such as hypoxic (low-oxygen) ones. Cancer can be inhibited by blocking the release or action of angiogenic factors or by otherwise altering the local environment to inhibit tumor angiogenesis. Natural compounds that inhibit tumor angiogenesis are discussed in Chapters 7 and 8.

6. *Inhibit invasion and metastasis.* Invasion requires enzymatic digestion of the healthy tissue surrounding the tumor. It also requires the migration of tumor cells. Invasion can be reduced by inhibiting enzymes that digest local tissues, by protecting normal tissues from the enzymes, and by reducing the ability of tumor cells to migrate. Natural compounds that inhibit invasion are discussed in Chapter 9. Metastasis requires that cells detach from the primary tumor, enzymatically digest blood vessel walls to gain access to and exit from the blood circulation, and evade the immune system while in the circulation. Thus metastasis can be checked by inhibiting any one of these processes. Natural compounds that do so are discussed in Chapter 10.

7. *Increase the immune response.* The immune response against cancer cells can be increased by stimulating the immune system and by reducing the

ability of cancer cells to evade immune attack. Both actions are best taken in tandem, since without prevention of immune evasion, immune stimulation will have little benefit; healthy, vital immune cells can destroy cancer cells, but only if the cancer cells can be recognized as foreign to the body. Chapters 11 and 12 discuss the use of natural compounds to stimulate the immune system and inhibit immune evasion.

When natural compounds are used in these strategies, some will directly inhibit cancer cells, causing them to die, revert to normalcy (a process called differentiation), or just stop proliferating. Others will inhibit cancer progression indirectly by inducing changes in the local environment that are unfavorable to angiogenesis, invasion, or metastasis. This might include, for example, inhibiting the enzymes produced by cancer cells that allow invasion. Thus we can group natural compounds into two broad categories of action: those that act directly on cancer cells to inhibit proliferation (called direct-acting compounds) and those that inhibit cancer progression by affecting tissues or compounds outside the cancer cell (called indirect-acting compounds). In addition, we can add a third category: compounds that inhibit cancer through stimulating the immune system. Although immune attack produces a direct cytotoxic effect against cancer cells, immune stimulants themselves generally do not.[a]

USING NATURAL COMPOUNDS IN COMBINATION

From the above discussions we begin to see why using combinations of natural compounds is so important. A well-designed combination of compounds will target all seven clusters of procancer events, a task a single compound could not perform. In addition, since most natural compounds inhibit several procancer events, a large combination of natural compounds will redundantly target all seven clusters of events. Redundant targeting is useful in that if one compound fails to perform its task, another is available to back it up. Redundancy is in fact common in stable systems. In nature, for example, biologic diversity provides redundant controls of insect pest populations.

---

[a] *By convention, we say that a cytotoxic effect occurs if cells are killed and a cytostatic effect occurs if cells are kept from proliferating. Cytotoxic and cytostatic effects can be readily studied in vitro. However, many in-vitro tests do not actually differentiate between the two, and in this book, I use the term* cytotoxic *to refer to both cytotoxic and cytostatic effects unless stated otherwise.*

Synergism in Combinations

The use of combinations provides one other important advantage: the possibility of additive or synergistic interactions. (For convenience, unless stated otherwise, the term *synergism* is used loosely to refer to either additive or synergistic interactions.) Synergism is important because it allows lower and safer doses of each compound to be used; in fact, it is more than important, it is required for our purposes. As discussed in Chapter 13, most direct-acting natural compounds, if used alone, would require excessive and unsafe doses to inhibit cancer. My colleagues and I have conducted preliminary research on large combinations of natural compounds, and other groups have conducted research on small combinations of natural compounds. The research as a whole strongly suggests that when used in combination, natural compounds can produce synergistic effects in vitro.[b] If synergistic effects are also produced in vivo, and there is reason to believe they would be, such interactions would make essentially all direct-acting natural compounds discussed in this book potentially effective when used at safe doses. This is true even if the interactions are additive rather than truly synergistic.

That most direct-acting natural compounds discussed here require synergism to be effective at safe doses is, ironically, related to the reason they are included in this book—they are milder than most chemotherapy drugs and less apt to produce adverse effects. Most of these compounds are on the average (geometric average) about 21-fold less toxic than most chemotherapy drugs.[1, c] Furthermore, the most toxic natural compound is about 270-fold less toxic than the most toxic chemotherapy drug.[d] However, they are also less toxic to can-

---

[b] *In vitro, literally, "in glass," refers to studies conducted in the test tube, and in vivo, literally, "in life," refers to studies conducted in animals.*

[c] *The geometric average is used at a few places in this book. It is the average of a group of* n *numbers as calculated by $(x_1 \cdot x_2 \cdot x_n)^{1/n}$ and is near the arithmetic average when the numbers are evenly dispersed. It is used instead of the arithmetic average primarily when the arithmetic average is heavily influenced by a relatively small number of extreme outlying points. In these cases, the geometric average can be a more meaningful descriptor.*

[d] *The geometric average of the oral lethal dose (LD_{50}) in rats predicted for 20 of the natural compounds discussed is 1.5 g/kg (see Table I.4 in Appendix I). This is in contrast to the 21-fold lower LD_{50} geometric average of 72 mg/kg for a representative sample of 17 chemotherapy drugs (NCI data obtained from the reference given). Furthermore, the lowest LD_{50} for the natural compounds is 270 mg/kg, whereas the lowest LD_{50} for the chemotherapy drugs is 1 mg/kg. The equivalent human doses are about 4.4 grams and 16 milligrams, respectively. Sixteen milligrams is a very small amount of material!*

cer cells than most chemotherapy drugs. Most of the natural compounds discussed are active in vitro at concentrations of about 1 to 50 µM. A target concentration of 15 µM is used in most of the dose calculations in later chapters. In contrast, standard chemotherapy drugs tend to be active at much lower concentrations. Based on a simple analysis of data from the National Cancer Institute, the average effective concentration (IC_{50}) for nine common chemotherapy drugs was 0.48 µM.[2, a] This is roughly 30-fold lower than the active concentrations of the natural compounds considered here.

Therefore, high concentrations are required to inhibit cancer, and this requires large doses. For roughly 65 percent of the direct-acting natural compounds, such high doses are likely to cause adverse effects. As previously stated, however, synergistic interactions will make essentially all of these direct-acting natural compounds potentially effective when used at safe doses.

Designing Combinations

Chapter 13, the introductory chapter to Part III, discusses how natural compounds might be chosen for use in combinations, but an overview of the process can provide some context for how the compounds discussed in Parts I and II might be used. Although compounds could be chosen for the particular procancer events they inhibit, it is more practical and probably just as useful to consider the design of combinations as a process of elimination; one that can be based on five constraints:

- Using a large number of compounds to assure redundancy, facilitate synergism, and target all seven clusters of procancer events. An ideal number of compounds might be 15 to 18, which means only about half the compounds discussed in this book would be used.

- Choosing compounds so that all three categories (direct acting, indirect acting, and immune stimulants) are represented. Since each compound tends to inhibit multiple procancer events, by using a large combination and compounds from all three categories, it is likely that all seven clusters of procancer events will be inhibited.

- To assure diversity, if a pair or group of compounds appear to act very similarly, using only one of the pair or a few of the group.

- Eliminating compounds that are not practical for whatever reason. For example, some compounds

discussed may not be commercially available at present.

- Eliminating compounds that do not appear to have strong anticancer effects relative to the other natural compounds.

The above process of elimination can be used to guide the initial design of a combination; after which it could be refined to meet the needs of a particular patient.

INTRODUCTION TO THE COMPOUNDS

Of the hundreds of natural compounds known to be active against cancer (at least in vitro), this book focuses primarily on only 38. This is clearly a very small percentage. Narrowing the focus was necessary for several reasons. For one thing, few data are available for most of those known to be active. For another, many would not be safe for human consumption. For these and other reasons, a set of criteria was used to narrow the focus; compounds were included that met most, if not all, of the following:

- They are not already approved as prescription drugs by the U.S. Food and Drug Administration. Furthermore, they are not patented or trade secret products, so their composition is known and they are not licensed to one manufacturer. Although such products can be useful, I will leave it to the manufacturers to argue their benefits.

- The compounds or their plant sources have a history of safe human use as food or in herbal medicine traditions.

- They are active at concentrations that are achievable in humans after oral administration. In many cases, this requires them to be used in synergistic combinations.

- They are expected to be nontoxic to the patient at the required dose. Again, this may require low doses and synergistic combinations.

- They are not excessively expensive.

- They are readily available commercially or could be readily available within the next few years.

- Sound theoretical reasoning exists to support the hypothesis that they may be useful in cancer treatment. For example, the means by which they may inhibit cancer cells is understood.

- They are suitable for long-term therapy because they are safe and can be administered orally.

Preference was also given to compounds that inhibit multiple procancer events. By affecting multiple events,

---

[a] *These are actually GI_{50} values rather than IC_{50} values. The GI_{50} is an adaptation of the IC_{50} by the National Cancer Institute to correct for cell count at time zero. The average value quoted here is based on data from sensitive cell lines.*

these compounds are more likely to inhibit a wider range of cancers under a greater variety of circumstances. The ability to inhibit multiple events also increases the chances that synergistic interactions will occur between compounds. In addition, preference was given to compounds with other desirable characteristics, such as dissimilarity to the other compounds, being of interest to the public, and being useful for instructive reasons. Although the compounds selected do include many of those already being used by cancer patients, not all in common use were included; it was not possible to discuss all compounds that may be of interest.

Some of the 38 compounds do not look as promising at this time as others. In particular, flaxseed, EGCG (from green tea), and hypericin (from St. John's wort) are all associated either with some uncertainties in safe or effective doses, or they are not likely to produce a strong anticancer effect relative to the other compounds. However, they are still discussed because of public interest in them, because it is instructive to see the problems associated with them, and because new research may remove the uncertainties and place them in a more promising light.

The primary compounds of interest are listed in Table 1.1. (Additional natural compounds are mentioned from time to time, but only in passing.) A detailed description of each is provided in Part III, and chemical information for most, including structural diagrams, is given in Appendix A. Note that thousands if not millions of natural compounds exist; but most of these do not inhibit cancer, and some are not safe for human ingestion. To avoid confusion, the term *natural compound* in this book refers only to those compounds listed in Table 1.1, unless specifically stated otherwise.

Most of the compounds in the table are available through supplement or herbal suppliers. They are formulated as pills, powders, liquids, or whole plant parts. Some formulations contain crude plant material and some contain extracts of various potencies. A small number are not yet commercially available, while a larger number are not yet available in the preferred form of high-potency standardized extracts. Such concentrated extracts are standardized to contain a specific amount of the active ingredient(s). It is likely that most will be available as standardized extracts in the future.[a]

As discussed earlier, natural compounds can be divided into three groups: those that inhibit cancer cell proliferation directly, those that act by indirect means to inhibit cancer progression, and those that stimulate the immune system. Table 1.2 lists them according to category. Of course, many compounds have multiple actions, and they could be placed in more than one category. Placing these in a single category is a judgment call. For example, melatonin has a beneficial effect on the immune system and can directly inhibit some types of cancer cells. The same could be said of ginseng. Here melatonin and ginseng are both characterized as immune stimulants. Judgment calls aside, the arrangement of natural compounds in this table is still a useful starting point for conceptualizing their behavior.

The natural compounds listed in Table 1.1 have received different amounts of in-vitro, animal, or human study. For some compounds, only a few studies involving cancer cells have been completed, whereas for others, there have been many dozens. Because a compound has received few studies does not mean it is ineffective. By the same token, because a compound has received many studies does not indicate it is highly effective. In fact, some studies could have reported negative results. Still, the number and type of studies roughly indicate how well the anticancer effect has been characterized. In this regard, human studies are, of course, the most useful in predicting effects in humans. Animal studies are less useful than human studies, and in-vitro studies are less useful still. On the other hand, in-vitro and animal studies can be the most useful in determining mechanisms of action. Thus all three types are useful and necessary.

To provide a rough estimate of how well the anticancer effects of different compounds have been characterized, compounds are ranked in Table 1.3 according to a scoring system that gives one point for each in-vitro study, three points for each animal study, and nine points for each human study. Although somewhat arbitrary, this system is useful in providing a very general ranking of how well different compounds have been characterized. The number of in-vitro, animal, and human studies listed is an estimate based on searches of the MEDLINE database of the National Library of Medicine. These searches covered the period between the mid-1960s and, depending on the compound, September–December of 2000. Other studies may exist that are not indexed in MEDLINE, and of course, new studies are being indexed on a regular basis. Also note that the studies listed do not include those that did not use cancer cells. For example, general studies on the inhibition of invasion enzymes are not listed unless the study specifically measured the ability of a compound to inhibit the invasion of cancer cells. Neither do they include cancer prevention studies or studies in which compounds were used in combination with chemotherapy drugs or radiotherapy (except for glutamine and

---

[a] *To learn about the latest availabilities, or to inform us of availability, please visit our web page at www.ompress.com.*

TABLE 1.1 NATURAL COMPOUNDS OF INTEREST	
COMPOUND	**BRIEF DESCRIPTION**
Anthocyanidins	Red-blue flavonoid pigments found in berries and other plants.
Apigenin	A flavonoid found in many plants.
Arctigenin	An active compound in burdock seeds (*Arctium lappa*).
Astragalus membranaceus	An herb used as an immunostimulant in Chinese herbal medicine.
Boswellic acid	An active compound in frankincense (*Boswellia carteri* or *B. serrata*).
Butcher's broom (*Ruscus aculeatus*)	An herb used to treat venous insufficiency.
Bromelain	A proteolytic enzyme obtained from pineapples.
Caffeic acid phenethyl ester (CAPE)	An active compound in bee propolis.
Centella asiatica	A tropical herb used to treat skin conditions. Also known as gotu kola.
Curcumin	An active compound in the spice turmeric (*Curcuma longa*).
EGCG (epigallocatechin gallate)	An active compound in green tea (*Camellia sinensis*).
Eleutherococcus senticosus	An herb with immunostimulant properties. Also known as Siberian ginseng and *Acanthopanax senticosus*.
Emodin	An active compound in the herb *Polygonum cuspidatum* and in other herbs.
EPA and DHA (eicosapentaenoic and docosahexaenoic acids)	Omega-3 fatty acids that are found together in fish oil. Of the two, EPA is of primary interest here.
Flaxseed (*Linum usitatissimum*)	A seed used as food and as a fiber agent.
Garlic (*Allium sativum*)	A medicinal herb and common flavoring agent. We are interested here mostly in its primarily metabolite, DADS (diallyl disulfide).
Ganoderma lucidum	A mushroom used in Chinese herbal medicine that has immunostimulating properties.
Genistein and daidzein	Isoflavonoids found in legumes such as soy.
Ginseng (*Panax ginseng*)	An herb with immunostimulant properties.
Glutamine	An amino acid that acts as a fuel for intestinal cells.
Horse chestnut (*Aesculus hippocastanum*)	An herb used to treat venous insufficiency.
Hypericin	An active compound in the herb St. John's wort (*Hypericum perforatum*).
Luteolin	A flavonoid found in many plants.
Melatonin	A hormone that is used clinically to induce sleep.
Monoterpenes	Fragrant essential oils. Monoterpenes include limonene, perillyl alcohol, and geraniol.
Parthenolide	An active compound in the herb feverfew (*Tanacetum parthenium*).
Proanthocyanidins	Flavonoids that are used to treat venous problems and other conditions.
PSP and PSK	Mushroom extracts (obtained from *Coriolus versicolor*) that have immunostimulant properties.
Quercetin	A flavonoid found in many plants.
Resveratrol	A compound found in wine and grapes, in the herb *Polygonum cuspidatum*, and in other herbs.
Selenium	A trace element that plays a role in the body's antioxidant system.
Shiitake (*Lentinus edodes*)	A mushroom that has immunostimulant properties.
Vitamin A (retinyl esters, retinol, and ATRA)	A vitamin important in vision, cell proliferation, and immune function. Retinol (as retinyl esters) is the dietary and supplement form of vitamin A, and ATRA (all-*trans* retinoic acid) is a primary active metabolite.
Vitamin C	An antioxidant vitamin that prevents scurvy and assists immune cells.
Vitamin D_3 (1,25-D_3)	A vitamin important in calcium uptake that has antitumor properties. 1,25-D_3 is its primary active metabolite.
Vitamin E (alpha-tocopherol)	An antioxidant vitamin that protects lipid membranes. Alpha-tocopherol is the form of vitamin E most used as a supplement.

PSP/PSK, which have primarily been studied in combination with chemotherapy).

Table 1.3 shows some interesting trends. First, there are a few compounds with very low scores, some having received only one study. Many of these low scores are

| TABLE 1.2   THERAPEUTIC CATEGORIES OF NATURAL COMPOUNDS ||
CATEGORY	COMPOUNDS
Immune stimulants	*Astragalus*, bromelain, *Eleutherococcus*, *Ganoderma*, ginseng, glutamine, melatonin, PSP/PSK, shiitake
Indirect-acting compounds	anthocyanidins, butcher's broom, horse chestnut, proanthocyanidins, vitamin C
Direct-acting compounds	apigenin, arctigenin, boswellic acid, CAPE, *Centella*, curcumin, EGCG, emodin, EPA/DHA, flaxseed, genistein and daidzein, garlic, hypericin, luteolin, monoterpenes, parthenolide, quercetin, resveratrol, selenium, vitamin A, vitamin D_3 (1,25-D_3), vitamin E

not surprising. For example, the three lowest-ranked compounds are indirect-acting ones. Most of the indirect-acting compounds listed in Table 1.2 have not generally been thought of as potential cancer treatment agents because they do not inhibit cancer cells in vitro at reasonable concentrations or they do not occur in the plasma at high concentrations after oral administration. A prime example would be horse chestnut. This book is among the first to argue that such compounds may still be useful in cancer treatment through their ability to protect the vasculature and reduce edema. *Centella* is another compound low on the list, having received only one in-vitro study and one animal study. Compounds quite similar to *Centella* have received more study, however, and it is reasonable to suppose it will produce comparable results. Clearly, all compounds in the list are still experimental, but those at the bottom of the list with a score of less than about 10, should be considered extremely so, relative to the others.

At the top of the list, a few compounds have received much study, including study in humans. For example, about 54 human studies have been conducted on PSK, and a relatively high number have also been conducted on melatonin. At least some of the human studies referenced in this list were randomized, placebo-controlled, double-blind studies. Thus it would be incorrect to say that natural compounds have not been studied in humans. Some clearly have been, but in all cases, additional study is still necessary, especially on their use in combinations.

PRACTICAL CONSIDERATIONS ON EFFECTIVE CONCENTRATIONS AND SCALING OF DOSES

We now turn to two practical considerations: identifying effective concentrations and scaling doses from animal studies. Both are mentioned here to give some context for understanding the concentrations and doses reported later in Parts I and II.

Effective Concentrations

Concentrations in this book are most commonly reported in micromolar (μM) units, the number of micromoles per liter of solution.[a] The text may indicate, for example, that a compound inhibits the proliferation of cancer cells at 30 μM. Commonly, this will be specified in the text by saying that the IC_{50} of a compound is 30 μM. The IC_{50} is the in-vitro concentration that inhibits the noted activity (such as cell proliferation) by 50 percent. Scientists use the IC_{50} as a convenient indicator of the concentration at which the compound is considered active.

To make sense of the reported concentrations, the reader should keep a few points in mind. First, most direct-acting natural compounds are active against cancer cells in vitro within the concentration range of about 1 to 50 μM. Second, for most of these compounds it is difficult to achieve in-vivo plasma concentrations much greater than 1 to 15 μM. Therefore, assuming that the concentration that is effective in vitro will also be effective in vivo, the required concentrations in vivo are often higher than the achievable concentrations. In other words, when used alone, the required dose for many compounds is higher than the safe dose. Although this is a problem if natural compounds are used singularly, it is reasonable to expect it will not be a problem if they are used in synergistic combinations. As stated above, synergistic interactions would make essentially all direct-acting natural compounds discussed potentially effective when used at safe doses. We can state as a general rule of thumb that compounds active in vitro at concentrations of 50 μM or less have good potential to be useful in vivo when they are used in synergistic combinations.

---

[a] *A 1 micromolar (μM) concentration is equal to 1×10^{-6} moles per liter, a 1 millimolar (mM) concentration is equal to 1×10^{-3} moles per liter, and a 1 nanomolar (nM) concentration is equal to 1×10^{-9} moles per liter. Research papers sometimes use the unit of micrograms/milliliter (μg/ml). To convert μg/ml to μM, multiply by 1,000 and divide by the molecular weight. Molecular weights for most natural compounds are provided in Appendix A.*

A few direct-acting compounds, specifically the monoterpenes, vitamin E, and diallyl disulfide (an active garlic compound), are effective at concentrations of 100 µM or greater. These compounds are still useful due to their favorable pharmacokinetic profiles, however. High plasma concentrations can be safely achieved after oral dosing. At the other extreme, only very low plasma concentrations can be achieved in vivo for a few other compounds, but this is also not a problem, since these compounds are also active at relatively low concentrations. An example is 1,25-D_3, the active metabolite of vitamin D_3.

Scaling Doses from Animal Studies

It is important to note that a dose (per kilogram body weight) that is effective in animals is not the same as the dose that would be effective in humans. Animals metabolize drugs at a different rate and sometimes in a different way than humans. In general, the rate of drug metabolism is related to body mass. A small animal will metabolize and excrete drugs much more quickly than a human. For this reason, the effective dose (per kilogram body weight) in an animal will be greater than that for a human. Stated another way, the dose required to produce a given plasma concentration in a small animal will be larger than the dose needed to produce the same plasma concentration in a human.

The scaling of doses between animals and humans is an uncertain science, and this is especially true of scaling oral (as opposed to intravenous) doses. In addition, note that a compound found effective in animals would not necessarily be so in humans. Nonetheless, animal studies are still useful to suggest compounds that may be effective in humans, and despite the uncertainties, scaling of animal doses to humans is commonly done.

Several generic methods have been devised to scale doses from animals to

TABLE 1.3 RANKING BASED ON THE NUMBER OF STUDIES CONDUCTED				
COMPOUND	IN VITRO	ANIMAL	HUMAN	SCORE
PSP and PSK[*]	16	39	54	619
EPA and DHA	57	66	12	363
Melatonin	14	13	28	305
Vitamin D_3 (1,25-D_3)	133	27	4	250
Glutamine[*]	7	21	17	223
Vitamin C	37	17	7	151
Genistein and daidzein	85	21	0	148
Vitamin A[†]	23	12	7	122
Ginseng	33	15	4	114
Bromelain	14	11	6	101
Astragalus	13	13	5	97
Selenium	35	20	0	95
Quercetin	73	4	0	85
Vitamin E[‡]	44	5	0	59
Eleutherococcus	4	8	3	55
Monoterpenes	15	7	2	54
EGCG and green tea	29	6	0	47
Boswellic acid	8	3	2	35
Apigenin and luteolin	26	2	0	32
Ganoderma and shiitake	2	9	0	29
Curcumin	19	3	0	28
Garlic	7	7	0	28
Emodin	14	3	0	23
Resveratrol	18	1	0	21
Flaxseed	7	3	0	16
Propolis and CAPE	11	1	0	14
Anthocyanidins	6	2	0	12
Hypericin[§]	9	0	0	9
Parthenolide	4	1	0	7
Arctigenin	7	0	0	7
Proanthocyanidins	5	0	0	5
Centella	1	1	0	4
Butcher's broom	1	0	0	1
Horse chestnut	1	0	0	1

[*] *Includes studies in conjunction with chemotherapy.*

[†] *Retinol or retinyl esters, but not ATRA.*

[‡] *Alpha-tocopherol and vitamin E succinate.*

[§] *Does not include studies on photoactivated hypericin.*

$$human\ dose\ (grams) = \frac{rat\ dose\ (mg/kg)}{61.7} = \frac{mouse\ dose\ (mg/kg)}{104}$$

Equation 1.1

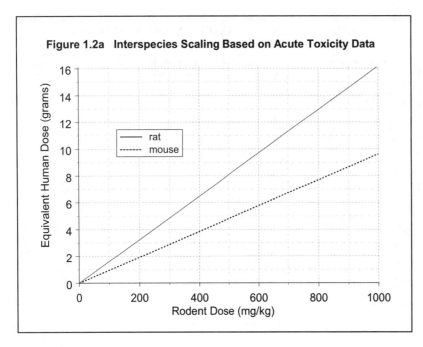

Figure 1.2a Interspecies Scaling Based on Acute Toxicity Data

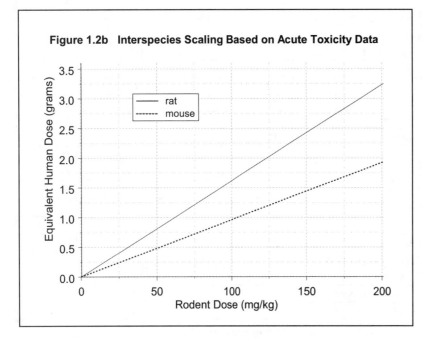

Figure 1.2b Interspecies Scaling Based on Acute Toxicity Data

methods provide only a rough approximation of the human dose. To be certain of that dose, we must do human studies.

Many of the animal doses in this book are reported both as the actual animal dose and as the estimated human equivalent, and therefore the reader need not keep referring to Equation 1.1 or the figures. In some cases, only the estimated equivalent human dose is reported. For example, a 100-mg/kg dose in rats might be reported as a "1.6-gram dose, as scaled to humans." Regardless of the reporting format, every conversion made in this book is based on Equation 1.1, with modifications for route of administration as discussed below.

Since we are interested in orally administered natural compounds, animal studies using the oral route most closely mimic the intended human use and are most valuable. Although many of the animal studies reported here did use the oral route, a good number used either the intraperitoneal route (injection into the intestinal cavity) or the subcutaneous route (injection below the skin). These routes of administration are not only physically different from the oral route but usually produce different results in terms of plasma concentrations and metabolism of the compound. It is useful to convert these doses to their oral equivalents but unfortunately, this sort of conversion is also an inexact science and has little precedent in the literature. Although it can be done, the results of such conversions provide only very rough approximations of an oral dose. The methods used to make these conversions and the reasoning behind them are explained in Appendix I.

humans. This book uses one common method based on data from acute toxicity studies, a method described in Appendix B. The result of this method is illustrated in Figures 1.2a and 1.2b (the latter is a blowup of the zero to 200-mg/kg dose range). A quick formula for the method is given in Equation 1.1.

This equation, like most equations and calculations used in this book, is based on a 70-kilogram (154 pound) human, a 0.2-kilogram rat, and a 0.025-kilogram mouse. Again, keep in mind that this and other scaling

REFERENCES

[1] Based on data from the U.S. National Toxicology Program online database 1999. http://ntp-server.niehs.nih.gov/

[2] Based on data from the Developmental Therapeutics Program online database, U.S. National Cancer Institute. 1999. http://dtp.nci.nih.gov/

PART I
CANCER AT THE CELLULAR LEVEL

Cancer cells are easy to kill using drug therapy; however, they are hard to kill without damaging normal cells. This is because cancer cells rely on processes that are fundamentally similar to the processes used by normal cells. Their differences are in activity, not function. It is like two clocks—one that keeps the right time and one that is fast. Both clocks use the same mechanisms, but one works at a higher speed. Any treatment that harms the structure of the fast clock, when given to the normal clock, would harm its structure as well.

Regarding the cellular level then, the best way to inhibit a cancer cell (and to spare normal cells) is not to destroy its structural properties but to normalize the signals that drive it. These signals derive from its genetic instability, abnormal expression of genes, abnormal sig-

nal transduction, and abnormal communication with healthy cells—the first four clusters of procancer events.

Part I is about these first four clusters and the natural compounds that inhibit them. Chapter 2 discusses the workings of DNA, the role of transcription factors in gene expression, and the causes of genetic instability. Chapter 3 presents the results hoped for from cancer treatment: cell death, lack of proliferation, or normalization of a cell's form and behavior. In Chapter 4, growth factors are discussed, as well as how growth-factor signals travel via signal transduction to reach the DNA. Chapter 5 reviews several transcription factors and the effects that oxidants and antioxidants have on them. Lastly, Chapter 6 discusses cell-to-cell communication.

MUTATIONS, GENE EXPRESSION, AND PROLIFERATION

Mutations—inheritable changes in the DNA—are central to the transformation of a normal cell into a cancer cell, to the development of malignant properties of cancer cells, and to cancer cells adaptation to their environment. The rate of genetic change is especially great when a cancer cell is faced with obstacles to its survival. Since mutations, along with proliferation, are so important to the survival of a cancer, this chapter discusses these events in some detail, starting with the basics: the structure and function of DNA and how cell proliferation occurs. After this, the mechanisms of genetic change are reviewed and therapies that might reduce the rate of this change are examined. Finally, the differences between chemotherapy drugs and natural compounds are explored, emphasizing how they affect DNA differently.

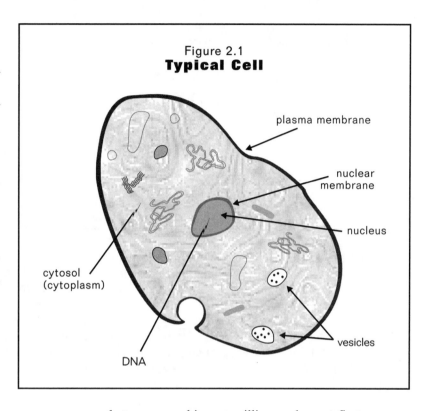

Figure 2.1
Typical Cell

plasma membrane

nuclear membrane

nucleus

cytosol (cytoplasm)

vesicles

DNA

DNA, RNA, AND GENE EXPRESSION

DNA (deoxyribonucleic acid) is like a library of cookbooks, with each book containing a recipe for one specific protein. Each book represents one gene, the gene being the functional unit of DNA. To make our analogy more accurate, we can say that each book is stacked end to end, and thus the library is an extremely long building. Each protein (whose "recipe" is contained in each gene) has an essential part to play in the life of the cell. By following the recipes, the cell produces countless numbers of different proteins, each at their appropriate time and each helping the cell perform a distinct function.

To make proteins, segments of DNA (i.e., genes) are first copied to form RNA (ribonucleic acid), which is a working copy of DNA. This copying process is called gene transcription and is initiated by the binding of transcription factors and other proteins to the affected gene. Once transcription is finished, the RNA is read and, based on its contents, proteins are built up, amino acid by amino acid. The process of reading RNA and making proteins is called translation. Using our analogy again, since the cookbook library (the DNA) does not allow its books to be checked out and does not have

photocopy machines, a willing cook must first copy, or transcribe, the book, letter by letter, then follow the copied version to create the dish. As the cook follows each word in the copied recipe to translate it into a new dish, so the cell follows each "word" in the RNA to translate it into a new protein. The entire process of transcription and translation that produces a new protein is called gene expression.

In cancer cells, the mutation of genes and the abnormal production or activity of transcription factors result in overexpression of genes that promote cancer and underexpression of genes that would otherwise inhibit cancer. By understanding how genes and transcription factors work, we can understand how natural compounds can be used to prevent their malfunction.

DNA and the Cell

The cell is of course where DNA resides. Figure 2.1 illustrates a typical cell. The outer surface of the cell, the plasma membrane, is sometimes called the lipid bilayer, since its basic structure is a dual layer of lipid molecules. Toward the center lies the nucleus, which contains the DNA. Like the cell as a whole, the nucleus is also surrounded by a membrane, called the nuclear membrane. The large space between the plasma mem-

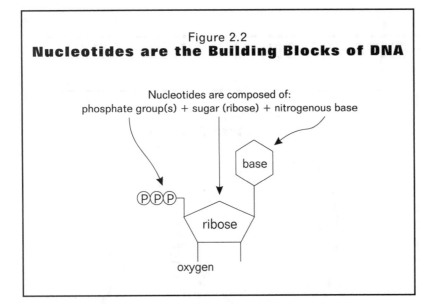

Figure 2.2
Nucleotides are the Building Blocks of DNA

Nucleotides are composed of:
phosphate group(s) + sugar (ribose) + nitrogenous base

base

ribose

oxygen

brane and the nucleus is called the cytoplasm; it contains many different cellular organs with a multitude of functions.

Nucleotides and the Structure of DNA

What is DNA? Using our analogy again, if each book in the DNA library is a gene, then each letter in each book is a nucleotide. Thus each gene is comprised of a series of nucleotides linked end to end, and DNA is comprised of a series of genes linked end to end. Each nucleotide is simply a compound made up of one or more phosphorous groups, a sugar core (ribose), and a nitrogenous base, as illustrated in Figure 2.2.

Each of the three elements comprising a nucleotide has a function within DNA.[a] The phosphorus groups link different nucleotides together to form DNA, the sugar molecules form the backbone of DNA and give it its structure, and the nitrogenous bases contain the actual code of information. These features are evident in the left inset of Figure 2.3. In our library analogy, the alphabet in which the books (genes) in the DNA library are written does not contain 26 letters, but only four. These four letters are the four choices of nitrogenous bases, after which the nucleotides are named: adenosine (having an adenine base), guanosine (having a guanine base), cytidine (having a cytosine base), and thymidine (having a thymine base). The actual structures of the bases and nucleotides are shown in Figures A.1 to A.7 of Appendix A. RNA, the working copy of DNA, is

also made up of nucleotides, but they are slightly different from the four listed above (one substitution is made).

As shown in the right insets of Figure 2.3, two strings of DNA are joined together by weak links between bases to form a ladderlike structure, and this structure is twisted to form a double helix. In the DNA ladder, the bases are always matched in specific pairs. Thymine is always matched with adenine, and cytosine is always matched with guanine.

Until now, we have been talking of DNA as if it occurs in one long string (one long DNA library). In actuality, it occurs in several groups of strings called chromosomes (several different libraries, each holding a duplicate set of its own books). In each chromosome, a long, double helix string of DNA is paired with a matching string. These strings are joined at the center, giving chromosomes their X-shaped structure; chromosomes thus contain four strands of DNA. Human cells have 46 chromosomes, each one different from the others. Certain genes appear on chromosome 1, for example, while other genes appear on chromosome 6. The reason chromosomes contain a set of matching double helix strings is that when the cell divides, it passes along one-half of the set to each daughter cell.

The total length of DNA in human cells is nearly two meters, containing about three billion base pairs. It is amazing that such a large amount of information can be packed into such a small space and even more amazing that this much information can be efficiently manipulated during cell division. DNA contains about 100,000 genes in total, with the average gene spanning about 10,000 to 20,000 base pairs. Not every gene is actually geared to producing proteins; some also code for the production of ribosomes that provide an intermediary function in protein synthesis, as will be discussed below.

RNA and Gene Expression

As stated previously, RNA is the working copy of DNA from which proteins are produced. During the life of a cell, many proteins must be manufactured to perform needed functions. To take two examples, during periods of oxidant stress a cell must manufacture the proteins needed to create antioxidant enzymes, and to start proliferation a cell must manufacture proteins that initiate division. Thus the need for specific proteins changes dynamically during the life of the cell.

---

[a] *Properly, we have to speak of nucleotides as the building blocks of DNA rather than genes, since some DNA sequences comprised of nucleotides are not genes themselves but serve as spacer sequences in DNA or serve other purposes.*

The process of gene transcription—copying a gene to form RNA—must occur without error for the cell to remain healthy. Unwanted gene transcription can be detrimental to the cell because it would lead to the production of unwanted proteins. For example, a cell would be harmed by manufacturing proteins that initiate proliferation if it were not ready to proliferate. The controls that govern gene transcription are therefore sophisticated. The enzyme that carries out transcription (RNA polymerase) will not bind to the DNA or begin transcription until a correct set of regulatory proteins have bound to the DNA and the enzyme. One important group of these regulatory proteins consists of transcription factors that bind to the DNA in the promoter region, which is a sequence of DNA located upstream of the transcription start point. Therefore, transcription factors play a crucial role in regulating protein synthesis as well as cell behavior. In cancer cells, abnormalities in the production or activity of transcription factors help the cell to survive, proliferate, and spread.

Once transcription starts, the DNA is copied base by base, with only one side of the DNA double strand being copied. The process of gene transcription is illustrated in the top inset of Figure 2.4.

Protein synthesis occurs when ribosomes, which are tiny intracellular organs, "read" the bases on RNA and match the coded message with appropriate free amino acids that are held in stock. To give an idea of how important this process is to the cell, human cells undergoing active protein synthesis contain about 10 million ribosomes. As the ribosomes read RNA, each group of three sequential bases they encounter informs them which amino acid is needed next for the protein recipe; then one by one, amino acids are strung together to form proteins in the process called translation (illustrated in the bottom inset of Figure 2.4). Using our library analogy one last time, we have said that the alphabet used to write the books (genes) contains only four letters (four nucleotides). These four letters are arranged in words, with each word, exactly three letters long, describing one amino acid. All the words in the book, when read sequentially, describe one protein.

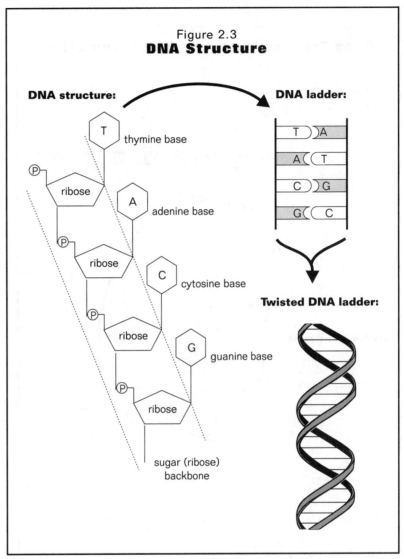

Figure 2.3
DNA Structure

DNA structure:

thymine base

ribose

adenine base

ribose

cytosine base

ribose

guanine base

ribose

sugar (ribose) backbone

DNA ladder:

Twisted DNA ladder:

The two-step process of transcription and translation, or gene expression, thus produces the protein that the gene has encoded. As we will see, some genes can be either underexpressed or overexpressed in cancer cells, giving the cancer cell a growth advantage.

CELL PROLIFERATION

In cancer treatment, we are greatly concerned with cell proliferation because a main reason cancer cells are so deadly is that they proliferate more during their lifetimes than do normal cells. The process of cellular proliferation takes place in a well-defined sequence of events called the cell cycle.

The Cell Cycle

In brief, the cell cycle is a series of events whereby a cell divides and shares one-half of each chromosome

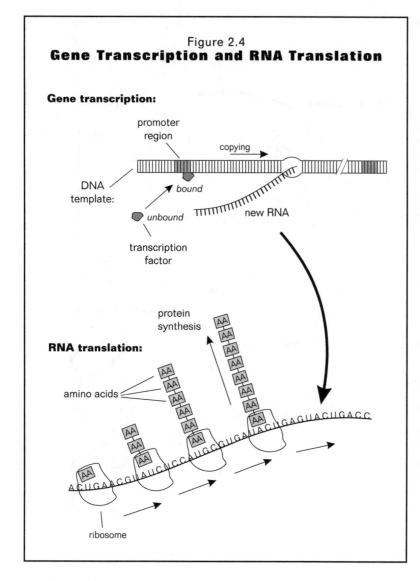

Figure 2.4
Gene Transcription and RNA Translation

Gene transcription:

promoter region

copying

DNA template:

bound

unbound   new RNA

transcription factor

RNA translation:

protein synthesis

amino acids

ribosome

up the middle (see bottom inset of Figure 2.5). A new double strand is then synthesized (through the actions of the enzyme DNA polymerase) to match the original double strand, all of which results in the needed pair of double strands (a complete chromosome).

3. A second gap phase (G_2) follows completion of DNA synthesis. This phase is a resting phase, at the end of which the cell is again checked for integrity.

4. Lastly, in the mitotic phase (M), the cell divides. Here the chromosomes are split, and an identical set of double-stranded DNA goes to each daughter cell. Before leaving the mitosis phase, the cell is checked once more for integrity.

Thus the integrity of all dividing cells is checked at least three times during the cell cycle, at the ends of the G_1, G_2, and M phases. During these checkpoints, the DNA is examined to make sure it is undamaged. If it is damaged, an otherwise healthy cell will stop the cycle and try to repair the lesions. If the lesions are irreparable, the cell cycle will stop and the cell will commit suicide via apoptosis to avoid passing on damaged DNA. Apoptosis, or programmed cell death, is an orderly way for cells to die. As we will see in the next chapter, many natural compounds induce cancer cells to undergo apoptosis.

with each offspring. Each offspring thus receives a double strand of DNA from each chromosome and uses it as a template to manufacture a new, matching double strand; with a complete set of chromosomes, it is then ready to divide itself. The cycle, which takes about 24 hours, is divided into four phases, as illustrated in Figure 2.5:

1. A gap phase (G_1) immediately follows the completion of mitosis (cell division). During this phase, there is active gene transcription and synthesis of proteins, which serve to meet the needs of the growing new cell. Before leaving this gap phase, the cell is checked for integrity.

2. A synthesis phase (S) follows G_1, in which DNA is replicated. After mitosis, the cell only contains half the DNA needed to divide again. During DNA replication, the coiled DNA is relaxed by enzymes called topoisomerases, and the double strand is split

Arrest at the G_1 checkpoint, and possibly others, is mediated by the p53 protein, a transcription factor produced by the *p53* gene.[a] We will discuss this gene and its protein in more detail later, but note here that the *p53* gene plays an extremely important role by inspecting and guarding DNA integrity. For this reason, the *p53* gene has been called the "guardian of DNA." We can imagine that the *p53* gene and its protein are like a perfectionist inspector in a parts factory, who searches for defective parts on the assembly line. If defective parts are found, he sends them in for repair, but if they cannot be repaired, he destroys the entire plant. What that means is that proper functioning of the gene and its

---

[a] *By convention, gene names are italicized, whereas the names of the proteins they produce are not. For example, the* p53 *gene produces the* p53 *protein.*

protein will destroy cancer cells, since cancer cells contain aberrant DNA. On the other hand, mutations in the *p53* gene, which are common in cancer cells, stop *p53* from performing its functions and allow cancer cells to continue to proliferate.

In addition to the four cell-cycle phases described above, a fifth phase also exists that is not part of the cell cycle proper. It is an initial gap phase, in which no proliferative activity takes place. In Figure 2.5, this resting phase is indicated by a box to the side of the cell cycle. Most cells spend the majority of their time in this gap phase, and only enter the cell cycle if they are properly stimulated. This stimulation generally takes place in four sequential steps:

1. One or more growth factors must bind to receptors on the cell surface.

2. The signal that is elicited by receptor binding must be transmitted to the cell's nucleus, the process of signal transduction.

3. "Early" genes must be activated to produce proteins. These genes include *fos, myc,* and *jun,* as described in Table 2.1.

4. The fos, myc, and jun proteins, which are transcription factors, must bind to the DNA on other genes to initiate the synthesis of proteins such as cyclins (discussed in Chapter 4) that drive the cell cycle proper.

Cancer cells are no different from normal cells in their need to be stimulated before entering the cell cycle, except that stimulation is excessive in cancer cells. This excessive stimulation provides a number of targets for inhibiting cancer cell proliferation. For example, drawing from the list above, proliferation can be inhibited by reducing any of these: the abnormal production of growth factors, the binding of growth factors to their receptors, abnormal signal transduction, abnormal expression of early genes, or the abnormal production or activity of transcription factors. As we will see, natural compounds can perform all of these tasks. In addition, natural compounds can affect processes in the cell cycle proper. For example, they can assist the expression of the *p53* gene (or the activity of the p53 protein) and so help it do its job as guardian of the DNA. Thus nearly every aspect of the cell cycle becomes a possible target in cancer treatment with natural compounds.

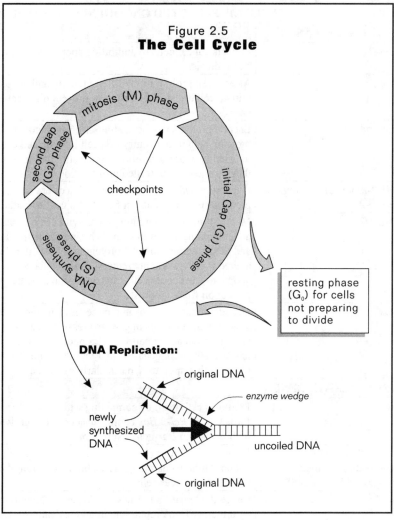

Figure 2.5
The Cell Cycle

MUTATIONS DURING CARCINOGENESIS AND PROGRESSION

Mutations play a critical role in both carcinogenesis and cancer progression, since mutations are the force that initiates a cancer cell, as well as the driving force for their survival and adaptation once formed. Two of the most important consequences of mutations are overexpression of certain genes called oncogenes (onco = cancer), which facilitate carcinogenesis and cancer progression, and underexpression of other genes called tumor suppressor genes, which inhibit carcinogenesis and cancer progression.

Oncogenes and Tumor Suppressor Genes

In healthy cells, the normal expression of oncogenes assists in various normal cell activities, including prolif-

TABLE 2.1 SELECTED ONCOGENES AND TUMOR SUPPRESSOR GENES	
ONCOGENES	**ACTION**
Bcl-2	Protects cancer cells by inhibiting apoptosis (programmed cell death) and by reducing damage from free radicals.
c-*myc*	Affects cell proliferation, differentiation, and apoptosis. Normal expression of the gene is needed to initiate cell division as well as to prevent differentiation. Members of this gene family also include n-*myc* and l-*myc*.
fos and *jun*	Encode proteins that act as transcription factors to facilitate proliferation and other activities. Their proteins help initiate entry of a cell into the cell cycle. In their normal form, these genes are transiently expressed following the stimulation of a cell by growth factors. When overexpressed, they promote uncontrolled proliferation.
HER-2/neu, also known as c-*erb-2*	Overexpressed in approximately 33% of breast cancers and associated with a poor prognosis. It produces proteins that can facilitate signal transduction and act in other ways to assist cancer cells.
MDM2	Mainly functions to inhibit *p53* activity. In normal cells, the MDM2 protein binds to the p53 protein and maintains p53 at low levels by increasing its destruction. When normal cells are under stress and the activity of the p53 protein is needed, the ability of MDM2 to bind to p53 is blocked or altered in a way that prevents MDM2-mediated degradation. As a result, p53 levels rise, causing apoptosis. In cancer cells, this oncogene is overexpressed, causing chronically low p53 levels and protection from apoptosis.
ras	Oncogenic forms of *ras* induce several changes in tumor cells, including changes in form and structure and changes in gene expression. The result is excessive DNA synthesis and an increase in chromosomal abnormalities. *Ras* oncogenes are thought to stimulate the production of enzymes (specifically, collagenases) that facilitate tumor invasion. Ras proteins may also protect cancer cells by inhibiting apoptosis, particularly by increasing the expression of *MDM2* genes.
SUPPRESSOR GENES	**ACTION**
Bax	Promotes cell death by competing with *Bcl-2*. While *Bax* acts as an inducer of apoptosis, the formation of *Bcl-2/Bax* conjugates evokes a survival signal for cells. The *p53* gene controls, in part, both *Bcl-2* and *Bax* gene expression.
genes that produce connexin proteins (e.g., *Cx32* and *Cx43*)	Form gap junctions (or portals) between neighboring cells. Communication through gap junctions not only inhibits carcinogenesis, but restoration of communication also normalizes malignant behavior of cancer cells.
p53	Called the "guardian of DNA." Whereas the wild-type (normal) *p53* gene suppresses tumor growth by initiating DNA repair and inducing death of irreparable cells, the mutant *p53* gene acts as an oncogene to allow proliferation of cells with DNA damage. Changes in the *p53* gene are one of the most common mutations found in human cancers.
Sources: References 2–11.	

eration. However, when overexpressed, that is, when too many of their proteins are produced or they are produced at the wrong times, oncogenes transform healthy cells into cancer cells or assist in cancer progression. Overexpression of oncogenes can be caused by exposure to carcinogens, radiation, or certain viruses. Overexpression can also be caused by free radicals, such as those produced during chronic inflammation.[1]

In contrast, tumor suppressor genes are ones that, when normally expressed, inhibit carcinogenesis. Thus, *p53* is a tumor suppressor gene. When they are underexpressed or when they mutate to nonfunctional forms, as is common in cancer, carcinogenesis and progression are facilitated.

Table 2.1 provides a list of oncogenes and tumor suppressor genes and briefly explains what they do. This list is not complete—more than 30 oncogenes and more

than 10 tumor suppressor genes have been discovered to date—but it does cover the primary oncogenes and tumor suppressor genes of interest to us.[11]

Classical DNA Mutations

The root cause of oncogene overexpression and tumor suppressor gene underexpression is gene mutations. In addition, mutations can lead to abnormal production or activity of transcription factors, abnormal signal transduction, or other events that exacerbate oncogene overexpression and tumor suppressor gene underexpression. To avoid both the direct and indirect effects, we must do all we can to prevent mutations.

In the sections below, we first discuss gene mutations as understood in classical genetics, where inheritable DNA damage is due to changes in DNA base sequences, that is, changes to the order in which bases normally occur within a gene. Later, we discuss epigenetic changes, in which the base sequences are not changed, but bases are still altered and the alterations are still inheritable. Hence, epigenetic changes, while not classical mutations, can be thought of as functional ones.

Base sequence changes are limited only by their toxicity to the cell. If the sequence change is not toxic and the cell does not repair it, the cell survives and the changes are passed on to subsequent generations. Sequence changes are relatively common, and most are repaired by the ever vigilant DNA repair system. If the repair system malfunctions, as is the case in some inherited disorders, the risk of developing cancer increases. Even when fully functional, however, the repair system is not perfect, and a small probability exists that damaged DNA will escape repair during any one cell division. Often this is a desirable fault, since slight changes in the DNA are required for evolution and adaptation of the species. Indeed, most species are programmed for a certain low level of ongoing mutations. If the damage is more than slight, however, or if it is in DNA sequences found in oncogenes or tumor suppressor genes, cancer may be initiated.

The sequence changes of classical mutations can be caused by a number of events. Some occur spontaneously, and some are due to external causes. One sequence change that can occur is the transformation of one base into another. Since the structures of the bases are quite similar, some bases are easily converted to others by simply adding or removing a few atoms (in particular, an amino group NH_2). The similarities in bases can be seen in Figures A.1 to A.5 of Appendix A. Other sequence changes are caused by external carcinogens, which alter a base in some way. For example, ultraviolet light can fuse two bases together; alkylating chemicals can add extra small molecules to a base (usually a methyl group, CH_3); free radicals can add an oxygen group to a base; and still other carcinogenic chemicals can add large molecules to a base. If the alteration does not cause the cell to die, the altered base is prone to being mismatched during DNA replication, resulting in a base sequence change.

Sequence changes can also be caused by base deletions or additions. Deletions can be large or small and can occur when a base is cleaved from DNA by a misplaced enzyme, or they can be the result of errors during DNA synthesis. Additions can be caused by viruses, which insert new DNA.

Free Radicals

Free radicals were mentioned above as playing a role in gene mutations and oncogene overexpression. Al-

though they will be discussed later, we introduce them here as molecules that are unstable because they contain an unpaired electron. When a free radical molecule contacts the electrons of a stable molecule, the free radical molecule gains or loses electrons to achieve a stable paired-electron configuration. In the process, however, the electron balance of the stable molecule is disturbed, and the stable molecule becomes a free radical molecule. In this manner, free radicals initiate a chain reaction of destruction. Free radicals can damage DNA, protein, and fats. Indeed, free radical damage has been implicated as a major contributor to cancer, as well as to other degenerative diseases such as aging, cardiovascular disease, immune dysfunction, brain dysfunction, and cataracts.[12]

Free radicals can be produced by a variety of means. They can be produced by external factors such as radiation and cigarette smoke, and by internal events such as immune cell activity and cellular respiration (cellular "breathing" of oxygen). In humans, up to 5 percent of oxygen taken in is converted to free radicals during cellular respiration.[13] During respiration, cells consume oxygen (O_2) and produce water (H_2O). Byproducts of this process include the superoxide radical ($O_2^{\bullet -}$), which can lead to the production of the very damaging hydroxyl radical ($OH^{\bullet}$). (The dot represents unpaired electrons.) The hydroxyl radical is the most toxic of all the oxygen-based free radicals.

Other important kinds of free radicals include the peroxyl and the alkoxyl radicals, both of which are involved in lipid peroxidation (oxidative damage to fats). In recent years, the term *reactive oxygen species* (ROS) has been adopted, since it includes the above-mentioned radicals plus hydrogen peroxide (H_2O_2) and molecular oxygen (O_2). While not free radicals in themselves, these two can easily become free radicals in the body.

The body maintains a variety of antioxidants as a multilevel defense against free radical damage. These include the enzymes superoxide dismutase, catalase, and glutathione peroxidase; antioxidants synthesized in the body, such as glutathione, proteins, and uric acid; and antioxidants obtained from the diet, such as flavonoids, vitamins C and E, and beta-carotene. Nevertheless, antioxidant defenses are not perfect, and DNA is damaged regularly. There may be as many as 10,000 oxidative hits to DNA per cell per day in humans.[12] The vast majority of these lesions are repaired by cellular enzymes. Those that are not repaired may progress toward neoplasia (the formation of cancer cells). Because of the continual bombardment of DNA and other tissues by free radicals, the body must obtain ample antioxidant supplies through the diet. Epidemiological studies support a protective role for dietary antioxidants by consistently reporting that populations who consume inadequate amounts of fresh fruits and vegetables are at a higher risk for cancer, heart disease, and other degenerative diseases.

Not only can free radicals initiate cancer, they can also facilitate cancer progression. And in fact, multiple human tumor cell lines have been reported to produce ROS (especially hydrogen peroxide) in vitro.[14] Under normal circumstances, few cells other than immune cells produce hydrogen peroxide. Free radical production by tumor cells may help them mutate or display other malignant properties such as tissue invasion. For example, superoxide radicals have been reported to increase the invasive capacity of rat liver cancer cells in vitro.[15]

To be clear though, free radicals are not always bad. Only when they are overproduced or the body's antioxidant system is overwhelmed do they cause problems. In Chapter 5, we discuss free radicals and antioxidants in more detail, explaining both their usefulness and destructiveness.

Epigenetic Changes in DNA

It has become clear in recent years that some inheritable characteristics of cancer cells are not due to changes in DNA sequence (classical mutations) but rather to functional changes in the otherwise normal DNA.[16] Unlike classical mutations, these "epigenetic" changes are reversible. This fact is quite important, since it suggests that some malignant characteristics may be normalized under the right circumstances. Epigenetic changes and their reversal are still poorly understood, but their study may one day lead to therapies that cause cancer cells to revert to more normal behavior. Metastasis, or the spread of tumor cells to distant locations, is one example of a process in which epigenetic events may play a crucial role. If genetic makeup were the only determinant in the production of metastatic cells, one would expect an exponential increase in metastases from previous metastases. This is generally not the case, however. Rather, it is likely that epigenetic changes play an important role in turning metastasis on and off.[17]

Epigenetic changes in DNA are characterized primarily by the attachment of a methyl (CH_3) group to a specific location in a cytosine base. This is illustrated simply in Figure 2.6, both for a single nucleotide and for a series of nucleotides in DNA. Cytosine methylation is illustrated in more detail in Figure A.8 of Appendix A.

Methylation of cytosine is actually the only known nonaberrant modification to DNA, and it plays a role in determining which genes are activated for transcription. Thus, methylation acts as an intelligent switching system to control the production of proteins needed at different times. In this regard, it is more like a long-term switching system than a short-term one, since methylation patterns are passed from generation to generation. The greater the amount of cytosine methylation in a gene, the less it is expressed. Therefore, depending on the needs of the cell, some genes may be lightly methylated (hypomethylated) and easily expressed, whereas others may be heavily methylated (hypermethylated) and silenced. A moderate amount of methylation is normal for most genes. As an analogy, we can think of the methyl groups added to a gene as a series of "do not disturb" signs. If the gene contains enough of these signs, the cell knows that the gene should not be expressed. For example, one way the body avoids expressing genes that contain virally inserted bases is to attach extra "do not disturb" methyl groups to it.[18]

Because cytosine methylation is not perceived as a DNA error by the body (unlike mutations, which are errors the body tries to repair), cytosine methylation patterns are purposefully passed on to the daughter cells when a cell divides. Methylation patterns are passed on in the synthesis phase of the cell cycle (see bottom inset of Figure 2.5), when the daughter cell is using its double strand of DNA as a template to manufacture a matching double strand. Specific enzymes recognize the methyl groups on the template DNA and add matching methyl groups to the new strands as they are being formed.

Abnormalities in cytosine methylation are very common in cancer cells, and they occur early in the carcinogenic process. Most genes in cancer cells tend to be hypomethylated and therefore overexpressed. This is particularly true of the many oncogenes that facilitate carcinogenesis. However, a smaller number of genes tend to be hypermethylated and therefore silenced. This is particularly true of the small number of tumor suppressor genes. One example is silencing the *p53* gene that inspects and protects DNA. Hypermethylation and silencing can occur in other genes also. For example, silencing of the gene controlling the production of transforming growth factor-beta (TGF-beta) can occur in cancer.[19] Like the proteins made from tumor suppressor genes, TGF-beta is a protein that represses cell proliferation. Therefore, silencing the TGF-beta gene can lead to increased cancer cell proliferation. As another example, hypermethylation and silencing of the gene that makes the estrogen receptor protein can occur in prostate cancer.[20] Estrogen inhibits prostate cancer growth, and a lack of estrogen receptors removes this inhibition. Lastly, hypermethylation and silencing of the genes that make cell-to-cell adhesion proteins (especially the gene controlling the adhesive protein E-cadherin) are also common in many types of cancer.[21] Reduced cell-to-cell communication, as we have discussed, can facilitate cancer progression.

Epigenetic changes and mutations work together to give cancer cells a growth advantage. In fact, epigenetic changes can lead to an increased rate of classical mutations in at least three ways. First, hypomethylation of oncogenes or hypermethylation of tumor suppressor genes make later mutations more likely. For example, hypermethylation and silencing of the *p53* gene allow mutations to occur with greater frequency, since DNA is not repaired and mutated cells are not forced to die. Second, when a methyl group is added to cytosine, the combination is easily converted to other bases besides cytosine, thereby producing base substitution mutations.[22] Third, the hypermethylation of genes interferes with their repair if they have been otherwise damaged.[23]

We see then that classical mutations and epigenetic changes are closely linked. This suggests that by reducing abnormal methylation, mutations may also be reduced. Antioxidants may help reduce abnormal methylation, since oxidative damage to DNA alters cytosine methylation patterns.[24, 25] As discussed at the end of this chapter, natural compounds that are methyl donors may also reduce abnormal methylation.

Mutator Phenotype Theory

Whether due to classic mutations or epigenetic changes, ongoing genetic alterations are crucial for the continued survival of cancer cells. Cancer cells live in a changing, hostile environment; among other things, immune cells and cancer treatments try to destroy them, the body in general tries to inhibit their activity in its attempts to maintain homeostasis, and since they overcrowd themselves, they must compete for nutrients and oxygen. Only the strongest cells survive, and as conditions change, cancer cells must also change.

The mutator phenotype theory proposes that surviving cancer cells exhibit two characteristics. First and most obvious, they contain specific mutations that allow them to survive the present adverse environment. Second and less obvious, they contain mutations that allow them to mutate easily. In other words, they contain mutations in genes that normally function to maintain genetic stability. Thus they have the characteristic, or phenotype, of

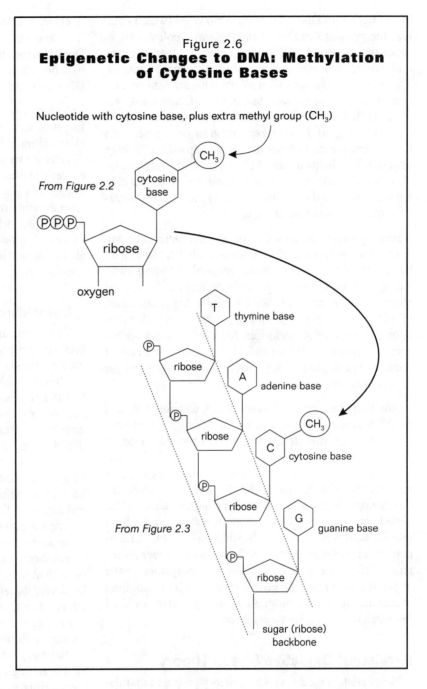

Figure 2.6
Epigenetic Changes to DNA: Methylation of Cytosine Bases

Nucleotide with cytosine base, plus extra methyl group (CH₃)

From Figure 2.2

CH₃

cytosine base

P P P

ribose

oxygen

T   thymine base

P

ribose

A   adenine base

P

ribose

CH₃

C   cytosine base

P

ribose

From Figure 2.3

G   guanine base

P

ribose

sugar (ribose) backbone

genetic instability.[26–30] The mutator phenotype theory helps explain why cancer cells have a much higher rate of gene mutations than normal cells. Proponents of this theory predict that as analytical techniques improve, perhaps thousands of gene mutations will be discovered in cancer cells.[31] Indeed, no single genetic change is found in 100 percent of any single type of cancer, but a bewildering number of gene mutations have so far been discovered.

According to the mutator phenotype theory, an early event in cancer progression is mutations in the genes that control genetic stability. These include mutations in the *p53* gene, in DNA polymerase enzymes (which catalyze the synthesis of DNA strands during replication), in genes that encode for DNA repair enzymes, and in genes that control chromosome segregation during mitosis. These genetic changes then allow a higher rate of random mutations, some fatal to cancer cells and some that promote their survival. Examples of the latter are mutations that lead to the overexpression of oncogenes. As tumors encounter new obstacles to expansion, a high mutation rate helps assure their survival. In fact, obstacles to expansion such as drug therapy and competition for nutrients and oxygen may actually increase the mutation rate as tumors attempt to adapt.[31, 32]

Some genetic changes that occur in cancer cells are epigenetic changes, and as discussed above, these may be reversible. Aside from reversal of epigenetic changes, it may also be possible to reduce the rate of classical mutations and thereby inhibit the progression of tumors.[27] Since it commonly takes about 20 years after exposure to a carcinogen for a solid tumor to become detectable, even a twofold decrease in the rate of mutations (and progression) would greatly reduce cancer deaths in adults.[26]

Mutations require two events: DNA damage and lack of DNA repair. One source of DNA damage that may play a primary role in supporting high mutation rates is reactive oxygen species (ROS). Because of inflammation and other factors, cancer cells normally exist in an environment that is rich in ROS. Indeed, chronic inflammatory diseases, which produce high levels of ROS, have been associated with genetic instability and a high incidence of cancer.[27, 33–35] In addition, chronic inflammation has been associated with increased cancer recurrence after surgery.[36] Some investigators have attempted to explain the involvement of ROS in ongoing mutations and cancer progression through what is called the persistent oxidative stress theory.

Persistent Oxidative Stress Theory

The persistent oxidative stress theory proposes that the chronically elevated levels of ROS to which cancer cells are exposed contribute to their survival and progression.[37–40] If extreme enough, oxidative conditions do stress cancer cell populations, killing a percentage of the cells. However, it is now well established that mild levels of ROS can stimulate cell proliferation and cancer progression.[41, 42, 43] For example, a recent study on patients with colorectal cancer reported that carcinoma cells, but not corresponding normal cells or benign tumors, were oxidatively stressed (as measured by oxidative modifications to DNA bases). This study also reported that cancer cell proliferation rates were posi-

tively correlated to oxidative stress levels.[38] Other studies have also reported that cancer cells exhibit more DNA damage than adjacent normal cells and that cancer patients show higher levels of ROS production and DNA damage than healthy subjects.[37, 44–46]

Clearly, one way by which oxidative conditions can facilitate cancer progression is by increasing the rate of classical mutations. Classical mutations can be induced directly by oxidative damage to DNA and indirectly via epigenetic changes, as discussed above. Oxidative conditions can also increase the proliferation of cancer cells through other means that will be discussed in later chapters. These include ROS-induced increases in the sensitivity of growth factor receptors and ROS-induced abnormalities in the production or activity of transcription factors.

Antioxidants in Cancer Treatment

We can see that oxidative stress could either inhibit or facilitate cancer cell proliferation, depending on the degree of stress. It is reasonable to suppose that supplementation with antioxidants could either inhibit or facilitate cancer cell proliferation, depending on the degree of oxidative stress and the antioxidant status of the individual. Based on the limited in-vivo data available, this does seem to be the case. Although this complex and rather controversial issue is discussed in detail in Chapter 15, I report here the conclusion that, depending on circumstances, antioxidants when used alone could produce beneficial, detrimental, or insignificant effects in cancer patients. When used in combination with other anticancer compounds (i.e., natural compounds or chemotherapy drugs), their effects are more likely to be beneficial or at least not harmful. Even when beneficial, however, the effects are likely to be mild for many patients. For these reasons, I regard antioxidants as supportive agents best used within larger combinations of cancer-inhibiting compounds. Natural compounds such as flavonoids that act as antioxidants but also inhibit cancer through other means have the potential to play a more primary role in treatment.

There is some concern that antioxidants may increase the success of metastasizing cells. This effect, which has been seen in some animal studies, will also be discussed in Chapter 15. It is likely, however, that this and any other disadvantages antioxidant use may pose could be reduced or eliminated by using antioxidants as only one part of an overall combination therapy, as this book recommends.

Some readers may question if cancer could successfully be treated by withholding antioxidants and in that way producing oxidative damage. Cancer inhibition was reported in such a study done in mice (see Chapter 15). Although it is true that cancer cells are susceptible to oxidative damage, it is almost assured that a certain number of cancer cells will survive oxidative therapies. It is reasonable to suppose from the above discussions that the surviving cells may be highly primed for mutations and that these therapies could therefore eventually produce more adaptable, more aggressive cancers that are not easily treated. In addition, restriction of antioxidant intake would likely cause adverse effects in healthy tissues. For these reasons, such a prooxidant therapy is not seen here as promising.

HOW NATURAL COMPOUNDS AND CHEMOTHERAPY DRUGS INHIBIT PROLIFERATION

Let us now pull together what has been presented about how natural compounds inhibit cancer cell proliferation and compare how natural compounds work to the way current chemotherapy drugs work, thus clarifying what natural compounds have to offer. As we will see, the cancer inhibitory effects of most natural compounds discussed are not due to direct DNA damage, whereas direct DNA damage is an important mechanism for many of the chemotherapy drugs used today. This distinction is important, in that natural compounds are therefore less likely than many chemotherapy drugs to induce DNA mutations in surviving cells. Moreover, natural compounds are more likely to act selectively on cancer cells and spare normal cells than are most chemotherapy drugs now in use.

Targets of Natural Compounds Versus Targets of Chemotherapy Drugs

Targets of Natural Compounds

Cancer cells can be likened to drug addicts. They need a regular fix to keep them going, and without it, they fall apart. Their fix is the abnormally high throughput of proliferation signals (and "do not die" signals). Without these signals, some cancer cells enter a quiescent period, and many, unable to survive without a fix, die via apoptosis. Normal cells, which do not depend on such a high throughput of signals (or self-originated signals), tend to be less susceptible. The natural compounds discussed here tend to inhibit the proliferation of cancer cells by removing the flow of signals that leads to cell proliferation and prevention of cell death.

Since cancer cells and normal cells work by the same mechanisms, the flow of signals that instructs both to proliferate is the same, except in cancer cells the signals

are more abundant and also largely self-originated. Therefore, if we were to eliminate these signals, normal cells would also suffer. The natural compounds I discuss do not have this strong an effect, however. Instead, at the plasma concentrations that are achievable with oral administration, they tend to reduce the signal flow to more normal levels.

The flow of information leading to cell proliferation is mediated through proteins, as illustrated in Figure 2.7. In the figure, abnormal gene expression is the most prominent feature, since such expression is central to the proliferation and malignant behavior of cancer cells. As shown, abnormal gene expression results in one of four types of protein signals that assist proliferation or malignant behavior. All four of these primary protein signals can be inhibited by natural compounds.

1. Errors in the *p53* gene can produce p53 proteins that fail to induce apoptosis in cells with DNA damage, resulting in increased DNA instability and unchecked proliferation. Errors in the *Bax* gene can produce proteins that also fail to induce apoptosis in cancer cells. Errors in the *Bcl-2* gene can produce excessive amounts of proteins that protect against apoptosis in cancer cells.

2. Abnormalities in some genes can produce excessive amounts of proteins that assist angiogenesis (the growth of new blood vessels), or assist in invasion, metastasis, or evasion of the immune system. Although these do not have direct effects on proliferation, they do affect proliferation or the rate of cell death indirectly.

3. Overexpression of oncogenes such as *fos*, *jun*, and *myc* can produce large amounts of fos, jun, and myc proteins. As discussed above, these proteins act as transcription factors to induce the expression of genes such as cyclin genes, whose proteins drive the cell cycle proper. In addition, overexpression of cyclin genes can directly produce excessive amounts of cyclin proteins.

4. Abnormal genes can produce several proteins that facilitate signal transduction. These proteins include growth factors, growth factor receptors, and kinase enzymes, ras proteins, and others. (These are discussed in Chapter 4.) Overproduction of these proteins results in increased signal transduction, which stimulates abnormal activity of transcription factors such as AP-1 and NF-κB (discussed in Chapter 5). Abnormal transcription factor activity stimulates gene expression, resulting in the overproduction of cyclin proteins that drive the cell cycle and the overproduction of other proteins that assist angiogenesis, invasion, and metastasis.

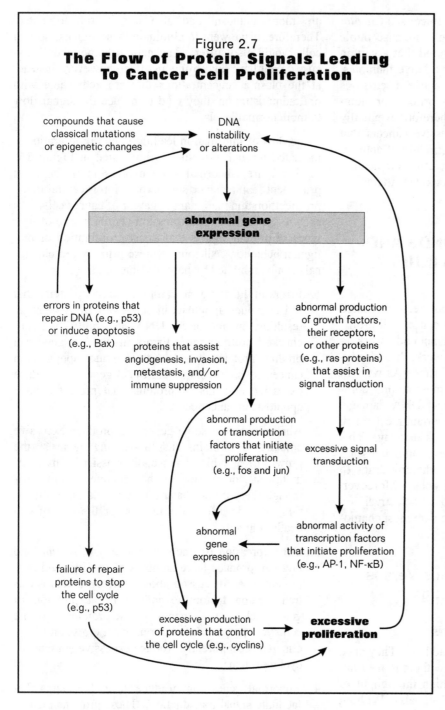

Figure 2.7
The Flow of Protein Signals Leading To Cancer Cell Proliferation

Natural compounds that inhibit signal transduction can play a dual role in inhibiting cancer. In addition to proliferation signals, cancer cells (like normal cells) also require "do not die" signals to prevent death through apoptosis. In cancer cells, these signals come in part from both growth factors and increased signal transduction. Therefore, natural compounds that reduce signal transduction not only can inhibit proliferation but can also induce cell death.

Targets of Chemotherapy Drugs

In contrast to natural compounds, the chemotherapy drugs in current use primarily target DNA. Several aspects of DNA are targeted, including the structure of individual nucleotides; the integrity of nucleotides or their bases within DNA; the main enzymes active in the synthesis phase (DNA polymerase and topoisomerases, which are active in DNA replication and in DNA unwinding, respectively); and the structures and enzymes active in the mitosis phase. By acting on these targets, these drugs prevent completion of the cell cycle. Their actions do not target cancer cells specifically but inhibit the proliferation of any cell in the cell cycle. This means that normal cells frequently in the cell cycle, such as hair cells, immune cells, and cells of the gastrointestinal lining, are harmed along with cancer cells. To give a clearer idea of how these drugs work, we consider these targets in more detail, starting with those that target nucleotide structure.

Natural compounds that inhibit these signals are discussed in Chapters 3 through 6. Their actions include lowering mutation rates by scavenging free radicals, normalizing *p53* activity, or both; inhibiting abnormal transcription factor activity; inhibiting kinases or other proteins involved in signal transduction; inhibiting the activity of cyclin proteins, which drive the cell cycle; and increasing cell-to-cell communication, which sends signals that normalize gene expression.

Targeting Nucleotides Structure

One way of inhibiting cancer cell proliferation is to inhibit the production of nucleotides. A number of chemotherapy drugs, classified as antimetabolites, act by this means. For example, folate, a B vitamin, is needed for the synthesis of some bases. Drugs such as methotrexate inhibit folate activity. Other drugs like fluorouracil, hydroxyurea, and cytarabine inhibit DNA synthesis in other ways. The latter inhibits DNA polymerase, the enzyme that makes new strands of DNA during replication. To some degree it also substitutes the sugar arabinose for ribose during DNA synthesis (functional nucleotides contain ribose).

Targeting Nucleotides Within DNA

A number of chemotherapy drugs act by altering the nucleotides within DNA once it is formed, thereby damaging the DNA and inhibiting its replication and transcription. Some drugs—for example, cyclophosphamide, carmustine, cisplatin, mitomycin, and busulfan—are alkylating agents, which means they add strings of hydrocarbon molecules to the nucleotides. These strings can bind DNA strands together or simply hang on single DNA strands, thereby interfering with DNA replication, transcription, or repair.

Other chemotherapy drugs, such as doxorubicin and bleomycin, are intercalating drugs, meaning they insert themselves between adjacent DNA base pairs. The flat structure of these drugs allows them to slip easily between base pairs. Some of these drugs, including doxorubicin and bleomycin, instigate free radical damage to bases once they are inserted. Intercalating drugs interfere with both DNA and RNA synthesis.

Targeting Topoisomerases

Topoisomerases are enzymes that unwind the DNA so that both DNA replication and gene transcription can take place. Some chemotherapy drugs, such as the natural compound camptothecin and the semisynthetic compound etoposide, act via topoisomerase inhibition.

Some natural compounds discussed here also have the capacity to inhibit topoisomerases. These include apigenin, ATRA (vitamin A), boswellic acid, genistein, luteolin, and quercetin (see Appendix C for details). These compounds are active in the concentration range of roughly 1 to 200 μM, with the IC_{50} for most of them tending to be greater than 30 μM. Two exceptions are boswellic acid and ATRA, which are reportedly active at concentrations between about 1 and 10 μM. This concentration of ATRA is similar to peak plasma concentrations normally produced during ATRA treatment of leukemia patients after high doses. All of these compounds, however, also inhibit cancer through other mechanisms and usually at lower concentrations than those just discussed. Therefore, topoisomerase inhibition is not likely to be a primary mode of cell inhibition for any of these compounds in vivo (after oral administration); other anticancer actions are likely to take precedence.

Targeting Mitosis

Compounds that inhibit the mitosis (M) phase in the cell cycle, called antimitotic compounds, prevent cell proliferation. Some chemotherapy drugs that are themselves natural compounds act as antimitotics, including vincristine and vinblastine. The natural compounds discussed in this book do not generally act in this way, however.

CYTOSINE METHYLATION AND DNA: A NOTE ON CANCER PREVENTION

As a concluding note, we discuss a promising approach to prevention (and perhaps eventually treatment) that is closely related to what has been covered so far. I already mentioned the possibility that antioxidants may help prevent abnormal methylation patterns. It seems likely that methyl donors have an important role to play in promoting normal methylation as well. (Information on a related topic, polyamine synthesis, is provided in Appendix C for those readers who want more information on other potential cancer prevention and treatment strategies.)

As a reminder, the genes of tumor cells tend to be hypomethylated (not enough "do not disturb" signs) and therefore overexpressed. This is particularly true of the oncogenes. A smaller number of genes, tumor suppressor genes, tend to be hypermethylated (too many "do not disturb" signs) and therefore silenced. As noted, these inheritable but potentially reversible changes in DNA structure are called epigenetic changes. Natural compounds that are methyl donors may affect methylation patterns in a way that prevents epigenetic changes, and so they may play a role in cancer prevention.

DNA methylation requires the presence of methyl groups, and the primary donor of methyl groups in the body is S-adenosylmethionine (SAM). Some readers will recognize SAM as a natural compound used experimentally to treat arthritis, inflammation, and depression.[47] (The structure of SAM is illustrated in Figure A.9 of Appendix A.) The SAM cycle is illustrated in Figure 2.8 (adapted from references 18 and 48).[a] Briefly, SAM is transformed into the amino acid homocysteine and then into the amino acid methionine. Methionine is then converted back into SAM. As shown, choline, vitamin B_{12}, and folate assist in this process. Because of their involvement in the SAM cycle, choline, folate, methionine, and vitamin B_{12} are considered the primary dietary sources of methyl donors. One donor,

---

[a] S-adenosylmethionine derives its name from being an adenosine molecule (a nucleotide) joined with a methionine molecule.

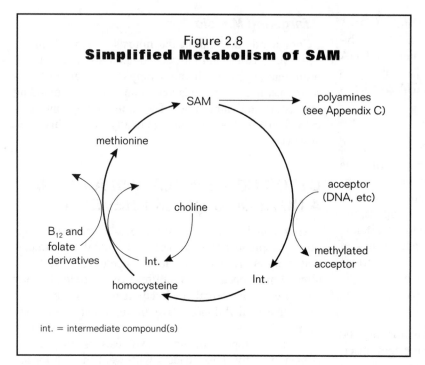

Figure 2.8
Simplified Metabolism of SAM

int. = intermediate compound(s)

Different methyl donors may have distinct effects. The methyl donor methionine, for example, has been reported to act as a promoting agent in some situations.[61] That methionine and SAM have variant effects was also suggested in a study where SAM administration reduced preneoplastic liver lesions in animals, but methionine administration had no effect.[62] The reasons for the dissimilar effects are not entirely clear but may be due to incomplete conversion of methionine to SAM.

Although methyl donors may be useful for cancer prevention, their usefulness in treating established cancers is more uncertain. For one thing, high SAM concentrations could theoretically facilitate hypermethylation and silencing of tumor suppressor genes. Second, high folate intake could assist nucleotide synthesis in cancer cells. In contrast, it is also possible that administration of methyl donors could be beneficial. For example, administration of SAM could lead to hypermethylation and silencing of oncogenes. The therapeutic use of SAM or other methyl donors as a treatment agent remains to be more fully investigated.

folate, is also required for nucleotide synthesis, as mentioned previously.

If the body does not have enough SAM, a variety of diseases can arise, including cancer. This is because an insufficient amount of SAM can result in hypomethylation and therefore overexpression of many genes, including oncogenes. In addition, low levels of SAM can increase the risk of spontaneous base substitutions, leading to mutations.

Since low levels of SAM can be produced by insufficient intake of methyl donors, the above discussion would suggest that methyl donors could be useful in cancer prevention. Although the data are somewhat conflicting, this does seem to be the case. Animals fed diets lacking in methyl groups (insufficient amounts of choline, methionine, folate, vitamin B_{12}, or all of these) are prone to developing hypomethylated genes (including *c-myc* and *c-fos* oncogenes) and to developing liver and other cancers.[49, 50, 51] Moreover, in a number of studies, intramuscular administration of SAM inhibited oncogene expression, normalized DNA methylation, reversed preneoplastic liver lesions, and provided long-term protection from cancer formation in animals treated with carcinogens.[52–55] In these studies, the few cancers that did form grew relatively slowly. Furthermore, adequate intake of the methyl donor folate appears to protect humans from some cancers, including cervical and colon cancer, although study results are inconsistent.[56–60] In one study, oral administration of folate was able to correct hypomethylation in the rectal cells of some but not all patients with colorectal cancer.[58]

CONCLUSION

Mutations are the central driving force behind transformation of a normal cell into a cancer cell and behind progression of the developing tumor. The mutations that give a cancer cell a proliferation advantage are those that lead to increased expression of oncogenes and decreased expression of tumor suppressor genes and those that lead to the production of proteins that otherwise assist proliferation.

Normal cells and cancer cells proliferate in response to the same signals. The distinguishing characteristic of cancer cells is the higher volume of proliferation signals (or the lower volume of "do not die" signals). Thus cancer cells are set apart by their extreme behavior, rather than by intrinsically foreign behavior. One characteristic that makes natural compounds attractive as anticancer agents is that they can be used to interrupt the flow of information that promotes extreme behavior and thus are generally not so damaging to normal cells as treatments that target DNA itself.

REFERENCES

[1] Ernst P. Review article: The role of inflammation in the pathogenesis of gastric cancer. Aliment Pharmacol Ther 1999 Mar; 13 Suppl 1:13–8.

[2] Bertino JR, ed. Encyclopedia of cancer. San Diego: Academic Press, 1997, pp. 419–431, 1481–1483, 1940–1953.

[3] Reed JC. Double identity for proteins of the Bcl-2 family. Nature 1977; 387:773–6.

[4] Haupt Y, Maya R, Kazaz A, Oren M. Mdm2 promotes the rapid degradation of p53. Nature 1977; 387:296.

[5] Marshall MS. Ras target proteins in eukaryotic cells. FASEB J 1995; 9:1311–1318.

[6] Steinman HM. The Bcl-2 oncoprotein functions as a pro-oxidant. J Biol Chem 1995 Feb 24; 270(8):3487–90.

[7] Fernandes RS, McGowan AJ, Cotter TG. Mutant H-ras overexpression inhibits drug and U.V. induced apoptosis. Anticancer Res 1996 Jul–Aug; 16(4A):1691–705.

[8] Smith AD, et al., eds. Oxford dictionary of biochemistry and molecular biology. Oxford: Oxford University Press, 1997.

[9] Ruch RJ. The role of gap junctional intercellular communication in neoplasia. Ann Clin Lab Sci 1994 May–Jun; 24(3):216–31.

[10] Momand J, Wu HH, Dasgupta G. MDM2—master regulator of the p53 tumor suppressor protein. Gene 2000 Jan 25; 242(1–2):15–29.

[11] Greenwald P, Kelloff G, Burch-Whitman C, et al. Chemoprevention. CA Cancer J Clin 1995; 45:31–49.

[12] Ames BN, Shigenaga MK, Hagen TM. Oxidants, antioxidants and the degenerative diseases of aging. Proc Natl Acad Sci USA 1993 Sep; 90:7915–22.

[13] Reiter RJ, Melchiorri D, Sewerynek E, Poeggeler B, et al. A review of the evidence supporting melatonin's role as an antioxidant. J Pineal Res 1995; 18(1):1–11.

[14] Szatrowski TP, Nathan CF. Production of large amounts of hydrogen peroxide by human tumor cells. Cancer Res 1991 Feb 1; 51(3):794–8.

[15] Shinkai K, Mukai M, Akedo H. Superoxide radical potentiates invasive capacity of rat ascites hepatoma cells in vitro. Cancer Letters 1986; 32:7–13.

[16] Rennie PS, Nelson CC. Epigenetic mechanisms for progression of prostate cancer. Cancer Metastasis Rev 1998–99; 17(4):401–9.

[17] Safarians S, Sternlicht MD, Freiman CJ, et al. The primary tumor is the primary source of metastasis in a human melanoma/SCID model. Implications for the direct autocrine and paracrine epigenetic regulation of the metastasis process. Int J Cancer 1996 Apr 10; 66(2):151–8.

[18] Zingg JM, Jones PA. Genetic and epigenetic aspects of DNA methylation on genome expression, evolution, mutation and carcinogenesis. Carcinogenesis 1997 May; 18(5):869–82.

[19] Kang SH, Bang YJ, Im YH, et al. Transcriptional repression of the transforming growth factor-beta type I receptor gene by DNA methylation results in the development of TGF-beta resistance in human gastric cancer. Oncogene 1999 Dec 2; 18(51):7280–6.

[20] Li LC, Chui R, Nakajima K, et al. Frequent methylation of estrogen receptor in prostate cancer: Correlation with tumor progression. Cancer Res 2000 Feb 1; 60(3):702–6.

[21] Tycko B. Epigenetic gene silencing in cancer. J Clin Invest 2000 Feb; 105(4):401–7.

[22] Gonzalgo ML, Jones PA. Mutagenic and epigenetic effects of DNA methylation. Mutat Res 1997 Apr; 386(2):107–18.

[23] Wachsman JT. DNA methylation and the association between genetic and epigenetic changes: Relation to carcinogenesis. Mutat Res 1997 Apr 14; 375(1):1–8.

[24] Weitzman SA, Turk PW, Milkowski DH, Kozlowski K. Free radical adducts induce alterations in DNA cytosine methylation. Proc Natl Acad Sci USA 1994 Feb 15; 91(4):1261–4.

[25] Cerda S, Weitzman SA. Influence of oxygen radical injury on DNA methylation. Mutat Res 1997 Apr; 386(2):141–52.

[26] Loeb KR, Loeb LA. Significance of multiple mutations in cancer. Carcinogenesis 2000 Mar; 21(3):379–385.

[27] Loeb LA. Cancer cells exhibit a mutator phenotype. Adv Cancer Res 1998; 72:25–56.

[28] Loeb LA, Christians FC. Multiple mutations in human cancers. Mutat Res 1996 Feb 19; 350(1):279–86.

[29] Christians FC, Newcomb TG, Loeb LA. Potential sources of multiple mutations in human cancers. Prev Med 1995 Jul; 24(4):329–32.

[30] Loeb LA. Mutator phenotype may be required for multistage carcinogenesis. Cancer Res 1991 Jun 15; 51(12):3075–9.

[31] Jackson AL, Loeb LA. The mutation rate and cancer. Genetics 1998 Apr; 148(4):1483–90.

[32] Ellison BJ, Rubin H. Individual transforming events in long-term cell culture of NIH 3T3 cells as products of epigenetic induction. Cancer Res 1992 Feb 1; 52(3):667–73.

[33] Ness RB, Cottreau C. Possible role of ovarian epithelial inflammation in ovarian cancer. J Natl Cancer Inst 1999 Sep 1; 91(17):1459–67.

[34] Tamatani T, Turk P, Weitzman S, Oyasu R. Tumorigenic conversion of a rat urothelial cell line by human polymorphonuclear leukocytes activated by lipopolysaccharide. Jpn J Cancer Res 1999 Aug; 90(8):829–36.

[35] Farinati F, Cardin R, Degan P, et al. Oxidative DNA damage accumulation in gastric carcinogenesis. Gut 1998 Mar; 42(3):351–6.

[36] Irani J, Goujon JM, Ragni E, et al. High-grade inflammation in prostate cancer as a prognostic factor for biochemical recurrence after radical prostatectomy. Urology 1999 Sep; 54(3):467–72.

[37] Toyokuni S, Okamoto K, Yodoi J, Hiai H. Persistent oxidative stress in cancer. FEBS Lett 1995 Jan 16; 358(1):1–3.

[38] Kondo S, Toyokuni S, Iwasa Y, et al. Persistent oxidative stress in human colorectal carcinoma, but not in adenoma. Free Radic Biol Med 1999 Aug; 27(3–4):401–10.

[39] Clutton SM, Townsend KM, Walker C, et al. Radiation-induced genomic instability and persisting oxidative stress in primary bone marrow cultures. Carcinogenesis 1996 Aug; 17(8):1633–9.

40 Dreher D, Junod AF. Role of oxygen free radicals in cancer development. Eur J Cancer 1996 Jan; 32A(1):30–8.

41 Arora-Kuruganti P, Lucchesi PA, Wurster RD. Proliferation of cultured human astrocytoma cells in response to an oxidant and antioxidant. J Neurooncol 1999; 44(3):213–21.

42 del Bello B, Paolicchi A, Comporti M, et al. Hydrogen peroxide produced during gamma-glutamyl transpeptidase activity is involved in prevention of apoptosis and maintainance of proliferation in U937 cells. FASEB J 1999 Jan; 13(1):69–79.

43 Burdon RH, Alliangana D, Gill V. Hydrogen peroxide and the proliferation of BHK-21 cells. Free Radic Res 1995 Nov; 23(5):471–86.

44 Li D, Zhang W, Sahin AA, Hittelman WN. DNA adducts in normal tissue adjacent to breast cancer: A review. Cancer Detect Prev 1999; 23(6):454–62.

45 Devi GS, Prasad MH, Saraswathi I, et al. Free radicals antioxidant enzymes and lipid peroxidation in different types of leukemias. Clin Chim Acta 2000 Mar; 293(1–2):53–62.

46 Matsui A, Ikeda T, Enomoto K, et al. Increased formation of oxidative DNA damage, 8-hydroxy-2'-deoxyguanosine, in human breast cancer tissue and its relationship to GSTP1 and COMT genotypes. Cancer Lett 2000 Apr 3; 151(1):87–95.

47 Stramentinoli G. Pharmacologic aspects of S-adenosylmethionine. Pharmacokinetics and pharmacodynamics. Am J Med 1987 Nov 20; 83(5A):35–42.

48 Chiang PK, Gordon RK, Tal J, et al. S-Adenosylmethionine and methylation. FASEB J 1996 Mar; 10(4):471–80.

49 Shivapurkar N, Wilson MJ, Hoover KL, et al. Hepatic DNA methylation and liver tumor formation in male C3H mice fed methionine- and choline-deficient diets. J Natl Cancer Inst 1986 Jul; 77(1):213–7.

50 Christman JK, Sheikhnejad G, Dizik M, et al. Reversibility of changes in nucleic acid methylation and gene expression induced in rat liver by severe dietary methyl deficiency. Carcinogenesis 1993 Apr; 14(4):551–7.

51 Wainfan E, Poirier LA. Methyl groups in carcinogenesis: Effects on DNA methylation and gene expression. Cancer Res 1992 Apr 1; 52(7 Suppl):2071s-2077s.

52 Gerbracht U, Eigenbrodt E, Simile MM, et al. Effect of S-adenosyl-L-methionine on the development of preneoplastic foci and the activity of some carbohydrate metabolizing enzymes in the liver, during experimental hepatocarcinogenesis. Anticancer Res 1993 Nov–Dec; 13(6A):1965–72.

53 Garcea R, Daino L, Pascale R, et al. Inhibition of promotion and persistent nodule growth by S-adenosyl-L-methionine in rat liver carcinogenesis: Role of remodeling and apoptosis. Cancer Res 1989 Apr 1; 49(7):1850–6.

54 Pascale RM, Marras V, Simile MM, et al. Chemoprevention of rat liver carcinogenesis by S-adenosyl-L-methionine: A long-term study. Cancer Res 1992 Sep 15; 52(18):4979–86.

55 Simile MM, Pascale R, De Miglio MR, et al. Correlation between S-adenosyl-L-methionine content and production of c-myc, c-Ha-ras, and c-Ki-ras mRNA transcripts in the early stages of rat liver carcinogenesis. Cancer Lett 1994 Apr 29; 79(1):9–16.

56 Clinical development plan: Folic acid. J Cell Biochem Suppl 1996; 26:100–13.

57 Childers JM, Chu J, Voigt LF, et al. Chemoprevention of cervical cancer with folic acid: A phase III Southwest Oncology Group Intergroup study. Cancer Epidemiol Biomarkers Prev 1995 Mar; 4(2):155–9.

58 Cravo ML, Pinto AG, Chaves P, et al. Effect of folate supplementation on DNA methylation of rectal mucosa in patients with colonic adenomas: Correlation with nutrient intake. Clin Nutr 1998 Apr; 17(2):45–9.

59 Grio R, Piacentino R, Marchino GL, Navone R. Antineoblastic activity of antioxidant vitamins: The role of folic acid in the prevention of cervical dysplasia. Panminerva Med 1993 Dec; 35(4):193–6.

60 Choi SW, Mason JB. Folate and carcinogenesis: An integrated scheme. J Nutr 2000 Feb; 130(2):129–32.

61 Duranton B, Freund JN, Galluser M, et al. Promotion of intestinal carcinogenesis by dietary methionine. Carcinogenesis 1999 Mar; 20(3):493–7.

62 Pascale RM, Simile MM, Satta G, et al. Comparative effects of L-methionine, S-adenosyl-L-methionine and 5'-methylthioadenosine on the growth of preneoplastic lesions and DNA methylation in rat liver during the early stages of hepatocarcinogenesis. Anticancer Res 1991 Jul–Aug; 11(4):1617–24.

RESULTS OF THERAPY AT THE CELLULAR LEVEL

As we explored in Chapter 2, gene mutations and the abnormal expression of genes play a central role in cancer. These abnormalities, in combination with a heavy flow of "do proliferate" and "do not die" signals, allow cancer cells to proliferate and avoid death. In this chapter we explore what happens when cancer cells fail to proliferate or fail to avoid death; that is, we explore at the cellular level the end results that anticancer therapies attempt to produce. We discuss results at this early point because by keeping the goal of treatment in mind, we are better able to evaluate the means needed to reach it. When planning a trip, one should know the intended destination before deciding the route to take. *Apoptosis*, a term used repeatedly in later chapters, is our most common "destination." The "route" taken to get there will involve inhibition of one or more of the seven clusters of procancer events.

There are four possible results of a successful therapy at the cellular level. A cancer cell may differentiate into a less malignant form, fail to enter the cell cycle and thus fail to proliferate, die through necrosis, or die through apoptosis.

CELL DIFFERENTIATION

Cell differentiation is a measure of the maturity of a cell. Cells that are fully differentiated (fully mature) resemble their parent cells in form and function, and they proliferate very slowly, if at all. In contrast, immature cells are poorly differentiated, do not yet resemble their parents, and are able to proliferate at a higher rate. Most cancer cells are less differentiated, less mature, than normal cells, allowing cancer cells to proliferate readily. The degree to which a cell differentiates is regulated by gene expression. Therefore, by manipulating gene expression, one can alter the degree of differentiation. A number of natural compounds, discussed below, can induce differentiation in cancer cells, thereby decreasing their proliferation rate and causing them to display fewer malignant characteristics.

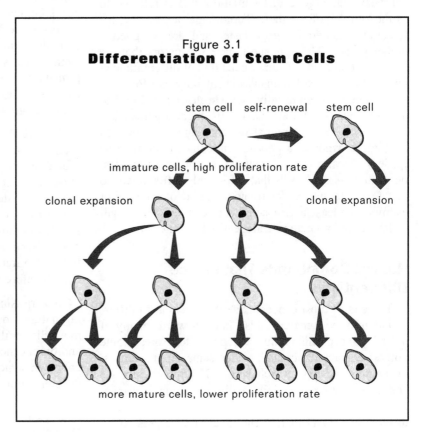

Figure 3.1
Differentiation of Stem Cells

stem cell   self-renewal   stem cell

immature cells, high proliferation rate

clonal expansion   clonal expansion

more mature cells, lower proliferation rate

Stem Cells

The least differentiated and most prolific cells within the body are called stem cells. In a healthy organism, stem cells act as a source of new cells during tissue repair, as illustrated in Figure 3.1 (adapted from reference 1). As shown in the figure, stem cells are capable of both self-renewal (self-replacement) and clonal expansion and so are virtually immortal. Not surprisingly, stem cells are present in high numbers in tissues that constantly renew their population, such as the bone marrow and intestinal lining. Bone marrow cells have a turnover rate of approximately five days, as opposed to several years for some vascular cells. Although stem cells in normal tissues have a high ability to proliferate, their proliferation is tightly regulated, occurring only under specific circumstances.

Small numbers of stem cells are also present in malignant tumors. Unlike stem cell proliferation in normal tissues, that in cancerous tissue is largely unregulated. Furthermore, the daughter cells do not fully differentiate (i.e., acquire the functions of more mature cells), and so the proliferation rate of the offspring remains high. For these reasons, stem cells are the prime targets of cyto-toxic chemotherapy and radiotherapy.

Tumors can be described by the degree to which their cells have undergone differentiation; this is referred to as the "grade" of a tumor. Tumors that are poorly differentiated generally grow faster and are assigned a higher grade. The opposite is true for tumors that are well differentiated. If tumor cells do not differentiate at all, the tumor is called anaplastic (literally, not formed). The grading system usually uses a scale of 1 to 3 or 1 to 4, with anaplastic tumors having the highest grade. For example, a well-differentiated tumor may be classified as grade 1, whereas a poorly differentiated one may be grade 4. Most tumors, except perhaps the most anaplastic, contain enough cells that sufficiently differentiate so that a pathologist can determine the tissue of origin. For example, at least a few cells from a bone cancer will differentiate into mature and identifiable bone cells.

Natural Compounds That Induce Differentiation

The cells of most cancers have the potential to differentiate into more mature cells. In other words, many, if not all, cancer cells retain the capacity to express some normal characteristics and, under some circumstances, to suppress malignant behavior.[2] Natural compounds and certain drugs can induce differentiation in cancer cells, although some cancers are more easily induced to differentiate than others. The greatest successes so far have been in inducing leukemia cells to differentiate.[3]

Cells must be in the cell cycle before they will respond to differentiating agents; that is, they must be actively dividing and not in the G_0 resting phase (see Figure 2.5). Leukemia cells are particularly sensitive to differentiating agents in large part because they have a high rate of proliferation relative to cells of other cancers. In contrast to leukemia and other fast-growing cancers, success in inducing the cells of most solid tumors to differentiate has been more sporadic.

We note here that, contrary to popular belief, cancer cells do not generally proliferate at a high rate relative to normal cells. Fast-growing cancers such as leukemias proliferate at roughly the rate of fast-growing normal cells such as bone marrow or hair cells. Fast-growing cancer cells and fast growing normal cells enter the cell cycle about once every two weeks or less, and in some cases once every few days. The cells of other cancers and those of most normal tissues proliferate much more slowly. Often, the rate of a tumor's growth is measured as its doubling time, the time required for it to double in

volume.[a] To provide some examples, the doubling rate of breast cancer is generally about 40 to 100 days, that of lung cancer about 60 to 270 days, of colorectal cancer about 630 days on the average, and that of prostate cancer is commonly greater than 740 days.[4–7] In general, tumors in younger patients have a faster doubling rate than those in older patients; likewise, tumors arising from metastases tend to have a faster doubling rate than primary tumors. All of these relatively slow-growing cancers are less susceptible to differentiating agents than the faster-growing ones.

We have then the seemingly contradictory result that drugs or other compounds that increase cancer cell proliferation can, when used in combination with differentiating agents, increase cell differentiation and in so doing, ultimately reduce proliferation. As we will later see, some chemotherapy drugs and natural compounds, apart from those that induce differentiation, may also be more effective at inhibiting cancer when cells are actively proliferating; agents that increase proliferation may therefore make these more effective too.

Not surprisingly, most of the differentiation studies using natural compounds have been conducted on leukemia cells. Still, melanoma, colon, breast, lung, bladder, and brain cancer cells have also been reported to differentiate in some cases.[8, 9] Natural compounds that induce differentiation in vitro are listed in Table 3.1. Of the compounds listed, ATRA (an active metabolite of vitamin A) and 1,25-D$_3$ (the active metabolite of vitamin D$_3$) have received the most research attention. The majority of compounds listed in Table 3.1 induce differentiation within the concentration range of roughly 1 to 50 μM, the exceptions being ATRA and 1,25-D$_3$, which induce differentiation within the concentration range of about 0.01 to 1 μM. This is still above the normal plasma concentrations for these two compounds, however.

Some of the compounds listed have also been reported to induce differentiation in vivo. For example, intraperitoneal administration of daidzein (at 25 to 50 mg/kg per day) reduced tumor volume and induced differentiation of leukemia cells held in chambers in mice.[10] The equivalent human oral dose is about 1.1 to 2.3 grams per day. The same intraperitoneal dose of boswellic acid also induced differentiation of leukemia cells in mice.[11, 12] The equivalent human oral dose is about 340 to 680 milligrams per day. Combinations of ATRA and

---

[a] *Note that actual proliferation rates of cancer cells are faster than tumor volume doubling times. Tumor volume doubling time is a function of both cell proliferation and cell death. The rate of cell death in many solid tumors may be 75 to 90 percent of the rate of cell proliferation.*

vitamin D_3 at high doses have also been reported to be effective in animals.[13, 14, 15]

FAILURE TO ENTER THE CELL CYCLE

The second possible result of successful treatment is causing cancer cells to stay out of the cell cycle. As discussed in Chapter 2 and illustrated in Figure 2.5, cells remain in the initial gap phase (G_0) until they are stimulated to proliferate. Generally, the required stimulation is initially due to the activity of growth factors. These stimulate the expression of the early genes in cell proliferation (*fos, myc,* and *jun*), which eventually results in increased expression of other genes that drive the cell cycle proper. Therefore, cells can be kept in the initial gap phase and out of the cell cycle by reducing the effects of growth factors. Natural compounds are capable of reducing these through at least two means. First, they can reduce signal transduction, a process growth factors rely on for their effects. Second, they can reduce abnormal transcription factor activity, which is the last step before growth factors cause gene expression. The use of natural compounds to inhibit growth factors by these means is discussed in Chapters 4 and 5.

In addition to preventing proliferation, keeping cells from entering the cell cycle may have the long-term effect of inducing apoptosis. When cells are not able to divide, they eventually die of old age. In most cases, cells that die of old age do so through apoptosis.

It is unlikely, however, that natural compounds will completely prevent cancer cells from leaving G_0 and entering the cell cycle. Those discussed here are more likely to slow down the rate of entry. Slowing down the proliferation rate may in fact be better than completely preventing cells from entering the cell cycle, since many natural compounds are more efficient at halting the cell cycle and inducing apoptosis once the cycle has begun. Once in the cycle, many events and stresses occur that make the cell vulnerable to injury. We might liken it to a woman being more vulnerable to injury while she is pregnant. As mentioned previously, differentiation agents and most chemotherapy drugs are also more effective on cells in the cycle. The same is true of radiotherapy.

APOPTOSIS AND NECROSIS

The last two possible results of successful treatment are cell death through apoptosis or necrosis. Of the two, apoptosis is the preferred form of death during therapy. Apoptosis is a rather new discovery (1972); before this, cell death was thought to occur only through necrosis.

TABLE 3.1 NATURAL COMPOUNDS THAT INDUCE DIFFERENTIATION IN VITRO
COMPOUND
Arctigenin
ATRA (vitamin A)
Boswellic acid
Bromelain and other proteolytic enzymes
CAPE
Flavonoids (including apigenin, luteolin, quercetin, genistein, and daidzein)
Emodin
EPA and DHA
Monoterpenes
Resveratrol
1,25-D_3 (vitamin D_3)
Note: See Table D.1 in Appendix D for details and references.

Apoptosis is programmed into the cell at birth and is triggered at old age or under other conditions where cell death benefits the organism as a whole. *Apoptosis* is a Greek word referring to the seasonal dropping of leaves from a tree. Like the seasonal dropping of leaves, apoptosis is a natural and necessary process in many types of human, animal, and even insect cells. For example, increased apoptosis allows rapid cell turnover during wound healing.

There are many differences between necrosis and apoptosis. Unlike necrosis, apoptosis affects scattered, individual cells, does not rupture the cell membrane, and does not produce inflammation; therefore, it does not damage adjacent cells. Immune cells ingest apoptotic cells before their plasma membranes rupture, and so the cell's contents spill into the extracellular space (the space outside and between cells). Apoptosis represents an orderly method of removing old, damaged, or otherwise unwanted cells. Necrosis, on the other hand, is a violent form of cell death, usually involving large numbers of cells. Since the plasma membrane of a necrotic cell ruptures and the cell's contents are spilled into the extracellular space, necrosis can easily lead to inflammation.

Both necrosis and apoptosis play a role in limiting tumor growth. Necrosis may occur, for example, in cells distanced from the blood supply. Until recently, induction of necrosis was thought to be the single goal in conventional anticancer therapy but it is now understood that anticancer agents commonly kill cancer cells via apoptosis. In fact, it appears that much of the cell death induced by chemotherapy drugs is due to apoptosis.

Although it may be possible under some conditions for natural compounds to induce necrosis, I do not advocate their use for this goal. For one thing, very high and probably unsafe doses of natural compounds would be required. Apoptosis can be induced by lower doses. Moreover, necrosis can induce inflammation, which can assist cancer progression through a variety of mechanisms. Finally, as compared to whole apoptotic cells, the contents of ruptured necrotic cells are not easily picked up by immune cells (macrophages). Therefore, the cancer's unique proteins are not efficiently presented to other immune cells (T cells), which need them to search out and destroy other cancer cells; T cells use antigens much like a dog uses a scent to identify what it tracks.

Apoptosis and Cancer

At any given moment for any given cell, apoptosis is either induced or not induced depending on the relative balance of "do die" and "do not die" signals. A growing body of evidence suggests that the default signal is "do die," meaning that apoptosis is an ever-present default pathway for all cells and cell survival is maintained only as long as cells receive the appropriate "do not die" survival signals (such as stimulation by growth factors).[16] Although not always successful, cancer cells have a gift for generating more "do not die" than "do die" signals, thereby preventing apoptosis. Fortunately, natural compounds can be used to readjust the balance in cancer cells to favor apoptosis.

"Do die" signals come from three primary sources. The first is through cellular damage, especially damage involving the DNA. The *p53* gene will attempt to repair DNA damage, and if the damage is irreparable, it will attempt to induce apoptosis. As we know, the *p53* gene is commonly mutated in cancer cells and so does not function properly.

A second source of "do die" signals comes from certain growth factors, or in this case, antigrowth factors. One such factor is transforming growth factor-beta (TGF-beta), which is discussed below. Cancer cells can avoid death by decreasing their sensitivity to the inhibitory effects of TGF-beta.

A third source of "do die" signals comes from within the cell itself. Certain "killer" genes such as the *Bax* gene, when activated, produce proteins that induce apoptosis. These killer genes can be mutated in cancer cells or can otherwise be underexpressed.

"Do not die" signals come from two primary sources. First, they can come from within the cell itself. Certain "protective" genes such as *bcl-2*, when activated, produce proteins that inhibit apoptosis. These protective genes can be overexpressed in cancer cells. Second, such signals come from growth factors and normal cell-to-cell communication. Unlike healthy cells, cancer cells commonly produce their own growth factors that not only stimulate proliferation but also mimic the "do not die" signals normally generated through cell-to-cell contact, thereby allowing cancer cells to detach from surrounding cells and migrate. In addition, cancer cells exhibit increased signal transduction that can magnify any "do not die" signals present.

The reduced rate of apoptosis in cancer cells is what makes cancer such a serious problem. In most solid tumors, growth occurs not so much because cancer cells proliferate rapidly as because cancer cells tend not to undergo apoptosis. Cancer cells live excessively long lives and are thus able to have many offspring. Nevertheless, the strategies cancer cells use to inhibit apoptosis are not able to protect all cells from death, and therefore apoptosis still plays a role in limiting net tumor growth.

Natural Compounds That Induce Apoptosis

Natural compounds can induce apoptosis in cancer cells by increasing "do die" signals and reducing "do not die" signals. The former can be increased through any of the following: cellular damage (which probably plays a larger role in in-vitro than in-vivo studies); increased function of the *p53* gene or its protein; and increased activity of antigrowth factors, such as TGF-beta. "Do not die" signals can be reduced by inhibiting growth factor activity and signal transduction. It is still unknown if natural compounds can directly affect killer genes or protective genes. Natural compounds known to induce apoptosis in cancer cells in vitro are listed in Table 3.2; the majority of these induce apoptosis within the concentration range of roughly 1 to 50 μM. One exception is 1,25-D$_3$, which is active at 10 to 100 nM; although this is a low concentration range, it is still above the normal plasma concentrations of this vitamin.

An important factor in translating in-vitro apoptosis data to in-vivo conditions is the mechanism by which apoptosis is induced. As we will see in Chapter 15, several compounds listed in Table 3.2 can induce apoptosis in vitro through prooxidant mechanisms (in other words, through oxidative damage to the cell). For example, this has been shown for curcumin, CAPE, and vitamin C. There are large differences in oxygen tension between in-vitro and in-vivo environments, however, not to mention differences in antioxidant enzymes and other antioxidant compounds. Thus cells in vitro may respond differently to some of these compounds than they do in vivo. Although evidence is still limited, it appears that compounds such as curcumin and CAPE can induce apoptosis in vivo but are likely to do so through mechanisms other than oxidative stress. Indeed, under most conditions these compounds probably act as antioxidants in vivo, rather than prooxidants. Still, the induction of apoptosis via oxidative stress is possible in vivo under some circumstances (e.g., vitamin C given intravenously at high doses), but such a prooxidant strategy is not recommended for the reasons summarized in Chapter 2.

Apoptosis and Transforming Growth Factor-beta

Some of the compounds listed in Table 3.2 may induce apoptosis in part by their effects on transforming growth factor-beta (TGF-beta). TGF-beta is a compound present in a variety of normal and neoplastic cells; it plays a role in regulating proliferation and differentiation. It is multifunctional and can either stimulate or inhibit cell proliferation, depending on the cell type and other conditions. For example, it induces apoptosis in cancer cells that are in the early stages of malignant transformation.[17, 18] In this respect, it can be thought of as an antigrowth factor that provides "do die" signals. In the cells of established cancers, however, TGF-beta can have a very different effect.

The cells of established cancers appear to lose their sensitivity to the growth-inhibiting effects of TGF-beta, either by underexpressing TGF-beta receptors or by otherwise exhibiting aberrant TGF-beta signaling.[19, 20, 21] Indeed, some cancers cells actually produce TGF-beta. Since TGF-beta also causes an immunosuppressive effect, these cancer cells can use TGF-beta to evade immune attack.[22, 23, 24] To some degree, production of TGF-beta can also stimulate cell proliferation, by binding to the receptors for other growth factors, and facilitate angiogenesis, in part by increasing the production of some growth factors.[25-29] Not surprisingly, inhibition of TGF-beta can inhibit growth and metastasis of established cancers in animal models.[30] Because of these effects, excessive production of TGF-beta is associated with poor prognosis in colorectal cancers, stomach cancers, and other neoplasms.[29, 31]

Some of the compounds in Table 3.2 induce apoptosis by normalizing the effects of TGF-beta, either by increasing TGF-beta receptor expression or by otherwise improving TGF-beta signaling. This has been shown, for example, for genistein, monoterpenes (especially perillyl alcohol), and ATRA.[32-35] By improving TGF-beta signaling, these compounds can induce apoptosis in both transforming and transformed cancer cells. Some natural compounds, including vitamin A, quercetin, curcumin, resveratrol, vitamin D_3 and melatonin, can increase TGF-beta production, yet they do not promote the progression of cancers in vivo.[36-41] At least for vitamin

TABLE 3.2   NATURAL COMPOUNDS THAT INDUCE APOPTOSIS IN VITRO
COMPOUND
1,25-D_3 (Vitamin D_3)
ATRA (vitamin A)
Boswellic acids
CAPE
Curcumin
EPA
Flavonoids (including apigenin, luteolin, genistein, quercetin, and EGCG)
Garlic
Hypericin
Leukotriene inhibitors (see Table 8.2)
Monoterpenes
Resveratrol
Selenium
Vitamin C
Vitamin E

Note: See Table D.2 in Appendix D for details and references.

A, this is probably because it improves TGF-beta signaling at the same time it increases TGF-beta production.

Other natural compounds are able to directly inhibit TGF-beta production or activity. For example, high-molecular-weight polysaccharides such as PSK can bind to and inactivate TGF-beta.[42, 43] By inhibiting TGF-beta activity, PSK can inhibit the progression of cancers that have lost sensitivity to TGF-beta's inhibitory effects. The ability of PSK to inactivate TGF-beta is in keeping with its role as an immune stimulant, since cancer cells can then no longer use TGF-beta to evade immune attack.

CONCLUSION

At the cellular level, successful anticancer therapies can have four possible outcomes. They can cause cancer cells to differentiate into cells that have more normal form and function, they can prevent cancer cells from entering the cell cycle, or they can induce cell death through necrosis or apoptosis. Of these, natural compounds are best suited for inducing differentiation (particularly in fast-growing cancers); preventing cells from entering the cell cycle; and inducing apoptosis. The induction of apoptosis is a primary goal of anticancer therapies using natural compounds because it is applicable to all types of cancer cells; it is the body's natural way of killing cancer cells; and it can be caused through several mechanisms that are sensitive to modification by natural compounds. These include increasing "do die" signals and decreasing "do not die" signals. Preventing cells from entering the cell cycle will also result in greater apoptosis rates, and can be caused by inhibiting "do proliferate" signals, such as those produced by the sequential effects of growth factors, signal transduction, and transcription factor activity.

REFERENCES

1 Tannock IF, Hill RP, eds. The basic science of oncology. 2nd ed. New York: McGraw-Hill, 1992, p. 140.

2 Bertino JR, ed. Encyclopedia of cancer. San Diego: Academic Press, 1997, p. 479.

3 Scott RE. Differentiation, differentiation/gene therapy and cancer. Pharmacol Ther 1997; 73(1):51–65.

4 Friberg S, Mattson S. On the growth rates of human malignant tumors: Implications for medical decision making. J Surg Oncol 1997 Aug; 65(4):284–97.

5 Spratt JS, Meyer JS, Spratt JA. Rates of growth of human neoplasms: Part II. J Surg Oncol 1996 Jan; 61(1):68–83.

6 Tannock IF, Hill RP, eds. The basic science of oncology. 2nd ed. New York: McGraw-Hill, 1992, p. 155.

7 Schlappack OK, Bush C, Delic JI, Steel GG. Growth and chemotherapy of a human germ-cell tumour line (GCT 27). Eur J Cancer Clin Oncol 1988 Apr; 24(4):777–81.

8 Marks PA, Rifkind RA. Differentiating factors. In *Biologic therapy of cancer*. DeVita Jr. VT, Hellman S, Rosenberg SA, eds. Philadelphia: JB Lippincott, 1991.

9 Bertino JR, ed. Encyclopedia of cancer. San Diego: Academic Press, 1997, p. 482.

10 Jing Y, Nakaya K, Han R. Differentiation of promyeloctic leukemia cells HL-60 induced by daidzen in vitro and in vivo. Anticancer Res 1993; 13(4):1049–54.

11 Jing Y, Xia L, Han R. Growth inhibition and differentiation of promyelocytic cells (HL-60) induced by BC-4, an active principle from Boswellia carterii Birdw. Chin Med Sci J 1992 Mar; 7(1):12–5.

12 Han R. Recent progress in the study of anticancer drugs originating from plants and traditional medicines in China. Chin Med Sci J 1994 Mar; 9(1):61–9.

13 Koshizuka K, Kubota T, Said J, et al. Combination therapy of a vitamin D3 analog and all-*trans* retinoic acid: Effect on human breast cancer in nude mice. Anticancer Res 1999 Jan–Feb; 19(1A):519–24.

14 Majewski S, Marczak M, Szmurlo A, et al. Retinoids, interferon alpha, 1,25-dihydroxyvitamin D3 and their combination inhibit angiogenesis induced by non-HPV-harboring tumor cell lines. RAR alpha mediates the antiangiogenic effect of retinoids. Cancer Lett 1995 Feb 10; 89(1):117–24.

15 Majewski S, Skopinska M, Marczak M, et al. Vitamin D3 is a potent inhibitor of tumor cell-induced angiogenesis. J Investig Dermatol Symp Proc 1996; 1(1):97–101.

16 Oppenheim RW. Related mechanisms of action of growth factors and antioxidants in apoptosis: An overview. Adv Neurol 1997; 72:69–78.

17 Panse J, Hipp ML, Bauer G. Fibroblasts transformed by chemical carcinogens are sensitive to intercellular induction of apoptosis: Implications for the control of oncogenesis. Carcinogenesis 1997 Feb; 18(2):259–64.

18 Bursch W, Oberhammer F, Jirtle RL, et al. Transforming growth factor-β1 as a signal for induction of cell death by apoptosis. Br. J Cancer 1993; 67:531–536.

19 Kim IY, Ahn HJ, Lang S, et al. Loss of expression of transforming growth factor-beta receptors is associated with poor prognosis in prostate cancer patients. Clin Cancer Res 1998 Jul; 4(7):1625–30.

20 Park K, Kim SJ, Bang YJ, et al. Genetic changes in the transforming growth factor beta (TGF-beta) type II receptor gene in human gastric cancer cells: Correlation with sensitivity to growth inhibition by TGF-beta. Proc Natl Acad Sci USA 1994 Sep 13; 91(19):8772–6.

21 Kim YS, Yi Y, Choi SG, Kim SJ. Development of TGF-beta resistance during malignant progression. Arch Pharm Res 1999 Feb; 22(1):1–8.

22 Chang NS. Transforming growth factor-beta protection of cancer cells against tumor necrosis factor cytotoxicity is counteracted by hyaluronidase (review). Int J Mol Med 1998 Dec; 2(6):653–9.

23 Lee C, Sintich SM, Mathews EP, et al. Transforming growth factor-beta in benign and malignant prostate. Prostate 1999 Jun 1; 39(4):285–90.

24 de Visser KE, Kast WM. Effects of TGF-beta on the immune system: Implications for cancer immunotherapy. Leukemia 1999 Aug; 13(8):1188–99.

25 Perez JR, Higgins-Sochaski KA, Maltese JY, Narayanan R. Regulation of adhesion and growth of fibrosarcoma cells by NF-kappa B RelA involves transforming growth factor beta. Mol Cell Biol 1994 Aug; 14(8):5326–32.

26 Jennings MT, Pietenpol JA. The role of transforming growth factor beta in glioma progression. J Neurooncol 1998 Jan; 36(2):123–40.

27 Reiss M. Transforming growth factor-beta and cancer: A love-hate relationship? Oncol Res 1997; 9(9):447–57.

28 Saito H, Tsujitani S, Oka S, et al. The expression of transforming growth factor-beta1 is significantly correlated with the expression of vascular endothelial growth factor and poor prognosis of patients with advanced gastric carcinoma. Cancer 1999 Oct 15; 86(8):1455–62.

29 Choi JH, Kim HC, Lim HY, et al. Detection of transforming growth factor-alpha in the serum of gastric carcinoma patients. Oncology 1999 Oct; 57(3):236–41.

30 Wojtowicz-Praga S. Reversal of tumor-induced immunosuppression: A new approach to cancer therapy. J Immunother 1997 May; 20(3):165–77.

31 Robson H, Anderson E, James RD, Schofield PF. Transforming growth factor beta 1 expression in human colorectal tumours: An independent prognostic marker in a subgroup of poor prognosis patients. Br J Cancer 1996 Sep; 74(5):753–8.

32 Kim H, Peterson TG, Barnes S. Mechanisms of action of the soy isoflavone genistein: Emerging role for its effects via transforming growth factor beta signaling pathways. Am J Clin Nutr 1998 Dec; 68(6 Suppl):1418S-1425S.

[33] Mills JJ, Chari RS, Boyer IJ, et al. Induction of apoptosis in liver tumors by the monoterpene perillyl alcohol. Cancer Res 1995 Mar 1; 55(5):979–83.

[34] Cohen PS, Letterio JJ, Gaetano C, et al. Induction of transforming growth factor beta 1 and its receptors during all-*trans* retinoic acid (RA) treatment of RA-responsive human neuroblastoma cell lines. Cancer Res 1995 Jun 1; 55(11):2380–6.

[35] Turley JM, Funakoshi S, Ruscetti FW, et al. Growth inhibition and apoptosis of RL human B lymphoma cells by vitamin E succinate and retinoic acid: Role for transforming growth factor beta. Cell Growth Differ 1995 Jun; 6(6):655–63.

[36] Sporn MB, Roberts AB, Wakefield LM, et al. Transforming growth factor-beta and suppression of carcinogenesis. Princess Takamatsu Symp 1989; 20:259–66.

[37] Sidhu GS, Singh AK, Thaloor D, et al. Enhancement of wound healing by curcumin in animals. Wound Repair Regen 1998 Mar–Apr; 6(2):167–77.

[38] Lu R, Serrero G. Resveratrol, a natural product derived from grape, exhibits antiestrogenic activity and inhibits the growth of human breast cancer cells. J Cell Physiol 1999 Jun; 179(3):297–304.

[39] Mercier T, Chaumontet C, Gaillard-Sanchez I, et al. Calcitriol and lexicalcitol (KH1060) inhibit the growth of human breast adenocarcinoma cells by enhancing transforming growth factor-beta production. Biochem Pharmacol 1996 Aug 9; 52(3):505–10.

[40] Molis TM, Spriggs LL, Jupiter Y, Hill SM. Melatonin modulation of estrogen-regulated proteins, growth factors, and proto-oncogenes in human breast cancer. J Pineal Res 1995 Mar; 18(2):93–103.

[41] Scambia G, Benedetti Panici P, Ranelletti FO, et al. Quercetin enhances transforming growth factor B1 secretion by human ovarian cancer cells. Int J Cancer 1994; 57:211–15.

[42] Matsunaga K, Hosokawa A, Oohara M, et al. Direct action of a protein-bound polysaccharide, PSK, on transforming growth factor-beta. Immunopharmacology 1998 Nov; 40(3):219–30.

[43] Habelhah H, Okada F, Nakai K, et al. Polysaccharide K induces Mn superoxide dismutase (Mn-SOD) in tumor tissues and inhibits malignant progression of QR-32 tumor cells: Possible roles of interferon alpha, tumor necrosis factor alpha and transforming growth factor beta in Mn-SOD induction by polysaccharide K. Cancer Immunol Immunother 1998 Aug; 46(6):338–44.

4

GROWTH FACTORS AND SIGNAL TRANSDUCTION

Growth factors and signal transduction play crucial roles in stimulating cell proliferation and in maintaining a cell's life. Briefly, growth factors are soluble extracellular proteins that bind to receptors on the outside of the cell. This binding elicits a chemical signal that is transferred to the cell's nucleus through a series of steps called signal transduction. The result is the activation of transcription factors and the initiation of gene expression. In addition to growth factors, cell-to-cell contact can also generate signals at the cell's surface that are again transferred to the nucleus via signal transduction. In normal cells, all these processes are tightly regulated. In cancer cells, however, the regulations fail, and growth factor activity and excessive signal transduction increase "do proliferate" and "do not die" signals, while decreasing "do die" signals. These changes in signals allow the cell to live a long life with many cell divisions.

In this chapter, we focus on how growth factors and signal transduction work and how natural compounds can be used to affect them. We discuss several important growth factors, then focus on three primary proteins that mediate signal transduction: protein tyrosine kinase (PTK), protein kinase C (PKC), and the ras protein. In addition, we briefly discuss other kinases involved in signal transduction, such as phosphatidylinositol kinase (PI kinase), as well as cyclin-dependent kinases that control the flow of signals as the cell moves through the cell cycle proper. All of these kinases and proteins can be inhibited by natural compounds.

This chapter starts with a brief recap of the differences in signals that occur between normal and cancer cells.

PROLIFERATION AND APOPTOSIS IN NORMAL CELLS VERSUS CANCER CELLS

All cells in the body at every moment are subject to the dynamic balance that exists between pro-life and pro-death signals. Two very basic pro-life signals are "do not die" and "do proliferate"; their counterpart pro-death signals are "do die" and "do not proliferate." All of these signals exist more or less simultaneously, and their relative strengths decide a cell's fate. Of these signals, "do die" and "do not proliferate" seem to be the defaults. That is, if cells are not told to live, they will undergo apoptosis, and if they are not told to proliferate, they will not enter the cell cycle.

The signals that tell a cell to live or to proliferate generally come from outside the cell, commonly from contact with growth factors and from contact, or lack of it, with other cells and tissues. To illustrate how these signals occur in normal tissues, consider the liver tissue of a healthy animal. The liver cells are in close contact with one another, both through actions of cell adhesion molecules on the surface of the cells and through gap junctions (portals) between cells. The liver cells do not undergo apoptosis, since contact with neighboring cells continually generates "do not die" signals. Also, they do not enter the cell cycle because there are few "do proliferate" signals.

Now imagine that the animal receives an injury that slices away a small section of its liver. The injured area soon becomes inflamed and steeped in growth factors. These factors, produced by immune cells, released from the blood, or derived from other sources, cause various types of cells to proliferate. For example, blood vessel cells proliferate to replace those damaged in the injury, and liver cells are also stimulated to proliferate by these growth factors. In addition, the reduced cell-to-cell contact at the edge of the healthy liver tissue signals that new liver cells are needed. In response to the growth factors and signals from reduced cell-to-cell contact, stem cells or other poorly differentiated cells in the liver enter the cell cycle and proliferate. The entire repair process and all the cell proliferation that goes on in it is wondrously orchestrated so that once tissue repair is complete, no new tissue is produced.

I stated previously that cell-to-cell contact is needed to generate "do not die" signals, but above I state that liver cells are stimulated to proliferate by lack of cell-to-cell contact. This apparent contradiction can be explained by considering that the growth factors present at the wound site provide signals that both stimulate proliferation and mimic the "do not die" signals normally originating from cell-to-cell contact. In addition, the liver cells at the edge of the injury are only partially separated from other liver cells.

The situation with cancer cells is both like and unlike the example of injured liver tissue. It is similar in that cancer cells, like liver cells, are stimulated to proliferate and not to undergo apoptosis. It is different in that the proliferation of cancer cells continues indefinitely. Moreover, the sources of "do proliferate" and "do not die" signals are also somewhat different. In both cases, inflammation results in the production or release of

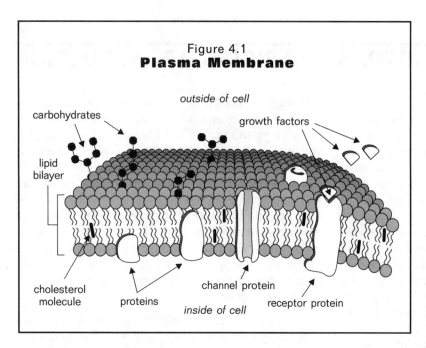

Figure 4.1
Plasma Membrane

outside of cell

carbohydrates

growth factors

lipid bilayer

cholesterol molecule

proteins

channel protein

inside of cell

receptor protein

GROWTH FACTORS

Figure 4.1 illustrates key features of the plasma membrane, including receptor proteins for growth factors. As shown, receptor proteins span the width of the plasma membrane and are therefore able to transfer the signal from growth factors outside the cell to structures within the cell.

Once inside the cell, the signal generated at the receptor is transferred to the cell's nucleus by kinase enzymes and other proteins. In many cases, the receptor itself is composed partly of a kinase enzyme. Kinases and other proteins relay the signal from the receptor to the nucleus in much the same way a baton is relayed from start to finish by different runners in a track race. This relay process is called signal transduction. Researchers commonly use a different analogy and speak of the relay process as a signal cascade, referring to the way water flows over a series of falls.

One feature common to the enzymes involved in signal transduction is that when the signal comes to them, they are energized by the attachment of phosphorus atoms. It is as if they receive a shock of energy, and this shock allows them to pass on phosphorus atoms to other carrier proteins, which then carry the signal to the next enzymes. The process of attaching phosphorus atoms to enzymes or other proteins is called protein phosphorylation. Phosphorus atoms are held tightly together by atomic bonds, and when a group of phosphorus atoms is split apart, a large amount of energy is released. The phosphorus groups needed for protein phosphorylation are delivered to the enzyme by ATP, the primary energy source in a cell.[a]

Table 4.1 provides a short description of several of the most important growth factors in cancer; the descriptions include the type of receptor protein each growth factor uses. As can be seen, the cellular receptors for most of these growth factors are protein tyrosine kinases (PTKs). PTKs are discussed in detail below, but note here that receptor PTKs can be produced by oncogenes and that an entire family of receptor PTKs exists, each

growth factors, but in cancer, the cells themselves also produce their own growth factors. In addition, cancer cells can get the most out of any available growth factors by producing excessive amounts of both the growth factor receptors and the proteins needed in signal transduction.

Cancer cells differ from injured liver cells in other ways. For one thing, cancer cells are generally less differentiated than liver cells. Since poorly differentiated cells are prone to proliferate, a relatively large population of cancer cells can enter the cell cycle in response to growth factor activity and signal transduction. In addition, oncogenes within cancer cells can directly produce proteins such as fos and jun that initiate the cell cycle, and ones such as cyclins that drive the cell cycle proper. Oncogenes are not overexpressed in liver cells.

Lastly, other gene derangements in cancer cells can lead to overproduction of proteins that protect against apoptosis (such as Bcl-2) and can lead to malfunctions or underproduction of proteins that induce apoptosis (such as p53 and Bax). These abnormalities do not occur in liver cells.

All the above factors allow cancer cells to override the complex controls that normally govern proliferation and survival. We can draw the analogy between cancerous and injured tissues; the environments of both allow increased cell proliferation, but the former acts as a wound that does not heal, and so its cell population expands without the limits inherent in the final stages of normal healing.

---

[a] *We can think of ATP (adenosine triphosphate) molecules as small batteries floating around in the cell; they give up their "charge" of phosphorus atoms to enzymes, thereby becoming ADP (adenosine diphosphate). ADP is later recharged to ATP through the process of burning glucose. ATP and ADP are nucleotides. Thus nucleotides play other roles in the cell besides the formation of DNA and RNA.*

TABLE 4.1 GROWTH FACTORS AND THEIR RECEPTORS[*]		
GROWTH FACTOR	**COMMENTS**	**RECEPTOR TYPE**
Epidermal growth factor (EGF)	The EGF receptor is overexpressed in many types of human cancers. It can be activated by at least five different growth factors, including EGF and TGF-alpha. EGF receptor binding can produce several effects, including increased cell proliferation, cell motility, invasion, and metastasis.	PTK
Fibroblast growth factors (FGF)	FGFs such as basic FGF (bFGF) can be overproduced by many types of tumor cells. They are heparan-binding growth factors, which allows them to be stored in the extracellular matrix, the connective tissue surrounding cells and tissues. FGFs stimulate proliferation of many cell types and are involved in angiogenesis.	PTK
Insulin-like growth factors (IGF)	IGFs stimulate cell proliferation and share many properties with insulin, except they do not stimulate glucose utilization. They can be overproduced by many types of tumor cells. IGF receptors occur on a variety of human tumors, including breast cancers.	PTK
Platelet-derived growth factor (PDGF)	PDGF stimulates the proliferation of epithelial cells and other cells. It is released by platelets to stimulate wound healing and can also be produced by tumor cells.	PTK
Transforming growth factor-alpha (TGF-alpha)	Like epidermal growth factor, TGF-alpha binds to EGF receptors. It is produced by macrophages, brain cells, and other cells. It induces angiogenesis in vivo.	PTK
Transforming growth factor-beta (TGF-beta)	TGF-beta is a multifunctional protein that controls proliferation, differentiation, and other cell activities. It can either increase or decrease proliferation, depending on the cell type and conditions. In the early stages of transformation, TGF-beta inhibits proliferation of several cell types; however, advanced cancers can become resistant to its growth-inhibitory actions. In these cancers, TGF-beta can promote invasion and metastasis, partly through its immunosuppressive effects.	comprised of three distinct proteins
Vascular endothelial growth factor (VEGF)	VEGF is also known as vascular permeability factor. It induces endothelial proliferation and vascular permeability and plays an important role in angiogenesis. It is related to PDGF and is produced by epithelial cells, macrophages, and smooth muscle cells.	PTK

Sources: References 1–4.

[*] *All growth factors listed are technically referred to as cytokines; however, I use the term* cytokine *to refer specifically to cytokines produced by immune cells that stimulate immune cell function or proliferation (for example, interleukins have this effect).*

with a slightly different function. By producing excessive amounts of PTKs or hypersensitive PTKs oncogenes can allow a cancer cell to become easily stimulated. In addition, oncogenes can also produce growth factors themselves or proteins that act as growth factors. In these ways, they help cancer cells proliferate even in environments that do not favor proliferation.

SIGNAL TRANSDUCTION

PTKs and Signal Transduction

Receptor PTKs are receptor-enzyme units that span the plasma membrane; in technical terms, they consist of an extracellular receptor domain, a transmembrane domain, and an intracellular tyrosine kinase domain. The intracellular portion consists of the kinase enzyme with a small attached tail. Both the tail and the enzyme itself can receive phosphorus groups from ATP, which, energize them. PTKs can also exist within the cell, in which case their structure is different, but here we are primarily discussing receptor PTKs. PTKs derive their name from the high concentration of the amino acid tyrosine in their intracellular portion.

The process of signal transduction by PTKs is illustrated in Figure 4.2 (adapted from reference 5). The figure shows a PTK consisting of a pair of protein chains. This is the structure for the insulin receptor, for example. Most other PTKs consist of only a single chain, but the process of activation is the same. Briefly, the extracellular portion of the receptor PTK is activated by binding to a growth factor. Binding activates the intracellular portion, where ATP gives up phosphorus groups to the enzyme, thereby producing ADP. The phosphorus signal is carried to another intracellular target, such as another kinase, by a carrier molecule.

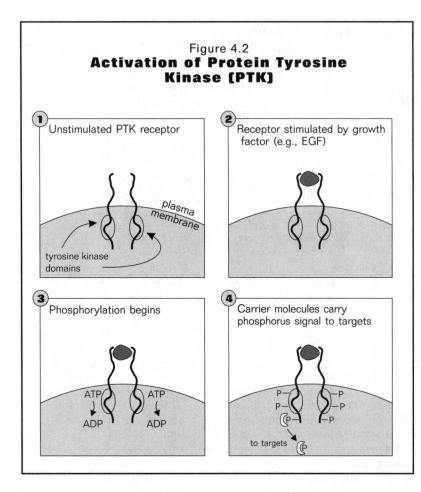

Figure 4.2
Activation of Protein Tyrosine Kinase (PTK)

inhibited receptor binding of growth factors (EGF and PDGF) to PTK receptors in human epidermoid carcinoma cells in vitro.[8]

Protein Kinase C and Signal Transduction

Like protein tyrosine kinase, protein kinase C (PKC) helps relay chemical signals through the cell, and a wide range of procancer events rely on abnormally high PKC activity for signal transduction. Unlike PTK, PKC resides totally within the cell and is activated by other membrane receptors such as PTK. PKC is found in almost all tissues, with the highest activity in the brain.[9]

PKC is a family of at least 12 related lipid-dependent enzymes, many of which are overexpressed in cancer cells. PKC becomes activated through a series of steps that are initiated when a stimulating agent, such as a growth factor, contacts the appropriate receptor on the cell surface. This process is illustrated in Figure 4.3 (adapted from references

A wide range of procancer events rely on abnormally high activity of protein tyrosine kinases for signal transduction. These include proliferation, cell migration, and angiogenesis, as well as avoidance of apoptosis and differentiation. Indeed, the PTK activity of squamous cell carcinomas, for example, can be from sixfold to eightfold higher than that in adjacent normal tissues.[6] Not surprisingly then, PTK inhibitors tend to reduce the proliferation of cancer cells more than that of normal cells.[7]

Table 4.2 lists the natural compounds that inhibit PTK activity. The compounds listed are active in the concentration range of roughly 1 to 100 μM, although the typical active concentration range is from 10 to 30 μM.[a] Another natural compound, resveratrol, is also a PTK inhibitor but is not listed in the table because activity has only been shown at high concentrations (greater than 110 μM) thus far.

Some natural compounds may inhibit the binding of growth factors to PTK receptors, rather than inhibiting PTK activity directly. For example, EGCG at 10 μM

TABLE 4.2 NATURAL COMPOUNDS THAT INHIBIT PROTEIN TYROSINE KINASES
COMPOUND
CAPE
Curcumin
Emodin
Flavonoids (including apigenin, luteolin, quercetin, genistein, and EGCG)
Hypericin (light-activated)
Parthenolide
Note: See Table E.1 in Appendix E for details and references.

10 and 11). In short, the signal generated by receptor binding activates a kinase such as a PTK. This in turn activates both cytosolic (within the cytosol, see Figure 2.1) and membrane PKC via compounds referred to as "second messengers." In addition, second messengers stimulate the movement of cytosolic PKC to the plasma membrane, where it can be phosphorylated. Like phosphorylation of PTK, phosphorylation of PKC allows high-energy phosphorus molecules to be transferred to other carrier molecules, thereby sending along the signal that originated at the surface receptor.

---

[a] *A notable exception is the photoactive compound hypericin and its companion compound pseudohypericin, which are effective at very low concentrations (less than 0.1 μM) when exposed to light.*

The details of these processes are complex and not essential to understand for our purposes, but I briefly describe them for readers who would like a more complete picture of what occurs. During cytosolic PKC activation, phosphorylation of the kinase receptor activates the enzyme phospholipase A_2 (PLA_2). This activated enzyme causes the release of arachidonic acid (AA) from the lipid bilayer. (Arachidonic acid will be discussed in Chapter 7.) The free arachidonic acid stimulates the phosphorylation of cytosolic PKC. One reason that fish oils rich in omega-3 fatty acids act as inhibitors of PKC is that these oils are not converted to arachidonic acid, and therefore the cell cannot use them to stimulate PKC.

During membrane PKC activation, phosphorylation of the kinase receptor activates the enzyme phospholipase C (PLC). PLC in turn, cleaves phosphatidyl inositol biphosphate (PIP_2), a membrane-bound compound, into two parts—its lipid tail, diacylglycerol (DAG), which remains in the membrane, and its nonlipid portion, inositol triphosphate (IP_3), which moves in the cell. IP_3 in turn stimulates the release of calcium ions that stimulate the movement of cytosolic PKC to the plasma membrane. PKC at the plasma membrane is then stimulated to undergo phosphorylation by DAG in conjunction with the phospholipid molecules in the membrane itself. Since they help relay the original signal, arachidonic acid, DAG, IP_3, and calcium are all referred to as second messengers of PKC.

PKC activity is commonly increased in cancer cells and plays a role in many cellular processes.[12–15] It is needed for angiogenesis and metastasis of some cell lines; highly metastatic lines contain more membrane-bound PKC than do weakly metastatic ones. PKC may also play a role in the activity of telomerase, an enzyme that has been associated with excessive life spans of cancer cells. Indeed, PKC inhibition has been reported to reduce telomerase activity in vitro.[16] PKC may also play a role in tumor cell invasion and multidrug resistance.[17, 18, 19] Note that in-vitro invasion can be suppressed in some cancer cells by using PKC inhibitors at low concentrations that do not inhibit cell proliferation.[20]

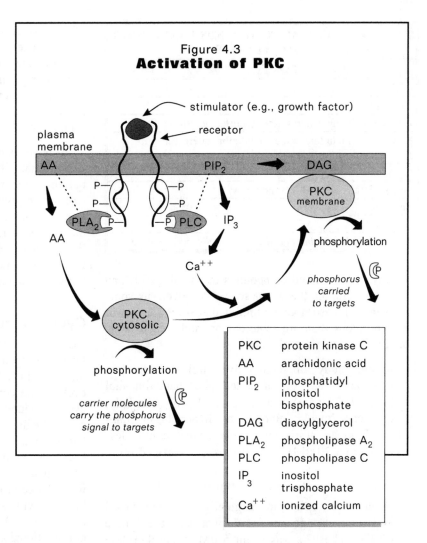

Figure 4.3
Activation of PKC

PKC	protein kinase C
AA	arachidonic acid
PIP_2	phosphatidyl inositol bisphosphate
DAG	diacylglycerol
PLA_2	phospholipase A_2
PLC	phospholipase C
IP_3	inositol trisphosphate
Ca^{++}	ionized calcium

PKC expression or activity is inhibited by a number of natural compounds, some of which are listed in Table 4.3. The compounds listed are active in the concentration range of roughly 1 to 50 μM. As with the PTK inhibitors, most are active in the range of about 10 to 30 μM.[a] Resveratrol may also inhibit PKC but is not listed because inhibition depends greatly on the PKC stimulus. In one study, the IC_{50} for PKC inhibition by resveratrol ranged from 30 to 300 μM.[21]

Other Kinases Involved in Signal Transduction

In addition to PTK and PKC, other kinases are involved in signal transduction and, when overactive, can facilitate cancer cell proliferation. In some cases, PTK or PKC activation occurs first, then the signal later passes through these kinases.

---

[a] *Again, hypericin and pseudohypericin are notable exceptions, since they are effective at very low concentrations when activated by light.*

TABLE 4.3   NATURAL COMPOUNDS THAT INHIBIT PROTEIN KINASE C
COMPOUND
CAPE
Curcumin
Emodin (although some studies reported no effect)
Flavonoids (including apigenin, luteolin, quercetin, and EGCG)
Hypericin
Omega-3 fatty acids (EPA and DHA)
Selenium
Vitamin E
Note: See Table E.2 in Appendix E for details and references.

Many of the natural compounds that inhibit PTK and PKC also inhibit these kinases. Moreover, in some cases these kinases may be inhibited at somewhat lower concentrations than are required for inhibition of PTK and PKC. Some examples are:

- In one study, apigenin only marginally inhibited PTK and PKC but inhibited phosphatidylinositol kinase (PI kinase) at an IC_{50} of 12 μM. Similarly, quercetin, luteolin, emodin, and hypericin all inhibited PI kinase at low micromolar concentrations (less than about 20 μM).[22-26] PI kinase is elevated up to fourfold in some types of cancers.[27] It is mentioned below in connection with ras proteins.

- In one study, curcumin marginally inhibited purified PKC but strongly inhibited phosphorylase kinase (PhK). The IC_{50} was about 5 μM. Phosphorylase kinase is a key regulatory enzyme involved in the intracellular metabolism of sugar (glycogen). In this way, PhK plays a central role in cell proliferation.[28] Quercetin also inhibited PhK, but it was tested only at high concentrations (100 μM).[29]

- Apigenin (at 12 to 50 μM) inhibited mitogen-activated protein kinase (MAPK).[30] Apigenin reversed *ras* transformation of rat fibroblast cells at 12 μM, apparently due to MAPK inhibition.[31] MAPK is mentioned below in connection with ras proteins.

- The ability of apigenin and quercetin to inhibit human prostate cancer cells in vitro was closely correlated with their ability to block activity of proline-directed protein kinase FA (PDPK FA). The IC_{50} for cell proliferation and kinase inhibition was about 6 to 18 μM. This kinase is associated with neoplastic transformation and cell proliferation.[32]

Why does the same group of natural compounds seem to inhibit so many different kinases? Their pluripotent activity is not surprising, since these compounds tend to affect similar targets in each enzyme. PTK, PKC, and other kinases all require ATP to donate phosphorus atoms for energy. If ATP is prevented from interacting with the enzyme, the enzyme cannot function. Several of the compounds discussed in this chapter inhibit ATP-enzyme interactions; these include flavonoids (genistein, apigenin and luteolin) and other phenolic compounds, such as emodin.[33, 34]

We have identified several kinases involved in signal transduction. Depending on the origin and type of signal, one or more of these kinases can be involved in the signal transduction pathway. Note that using combinations of compounds to inhibit multiple kinases can produce synergistic effects. For example, a recent study on liver cancer cells reported that a combination of genistein and quercetin synergistically inhibited signal transduction and cell proliferation.[35]

Cyclin-Dependent Kinases

Cyclin-dependent kinases are not involved with transferring a signal from surface receptors to the nucleus, but they do help control the signals that drive the cell cycle. The cell cycle is regulated in part through the cyclic production and destruction of a family of proteins called cyclins. They derive their name from their oscillatory nature. These proteins help instruct the cell to begin the mitosis phase (see Figure 2.5), and they instruct it to move through other cell cycle transitions as well. Once produced, cyclins become activated through binding with specific kinases called cyclin-dependent kinases (Cdks). Without activation by Cdks, cyclins are nonfunctional and cannot drive cell proliferation.

In healthy cells, the ability of Cdks to activate cyclins is held in check by a family of cyclin-dependent kinase inhibitors. Primary Cdk inhibitors include the protein p21 and the closely related p27.[36, 37, a] p21 is of particular interest, since its production is induced by the p53 protein. Induction of p21 protein is one way that p53 halts the cell cycle in injured cells. Induction of p21 stops cell proliferation but still allows DNA repair to proceed. p21 can also be induced independently of the p53 protein.

Among other beneficial effects, the p27 protein seems to be involved in mediating the growth-inhibitory effects of TGF-beta. Not surprisingly, mice lacking the *p27* gene are prone to developing cancer. Furthermore, loss of *p27* activity has been associated with poor prognosis for prostate and colorectal cancer patients.[38, 39]

---

[a] *The p21 protein is sometimes referred to as p21^{Cip1} or p21^{WAF1}. Like p21, the p27 protein also belongs to the Cip/Kip family of proteins.*

Cancer cells commonly underexpress *p21* or *p27* genes or both. Many natural compounds can induce *p21* and/or *p27* gene activity and so lead to restoration of normal levels of p21 and p27 proteins. Some of these compounds act by inducing *p53* gene expression, while others act by alternate means and so can induce *p21* or *p27* activity even in cancer cells that contain mutated *p53* genes. For example, vitamin D_3 (1,25-D_3), vitamin E, antioxidants, and genistein can induce *p21* expression independent of *p53*. Table 4.4 lists compounds that can induce *p21* or *p27* activity.

The vitamin E study referred to in Table 4.4 is of special interest, since it suggested that antioxidants in general might induce *p21* independent of *p53*. Other studies on the amino acid *N*-acetyl-cysteine, which has antioxidant properties, further support this concept.[40] Again, compounds that induce *p21* or *p27* expression independent of the *p53* gene are valuable because *p53* is commonly mutated in cancer cells. So far however, induction has only been reported at high antioxidant concentrations in vitro, and since these concentrations cannot be achieved in vivo after oral administration, it is not certain that antioxidants would produce this effect in vivo. Thus while antioxidants could be useful in vivo for many reasons, induction of *p21* independent of *p53* may not be one of them.

Lastly, note that cyclin-dependent kinases may be inhibited by means other than expression of *p21* or *p27*. For example, PKC has been reported to be an upstream inducer of cyclin-dependent kinases in some cancer cells. In one study, inhibition of PKC activity (by selenium compounds) markedly reduced cyclin-dependent kinase activity in mouse breast cancer cells.[41] Other natural compounds that are not PKC inhibitors, such as *Eleuthero-coccus*, have also been reported to inhibit cyclin-dependent kinases in cancer cells, apparently by some other mechanism.[42]

Ras Proteins and Signal Transduction

Like PTK and PKC, ras proteins also play a role in signal transduction and are commonly overproduced in cancer cells. Oncogenic forms of the *ras* gene have been observed in 20 to 30 percent of human cancers. Their appearance is most frequent in pancreatic cancer

TABLE 4.4 NATURAL COMPOUNDS THAT INDUCE *p21* OR *p27* ACTIVITY
COMPOUND
ATRA (vitamin A)
Flavonoids (including apigenin, genistein, and EGCG)
Silymarin
Vitamin D_3 (1,25-D_3)
Vitamin E*

* *Water soluble analog of vitamin E*
Note: *See Table E.3 in Appendix E for details and references.*

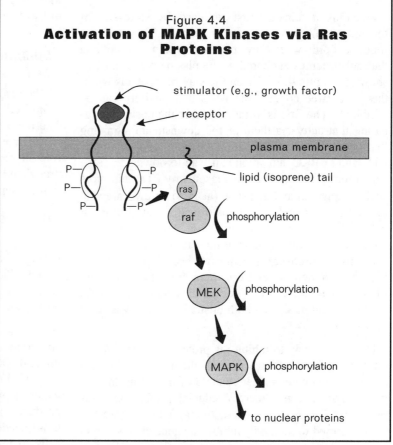

Figure 4.4
Activation of MAPK Kinases via Ras Proteins

(greater than 80 percent of patients) and colon cancer (greater than 50 percent).[43]

Ras proteins play a primary role in the MAPK signal transduction cascade illustrated in Figure 4.4. Briefly, phosphorylation of a surface receptor such as a receptor PTK stimulates the membrane-bound ras protein. Activation of ras, in turn, stimulates the phosphorylation of the kinase series raf, MEK, and MAPK. MAPK activation plays a central role in initiating cell proliferation, as it can directly interact with nuclear transcription factors. The ras protein also plays a role in initiating a number of other signal transduction cascades, including activation of PI kinase (mentioned above) and activation of PKC.[44] Since the ras protein is overexpressed in a large number of cancers and it plays an important role in multiple signal transduction cascades, inhibition of ras action is now considered an important goal in cancer treatment.[45] Moreover, inhibition of ras action is important because the ras protein, via stimulation of the MAPK signal transduction cascade, induces the expression of the *MDM2* gene, whose protein serves to inhibit the activity of the p53 protein (see Table 2.1 for more information on the *MDM2* gene). In this way, ras activity reduces the ability of the p53 protein to induce apoptosis in cancer cells.[46]

When ras proteins are first produced (by expression of the *ras* gene), they are not functional. They become functional only when they are joined with a lipid tail and that tail becomes anchored in the plasma membrane, as shown in Figure 4.4.[a] Given the way ras proteins work, there are three conceivable ways their activity can be inhibited. The first is to inhibit either the upstream signaling that activates them or the downstream signaling that occurs after ras activation, or both. For example, PTK and/or PKC activation can lead to downstream ras activation. This may be one reason why PTK inhibitors such as apigenin and genistein (at 12 to 25 µM) are able to reverse *ras*-induced transformation of fibroblast cells.[47, 48] Remember (from Table 2.1) that *ras* is an oncogene, capable of transforming normal cells to cancer cells. Moreover, apigenin has been reported to inhibit MAPK activity and can therefore act downstream of ras activation. Natural compounds such as apigenin may then inhibit signals both upstream and downstream of ras proteins.

The second way to inhibit ras protein activity is to inhibit production of the proteins themselves. Several natural compounds appear capable of inhibiting the expression of *ras* genes, thereby reducing production of ras proteins. For example, quercetin (at 5 to 10 µM) has been reported to markedly inhibit *ras* gene expression in human colon cancer cells and human leukemia cells.[49, 50] This effect appeared to be specific for *ras* expression in cancer cells, as normal cells were not affected.[51] (Normal cells transiently express but not overexpress *ras* genes.) ATRA, vitamin E (vitamin E succinate), and vitamin D$_3$ can also inhibit the expression of the *ras*

gene in cancer cells under some conditions.[52–56] However, it is not clear whether these vitamins inhibit *ras* expression directly or whether inhibition comes indirectly, as a consequence of other inhibitory actions.

The third way of inhibiting ras protein activity is to reduce production of the lipid tail necessary for the protein to function. The lipid tail that attaches to ras proteins is composed of isoprene units. We will go into some detail on what isoprene units are and how their synthesis can be decreased because some natural compounds that inhibit isoprene synthesis have been reported to inhibit cancer cell proliferation in vitro and in vivo, either by inhibiting production of the lipid tail (and ras function) or by other means discussed below.

Inhibiting Production of the Lipid (Isoprene) Tail

When isoprene units join with the ras protein to give it a lipid tail, the protein is said to become isoprenylated. The ras protein is the primary isoprenylated protein we will discuss, but we briefly mention others that play a role in cancer progression. The function of all isoprenylated proteins can be reduced by inhibiting production of isoprene synthesis.

Isoprene Synthesis

Cells produce isoprenes (also known as isoprenoids) through the same pathway by which cholesterol is produced. This pathway is important for other reasons besides ras activation and so is worthy of detailed discussion.

Isoprenoids and their derivatives are a large family of compounds that occur in both animals and plants; more than 20,000 isoprene compounds are known. Many isoprenoid products are familiar, including cholesterol, which is produced in animal cells, and rubber, which is produced in plant cells. Certain isoprenoids, such as those needed for the ras tail, are needed for some cancer cells to proliferate. Other isoprenoid compounds, including such well-known compounds as vitamins A and E, may inhibit cancer through a number of other mechanisms. Chapters 21 and 22 are devoted to isoprenoids and isoprenoid-related compounds that show promise in cancer treatment. Other common isoprenoid compounds include sex hormones, plant monoterpenes (essential oils), beta-carotene, and coenzyme Q10. Some of these, like vitamins A and E, consist of isoprene side chains attached to non-isoprene units.

In spite of their diversity, the starting material of all plant and mammalian isoprenoids is acetate. Through a series of steps that are largely regulated by the enzyme HMGR (hydroxymethylglutaryl-coenzyme A reductase),

---

[a] *The ras protein belongs to a large family of small GTP-binding proteins. GTP is the nucleotide guanine triphosphate. Ras proteins are activated when they bind with GTP and are inactivated when GTP is exchanged for GDP (guanine diphosphate). Special regulatory proteins force this exchange to occur, thereby allowing only momentary activation of ras proteins. Cancer cells, however, often produce deranged regulatory proteins, thereby allowing ras proteins to remain activated for longer periods of time.*

acetate is transformed into the basic isoprene unit. Basic isoprene units are then
combined, like links in a chain, to form
increasingly complex isoprenoid compounds. The formation of isoprenoid
compounds from acetate is shown in
Figure 4.5 (adapted from references
57–60 and 65).

This figure illustrates several important points. It shows that the enzyme
HMGR plays an early role in the formation of all isoprenoid compounds and in
addition, that the actions of HMGR are
controlled through two negative feedback loops, one from cholesterol (in animals) and one from monoterpenes and
possibly sesquiterpenes or other
isoprenoids (in plants). Cholesterol accounts for over 90 percent of all isoprenoids produced in animals, and when its
concentration gets too high, it serves to
inhibit its own production through the
negative feedback loop. This regulatory
system becomes deranged in cancer
cells, which can produce excessive
amounts of cholesterol and other isoprenoids, including the isoprenoids needed
to make the tail required by the ras protein.[61–65] Fortunately, monoterpenes,
even though produced in plants, can still
be used in animals to inhibit the activity
of HMGR, and inhibition by monoterpenes works even when the negative
feedback loop for cholesterol does not.

Figure 4.5 implies that the core isoprenoids—IPP, GPP, FPP, and GGPP—are
built up by adding basic isoprene units to one another
(note the structure of the basic isoprene unit). IPP contains one basic unit, GPP contains two basic units, and
so on. These core isoprenoids are then combined, again
like links in a chain, to form more complex compounds.
For example, looking at FPP in the figure, one FPP unit
is used to make sesquiterpenoids (sesquiterpenes) and
two FP units are combined to make triterpenoids and
steroids.

The figure also shows that ras proteins are produced
from FPP via the actions of an enzyme called farnesyl
protein transferase (FPTase). For this reason, ras proteins are sometimes referred to as farnesylated proteins.
Although there are several farnesylated proteins involved in cancer, the most studied of these are the ras
proteins.

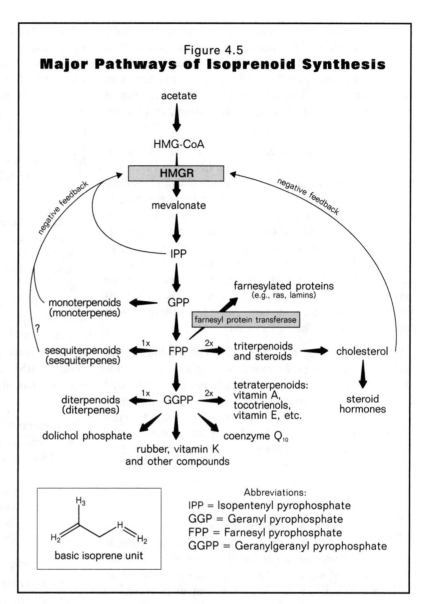

Figure 4.5
Major Pathways of Isoprenoid Synthesis

Inhibition of Isoprenoid Synthesis and Cancer

A number of natural compounds inhibit isoprene synthesis, primarily by inhibiting the synthesis of HMGR.
For example, one drug, Lovastatin, which is a natural
compound derived from a fungus, has been reported to
reduce HMGR activity and the proliferation of a wide
variety of cancer cell lines in vitro.[66, 67] Monoterpenes
(discussed in Chapter 21) also inhibit HMGR, as well as
cancer cells in vitro and in vivo. In addition to inhibiting HMGR, some natural compounds may also directly
reduce ras protein activity by inhibiting farnesyl protein
transferase, the enzyme that attaches isoprene units to
ras to form the lipid tail (see Figure 4.5).

Aside from their effects on ras proteins, HMGR inhibitors and those of FPTase may also reduce cancer cell
proliferation by reducing the attachment of lipid tails to
the lamin family of proteins (see Figure 4.5). Lamins

are farnesylated proteins that form the lamina (thin wall) at the inner side of the nuclear membrane (see Figure 2.1). An intact lamina is required for cell division. Like ras proteins, lamins need a lipid tail in order to function. At the time of division, the nuclear lamina is broken down and re-formed in a regulated manner, and lamins are needed for this process.

Another conceivable mechanism by which HMGR inhibitors may reduce cancer cell proliferation is by decreasing the synthesis of the isoprene dolichol phosphate (see Figure 4.5). This isoprene has a critical function in the assembly of glycoproteins such as growth factors, enzymes, growth factor receptors, and membrane components. Decreased production of any of these could reduce cellular proliferation. For example, HMGR inhibitors reduced dolichol phosphate synthesis and the proliferation of melanoma cells in vitro. The effect appeared due to decreased numbers of insulin-like growth factor receptors at the cell's surface.[68]

One last mechanism by which HMGR inhibitors may reduce cancer cell proliferation is by inhibiting the production of cholesterol itself. Cholesterol is a required component of cell membranes, and limiting cholesterol uptake or synthesis in cancer cells can damage their membranes. For example, cholesterol is needed for membrane rigidity (see Figure 4.1). In one study, reducing membrane cholesterol content by 50 percent doubled the toxicity of a fluorescent dye to leukemia and neuroblastoma cells.[62]

Natural Agents That Inhibit Isoprene Synthesis

Regardless of their exact mechanism of action, HMGR inhibitors do produce an antiproliferative effect in a variety of normal and cancer cells, and they do produce an antitumor effect in vivo. Moreover, cancer cells tend to be more sensitive to these effects than normal cells. Clearly, the disruption of isoprene synthesis by HMGR inhibitors is a promising treatment strategy. Natural compounds discussed in this book that inhibit HMGR include monoterpenes, garlic compounds, and omega-3 fatty acids.

Monoterpenes

Monoterpenes that inhibit HMGR include limonene, perillyl alcohol, and geraniol. As would be expected of a compound that inhibits isoprene synthesis, monoterpenes also moderately reduce plasma cholesterol levels.[69, 70, a] Of the monoterpenes, limonene and perillyl alcohol have been most extensively studied. Both compounds inhibit a variety of cancers in rodents, including stomach, lung, skin, and liver cancers (see Chapter 21).

Monoterpenes appear to have two actions: at lower concentrations they inhibit HMGR activity, and at higher concentrations (greater than 1 mM) they also reduce protein isoprenylation by inhibiting FPTase.[71, 72, b] The result at high concentrations is inhibition of the isoprenylation of both ras proteins and the nuclear lamin proteins required for cell proliferation.[73, 74, 75] Monoterpenes may also interfere with the synthesis of glycoproteins such as IGF-1 receptors, probably from inhibiting the isoprene dolichol phosphate.[76]

Garlic

Garlic (*Allium sativum*) also inhibits HMGR and has been reported to reduce plasma cholesterol levels in humans. The compounds responsible include allicin, ajoene, diallyl disulfide (DADS), and possibly other sulfur-containing compounds.[77–82] Both allicin and ajoene have been reported to reduce HMGR in healthy liver and intestinal tissue, as well as in human liver cancer cells in vitro.[79, 83] Allicin has also been reported to decrease isoprenylation of GGPP products at an IC_{50} of about 43 μM.[84] (One GGPP product that facilitates cancer and has already been discussed is dolichol phosphate.)

Garlic compounds have shown activity in vivo. In one study, oral administration of high doses of diallyl disulfide (190 mg/kg three times per week) delayed tumor growth, decreased tumor volume, and decreased tumor weight in mice injected with *ras*-transformed cancer cells. Furthermore, the treatment reduced HMGR activity by nearly 80 percent in both liver and tumor tissue as compared with control mice.[43]

Omega-3 Fatty Acids

EPA (eicosapentaenoic acid), an omega-3 fatty acid from fish oil, can also inhibit HMGR and ras activation. For example, in one study on rats, oral administration of omega-3 fatty acids (at 20 percent of diet) reduced FPTase expression, ras function, and colon cancer development. In contrast, omega-6 fatty acids, such as those in most vegetable oils used for cooking, had the opposite effect.[85] These fatty acids have been implicated in increased cancer risk. In another study on rats, oral administration of omega-3 fatty acids reduced ras protein levels in rat mammary glands, whereas omega-6 fatty acids raised the levels.[86] In two other rat studies, oral administration of omega-3 fatty acids (at 7 percent of diet) reduced the expression of HMGR in breast tissue compared with administration of omega-6 fatty acids.[87, 88]

---

[a] *Another isoprene product whose synthesis is inhibited by monoterpenes is ubiquinone, coenzyme Q10.*

[b] *At high concentrations, curcumin derivatives may also inhibit FPTase activity.*

CONCLUSION

To avoid apoptosis and promote proliferation, cancer cells override the controls that normally regulate these processes in healthy cells. Cancer cells use several interrelated and complementary means to override these controls, two important parts of which are increased growth factor activity and increased signal transduction. Indeed, cancer cells commonly produce their own growth factors, and the enzymes and proteins that are active in signal transduction tend to occur at abnormally high concentrations in cancer cells. Growth factor activity and signal transduction enzymes and proteins provide targets for inhibiting cancer with natural compounds. Discussed in detail in Part III, natural compounds that inhibit signal transduction have already been reported to produce antitumor effects in animals.

REFERENCES

[1] Smith AD, et al., eds. Oxford dictionary of biochemistry and molecular biology. Oxford: Oxford University Press, 1997.

[2] Tannock IF, Hill RP, eds. The basic science of oncology. 2nd ed. New York: Mc Graw-Hill, 1992, pp. 148–52.

[3] Korutla L, Kumar R. Inhibitory effect of curcumin on epidermal growth factor receptor kinase activity in A431 cells. Biochimica Biophysica Acta 1994; 1224:597–600.

[4] Wojtowicz-Praga S. Reversal of tumor-induced immunosuppression: A new approach to cancer therapy [see comments]. J Immunother 1997 May; 20(3):165–77.

[5] Bertino JR, ed. Encyclopedia of cancer. San Diego: Academic Press, 1997, p. 1632.

[6] Rydell EL, Olofsson J, Hellem S, Axelsson KL. Tyrosine kinase activities in normal and neoplastic epithelia tissue of the human upper aero-digestive tract. Second Messengers Phosphoproteins 1991; 13(4):217–29.

[7] Powis G, Abraham RT, Ashendel CL, et al. Anticancer drugs and signalling targets: Principles and examples. International Journal of Pharmacognosy 1995; 33 Supplement:17–26.

[8] Liang YC, Chen YC, Lin YL, et al. Suppression of extracellular signals and cell proliferation by the black tea polyphenol, theaflavin-3,3'-digallate. Carcinogenesis 1999 Apr; 20(4):733–6.

[9] Niles RM. Interactions between retinoic acid and protein kinase C in induction of melanoma differentiation. Adv Exp Med Biol 1994; 354:37–57.

[10] Blobe GC, Obeid LM, Hannun YA. Regulation of protein kinase C and role in cancer biology. Cancer Metastasis Rev 1994 Dec; 13(3–4):411–31.

[11] Blobe GC, Khan WA, Hannun YA. Protein kinase C: Cellular target for the second messenger arachidonic acid? Prostag Leukotrienes Essen Fatty Acids 1995; 52:129–135.

[12] Davidson NE, Kennedy MJ. Protein kinase C and breast cancer. Cancer Treat Res 1996; 83:91–105.

[13] Alessandro R, Spoonster J, Wersto RP, Kohn EC. Signal transduction as a therapeutic target. Curr Top Microbiol Immunol 1996; 213 (Pt3):167–88.

[14] Rose DP, Hatala MA. Dietary fatty acids and breast cancer invasion and metastasis. Nutr Cancer 1994; 21(2):103–11.

[15] Philip PA, Harris AL. Potential for protein kinase C inhibitors in cancer therapy. Cancer Treat Res 1995; 78:3–27.

[16] Ku WC, Cheng AJ, Chien T, Wang V. Inhibition of telomerase activity by PKC inhibitors in human nasopharyngeal cancer cells in culture. Biochem Biophys Res Commun 1997; 241:730–736.

[17] McCarty MF. Fish oil may impede tumour angiogenesis and invasiveness by down-regulating protein kinase C and modulating eicosanoid production. Med Hypotheses 1996 Feb; 46(2):107–15.

[18] O'Brian CA, Ward NE, Gravitt KR, Fan D. The role of protein kinase C in multidrug resistance. Cancer Treat Res 1994; 73:41–55.

[19] Dumont JA, Jones WD, Bitonti AJ. Inhibition of experimental metastasis and cell adhesion of B16F1 melanoma cells by inhibitors of protein kinase C. Cancer Res 1992; 52:1195–1200.

[20] Schwartz GK, Jiang J, Kelsen D, Albino AP. Protein kinase C: A novel target for inhibiting gastric cancer cell invasion. J Natl Cancer Inst 1993 Mar 3; 85(5):402–7.

[21] Garcia-Garcia J, Micol V, de Godos A, et al. The cancer chemopreventive agent resveratrol is incorporated into model membranes and inhibits protein kinase C alpha sctivity. Arch Biochem Biophys 1999 Dec 15; 372(2):382–388.

[22] Agullo G, Gamet-Payrastre L, Maneti S, et al. Relationship between flavonoid structure and inhibtion of phosphatidylinositol 3-kinase: A comparison with tyrosine kinase and protein kinase C inhibition. Biochem Pharmacol 1997; 53(11):1649–1657.

[23] Frew T, Powis G, Berggren M, et al. A multiwell assay for inhibitors of phosphatidylinositol-3-kinase and the identification of natural product inhibitors. Anticancer Res 1994 Nov–Dec; 14(6B):2425–8.

[24] Vlahos CJ, Matter WF, Hui KY, Brown RF. A specific inhibitor of phosphatidylinositol 3-kinase, 2-(4-morpholinyl)-8-phenyl-4H-1-benzopyran-4-one (LY294002). J Biol Chem 1994 Feb 18; 269(7):5241–8.

[25] Matter WF, Brown RF, Vlahos CJ. The inhibition of phosphatidylinositol 3-kinase by quercetin and analogs. Biochem Biophys Res Commun 1992 Jul 31; 186(2):624–31.

[26] Singhal RL, Yeh YA, Praja N, et al. Quercetin down-regulates signal transduction in human breast carcinoma cells. Biochem Biophys Res Commun 1995 Mar 8; 208(1):425–31.

[27] Weber G, Shen F, Prajda N, et al. Increased signal transduction activity and down-regulation in human cancer cells. Anticancer Res 1996 Nov–Dec; 16(6A):3271–82.

[28] Reddy S, Aggarwal BB. Curcumin is a non-competitive and selective inhibitor of phosphorylase kinase. FEBS 1994; 341:19–22.

[29] Srivastava AK. Inhibition of phosphorylase kinase, and tyrosine protein kinase activities by quercetin. Biochem Biophys Res Commun 1985 Aug 30; 131(1):1–5.

[30] Yin F, Giuliano AE, Van Herle AJ. Signal pathways involved in apigenin inhibition of growth and induction of apoptosis of human anaplastic thyroid cancer cells. Anticancer Res 1999 Sep–Oct; 19(5B):4297–303.

[31] Kuo ML, Yang NC. Reversion of v-H-ras-transformed NIH 3T3 cells by apigenin through inhibiting mitogen activated protein kinase and its downstream oncogenes. Biochem Biophys Res Comm 1995; 212(3):767–775.

[32] Lee SC, Kuan CY, Yang CC, et al. Bioflavonoids commonly and potently induce tyrosine dephosphorylation/inactivation of oncogenic proline-directed protein kinase FA in human prostate carcinoma cells. Anticancer Res 1998 Mar–Apr; 18(2A):1117–21.

[33] Akiyama T, Ishida J, Nakagawa S, et al. Genistein, a specific inhibitor of tyrosine-specific protein kinases. J Biol Chem 1987; 262(12):5592–5595.

[34] Jayasuriya H, Koonchanok NM, Geahlen RL, et al. Emodin, a protein tyrosine kinase inhibitor from Polygonum cuspidatum. J Nat Prod 1992; 55(5):696–8.

[35] Weber G, Shen F, Yang H, et al. Regulation of signal transduction activity in normal and cancer cells. Anticancer Res 1999 Sep–Oct; 19(5A):3703–9.

[36] Johnson DG, Walker CL. Cyclins and cell cycle checkpoints. Annu Rev Pharmacol Toxicol 1999; 39:295–312.

[37] Gartel AL, Tyner AL. The growth-regulatory role of p21 (WAF1/CIP1). Prog Mol Subcell Biol 1998; 20:43–71.

[38] Macri E, Loda M. Role of p27 in prostate carcinogenesis. Cancer Metastasis Rev 1998–99; 17(4):337–44.

[39] Loda M, Cukor B, Tam SW, et al. Increased proteasome-dependent degradation of the cyclin-dependent kinase inhibitor p27 in aggressive colorectal carcinomas. Nat Med 1997 Feb; 3(2):231–4.

[40] Liu M, Wikonkal NM, Brash DE. Induction of cyclin-dependent kinase inhibitors and G(1) prolongation by the chemopreventive agent N-acetylcysteine. Carcinogenesis 1999 Sep; 20(9):1869–72.

[41] Sinha R, Kiley SC, Lu JX, et al. Effects of methylselenocysteine on PKC activity, cdk2 phosphorylation and gadd gene expression in synchronized mouse mammary epithelial tumor cells. Cancer Lett 1999 Nov 15; 146(2):135–45.

[42] Shan BE, Zeki K, Sugiura T, et al. Chinese medicinal herb, Acanthopanax gracilistylus, extract induces cell cycle arrest of human tumor cells in vitro. Jpn J Cancer Res 2000 Apr; 91(4):383–389.

[43] Singh SV, Mohan RR, Agarwal R, et al. Novel anti-carcinogenic activity of an organosulfide from garlic: Inhibition of H-RAS oncogene transformed tumor growth in vivo by diallyl disulfide is associated with inhibition of p21H-ras processing. Biochem Biophys Res Commun 1996 Aug 14; 225(2):660–5.

[44] Pincus MR, Brandt-Rauf PW, Michl J, et al. ras-p21-induced cell transformation: Unique signal transduction pathways and implications for the design of new chemotherapeutic agents. Cancer Invest 2000; 18(1):39–50.

[45] Rowinsky EK, Windle JJ, Von Hoff DD. Ras protein farnesyltransferase: A strategic target for anticancer therapeutic development. J Clin Oncol 1999 Nov; 17(11):3631–52.

[46] Ries S, Biederer C, Woods D, et al. Opposing effects of Ras on p53: Transcriptional activation of mdm2 and induction of p19ARF. Cell 2000 Oct 13; 103(2):321–30.

[47] Kuo ML, Lin JK, Huang TS, Yang NC. Reversion of the transformed phenotypes of v-H-ras NIH3T3 cells by flavonoids through attenuating the content of phosphotyrosine. Cancer Letters 1994; 87:91–97.

[48] Lin JK, Chen YC, Huang YT, Lin-Shiau SY. Suppression of protein kinase C and nuclear oncogene expression as possible molecular mechanisms of cancer chemoprevention by apigenin and curcumin. J Cell Biochem Suppl 1997; 28/29:39–48.

[49] Ranelletti FO, Maggiano N, Serra FG, et al. Quercetin inhibits p21-RAS expression in human colon cancer cell lines and in primary colorectal tumors. Int J Cancer 2000 Feb 1; 85(3):438–45.

[50] Csokay B, Prajda N, Weber G, Olah E. Molecular mechanisms in the antiproliferative action of quercetin. Life Sci 1997; 60(24):2157–63.

[51] Avila MA, Cansado J, Harter KW, et al. Quercetin as a modulator of the cellular neoplastic phenotype. Effects on the expression of mutated H-ras and p53 in rodent and human cells. Adv Exp Med Biol 1996; 401:101–10.

[52] Spina A, Chiosi E, Naviglio S, et al. Treatment of v-Ki-ras-transformed SVC1 cells with low retinoic acid induces malignancy reversion associated with ras p21 down-regulation. Biochim Biophys Acta 2000 Apr 17; 1496(2–3):285–95.

[53] Prasad KN, Cohrs RJ, Sharma OK. Decreased expressions of c-myc and H-ras oncogenes in vitamin E succinate induced morphologically differentiated murine B-16 melanoma cells in culture. Biochem Cell Biol 1990 Nov; 68(11):1250–5.

[54] Cohrs RJ, Torelli S, Prasad KN, et al. Effect of vitamin E succinate and a cAMP-stimulating agent on the expression of c-myc and N-myc and H-ras in murine neuroblastoma cells. Int J Dev Neurosci 1991; 9(2):187–94.

[55] Prasad KN, Edwards-Prasad J, Kumar S, Meyers A. Vitamins regulate gene expression and induce differentiation and growth inhibition in cancer cells. Their relevance in cancer prevention. Arch Otolaryngol Head Neck Surg 1993 Oct; 119(10):1133–40.

[56] Prasad KN, Edwards-Prasad J. Expressions of some molecular cancer risk factors and their modification by vitamins. J Am Coll Nutr 1990 Feb; 9(1):28–34.

[57] Bruneton J. Pharmacognosy, phytochemistry, medicinal plants. Secaucus, NY: Lavoisier Publishing c/o Springer-Verlag, 1995, p. 388.

[58] Robbers JE, Speedie MK, Tyler VE. Pharmacognosy and pharmacobiotechnology. Baltimore: Williams & Wilkins, 1996, p. 82.

[59] Hohl RJ. Monoterpenes as regulators of malignant cell proliferation. Adv Exp Med Biol 1996; 401:137–146.

[60] Kohl NE, Conner MW, Gibbs JB, et al. Development of inhibitors of protein farnesylation as potential chemotherapeutic agents. J Cell Biochem Suppl 1995; 22:145–150.

[61] Rao KN. The significance of the cholesterol biosynthetic pathway in cell growth and carcinogenesis (review). Anticancer Res 1995 Mar–Apr; 15(2):309–14.

[62] Lenz M, Miehe WP, Vahrenwald F, et al. Cholesterol based antineoplastic strategies. Anticancer Res 1997 Mar–Apr; 17(2A):1143–6.

[63] Coleman PS, Chen LC, Sepp-Lorenzino L. Cholesterol metabolism and tumor cell proliferation. Subcell Biochem 1997; 28:363–435.

[64] Goel R, Varma S, Kaul D. Sterol dependent LDL-receptor gene transcription in lymphocytes from normal and CML patients. Cancer Lett 1996 Oct 22; 107(2):193–8.

[65] Larsson O. HMG-CoA reductase inhibitors: Role in normal and malignant cells. Crit Rev Oncol Hematol 1996 Apr; 22(3):197–212.

[66] Addeo R, Altucci L, Battista T, et al. Stimulation of human breast cancer MCF-7 cells with estrogen prevents cell cycle arrest by HMG-CoA reductase inhibitors. Biochem Biophys Res Commun 1996 Mar 27; 220(3):864–70.

[67] Nordenberg J, Goldwasser I, Zoref-Shani E, et al. Inhibition of B16 melanoma cell proliferation and alterations in p21 ras expression induced by interceptors of signal transduction pathways. Isr J Med Sci 1996 Dec; 32(12):1153–7.

[68] Carlberg M, Dricu A, Blegen H, et al. Mevalonic acid is limiting for N-linked glycosylation and translocation of the insulin-like growth factor-1 receptor to the cell surface. Evidence for a new link between 3-hydroxy-3-methylglutaryl-coenzyme a reductase and cell growth. J Biol Chem 1996 Jul 19; 271(29):17453–62.

[69] Elegbede JA. Prospective roles of plant secondary metabolites in the treatment of mammary cancer. Diss Abstr Int 1985; 46(6):1874.

[70] Elson CE, Yu SG. The chemoprevention of cancer by mevalonate-derived constituents of fruits and vegetables. J Nutr 1994 May; 124(5):607–14.

[71] Chen X, Hasuma T, Yano Y, et al. Inhibition of farnesyl protein transferase by monoterpene, curcumin derivatives and gallotannin. Anticancer Res 1997 Jul–Aug; 17(4A):2555–64.

[72] Elson CE. Suppression of mevalonate pathway activities by dietary isoprenoids: Protective roles in cancer and cardiovascular disease. J Nutr 1995; 125:1666S-1672S.

[73] Yu SG, Hildebrandt LA, Elson CE. Geraniol, an inhibitor of mevalonate biosynthesis, suppresses the growth of hepatomas and melanomas transplanted to rats and mice. J Nutr 1995 Nov; 125(11):2763–7.

[74] Karlson J, Borg-Karlson AK, Unelius R, et al. Inhibition of tumor cell growth by monoterpenes in vitro: Evidence of a ras-independent mechanism of action. Anticancer Drugs 1996 Jun; 7(4):422–9.

[75] Ruch RJ, Sigler K. Growth inhibition of rat liver epithelial tumor cells by monoterpenes does not involve ras plasma membrane association. Carcinogenesis 1994; 15(4):787–89.

[76] Carlberg M, Dricu A, Blegen H, et al. Mevalonic acid is limiting for N-linked glycosylation and translocation of the insulin-like growth factor-1 receptor to the cell surface. Evidence for a new link between 3-hydroxy-3-methylglutaryl-coenzyme a reductase and cell growth. J Biol Chem 1996 Jul 19; 271(29):17453–62.

[77] Qureshi AA, Crenshaw TD, Abuirmeileh N, et al. Influence of minor plant constituents on porcine hepatic lipid metabolism. Impact on serum lipids. Atherosclerosis 1987 Apr; 64(2–3):109–15.

[78] Gebhardt R. Multiple inhibitory effects of garlic extracts on cholesterol biosynthesis in hepatocytes. Lipids 1993 Jul; 28(7):613–9.

[79] Gebhardt R, Beck H, Wagner KG. Inhibition of cholesterol biosynthesis by allicin and ajoene in rat hepatocytes and HepG2 cells. Biochim Biophys Acta 1994 Jun 23; 1213(1):57–62.

[80] Sheela CG, Augusti KT. Effects of S-allyl cysteine sulfoxide isolated from Allium sativum Linn and gugulipid on some enzymes and fecal excretions of bile acids and sterols in cholesterol fed rats. Indian J Exp Biol 1995 Oct; 33(10):749–51.

[81] Sheela CG, Augusti KT. Antidiabetic effects of S-allyl cysteine sulphoxide isolated from garlic Allium sativum Linn. Indian J Exp Biol 1992 Jun; 30(6):523–6.

[82] Kumar RV, Banerji A, Kurup CK, Ramasarma T. The nature of inhibition of 3-hydroxy-3-methylglutaryl CoA reductase by garlic-derived diallyl disulfide. Biochim Biophys Acta 1991 Jun 24; 1078(2):219–25.

[83] Gebhardt R, Beck H. Differential inhibitory effects of garlic-derived organosulfur compounds on cholesterol biosynthesis in primary rat hepatocyte cultures. Lipids 1996 Dec; 31(12):1269–76.

[84] Lee S, Park S, Oh JW, Yang C. Natural inhibitors for protein prenyltransferase. Planta Med 1998 May; 64(4):303–8.

[85] Singh J, Hamid R, Reddy BS. Dietary fish oil inhibits the expression of farnesyl protein transferase and colon tumor development in rodents. Carcinogenesis 1998 Jun; 19(6):985–9.

[86] Badawi AF, El-Sohemy A, Stephen LL, et al. The effect of dietary n-3 and n-6 polyunsaturated fatty acids on the expression of cyclooxygenase 1 and 2 and levels of p21ras in rat mammary glands. Carcinogenesis 1998 May; 19(5):905–10.

[87] El-Sohemy A, Archer MC. Regulation of mevalonate synthesis in rat mammary glands by dietary n-3 and n-6 polyunsaturated fatty acids. Cancer Res 1997 Sep 1; 57(17):3685–7.

[88] El-Sohemy A, Archer MC. Regulation of mevalonate synthesis in low density lipoprotein receptor knockout mice fed n-3 or n-6 polyunsaturated fatty acids. Lipids 1999 Oct; 34(10):1037–43.

5

TRANSCRIPTION FACTORS AND REDOX SIGNALING

Transcription factors bind to the regulatory portion of a gene and directly serve to initiate gene transcription (see Figure 2.4). In this way, they have final control over production of all proteins within a cell, and therefore they control much of a cell's behavior. In order to do their job, they must be present in sufficient quantity and must be activated to bind to their target gene. Their quantity is dependent on gene expression, since transcription factors are themselves protein products of genes. Their activation, on the other hand, is usually dependent on signal transduction, which is initiated by growth factors, cell-to-cell interactions, or some other stimulus such as cell damage.

The amount and activation of transcription factors is often abnormal in cancer cells. These abnormalities favor the production of proteins that allow cancer cells to proliferate, invade, and metastasize, as well as avoid apoptosis. For example, oncogenes such as *fos*, *jun* and *myc* produce excessive amounts of fos, jun and myc proteins. These proteins serve as transcription factors to initiate the expression of genes that drive the cell cycle (such as cyclin genes). Other genes, when abnormally expressed, produce excessive amounts of transcription factors that stimulate the expression of genes that control other aspects of cancer progression, such as invasion and metastasis. At the same time excessive amounts of transcription factors are being produced, excessive signal transduction is also occurring, which serves to activate available transcription factors.

Although many kinds of transcription factors exist, in this chapter we take a closer look at three that play a crucial role in cancer: the p53 protein, NF-κB (nuclear factor-kappa B), and AP-1 (activator protein-1). The p53 protein binds to the regulatory portion of a variety of genes, thus acting as a multifunctional transcription factor. For example, it binds to the regulatory portion of the *p21* gene, discussed in the previous chapter, thereby controlling progression of a cell through the cell cycle. The other two transcription factors, NF-κB and AP-1, also play a role in cell proliferation, as well as in a variety of other processes such as inflammation, angiogenesis, cancer cell invasion, and apoptosis. Like the p53 protein, the NF-κB protein also binds to several genes and is thus multifunctional.

In Chapter 4 we discussed how kinases and ras proteins influence signal transduction. The signal transduction related to these proteins is dependent upon the propagated movement of high-energy phosphorus groups (a process involving protein phosphorylation). This process is not the only means by which signals travel within cells, however. In the last decade, researchers have discovered that signal transduction also occurs via free radicals in a process called redox (reduction-oxidation) signaling. This discovery lagged behind that of protein phosphorylation because of the inherently transient nature of free radicals and the difficulty of tracking them. It is now clear that a dynamic balance of oxidants and antioxidants exists within a healthy cell. Fluctuating concentrations of free radicals serve to switch on and off a variety of cellular activities, including enzyme activation and, via transcription factors, gene expression.[1] Although more ephemeral, this form of signal transduction is as important as that of protein phosphorylation. And like signal transduction due to protein phosphorylation, redox signaling is also abnormal in cancer cells, providing them with survival advantages.

Because redox signaling plays a large role in activating transcription factors, this chapter starts with a general introduction to redox reactions. Not all the information presented will be used in discussing transcription factors, but it will come into play in later discussions such as those on the role of iron and copper in cancer progression and the use of selenium in cancer treatment.

INTRODUCTION TO REDOX REACTIONS

Definition of Terms

First, it will help to define terms. *Oxidants* (sometimes called prooxidants) are compounds that accept one or more electrons in a redox reaction; they play a coupled role with their opposites, *reductants*, which are compounds that lose one or more electrons in a redox reaction. *Redox reactions*, then, are reactions in which the gain of electrons by an oxidant is coupled with the loss of electrons from a reductant. Similarly, the *redox state* of a cell refers to the moment-to-moment balance that exists between its oxidant and reductive forces.

The term *redox reaction* is shorthand for coupled reduction-oxidation reaction. In the process of reduction, one compound (the oxidant) gains an electron. In the process of oxidation, the other compound (the reductant) loses an electron. Oxidation is the well-known process that turns metal to rust or browns an apple after it has

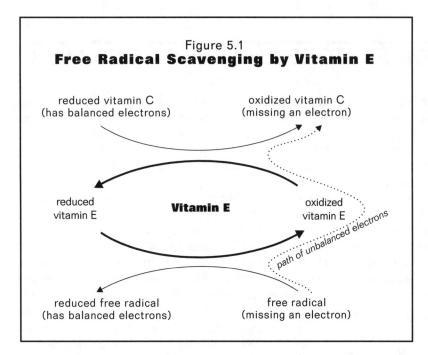

Figure 5.1
Free Radical Scavenging by Vitamin E

reduced vitamin C
(has balanced electrons)

oxidized vitamin C
(missing an electron)

reduced
vitamin E

Vitamin E

oxidized
vitamin E

path of unbalanced electrons

reduced free radical
(has balanced electrons)

free radical
(missing an electron)

been sliced. In all redox reactions, we say that the oxidant is reduced and the reductant is oxidized.

Antioxidants are, simply enough, compounds that oppose oxidation. They can do this through a number of means; for example, some antioxidants bind iron or copper, keeping them from participating in redox reactions. (As we will see, iron and copper are needed to catalyze many types of redox reactions.) These types of antioxidants need not participate in electron exchange at all. More commonly though, when we use the term *antioxidant*, we are referring to a compound that offers itself as a sacrificial reductant, thereby giving up one of its electrons to spare or replace electron loss from other compounds, such as DNA and fatty acids, that would be damaged by such a loss. These types of antioxidants are often referred to as *free radical scavengers*. Free radicals are compounds that have an uneven number of electrons and are therefore unbalanced and reactive. They act as oxidants, attempting to gain stability (an even number of electrons) by stealing an electron from the compounds they encounter. Antioxidants offer this electron to free radicals, thereby neutralizing their destructive nature. We can say then that free radical-antioxidant reactions are a subset of reduction-oxidation reactions.

One last general point is that redox reactions often involve the transfer of hydrogen atoms, since hydrogen is the only atom with a single electron. During oxidation, a hydrogen atom is commonly lost, and during reduction, one is commonly gained. This can be seen in Figures A.19 and A.20 of Appendix A, which show the loss

of a hydrogen atom when vitamin C (ascorbate) is oxidized.

Cycling of Antioxidants

Because free radical scavenging antioxidants are of great interest to us, we now look at how they participate in redox reactions, focusing attention on vitamin E as an example. Vitamin E is a fat-soluble antioxidant that protects fatty acids, such as those in the plasma membrane, from oxidation. To prevent the electrons of fatty acids from being lost to an oxidant or to replace them after they are lost, vitamin E sacrifices its electrons. This creates a vitamin E molecule that is now itself a free radical (i.e., it is missing an electron). Other antioxidants, commonly vitamin C, sacrifice an electron to the vitamin E radical, thus becoming free radicals themselves but regenerating vitamin E so that it can act again as an antioxidant. In a chain reaction of electron transport, the unbalance in electrons that started with the invading free radical moved first to vitamin E, then to vitamin C, and finally to NADH, the fundamental electron source within cells.[a] The electrons for NADH are regenerated by burning glucose. Thus glucose is the ultimate source of antioxidant energy within a cell. This process for vitamin E is illustrated in Figure 5.1; in it, vitamin E cycles between a reduced (antioxidant) state and an oxidized (free radical) state.

Sources of Free Radicals

Many of the free radicals we are concerned with are grouped under the term *reactive oxygen species* (ROS). As discussed in Chapter 2, these are either free radicals themselves (for example, the hydroxyl radical) or easily converted into free radicals (molecular oxygen and hydrogen peroxide). The primary source of ROS in a cell is molecular oxygen (O_2), which is converted to free radicals or other ROS during cell respiration, immune activity, and redox reactions with trace metals. ROS can also be introduced from sources outside the body, such

[a] *NADH (reduced nicotinamide adenine dinucleotide) is comprised of two nucleotides joined together. One has an adenine base and the other a nicotinamide base (nicotinamide is formed from niacin, vitamin B_3.). After donating electrons, NADH becomes NAD^+ (oxidized nicotinamide adenine dinucleotide), which is converted back to NADH through the burning of glucose. In some cases, NADH carries an extra phosphate group, in which case it is called NADPH. It functions in the same way as NADH and is interchangeable in many reactions.*

as intake of oxidized (rancid) fatty acids. ROS production by immune cells and ROS production via trace metal reactions play an important role in cancer; since both will be mentioned again in later chapters, we discuss these two sources of ROS in more detail below.

ROS from Immune Cells

Immune cells like macrophages destroy invading pathogens and cancer cells by spitting out noxious chemicals. These chemicals include ROS such as the superoxide radical ($O_2^{\bullet -}$), which is easily converted to the more damaging hydroxyl radical (OH $^{\bullet}$). (The dot signifies a free radical.) In addition, macrophages produce nitric oxide (NO$^{\bullet}$), a free radical based on nitrogen rather than oxygen. Thus the environment surrounding an activated macrophage is rich in free radicals.

Although free radical production by immune cells is generally beneficial, it can be detrimental if it is part of a chronic inflammatory response. In this case, there is no resolution to the inflammation and free radical generation and subsequent tissue destruction can occur. In addition, as noted, chronic inflammation can lead to the transformation of normal cells into cancer cells and can assist the progression of cancer cells.

ROS from Trace Metal Reactions

Redox reactions with trace metals, especially iron and copper, can easily generate free radicals. A limited amount of free radical generation by this means can be beneficial, but excessive production is usually harmful. For example, high stores of iron in the body, which lead to increased free radical production, have been linked to increased risk of both heart disease and cancer.[2, 3, 4]

To produce free radicals from iron or copper usually requires the presence of an antioxidant, and some antioxidants are particularly prone to react with these metals. This is true for vitamin C (see Chapter 15). Briefly, vitamin C can participate in the first of two linked reactions that are important:

$$ascorbate + O_2^{\bullet -} \rightarrow ascorbate\ radical + H_2O_2$$

$$copper^{+1} + H_2O_2 \rightarrow copper^{+2} + OH^{\bullet} + OH^{-}$$

Although the shorthand symbols may be unfamiliar to some readers, their meaning is rather straightforward. In the first reaction, vitamin C (called ascorbate when in solution) reacts with the superoxide radical to produce the ascorbate free radical and hydrogen peroxide (H_2O_2). Hydrogen peroxide is a very mobile type of ROS; it can easily pass through membranes to reach any intracellular compartment.[5] In the second reaction, the hydrogen peroxide produced in the first reaction (or elsewhere)

reacts with reduced copper (copper^{+1}) to form oxidized copper (copper^{+2}) and, most important, the hydroxyl radical (OH$^{\bullet}$). The hydroxyl radical is a very potent free radical that can easily damage DNA and other cellular components.

What is important in these reactions is that some antioxidants can react with ROS to make hydrogen peroxide, and hydrogen peroxide can react with copper or iron to produce the hydroxyl radical. In other words, in the presence of iron or copper, some antioxidants can lead to the production of the damaging hydroxyl radical. This is in contrast to the popular view that antioxidants always act as free radical scavengers. Although under most in-vivo conditions antioxidants do scavenge free radicals, antioxidants can still produce hydroxyl radicals in some situations. This possibility is discussed in more detail in Chapter 15.

Antioxidant Enzymes

Although the relatively small-sized antioxidants, vitamin C, vitamin E, and glutathione, have received the most public attention, large antioxidant enzymes in the cell also perform a vital role in neutralizing free radicals.[a] In fact, they act more efficiently than the small antioxidant compounds because they directly catalyze the conversion of free radicals to other, less harmful free radicals or to inert or useful compounds such as water and reduced glutathione. Unlike the small antioxidant compounds, antioxidant enzymes do not become free radicals that need to be regenerated. The conversion of free radicals by antioxidant enzymes is illustrated in Figure 5.2.

The left side of the figure shows how oxygen (O_2) loses an electron to produce the superoxide radical ($O_2^{\bullet -}$). Superoxide is then converted to hydrogen peroxide by the enzyme SOD. Hydrogen peroxide is converted to harmless water (H_2O) by the enzymes catalase, glutathione peroxidase, or both, with glutathione peroxidase requiring the presence of glutathione to be effective. The right side of the figure shows that the enzyme glutathione reductase converts oxidized glutathione to reduced glutathione. Reduced glutathione either can scavenge free radicals itself, or it can act with glutathione peroxidase as shown.

Interestingly, cancer cells are frequently deficient in the enzymes catalase and SOD, a deficiency that would have the effect of producing extra superoxide radicals and hydrogen peroxide, as long as glutathione peroxi-

---

[a] *A number of other relatively large protein compounds act as antioxidants, including uric acid and albumin, but will not be treated here.*

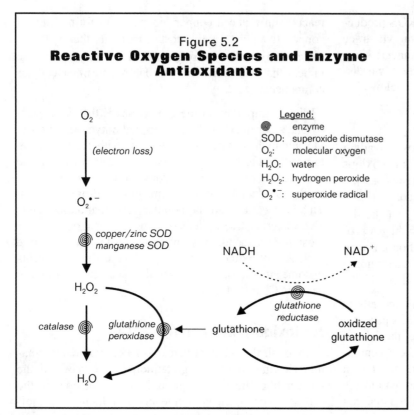

Figure 5.2
Reactive Oxygen Species and Enzyme Antioxidants

bridge, is illustrated in Figure 5.3. The disulfide bridge is broken when the cysteine molecules are reduced, as when, for example, they contact an antioxidant. Breaking this bridge is like throwing the on switch for the protein.

One simple example of a redox-active protein, or in this case, a redox-active peptide, has already been mentioned.[a] The amino acid glutathione acts as an antioxidant in its reduced form. Glutathione is actually a tripeptide made up of three amino acids, one of which is cysteine. When glutathione is oxidized, it loses a hydrogen atom from its cysteine component. Thus unbalanced, it bonds with another oxidized glutathione molecule via a disulfide bridge. In this state, it cannot act as an antioxidant (i.e., it is turned off). Once it is reduced again, by NADH for example, the disulfide bridge breaks and the glutathione molecule can again act as an antioxidant (it is turned on).

dase is not increased. Indeed, cancer cells are known to produce large quantities of hydrogen peroxide, as discussed in Chapter 2. Superoxide concentrations are also commonly increased at cancer sites. Increased production of these ROS may give cancer cells certain survival advantages, some of which are discussed below.

Redox Activation and Deactivation of Proteins

We have discussed what free radicals are and how they are produced and neutralized; now we turn to one primary means by which free radicals activate or deactivate proteins, thus returning to turn back to the primary topic of this chapter, transcription factors. Transcription factors, being proteins, can be affected by free radicals through this mechanism.

Like trace metals and antioxidants, proteins can undergo redox reactions. This is especially true for proteins containing the amino acid cysteine. Such redox reactions alter cysteine molecules in a way that activates or deactivates the protein, much as if the cysteine portion of the protein were an on-off switch. The off mode comes into play when the sulfur atom in cysteine is oxidized (i.e., loses a hydrogen atom). When oxidation occurs for two sulfur atoms in adjacent cysteine molecules, the resulting unbalanced sulfur atoms can bond with one another. This bond, aptly called a disulfide

Protein interactions with free radicals are actually more complex than this basic sketch suggests. In addition to linking separate proteins, disulfide bonds play a role in maintaining the three-dimensional structure of complex proteins. We have focused on the concept of cysteine reduction/oxidation acting as an on-off switch because similar actions play a role in many biological processes, and it illustrates well how proteins can be affected by redox states.

TRANSCRIPTION FACTORS

We now turn to three transcription factors (p53 protein, NF-κB, and AP-1) that play a vital role in both healthy and cancerous cells. Cancerous cells gain a survival advantage by producing insufficient or nonfunctional p53 proteins and by producing excessive amounts of NF-κB and AP-1. Many references to redox reactions and redox signaling occur in the following, since these have an effect on all three transcription factors.

p53 Protein as a Transcription Factor

The *p53* gene acts as the guardian of DNA, and in the event of DNA damage it performs three crucial functions. First, it halts the cell cycle, for example, by in-

---

[a] *Peptides consist of a few amino acids joined together and proteins consist of many joined together.*

creasing the expression of the *p21* gene. Second, it initiates DNA repair. Third, if the DNA cannot be repaired, it initiates apoptosis, for example, by increasing the expression of the *Bax* gene. To perform these diverse functions, the p53 protein acts as a transcription factor, binding to and initiating the expression of multiple genes.

Because of its role in protecting DNA and halting the cell cycle, a functional *p53* gene protects against cancer. Not surprisingly then, mutations of the *p53* gene are very common in cancer cells. The mutated *p53* gene is unable to perform its normal functions, thereby allowing cancer cells to proliferate and increasing the possibility of additional mutations by allowing cells with a mutator phenotype to survive (see Chapter 2). Moreover, the mutated *p53* gene can produce abnormal proteins that in and of themselves facilitate cancer progression.[6] Mutations in the *p53* gene are associated with increased tumor grade, stage, and proliferation, as well as poor prognosis.[7–11]

In addition to the outright mutations of the *p53* gene in cancer cells and, subsequently, the production of abnormal p53 proteins, the p53 protein can also be made nonfunctional after its production. The functionality of the p53 protein is regulated by *ras* activity (via the effects of ras proteins on *MDM2* expression; see Chapter 4) and by both the redox status of the cell and trace metal concentrations in the cell.[12–15]

The p53 protein contains 10 different cysteine residues, and although disulfide bonds do not actually form between these cysteine residues, a similar type of bond does form, based on the insertion of zinc atoms between the sulfur atoms. These bonds, which help to maintain the active three-dimensional structure of the protein, are redox-sensitive and are altered by oxidants. Indeed, nitric oxide and other free radicals that bind to cysteine can change the structure of the p53 protein, making it inactive.[16] As discussed in Chapter 2, cancer cells tend to be in a prooxidant state, and the excess oxidants in such a state may thus help reduce p53 activity.

The trace metal cadmium can also inhibit the p53 protein by substituting for zinc. The same effect can be caused by copper. In addition, copper can induce the production of free radicals, as discussed above. This

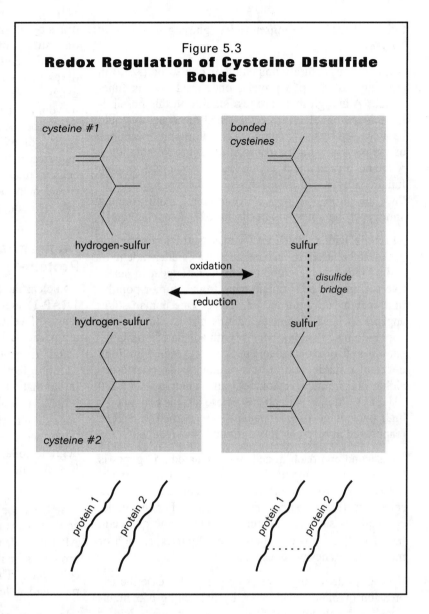

Figure 5.3
Redox Regulation of Cysteine Disulfide Bonds

partly explains both why cadmium and copper are carcinogenic and also why zinc deficiency is carcinogenic.

Effect of Natural Compounds on p53 and Its Protein

There are two basic situations to consider when speaking of the effects of natural compounds on the *p53* gene: when it is not mutated and when it is. Both situations can occur within the same tumor. In general, some cells within a tumor contain mutated *p53* genes and some do not, although many tumors will contain a high percentage of one cell type or the other.

In cancer cells with normal *p53* genes, natural compounds can stimulate the expression of that gene, leading to apoptosis. This has been reported, for example, with melatonin (at 1 nM), curcumin (at 50 μM), resveratrol (at 50 μM), and ginsenosides (ginseng saponins, at 10 μM).[17–20]

In addition, natural compounds may also be useful in assuring that the p53 protein, once produced, is functional. Although there are few studies on this possibility, it is reasonable to expect that p53 functionality could be increased by using compounds that inhibit the actions of ras proteins and by using antioxidants to maintain a reducing environment in the cell. Also, p53 protein functionality might be increased by preventing high intracellular iron or copper concentrations. Anti-iron and anticopper therapies will be discussed in later chapters.

In cells with mutated *p53* genes, natural compounds can still be used to induce apoptosis, independent of *p53*. Indeed, some natural compounds appear to selectively eliminate *p53* mutant cells from a tumor population, leaving only normal *p53* cells. One human study appears to have demonstrated this effect. In a small, nonrandomized study, patients with advanced premalignant lesions of the head and neck were treated with high doses of retinoic acid (13-cis-retinoic acid), interferon-alpha (an immune cytokine), and vitamin E (1,200 I.U./day). In half the patients whose lesions contained a high percentage of *p53* mutants, the normal *p53* gene reappeared in biopsies after 12 months of treatment.[21]

A second approach in cells with mutated *p53* genes is to use natural compounds to inhibit production of abnormal p53 proteins, since such proteins can by themselves facilitate cancer progression. For example, antioxidants such as vitamin E succinate and quercetin (at 23 μM) have been reported to inhibit expression of mutant *p53* genes in cancer cells.[22, 23, 24]

As an aside, methyl donors may help decrease the expression of mutant *p53* genes by preventing *p53* mutations. For example, rat diets deficient in folate and/or other methyl donors have been reported to cause DNA strand breaks within the *p53* gene.[25, 26, 27] Supplementation with methyl donors may be more applicable to cancer prevention than cancer treatment, as discussed at the end of Chapter 2, but it would be interesting to investigate the effects of methyl donors such as SAM on established cancers. Currently, the effects are unknown.

Although the preponderance of evidence suggests that *p53* mutations are detrimental to the cancer patient, some evidence implies that *p53* mutant cells may be more susceptible to cancer treatment. This is not surprising since *p53* mutant cells are less able to repair themselves and thus are more easily destroyed.[28] For example, one study demonstrated that genistein (at 10 μM) inhibited cell proliferation to a greater extent in *p53* mutant melanoma cells than in *p53* normal melanoma cells. In addition, increased sensitivity to chemotherapy

drugs by *p53* mutants has been demonstrated in vivo. In one study, breast cancer patients with *p53* mutants showed a better response to a variety of chemotherapy drugs than patients whose cancer cells had *p53* normal genes.[29] Nevertheless, based on the available evidence, it would not seem prudent to try to induce *p53* mutations, nor does it seem unreasonable to inhibit the proliferation of *p53* mutant cells. Indeed, even though *p53* mutation may increase the initial sensitivity of cancer cells to treatment, the high mutation rate of these cells would help them over time to develop resistance to the therapy being used.

Nuclear Factor-kappa B and Activator Protein-1

Nuclear factor-kappa B (NF-κB) and activator protein-1 (AP-1) are transcription factors that control a wide range of cellular activities. Both transcription factors are particularly important to the functioning of immune cells. In general, NF-κB can be thought of as a transcription factor whose activity leads to immune activity, inflammation, and cell proliferation.[30, 31] Like the p53 protein, it binds to and helps regulate several different genes. NF-κB helps regulate the genes that produce tumor necrosis factor (TNF), collagenases (enzymes that degrade collagen), cell adhesion molecules (VCAM and ICAM), and immunostimulating proteins (interleukins 1, 2, 6, and 8).[32, 33, 34, a]

AP-1 can be thought of as a transcription factor whose activity leads primarily to cell proliferation.[34] Actually, AP-1 is made up of a pair of fos and jun proteins. These proteins stimulate the expression of genes that drive the cell cycle. Thus the actions of fos and jun proteins are mediated, at least in part, through AP-1 activity.

In cancer cells, the amount and activity of AP-1 and NF-κB are commonly excessive, providing the cells with a proliferation and survival advantage. For example, one study observed excessive activation of NF-κB in 93 percent of childhood acute lymphoblastic leukemia patients.[35] Another study observed that the basal expression of NF-κB was fourfold higher in metastatic melanoma cells compared to normal cells and that oxidative stress (created by hydrogen peroxide) stimulated a greater expression of NF-κB in melanoma cells compared to normal cells.[36]

---

a NF-κB is also important in the progression of AIDS, since the DNA sequences affected by the virus contain binding sites for the transcription factor. Inhibitors of NF-κB have been studied as anti-AIDS drugs.

By producing excessive amounts of NF-κB and AP-1 or by excessively activating them, or both, cancers cells profit in three ways. First, their proliferation is stimulated. Second, apoptosis is reduced. Third, the inflammation that NF-κB causes is of general use to cancer cells. For example, as will be discussed in Chapters 7 and 8, inflammation can facilitate angiogenesis. Indeed, preliminary experiments have reported that excessive NF-κB activity in cancer cells is correlated to invasiveness, metastasis, and poor prognosis.[37, 38] In one in-vivo study, partial inhibition of NF-κB activity (by RNA manipulation) produced both an antimetastatic and antiproliferative response in cancer-bearing rodents.[39, 40] Moreover, at doses that inhibited tumor growth in vivo, NF-κB inhibitors did not cause serious adverse effects in the rodents. This is probably because cancer cells rely on a higher volume of NF-κB activity than do normal cells.

As stated above, NF-κB activity plays a central role in inflammation. Indeed, it may be one of the key regulators of inflammation. Not surprisingly then, a variety of anti-inflammatory drugs, such as aspirin, produce their effects in part by inhibiting NF-κB activity. This can occur in at least two ways. First, NF-κB can be stimulated by redox signals, and some anti-inflammatory drugs may act through attenuation of these signals. For example, gold thiolate, an anti-inflammatory drug used in treating arthritis, may inhibit NF-κB partly through its antioxidant capabilities.

Second, some anti-inflammatory drugs may inhibit NF-κB by preventing its disassociation with NF-κB inhibitor, a compound referred to as I-κB. NF-κB normally resides inactive within the cell, bound to I-κB. Upon activation (by protein phosphorylation), the two proteins are dissociated and NF-κB travels to the nucleus, where it controls gene expression. The anti-inflammatory glucocorticoids (for example, cortisone) may act in part by preventing the dissociation of NF-κB from I-κB.

Pathways of NF-κB and AP-1 Activation

Although it is now receiving intense research, the relationship between NF-κB and AP-1 on the one hand and free radicals, inflammation, cell proliferation, and apoptosis on the other, is still poorly understood. Clearly, any pathways controlling proliferation, inflammation, and cell death must be tightly regulated if an organism is to remain healthy. These complex relationships contain internal feedback loops and other components not discussed here. Nonetheless, trends are being discovered that have clinical significance. A preliminary schematic of relationships is presented in Figure 5.4 (based on references 1 and 41–52). The pathways shown in the figure are active in both cancer cells and normal cells such as immune cells. The difference is, the pathways are excessively active in cancer cells.

A few new terms are used in Figure 5.4. Caspases are enzymes that mediate the final stages of apoptosis. IL-1 is the immune cytokine interleukin-1. TNF is tumor necrosis factor, an immune cytokine that promotes angiogenesis but in high concentrations is toxic to cancer cells. Cytokines will be discussed in more detail in the chapters on the immune system. Lastly, as a reminder, CAMs are cell adhesion molecules, which keep cells in contact with one another and the surrounding extracellular matrix. We discuss CAMs in the next chapter.

Briefly, the figure shows that external stimulants like growth factors initiate a signal at the membrane receptor. Reactive oxygen species (ROS) can affect surface receptors (e.g., a receptor PTK), either by making them more sensitive to activation by growth factors or by making them less easy to turn off after activation.[53] The latter effect appears to involve inhibition of protein tyrosine phosphatases, the enzymes that serve to "reset" and inactivate kinases.[54, 55] In similar ways, ROS can also sensitize other kinases that act inside the cell, such as PKC.[56]

Activation of the surface receptor (or internal kinases) can be blocked by kinase inhibitors. Likewise, ROS signals originating from activated receptors (or internal kinases or ras proteins) can be blocked by antioxidants. If not blocked, the signals stimulate NF-κB and/or AP-1 activity, which in turn stimulate gene transcription. Gene transcription leads to additional inflammation, proliferation, and cell migration.

We see then that redox status is linked with signal transduction via the protein phosphorylation pathways in at least two ways. First, surface receptor activity and the activity of internal kinases are sensitive to ROS. Second, activation of these kinases, and ras proteins, produce ROS. These internally produced ROS, in conjunction with ROS that enter the cell from outside, affect the activity of transcription factors.[57, 58] We note, however, that the role of ROS in the activation of NF-κB and AP-1 is still being debated. It is possible the effects may be limited to specific cell types and conditions, and some effects certainly occur through poorly understood mechanisms.[59] Quite likely, ROS are not the driving force behind NF-κB and AP-1 activation. Rather, their role is probably a supportive one.[60] Also note that if concentrations of ROS are too high, they will not participate in signal transduction and will only damage the cell, inducing apoptosis or necrosis.

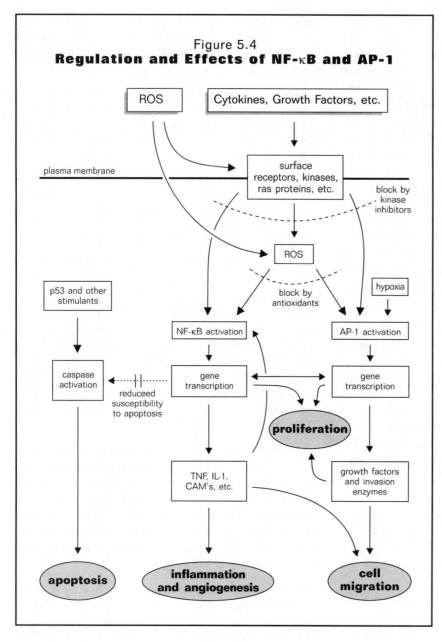

Figure 5.4
Regulation and Effects of NF-κB and AP-1

clear concentrations of glutathione are very tightly regulated, since glutathione is needed to protect the DNA from damage. Indeed, genes such as *Bcl-2* protect against apoptosis in part by redistributing glutathione to the nucleus.[61, 62] Nonetheless, antioxidants are still able to inhibit the binding of NF-κB and AP-1 to DNA, even though antioxidants help assure a reducing environment.[63] How this works is still not clear. Perhaps antioxidants alter the structure of NF-κB and AP-1 so that they are no longer active, or perhaps some antioxidants actually act by nonredox means to affect DNA binding.[64]

Note in Figure 5.4 that hypoxia (a low-oxygen environment) helps stimulate AP-1. For immune cells, this is useful, since wounds contain hypoxic areas. In this way, immune cell activity can be stimulated in wounds. Hypoxia-induced AP-1 stimulation is also useful for cancer cells. Solid tumors contain hypoxic areas due to their poorly developed and chaotic arrangement of blood vessels. Hence much of the tissue within the tumor mass fluctuates between oxygenated and hypoxic conditions. During mild hypoxia, AP-1 is stimulated, and during reoxygenation, free radicals are produced and NF-κB is stimulated. This push-pull arrangement facilitates continued proliferation.

Redox reactions affect one other aspect of nuclear factor activity that can be altered with natural compounds. As with many if not most transcription factors, the ability of NF-κB and AP-1 to bind to DNA and initiate gene transcription is controlled in part through redox status. The mechanisms that control transcription-factor binding to DNA are complex. On the one hand, oxidative conditions in the cytosol can initiate NF-κB activity, as discussed above. On the other hand, a reducing environment is needed in the nucleus in order for NF-κB to bind to DNA. This fits into the way that intracellular concentrations of antioxidants such as glutathione are controlled. Cytosolic concentrations of glutathione are allowed to fluctuate widely, and such fluctuations do not generally cause much cellular damage. In contrast, nu-

It is important to note that the pathways shown in Figure 5.4 are actually circular in nature. The end results, particularly growth factor production and inflammation (and associated ROS) start the process all over again. This self-generating movement through the pathways helps immune cells to proliferate and mount an attack on invading pathogens or other tissues perceived as foreign. If the condition is not readily resolved, however, it can also result in chronic inflammatory conditions, which are detrimental.[65] The situation with cancer cells is similar to that of chronic inflammation, only worse because fewer controls function in cancer cells. The circular pathway feeds on itself, producing more and more proliferation and more and more inflammation, ROS, and growth factors.

Not surprisingly, researchers have found that NF-κB and AP-1 activity can protect cells from apoptosis induced by free radicals or other noxious compounds.[37, 66] This protective effect is very useful for immune cells that must survive in an inflamed environment rich in ROS. However, it is also useful for cancer cells that must survive in the same inhospitable environment. A variety of cancer cell lines exhibit increased free radical generation and NF-κB activity but reduced apoptosis.[47, 75]

Natural Compounds That Inhibit NF-κB and AP-1 Activity

Natural compounds that inhibit NF-κB and AP-1 activity can be roughly divided into two groups: those that act through antioxidant means and those that act through nonantioxidant ones. Most of the studies on NF-κB and AP-1 inhibition have involved antioxidants. However, natural compounds that act through nonantioxidant means may actually be the most useful clinically. One reason for the more limited potency of antioxidant compounds is that ROS are probably not the driving force behind activation of NF-κB and AP-1 activity, as mentioned above. Instead, signal transduction through protein phosphorylation probably plays the primary role.

Antioxidants as Inhibitors of NF-κB and AP-1

Inhibition of NF-κB and AP-1 activity, and especially NF-κB activity, has been demonstrated in vitro by a number of different antioxidants. Table 5.1 lists some of these in order of decreasing potency. As the table indicates, the ability of antioxidants to affect NF-κB activity varies greatly. Whereas moderately lipophilic (fat-soluble) antioxidants such as melatonin more strongly affect NF-κB activity, water-soluble antioxidants like vitamin C and strongly lipophilic antioxidants like vitamin E are substantially weaker.[33, 72–74, a]

Antioxidants may act at various stages of nuclear factor activation. For example, some extracellular antioxidants may neutralize ROS before they enter the cell. Antioxidants can also act within the cell by attenuating the ROS signal produced by activation of kinases (e.g., PKC) or by activation of ras proteins.[1, 75, 76]

TABLE 5.1 INHIBITION OF NF-κB ACTIVITY BY ANTIOXIDANTS IN VITRO		
COMPOUND	**CONCENTRATION***	**REFERENCES**
Melatonin	10 μM and higher	67
Vitamin E succinate[†]	100 to 1,000 μM	74
Vitamin E	> 1 mM	74
Alpha-lipoic acid	1 to 4 mM	68, 69, 70
Vitamin C	5 to 20 mM	71
N-acetylcysteine (NAC)	20 mM	68

* Since different types of assays were used to determine these values, the values only provide rough comparisons of active concentrations.
† A water-soluble form of vitamin E.

In spite of their activity in vitro, it is unlikely that these antioxidants strongly inhibit NF-κB activity in vivo, at least when used alone. The concentrations at which antioxidants are active in vitro are greater than those normally present in the body, even after supplementation. For example, the plasma concentration of melatonin in humans after an extremely large (100-milligram) dose is only about 440 nM.[77] This is 23-fold lower than the effective concentration listed in Table 5.1. Moreover, the normally achievable plasma levels of vitamin E are probably about 10-fold lower than the effective concentration listed in the table.

It should not be surprising that these antioxidants are weak inhibitors of NF-κB activity in vivo, since they are not known to produce potent anti-inflammatory effects in vivo. Nonetheless, some antioxidants, including vitamin E, combinations of antioxidants, and high doses of melatonin (13 to 50 mg/kg intraperitoneal in rats), can produce weak to moderate anti-inflammatory effects in rodents and humans, part of which may be due to NF-κB inhibition.[78–80, b] Thus while antioxidants may not be highly potent at inhibiting NF-κB activity in vivo, they may still be useful in supporting other more potent natural compounds. Also, the ability of antioxidants to inhibit NF-κB is likely to increase when they are used in combination.

Nonantioxidants as Inhibitors of NF-κB and AP-1

The primary means by which nonantioxidant compounds inhibit NF-κB and AP-1 activity is by inhibiting kinase activation, ras protein activation, or other aspects of signal transduction. This is as expected, since signal transduction via protein phosphorylation is probably the primary stimulus for inducing NF-κB and AP-1 activity.

---

a The ability of alpha-lipoic acid to inhibit NF-κB activity is not related to its ability to increase intracellular reduced glutathione. Similarly, vitamin C, which also increases intracellular glutathione, is a weak inhibitor of NF-κB activity.

---

b This intraperitoneal dose of melatonin is equal to a human oral dose of about 210 to 810 milligrams. This is much higher than the normal human dose of 3 to 10 milligrams.

TABLE 5.2   INHIBITION OF NF-κB AND AP-1 ACTIVITY BY NONANTIOXIDANT COMPOUNDS IN VITRO

COMPOUND	CONCENTRATION AND COMMENTS*	REFERENCES
NF-κB		
1,25-D₃	20 nM (weak)	81, 82
Apigenin	10 µM; prevents IκB degradation	83, 84, 85
Curcumin	5 to 150 µM; complete inhibition of DNA binding at 25 µM in one study	86–91, 121
CAPE	90 µM (weak)	92
EGCG	10 µM to 100 mM (dependent on cell line and conditions); prevents IκB degradation	93, 94, 95
Emodin	185 µM (weak)	96
Genistein	30 to 150 µM	72, 97–99
Hypericin	2 µM	100
Leukotriene inhibitors (see Table 8.2)	inhibits NF-κB	101, 102
Luteolin	25 µM	83, 84
Parthenolide	5 µM	103, 104
PTK and PKC inhibitors (see Tables 4.2 and 4.3)	inhibits NF-κB	discussed in text
Proanthocyanidins	35 to 110 µM	105
Quercetin	10 to 50 µM; prevents IκB degradation	106, 107, 108
Resveratrol†	30 µM	109
AP-1		
Curcumin	20 to 50 µM	90, 110, 111
EGCG	typically 5 to 20 µM	112, 113
Genistein	15 to 74 µM	114, 115, 116
PTK inhibitors (see Table 4.2)	inhibits AP-1	116
Quercetin	10 to 50 µM	117
Selenium	1 to 10 µM	118, 119

* Since different types of assays were used to determine these values, they provide only rough comparisons of active concentrations.

† Other authors reported that resveratrol does not affect lipopolysaccharide-induced NF-κB activation, as suggested here.[120]

1,25-D₃

Other mechanisms of inhibition may be possible. For example, leukotriene inhibitors may reduce NF-κB activity, in part by reducing the signal transduction initiated by leukotrienes. Leukotrienes are natural inflammatory compounds that act somewhat like growth factors; hence their ability to stimulate NF-κB activity is not surprising. Many natural compounds inhibit leukotriene production or activity (discussed in Chapter 8).

Table 5.2 lists nonantioxidant compounds that inhibit NF-κB and AP-1 activity. Note that these compounds may be effective in some cell lines and circumstances but not in others. Many of these actually are antioxidants, but they appear to inhibit NF-κB and AP-1 primarily by nonantioxidant means. Many are also leukotriene inhibitors, and some inhibit both PTK and PKC. Because most natural compounds have multiple effects, the exact method of NF-κB inhibition is often not clear. For example, apigenin, curcumin, EGCG, and luteolin are all antioxidants, as well as inhibitors of PTK, PKC, and leukotrienes.

Most of the NF-κB inhibitors listed produce an anti-inflammatory effect and/or affect cell adhesion molecules in vivo. Furthermore, many inhibit the production of TNF by immune cells as well as TNF-induced cell adhesion.[86, 121] (TNF and CAMs are produced via NF-κB activity, as illustrated in Figure 5.4.) The fact that most of these compounds produce an anti-inflammatory effect in vivo supports the possibility they may be acting through inhibition of NF-κB and/or AP-1 activity. As with antioxidant compounds, it is likely that the effects of these compounds could be maximized by using synergistic combinations.

MECHANISMS OF REDOX MODULATION

In this chapter, we have stated that redox status could affect signal transduction, gene transcription, and cell

Also, as mentioned previously, NF-κB must disassociate from its inhibitory carrier I-κB to become active. This dissociation appears to be controlled in large part through kinase activity, probably through the activity of a kinase called IKK, inhibitor of NF-κB kinase.[59] As mentioned in Chapter 4, the natural compounds discussed here tend to inhibit multiple kinases, rather than being specific for only one. Therefore, some natural compounds that are inhibitors of PTK, PKC, or other kinases probably affect IKK as well.

activity; therefore, a brief discussion on the means by which redox status may be altered in or around cancer cells seems appropriate.

Cancer cells generally exist under oxidative stress; which assists cancer cell proliferation and survival in several ways. First, it damages DNA. As long as the stress level is not so high that it causes cell death, this can lead to higher mutation rates, which is generally beneficial to the cancer cell. Second, oxidative stress can increase some types of redox signaling, and it can inactivate certain transcription factors (such as the p53 protein) that limit cell proliferation. Lastly, oxidative stress impedes cell-to-cell contact, thereby facilitating cancer progression.

Based on the available evidence, it appears that cancer cells may have some control over their redox environment and their ability to withstand oxidative stress.[122] In general, cancer cells appear to be more susceptible to free radical damage than normal ones, yet they tend to exist in a prooxidant state. Thus in some way cancer cells must develop a balance between ROS-induced apoptosis on the one hand and ROS-induced mutations and other alterations in biology that favor survival on the other. Several mechanisms lead to production of or protection from ROS:

1. Immune cells, and especially macrophages, are significant sources of ROS. If they produce a sufficient quantity of ROS they will kill cancer cells. However, cancer cells can minimize macrophage activity by producing immunosuppressive compounds like IL-10, TGF-beta, and PGE$_2$.[123, 124] A subdued immune response may then produce mild ROS concentrations, suitable for cancer progression. For example, in a recent mouse study, weakly tumorigenic fibrosarcoma cells injected subcutaneously were unable to grow; however, when co-implanted with a foreign body (a piece of sponge) that generated an immune response, the cancer cells exhibited increased DNA mutations and subsequently formed aggressive tumors. In addition, this response was associated with a decline in tumor-cell antioxidant enzymes.[125] Note that the immune response was not directly targeted to the cancer cells in this study; thus it was not intense enough to effectively eliminate the cancer cells.

2. ROS can be produced through reactions between reducing agents (antioxidants) and copper or iron. The inflammation surrounding tumors may increase the rate of these reactions, since the tissue damage associated with inflammation leads to the release of free (unbound) metal ions capable of redox reactions.

3. ROS can be produced by overexpression of *ras* family oncogenes. This may lead to both elevated ROS production and elevated protection from ROS.[126, 127] ROS may also be produced during kinase activity, such as that of PTK or PKC.[128]

4. ROS can be produced by NF-κB activation. NF-κB leads to the production of TNF and other inflammatory substances. TNF itself can cause marked increases in hydrogen peroxide production by normal cells.[129]

5. Ironically, ROS can be produced during glutathione synthesis. The tripeptide glutathione is poorly transported across the cell membrane. To maintain intracellular glutathione concentrations, extracellular glutathione is split apart by GGT (gamma-glutamyl transpeptidase) enzymes located on the outside of the cell. The amino acid fragments are then transported into the cell, where glutathione is reassembled. In the process of splitting glutathione, however, GGT produces a significant amount of ROS; enough to stimulate cancer cell proliferation in vitro or in some cases to induce apoptosis.[130, 131]

6. Protection from high ROS levels may be mediated through alterations in membrane lipids. The low omega-6 and, more important, the low omega-3 content found in the membranes of many cancer cells help decrease lipid peroxidation because these fatty acids are easily subject to free radical damage.

7. Protection from apoptosis caused by high ROS levels may be mediated through increased expression of antioxidant genes (including the *Bcl-2* gene) as well as *ras* genes and those that control the production of antioxidant enzymes.

CONCLUSION

The transcription factors p53, NF-κB, and AP-1 play an important role in the proliferation and activity of both healthy cells and cancer cells. The differences are that cancer cells rely on abnormally low p53 protein activity and abnormally high NF-κB and AP-1 activity. Since these transcription factors play an important role in proliferation and cell activity, their regulation is necessarily complex; partly they are regulated by both protein phosphorylation and redox signaling. Redox signaling is in itself both complex and subtle. Nonetheless, it is clear at this early stage of research that a number of natural compounds are able to influence transcription factors in ways that can inhibit cancer cell proliferation and activity. Since cancer cells need extreme alterations in transcription factor activity, they are likely to be more sensitive than healthy cells to these natural compounds.

REFERENCES

[1] Powis G, Gasdaska JR, Baker A. Redox signaling and the control of cell growth and death. Advances in Pharmacology 1997; 38:329–359.

[2] Deneo-Pellegrini H, De Stefani E, Boffetta P, et al. Dietary iron and cancer of the rectum: A case-control study in Uruguay. Eur J Cancer Prev 1999 Dec; 8(6):501–8.

[3] Weinberg ED. The development of awareness of the carcinogenic hazard of inhaled iron. Oncol Res 1999; 11(3):109–13.

[4] de Valk B, Marx JJ. Iron, atherosclerosis, and ischemic heart disease. Arch Intern Med 1999 Jul 26; 159(14):1542–8.

[5] Toyokuni S, Okamoto K, Yodoi J, Hiai H. Persistent oxidative stress in cancer. FEBS Lett 1995 Jan 16; 358(1):1–3.

[6] Lanyi A, Deb D, Seymour RC, et al. "Gain of function" phenotype of tumor-derived mutant p53 requires the oligomerization/nonsequence-specific nucleic acid-binding domain. Oncogene 1998 Jun 18; 16(24):3169–76.

[7] Kahlenberg MS, Stoler DL, Rodriguez-Bigas MA, et al. p53 tumor suppressor gene mutations predict decreased survival of patients with sporadic colorectal carcinoma. Cancer 2000 Apr 15; 88(8):1814–9.

[8] Blaszyk H, Hartmann A, Cunningham JM, et al. A prospective trial of midwest breast cancer patients: A p53 gene mutation is the most important predictor of adverse outcome. Int J Cancer 2000 Jan 20; 89(1):32–8.

[9] Ireland AP, Shibata DK, Chandrasoma P, et al. Clinical significance of p53 mutations in adenocarcinoma of the esophagus and cardia. Ann Surg 2000 Feb; 231(2):179–87.

[10] Symonds H, Krall L, Remington L, et al. p53-dependent apoptosis suppresses tumor growth and progression in vivo. Cell 1994 Aug 26; 78(4):703–11.

[11] Geisler JP, Geisler HE, Miller GA, et al. p53 and bcl-2 in epithelial ovarian carcinoma: Their value as prognostic indicators at a median follow-up of 60 months. Gynecol Oncol 2000 May; 77(2):278–82.

[12] Meplan C, Verhaegh G, Richard MJ, Hainaut P. Metal ions as regulators of the conformation and function of the tumour suppressor protein p53: Implications for carcinogenesis. Proc Nutr Soc 1999 Aug; 58(3):565–71.

[13] Verhaegh GW, Richard MJ, Hainaut P. Regulation of p53 by metal ions and by antioxidants: Dithiocarbamate down-regulates p53 DNA-binding activity by increasing the intracellular level of copper. Mol Cell Biol 1997 Oct; 17(10):5699–706.

[14] Meplan C, Richard MJ, Hainaut P. Redox signalling and transition metals in the control of the p53 pathway. Biochem Pharmacol 2000 Jan 1; 59(1):25–33.

[15] Wu HH, Momand J. Pyrrolidine dithiocarbamate prevents p53 activation and promotes p53 cysteine residue oxidation. J Biol Chem 1998 Jul 24; 273(30):18898–905.

[16] Sun Y, Oberley LW. Redox regulation of transcriptional activators. Free Radic Biol Med 1996; 21(3):335–48.

[17] Mediavilla MD, Cos S, Sanchez-Barcelo EJ. Melatonin increases p53 and p21WAF1 expression in MCF-7 human breast cancer cells in vitro. Life Sci 1999; 65(4):415–20.

[18] Jee SH, Shen SC, Tseng CR, et al. Curcumin induces a p53-dependent apoptosis in human basal cell carcinoma cells. J Invest Dermatol 1998 Oct; 111(4):656–61.

[19] Kim SE, Lee YH, Park JH, Lee SK. Ginsenoside-Rs4, a new type of ginseng saponin concurrently induces apoptosis and selectively elevates protein levels of p53 and p21WAF1 in human hepatoma SK-HEP-1 cells. Eur J Cancer 1999 Mar; 35(3):507–11.

[20] Hsieh TC, Juan G, Darzynkiewicz Z, Wu JM. Resveratrol increases nitric oxide synthase, induces accumulation of p53 and p21(WAF1/CIP1), and suppresses cultured bovine pulmonary artery endothelial cell proliferation by perturbing progression through S and G2. Cancer Res 1999 Jun 1; 59(11):2596–601.

[21] Shin DM, Mao L, Papadimitrakopoulou VM, et al. Biochemopreventive therapy for patients with premalignant lesions of the head and neck and p53 gene expression. J Natl Cancer Inst 2000 Jan 5; 92(1):69–73.

[22] Shklar G. Mechanisms of cancer inhibition by anti-oxidant nutrients. Oral Oncol 1998 Jan; 34(1):24–9.

[23] Avila MA, Velasco JA, Cansado J, Notario V. Quercetin mediates the down-regulation of mutant p53 in the human breast cancer cell line MDA-MB468. Cancer Res 1994 May 1; 54(9):2424–8.

[24] Avila MA, Cansado J, Harter KW, et al. Quercetin as a modulator of the cellular neoplastic phenotype. Effects on the expression of mutated H-ras and p53 in rodent and human cells. Adv Exp Med Biol 1996; 401:101–10.

[25] Kim YI, Pogribny IP, Basnakian AG, et al. Folate deficiency in rats induces DNA strand breaks and hypomethylation within the p53 tumor suppressor gene. Am J Clin Nutr 1997 Jan; 65(1):46–52.

[26] Pogribny IP, Basnakian AG, Miller BJ, et al. Breaks in genomic DNA and within the p53 gene are associated with hypomethylation in livers of folate/methyl-deficient rats. Cancer Res 1995 May 1; 55(9):1894–901.

[27] Kim YI, Pogribny IP, Salomon RN, et al. Exon-specific DNA hypomethylation of the p53 gene of rat colon induced by dimethylhydrazine. Modulation by dietary folate. Am J Pathol 1996 Oct; 149(4):1129–37.

[28] Wallace-Brodeur RR, Lowe SW. Clinical implications of p53 mutations. Cell Mol Life Sci 1999 Jan; 55(1):64–75.

[29] Elledge RM, Gray R, Mansour E, et al. Accumulation of p53 protein as a possible predictor of response to adjuvant combination chemotherapy with cyclophosphamide, methotrexate, fluorouracil, and prednisone for breast cancer. J Natl Cancer Inst 1995 Aug 16; 87(16):1254–6.

[30] Biswas DK, Cruz AP, Gansberger E, Pardee AB. Epidermal growth factor-induced nuclear factor kappa B activation: A major pathway of cell-cycle progression in estrogen-receptor negative breast cancer cells. Proc Natl Acad Sci USA 2000 Jul 18; 97(15):8542–7.

[31] Kim DW, Sovak MA, Zanieski G, et al. Activation of NF-kappaB/Rel occurs early during neoplastic transformation of mammary cells. Carcinogenesis 2000 May; 21(5):871–9.

[32] Conner EM, Grisham MB. Inflammation, free radicals, and antioxidants. Nutrition 1996 Apr; 12(4):274–7.

33 Allison AC. Antioxidant drug targeting. Advances in Pharmacology 1997; 38:273–291.

34 Winyard PG, Blake DR. Antioxidants, redox-regulated transcription factors, and inflammation. Advances in Pharmacology 1997; 38:403–421.

35 Kordes U, Krappmann D, Heissmeyer V, et al. Transcription factor NF-kappaB is constitutively activated in acute lymphoblastic leukemia cells. Leukemia 2000 Mar; 14(3):399–402.

36 Meyskens FL Jr, Buckmeier JA, McNulty SE, Tohidian NB. Activation of nuclear factor-kappa B in human metastatic melanomacells and the effect of oxidative stress. Clin Cancer Res 1999 May; 5(5):1197–202.

37 Bours V, Dejardin E, Goujon-Letawe F, et al. The NF-kappa B transcription factor and cancer: High expression of NF-kappa B- and I kappa B-related proteins in tumor cell lines. Biochem Pharmacol 1994 Jan 13; 47(1):145–9.

38 Nakshatri H, Bhat-Nakshatri P, Martin DA, et al. Constitutive activation of NF-kappaB during progression of breast cancer to hormone-independent growth. Mol Cell Biol 1997 Jul; 17(7):3629–39.

39 Sharma HW, Narayanan R. The NF-kappaB transcription factor in oncogenesis. Anticancer Res 1996 Mar–Apr; 16(2):589–96.

40 Narayanan R. Antisense therapy of cancer. In Vivo 1994 Nov–Dec; 8(5):787–93.

41 Aggarwal BB. Personal communication. October, 1997.

42 Bustamante J, Slater AF, Orrenius S. Antioxidant inhibition of thymocyte apoptosis by dihydrolipoic acid. Free Radic Biol Med 1995 Sep; 19(3):339–47.

43 Sanchez A, Alvarez AM, Benito M, Fabregat I. Apoptosis induced by transforming growth factor-beta in fetal hepatocyte primary cultures: Involvement of reactive oxygen intermediates. J Biol Chem 1996 Mar 29; 271(13):7416–22.

44 Xu Y, Nguyen Q, Lo DC, Czaja MJ. c-myc-Dependent hepatoma cell apoptosis results from oxidative stress and not a deficiency of growth factors. J Cell Physiol 1997 Feb; 170(2):192–9.

45 Van Antwerp DJ, Martin SJ, Kafri T, et al. Suppression of TNF-α-induced apoptosis by NF-κB. Science 1996; 274:787–789.

46 Wang CY, Mayo MW, Baldwin AS. TNF- and cancer therapy-induced apoptosis: Potentiation by inhibition of NF-κB. Science 1996; 274:784–787.

47 Beg AA, Baltimore D. An essential role for NF-κB in preventing TNF-α-induced cell death. Science 1996; 274:782–784.

48 Barinaga M. Life-death balance within the cell [comment]. Science 1996; 274:724.

49 Liu ZG, Hsu H, Goeddel DV, Karin M. Dissection of TNF receptor 1 effector functions: JNK activation is not linked to apoptosis while NF-kappaB activation prevents cell death. Cell 1996 Nov 1; 87(3):565–76.

50 Rupec RA, Baeuerle PA. The genomic response of tumor cells to hypoxia and reoxygenation. Differential activation of transcription factors AP-1 and NF-kappa B. Eur J Biochem 1995 Dec 1; 234(2):632–40.

51 Wissing D, Mouritzen H, Egeblad M, et al. Involvement of caspase-dependent activation of cytosolic phospholipase A2 in tumor necrosis factor-induced apoptosis. Proc Natl Acad Sci USA 1997 May 13; 94(10):5073–7.

52 Wyllie AH. Apoptosis and carcinogenesis. Eur J Cell Biol 1997 Jul; 73(3):189–97.

53 Peranovich TM, da Silva AM, Fries DM, et al. Nitric oxide stimulates tyrosine phosphorylation in murine fibroblasts in the absence and presence of epidermal growth factor. Biochem J 1995 Jan 15; 305 (Pt 2):613–9.

54 Herrlich P, Bohmer FD. Redox regulation of signal transduction in mammalian cells. Biochem Pharmacol 2000 Jan 1; 59(1):35–41.

55 Goldman R, Ferber E, Zor U. Involvement of reactive oxygen species in phospholipase A2 activation: Inhibition of protein tyrosine phosphatases and activation of protein kinases. Adv Exp Med Biol 1997; 400A:25–30.

56 Gopalakrishna R, Jaken S. Protein kinase C signaling and oxidative stress. Free Radic Biol Med 2000 May 1; 28(9):1349–61.

57 Vepa S, Scribner WM, Parinandi NL, et al. Hydrogen peroxide stimulates tyrosine phosphorylation of focal adhesion kinase in vascular endothelial cells. Am J Physiol 1999 Jul; 277(1 Pt 1):L150–8.

58 Lelkes PI, Hahn KL, Sukovich DA, et al. On the possible role of reactive oxygen species in angiogenesis. Adv Exp Med Biol 1998; 454:295–310.

59 Renard P, Raes M. The proinflammatory transcription factor NFkappaB: A potential target for novel therapeutical strategies. Cell Biol Toxicol 1999; 15(6):341–4.

60 Bowie A, O'Neill LA. Oxidative stress and nuclear factor-kappaB activation: A reassessment of the evidence in the light of recent discoveries. Biochem Pharmacol 2000 Jan 1; 59(1):13–23.

61 Jevtovic-Todorovic V, Guenthner TM. Depletion of a discrete nuclear glutathione pool by oxidative stress, but not by buthionine sulfoximine. Correlation with enhanced alkylating agent cytotoxicity to human melanoma cells in vitro. Biochem Pharmacol 1992 Oct 6; 44(7):1383–93.

62 Voehringer DW, McConkey DJ, McDonnell TJ, et al. Bcl-2 expression causes redistribution of glutathione to the nucleus. Proc Natl Acad Sci USA 1998 Mar 17; 95(6):2956–60.

63 Ripple MO, Henry WF, Schwarze SR, et al. Effect of antioxidants on androgen-induced AP-1 and NF-kappaB DNA-binding activity in prostate carcinoma cells. J Natl Cancer Inst 1999 Jul 21; 91(14):1227–32.

64 Azzi A, Boscoboinik D, Fazzio A, et al. RRR-alpha-tocopherol regulation of gene transcription in response to the cell oxidant status. Z Ernahrungswiss 1998; 37 Suppl 1:21–8.

65 Rosenfeld ME. Inflammation, lipids, and free radicals: Lessons learned from the atherogenic process. Semin Reprod Endocrinol 1998; 16(4):249–61.

66 Karin M, Liu ZG, Zandi E. AP-1 function and regulation. Curr Opin Cell Biol 1997; 9(2):240–6.

67 Mohan N, Sadeghi K, Reiter RJ, Meltz ML. The neurohormone melatonin inhibits cytokine, mitogen and ionizing radiation induced NF-kappa B. Biochem Mol Biol Int 1995 Dec; 37(6):1063–70.

[68] Suzuki YJ, Aggarwal BB, Packer L. Alpha-lipoic acid is a potent inhibitor of NF-kappa B activation in human T cells. Biochem Biophys Res Commun 1992 Dec 30; 189(3):1709–15.

[69] Packer L, Suzuki YJ. Vitamin E and alpha-lipoate: Role in antioxidant recycling and activation of the NF-kappa B transcription factor. Mol Aspects Med 1993; 14(3):229–39.

[70] Packer L, Roy S, Sen CK. α-Lipoic acid: A metabolic antioxidant and potential redox modulator of transcription. Advances in Pharmacology 1997; 38:79–101.

[71] Bowie A, O'Neill LA. Vitamin C inhibits NF kappa B activation in endothelial cells. Biochem Soc Trans 1997; 25(1):131S.

[72] Eugui EM, DeLustro B, Rouhafza S, et al. Some antioxidants inhibit, in a co-ordinate fashion, the production of tumor necrosis factor-alpha, IL-beta, and IL-6 by human peripheral blood mononuclear cells. Int Immunol 1994; 6(3):409–22.

[73] Sen CK, Packer L. Antioxidant and redox regulation of gene transcription [see comments]. FASEB J 1996 May; 10(7):709–20.

[74] Traber MG, Packer L. Vitamin E: Beyond antioxidant function. Am J Clin Nutr 1995 Dec; 62(6 Suppl):1501S–1509S.

[75] Irani K, Xia Y, Zweier JL, et al. Mitogenic signaling mediated by oxidants in ras-transformed fibroblasts [see comments]. Science 1997 Mar 14; 275(5306):1649–52.

[76] Pennisi E. Superoxides relay ras protein's oncogenic message [comment]. Science 1997 Mar 14; 275(5306):1567–8.

[77] Vakkuri O, Leppaluto J, Kauppila A. Oral administration and distribution of melatonin in human serum, saliva and urine. Life Sci 1985 Aug 5; 37(5):489–95.

[78] Grimble RF. Nutritional antioxidants and the modulation of inflammation: Theory and practice. New Horiz 1994 May; 2(2):175–85.

[79] Uden S, Bilton D, Nathan L, et al. Antioxidant therapy for recurrent pancreatitis: Placebo-controlled trial. Aliment Pharmacol Ther 1990 Aug; 4(4):357–71.

[80] Cuzzocrea S, Costantino G, Mazzon E, Caputi AP. Regulation of prostaglandin production in carrageenan-induced pleurisy by melatonin. Pineal Res 1999 Aug; 27(1):9–14.

[81] Harant H, Wolff B, Lindley JD. 1Alpha,25-dihydroxyvitamin D3 decreases DNA binding of nuclear factor-kappaB in human fibroblasts. FEBS Lett 1998 Oct 9; 436(3):329–34.

[82] Harant H, Andrew PJ, Reddy GS, et al. 1alpha,25-dihydroxyvitamin D3 and a variety of its natural metabolites transcriptionally repress nuclear-factor-kappaB-mediated interleukin-8 gene expression. Eur J Biochem 1997 Nov 15; 250(1):63–71.

[83] Gerritsen ME, Carley WW, Ranges GE, et al. Flavonoids inhibit cytokine-induced endothelial cell adhesion protein gene expression. Am J Pathology 1995; 147(2):278–292.

[84] Read MA. Flavonoids: Naturally occurring anti-inflammatory agents [comment]. Am J Pathol 1995 Aug; 147(2):235–7.

[85] Liang YC, Huang YT, Tsai SH, et al. Suppression of inducible cyclooxygenase and inducible nitric oxide synthase by apigenin and related flavonoids in mouse macrophages. Carcinogenesis 1999 Oct; 20(10):1945–52.

[86] Kumar A, Dhawan S, Hardegen NJ, Aggarwal BB. Curcumin (Diferuloylmethane) inhibition of tumor necrosis factor (TNF)-mediated adhesion of monocytes to endothelial cells by suppression of cell surface expression of adhesion molecules and of nuclear factor-kappaB activation. Biochem Pharmacol 1998 Mar 15; 55(6):775–83.

[87] Singh S, Aggarwal BB. Activation of transcription factor NF-kappa B is suppressed by curcumin (diferuloylmethane) [corrected]. J Biol Chem 1995 Oct 20; 270(42):24995–5000.

[88] Wang W, Abbruzzese JL, Evans DB, et al. The nuclear factor-kappaB RelA transcription factor is constitutively activated in human pancreatic adenocarcinoma cells. Clin Cancer Res 1999 Jan; 5(1):119–27.

[89] Brennan P, O'Neill LA. Inhibition of nuclear factor kappaB by direct modification in whole cells—mechanism of action of nordihydroguaiaritic acid, curcumin and thiol modifiers. Biochem Pharmacol 1998 Apr 1; 55(7):965–973.

[90] Bierhaus A, Zhang Y, Quehenberger P, et al. The dietary pigment curcumin reduces endothelial tissue factor gene expression by inhibiting binding of AP-1 to the DNA and activation of NF-kappa B. Thromb Haemost 1997 Apr; 77(4):772–82.

[91] Plummer SM, Holloway KA, Manson MM, et al. Inhibition of cyclo-oxygenase 2 expression in colon cells by the chemopreventive agent curcumin involves inhibition of NF-kappaB activation via the NIK/IKK signalling complex. Oncogene 1999 Oct 28; 18(44):6013–6020.

[92] Natarajan K, Singh S, Burke TH, et al. Caffeic acid phenethyl ester is a potent and specific inhibitor of activation of nuclear transcription factor NF-κB. Proc Natl Acad Sci 1996; 93:9090–9095.

[93] Yang F, De Villiers WJS, McClain CJ, Varilek GW. Green tea polyphenols block endotoxin-induced tumor necrosis factor-production and lethality in a murine model. J Nutr 1998 Dec; 128(12):2334–40.

[94] Okabe S, Ochiai Y, Aida M, et al. Mechanistic aspects of green tea as a cancer preventive: Effect of components on human stomach cancer cell lines. Jpn J Cancer Res 1999 Jul; 90(7):733–9.

[95] Lin YL, Lin JK. (-)-Epigallocatechin-3-gallate blocks the induction of nitric oxide synthase by down-regulating lipopolysaccharide-induced activity of transcription factor nuclear factor-kappaB. Mol Pharmacol 1997 Sep; 52(3):465–72.

[96] Kumar A, Dhawan S, Aggarwal BB. Emodin (3-methyl-1,6,8-trihydroxyanthraquinone) inhibits TNF-induced NF-kappaB activation, IkappaB degradation, and expression of cell surface adhesion proteins in human vascular endothelial cells. Oncogene 1998 Aug 20; 17(7):913–8.

[97] Weber C, Negrescu E, Erl W, et al. Inhibitors of protein tyrosine kinase suppress TNF-stimulated induction of endothelial cell adhesion molecules. J Immunol 1995 Jul 1; 155(1):445–51.

[98] Natarajan X, Manna SK, Chaturvedi MM, Aggarwal BB. Portein tyrosine kinase inhibitors block tumor necrosis factor-induced activation of nuclear factor-κB, degradation of IKBα, nuclear translocation of p65, and subsequent gene expression. Archives of Biochem Biophys 1998; 352(1):59–70.

[99] Davis JN, Kucuk O, Sarkar FH. Genistein inhibits NF-kappa B activation in prostate cancer cells. Nutr Cancer 1999; 35(2):167–74.

[100] Bork PM, Bacher S, Schmitz ML, et al. Hypericin as a non-antioxidant inhibitor of NF-κB. Planta Medica 1999; 65:297–300.

[101] Lee S, Felts KA, Parry GC, et al. Inhibition of 5-lipoxygenase blocks IL-1 beta-induced vascular adhesion molecule-1 gene expression in human endothelial cells. J Immunol 1997 Apr 1; 158(7):3401–7.

[102] Faux SP, Howden PJ. Possible role of lipid peroxidation in the induction of NF-kappa B and AP-1 in RFL-6 cells by crocidolite asbestos: Evidence following protection by vitamin E. Environ Health Perspect 1997 Sep; 105 Suppl 5:1127–30.

[103] Hehner SP, Heinrich M, Bork PM, et al. Sesquiterpene lactones specifically inhibit activation of NF-kappa B by preventing the degradation of I kappa B-alpha and I kappa B-beta. J Biol Chem 1998 Jan 16; 273(3):1288–97.

[104] Bork PM, Schmitz ML, Kuhnt M, et al. Sesquiterpene lactone containing Mexican Indian medicinal plants and pure sesquiterpene lactones as potent inhibitors of transcription factor NF-kappaB. FEBS Lett 1997 Jan 27; 402(1):85–90.

[105] Peng Q, Wei Z, Lau BH. Pycnogenol inhibits tumor necrosis factor-alpha-induced nuclear factor kappa B activation and adhesion molecule expression in human vascular endothelial cells. Cell Mol Life Sci 2000 May; 57(5):834–41.

[106] Musonda CA, Chipman JK. Quercetin inhibits hydrogen peroxide (H2O2)-induced NF-kappaB DNA binding activity and DNA damage in HepG2 cells. Carcinogenesis 1998 Sep; 19(9):1583–9.

[107] Rangan GK, Wang Y, Tay YC, Harris DC. Inhibition of NFkappaB activation with antioxidants is correlated with reduced cytokine transcription in PTC. Am J Physiol 1999 Nov; 277(5 Pt 2):F779–89.

[108] Peet GW, Li J. IkappaB kinases alpha and beta show a random sequential kinetic mechanism and are inhibited by staurosporine and quercetin. J Biol Chem 1999 Nov 12; 274(46):32655–61.

[109] Tsai SH, Lin-Shiau SY, Lin JK. Suppression of nitric oxide synthase and the down-regulation of the activation of NFkappaB in macrophages by resveratrol. Br J Pharmacol 1999 Feb; 126(3):673–80.

[110] Huang TS, Lee SC, Lin JK. Suppression of c-jun/AP-1 activation by an inhibitor of tumor promotion in mouse fibroblast cells. Proc Natl Acad Sci 1991; 88:5292–5296.

[111] Sikora E, Bielak-Zmijewska A, Piwocka K, et al. Inhibition of proliferation and apoptosis of human and rat T lymphocytes by curcumin, a curry pigment. Biochem Pharmacol 1997 Oct 15; 54(8):899–907.

[112] Dong Z, Ma W, Huang C, Yang CS. Inhibition of tumor promoter-induced activator protein 1 activation and cell transformation by tea polyphenols, (-)-epigallocatechin gallate, and theaflavins. Cancer Res 1997 Oct 1; 57(19):4414–9.

[113] Barthelman M, Bair WB 3rd, Stickland KK, et al. (-)-Epigallocatechin-3-gallate inhibition of ultraviolet B-induced AP-1 activity. Carcinogenesis 1998 Dec; 19(12):2201–4.

[114] El-Dahr SS, Dipp S, Baricos WH. Bradykinin stimulates the ERK-->Elk-1-->Fos/AP-1 pathway in mesangial cells. Am J Physiol 1998 Sep; 275(3 Pt 2):F343–52.

[115] Chen Y, Sun AY. Activation of transcription factor AP-1 by extracellular ATP in PC12 cells. Neurochem Res 1998 Apr; 23(4):543–50.

[116] Zhu Y, Lin JH, Liao HL, et al. LDL induces transcription factor activator protein-1 in human endothelial cells. Arterioscler Thromb Vasc Biol 1998 Mar; 18(3):473–80.

[117] Kobuchi H, Roy S, Sen CK, et al. Quercetin inhibits inducible ICAM-1 expression in human endothelial cells through the JNK pathway. Am J Physiol 1999 Sep; 277(3 Pt 1):C403–11.

[118] Handel ML, Watts CK, deFazio A, et al. Inhibition of AP-1 binding and transcription by gold and selenium involving conserved cysteine residues in Jun and Fos. Proc Natl Acad Sci USA 1995 May 9; 92(10):4497–501.

[119] Spyrou G, Bjornstedt M, Kumar S, et al. AP-1 DNA-binding activity is inhibited by selenite and selenodiglutathione. FEBS Lett 1995 Jul 10; 368(1):59–63.

[120] Wadsworth TL, Koop DR. Effects of the wine polyphenolics quercetin and resveratrol on pro-inflammatory cytokine expression in RAW 264.7 macrophages. Biochem Pharmacol 1999 Apr 15; 57(8):941–9.

[121] Chan MM. Inhibition of tumor necrosis factor by curcumin, a phytochemical. Biochem Pharmacol 1995 May 26; 49(11):1551–6.

[122] Saintot M, Astre C, Pujol H, Gerber M. Tumor progression and oxidant-antioxidant status. Carcinogenesis 1996 Jun; 17(6):1267–71.

[123] Sica A, Saccani A, Bottazzi B, et al. Autocrine production of IL-10 mediates defective IL-12 production and NF-kappa B activation in tumor-associated macrophages. J Immunol 2000 Jan 15; 164(2):762–7.

[124] Stolina M, Sharma S, Lin Y, et al. Specific inhibition of cyclooxygenase 2 restores antitumor reactivity by altering the balance of IL-10 and IL-12 synthesis. J Immunol 2000 Jan 1; 164(1):361–70.

[125] Okada F, Nakai K, Kobayashi T, et al. Inflammatory cell-mediated tumour progression and minisatellite mutation correlate with the decrease of antioxidative enzymes in murine fibrosarcoma cells. Br J Cancer 1999 Feb; 79(3–4):377–85.

[126] Irani K, Goldschmidt-Clermont PJ. Ras, superoxide and signal transduction. Biochem Phaol 1998 May 1; 55(9):1339–46.

[127] Miller AC, Samid D. Tumor resistance to oxidative stress: Association with ras oncogene expression and reversal by lovastatin, an inhibitor of p21ras isoprenylation. Int J Cancer 1995 Jan 17; 60(2):249–54.

[128] Vladimirova O, Lu FM, Shawver L, Kalman B. The activation of protein kinase C induces higher production of reactive oxygen species by mononuclear cells in patients with multiple sclerosis than in controls. Inflamm Res 1999 Jul; 48(7):412–6.

[129] Okamoto M, Oyasu R. Transformation in vitro of a nontumorigenic rat urothelial cell line by tumor necrosis factor-alpha. Lab Invest 1997 Aug; 77(2):139–44.

[130] Perego P, Paolicchi A, Tongiani R, et al. The cell-specific anti-proliferative effect of reduced glutathione is mediated by gamma-glutamyl transpeptidase-dependent extracellular pro-oxidant reactions. Int J Cancer 1997 Apr 10; 71(2):246–50.

[131] del Bello B, Paolicchi A, Comporti M, et al. Hydrogen peroxide produced during gamma-glutamyl transpeptidase activity is involved in prevention of apoptosis and maintainance of proliferation in U937 cells. FASEB J 1999 Jan; 13(1):69–79.

6

CELL-TO-CELL COMMUNICATION

Cell-to-cell communication is our last topic in Part I. Since cell-to-cell communication obviously involves interactions between a cell and its surroundings, this chapter forms a natural bridge between Part I, which is concerned with the behavior of individual cells, and Part II, which examines how a population of cancer cells interacts with the organism in which it grows.

This chapter considers how a cell communicates with adjacent cells and how it interacts with the extracellular matrix (ECM), the ground substance that surrounds cells and tissues and holds them in place. Cell-to-cell and cell-matrix communication occurs in two ways: through cell adhesion molecules (CAMs), the surface proteins that bind cells to one another and to the ECM, and through direct cell-to-cell exchange of compounds through gap junctions, the portals that form between adjacent cells.

In healthy cells, cell-to-cell and cell-matrix interactions are extremely important, as they help regulate a wide range of cellular activities, including proliferation and movement. Cancer cells, on the other hand, tend to detach from surrounding cells and from the matrix, thereby freeing themselves from signals that would restrict their proliferation and activity. At the same time, since contact with other cells and the matrix also provides "do not die" signals, cancer cells have evolved ways to mimic these signals, chiefly through growth factor production and increased signal transduction, thereby assuring they can survive as detached cells.

Cell-to-cell communication is a dynamic, complex process. At least four large families of CAMs are involved, each with members that play somewhat distinct roles. In addition, several other proteins are involved in assuring cell-to-cell communication via gap junctions. Moreover, the signals generated by CAMs and the signals that control them travel to and from the nucleus via protein phosphorylation. For this reason, PTK, PKC, and other proteins involved in signal transduction, as well as free radicals, can affect CAM function and behavior. Any or all of these mediators of cell-to-cell communication can be abnormal in cancer cells. Despite the complexities, however, many natural compounds help restore normal cell-to-cell communication in such a way as to induce apoptosis or inhibit cancer cell migration, invasion, metastasis, or proliferation. For instance, PTK inhibitors can reduce the invasion of cancer cells through mechanisms related to cell-to-cell communication. Most of the natural compounds discussed in this chapter can affect cell-to-cell communication in more than one way. Some of their effects, such as improved gap junction communication and improved activity of E-cadherin (a particular type of CAM), are clearly useful in inhibiting cancer. Other effects, such as inhibition of other CAM families, are probably, but not positively, useful in inhibiting cancer.

CELL ADHESION MOLECULES

Cell adhesion molecules are specialized proteins located on the outside of the plasma membrane. Due to recent advances in laboratory techniques, research on CAMs has flourished and the pivotal role they play is understood more completely. Through interactions with the ECM and other cells, CAMs regulate proliferation, architecture, cell migration, differentiation, apoptosis, angiogenesis, and invasion.[1-5] We can think of CAMs as the fingers of a cell, but instead of 10 fingers, cells have many hundreds, each lasting only for a few hours. Depending on the type of CAM, they generally have three functions. First, they grasp molecules on other cells or on the matrix. In some cases, this grasping helps a cell move and in others, helps it stay in place. Second, they send signals to the nucleus telling it what they feel. Third, they, or associated proteins, receive signals back from the nucleus that alters CAM behavior. We see then that signal transduction mediates messages both to and from CAMs, and compounds that affect signal transduction, such as PTK and PKC inhibitors, can greatly affect CAM expression and activity. In addition to sending signals to alter CAM behavior, the nucleus can also increase or decrease the production of different CAMs, depending on the signals it receives.

Four families of CAMs are discussed here: integrins, cadherins, selectins, and the immunoglobulin superfamily of adhesion molecules (see Figure 6.1; adapted from references 6 and 7). Although each of these CAMs plays complex roles, in general the cadherins hold tissues tightly together and the other three help in cell migration, especially that of immune cells. One other CAM family, the CD44 surface molecule, also helps cells to migrate; it is discussed in Chapter 9 in relation to cancer invasion.

The first three families of CAMs we discuss are integrins, selectins, and the immunoglobulin superfamily of adhesion molecules. Because all of these play a role in immune cell migration, it is useful to outline how these CAMs allow leukocytes (immune cells) to attach

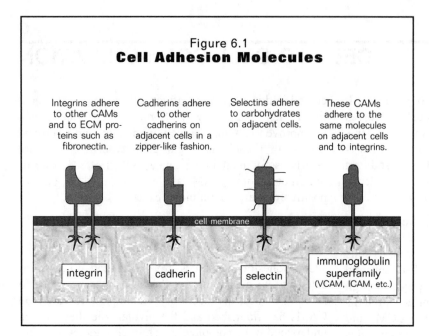

Figure 6.1
Cell Adhesion Molecules

Integrins adhere to other CAMs and to ECM proteins such as fibronectin.

Cadherins adhere to other cadherins on adjacent cells in a zipper-like fashion.

Selectins adhere to carbohydrates on adjacent cells.

These CAMs adhere to the same molecules on adjacent cells and to integrins.

cell membrane

integrin

cadherin

selectin

immunoglobulin superfamily (VCAM, ICAM, etc.)

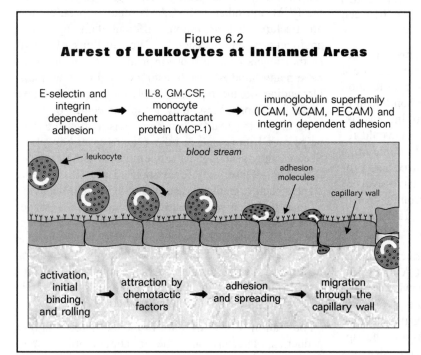

Figure 6.2
Arrest of Leukocytes at Inflamed Areas

E-selectin and integrin dependent adhesion → IL-8, GM-CSF, monocyte chemoattractant protein (MCP-1) → imunoglobulin superfamily (ICAM, VCAM, PECAM) and integrin dependent adhesion

blood stream

leukocyte

adhesion molecules

capillary wall

activation, initial binding, and rolling → attraction by chemotactic factors → adhesion and spreading → migration through the capillary wall

(c) interactions between the immunoglobulin superfamily of adhesion molecules (ICAMs, VCAMs, PECAMs) and integrins that induce the cells to arrest (stop at a particular place on the cell wall), spread, and finally migrate through the vascular wall. (In the figure, IL-8 stands for interleukin-8 and GM-CSF stands for granulocyte macrophage-colony stimulating factor, both of which are immune cytokines. Immune cytokines will be discussed in later chapters and are shown here only for completeness.)

The process illustrated in Figure 6.2 is of interest not only because it is important in the immune response, but also because it is likely that blood-borne tumor cells bind, creep, and stop at a metastatic site in a similar fashion. In other words, integrins, selectins, and the immunoglobulin superfamily of adhesion molecules all likely play a role in cancer metastasis. The exact role they play in cancer is complex; but in general, these CAMs tend to be overexpressed in cancer cells, and the natural compounds discussed here tend to inhibit their expression or activity and thus cancer metastasis.

Integrins

Integrins bind to a number of ECM proteins, including collagen, laminin, and fibronectin, and they are receptors for certain selectins and immunoglobulin superfamily adhesion molecules, including intercellular adhesion molecules (ICAMs). Like other CAMs, the intracellular root of integrins is attached to the cell's internal (actin) cytoskeleton. Through these connections, integrins and other CAMs can affect signal transduction and cellular structure.

Integrins are the most ubiquitous and versatile of all adhesion receptors.[9] Of all the CAMs, they are the ones most responsible for anchoring cells to the ECM. Their expression and regulation is controlled in a complex, dynamic fashion involving feedback from cell-cell, cell-matrix, and cell-growth factor interactions. At different stages in a cell's life and/or in response to changes in their microenvironment, various integrins are expressed

to and migrate through a vessel wall during an immune response. After floating in the bloodstream and arriving at a target location such as an infected area, leukocytes must attach to the inner vascular wall, then slip through the vascular tissue. This three-part process (see Figure 6.2; adapted from reference 8) consists of (a) transient interactions between selectins and integrins on the leukocytes and vascular cells, which pull leukocytes from the circulation and initiate their rolling along the vascular wall; (b) interactions with chemotactic proteins secreted by vascular cells, which cause leukocytes to creep along the vascular wall toward the site of infection; and to allow necessary growth, architectural changes, movement, and function.

Quantitative and qualitative changes in integrin expression have been observed in a large number of human tumors.[9] Numerous integrins can be affected, and the effects may be complex. In some cases, integrin binding can prevent cancer progression by keeping cells in contact with the matrix. Indeed, in some highly metastatic human tumors, the synthesis of specific integrins is reduced.[10] In general, however, integrins tend to be overexpressed in cancer cells, a situation that leads to increased arrest of the cells on the vascular lining during metastasis (see Figure 6.2).[11, 12] For example, human prostate cancer cells express a large number of integrins, and blocking these integrins reduces their invasion through vessel membranes in vitro.[13] In fact, highly metastatic cells tend to adhere more easily to the vascular lining than low or nonmetastatic cells—an effect due in part to excess integrin expression.[14]

Because of the complexities in the function and activity of integrins, some uncertainties exist about the potential role for integrin manipulation in cancer treatment. Nevertheless, inhibition of integrin expression does seem to inhibit cancer progression. Indeed, a number of natural compounds do inhibit integrin expression, and their actions generally lead to antiproliferation, antiinvasion, or antimetastatic effects, or all three.

Effects of Natural Compounds on Integrin Activity

As we know, signal transduction in cancer cells via PTK, PKC, and other proteins is generally greater than in healthy cells. This serves two functions with regard to integrins. First, the "do not die" signals provided by contact with other cells and the matrix appear to be mediated through integrin-induced stimulation of such kinases. For example, integrin activity increases, via signal transduction, expression of the antiapoptotic *Bcl-2* gene, thus providing "do not die" signals.[15] Cancer cells, being detached from other cells and the matrix, miss this source of "do not die" signals. They compensate by relying heavily on excessive signal transduction, thereby mimicking contact with other cells and the matrix. Kinase inhibitors, then, can reduce the "do not die" signals in cancer cells, causing apoptosis.

Second, excess signal transduction stimulates integrin expression and activity, resulting in increased migration and invasion. For example, stimulation of PKC can increase integrin expression on human prostate cancer cells and human melanoma cells, as well as their adhesion to matrix components.[13, 16] Not surprisingly then, kinase inhibitors can reduce cell adhesion and the events

that depend on it, such as migration and invasion. For example, genistein (at 20 to 100 µM) markedly reduced the invasion of mouse melanoma cells in vitro, apparently due to interruption of integrin activity.[17, 18] Genistein also reduced melanoma cell adhesion to ECM components, an event also likely due to interruption of integrin activity.[19] PKC inhibitors can also reduce tumor cell motility, invasion, and metastasis.[20–28] In one study, PKC inhibition increased the life span of rats with liver cancer, an effect apparently mediated by a reduction of integrin expression and tumor cell adhesion.[29] In another study, PKC inhibition reduced both the expression of integrins on liver cancer cells and their adhesion.[30, 31] Lastly, both PKC and PTK inhibitors reduced the migration of ovarian cancer cells and the attachment of lung cancer cells to endothelial cells in vitro.[12, 32] Although the above studies did not always use natural compounds to reduce PTK or PKC activity, natural compounds that inhibit these kinases could be expected to produce a similar effect.

Leukotriene inhibitors may have a similar inhibitory effect on integrin binding.[33, 34] Leukotrienes (discussed in Chapter 7) are hormone-like compounds that act like growth factors to cause inflammation and other events. Highly metastatic cell lines are associated with increased PKC activity and increased production of or sensitivity to leukotrienes. The omega-3 fatty acids EPA and DHA, which inhibit PKC activity and leukotriene production, have been reported to reduce the expression of integrins and other CAMs on cancer cells and other cells.[35–39] In several studies, diets high in EPA and DHA inhibited the growth of human breast and colon cancer cells and metastasis in mice.[40, 41, 42] Similar inhibition of invasion and metastasis was seen in vitro and in vivo in studies using melanoma and fibrosarcoma cells.[43]

Other natural compounds may interact directly with nuclear receptors to inhibit integrin expression. For example, vitamin D_3 (1,25-D_3) reduced cell proliferation and the production of integrins in human melanoma cells and human leukemia cells.[44, 45] This effect probably occurred from direct interactions with nuclear receptors.

Lastly, since integrins sense the conditions outside the cell and then eventually respond to these conditions, changes in the composition of the ECM can affect integrin gene expression.[46] Therefore, natural compounds that protect matrix integrity have the potential to normalize integrin expression. These will be discussed in Chapter 9.

Selectins

The selectin family consists of three members, named for the cells on which they were first discovered. L-selectin is expressed on leukocytes and attaches to activated endothelial cells. E-selectin is produced by endothelial cells and attaches to leukocytes. P-selectin is preformed, then stored in platelets and some endothelial cells; it attaches to the same cells as E-selectin. The junctions produced by selectin binding are relatively weak. Hence E-selectin plays a role in leukocyte rolling (see Figure 6.2). When overexpressed in cancer, selectins, like integrins, tend to help metastatic cancer cells arrest at locations in the vasculature, where they can then begin new colonies.

Each selectin molecule contains strings of proteins called lectins that are devoid of sugar chains. These proteins bind sugars (carbohydrates) on adjacent cells in a "lock and key" fashion. They can also bind with integrins in a similar fashion. In addition, these proteins can bind to free sugars. If all the sugar-binding sites are filled with free sugars, the selectin is not able to bind to other cells. Based on recent studies, it may be possible to saturate the proteins through oral administration of certain sugars. In regard to cancer, this would reduce the initial binding of tumor cells to the vascular wall as they travel through the circulation. One sugar that has been studied is modified citrus pectin. Oral administration of modified citrus pectin inhibited metastasis of melanoma cells in mice and prostate cancer cells in rats.[47, 48, 49] Moreover, given orally to mice at a daily dose of 310 and 620 milligrams it reduced the growth of transplanted colon cancer cells by 38 and 70 percent, respectively.[50]

Selectins and NF-κB

Recall from Chapter 5 that NF-κB produces an inflammatory effect in part by upregulating the synthesis of CAMs. These CAMs include E-selectin and the immunoglobulin superfamily adhesion molecules ICAM and VCAM. Therefore, inhibitors of NF-κB can decrease expression of E-selectin and other CAMs. Indeed, several NF-κB inhibitors, including antioxidants, PTK inhibitors, and PKC inhibitors, have been reported to reduce production of CAMs.[8] For example, in one study vitamin E was effective at inhibiting the synthesis of E-selectin and the adhesion of immune cells to vascular tissue.[51] In another study, resveratrol (at 0.1 to 1 μM) inhibited ICAM and VCAM expression on stimulated human endothelial cells.[52] Flavonoids may also effect CAM expression via inhibition of NF-κB. One study reported that quercetin (at 10 to 50 μM) inhibited ICAM expression in vascular cells in vitro.[53] In another

study on more than 18 flavonoids and isoflavonoids, apigenin (at 10 μM) was the most potent at inhibiting the expression of E-selectin, ICAM, and VCAM on vascular cells in vitro. Luteolin (at 25 μM) was also effective. Apigenin was also reported to be effective in vivo—an anti-inflammatory effect, apparently due to inhibition of ICAM, VCAM, or other cell adhesion molecules, was produced in rats after an intraperitoneal dose of 50 mg/kg.[54, 55] The equivalent human oral dose is about 4.1 grams per day. Another study also demonstrated inhibition of ICAM expression by apigenin in rats.[56]

These studies measured the ability of natural compounds to inhibit E-selectin, ICAM, and VCAM on immune cells and vascular cells. However, since interactions of these same CAMs between cancer cells and vascular cells may also be involved in tumor cell arrest at a metastatic site, inhibition of NF-κB activity may also reduce tumor cell adhesion and metastasis. At least one study has supported this possibility: aspirin and high concentrations of the thiol antioxidant *N*-acetylcysteine (NAC) reduced the adhesion of tumor cells to human veins in vitro.[57] Both aspirin and NAC, at high concentrations, can inhibit NF-κB activity.

Immunoglobulin Superfamily of Adhesion Molecules

The immunoglobulin superfamily of cell adhesion molecules contains the evolutionary precursors of the immune system. The most studied groups of immunoglobulin adhesion molecules are N-CAMs (found in nervous tissue), intercellular cell adhesion molecules (ICAMs), vascular cell adhesion molecules (VCAMs), and platelet endothelial cell adhesion molecules (PE-CAMs). All of these play a role in assisting immune cells and cancer cells to arrest at a target location on the vascular wall. The synthesis of many of these is upregulated by NF-κB, as discussed above, and inhibitors of NF-κB may reduce their expression.

Cadherins

In contrast to the three families of CAMs discussed above that play a role in immune cell migration, cadherins play a role in maintaining the structure of tissues. Cadherins are a family of calcium-dependent adhesion molecules. As indicated in Figure 6.1, they bind to other cadherins on adjacent cells in a zipperlike fashion, forming a tight bond between cells, the tightest formed by any cell adhesion molecule. Cadherins are named for the tissues in which they were first found. The various types include E-cadherin (epithelial cells), N-cadherin (nerve cells), and P-cadherin (placental cells).

E-cadherin deserves special mention here because its expression is closely related to the degree of cellular differentiation. Cancer cells, being relatively poorly differentiated, commonly display a decreased number of E-cadherin molecules or a decrease or malfunction in catenin molecules, which are the proteins that attach cadherins to the intracellular actin cytoskeleton. Reduced cadherin expression or function allows cancer cells to detach from adjacent cells. Not surprisingly then, E-cadherin activity appears to act reliably and consistently to suppress invasion of cancer cells. Moreover, underexpression of E-cadherin has been associated with poor prognosis, decreased differentiation, and increased tumor invasion and metastasis in a wide range of human tumors.[58, 59] Consequently, stimulation of E-cadherin expression or function may present an ideal target for cancer therapy.

A number of natural compounds can stimulate E-cadherin expression or function. First, since PTK activity rapidly downregulates E-cadherin function, PTK inhibitors may maintain its function.[60] In addition, since E-cadherin expression is related to cell differentiation, most compounds that induce differentiation are likely to induce E-cadherin expression. For example, ATRA, which induces differentiation, can increase the expression of E-cadherin in cancer cells.[61, 62] Lastly, one study reported that melatonin at near-normal concentrations (1 nM) inhibited invasion of human breast cancer cells and increased the expression of E-cadherin in vitro.[63] The mechanism by which it acted was uncertain, but it could have involved antioxidant interference with PTK signaling.

GAP JUNCTIONS

The last form of cell-to-cell communication discussed is intercellular communication through gap junctions. Such communication almost universally maintains tissue health and inhibits cancer progression. Gap junctions, which are portal structures between adjacent cells (see Figure 1.1), allow cells to exchange ions and small molecules directly, including ions and molecules used in signal transduction.[a] For example, calcium ions, which act as second messengers during PKC activation, can be exchanged through gap junctions. Indeed, waves of ions can pass among cells of a tissue through gap junctions. This wave can actually be seen visually, since gap junctions will also transfer a dye between cells of a tissue. Gap junctions can also transfer toxins, thus allowing a toxin to be distributed over many cells; such spreading

and dilution of a toxin can help prevent cell death. Gap junctions themselves are comprised of proteins called connexins. We can envision connexins as short rods that, when arranged in a circle, form a tube. The tube in one cell then links up with the tube in an adjacent cell, thereby forming the gap junction.

As discussed in Chapter 1, when cells become cancerous, they detach from neighboring cells. This occurs in part through downregulation of connexin genes. In fact, many if not all tumor-promoting agents reduce gap junction communication.[64] Normal gap junction communication has the opposite effect of tumor promoting agents—it decreases malignant behavior. Furthermore, restoring gap junction communication between cancer cells (by gene transfection) has been reported to cause them to behave more like normal cells.[65] Therefore, in recent years connexin genes have become viewed as a family of tumor suppressor genes. Connexin genes are usually not mutated in cancer cells but are generally silenced via hypermethylation (see Chapter 2), and/or their protein products are altered after production so as to make them nonfunctional.[66, 67, 68] Connexin proteins can be rendered nonfunctional through abnormal protein phosphorylation, including abnormal PKC activity.[69] Lack of cell adhesion molecules and, especially, E-cadherin can also render connexin proteins nonfunctional.[70, 71]

A variety of natural compounds foster gap junction intercellular communication (GJIC) and prevent its disruption (see Table 6.1). It is likely that many other natural compounds discussed in this book will also improve GJIC, but they have not yet been tested. Note that the dose of natural compound given greatly affects the result. Whereas moderate doses may be beneficial, doses that induce oxidative or other damage may be detrimental. For example, in a study on rats, oral administration of beta-carotene and lycopene inhibited gap junction communication in liver cells when given at 810 milligrams per day (as scaled to humans) but improved gap junction communication when given at 81 milligrams per day (as scaled to humans).[72] The common dose of beta-carotene during supplementation is about 15 mg (25,000 I.U.).[73] A dose-responsive effect was also seen with melatonin, as indicated in the table. Also note that antioxidants in general may prevent loss of gap junction communication, since oxidants can stimulate PKC activity.[74] In addition, since tumor necrosis factor can decrease gap junction communication, inhibitors of NF-κB (which reduce TNF production) may prevent communication loss. Vitamin C (at 10 μM), vitamin E (at 1 μM), and glutathione (at 1 mM) all inhibited TNF-induced loss of gap junction communication in smooth muscle

---

[a] *Gap junctions can exchange compounds of molecular weight below about 1,000 grams/mole.*

TABLE 6.1   NATURAL COMPOUNDS THAT FACILITATE GAP JUNCTION INTERCELLULAR COMMUNICATION (GJIC)

COMPOUND	EFFECTS
Apigenin	• At 25 µM, apigenin induced GJIC in epithelial cells.[76] • At 25 µM, apigenin inhibited loss of GJIC by tumor promoters in epithelial cells.[77]
ATRA	• At 1 µM, ATRA induced GJIC in fibroblasts.[78]
CAPE	• At 18 µM, CAPE restored GJIC in cancer cells.[79]
Genistein	• At 10 µM, genistein inhibited loss of GJIC due to oxidants in vascular cells.[80]
EGCG (studied as green tea)	• Oral administration of green tea extract prevented loss of GJIC in liver cells of mice given a tumor-promoting agent.[81]
Melatonin	• At 10 pM to 100 pM, melatonin induced GJIC in fibroblasts. These are normal concentrations seen in vivo. Melatonin was not effective at concentrations greater than 100 pM.[82]
Resveratrol	• At 17 to 50 µM, resveratrol inhibited loss of GJIC by tumor promoters in epithelial cells.[83]
Selenium	• At 0.1 to 1 µM, selenite inhibited loss of GJIC due to toxins in epithelial cells.[84]
Vitamin D_3	• At 0.01 and 1 µM, vitamin D_3 induced GJIC in fibroblasts.[78] • At 0.1 µM, 1,25-D_3 induced GJIC in fibroblasts.[85]

cells in vitro.[75] A similar effect would be expected with cancer cells.

CONCLUSION

Cells do not exist distinct from their environment. Intercellular communication and cell-matrix interactions are vital processes that link a cell to its environment and so play an important role in the life of a healthy cell. Cancer cells commonly exhibit aberrant forms of cell-cell and cell-matrix communication, and this aberrant communication is one factor that allows them to act independently and malignantly. Natural compounds can normalize and protect cell-cell and cell-matrix interactions through their inhibitory effects on PTK, PKC, and NF-κB and through other ways discussed. Although the exact role of some CAMs in cancer progression is still uncertain, we do know that increasing E-cadherin expression and increasing gap junction communication will be useful strategies in cancer treatment. The natural compounds discussed here tend to normalize many aspects of cell-to-cell communication, including the two just mentioned, and in so doing can inhibit the proliferation, invasion, and metastasis of cancer cells.

REFERENCES

[1] Roth J. Tumors—disorders of cell adhesion. Verh Dtsch Ges Pathol 1994; 78:22–5.

[2] Agrez MV, Bates RC. Colorectal cancer and the integrin family of cell adhesion receptors: Current status and future directions. Eur J Cancer 1994; 30A(14):2166–70.

[3] Pignatelli M, Vessey CJ. Adhesion molecules: Novel molecular tools in tumor pathology. Hum Pathol 1994; 25(9):849–56.

[4] Juliano RL, Varner JA. Adhesion molecules in cancer: The role of integrins. Curr Opin Cell Biol 1993; 5(5):812–8.

[5] Brooks PC. Role of Integrins in angiogenesis. Eur J Cancer 1996; 32A(14):2423–2429.

[6] http://bioag.byu.edu/Zoology/Zoology_373/Zoology373.htm

[7] http://arbl.cvmbs.colostate.edu/hbooks/cmb/cells/cells.html

[8] Manning AM, Anderson DC. Transcription factor NF-κB: An emerging regulator of inflammation. Annu Rep Med Chem 1994; 29:235–244.

[9] Pignatelli M, Stamp G. Integrins in tumour development and spread. Cancer Surveys 1995; 24:113–127.

[10] Malik RK, Parsons JT. Integrin-mediated signaling in normal and malignant cells: A role of protein tyrosine kinases. Biochim Biophys Acta 1996 Jun 7; 1287(2–3):73–6.

[11] Miloszewska J, Kowalczyk D, Janik P. Migration induction of contact inhibited C3H 10T1/2 cells by protein kinase C (PKC) dependent process. Neoplasma 1998; 45(2):77–80.

[12] Carreiras F, Rigot V, Cruet S, et al. Migration properties of the human ovarian adenocarcinoma cell line IGROV1: Importance of alpha(v)beta3 integrins and vitronectin. Int J Cancer 1999 Jan 18; 80(2):285–94.

[13] Trikha M, Timar J, Lundy SK, et al. Human prostate carcinoma cells express functional alphaIIb(beta)3 integrin. Cancer Res 1996 Nov 1; 56(21):5071–8.

14 Koike C, Oku N, Watanable M, et al. Real-time PET analysis of metastatic tumor cell trafficking in vivo and its relation to adhesion properties. Biochim Biophys Acta 1995 Sep 13; 1238(2):99–106.

15 Ruoslahti E. Integrins as signaling molecules and targets for tumor therapy. Kidney Int 1997 May; 51(5):1413–7.

16 Trikha M, Timar J, Lundy SK, et al. The high affinity alphaIIb beta3 integrin is involved in invasion of human melanoma cells. Cancer Res 1997 Jun 15; 57(12):2522–8.

17 Yan C, Han R. Genistein suppresses adhesion-induced protein tyrosine phosphorylation and invasion of B16-BL6 melanoma cells. Cancer Lett 1998 Jul 3; 129(1):117–24.

18 Yan C, Han R. Suppression of adhesion-induced protein tyrosine phosphorylation decreases invasive and metastatic potentials of B16-BL6 melanoma cells by protein tyrosine kinase inhibitor genistein. Invasion Metastasis 1997; 17(4):189–98.

19 Smith TW, Menter DG, Nicholson GL, McIntire LV. Regulation of melanoma cell adhesion stabilization to fibronectin. Melanoma Res 1996 Oct; 6(5):351–62.

20 Rao CV, Simi B, Reddy BS. Inhibition by dietary curcumin of azoxymethane-induced ornithine decarboxylase, tyrosine protein kinase, arachidonic acid metabolism and aberrant crypt foci formation in the rat colon. Carcinogenesis 1993; 14(11):2219–2225.

21 Timar J, Raso E, Fazakas ZS, et al. Multiple use of a signal transduction pathway in tumor cell invasion. Anticancer Res 1996 Nov–Dec; 16(6A):3299–306.

22 Ways DK, Kukoly CA, deVente J, et al. MCF-7 breast cancer cells transfected with protein kinase C-alpha exhibit altered expression of other protein kinase C isoforms and display a more aggressive neoplastic phenotype. J Clin Invest 1995 Apr; 95(4):1906–15.

23 Schwartz GK, Redwood SM, Ohnuma T, et al. Inhibition of invasion of invasive human bladder carcinoma cells by protein kinase C inhibitor staurosporine. J Natl Cancer Inst 1990 Nov 21; 82(22):1753–6.

24 Schwartz GK, Jiang J, Kelsen D, Albino AP. Protein kinase C: A novel target for inhibiting gastric cancer cell invasion. J Natl Cancer Inst 1993 Mar 3; 85(5):402–7.

25 Honn KV, Timar J, Rozhin J, et al. A lipoxygenase metabolite, 12-(S)-HETE, stimulates protein kinase C-mediated release of cathepsin B from malignant cells. Exp Cell Res 1994 Sep; 214(1):120–30.

26 Honn KV, Grossi IM, Steinert BW, et al. Lipoxygenase regulation of membrane expression of tumor cell glycoproteins and subsequent metastasis. Adv Prostaglandin Thromb Leukotriene Res 1989; 19:439–443.

27 Dumont JA, Jones WD, Bitonti AJ. Inhibition of experimental metastasis and cell adhesion of B16F1 melanoma cells by inhibitors of protein kinase C. Cancer Res 1992; 52:1195–1200.

28 Blobe GC, Obeid LM, Hannun YA. Regulation of protein kinase C and role in cancer biology. Cancer Metastasis Rev 1994 Dec; 13(3–4):411–31.

29 Nomura M, Sugiura N, Miyamoto K. A protein kinase C inhibitor NA-382 prolongs the life span of AH66F-bearing rats as well as inhibiting leukocyte function-associated antigen-1

30 Nomura M, Sugiura N, Moritani S, Miyamoto K. Inhibition by protein kinase C inhibitor of expression of leukocyte function-associated antigen-1 molecules in rat hepatoma AH66F cells. Jpn J Cancer Res 1997 Mar; 88(3):267–72.

31 Nomura M, Yamamoto H, Sugiura N, Miyamoto K. Leukocyte function-associated antigen 1-dependent adhesion of rat hepatoma AH66F cells and inhibition by protein kinase C inhibitors. Biochem Pharmacol 1997 May 9; 53(9):1333–7.

32 Sheski FD, Natarajan V, Pottratz ST. Tumor necrosis factor-alpha stimulates attachment of small cell lung carcinoma to endothelial cells. J Lab Clin Med 1999 Mar; 133(3):265–73.

33 Boike GM, Sloane BF, Deppe G, et al. The role of calcium and arachidonic acid in the chemotaxis of a new murine tumor line. Proceedings of the Am Assoc Cancer Res 1987; 28:82.

34 Timar J, Chen YQ, Liu B, et al. The lipoxygenase metabolite 12(S)-HETE promotes αIIbβ3 integrin-mediated tumor-cell spreading on fibronectin. Int J Cancer 1992; 52:594–603.

35 De Caterina R, Libby P. Control of endothelial leukocyte adhesion molecules by fatty acids. Lipids 1996 Mar; 31 Suppl:S57–63.

36 De Caterina R, Cybulsky MI, Clinton SK, et al. The omega-3 fatty acid docosahexaenoate reduces cytokine-induced expression of proatherogenic and proinflammatory proteins in human endothelial cells. Arterioscler Thromb 1994; 14:1829–1836.

37 Weber C, Erl W, Pietsch A. Docosahexaenoic acid selectivity attenuates induction of vascular cell adhesion molecule-1 and subsequent monocytic cell adhesion to human endothelial cells stimulated by tumor necrosis factor-α. Arterioscler Thromb Vasc Biol 1995; 15:622–628.

38 German NS, Johanning GJ. Eicosapentaenoic acid and epidermal growth factor modulation of human breast cancer cell adhesion. Cancer Letters 1997; 118:95–100.

39 Collie-Duguid ES, Wahle KW. Inhibitory effect of fish oil N-3 polyunsaturated fatty acids on the expression of endothelial cell adhesion molecules. Biochem Biophys Res Commun 1996 Mar 27; 220(3):969–74.

40 Rose DP, Rayburn J, Hatala MA, Connolly JM. Effects of dietary fish oil on fatty acids and eicosanoids in metastasizing human breast cancer cells. Nutr Cancer 1994; 22:131–141.

41 Rose DP, Connolly JM. Effects of dietary omega-3 fatty acids on human breast cancer growth and metastasis in nude mice. J Natl Cancer Inst 1993; 85:1743–1747.

42 Iigo M, Nakagawa T, Ishikawa C, et al. Inhibitory effects of docosahexaenoic acid on colon carcinoma 26 metastasis to the lung. Br J Cancer 1997; 75(5):650–5.

43 Reich R, Royce L, Martin GR. Eicosapentaenoic acid reduces the invasive and metastatic activities of malignant tumor cells. Biochem Biophys Res Commun 1989; 160(2):559–564.

44 Hansen CM, Madsen MW, Arensbak B, et al. Down-regulation of laminin-binding integrins by 1 alpha,25-dihydroxyvitamin D3 in human melanoma cells in vitro. Cell Adhes Commun 1998; 5(2):109–20.

45 Kaneko A, Suzuki S, Hara M, et al. 1,25-Dihydroxyvitamin D3 suppresses the expression of the VCAM-1 receptor, VLA-4

(LFA-1)-dependent adhesion of the cells. Biol Pharm Bull 1996 Dec; 19(12):1611–3.

human leukemic HL-60 cells. Biochem Biophys Res Commun 1999 Feb 16; 255(2):371–6.

46 Stetler-Stevenson WG, Aznavoorian S, Liotta LA. Tumor cell interactions with the extracellular matrix during invasion and metastasis. Annu Rev Cell Biol 1993; 9:541–73.

47 Pienta KJ, Naik H, Akhtar A, et al. Inhibition of spontaneous metastasis in a rat prostate cancer model by oral administration of modified citrus pectin. J Natl Cancer Inst 1995 Mar 1; 87(5):348–53.

48 Inohara H, Raz A. Effects of natural complex carbohydrate (citrus pectin) on murine melanoma cell properties related to galectin-3 functions. Glycoconj J 1994 Dec; 11(6):527–32.

49 Platt D, Raz A. Modulation of the lung colonization of B16-F1 melanoma cells by citrus pectin. J Natl Cancer Inst 1992; 84(6):438–42.

50 Hayashi A, Gillen AC, Lott JR. Effects of daily oral administration of quercetin chalcone and modified citrus pectin. Altern Med Rev 2000 Dec; 5(6):546-552.

51 Traber MG, Packer L. Vitamin E: Beyond antioxidant function. Am J Clin Nutr 1995 Dec; 62(6 Suppl):1501S-1509S.

52 Ferrero ME, Bertelli AAE, Fulgenzi A, et al. Activity in vitro of resveratrol on granulocyte and monocyte adhesion to endothelium. Am J Clin Nutr 1998 Dec; 68(6):1208–14.

53 Kobuchi H, Roy S, Sen CK, et al. Quercetin inhibits inducible ICAM-1 expression in human endothelial cells through the JNK pathway. Am J Physiol 1999 Sep; 277(3 Pt 1):C403–11.

54 Gerritsen ME, Carley WW, Ranges GE, et al. Flavonoids inhibit cytokine-induced endothelial cell adhesion protein gene expression. Am J Pathology 1995; 147(2):278–292.

55 Read MA. Flavonoids: Naturally occurring anti-inflammatory agents [comment]. Am J Pathol 1995 Aug; 147(2):235–7.

56 Panes J, Gerritsen ME, Anderson DC, et al. Apigenin inhibits tumor necrosis factor-induced intercellular adhesion molecule-1 upregulation in vivo. Microcirculation 1996; 3(3):279–286.

57 Tozawa K, Sakurada S, Kohri K, Okamoto T. Effects of anti-nuclear factor kappa B reagents in blocking adhesion of human cancer cells to vascular endothelial cells. Cancer Res 1995 Sep 15; 55(18):4162–7.

58 Bracke ME, Van Roy FM, Mareel MM. The E-cadherin/catenin complex in invasion and metastasis. Curr Top Microbiol Immunol 1996; 213(Pt 1):123–61.

59 Heimann R, Lan F, McBride R, Hellman S. Separating favorable from unfavorable prognostic markers in breast cancer: The role of E-cadherin. Cancer Res 2000 Jan 15; 60(2):298–304.

60 Akimoto S, Ochiai A, Inomata M, et al. Expression of cadherin-catenin cell adhesion molecules, phosphorylated tyrosine residues and growth factor receptor-tyrosine kinases in gastric cancers. Jpn J Cancer Res 1998 Aug; 89(8):829–36.

61 Wu H, Lotan R, Menter D, et al. Expression of E-cadherin is associated with squamous differentiation in squamous cell carcinomas. Anticancer Res 2000 May–Jun; 20(3A):1385–90.

62 Schmutzler C, Kohrle J. Retinoic acid redifferentiation therapy for thyroid cancer. Thyroid 2000 May; 10(5):393–406.

63 Cos S, Fernandez R, Guezmes A, et al. Influence of melatonin on invasive and metastatic properties of MCF-7 human breast cancer cells. Cancer Res 1998 Oct 1; 58(19):4383–90.

64 Yamasaki H, Krutovskikh V, Mesnil M, Omori Y. Connexin genes and cell growth control. Arch Toxicol Suppl 1996; 18:105–14.

65 Ruch RJ. The role of gap junctional intercellular communication in neoplasia. Ann Clin Lab Sci 1994 May–Jun; 24(3):216–31.

66 Yamasaki H, Omori Y, Krutovskikh V, et al. Connexins in tumour suppression and cancer therapy. Novartis Found Symp 1999; 219:241–54; discussion 254–60.

67 Yamasaki H, Omori Y, Zaidan-Dagli ML, et al. Genetic and epigenetic changes of intercellular communication genes during multistage carcinogenesis. Cancer Detect Prev 1999; 23(4):273–9.

68 Piechocki MP, Burk RD, Ruch RJ. Regulation of connexin32 and connexin43 gene expression by DNA methylation in rat liver cells. Carcinogenesis 1999 Mar; 20(3):401–6.

69 Cesen-Cummings K, Warner KA, Ruch RJ. Role of protein kinase C in the deficient gap junctional intercellular communication of K-ras-transformed murine lung epithelial cells. Anticancer Res 1998 Nov–Dec; 18(6A):4343–6.

70 Yamasaki H, Mesnil M, Omori Y, et al. Intercellular communication and carcinogenesis. Mutat Res 1995 Dec; 333(1–2):181–8.

71 Holder JW, Elmore E, Barrett JC. Gap junction function and cancer. Cancer Res 1993 Aug 1; 53(15):3475–85

72 Krutovskikh V, Asamoto M, Takasuka N, et al. Differential dose-dependent effects of alpha-, beta-carotenes and lycopene on gap-junctional intercellular communication in rat liver in vivo. Jpn J Cancer Res 1997 Dec; 88(12):1121–4.

73 Murray M. Encyclopedia of nutritional supplements. Rocklin, CA: Prima Publishing, 1996, p. 36.

74 Hu J, Speisky H, Cotgreave IA. The inhibitory effects of boldine, glaucine, and probucol on TPA-induced down regulation of gap junction function. Relationships to intracellular peroxides, protein kinase C translocation, and connexin 43 phosphorylation. Biochem Pharmacol 1995 Nov 9; 50(10):1635–43.

75 Mensink A, de Haan LH, Lakemond CM, et al. Inhibition of gap junctional intercellular communication between primary human smooth muscle cells by tumor necrosis factor alpha. Carcinogenesis 1995 Sep; 16(9):2063–7.

76 Chaumontet C, Bex V, Gaillard-Sanchez I, et al. Apigenin and tangeretin enhance gap junctional intercellular communication in rat liver epithelial cells. Carcinogenesis 1994 Oct; 15(10):2325–30.

77 Chaumontet C, Droumaguet C, Bex V, et al. Flavonoids (apigenin, tangeretin) counteract tumor promoter-induced inhibition of intercellular communication of rat liver epithelial cells. Cancer Lett 1997 Mar 19; 114(1–2):207–10.

78 Stahl W, Nicolai S, Hanusch M, Sies H. Vitamin D influences gap junctional communication in C3H/10T 1/2 murine fibroblast cells. FEBS Lett 1994 Sep 19; 352(1):1–3.

79 Na H, Wilson MR, Kang K, et al. Restoration of gap junctional intercellular communication by caffeic acid phenethyl ester

(CAPE) in a ras-transformed rat liver epithelial cell line. Cancer Lett 2000 Aug 31; 157(1):31–38.

80 Zhang YW, Morita I, Nishida M, Murota SI. Involvement of tyrosine kinase in the hypoxia/reoxygenation-induced gap junctional intercellular communication abnormality in cultured human umbilical vein endothelial cells. J Cell Physiol 1999 Sep; 180(3):305–13.

81 Sai K, Kanno J, Hasegawa R, et al. Prevention of the down-regulation of gap junctional intercellular communication by green tea in the liver of mice fed pentachlorophenol. Carcinogenesis 2000 Sep; 21(9):1671–6.

82 Ubeda A, Trillo MA, House DE, Blackman CF. Melatonin enhances junctional transfer in normal C3H/10T1/2 cells. Cancer Lett 1995 May 8; 91(2):241–5.

83 Nielsen M, Ruch RJ, Vang O. Resveratrol reverses tumor-promoter-induced inhibition of gap-junctional intercellular communication. Biochem Biophys Res Commun 2000 Sep 7; 275(3):804–9.

84 Sharov VS, Briviba K, Sies H. Peroxynitrite diminishes gap junctional communication: Protection by selenite supplementation. IUBMB Life 1999 Oct; 48(4):379–84.

85 Clairmont A, Tessman D, Stock A, et al. Induction of gap junctional intercellular communication by vitamin D in human skin fibroblasts is dependent on the nuclear vitamin D receptor. Carcinogenesis 1996 Jun; 17(6):1389–91.

Part II
CANCER AT THE LEVEL OF THE ORGANISM

Part II focuses on the procancer events that occur at the level of the organism and the natural compounds that may inhibit them. These events, which consist of interactions between a population of cancer cells and the body, fall into three primary clusters: events that facilitate angiogenesis, invasion and metastasis, and immune evasion.

In Chapter 7 we discuss the basics of angiogenesis, the growth of new blood vessels. These vessels provide the cells of a tumor not only nutrition and oxygen but also access to the circulation, thereby allowing metastasis. Natural compounds that inhibit angiogenesis are discussed in Chapter 8. In Chapters 9 and 10 we turn our attention to cancer invasion—the spread of cancer cells into adjacent areas—and metastasis—the spread of cancer cells into distant locations via the blood or lymph. We then consider the immune response against cancer, discussing the basics of the immune system in Chapter 11 and natural compounds that affect it in Chapter 12.

As in Part I, we see in Part II that the difference between cancer cells and healthy cells is not that the former have unique ways of acting but that the extent and timing of their actions are abnormal. Angiogenesis, invasion, metastasis, and immune response are all normal processes that occur apart from cancer. For example, wound healing requires angiogenesis and an immune response, and during an immune response, immune cells must invade injured tissues. Similarly, immune cells perform a type of metastasis when they travel from one part of the body to distant parts (although this is not commonly referred to as metastasis). Cancer cells have devised ways to co-opt all these normal processes for their own benefit. There are many parallels between wound healing and immune cell activity on one hand, and cancer cell activity on the other. The analogy between tumors and nonhealing wounds was first mentioned in Chapter 4 with respect to cell proliferation. The analogy between cancer cells and immune cells was first discussed in Chapter 5 with respect to their reliance on activation of the transcription factors NF-κB and AP-1. In Chapter 7 and 8 we see how tumors act like nonhealing wounds to facilitate angiogenesis, and in Chapter 9 we examine similarities between immune cell and cancer cell migration.

The abnormal behavior of cancer cells relies largely on the abnormal signaling discussed in detail in Part I, which focused on how abnormal signaling helps cancer cells proliferate and avoid apoptosis. Cancer angiogenesis, invasion, and metastasis also rely in part on several kinds of abnormal signaling, including production of growth factors; activity of PTK, PKC, ras proteins, and transcription factors; and production of free radicals. Thus many of the natural compounds identified in Part I as inhibitors of cellular activity will also be discussed in Part II as inhibitors of angiogenesis, invasion, and metastasis. Moreover, because Part II reviews interactions between cancer and the body, we will introduce additional compounds that principally affect normal cells, allowing them to resist cancer invasion or, in the case of immune cells, to attack cancer.

7

OVERVIEW OF ANGIOGENESIS

Angiogenesis, the growth of new blood vessels, is needed anywhere new tissue is growing. Thus it not only occurs in benign and malignant tumors but also in wound healing, ovulation, menstruation, and pregnancy. Abnormal angiogenesis also takes place in other diseases, including rheumatoid arthritis, psoriasis, and atherosclerosis.

Researchers believe that if angiogenesis can be inhibited in cancer patients, tumor growth will be inhibited or even reversed. Although inhibition of tumor angiogenesis is a very promising anticancer therapy, it is not without challenges. The same factors and environments that drive angiogenesis during cancer also drive angiogenesis during wound healing and other normal conditions in which it occurs. Since wound healing and other normal angiogenic processes are so vital for survival, the body employs redundant mechanisms to assure that angiogenesis occurs when needed. Overriding these mechanisms to stop tumor angiogenesis is not trivial. Nonetheless, because a number of natural compounds have been reported to inhibit tumor angiogenesis in vitro, and some of these inhibit it in animals, the prospects of doing so in humans look hopeful.

Since angiogenesis is a normal, necessary process in healthy humans, the goal in antiangiogenic therapy is to inhibit blood vessel growth as much as possible at the tumor site while allowing it to continue as necessary elsewhere.[1] Such selective inhibition seems possible. Natural compounds, by reducing the excessive signaling needed by cancer cells, are likely to selectively inhibit tumor angiogenesis. Moreover, even the use of experimental antiangiogenic drugs appears to be safe, at least in the short term. The kind of adverse effects one might expect from inhibition of normal angiogenesis have not yet been reported in rodent or human trials that studied antiangiogenic therapies.[2–10] For one thing, the need for angiogenesis in most adults is small and of short duration relative to the tumor's need. For another, the body attempts to limit aberrant angiogenesis whenever it can, and antiangiogenic therapies can assist the body in this endeavor.

MECHANICS OF ANGIOGENESIS

Although it has been known for over a hundred years that tumors contain an abnormally dense blood vessel network, it was not until the 1960s that investigators realized tumors induce their own blood supply. In the 1970s investigators found that the growth of solid tumors is dependent upon the growth of new blood vessels.[a] The blood vessels formed during angiogenesis supply the tumor with oxygen and nutrients and provide access to the circulation for metastasizing cells. In their landmark 1972 study, Folkman and Hochberg reported that tumors implanted in the eyes of rabbits grew only to a size of approximately one cubic millimeter before developing their own blood supply.[11] Thus antiangiogenic therapies may severely limit tumor growth and metastasis.

Growth in experimental tumors is slow and gradual before angiogenesis but explosive afterward. The proliferation rate of individual cells may be similar before and after angiogenesis, but the high rate of tumor growth after angiogenesis appears to be due to a severe reduction of apoptosis.[12] In tumors with active angiogenesis, cells do not die when they should, and therefore more cells are alive to proliferate. As mentioned in Chapter 3, cancer cells die by apoptosis unless exposed to growth factors or similar stimuli. Angiogenesis occurs in and produces an environment steeped in growth factors.

Angiogenesis is a complex process in which existing mature blood vessels generate sprouts, and these sprouts develop into complete new vessels. During angiogenesis, vascular cells proliferate at abnormally rapid rates. Whereas under normal circumstances capillary cells divide approximately once every 7 years, capillary cells in experimental tumors may divide once every 7 to 10 days.[13]

Angiogenesis within tumors or wounds involves at least four steps:[14, 15]

1. Cancer cells (or adjacent tissues) secrete angiogenic factors.

2. The basement membrane surrounding a mature capillary vessel dissolves, and a bud begins to grow (see Figure 7.1). The basement membrane is a layer of specialized connective tissue that encircles capillaries and serves as the connection point between the extracellular matrix (ECM), the ground substance surrounding cells and tissues and holding them in place, and the capillary itself. The basement membrane also provides structural support to the capillary.

---

[a] Recent studies indicate that several leukemias and lymphomas also depend on angiogenesis.

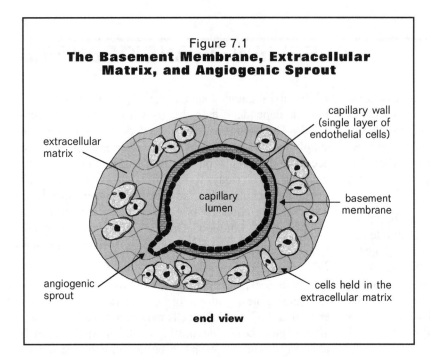

Figure 7.1
The Basement Membrane, Extracellular Matrix, and Angiogenic Sprout

extracellular matrix

capillary wall (single layer of endothelial cells)

capillary lumen

basement membrane

angiogenic sprout

cells held in the extracellular matrix

end view

3. Vascular (endothelial) cells proliferate and migrate from the bud toward the angiogenic stimulus—often that means toward a low-oxygen (hypoxic) environment.

4. The sprout eventually forms a hollow tube (lumen) and joins its end with another sprout to form a new capillary vessel.

Further budding from the newly formed capillary follows as the process repeats itself. Angiogenesis is a relatively rapid process; buds can form within 48 hours of exposure to an angiogenic factor.[16]

In spite of active angiogenesis, the blood supply in a solid tumor is relatively limited compared to that of normal tissue. Tumor angiogenesis results in chaotic vessel growth, and the new vessels are surrounded by poorly developed basement membranes. Because of their abnormal basement membranes, the vessels tend to be thin-walled and leaky. Some sprouts may not fuse with others, and they become dead-end sacs. These factors, in conjunction with a lack of tumor lymph vessels, lead to the creation of pressure gradients within tumors. Pressure gradients, in turn, compress the vessels and further restrict or occlude blood flow. A lack of circulation appears to be a primary cause of the central necrosis found in many large tumors. Although this process does destroy some cancer cells, the increased pressure also limits the uptake of treatment agents and immune cells into the tumor.[17]

ANGIOGENIC FACTORS AND ANGIOGENESIS INHIBITION

Recent studies indicate that due to a variety of angiogenic factors, healthy vascular endothelial cells are perpetually poised to proliferate and that they are restrained from doing so by elaborate machinery.[18] Endothelial cells are literally steeped in angiogenic factors, yet they proliferate only under tightly controlled conditions. In experimental conditions, angiogenesis is not easily sustained. When angiogenic factors are used to stimulate angiogenesis, angiogenesis halts when the factors are removed. In contrast, pathologic angiogenesis in vivo is difficult to stop, which suggests that in diseases like cancer, the normal machinery that inhibits vascular growth is somehow deranged.

Thus we have two possible therapeutic routes by which we can reduce angiogenesis. First, we can normalize the machinery that restrains angiogenesis. This machinery in normal tissues includes the following:

•   *Mechanical forces.* In some cases, mechanical forces are necessary for growth factors to function. These forces are generated through the tension that exists between the cell and the ECM and are mediated by CAMs. Endothelial cells are resistant to growth factors and angiogenesis if they have no room to stretch or spread. For this reason, it is possible that vasodilation (that is, expansion of the blood vessels, such as occurs in inflammation) is necessary to make endothelial cells susceptible to growth factors.

•   *Angiogenic substances may be bound in the extracellular matrix.* As discussed below, the ECM can bind various growth factors and make them inaccessible to endothelial cells.

•   *Angiogenesis suppressor genes.* Tumor suppressor genes such as *p53* may inhibit angiogenesis. Mutated genes would not fulfill this function.

•   *Antiangiogenic compounds.* A number of negative regulators of angiogenesis exist within the body, including angiostatin and thrombospondin.[19] In some human cells, thrombospondin is under the control of the *p53* tumor suppressor gene.

Natural compounds could be used to affect most of the above factors. For example, those that promote proper cell-to-cell and cell-matrix connections (see Chapter 6) and those that inhibit inflammation (discussed below) may reduce angiogenesis by maintaining proper tension between cells. Natural compounds that inhibit invasion enzymes (discussed in Chapter 9) may reduce angiogenesis by maintaining the safe storage of growth factors in the extracellular matrix. Natural compounds that support *p53* function (see Chapter 5) may also reduce angiogenesis.

The second route available for reducing angiogenesis is to inhibit the factors that stimulate it. This route is the primary focus here. Some of the more important factors that stimulate angiogenesis are listed in Table 7.1, each of which can be inhibited by natural compounds. In order to understand the effects of natural compounds on angiogenesis, we describe the role these factors play in causing it to occur.

Of the compounds listed in the table, VEGF (vascular endothelial growth factor) and bFGF (basic fibroblast growth factor) are considered primary angiogenic compounds, whereas the others are considered secondary, since they play a more complementary or initiating role. Many other factors stimulate or help stimulate angiogenesis, but these are discussed here only in passing. These include kinins, platelet activating factor (PAF), epidermal growth factor (EGF), platelet-derived growth factor (PDGF), interleukins-1, -6, and -8, elastase, collagenase, urokinase plasminogen activator (uPA), and transforming growth factor-alpha and -beta (TGF-alpha, TGF-beta).[14, 53] Because many of these factors can be inhibited by natural compounds, they provide yet another means by which these compounds might act when they inhibit angiogenesis.

SIMILARITY OF ANGIOGENESIS IN WOUND HEALING AND CANCER

Wound healing is a normal process we are all familiar with, and the factors that stimulate angiogenesis in wound healing and cancer are the same.[23] Indeed, the surgical wounding of tissues next to implanted tumors has been reported to increase tumor growth and angiogenesis in mice.[24] In addition, wound fluid itself stimulates tumor angiogenesis as well as cell proliferation in vivo.[23] Angiogenesis during wound healing and angiogenesis during cancer are so similar that some researchers have described cancer as a "wound that will not heal." [25, 26] Not surprisingly, one study observed that when tumor cells were implanted into injured tissue in rodents, normal wound healing was inhibited, and an open, persistent wound developed that continued to form blood vessels.[23] The primary difference between tumor angiogenesis and wound angiogenesis is that the former is driven by abnormal signals and continues unabated,

TABLE 7.1   PARTIAL LISTING OF ANGIOGENIC FACTORS
ANGIOGENIC FACTOR
Basic fibroblast growth factor (bFGF)
Detrimental eicosanoids (such as prostaglandin E_2)
Fibrin (and plasmin)
Histamine
Insulin
Lactic acid
Tumor necrosis factor (TNF) (at low concentrations)
Vascular endothelial growth factor (VEGF)
Sources: References 14, 20–22, and 53.

whereas the latter is driven by normal fluctuations in signals and terminates when it is no longer needed in the healing process.

WOUND HEALING AND ANGIOGENIC FACTORS

The repair of wounds involves blood coagulation (blood clot formation), inflammation, and the formation of new connective tissue. Each of these processes produces factors that stimulate angiogenesis. To better understand the role of these processes in angiogenesis, we consider their role in wound healing, referring to their role tumor angiogenesis when appropriate.

For convenience, we can consider wound healing to occur in four separate stages with some overlaps:

1. In the first stage, activated platelets form a temporary plug to stop blood flow. In addition, inflammation is induced by compounds that escape from the blood, are produced by damaged tissues, or are produced by local immune cells (mostly basophils).

2. In the second stage, additional immune cells are recruited to the wound site, first neutrophils and then macrophages. Immune cells are attracted by the inflammatory compounds present, and their movement is aided by the edema and increased vascular permeability produced as part of inflammation. Subsequently, compounds released from the recruited neutrophils and macrophages further promote inflammation. Angiogenesis begins in this second stage, partly due to compounds released by macrophages.

3. In the third stage, the effects of fibrin deposition become prominent. Fibrin is a fibrous protein that strengthens the platelet blood clot. Inflammation and angiogenesis continue through this third stage.

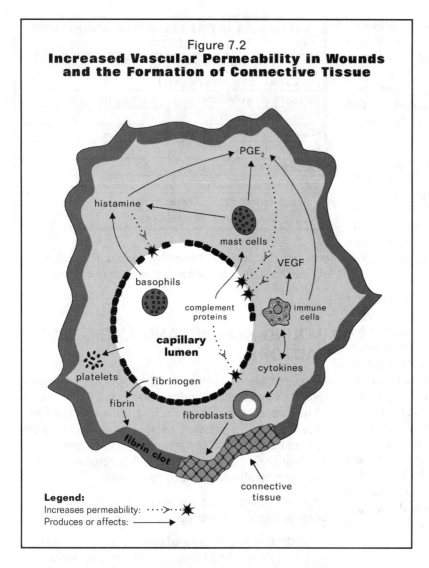

Figure 7.2
Increased Vascular Permeability in Wounds and the Formation of Connective Tissue

Legend:
Increases permeability: ·····>···✳
Produces or affects: ————>

illaries become "leaky" and allow certain blood components to escape into the extracellular space. This creates localized swelling, or edema. Increased vascular permeability is a very important requirement for angiogenesis and in fact may be its rate-limiting step. Increased vascular permeability is initially induced by the release of histamine from circulating immune cells (basophils) and ruptured or activated mast cells. (Mast cells are basophils that reside in connective tissue.) Increased permeability is further induced by blood components that leave the vessel to enter the extracellular space. One group of these blood components consists of proteins of the complement system, a series of proteins produced during an immune response that help immune cells search out and destroy foreign particles. In so doing, they stimulate mast cells to release more histamine.

As edema progresses, additional compounds are released that further increase vascular permeability. Figure 7.2 shows some of these compounds, as well as the formation of a fibrin clot and connective tissue that will be discussed later. Two of these compounds, VEGF and prostaglandin E_2 (PGE$_2$), are treated in more detail below, along with other eicosanoids (compounds related to PGE$_2$).

4. In the fourth stage, connective tissue replaces the fibrin clot, inflammation recedes, and angiogenesis stops. The new blood vessels formed in the previous two stages supply the new tissues with nutrients and oxygen.

A somewhat similar scenario occurs at tumor sites; however, the healing process there becomes stuck in the second and third stages. Under these conditions, immune reaction and inflammation are chronic and promote excessive angiogenesis and tumor progression, especially if the immune response is muted by tumor-induced immunosuppressive compounds, which it usually is. Since the healing process does not fully proceed to the fourth stage, angiogenesis continues indefinitely. All four stages are now discussed in more detail.

First Stage of Wound Healing

During the first stage of inflammation, blood vessels dilate and vascular permeability increases. That is, cap-

VEGF

Vascular endothelial growth factor is a protein 50,000 times more active than histamine in enhancing vascular permeability.[25] VEGF is very similar to, if not identical with, vascular permeability factor (VPF), and it is one of the most potent and important mediators of increased vascular permeability during angiogenesis.[13, 25] In a series of studies, antibodies specific to VEGF reduced angiogenesis and almost completely inhibited the growth and metastasis of transplanted human tumors in mice.[27, 28] In addition to production by activated immune cells, some cancers can make VEGF, as has been demonstrated in human colorectal cancers.[29] Recent studies suggest that high plasma concentrations of VEGF can be used to diagnose some forms of cancer or their recurrence.[30]

PGE₂ and Other Eicosanoids

Eicosanoids are 20-carbon polyunsaturated fatty acids such as arachidonic acid, EPA (from fish oil), and their derivatives. We are interested here in their derivatives—the prostanoids and leukotrienes, and the term *eicosanoids* will hereafter refer exclusively to these two.

The body produces a variety of prostanoids and leukotrienes that affect a wide range of functions: blood pressure, gastric secretion, platelet aggregation, tension of the intestinal and uterine muscles, inflammation, hormone production, pain sensation, and induction of labor. Eicosanoids are very potent substances—as little as one billionth of a gram can have measurable biological effects. Eicosanoids are actually produced by many cell types according to their immediate need and are not stored. Once synthesized, they quickly degrade in the body, which means they can act only on nearby cells. The production of many eicosanoids is initiated in response to inflammatory stimuli, such as the histamine and cytokines produced by immune cells.

Prostanoids include prostaglandins and thromboxanes. Prostaglandins, the first eicosanoids to be recognized, derive their name from the prostate gland, where scientists at first thought they were produced. Some prostaglandins, particularly prostaglandin E₂ (PGE₂), potently increase vascular permeability. PGE₂ also suppresses immune cell activity, probably as a negative feedback mechanism to prevent excessive immune response and resultant tissue damage. Solid tumors are known to produce excessive amounts of PGE₂, which may help them induce angiogenesis, proliferate, and evade immune attack. Thromboxanes, the other type of prostanoid, function in blood clotting (platelet aggregation). Most leukotrienes, the other type of eicosanoid, also induce inflammation, and they too can be produced by tumor cells.

Eicosanoid (Prostanoid and Leukotriene) Synthesis

Eicosanoids are produced by enzymes acting on the fatty acids stored in the lipid bilayer, the plasma membrane of cells (see Figure 2.1). One group of enzymes

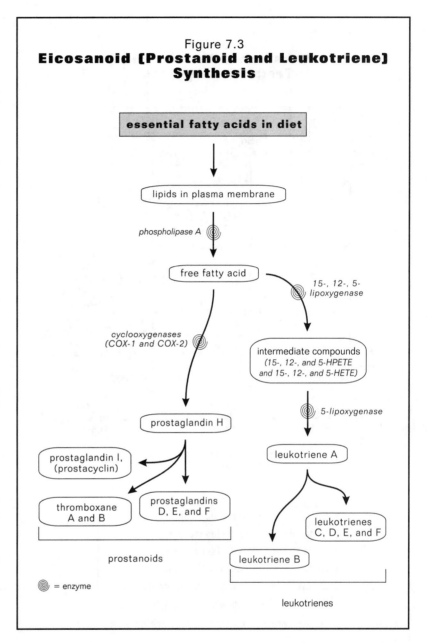

Figure 7.3
Eicosanoid [Prostanoid and Leukotriene] Synthesis

(phospholipases) releases the fatty acids from the cell wall, then other enzyme groups (cyclooxygenases and lipoxygenases) convert the free fatty acids either to prostanoids or leukotrienes. This process is illustrated in Figure 7.3 (adapted from reference 31). Although many different prostanoids and leukotrienes appear in the figure, the figure's primary purpose is simply to show that cyclooxygenases and lipoxygenases produce prostanoids and leukotrienes, respectively, from free fatty acids liberated from the cell membrane.

Note that two forms of cyclooxygenase exist, referred to as cyclooxygenase 1 and 2 (COX-1 and COX-2). Whereas COX-1 mostly produces prostanoids that regulate normal tissue homeostasis, including gastrointestinal homeostasis, COX-2 produces prostanoids that

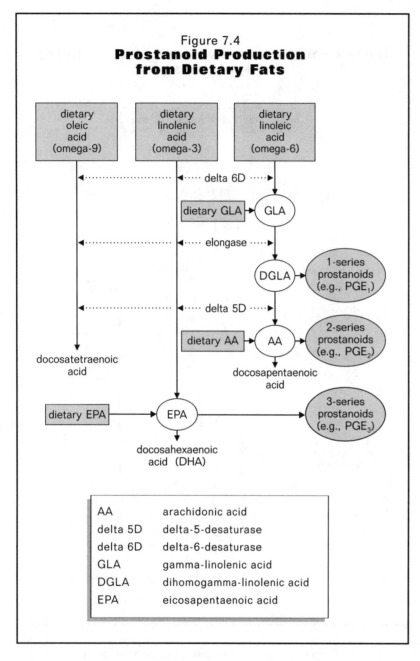

Figure 7.4
**Prostanoid Production
from Dietary Fats**

AA	arachidonic acid
delta 5D	delta-5-desaturase
delta 6D	delta-6-desaturase
GLA	gamma-linolenic acid
DGLA	dihomogamma-linolenic acid
EPA	eicosapentaenoic acid

fatty acids and the omega-3 fatty acids, both of which are discussed more in Chapter 17.

Omega-6 fatty acids include arachidonic acid, which is obtained from animal fats, and linoleic acid, which is obtained from most vegetable oils (corn oil, for example). The prostanoids that form from arachidonic acid are given the subscript 2 (for example, PGE_2), and the leukotrienes are given the subscript 4 (LTB_4). These eicosanoids tend to be inflammatory, and many can promote angiogenesis and progression. Since linoleic acid can be converted to arachidonic acid in vivo, linoleic acid can also produce 2-series prostanoids and 4-series leukotrienes and can promote angiogenesis and cancer progression.

Omega-3 fatty acids include alpha-linolenic from flaxseed oil and EPA from fish oil. The prostanoids that form from omega-3 fatty acids have the subscript 3 (PGE_3), and leukotrienes, the subscript 5 (LTB_5). In contrast to those produced from arachidonic acid and linoleic acid, these eicosanoids tend to be anti-inflammatory (or much less inflammatory than those from arachidonic acid), and they tend to inhibit angiogenesis and cancer progression.[33]

The production of eicosanoids from different fatty acids and the enzymes that form them are illustrated in Figure 7.4 (adapted from references 34 and 35). Note that omega-9 fatty acids, such as found in olive oil, do not contribute to prostanoid production. Unlike omega-6 fatty acids, omega-9 fatty acids have not been linked to cancer progression, but they also do not appear to inhibit cancer, as do omega-3 fatty acids. Their effects on cancer are therefore considered neutral. Although the production of leukotrienes is not shown in the figure, arachidonic acid produces 4-series leukotrienes and EPA produces 5-series ones.

Since the eicosanoids produced from omega-3 fatty acids reduce inflammation and inhibit angiogenesis and other aspects of cancer progression, therapies that favor production of 3-series prostanoids and 5-series leukotrienes, as well as therapies that inhibit production of 2-series prostanoids and 4-series leukotrienes, appear to be useful. These therapies primarily consist of increasing the intake of omega-3 fatty acids and decreasing the in-

induce inflammation.[32] Because of its role in inflammation and cancer initiation and progression, we are most interested here in the effects of COX-2. Selective COX-2 inhibitors are preferable to those that inhibit both enzymes, since COX-1 inhibition can produce adverse gastrointestinal effects similar to those produced by nonselective anti-inflammatory drugs such as aspirin.

As mentioned above, fatty acids in the cell wall act as the building material for eicosanoids. Each type of fatty acid will produce a distinct series of eicosanoids, and depending on the series, some will promote angiogenesis and cancer progression, and others will inhibit angiogenesis and cancer progression. We are most interested in eicosanoids produced from the omega-6 take of arachidonic acid and other omega-6 fatty acids. In addition, inhibition of prostanoid and leukotriene synthesis in general can be produced by inhibitors of the cyclooxygenase and lipoxygenase enzymes. For example, drugs like aspirin and ibuprofen produce an anti-inflammatory effect in part by inhibiting cyclooxygenase. Natural compounds have been reported to inhibit cyclooxygenase or lipoxygenase or both. Their potential use in inhibiting angiogenesis is discussed in Chapter 8.

To return to the role of eicosanoids in wound healing, inflammatory eicosanoids produced from omega-6 fatty acids help attract immune cells to the wound and induce inflammation, thereby assisting the angiogenic process. Again, the production of these inflammatory eicosanoids is tightly regulated in normal angiogenesis but excessive and long lasting in tumor angiogenesis.

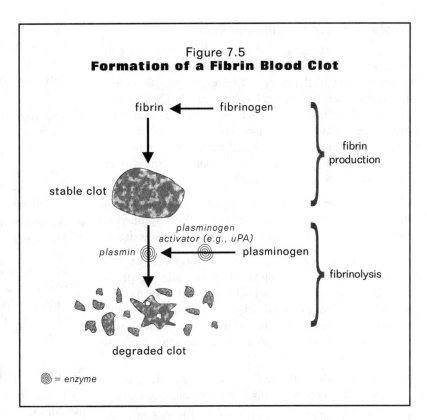

Figure 7.5
Formation of a Fibrin Blood Clot

Second Stage of Wound Healing

After dilation of blood vessels and formation of edema, the second stage in wound healing is immune cell migration, in particular migration of neutrophils and macrophages. Within an hour after the inflammatory response begins, neutrophils migrate toward the injury site. They are attracted partly by the previous release of prostanoids and leukotrienes. Neutrophils predominate in early stages of inflammation but tend to die off early. They are replaced by macrophages, which are large enough to engulf invading microbes, dead neutrophils, and necrotic tissue; macrophages are the most active and effective of the immune phagocytes (debris-eating cells).

The fact that macrophages predominate in this stage is important because they also produce TNF (tumor necrosis factor), growth factors, enzymes, and other related compounds. In normal wound healing, these compounds help kill pathogens, degrade damaged tissue, and stimulate the growth of vascular (endothelial) cells required for normal angiogenesis. In the case of cancer, however, these compounds can stimulate cancer cell proliferation, angiogenesis, invasion, and metastasis. Indeed, one study reported an increased risk of melanoma metastasis in mice after an intense inflammatory reaction.[36] In the next chapter, we discuss ways to inhibit the angiogenic effects of TNF and other growth factors produced by macrophages.

Third Stage of Wound Healing

In the first stage of wound healing, vascular permeability increased and blood platelets formed a temporary plug that inhibited bleeding. In the third stage, the platelet clot is reinforced by deposition of fibrin, a sticky fibrous protein that gives a blood clot strength. Fibrin deposition actually begins in the first stage of healing, but not until the third stage does it accumulate enough to become the major component of the clot. The process of blood clot formation during wound healing is complex, and only a few points critical to understanding angiogenesis are discussed below.

Fibrin is formed from the protein fibrinogen and is destroyed by the enzyme plasmin, which is formed from plasminogen (see Figure 7.5). The increased permeability of inflamed tissues allows fibrinogen to escape from the blood and enter the wound area, where it can form into a fibrin clot. The proteolytic enzyme plasmin breaks down the fibrin clot in a process called fibrinolysis. If all is working correctly, fibrinolysis and fibrin formation exist in a dynamic balance. Fibrin production prevails in the early stages of clot formation and fibrinolysis in the later stages, as new connective tissue forms to replace the fibrin clot.

Role of Fibrin in Angiogenesis

Recent research suggests that fibrin may play a role in wound-induced angiogenesis. Fibrin deposition occurs within minutes of the entry of fibrinogen and other clotting factors into the extracellular space. While fibrin is forming, the fibrinolytic system is stimulated and substantial destruction of fibrin occurs. In spite of this, fibrin production prevails, and sufficient fibrin eventually accumulates to produce a provisional fibrin stroma (structural framework) surrounding the wound.

The formation and eventual degradation of the fibrin stroma during the four stages of wound healing plays a role in at least three processes related to angiogenesis:

- The ongoing degradation of the fibrin clot by the enzyme plasmin produces fibrin degradation products (fibrin fragments) that stimulate angiogenesis.[37–43] As might be expected, angiogenesis is associated with increased production of urokinase plasminogen activator (uPA), an enzyme that facilitates plasmin production (see Figure 7.5).

- Immune cells infiltrate the stroma, and the growth factors they produce further stimulate angiogenesis.

- In the last stage of wound healing, fibroblasts infiltrate the stroma, and the connective tissue they produce replaces the fibrin that is being degraded. The presence of mature connective tissue, along with the lack of new fibrin deposition, helps create the correct conditions for angiogenesis finally to stop.

Formation of a fibrin stroma may be one of the most important preconditions for wound angiogenesis. Studies have reported that the removal of fibrin through severe fibrinolysis terminates wound angiogenesis.[43]

As in wound healing, a provisional fibrin stroma forms around a tumor, where it also facilitates angiogenesis.[25, 44, 45] Unlike normal wound healing, however, at a tumor site inflammation as well as fibrin production and degradation continue chronically. Instead of evolving into mature connective tissue, the fibrin stroma surrounding a tumor transforms into a chaotic mass of fibrin, immature blood vessels, and connective tissue in which fibrinolysis and angiogenesis persist. In fact, the levels of both fibrin formation and fibrin destruction are consistently elevated in patients with a variety of cancers.[46]

The ongoing production of the stroma may facilitate tumor growth in at least four ways:

- The fibrin stroma provides a structure that physically supports the tumor.[25] In the early stages of tumor growth, the fibrin stroma encases individual tumor cells or clumps of tumor cells. This process is seen even in nonsolid tumors such as lymphomas. These clumps remain discrete units as the tumor grows. Newer stroma is deposited on the periphery of the tumor as it grows. In total, the stroma in some tumors can comprise up to 90 percent of a tumor's mass.

- The fibrin stroma may shield the tumor cells from immune attack and therapeutic intervention.[47]

- The fibrin deposited on cancer cells helps promote successful metastasis. A sticky fibrin coating helps metastasizing cells adhere more securely to distant vasculature.

- As stated above, products of partial fibrin degradation stimulate angiogenesis. Tumor concentrations of uPA, an enzyme that promotes fibrin degradation and angiogenesis and is produced by both macrophages and tumor cells, is an independent prognostic indicator for breast cancer as well as stomach, colorectal, esophageal, kidney, endometrial, and ovarian cancers.[48]

Fourth Stage of Wound Healing

After a fibrin clot forms around a wound and foreign material is removed by macrophages, the clot is slowly dissolved by plasmin and replaced by connective tissue. Connective tissue is produced by cells called fibroblasts when they are stimulated by basic fibroblast growth factor (bFGF) and other factors. Since connective tissue is essential to produce new basement membranes for growing capillaries, bFGF is also a potent angiogenic factor. In fact, there appear to be at least two distinct routes of angiogenesis stimulation. The first is mediated primarily through bFGF and the second primarily through VEGF (although the other angiogenic factors discussed here also play a role).[49, 50] In addition to its effects on angiogenesis, bFGF is also a growth factor for cancer cell proliferation.[51]

As mentioned, tumors do not fully enter this fourth stage of wound healing; they remain as chronic wounds, and the damaged tissues surrounding them are not replaced by new, healthy, connective tissue. Nonetheless, bFGF does have a role in tumor angiogenesis; it can be released by tissue injury, including injury caused by enzymes freed during inflammation and tumor invasion. Current research suggests that before tissue injury, bFGF and many other angiogenic factors are safely bound within the extracellular matrix (ECM). Tissue injury stimulates the secretion of enzymes that degrade the ECM and thereby liberate the bound factors.[20, 52, 53] In fact, nearly 37 percent of cancer patients have bFGF levels 100 to 200 times higher than normal.[54] The binding and release of bFGF from the ECM is illustrated in

Figure 7.6. In some cases, bFGF may also be secreted directly by immune cells and tumor cells.

One of the primary matrix components that binds bFGF and other angiogenic factors is heparan sulfate. The binding of bFGF and other angiogenic factors by heparan sulfate or other ECM components is important, because natural compounds can be used to maintain proper binding. For example, they can be used to strengthen the ECM against enzymatic degradation, to inhibit the enzymes that degrade the ECM, and to inhibit inflammation that may facilitate the release of bound growth factors. By preventing the release of bound growth factors, natural compounds have the potential not only to inhibit angiogenesis but also invasion and cancer cell proliferation. Natural compounds that protect the ECM or inhibit ECM-degrading enzymes are discussed in Chapter 9.

Lactic Acid, Insulin, and Angiogenesis

We end this chapter with a brief discussion of the relationship between lactic acid, insulin, and angiogenesis in wound healing and cancer. As mentioned earlier, vascular cells proliferate and migrate toward an angiogenic stimulus, usually toward a low-oxygen (hypoxic) environment. In wound healing, hypoxia occurs from a lack of blood circulation in the traumatized area. In tumors, hypoxic conditions occur both through inflammation, which reduces blood flow, and the chaotic development of blood vessels within tumors.

Hypoxic environments alter the pathway by which immune cells and tumor cells burn fuel (specifically, glucose) for energy. The result of hypoxia is that affected cells produce excessive lactic acid, which is an angiogenic factor. Under aerobic, or oxygen-rich, conditions, glucose is burned in an efficient process that produces a maximal amount of energy and a minimal amount of lactic acid. Under hypoxic conditions, however, glucose is burned in an inefficient process that produces a small amount of energy and a large amount of lactic acid (see Figure 7.7). Note that lactic acid is an angiogenic factor because it causes macrophages to secrete other angiogenic factors.[55]

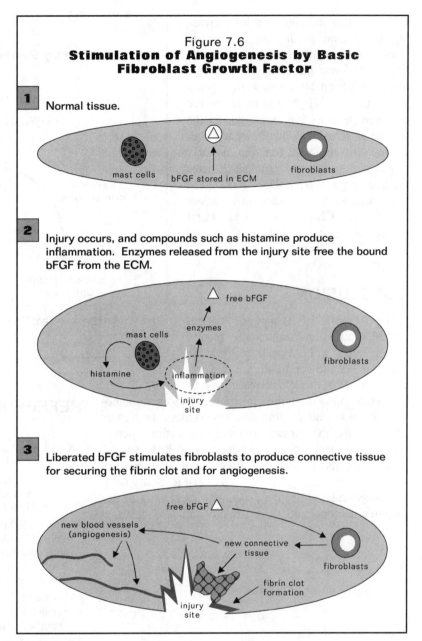

Figure 7.6
Stimulation of Angiogenesis by Basic Fibroblast Growth Factor

1 Normal tissue.

mast cells   bFGF stored in ECM   fibroblasts

2 Injury occurs, and compounds such as histamine produce inflammation. Enzymes released from the injury site free the bound bFGF from the ECM.

free bFGF

enzymes

mast cells

histamine   inflammation   fibroblasts

injury site

3 Liberated bFGF stimulates fibroblasts to produce connective tissue for securing the fibrin clot and for angiogenesis.

free bFGF

new blood vessels (angiogenesis)

new connective tissue

fibroblasts

fibrin clot formation

injury site

In tumor cells, the chronic hypoxic conditions cause excessive production of lactic acid and a prolonged inefficient utilization of glucose. The reduced energy output stimulates tumor cells to burn more glucose, which makes even more lactic acid. Thus the glycolysis (glucose-burning) pathway is greatly stimulated in tumor cells. Tumor cells consume glucose at a rate three to five times higher than normal cells.[56, 57] Not only can this waste the energy reserves of a cancer patient, but as stated, the lactic acid produced can stimulate macrophages to produce more angiogenic factors.[20]

One growth factor that is intimately involved in glycolysis is insulin. Insulin stimulates not only glycolysis but also proliferation of many cancer cell lines.[54, 58–60] It may facilitate angiogenesis by increasing lactic acid production in hypoxic tumor cells and by stimulating the proliferation of vascular cells. For example, insulin injection can increase angiogenesis in mice.[61] High insulin levels are common in cancerous tissue and in the plasma of cancer patients.[62] In addition, the high insulin levels found in the early stages of non-insulin-dependent diabetes mellitus type II (NIDDM) have been implicated as a risk factor for a variety of cancers.[63] Chapter 8 discusses natural compounds that can reduce lactic acid and insulin production.

CONCLUSION

Angiogenesis is a part of natural wound healing, and tumors also require angiogenesis. In both cases, many of the same factors and conditions are at work; central to all of these is increased vascular permeability and inflammation. However, angiogenesis in wound healing and angiogenesis in tumors differ in that the former lasts only for a finite period while tumor angiogenesis proceeds unchecked. By understanding the factors that drive tumor angiogenesis, we can begin to design therapies that halt it. Many natural compounds inhibit the production or activity of angiogenic factors, and these are the topic of the next chapter.

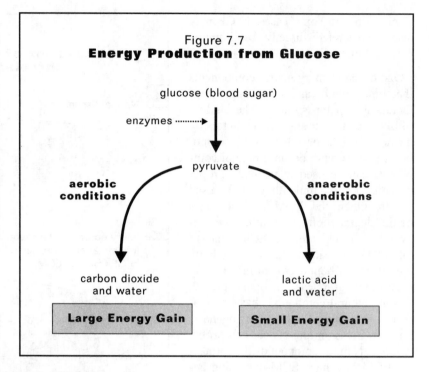

Figure 7.7
Energy Production from Glucose

REFERENCES

[1] Kerbel RS. Tumor angiogenesis: Past, present and the near future. Carcinogenesis 2000 Mar; 21(3):505–15.

[2] Brewer GJ, Dick RD, Grover DK, et al. Treatment of metastatic cancer with tetrathiomolybdate, and anticopper, antiangiogenic agent: Phase I study. Clin Cancer Res 2000; 6:1–10.

[3] Majewski S, Marczak M, Szmurlo A, et al. Retinoids, interferon alpha, 1,25-dihydroxyvitamin D3 and their combination inhibit angiogenesis induced by non-HPV-harboring tumor cell lines. RAR alpha mediates the antiangiogenic effect of retinoids. Cancer Lett 1995 Feb 10; 89(1):117–24.

[4] Majewski S, Skopinska M, Marczak M, et al. Vitamin D3 is a potent inhibitor of tumor cell-induced angiogenesis. J Investig Dermatol Symp Proc 1996; 1(1):97–101.

[5] Zhou JR, Mukherjee P, Gugger ET, et al. Inhibition of murine bladder tumorigenesis by soy isoflavones via alterations in the cell cycle, apoptosis, and angiogenesis. Cancer Res 1998 Nov 15; 58(22):5231–8.

[6] Joseph IB, Isaacs JT. Macrophage role in the anti-prostate cancer response to one class of antiangiogenic agents. J Natl Cancer Inst 1998 Nov 4; 90(21):1648–53.

[7] Bhargava P, Marshall JL, Rizvi N, et al. A phase I and pharmacokinetic study of TNP-470 administered weekly to patients with advanced cancer. Clin Cancer Res 1999 Aug; 5(8):1989–95.

[8] Kudelka AP, Levy T, Verschraegen CF, et al. A phase I study of TNP-470 administered to patients with advanced squamous cell cancer of the cervix. Clin Cancer Res 1997 Sep; 3(9):1501–5.

[9] Joseph IB, Vukanovic J, Isaacs JT. Antiangiogenic treatment with linomide as chemoprevention for prostate, seminal

vesicle, and breast carcinogenesis in rodents. Cancer Res 1996 Aug 1; 56(15):3404–8.

[10] Eckhardt SG, Burris HA, Eckardt JR, et al. A phase I clinical and pharmacokinetic study of the angiogenesis inhibitor, tecogalan sodium. Ann Oncol 1996 Jul; 7(5):491–6.

[11] Folkman J, Hochberg M. Self-regulation of growth in three dimensions. J Exp Med 1973 Oct 1; 138(4):745-53.

[12] Lu C, Tanigawa N. Spontaneous apoptosis is inversely related to intratumoral microvessel density in gastric carcinoma. Cancer Research 1997 Jan 15; 57:221–224.

[13] Scott PA, Harris A. Current approaches to targeting cancer using antiangiogenesis therapies. Cancer Treatment Reviews 1994; 20:393–412.

[14] Denekamp J. Review article: Angiogenesis, neovascular proliferation and vascular pathophysiology as targets for cancer therapy. British Journal of Radiology 1993; 66:181–96.

[15] Paper DH. Natural products as angiogenesis inhibitors. Planta Medica 1998; 64:686–695.

[16] Folkman J. The vascularization of tumors. Sci Amer 1976; 234(5):58–64, 70–3.

[17] Jain RK. Vascular and interstitial barriers to delivery of therapeutic agents in tumors. Cancer Metastasis Rev 1990 Nov; 9(3):253–66.

[18] Folkman J. Angiogenesis and angiogenesis inhibition: An overview. EXS 1997; 79:1–8.

[19] Folkman J. Angiogenesis in cancer, vascular, rheumatoid and other disease. Nat Med 1995 Jan; 1(1):27–31.

[20] Folkman J. Tumor angiogenesis. In *Cancer medicine*. 3rd ed. Holland JF, Frei E, Bast RG, et al., eds. Philadelphia: Lea & Febiger, 1993, pp. 153–170.

[21] Polverini PJ. The pathophysiology of angiogenesis. Crit Rev Oral Biol Med 1995; 6(3):230–47.

[22] Yamagishi S, Kawakami T, Fujimori H, et al. Insulin stimulates the growth and tube formation of human microvascular endothelial cells through autocrine vascular endothelial growth factor. Microvasc Res 1999 May; 57(3):329–39.

[23] Abramovitch R, Marikovsky M, Meir G, Neeman M. Stimulation of tumour growth by wound-derived growth factors. Br J Cancer 1999 Mar; 79(9–10):1392–8.

[24] Abramovitch R, Marikovsky M, Meir G, Neeman M. Stimulation of tumour angiogenesis by proximal wounds: Spatial and temporal analysis by MRI. Br J Cancer 1998; 77(3):440–7.

[25] Nagy JA, Brown LF, Senger DR, et al. Pathogenesis of tumor stroma generation: A critical role for leaky blood vessels and fibrin deposition. Biochim Biophys Acta 1989; 948(3):305–26.

[26] Haddow A. Molecular repair, wound healing, and carcinogenesis: Tumor production a possible overhealing? Adv Cancer Res 1972; 16:181–234.

[27] Kim KJ, Li B, Winer J, et al. Inhibition of vascular endothelial growth factor-induced angiogenesis suppresses tumour growth in vivo. Nature 1993; 362:841–4.

[28] Asano M, Yukita A, Matsumoto T, et al. Inhibition of tumor growth and metastasis by an immunoneutralizing monoclonal antibody to human vascular endothelial growth factor/vascular permeability factor 121. Cancer Research 1995 Nov 15; 55:5296–5301.

[29] Nakata S, Ito K, Fujimori M, et al. Involvement of vascular endothelial growth factor and urokinase-type plasminogen activator receptor in microvessel invasion in human colorectal cancers. Int J Cancer 1998 Apr 17; 79(2):179–86.

[30] Fuhrmann-Benzakein E, Ma MN, Rubbia-Brandt L, et al. Elevated levels of angiogenic cytokines in the plasma of cancer patients. Int J Cancer 2000 Jan 1; 85(1):40–5.

[31] Hostettmann K, et al., eds. Phytochemistry of plants used in traditional medicine. New York: Oxford University Press, 1995. Figure 6.3.

[32] Lipsky PE. Specific COX-2 inhibitors in arthritis, oncology, and beyond: Where is the science headed? J Rheumatol 1999 Apr; 26 Suppl 56:25–30.

[33] Hammarstrom S. Leukotriene C5: A slow reacting substance derived from eicosapentaenoic acid. J Biol Chem 1980 Aug 10; 255(15):7093–4.

[34] Booyens J, Maguire. Dietary fats and cancer. Med Hypotheses 1985; 17:351–362.

[35] Linder MC, ed. Nutritional biochemistry and metabolism. 2nd ed. New York: Elsevier Science, 1991, p. 60.

[36] Ellis LM, Fidler IJ. Angiogenesis and metastasis. European J Cancer 1996; 32A(14):2451–2460.

[37] Thompson WD, Smith EB, Stirk CM, et al. Angiogenic activity of fibrin degradation products is located in fibrin fragment E. UK J Pathol 1992; 168(1):47–53.

[38] Thompson WD, Harvey JA, Kazmi MA, et al. Fibrinolysis and angiogensis in wound healing. UK J Pathol 1991; 165(4):311–8.

[39] Thompson WD, Smith EB, Stirk CM, et al. Atherosclerotic plaque growth: Presence of stimulatory fibrin degradation products. Blood Caogul Fibrinolysis 1990; 1(4–5):489–93.

[40] Thompson WD, Smith EB, Stirk CM, et al. Factors relevant to stimulatory activity of fibrin degradation products in vivo. Blood Coagul Fibrinolysis 1990; 1(4–5):517–20.

[41] Liu HM, Wang DL, Liu CY. Interactions between fibrin, collagen and endothelial cells in angiogenesis. Adv Exp Med Biol 1990; 281:3 19–31.

[42] Dvorak HF, Harvey VS, Estrella P, et al. Fibrin containing gels induce angiogenesis. Lab Invest 1987; 57 (6):673–86.

[43] Liu HM. Wound chamber study of nerve and blood vessel growth. Proc Natl Sci Counc Repub China 1992; 16(1):65–9.

[44] Brown LF, Dvorak AM, Dvorak HF, et al. Leaky vessels, fibrin deposition, and fibrosis: A sequence of events common to solid tumors and to many other types of disease. Am Rev Respir Dis 1989; 140(4):1104–7.

[45] Beranek JT. Ingrowth of hypoplastic capillary sprouts into fibrin clots: Further evidence in favor of the angiogenic hypothesis of repair and fibrosis. Med Hypotheses 1989; 28(4):271–3.

[46] Sagripanti A, Carpi A, Baicchi U, Grassi B. Plasmatic parameters of fibrin formation and degradation in cancer patients: Correlation between fibrinopeptide A and D-dimer. Biomed Pharmacother 1993; 47(6–7):235–9.

[47] Gasic GJ. Role of plasma, platelets, and endothelial cells in tumor metastasis. Cancer Metastasis Rev 1984; 3(2):99–114.

[48] Duffy MJ, Maguire TM, McDermott EW, O'Higgins N. Urokinase plasminogen activator: A prognostic marker in multiple types of cancer. J Surg Oncol 1999 Jun; 71(2):130–5.

[49] Friedlander M, Brooks PC, Shaffer RW, et al. Definition of two angiogenic pathways by distinct alpha v integrins. Science 1995 Dec 1; 270(5241):1500–2.

[50] Samoto K, Ikezaki K, Ono M, et al. Expression of vascular endothelial growth factor and its possible relation with neovascularization in human brain tumors. Cancer Res 1995 Mar 1; 55(5):1189–93.

[51] Liuzzo JP, Moscatelli D. Human leukemia cell lines bind basic fibroblast growth factor (FGF) on FGF receptors and heparan sulfates: Downmodulation of FGF receptors by phorbol ester. Blood 1996 Jan 1; 87(1):245–55.

[52] Folkman J, Klagsburn M. Angiogenic factors. Science 1987; 235:442–7.

[53] Norrby K. Angiogenesis: New aspects relating to its initiation and control. APMIS 1997; 105:417–437.

[54] Lupulescu A. The role of hormones, growth factors and vitamins in carcinogenesis. Crit Rev Oncol Hematol 1996 Jun; 23(2):95–130.

[55] Jensen JA, Hunt TK, Scheuenstuhl H, Banda MJ. Effect of lactate, pyruvate, and pH on secretion of angiogenesis and mitogenesis factors by macrophages. Lab Invest 1986 May; 54(5):574–8.

[56] Mahnensmith RL, Aronson PS. The plasma membrane sodium-hydrogen exchanger and its role in physiological and pathophysiological processes. Circ Res 1985; 56(6):773–88.

[57] Demetrakopoulos GE, Brennan MF. Tumoricidal potential of nutritional manipulations. Cancer Res (Suppl) 1982; 42:756s-65s.

[58] Lupulescu AP. Hormones, vitamins, and growth factors in cancer treatment and prevention. A critical appraisal. Cancer 1996 Dec 1; 78(11):2264–80.

[59] Corpet DE, Jacquinet C, Peiffer G, Tache S. Insulin injections promote the growth of aberrant crypt foci in the colon of rats. Nutrition and Cancer 1997; 27(3):316–320.

[60] Pearline RV, Lin YZ, Shen KJ, et al. Alterations in enzymatic functions in hepatocytes and hepatocellular carcinomas from Ras-transduced livers resemble the effects of insulin. Hepatology 1996 Oct; 24(4):838–48.

[61] Kimura M, Amemiya K, Suzuki J. Insulin-induced granuloma tissue formation and angiogenesis in alloxan-treated diabetic mice. Endocrinol Jpn 1987 Feb; 34(1):55–63.

[62] Yam D, Ben-Hur H, Dgani R, et al. Subcutaneous, omentum and tumor fatty acid composition, and serum insulin status in patients with benign or cancerous ovarian or endometrial tumors. Do tumors preferentially utilize polyunsaturated fatty acids? Cancer Letters 1997; 111:179–185.

[63] Moore MA, Park CB, Tsuda H. Implications of the hyperinsulinaemia-diabetes-cancer link for preventive efforts. Eur J Cancer Prev 1998; 7(2):89–107.

8

NATURAL INHIBITORS OF ANGIOGENESIS

After examining the basic mechanisms of angiogenesis in Chapter 7 and identifying a number of angiogenic factors, this chapter discusses the role that natural compounds could play in reducing tumor angiogenesis. Several angiogenic factors produce increased vascular permeability and/or inflammation, and both these events, in turn, increase production or release of other angiogenic factors. Angiogenic factors include vascular endothelial growth factor (VEGF); eicosanoids such as PGE_2 that derive from omega-6 fatty acids; tumor necrosis factor (TNF); fibrin; basic fibroblast growth factor (bFGF); and histamine, insulin, and lactic acid. Here we identify a number of natural compounds that block the abnormal production or activity of angiogenic factors; many of these compounds also decrease vascular permeability and inflammation. We also discuss natural compounds that inhibit angiogenesis by still other means.

INHIBITION OF ANGIOGENIC FACTORS

Vascular Endothelial Growth Factor

As mentioned in Chapter 7, the rate-limiting step in angiogenesis seems to be increased vascular permeability, and vascular endothelial growth factor (VEGF), one of the most potent inducers of permeability known, plays a key role in angiogenesis. Not surprisingly, some studies have reported that plasma concentrations of VEGF are predictive of recurrence and survival in cancer patients.[1] In addition to increased angiogenesis, high concentrations of VEGF have also been associated with increased metastasis of a variety of cancers.[2, 3, 4] Increased metastasis is likely a byproduct of increased angiogenesis, since metastasis will not happen until angiogenesis has occurred.

There are two conceivable means to reduce VEGF-mediated angiogenesis. The first is to reduce VEGF production, and the second is to reduce the end effect of VEGF, which is increased vascular permeability itself.

Inhibition of VEGF Production

VEGF is produced in response to hypoxic (low-oxygen) conditions, which are prevalent within tumors. It is also produced secondarily in response to the production of other growth factors, such as platelet-derived growth factor (PDGF), epidermal growth factor (EGF), tumor necrosis factor (TNF), and transforming growth factor-beta (TGF-beta).[5–10] Indeed, one study reported that wound fluid stimulated tumor growth and angiogenesis in vivo, and that PDGF and EGF contained in the fluid were apparently responsible for the effect.[11] Most likely, PDGF and EGF stimulated the production of VEGF, which led to angiogenesis. Thus by inhibiting the production or activity of PDGF, EGF, TNF, or TGF-beta, it may be possible to decrease production of VEGF and its stimulating effect on angiogenesis.

A major source of PDGF, EGF, and TNF within solid tumors is macrophages. The production of these and other growth factors by macrophages is discussed later in this chapter, as well as the effects of hypoxia on macrophages and VEGF production, but note here that antioxidants, PTK inhibitors, PKC inhibitors, and leukotriene inhibitors may all reduce production of VEGF by macrophages or other cells in response to growth factors or hypoxia. In addition, inhibitors of AP-1 may also block VEGF production, as has been reported for curcumin.[12]

Reduced production of VEGF has been reported, for example, with genistein, a PTK inhibitor, and EPA, a PKC inhibitor, in vitro and ex vivo.[13–18, a] Reduced production of VEGF has been reported in vivo with selenium, a PKC inhibitor. In one study, oral administration of about 3.6 milligrams of selenium per day (as scaled to humans) for seven weeks reduced angiogenesis in rats with breast cancer.[19] VEGF concentrations in tumor tissue were reduced, presumably due to reduced production by macrophages. In support of the types of synergistic combinations discussed in this book, recent evidence suggests that combinations of VEGF inhibitors, for example, PTK and PKC inhibitors, may be more effective than single therapies at reducing VEGF production.[20]

It should come as no surprise that PTK inhibitors would reduce the stimulatory effects of growth factors such as EGF and PDGF on VEGF production. Recall from Table 4.1 that receptors for most growth factors, including EGF and PDGF, are protein tyrosine kinases. Indeed, PTK inhibitors such as EGCG, curcumin, CAPE, and genistein have been reported to reduce EGF and PDGF signaling in a variety of cells.[21–27]

---

[a] *In ex-vivo studies, compounds are administered in vivo, then the blood or blood cells are withdrawn and tested in vitro.*

TABLE 8.1 NATURAL COMPOUNDS THAT INHIBIT INCREASED VASCULAR PERMEABILITY
COMPOUND
Anthocyanidins
Butcher's broom
Centella asiatica
Horse chestnut
Proanthocyanidins
Note: See Table F.1 in Appendix F for details and references.

Some studies have looked specifically at the anti-angiogenic properties of genistein. Genistein (at 13 µM) is an effective inhibitor of endothelial cell proliferation (vascular cells are endothelial cells).[28] Also, genistein was identified as the most potent compound in the angiogenesis-inhibiting urine of healthy humans who consumed a plant-based diet.[29, 30] At least three animal studies have reported that genistein can inhibit angiogenesis and tumor growth in vivo.[31, 32, 33] One, an oral study, also reported that genistein reduced the number of tumor-associated macrophages.[32] It is likely this effect played a role in reducing angiogenesis, since this would reduce the source of many angiogenic factors. In another in-vivo study, a combination of genistein (at 100 mg/kg intraperitoneal) and an antiangiogenic drug (TNP-470), along with a variety of cytotoxic chemotherapy drugs and radiotherapy, was more effective at inhibiting tumor growth in mice with implanted lung tumors than either genistein or TNP-470 used separately with chemotherapy or radiotherapy. Even without TNP-470, genistein reduced angiogenesis in the tumors by about 35 to 51 percent.[34, 35] The human oral equivalent of the genistein dose is about 4.5 grams per day.

Other flavonoids, which are also PTK inhibitors, may be as potent as genistein. At 10 µM, genistein, luteolin, and apigenin inhibited in-vitro angiogenesis by 60 to 75 percent. The IC_{50} for inhibition of endothelial cell proliferation was about 2 to 7 µM.[36]

As with PTK inhibitors, it is not surprising that PKC inhibitors would reduce the stimulatory effects of growth factors such as EGF and PDGF on VEGF production. As discussed in Chapter 4 (see Figure 4.3), signal transduction cascades tend to be interrelated. For example, stimulation of a PTK receptor on the cell surface (such as the EGF or PDGF receptor) can later stimulate PKC within the cell. Thus inhibitors of PKC can block some effects of PTK receptor activity. For example, EPA reduced EGF and PDGF signaling and reduced angiogenesis in vitro.[13, 37–40]

PKC and PTK inhibitors may also act through other means to reduce angiogenesis, apart from decreasing

VEGF production, since PKC and PTK signaling control many aspects of cell behavior. For example, PKC inhibitors may reduce angiogenesis in part by lowering production of collagenases, which are enzymes involved in tumor invasion (discussed in Chapter 9).[41] Other types of collagenase inhibitors also reduce angiogenesis.[42, 43] They are effective because both invasion and angiogenesis have some events in common (vascular cells must invade through tissues during angiogenesis).[44, 45] Lastly, PKC inhibitors may also reduce angiogenesis by decreasing histamine release by mast cells and by lowering insulin resistance, as is discussed below.

Before leaving this discussion on VEGF and the growth factors that stimulate its production, note that some natural compounds may directly interfere with growth factors or their receptors. For example, EGCG inhibited the binding of EGF to its receptors, and high-molecular-weight polysaccharides such as PSK inhibited the binding of TGF-beta to its receptors.[24, 46] In addition, EPA inhibited the binding of PDGF to its receptor.[47]

Normalization of Vascular Permeability

A second possible method to reduce VEGF-induced angiogenesis is to minimize the primary effect of VEGF: increased vascular permeability. Again, increased vascular permeability at tumor sites facilitates inflammation and the release or eventual production of angiogenic compounds. Numerous natural compounds have been reported to decrease vascular permeability in animals and humans. Some of these compounds are listed in Table 8.1. Although this approach of normalizing vascular permeability seems reasonable, it has not been investigated in any depth; this book is one of the first to suggest it may be useful.

Eicosanoids (Prostanoids and Leukotrienes)

Eicosanoids were introduced in Chapter 7. There we focused on how prostanoids and leukotrienes are produced from fatty acids, namely via the cyclooxygenase and lipoxygenase pathways, respectively. We also looked at how different fatty acids in the membrane produce different series of prostanoids and leukotrienes, then noted that eicosanoids derived from omega-6 fatty acids facilitate cancer progression and eicosanoids from omega-3 fatty acids inhibit it. We focus here on the role eicosanoids play in angiogenesis and other aspects of cancer progression, as well as on natural compound's ability to inhibit the production of detrimental eicosanoids or increase that of beneficial ones.

When produced in appropriate amounts and at appropriate times, eicosanoids play a positive role in the body; when they are produced inappropriately, however, they can play a variety of roles in the initiation, promotion, and progression of cancer. Some observed relationships between eicosanoids and cancer include:[48–54]

- Malignant cells synthesize excessive levels of prostaglandins, especially PGE_2. Elevated levels of prostaglandins have been detected in the blood and urine of tumor-bearing animals. This not only increases inflammation and angiogenesis but can also increase cancer cell proliferation.

- Diets high in omega-6 fatty acids (for example, those high in vegetable oil) promote prostaglandin (PGE_2) synthesis and stimulate tumor progression. The tumor-promoting effects of high-fat diets can be reduced by inhibitors of prostaglandin synthesis.[55, 56]

- Prostanoids may mediate angiogenesis. Cyclooxygenase inhibitors reduced angiogenesis and tumor progression in vivo, apparently by blocking VEGF and bFGF production.[57–60] The ability of COX-2 inhibitors to reduce angiogenesis is particularly apparent.[61] Moreover, tumor cells lacking the ability to express COX-2 proliferate very slowly in vivo.[62]

- Leukotrienes may be critical intermediates in regulating growth-factor-induced angiogenesis, and they have been reported to stimulate angiogenesis in some tissues without the assistance of growth factors.[63, 64] They may induce angiogenesis in part by inducing NF-κB; therefore inhibition of leukotriene activity may reduce NF-κB-induced angiogenesis. Conversely, NF-κB activity may induce angiogenesis, in part by promoting leukotriene production. (NF-κB can act as a transcription factor for the genes that control lipoxygenase and cyclooxygenase production.[65])

- PGE_2 and leukotrienes can stimulate cancer cell proliferation. For example, PGE_2 stimulated the proliferation of human colon cancer cells in vitro.[66, 67] In some cases, leukotrienes may play an even more important role than PGE_2 in stimulating proliferation.[66, 68–72] For example, in two studies, lipoxygenase inhibitors reduced the proliferation of human brain cancer cells and human leukemia cells in vitro, whereas cyclooxygenase inhibitors (PGE_2 inhibitors) had no effect.[73, 74] Moreover, the leukotriene 5-HETE is a potent survival factor for some cancer cells, including human prostate cancer cells, and can protect them from apoptosis.[75] Arachidonic acid and other omega-6 fatty acids can stimulate the proliferation of prostate cancer cells through the production of 5-HETE.[76, 77] (See Figure 7.3 for an illustration of

TABLE 8.2   NATURAL COMPOUNDS THAT BENEFICIALLY EFFECT PROSTANOID AND LEUKOTRIENE SYNTHESIS
COMPOUND
Boswellic acids
CAPE and bee propolis
Curcumin
EPA and DHA
Flavonoids (including genistein, apigenin, luteolin, quercetin, and EGCG)
Garlic
Glutathione-enhancing agents
Melatonin
NF-κB Inhibitors (see Tables 5.1 and 5.2)
Parthenolide
PTK inhibitors (see Table 4.2)
Resveratrol
Vitamin E
Note: See Table F.2 in Appendix F for details and references.

the role of lipoxygenases and cyclooxygenases in the production of eicosanoids.)

Natural compounds that inhibit the production of eicosanoids derived from omega-6 fatty acids (detrimental eicosanoids) or increase the production of eicosanoids derived from omega-3 fatty acids (beneficial eicosanoids) are listed in Table 8.2. Although most studies on these compounds were conducted in vitro, a few were also done in vivo. Compounds reported to beneficially affect eicosanoid production in vivo include CAPE, curcumin, EPA/DHA, flavonoids, and vitamin E. Many of the compounds listed in the table have also been reported to inhibit COX-2 (and hence PGE_2 production) in vitro. These compounds include CAPE, curcumin, EPA/DHA, flavonoids, parthenolide, and resveratrol (see Table F.2 for details).

Reducing the intake of omega-6 fatty acids (such as most vegetable oils) is also important. Reduced intake not only provides less material to make detrimental eicosanoids but also helps cells use omega-3 fatty acids to make beneficial eicosanoids.

Macrophages as Inducers and Inhibitors of Angiogenesis

Although it is a common belief that immune activity will inhibit cancer, this simplistic view does not accurately describe what occurs in the body, at least not for macrophages. Macrophages, the predominant immune cell at tumor sites, can both induce and inhibit angiogenesis and tumor progression, depending on the circumstances. That macrophages play a dual role in tumor angiogenesis is not surprising—they also do so in wound angiogenesis. Macrophages are the predominant immune cell at wound sites, acting not only as phagocytes, engulfing debris and foreign cells, but also as small chemical factories, producing compounds that guide the healing process. As we saw in Chapter 7, the healing process has several stages; the early ones require angiogenesis and the last stage requires it to end. Macrophages produce different compounds, according to the healing stage. In this way, they promote angiogenesis in early stages and halt or at least do not promote it in the final stage.[78, 79] As also discussed there, tumors become stuck in the second and third stages of the healing process, where active angiogenesis occurs, and thus tumors behave like nonhealing wounds. In cancer treatment then, our goal is to create an environment that favors movement to the fourth and final stage of healing, so that angiogenesis can cease. To help achieve this goal, natural compounds can be used to reduce the signals that tell macrophages they are in the second and third stages, thereby easing entry into the fourth stage.

Macrophages play an essential role in the immune response by engulfing dead bacteria and other debris and by producing noxious compounds, such as free radicals and TNF, that kill invading pathogens. If produced in sufficient quantity, these same noxious compounds can also kill cancer cells. If macrophages produce only low concentrations, however, these same compounds can facilitate tumor proliferation and angiogenesis.[80] Macrophages can also produce or activate various factors that inhibit angiogenesis, such as angiostatin and thrombospondin-1.

In many cases the overall effect of macrophages is promotion of angiogenesis and tumor progression.[81, 87] For example, a significant positive correlation has been reported between macrophage infiltration, angiogenesis, tumor stage, reduced relapse-free survival, and/or reduced overall survival in breast cancer and melanoma patients.[82, 83, 84] For these reasons, inhibitors of tumor-associated macrophage activity are being studied as potential anticancer agents.[85]

The ability of macrophages to mediate angiogenesis results from a complex interplay between opposing macrophage regulators.[86] During normal wound healing, macrophages may switch from an initial angiogenesis-promoting mode to a later angiogenesis-inhibiting mode. At tumor sites, however, the signals that cause them to switch modes appear to be lacking, and the initial promoting mode prevails.[87]

Macrophages produce various compounds that stimulate angiogenesis, and of these, TNF may be the most active. We are speaking here of mild to moderate TNF concentrations since, as stated above, high concentrations can kill cancer cells. The effects of TNF on angiogenesis may be related to its ability to stimulate production of other angiogenic factors, such as VEGF and bFGF, by macrophages or other cells. In-vitro studies suggest that TNF-induced angiogenesis can be prevented by inhibiting VEGF and bFGF activity.[88] This is not to say that TNF is the only important angiogenesis factor produced by macrophages. In total, macrophages secrete over a hundred different molecules; more than twenty of these can stimulate endothelial cell proliferation and migration.[89] In addition to producing TNF, VEGF, and bFGF, macrophages are also capable of producing copious amounts of other angiogenic factors, including PDGF and EGF, which can stimulate production of VEGF and the proliferation of some tumor cells.[81, 90]

There are at least three conceivable ways natural compounds could be employed to favor the antiangiogenic and antitumor mode of macrophages; all three are likely to be most effective when used together. First, natural compounds could be used to inhibit inflammation and the factors that help drive angiogenesis. In addition to those discussed in this chapter, ways to reduce inflammation and TNF production were given in Chapter 5 with reference to inhibition of NF-κB. When angiogenesis and inflammation are inhibited, macrophages at tumor sites will get the message that the fourth stage of healing has begun, and we can expect them to switch to the antiangiogenic mode.

Second, natural compounds could be used to stimulate macrophage (and other immune cell) activity and to reduce immune evasion. Stimulated macrophages may produce greater amounts of TNF, and as we have stated, high concentrations of TNF are lethal rather than proangiogenic. Immunosuppressive compounds such as PGE_2 that are produced by cancer cells keep macrophages and other immune cells in a state of low activity, thereby helping to assure that lower concentrations of TNF, free radicals, and other compounds are produced. If we reduce production of immunosuppressive compounds, macrophages and other immune cells will be more capable of producing lethal concentrations of antitumor compounds.

Since inflammation is part of the immune response, one might think that using compounds that reduce inflammation would be incompatible with using ones that stimulate the immune system. However, for reasons discussed in Chapter 12, it seems probable that both types of compounds could be used together to produce benefit.

Third, natural compounds could promote the antiangiogenic mode of macrophages by reducing the signals that tell macrophages angiogenesis is necessary. One primary source of these signals is hypoxic conditions and, along with them, high lactic acid concentrations, a byproduct of such conditions. To make clear how cutting down the flow of signals caused by hypoxia will be useful, we look more closely at hypoxia's role in wound angiogenesis.

Because hypoxic tissues in wounds are in great need of angiogenesis, the body contains redundant mechanisms to ensure that angiogenesis in these locations is successful. Some of these mechanisms involve macrophages. For example, macrophages cultured under hypoxic environments are reported to produce abundant amounts of angiogenesis factors, but they produce little once they have been put under normal oxygen conditions.[91] Because macrophages comprise 10 to 30 percent of the cells in a solid tumor and solid tumors commonly contain hypoxic areas, hypoxia-stimulated macrophages are likely to produce substantial quantities of angiogenesis factors. Hypoxic conditions also stimulate fibroblasts to produce more collagen, which also facilitates angiogenesis since collagen synthesis is needed to produce the basement membranes for new blood vessels.[92]

The chronic hypoxic conditions at tumor sites are created in large part by the chaotic and faulty development of blood vessels during tumor angiogenesis. If extreme, hypoxia causes cell death, which accounts for the common observation of dead cells at the center of solid tumors (central necrosis). In contrast, moderate or transient hypoxia stimulates angiogenesis. One way that hypoxia drives macrophages toward a pro-angiogenic mode is by inducing macrophages (and cancer cells and vascular cells) to produce greater quantities of angiogenesis factors such as VEGF.[93, 94] The production of VEGF by macrophages may also be stimulated by the oxygen reperfusion that occurs in moderately hypoxic tissues after reexposure to oxygen. Oxygen reperfusion produces a high concentration of free radicals, which in turn stimulates VEGF production by various cells.[95]

From the above, we can see at least two possible ways natural compounds could reduce the signaling caused by hypoxia and oxygen reperfusion. First, natural compounds that are antioxidants could scavenge the free radicals produced during reperfusion. Indeed, in-vitro studies have reported that antioxidants can successfully inhibit VEGF production or macrophage-induced angiogenesis or both.[96–99] Some antioxidants also appear to be effective in vivo. For example, vitamin E (given orally at about 92 I.U. per day in the succinate form, as scaled to humans) inhibited angiogenesis in oral tumors in hamsters.[100]

Second, natural compounds can be used to inhibit the signal transduction pathways that transport the hypoxia signal from outside the cell to the nucleus. The signals induced by hypoxia travel to the nucleus by multiple pathways, some of which involve protein kinase C; inhibitors of PKC can reduce the synthesis of VEGF in hypoxic environments and can inhibit VEGF-induced endothelial cell proliferation in vitro.[101, 102] PTK may also be involved. For example, the PTK inhibitor genistein reportedly blocked the inducing effect of hypoxia on VEGF production in vitro.[103] In one study, the IC_{50} for genistein was about 36 μM.[104]

In summary, natural compounds that are anti-inflammatory, antiangiogenic, antioxidants, or inhibitors of signal transduction may all help drive macrophages toward an antiangiogenic mode. These compounds may inhibit hypoxia-induced VEGF production as well as production of TNF, and subsequently VEGF. A recent review reported that the following natural compounds inhibited TNF secretion by macrophages and/or inhibited TNF function: ATRA, caffeic acid, curcumin, EGCG, emodin, EPA, hypericin, luteolin, parthenolide, quercetin, and resveratrol.[105] All of these are antioxidants, inhibitors of PTK or PKC, and/or inhibitors of NF-κB. In addition, it may be possible to increase TNF production by macrophages by using natural compounds that stimulate the immune system or inhibit immune evasion; high TNF concentrations are lethal to cancer cells. Producing an anti-inflammatory effect while increasing the immune response may seem contradictory but still should be possible (see Chapter 12).

Fibrin

As discussed in Chapter 7, a fibrin stroma forms around developing tumors. Fibrin deposition and stroma formation may assist tumor progression by providing a physical support, by shielding the tumor from immune attack, and by promoting metastasis. In addition, fibrin degradation products may act as angiogenic factors. Therefore, agents that induce fibrinolysis could inhibit tumor progression but also might increase angiogenesis by producing more fibrin fragments. Indeed, preliminary evidence suggests that high intravenous doses of fibrinolytic agents may promote tumor angiogenesis.[106] However, oral doses of fibrinolytic agents, which produce lower plasma concentrations, are much less likely to increase angiogenesis and do appear to inhibit tumor metastasis.[107, 108] Orally administered fibrinolytic agents could also facilitate perfusion of anticancer agents into solid tumors. It appears that at least some natural compounds that possess fibrinolytic activity produce an overall anticancer effect when given orally. Natural compounds that inhibit fibrin production and/or stimu-

TABLE 8.3 NATURAL COMPOUNDS THAT INHIBIT MAST CELL GRANULATION IN VITRO
COMPOUND
Eleutherococcus senticosus
Flavonoids (including apigenin, luteolin, genistein, quercetin, EGCG, and proanthocyanidins)
Vitamin C
Note: See Table F.3 in Appendix F for details and references.

late fibrinolysis include bromelain and garlic. Bromelain has been reported to stimulate plasmin production and fibrinolysis in vitro and in vivo.[109, 110] Multiple studies have reported that daily ingestion of garlic by humans increases fibrinolysis, in part by increasing plasmin activity via increased plasminogen (see Figure 7.5).[111–115] Bromelain has shown promising effects in cancer patients (discussed in Chapter 18). Garlic has also shown antitumor effects in animals, but mostly these were at high doses and may have been related to other mechanisms. Still, a fibrinolytic effect would have been produced, and no increase in angiogenesis was seen. Studies on garlic also are discussed in Chapter 18.

Basic Fibroblast Growth Factor

Basic fibroblast growth factor (bFGF), like VEGF, is a potent angiogenic factor. Excessive concentrations of bFGF have been identified in the plasma, urine, and/or tumor tissues of patients with a variety of cancers, including those of the uterus, prostate, kidney, liver, endometrium, and stomach. Its presence has also been positively correlated with reduced survival of patients with breast, kidney, and uterine cancer.[116, 117]

Unfortunately, few studies on bFGF inhibition by natural compounds have been conducted. Studies on the polysaccharide PSK reported it may inhibit production of bFGF in rat prostate cancer cells.[118, 119] One study on curcumin reported that oral administration of about 1.2 grams per day (as scaled to humans) inhibited angiogenesis induced by fibroblast growth factor-2 (FGF-2) in the corneas of mice.[120] FGF-2 is similar to bFGF. This mouse study, and another, also reported that direct treatment of the cornea with curcumin inhibited angiogenesis induced by FGF-2 or bFGF.[121]

Given what we already know about the actions of natural compounds, it seems likely that many could be useful in inhibiting bFGF activity indirectly. Conceivably, this could be accomplished in two ways. First, the extracellular matrix (ECM) could be protected from enzymatic degradation. As discussed in the previous chapter, bFGF is safely stored in the ECM until it is released through enzymatic action. Natural compounds that in-

hibit these enzymes or otherwise stabilize the ECM are discussed in Chapter 9. Second, inhibition of TNF production could help, since TNF can stimulate bFGF production by macrophages and other cells.

Histamine—The Role of Mast Cells

Histamine is generated by mast cells in response to tissue injury and other factors.[a] Mast cells migrate toward tumors in response to growth factor production, and once at the site, the histamine they release increases vascular permeability and stimulates angiogenesis.[122, 123]

Numerous natural compounds inhibit the release of histamine from mast cells. This release is referred to as mast cell "granulation," since histamine is stored in intracellular pouches called granules. Natural compounds that inhibit mast cell granulation are listed in Table 8.3. Note that many of these compounds occur in traditional herbal formulas used to treat asthma and allergies, which are diseases mediated by histamine release. Some compounds listed in the table are PTK inhibitors, which have been reported to inhibit histamine release from mast cells in some circumstances.[124, 125] PKC inhibitors may also inhibit histamine release.[126] Apigenin, luteolin, and EGCG are PTK and PKC inhibitors, and genistein inhibits PTK.

A second method of reducing histamine secretion is to inhibit mast cell migration. This prevents mast cells from reaching an inflamed area and releasing histamine there. Mast cells are attracted to growth factors such as VEGF, PDGF, EGF, and bFGF, so again, inhibitors of these compounds may reduce angiogenesis. Mast cell migration can also be reduced by compounds that inhibit NF-κB activation and PTK activity, both of which inhibit VEGF, PDGF, EGF, and/or bFGF production.

Lactic Acid and Insulin

As mentioned, under hypoxic conditions lactic acid may stimulate production of angiogenic factors by macrophages. Unfortunately, few natural compounds have been tested for their effects on lactic acid generation in cancer cells. In one study, apigenin and luteolin inhibited both proliferation and lactic acid release from a human adenocarcinoma cell line in vitro.[127] In other studies, the flavonoid quercetin reduced the production of lactic acid in healthy rat cells, probably by blocking the transport of lactic acid out of the cell.[128, 129] Antioxidants may also inhibit lactic acid production. For example, vitamin C has been reported to increase oxy-

---

[a] *Mast cells derive from basophils and reside in a variety of tissues.*

gen consumption and reduce lactic acid production in tumor and normal cell cultures.[130, 131]

Insulin may stimulate cell proliferation and angiogenesis. Among its effects, insulin stimulates hypoxic cells to produce greater amounts of lactic acid. One way to regulate insulin production is through dietary modifications. When food is digested, its carbohydrate content is converted to glucose, and elevated plasma concentrations of glucose stimulate the secretion of insulin. Foods that are slowly converted to glucose raise insulin levels less dramatically than foods that contain glucose or are easily converted to glucose. The ability of foods to increase insulin concentrations is referred to as their glycemic index. Thus, insulin secretion can be kept to a minimum by eating foods that have a low glycemic index, such as vegetables and protein and, to a lesser extent, whole grains and beans. The glycemic index has been used extensively by diabetic patients to control their insulin requirements.

Some natural compounds have also been reported to inhibit the cancer-promoting effects of insulin. For example, genistein inhibited insulin-induced proliferation of human breast cancer cells in vitro.[132] This likely occurred via inhibition of PTK activity. In addition, some natural compounds may be able to reduce insulin production by reducing insulin resistance. Insulin resistance occurs when cells are no longer sensitive to insulin and thus more is produced in an effort to reduce blood glucose levels. Insulin resistance has been implicated as a risk factor for breast cancer.[133, 134, 135] Diets high in omega-6 fatty acids promote insulin resistance, possibly via chronic activation of PKC.[136, 137, 138] Natural compounds that can reduce insulin resistance include omega-3 fatty acids and other PKC inhibitors.[139–142]

Omega-3 fatty acids have been reported to effectively reduce both lactic acid and insulin production in vivo. For example, in a randomized, double-blind, placebo-controlled study, a diet containing about 6 percent fish oil (containing omega-3 fatty acids) and 3 percent arginine (an amino acid) enhanced the antitumor effect of doxorubicin in dogs with spontaneous lymphoma. The treatment reduced plasma concentrations of insulin and lactic acid, and low lactic acid concentrations were associated with greater survival.[143]

ADDITIONAL NATURAL COMPOUNDS THAT MAY INHIBIT ANGIOGENESIS

Vitamins A and D$_3$

Vitamins A (ATRA) and D$_3$ (1,25-D$_3$) have been reported to inhibit angiogenesis in vitro and in vivo, probably through their direct effects on nuclear receptors.[144–149] Three in-vivo examples follow:

- A combination of 1,25-D$_3$ (at 0.5 µg/kg intraperitoneal) and ATRA (at 2.5 mg/kg intraperitoneal) synergistically inhibited tumor-induced angiogenesis in vitro and in mice.[150, 151] Angiogenesis was also inhibited by 1,25-D$_3$ alone. The equivalent human oral doses are about 7.2 micrograms of 1,25-D$_3$ and 36 milligrams of ATRA.

- Subcutaneous administration of 1 and 2.1 µg/kg of 1,25-D$_3$ or vitamin D$_3$ inhibited angiogenesis induced by transplanted kidney cancer cells in mice.[152] The equivalent human oral dose is about 19 and 39 micrograms.

- Subcutaneous administration of 0.21 µg/kg 1,25-D$_3$ inhibited angiogenesis in transplanted breast cancer cells in mice.[153] The equivalent human oral dose is about 3.9 micrograms.

In addition to the above, treatment with similar doses of 1,25-D$_3$ (1.7 µg/kg intraperitoneal) also prevented increased vascular permeability in experimentally induced edema in rodents.[148, 150, 151, 154–156]

Anticopper Compounds

Another approach to inhibiting angiogenesis depends on reducing copper concentrations in the body. In normal functioning, copper is needed for proper formation of vascular components, and it induces the proliferation and migration of endothelial cells.[157, 158] Copper levels are commonly elevated in cancer tissues, as well as in the plasma of cancer patients, and there it contributes to uncontrolled angiogenesis.[159, 160, 161] Copper may also facilitate angiogenesis by increasing the binding of angiogenic factors to endothelial cells and by increasing the production of free radicals.[162]

A recent phase I study in humans has reported that angiogenesis can be reduced by lowering plasma copper concentrations.[a] This study used tetrathiomolybdate (a derivative of the trace metal molybdenum) to reduce copper levels. A reduction of plasma copper concentrations to about 20 percent of baseline for 90 days or more stopped the growth of advanced cancers in five of six patients. Side effects were minimal.[163] Molybdenum acts by forming complexes with copper in the intestines and plasma, thereby preventing copper absorption and

---

[a] *In phase I studies, a drug is given to a small group of patients to determine the maximum tolerated dose and identify the types of adverse effects caused. Low doses are given first, and the dose is increased over time until toxicity begins to occur. Phase I studies are not designed to produce an anticancer effect, although this . does sometimes happen.*

activity.[164, 165] Similar results were seen in studies on rats and rabbits, where administration of a copper-chelating agent (penicillamine) in combination with a copper-depleted diet reduced tumor copper concentrations and invasion, angiogenesis, and the growth of transplanted brain cancer cells.[161, 166, 167] (A copper-chelating agent is one that binds with and reduces the bioavailability of copper.) Another copper-chelating agent (diethyldithiocarbamate) has also been reported effective in inhibiting angiogenesis in rodent models.[168]

In addition to molybdenum compounds, other natural compounds may be useful in anticopper therapies. For example, a number of natural compounds are known to chelate copper and reduce its prooxidant effect. These include luteolin, alpha-lipoic acid, green tea catechins such as EGCG, protocatechuic acid (a flavonoid metabolite produced in vivo), proanthocyanidins, and resveratrol.[169–177]

CONCLUSION

This chapter has discussed angiogenic factors and the natural compounds that may inhibit them. Since the body uses multiple factors to assure angiogenesis, it would seem that multiple natural compounds might be needed to inhibit angiogenesis. Such combinations would target inflammation and increased vascular permeability in general and production of detrimental eicosanoids, VEGF, bFGF, and other angiogenic factors specifically. These combinations would likely include antioxidants and inhibitors of PTK, PKC, NF-κB, COX-2, and lipoxygenases, as well as anticopper compounds and vitamins A and D_3. Only a few studies have been conducted on combinations of multiple angiogenesis inhibitors or combinations of angiogenesis inhibitors and other types of antitumor agents. Such studies on genistein combined with other angiogenesis inhibitors have reported promising results, and the use of combinations is definitely worth exploring further.

REFERENCES

[1] Yoshikawa T, Tsuburaya A, Kobayashi O, et al. Plasma concentrations of VEGF and bFGF in patients with gastric carcinoma. Cancer Lett 2000 May 29; 153(1–2):7–12.

[2] Salven P, Manpaa H, Orpana A, et al. Serum vascular endothelial growth factor is often elevated in disseminated cancer. Clin Cancer Res 1997 May; 3(5):647–51.

[3] Valtola R, Salven P, Heikkila P, et al. VEGFR-3 and its ligand VEGF-C are associated with angiogenesis in breast cancer. Am J Pathol 1999 May; 154(5):1381–90.

[4] Salven P, Perhoniemi V, Tykka H, et al. Serum VEGF levels in women with a benign breast tumor or breast cancer. Breast Cancer Res Treat 1999 Jan; 53(2):161–6.

[5] Gille J, Swerlick RA, Caughman SW. Transforming growth factor-alpha-induced transcriptional activation of the vascular permeability factor (VPF/VEGF) gene requires AP-2-dependent DNA binding and transactivation. EMBO J 1997 Feb 17; 16(4):750–9.

[6] Jensen RL. Growth factor-mediated angiogenesis in the malignant progression of glial tumors: A review. Surg Neurol 1998 Feb; 49(2):189–95.

[7] Petit AM, Rak J, Hung MC, et al. Neutralizing antibodies against epidermal growth factor and ErbB-2/neu receptor tyrosine kinases down-regulate vascular endothelial growth factor production by tumor cells in vitro and in vivo: Angiogenic implications for signal transduction therapy of solid tumors. Am J Pathol 1997 Dec; 151(6):1523–30.

[8] Tsai JC, Goldman CK, Gillespie GY. Vascular endothelial growth factor in human glioma cell lines: Induced secretion by EGF, PDGF-BB, and bFGF. J Neurosurg 1995 May; 82(5):864–73.

[9] Goldman CK, Kim J, Wong WL, et al. Epidermal growth factor stimulates vascular endothelial growth factor production by human malignant glioma cells: A model of glioblastoma multiforme pathophysiology. Mol Biol Cell 1993 Jan; 4(1):121–33.

[10] Harmey JH, Dimitriadis E, Kay E, et al. Regulation of macrophage production of vascular endothelial growth factor (VEGF) by hypoxia and transforming growth factor beta-1. Ann Surg Oncol 1998 Apr–May; 5(3):271–8.

[11] Abramovitch R, Marikovsky M, Meir G, Neeman M. Stimulation of tumour growth by wound-derived growth factors. Br J Cancer 1999 Mar; 79(9–10):1392–8.

[12] Matsushita K, Motani R, Sakuta T, et al. Lipopolysaccharide enhances the production of vascular endothelial growth factor by human pulp cells in culture. Infect Immun 1999 Apr; 67(4):1633–9.

[13] Morita I. [Regulation of angiogenesis-expression of VEGF receptors.] Hum Cell 1998 Dec; 11(4):215–20.

[14] Alvarez Arroyo MV, Arroyo MV, Castilla MA, et al. Role of vascular endothelial growth factor on erythropoietin-related endothelial cell proliferation. J Am Soc Nephrol 1998 Nov; 9(11):1998–2004.

[15] Yang SP, Morita I, Murota SI. Eicosapentaenoic acid attenuates vascular endothelial growth factor-induced proliferation via inhibiting Flk-1 receptor expression in bovine carotid artery endothelial cells. J Cell Physiol 1998 Aug; 176(2):342–9.

[16] Mukhopadhyay D, Tsiokas L, Sukhatme VP. High cell density induces vascular endothelial growth factor expression via protein tyrosine phosphorylation. Gene Expr 1998; 7(1):53–60.

[17] White FC, Benehacene A, Scheele JS, et al. VEGF mRNA is stabilized by ras and tyrosine kinase oncogenes, as well as by UV radiation—evidence for divergent stabilization pathways. Growth Factors 1997; 14(2–3):199–212.

[18] Baumann KH, Hessel F, Larass I, et al. Dietary omega-3, omega-6, and omega-9 unsaturated fatty acids and growth factor and cytokine gene expression in unstimulated and

stimulated monocytes. A randomized volunteer study. Arterioscler Thromb Vasc Biol 1999 Jan; 19(1):59–66.

19 Jiang C, Jiang W, Ip C, et al. Selenium-induced inhibition of angiogenesis in mammary cancer at chemopreventive levels of intake. Mol Carcinog 1999 Dec; 26(4):213–225.

20 Gruden G, Thomas S, Burt D, et al. Mechanical stretch induces vascular permeability factor in human mesangial cells: Mechanisms of signal transduction. Proc Natl Acad Sci USA 1997 Oct 28; 94(22):12112–6.

21 Ahn HY, Hadizadeh KR, Seul C, et al. Epigallocathechin-3 gallate selectively inhibits the PDGF-BB-induced intracellular signaling transduction pathway in vascular smooth muscle cells and inhibits transformation of sis-transfected NIH 3T3 fibroblasts and human glioblastoma cells (A172). Mol Biol Cell 1999 Apr; 10(4):1093–104.

22 Shao ZM, Wu J, Shen ZZ, et al. Genistein inhibits both constitutive and EGF-stimulated invasion in ER-negative human breast carcinoma cell lines. Anticancer Res 1998 May–Jun; 18(3A):1435–9.

23 Nakanishi H, Yamanouchi K, Gotoh Y, et al. The association of platelet-derived growth factor (PDGF) receptor tyrosine phosphorylation to mitogenic response of human osteoblastic cells in vitro. Oral Dis 1997 Dec; 3(4):236–42.

24 Liang YC, Lin-shiau SY, Chen CF, et al. Suppression of extracellular signals and cell proliferation through EGF receptor binding by (-)-epigallocatechin gallate in human A431 epidermoid carcinoma cells. J Cell Biochem 1997 Oct 1; 67(1):55–65.

25 Yang EB, Wang DF, Mack P, Cheng LY. Genistein, a tyrosine kinase inhibitor, reduces EGF-induced EGF receptor internalization and degradation in human hepatoma HepG2 cells. Biochem Biophys Res Commun 1996 Jul 16; 224(2):309–17.

26 Korutla L, Cheung JY, Mendelsohn J, et al. Inhibition of ligand-induced activation of epidermal growth factor receptor tyrosine phosphorylation by curcumin. Carcinogenesis 1995 Aug; 16(8):1741–5.

27 Zheng ZS, Xue GZ, Grunberger D, et al. Caffeic acid phenethyl ester inhibits proliferation of human keratinocytes and interferes with the EGF regulation of ornithine decarboxylase. Oncol Res 1995; 7(9):445–52.

28 Koroma BM, de Juan E Jr. Inhibition of protein tyrosine phosphorylation in endothelial cells: Relationship to antiproliferative action of genistein. Biochem Soc Trans 1997 Feb; 25(1):35–40.

29 Fotsis T, Pepper M, Adlercreutz H, Fleischmann G, et al. Genistein, a dietary-derived inhibitor of in vitro angiogenesis. Proc Natl Acad Sci USA 1993; 90(7):2690–4.

30 Fotsis T, Pepper M, Adlercreutz H, et al. Genistein, a dietary ingested isoflavonoid, inhibits cell proliferation and in vitro angiogenesis. J Nutr 1995 Mar; 125(3 Suppl):790S–797S.

31 Zhou JR, Mukherjee P, Gugger ET, et al. Inhibition of murine bladder tumorigenesis by soy isoflavones via alterations in the cell cycle, apoptosis, and angiogenesis. Cancer Res 1998 Nov 15; 58(22):5231–8.

32 Joseph IB, Isaacs JT. Macrophage role in the anti-prostate cancer response to one class of antiangiogenic agents. J Natl Cancer Inst 1998 Nov 4; 90(21):1648–53.

33 Shao ZM, Wu J, Shen ZZ, Barsky SH. Genistein exerts multiple suppressive effects on human breast carcinoma cells. Cancer Res 1998 Nov 1; 58(21):4851–7.

34 Kakeji Y, Teicher BA. Preclinical studies of the combination of angiogenic inhibitors with cytotoxic agents. Invest New Drugs 1997; 15(1):39–48.

35 Teicher BA, Holden SA, Ara G, et al. Comparison of several antiangiogenic regimens alone and with cytotoxic therapies in the Lewis lung carcinoma. Cancer Chemother Pharmacol 1996; 38(2):169–77.

36 Fotsis T, Pepper MS, Aktas E, et al. Flavonoids, dietary-derived inhibitors of cell proliferation and in vitro angiogenesis. Cancer Res 1997; 57(14):2916–2921.

37 Mizutani M, Asano M, Roy S, et al. Omega-3 polyunsaturated fatty acids inhibit migration of human vascular smooth muscle cells in vitro. Life Sci 1997; 61(19):PL269–74.

38 Nitta K, Uchida K, Tsutsui T, et al. Eicosapentaenoic acid inhibits mitogen-induced endothelin-1 production and DNA synthesis in cultured bovine mesangial cells. Am J Nephrol 1998; 18(2):164–70.

39 Kaminski WE, Jendraschak E, Kiefl R, et al. Dietary omega-3 fatty acids lower levels of platelet-derived growth factor mRNA in human mononuclear cells. Blood 1993 Apr 1; 81(7):1871–9.

40 Terano T, Shiina T, Saito J, et al. Eicosapentaenoic acid suppressed the proliferation of vascular smooth muscle cells through modulation of binding of growth factor. Jpn J Pharmacol 1992; 58 Suppl 2:286P.

41 McCarty MF. Fish oil may impede tumour angiogenesis and invasiveness by down-regulating protein kinase C and modulating eicosanoid production. Med Hypotheses 1996 Feb; 46(2):107–15.

42 Wojtowicz-Praga SM, Dickson RB, Hawkins MJ. Matrix metalloproteinase inhibitors. Invest New Drugs 1997; 15(1):61–75.

43 Hiraoka N, Allen E, Apel IJ, et al. Matrix metalloproteinases regulate neovascularization by acting as pericellular fibrinolysins. Cell 1998 Oct 30; 95(3):365–77.

44 Pluda JM, Parkinson DR. Clinical implications of tumor-associated neovascularization and current antiangiogenic strategies for the treatment of malignancies of pancreas. Cancer 1996; 78:680–7.

45 Alessandro R, Kohn EC. Molecular genetics of cancer. Cancer 1995; 76(10):1874–1877.

46 Matsunaga K, Hosokawa A, Oohara M, et al. Direct action of a protein-bound polysaccharide, PSK, on transforming growth factor-beta. Immunopharmacology 1998 Nov; 40(3):219–30.

47 Terano T, Shiina T, Tamura Y. Eicosapentaenoic acid suppressed the proliferation of vascular smooth muscle cells through modulation of various steps of growth signals. Lipids 1996 Mar; 31 Suppl:S301–4.

48 Fischer S, Slaga T. Arachidonic acid metabolism and tumor promotion. Boston: Martinus Nijhoff Publishing, 1985, pp. 42, 174.

49 Jaffe BM, Santoro MG. Prostaglandin production by tumors. In Prostaglandins in cancer research. Garaci E, Paoletti R, Santoro MG, eds. Berlin: Springer-Verlag, 1987.

50 Levine L. Tumor promoters, growth factors and arachidonic acid. In *Prostaglandins in cancer research*. Garaci E, Paoletti R, Santoro MG, eds. Berlin: Springer-Verlag, 1987.

51 Breitman TR. The role of prostaglandins and other arachidonic acid metabolites in the differentiation of HL-60. In *Prostaglandins in cancer research*. Garaci E, Paoletti R, Santoro MG, eds. Berlin: Springer-Verlag, 1987.

52 Favalli C, Mastino A, Garaci E. Prostaglandins in immunotherapy of cancer. In *Prostaglandins in cancer research*. Garaci E, Paoletti R, Santoro MG, eds. Berlin: Springer-Verlag, 1987.

53 Waymack PJ, Chance WT. Effect of prostaglandin E in multiple experimental models; V effect on tumor/host interaction. Journal of Surgical Oncology 1990; 45:110–16.

54 Wojtowicz-Praga S. Reversal of tumor-induced immunosuppression: A new approach to cancer therapy [see comments]. J Immunother 1997 May; 20(3):165–77.

55 Carter CA, Milholland RJ, Shea W, Ip MM. Effect of the prostaglandin synthetase inhibitor indomethacin on 7,12-dimethylbenz(a)anthracene-induced mammary tumorigenesis in rats fed different levels of fat. Cancer Res 1983; 43:3559–3562.

56 Kollmorgen GM, King MM, Kosanke SD, Do C. Influence of dietary fat and indomethacin on the growth of transplantable mammary tumors in rats. Cancer Res 1983; 43:4714–4719.

57 Sawaoka H, Tsuji S, Tsujii M, et al. Cyclooxygenase inhibitors suppress angiogenesis and reduce tumor growth in vivo. Lab Invest 1999 Dec; 79(12):1469–77.

58 Masferrer JL, Leahy KM, Koki AT, et al. Antiangiogenic and antitumor activities of cyclooxygenase-2 inhibitors. Cancer Res 2000 Mar 1; 60(5):1306–11.

59 Williams CS, Tsujii M, Reese J, et al. Host cyclooxygenase-2 modulates carcinoma growth. J Clin Invest 2000 Jun; 105(11):1589–94.

60 Bamba H, Ota S, Kato A, et al. Prostaglandins up-regulate vascular endothelial growth factor production through distinct pathways in differentiated U937 cells. Biochem Biophys Res Commun 2000 Jul 5; 273(2):485–491.

61 Prescott SM. Is cyclooxygenase-2 the alpha and the omega in cancer? J Clin Invest 2000; 105(11):1511–1513.

62 Zhang X, Morham SG, Langenbach R, et al. Lack of cyclooxygenase-2 inhibits growth of teratocarcinomas in mice. Exp Cell Res 2000 Feb 1; 254(2):232–40.

63 Dethlefsen SM, Shepro D, D'Amore PA. Arachidonic acid metabolites in bFGF-, PDGF-, and serum-stimulated vascular cell growth. Exp Cell Res 1994; 212(2):262–73.

64 Stoltz RA, Abraham NG, Laniado-Schwartzman M. The role of NF-kappaB in the angiogenic response of coronary microvessel endothelial cells. Proc Natl Acad Sci USA 1996 Apr 2; 93(7):2832–7.

65 Renard P, Raes M. The proinflammatory transcription factor NFkappaB: A potential target for novel therapeutical strategies. Cell Biol Toxicol 1999; 15(6):341–4.

66 Bortuzzo C, Hanif R, Kashfi K, et al. The effect of leukotrienes B and selected HETEs on the proliferation of colon cancer cells. Biochim Biophys Acta 1996 May 20; 1300(3):240–6.

67 Qiao L, Kozoni V, Tsioulias GJ, et al. Selected eicosanoids increase the proliferation rate of human colon carcinoma cell lines and mouse colonocytes in vivo. Biochim Biophys Acta 1995 Sep 14; 1258(2):215–23.

68 Rose DP, Connolly JM, Rayburn J, Coleman M. Influence of diets containing eicosapentaenoic or docosahexaenoic acid on growth and metastasis of breast cancer cells in nude mice. Journal of the National Cancer Institute 1995 Apr 19; 87(8):587–592.

69 Noguchi M, Earashi M, Minami M, et al. Effects of eicosapentaenoic and docosahexaenoic acid on cell growth and prostaglandin E and leukotriene B production by a human breast cancer cell line (MDA-MB-231). Oncology 1995; 52:458–464.

70 Tang DG, Chen YQ, Honn KV. Arachidonate lipoxygenases as essential regulators of cell survival and apoptosis. Proc Natl Acad Sci USA 1996 May 28; 93(11):5241–6.

71 Heidenreich S, Otte B, Lang D, Schmidt M. Infection by Candida albicans inhibits apoptosis of human monocytes and monocytic U937 cells. J Leukoc Biol 1996 Dec; 60(6):737–43.

72 Brown DM, Phipps RP. Bcl-2 expression inhibits prostaglandin E2-mediated apoptosis in B cell lymphomas. J Immunol 1996 Aug 15; 157(4):1359–70.

73 Blomgren H, Kling-Andersson G. Growth inhibition of human malignant glioma cells in vitro by agents which interfere with biosynthesis of eicosanoids. Anticancer Res 1992 May–Jun; 12(3):981–6.

74 Snyder DS, Castro R, Desforges JF. Antiproliferative effects of lipoxygenase inhibitors on malignant human hematopoietic cell lines. Exp Hematol 1989; 17(1):6–9.

75 Myers CE, Ghosh J. Lipoxygenase inhibition in prostate cancer. Eur Urol 1999; 35(5–6):395–8.

76 Ghosh J, Myers CE. Inhibition of arachidonate 5-lipoxygenase triggers massive apoptosis in human prostate cancer cells. Proc Natl Acad Sci USA 1998 Oct 27; 95(22):13182–7.

77 Ghosh J, Myers CE. Arachidonic acid stimulates prostate cancer cell growth: Critical role of 5-lipoxygenase. Biochem Biophys Res Commun 1997 Jun 18; 235(2):418–23.

78 Sunderkotter C, Steinbrink K, Goebeler M, et al. Macrophages and angiogenesis. J Leukoc Biol 1994 Mar; 55(3):410–22.

79 Polverini PJ. The pathophysiology of angiogenesis. Crit Rev Oral Biol Med 1995; 6(3):230–47.

80 DiPietro LA. Personal communication. 1997.

81 Mantovani A. Tumor-associated macrophages in neoplastic progression: A paradigm for the in vivo function of chemokines. Lab Invest 1994 Jul; 71(1):5–16.

82 Leek RD, Lewis CE, Whitehouse R, et al. Association of macrophage infiltration with angiogenesis and prognosis in invasive breast carcinoma. Cancer Res 1996 Oct 15; 56(20):4625–9.

83 Hildenbrand R, Dilger I, Horlin A, Stutte HJ. Urokinase and macrophages in tumour angiogenesis. Br J Cancer 1995 Oct; 72(4):818–23.

84 Torisu H, Ono M, Kiryu H, et al. Macrophage infiltration correlates with tumor stage and angiogenesis in human malignant melanoma: Possible involvement of TNFalpha and IL-1alpha. Int J Cancer 2000 Jan 15; 85(2):182–8.

85 Wahl LM, Kleinman HK. Tumor-associated macrophages as targets for cancer therapy. J Natl Cancer Inst 1998; 90(21):1583–4.

86 DiPietro LA, Polverini PJ. Angiogenic macrophages produce the angiogenic inhibitor thrombospondin 1. Am J Pathol 1993 Sep; 143(3):678–84.

87 Polverini PJ. How the extracellular matrix and macrophages contribute to angiogenesis-dependent diseases. Eur J Cancer 1996 Dec; 32A(14):2430–7.

88 Yoshida S, Ono M, Shono T, et al. Involvement of interleukin-8, vascular endothelial growth factor, and basic fibroblast growth factor in tumor necrosis factor alpha-dependent angiogenesis. Mol Cell Biol 1997 Jul; 17(7):4015–23.

89 Polverini PJ. Role of the macrophage in angiogenesis-dependent diseases. EXS 1997; 79:11–28.

90 Lewis CE, Leek R, Harris A, McGee JO. Cytokine regulation of angiogenesis in breast cancer: The role of tumor-associated macrophages. J Leukoc Biol 1995 May; 57(5):747–51.

91 Knighton DR, Hunt TK, Scheuenstuhl H, et al. Oxygen tension regulates the expression of angiogenesis factor by macrophages. Science 1983; 221:1283–5.

92 Gailit J, Clark RA. Wound repair in the context of extracellular matrix. Current Opinion in Cell Biology 1994; 6:717–725.

93 Levy AP, Levy NS, Goldberg MA. Post-transcriptional regulation of vascular endothelial growth factor by hypoxia. J Biol Chem 1996 Feb 2; 271(5):2746–53.

94 Griffiths L, Dachs GU, Bicknell R, et al. The influence of oxygen tension and pH on the expression of platelet-derived endothelial cell growth factor/thymidine phosphorylase in human breast tumor cells grown in vitro and in vivo. Cancer Research 1997 Feb 15; 57:570–572.

95 Brauchle M, Funk JO, Kind P, Werner S. Ultraviolet B and H2O2 are potent inducers of vascular endothelial growth factor expression in cultured keratinocytes. J Biol Chem 1996 Sep 6; 271(36):21793–7.

96 Kuroki M, Voest EE, Amano S, et al. Reactive oxygen intermediates increase vascular endothelial growth factor expression in vitro and in vivo. J Clin Invest 1996 Oct 1; 98(7):1667–75.

97 Monte M, Davel LE, de Lustig ES. Inhibition of lymphocyte-induced angiogenesis by free radical scavengers. Free Radic Biol Med 1994 Sep; 17(3):259–66.

98 Koch AE, Cho M, Burrows JC, et al. Inhibition of production of monocyte/macrophage-derived angiogenic activity by oxygen free-radical scavengers. Cell Biology Int Reports 1992; 16(5):415–25.

99 Koch AE, Burrows JC, Polverini PJ, Cho M, Leibovich SJ. Thiol-containing compounds inhibit the production of monocyte/macrophage-derived angiogenic activity. Agents Actions 1991 Nov; 34(3–4):350–7.

100 Shklar G, Schwartz JL. Vitamin E inhibits experimental carcinogenesis and tumour angiogenesis. Eur J Cancer B Oral Oncol 1996 Mar; 32B(2):114–9.

101 Levy AP, Levy NS, Iliopoulos O, et al. Regulation of vascular endothelial growth factor by hypoxia and its modulation by the von Hippel-Lindau tumor suppressor gene. Kidney Int 1997 Feb; 51(2):575–8.

102 Takahashi T, Ueno H, Shibuya M. VEGF activates protein kinase C-dependent, but Ras-independent Raf-MEK-MAP kinase pathway for DNA synthesis in primary endothelial cells. Oncogene 1999 Apr 1; 18(13):2221–30.

103 Okuda Y, Tsurumaru K, Suzuki S, et al. Hypoxia and endothelin-1 induce VEGF production in human vascular smooth muscle cells. Life Sci 1998; 63(6):477–84.

104 Mukhopadhyay D, Tsiokas L, Zhou XM, et al. Hypoxic induction of human vascular endothelial growth factor expression through c-Src activation. Nature 1995 Jun 15; 375(6532):577–81.

105 Habtemariam S. Natural inhibitors of tumour necrosis factor-alpha production, secretion and function. Planta Med 2000 May; 66(4):303–13.

106 Teuscher E, Pester E. A possible explanation of mechanisms inducing inhibition of vascularization of tumours by antifibrinolytic drugs—the influence of migratory behaviour of endothelial cells. Biomed Biochim Acta 1984; 43(4):447–56.

107 Batkin S, Taussig S, Szekerczes J. Modulation of pulmonary metastasis (Lewis lung carcinoma) by bromelain, an extract of the pineapple stem (Ananas comosus) [letter]. Cancer Invest 1988; 6(2):241–2.

108 Riggs DR, DeHaven JI, Lamm DL. Allium sativum (garlic) treatment for murine transitional cell carcinoma. Cancer 1997; 79:1987–94.

109 Klaschka, F. Oral enzymes in oncology. MUCOS Pharma GmbH, 1997. http://www.mucos.de

110 Kelly GS. Bromelain: A literature review and discussion of its therapeutic applications. Alt Med Rev 1996; 1(4):243–257.

111 Ernst E. Garlic therapy? Theories of a folk remedy (author's translation). MMW Munch Med Wochenschr 1981; 123(41):1537–8.

112 Arora RC, Arora S, Gupta RK. The long-term use of garlic in ischemic heart disease—an appraisal. Atherosclerosis 1981; 40(2):175–9.

113 Chang HM, But PPH. Pharmacology and applications of Chinese materia medica. Vol. 1. Teaneck, NJ: World Scientific, 1986, p. 90.

114 Katiyar SK, Agarwal R, Mukhtar H. Inhibition of tumor promotion in SENCAR mouse skin by ethanol extract of Zingiber officinale rhizome. Cancer Res 1996 Mar 1; 56(5):1023–30.

115 Legnani C, Frascaro M, Guazzaloca G, et al. Effects of dried garlic preparations on fibrinolysis and platelet aggregation in healthy subjects. Arzneim Forsch 1993; 43(2):119–122.

116 Scott PA, Harris A. Current approaches to targeting cancer using antiangiogenesis therapies. Cancer Treatment Reviews 1994; 20:393–412.

117 Fujimoto J, Ichigo S, Hori M, et al. Expression of basic fibroblast growth factor and its mRNA in advanced uterine cervical cancers. Cancer Letters 1997; 111:21–26.

118 Kanoh T, Matsunaga K, Saito K, Fujii T. Suppression of in vivo tumor-induced angiogenesis by the protein-bound polysaccharide PSK. In Vivo 1994 Mar–Apr; 8(2):247–50.

119 Mickey DD. Alteration of gene expression in prostatic tumor by PSK. J Cancer Res Clin Oncol 1990; 116:871.

[120] Mohan R, Sivak J, Ashton P, Russo LA, et al. Curcuminoids inhibit the angiogenic response stimulated by fibroblast growth factor-2, including expression of matrix metalloproteinase gelatinase B. J Biol Chem 2000 Apr 7; 275(14):10405–12.

[121] Arbiser JL, Klauber N, Rohan R, et al. Curcumin is an in vivo inhibitor of angiogenesis. Mol Med 1998 Jun; 4(6):376–83.

[122] Gruber BL, Marchese MJ, Kew R. Angiogenic factors stimulate mast-cell migration. Blood 1995 Oct 1; 86(7):2488–2493.

[123] Folkman J, Klagsburn M. Angiogenic factors. Science 1987; 235:442–7.

[124] Lavens-Phillips SE, Mockford EH, Warner JA. The effect of tyrosine kinase inhibitors on IgE-mediated histamine release from human lung mast cells and basophils. Inflamm Res 1998 Mar; 47(3):137–43.

[125] Frew A, Chan H, Salari H, et al. Is tyrosine kinase activation involved in basophil histamine release in asthma due to western red cedar? Allergy 1998 Feb; 53(2):139–43.

[126] Middleton E, Ferriola P. Effect of flavonoids on protein kinase C: Relationship to inhibition of human basophil histamine release. In *Plant flavonoids in biology and medicine II*. Alan R. Liss Inc., 1988, pp. 251–266.

[127] Agullo G, Gamet-Payrastre L, Fernandez Y, et al. Comparative effects of flavonoids on the growth, viability and metabolism of a colonic adenocarcinoma cell line (HT29 cells). Cancer Lett 1996 Jul 19; 105(1):61–70.

[128] Trejo R, Valadez-Salazar A, Delhumeau G. Effects of quercetin on rat testis aerobic glycolysis. Can J Physiol Pharmacol 1995 Nov; 73(11):1605–15.

[129] Volk C, Kempski B, Kempski OS. Inhibition of lactate export by quercetin acidifies rat glial cells in vitro. Neurosci Lett 1997 Feb 21; 223(2):121–4.

[130] Cameron E, Pauling L, Leibovitz B. Ascorbic acid and cancer: A review. Cancer Research 1979 March; 39:663–681.

[131] Alcain FJ, Buron MI. Ascorbate on cell growth and differentiation. J Bioenerg Biomembr 1994 Aug; 26(4):393–8.

[132] Panno ML, Salerno M, Pezzi V, et al. Effect of oestradiol and insulin on the proliferative pattern and on oestrogen and progesterone receptor contents in MCF-7 cells. J Cancer Res Clin Oncol 1996; 122(12):745–9.

[133] Stoll BA. Western nutrition and the insulin resistance syndrome: A link to breast cancer. Eur J Clin Nutr 1999 Feb; 53(2):83–7.

[134] Stoll BA. Essential fatty acids, insulin resistance, and breast cancer risk. Nutr Cancer 1998; 31(1):72–7.

[135] Koohestani N, Tran TT, Lee W, et al. Insulin resistance and promotion of aberrant crypt foci in the colons of rats on a high-fat diet. Nutr Cancer 1997; 29(1):69–76.

[136] Schmitz-Peiffer C, Browne CL, Oakes ND, et al. Alterations in the expression and cellular localization of protein kinase C isozymes epsilon and theta are associated with insulin resistance in skeletal muscle of the high-fat-fed rat. Diabetes 1997 Feb; 46(2):169–78.

[137] Avignon A, Yamada K, Zhou X, et al. Chronic activation of protein kinase C in soleus muscles and other tissues of insulin-resistant type II diabetic Goto-Kakizaki (GK), obese/aged, and obese/Zucker rats. A mechanism for inhibiting glycogen synthesis. Diabetes 1996 Oct; 45(10):1396–404.

[138] Shmueli E, Alberti KG, Record CO. Diacylglycerol/protein kinase C signaling: A mechanism for insulin resistance? J Intern Med 1993 Oct; 234(4):397–400.

[139] Chicco A, D'Alessandro ME, Karabatas L, et al. Effect of moderate levels of dietary fish oil on insulin secretion and sensitivity, and pancreas insulin content in normal rats. Ann Nutr Metab 1996; 40(2):61–70.

[140] Luo J, Rizkalla SW, Boillot J, et al. Dietary (n-3) polyunsaturated fatty acids improve adipocyte insulin action and glucose metabolism in insulin-resistant rats: Relation to membrane fatty acids. J Nutr 1996 Aug; 126(8):1951–8.

[141] Raheja BS, Sadikot SM, Phatak RB, Rao MB. Significance of the N-6/N-3 ratio for insulin action in diabetes. Ann N Y Acad Sci 1993 Jun 14; 683:258–71.

[142] Storlien LH, Jenkins AB, Chisholm DJ, et al. Influence of dietary fat composition on development of insulin resistance in rats. Relationship to muscle triglyceride and omega-3 fatty acids in muscle phospholipid. Diabetes 1991 Feb; 40(2):280–9.

[143] Ogilvie GK, Fettman MJ, Mallinckrodt CH, et al. Effect of fish oil, arginine, and doxorubicin chemotherapy on remission and survival time for dogs with lymphoma: A double-blind, randomized placebo-controlled study. Cancer 2000 Apr 15; 88(8):1916–28.

[144] Braunhut SJ, Palomares M. Modulation of endothelial cell shape and growth by retinoids. Microvasc Res 1991 Jan; 41(1):47–62.

[145] Paige K, Palomares M, D'Amore PA, et al. Retinol-induced modification of the extracellular matrix of endothelial cells: Its role in growth control. In Vitro Cell Dev Biol 1991; 27A(2):151–7.

[146] Oikawa T, Hirotani K, Nakamura O, Shudo K, et al. A highly potent antiangiogenic activity of retinoids. Cancer Lett 1989 Nov 30; 48(2):157–62.

[147] Ingber D, Folkman J. Inhibition of angiogenesis through modulation of collagen metabolism. Lab Invest 1988 Jul; 59(1):44–51.

[148] Bollag W, Majewski S, Jablonska S. Cancer combination chemotherapy with retinoids: Experimental rationale. Leukemia 1994 Sep; 8(9):1453–7.

[149] Bollag W. Experimental basis of cancer combination chemotherapy with retinoids, cytokines, 1,25-dihydroxyvitamin D3, and analogs. J Cell Biochem 1994 Dec; 56(4):427–35.

[150] Majewski S, Marczak M, Szmurlo A, et al. Retinoids, interferon alpha, 1,25-dihydroxyvitamin D3 and their combination inhibit angiogenesis induced by non-HPV-harboring tumor cell lines. RAR alpha mediates the antiangiogenic effect of retinoids. Cancer Lett 1995 Feb 10; 89(1):117–24.

[151] Majewski S, Skopinska M, Marczak M, et al. Vitamin D3 is a potent inhibitor of tumor cell-induced angiogenesis. J Investig Dermatol Symp Proc 1996; 1(1):97–101.

[152] Fujioka T, Hasegawa M, Ishikura K, et al. Inhibition of tumor growth and angiogenesis by vitamin D3 agents in murine renal cell carcinoma. J Urol 1998; 160:247–251.

[153] Mantell DJ, Owens PE, Bundred NJ, et al. 1 alpha,25-dihydroxyvitamin D(3) inhibits angiogenesis in vitro and in vivo. Circ Res 2000 Aug 4; 87(3):214–20.

[154] Majewski S, Szmurlo A, Marczak M, Jablonska S, Bollag W. Inhibition of tumor cell-induced angiogenesis by retinoids, 1,25-dihydroxyvitamins D3 and their combination. Cancer Lett 1993 Nov 30; 75(1):35–9.

[155] Oikawa T, Hirotani K, Ogasawara H, Katayama T, et al. Inhibition of angiogenesis by vitamin D3 analogues. Eur J Pharmacol 1990 Mar 20; 178(2):247–50.

[156] Chen SF, Ruan YJ. 1α,25-Dihydroxyvitamin D$_3$ decreases scalding- and platelet-activating factor-induced high vascular permeability and tissue oedema. Pharmacology & Toxicology 1995; 76:365–367.

[157] Rabinovitz M. Angiogenesis and its inhibition: The copper connection. J Natl Cancer Inst 1999 Oct 6; 91(19):1689–90.

[158] Hu GF. Copper stimulates proliferation of human endothelial cells under culture. J Cell Biochem 1998 Jun 1; 69(3):326–35.

[159] Huang YL, Sheu JY, Lin TH. Association between oxidative stress and changes of trace elements in patients with breast cancer. Clin Biochem 1999 Mar; 32(2):131–6.

[160] Yoshida D, Ikeda Y, Nakazawa S. Quantitative analysis of copper, zinc and copper/zinc ratio in selected human brain tumors. J Neurooncol 1993 May; 16(2):109–15.

[161] Yoshida D, Ikeda Y, Nakazawa S. Copper chelation inhibits tumor angiogenesis in the experimental 9L gliosarcoma model. Neurosurgery 1995 Aug; 37(2):287–92; discussion 292–3.

[162] Soncin F, Guitton JD, Cartwright T, Badet J. Interaction of human angiogenin with copper modulates angiogenin binding to endothelial cells. Biochem Biophys Res Commun 1997 Jul 30; 236(3):604–10.

[163] Brewer GJ, Dick RD, Grover DK, et al. Treatment of metastatic cancer with tetrathiomolybdate, an anticopper, antiangiogenic agent: Phase I study. Clin Cancer Res 2000; 6:1–10.

[164] Murray M, Pizzorno J. Encyclopedia of natural medicine. Rocklin, CA: Prima Publishing, 1991, pp. 220–1.

[165] Turnlund JR. Copper nutriture, bioavailability, and the influence of dietary factors. J Am Diet Assoc 1988 Mar; 88(3):303–8.

[166] Brem S, Tsanaclis AM, Zagzag D. Anticopper treatment inhibits pseudopodial protrusion and the invasive spread of 9L gliosarcoma cells in the rat brain. Neurosurgery 1990 Mar; 26(3):391–6.

[167] Brem SS, Zagzag D, Tsanaclis AM, et al. Inhibition of angiogenesis and tumor growth in the brain. Suppression of endothelial cell turnover by penicillamine and the depletion of copper, an angiogenic cofactor. Am J Pathol 1990 Nov; 137(5):1121–42.

[168] Ambrus JL, Ambrus CM, Forgach P, et al. Studies on tumor induced angiogenesis. EXS 1992; 61:436–44.

[169] Brown JE, Rice-Evans CA. Luteolin-rich artichoke extract protects low density lipoprotein from oxidation in vitro. Free Radic Res 1998 Sep; 29(3):247–55.

[170] Brown JE, Khodr H, Hider RC, Rice-Evans CA. Structural dependence of flavonoid interactions with Cu2+ ions: Implications for their antioxidant properties. Biochem J 1998 Mar 15; 330 (Pt 3):1173–8.

[171] Ou P, Tritschler HJ, Wolff SP. Thioctic (lipoic) acid: A therapeutic metal-chelating antioxidant? Biochem Pharmacol 1995 Jun 29; 50(1):123–6.

[172] Lodge JK, Traber MG, Packer L. Thiol chelation of Cu2+ by dihydrolipoic acid prevents human low density lipoprotein peroxidation. Free Radic Biol Med 1998 Aug; 25(3):287–97.

[173] Guo Q, Zhao B, Li M, et al. Studies on protective mechanisms of four components of green tea polyphenols against lipid peroxidation in synaptosomes. Biochim Biophys Acta 1996 Dec 13; 1304(3):210–22.

[174] Da Silva EL, Piskula M, Terao J. Enhancement of antioxidative ability of rat plasma by oral administration of (-)-epicatechin. Free Radic Biol Med 1998 May; 24(7–8):1209–16.

[175] Ueda J, Saito N, Shimazu Y, Ozawa T. A comparison of scavenging abilities of antioxidants against hydroxyl radicals. Arch Biochem Biophys 1996 Sep 15; 333(2):377–84.

[176] Belguendouz L, Fremont L, Linard A. Resveratrol inhibits metal ion-dependent and independent peroxidation of porcine low-density lipoproteins. Biochem Pharmacol 1997 May 9; 53(9):1347–55.

[177] Packer L, Rimbach G, Virgili F. Antioxidant activity and biologic properties of a procyanidin-rich extract from pine (Pinus maritima) bark, pycnogenol. Free Radic Biol Med 1999 Sep; 27(5–6):704–24.

Invasion is the spread of cancer cells into adjacent tissues. Along with metastasis, the spread of cells to distant sites, it is one of the distinguishing features of malignancy. Invasion and metastasis are in fact related—cancer cells must generally invade the connective tissue surrounding blood vessels (the basement membrane) for metastasis to be successful. This chapter and the next then form a pair; in this one, we focus on the central role that tumor-induced protease (protein-degrading) and glycosidase (glycoside-degrading) enzymes play in invasion. These enzymes provide the means by which tumors digest the extracellular matrix, thereby allowing local spread. Since invasion takes place in the ECM environment, we also discuss in some depth its makeup and function. In addition, we discuss natural compounds that can inhibit these enzymes or stabilize the ECM. By performing these functions, natural compounds can help prevent destruction of tissue and reduce invasion.

To put our discussion in context, note that these types of enzymes are active in a wide variety of normal biological processes in addition to their role in cancer invasion. Various enzymes are produced both inside the digestive tract, where they digest food proteins and starches, and outside of it, where they play important roles in numerous body functions. For example, proteolytic enzymes are active in normal wound healing because immune cells (e.g., macrophages) secrete proteolytic enzymes that dissolve damaged tissue. The source of some ECM-degrading enzymes in cancer invasion may actually be stimulated immune cells. As with angiogenesis, enzyme activity at cancer sites is another natural, beneficial process gone awry, and natural compounds can be used to help restore it to normal.

CONNECTIVE TISSUE AND THE EXTRACELLULAR MATRIX

Cells in the body are held together and supported by connective tissue, the most common tissue in the body. Connective tissue lies between and supports other tissues, and it consists of a limited number of cells embedded in a large amount of extracellular matrix. We include under the term *connective tissue* tendons, bones, cartilage, reticular tissue (the tissue that forms the structure of organs), and most important for our purposes, the extracellular matrix itself. Because the ECM is the first barrier to tumor invasion and its properties govern the

function and proliferation of cells within it, it is of prime importance to any discussion on cancer.

The ground substance of the ECM is a complex, gelatinous material composed of a variety of interlacing glycosaminoglycans (GAGs), most of which are proteoglycans (GAGs bound to a central protein core).[a] GAGs are large spongelike, hydrophilic (water-loving) molecules that consist of repeated sugar chains. GAGs form a viscous mesh through which all nutrients and waste products make their way to and from the cell surface. This mesh is a conduit for the transfer of electrolytes, metabolites, dissolved gases, trace elements, vitamins, hormones, growth factors, enzymes, carbohydrates, fats, and proteins. In addition to its role as conduit, the GAG mesh is also a storage repository for some compounds, including many growth factors.

Extracellular matrix GAGs exist in four forms: heparan sulfate, chondroitin sulfate, keratin sulfate, and hyaluronic acid. The first three are proteoglycans, and the last is a pure GAG. Each of these GAGs, but in particular the sulfated GAGs, carry a strong negative charge that causes positively charged molecules like growth factors to bind tightly to them. For example, as mentioned in Chapter 7, heparan sulfate binds and stores basic fibroblast growth factor (bFGF) until it is needed for wound repair or other functions.

The ECM also contains a network of microscopic protein fibers that provides structure and ensures its integrity. Most of these fibers are made of collagen, but other fibrous proteins such as elastin and fibronectin are also present.[b] Some of these collagen fibers are cross-linked together by GAG chains and hydrogen bonds to form visible collagen "ropes." Cross-linked collagen fibers reinforce the ECM in much the same way that rebar reinforces a concrete wall.

THE ECM AND CANCER

The ECM not only provides a barrier to tumor invasion, it also governs the behavior of the cells it surrounds. The makeup of the ECM varies in gross or

---

[a] *Proteoglycans are a subset of glycoproteins. Glycoproteins are proteins bound to glucose residues.*

[b] *Fibronectin is an adhesive glycoprotein found on the surface of cells and in the ECM. It binds to cell surfaces, collagen, fibrin, and other components, and it is involved in cell adhesion, cell motility, and other processes.*

subtle ways in different body tissues. These differences partly govern not only the architecture of the tissue but also the function and proliferation of the tissue's cells. The production and maintenance of the ECM is a dynamic process, and ECM GAGs are renewed and replaced rapidly, usually within a month's time. Since the source of GAG synthesis is the cells themselves, a complex, two-way regulatory loop exists. Cells affect ECM formation and ECM formation affects cells. Because of this intimate relationship, cells cannot be adequately discussed apart from their immediate environment. For example, most normal cells undergo apoptosis when they become detached from the ECM.[1] Recall from Chapter 3 that apoptosis may be an ever-present default pathway and that cell survival is maintained only so long as cells receive the appropriate antiapoptotic survival signals; these signals can be produced partly through cell-matrix interactions. In contrast, most cancer cells do not undergo apoptosis when they become detached from the ECM; instead, they exhibit an increased tendency to proliferate. In part, prevention of apoptosis may be due to the ability of cancer cells to self-stimulate the signal transduction pathways that would normally be activated through cell-matrix (or cell-cell) interactions.

Cancer cells can in fact produce matrix components that favor their migration and proliferation. In particular, a number of cancer cell lines do not assemble a functioning matrix. Although they do produce the proteoglycan components, the components tend to be in an under-sulfated form.[2-5] Such altered proteoglycans are less capable of gluing collagen and other protein fibers to one another, of maintaining cell attachment, and of binding growth factors. These characteristics facilitate increased invasion and proliferation.

In addition to producing chemically altered matrix components, some cancer cells produce an abnormally large volume of matrix components. This is especially true with cancer cells that have a high ability to invade and metastasize.[6-10] Matrix synthesis may occur within the cancer cell itself or within fibroblasts stimulated by the cancer cell.[11] In either case, insulin and other growth factors may provide the stimulatory signals for excessive matrix synthesis.[12] Not surprisingly, elevated levels of hyaluronic acid (a GAG extracellular matrix component) have been observed in the blood of cancer patients. For example, one study reported that patients with lymphoma exhibited increased plasma levels of hyaluronic acid, and the highest levels were found in patients with relapsing or resistant disease.[13] Increased plasma levels of hyaluronic acid have also been found in lung cancer patients.[14] Therefore, hyaluronic acid, especially its low-molecular-weight fragments, has been proposed as a plasma diagnostic marker to measure cancer progression.[13, 15, 16, 19]

Theoretically, it might seem that hyaluronic acid production could inhibit tumor progression, for example, hyaluronic acid synthesis is needed to repair the damaged ECM during wound healing. It is much more likely, however, that it facilitates cancer progression. For one thing, the excess hyaluronic acid produced during cancer is probably not of the normal type, or it is produced in relative imbalance to other ECM components such as collagen and fibronectin. As discussed below, this type of imbalance (high GAG production and low collagen production) occurs in the dysfunctional matrix produced around varicose veins, a condition that has some similarities to cancer invasion.

Even if the excess hyaluronic acid produced by cancer cells is of a normal type, it may still facilitate tumor progression. For example, normal hyaluronic acid facilitated invasion of brain cancer cells in vitro.[17] It is not clear exactly how this occurs, but hyaluronic acid is produced on the leading edge of invading tumors and could assist tumor cell migration by opening up spaces in the ECM for tumor cell movement (recall that hyaluronic acid has a spongelike quality). In addition, hyaluronic acid could further promote cell migration by providing a path tumor cells can "walk" on. Furthermore, hyaluronic acid forms a "halo" around invading tumor cells, which could protect them from immune recognition and attack.[19] Lastly, the production of hyaluronic acid could indirectly facilitate angiogenesis. As the newly formed hyaluronic acid is overcome by the leading edge of the invading tumor mass, it is digested by tumor-generated hyaluronidases, which produce hyaluronic acid fragments. These fragments can act as angiogenic factors, not unlike the fibrin breakdown products discussed in Chapter 7.[18, 19, 20]

We see then that cancer cells can alter their relationship with the ECM to their own benefit. They can produce abnormal ECM components or produce an excessive volume or abnormal mix of ECM components, or any of these. Natural compounds can reduce the degree to which these processes occur. For one thing, natural compounds can reduce the growth factor-induced signal transduction that allows excessive production of ECM components. Protein tyrosine kinase inhibitors like genistein can inhibit increases in hyaluronic acid production induced by growth factors, and they can inhibit cell migration.[21, 22] In one study genistein (at 37 μM) inhibited hyaluronic acid production by fibroblast cells that were stimulated by the growth factors EGF, IGF, and PDGF.[23] Moreover, PTK inhibitors may be useful in blocking the ability of hyaluronic acid degradation fragments to induce vascular cell proliferation and angiogenesis. This effect was demonstrated for genistein at 10 μM.[24]

Natural compounds can also inhibit production of GAGs by other means. For example, boswellic acid is not a kinase inhibitor, but it can reduce GAG synthesis in vitro.[25] Perhaps its ability to do so is related to its anti-inflammatory action.

GLYCOSIDASES, PROTEASES, AND CANCER

As discussed previously, the strength and structure of the ECM is provided by collagen fibers linked together by GAG chains. To break free of the ECM, cancer cells (or cancer-stimulated immune cells) produce enzymes that degrade these ECM components. These enzymes include glycosidases, which break apart GAG chains, and proteases, which break apart protein structures. Many different types of proteases and glycosidases may be involved in cancer invasion, but only two primary ones are discussed here: collagenases, proteases that digest the protein collagen, and hyaluronidases, a family of glycosidases that digest hyaluronic acid. Other enzymes will be discussed more briefly.[a]

Proteases and glycosidases appear to mediate at least five processes that influence cancer progression. Proteases can stimulate inflammation, cell proliferation, invasion, metastasis, and angiogenesis. It follows that inhibitors of these enzymes could impede all these processes, described below:

- *Inflammation.* The inflammatory response, including that associated with cancer, involves the release of histamine, free radicals, eicosanoids, and proteases such as collagenases. It appears that each individual product of inflammation affects the release of others; for example, some proteases may cause stimulated macrophages to produce two to six times more free radicals.[26] Similarly, various proteases increase PGE_2 synthesis, and a variety of protease inhibitors inhibit PGE_2 synthesis.

- *Cell proliferation.* Some proteases have been reported to stimulate cell proliferation.[27]

- *Invasion.* Invasion requires a delicate balance between conditions that stabilize the ECM (enzyme inhibition and matrix synthesis) and conditions that destabilize it (enzyme production and abnormal matrix synthesis). When the ECM is highly stable, it is

difficult for tumor cells to break loose and invade. Similarly, when the ECM is highly unstable, it is difficult for tumor cells to use the ECM as a track for movement.

- *Metastasis.* For successful metastasis, cancer cells must generally penetrate the basement membrane surrounding capillaries to obtain access to and exit from the circulation. Because the basement membrane is a collagen-rich form of the ECM, collagenases are required for this process.

- *Angiogenesis.* Proteases may facilitate angiogenesis by inducing inflammation and increases in capillary permeability, and by freeing other angiogenic factors stored in the extracellular matrix. In addition, glycosidases produce hyaluronic acid fragments, and these may directly stimulate angiogenesis, as discussed.

ENZYME INHIBITORS

GAGs provide the ground substance of the ECM, and hyaluronic acid is one of the most ubiquitous of GAGs; thus our discussions on enzyme inhibitors start with inhibitors of hyaluronidase, the enzyme that degrades hyaluronic acid. We also discuss inhibitors of other enzymes involved in GAG degradation, then turn to inhibitors of heparanases and finally, those of collagenase.

Hyaluronidase and Its Inhibitors

Hyaluronidase is capable of cutting channels through the ECM. It follows that the hyaluronidase produced by cancer cells helps them invade surrounding tissues. In much the same way, the hyaluronidase in snake and bee venoms allows the rapid spread of their poisons through the extracellular matrix. Moreover, injections of hyaluronidase have been shown useful in enhancing the antitumor effects of locally applied chemotherapy drugs, by helping the drugs spread to tumor tissues.[28, 29, 30]

Hyaluronic acid is actually degraded, or digested, in a two-step process. In step one, it is converted to medium-length sugar chains by hyaluronidase. In step two, these chains are further shortened by the enzymes beta-glucuronidase and N-acetyl-beta-glucosaminidase. N-acetyl-beta-glucosaminidase activity is elevated in the plasma of patients with a variety of cancers, including those of the breast, stomach, liver, pancreas, and colorectum.[31, 32] It is also excessively secreted by human ovarian cancer cells in vitro and increases their ability to degrade ECM components.[33, 34] Elevated beta-glucuronidase levels have been observed in the urine of patients with bladder and kidney cancers.[35, 36] It appears to be less sensitive than N-acetyl-beta-glucosaminidase as a diagnostic marker for cancer, however.

---

[a] *One enzyme active in tumor cell invasion is urokinase plasminogen activator (uPA, see Figure 7.5). uPA is produced by macrophages and tumor cells, in some cases as a result of production of VEGF and other growth factors.*

TABLE 9.1 NATURAL COMPOUNDS THAT INHIBIT HYALURONIDASE, ITS ASSISTANT ENZYMES, OR ELASTASE				
COMPOUND	HYALURONIDASE	BETA-GLUCURONIDASE	NABG[*]	ELASTASE
Apigenin	weak	x		
Boswellic acids		in vivo	in vivo	x
Centella asiatica		in vivo		
Escin, from horse chestnut	weak			
Luteolin	weak	x		
Proanthocyanidins	weak	x		x
Resveratrol		x		x
Ruscogenin, from butcher's broom				weak
Vitamin C		in vivo	x	

[*] *NABG = N-acetyl-beta-glucosaminidase*
Note: See Table G.1 in Appendix G for details and references.

Like hyaluronidase and its assistant enzymes, the enzyme elastase is also involved in matrix destruction and invasion. It is produced by a variety of cells, including macrophages and tumor cells. Elastase degrades components of the extracellular matrix, including elastin, collagen, and other proteoglycans; it also degrades fibronectin. Table 9.1 lists some natural compounds that inhibit hyaluronidase, its assistant enzymes, or elastase. The studies on which the table is based were mostly conducted in vitro, the few in-vivo studies being noted. Compounds that produced an inhibitory effect at concentrations of 50 μM or greater are marked as "weak" in the table.

It was possible to construct Table 9.1 from the available evidence, but in fact, few studies have actually been conducted and it is quite likely future studies will report additional effects. For example, we see from the table that escin and ruscogenin have only weak effects on a limited number of enzymes (and they are not reported to affect collagenase).   Horse chestnut extract and butcher's broom extract, however, are both effective in preventing increased capillary permeability after oral administration in humans and animals (see Table F.1 in Appendix F). Escin and ruscogenin are thought to be the primary active ingredients in these extracts, and their effects on vascular health are likely mediated, at least in part, through inhibition of one or more of the four enzymes listed, or inhibition of collagenase. Thus escin and ruscogenin and the other compounds listed in the table may inhibit more enzymes than shown or may inhibit them at lower concentrations.

Although not listed specifically in the table, prostaglandin inhibitors may reduce hyaluronidase activity. The potent prostaglandin inhibitor and anti-inflammatory drug indomethacin markedly reduced plasma hyaluronidase activity in rodents when used at normal doses.[37] Natural prostaglandin inhibitors (see Chapter 8) could also have this effect.

Heparanases and Their Inhibitors

Heparan sulfate is a prominent component of the ECM, and enzymes that digest heparan sulfate (heparanases) may play a role in invasion and metastasis. A variety of sulfated polysaccharides capable of inhibiting heparanase have been reported to inhibit metastasis of breast and liver tumors in rats.[38, 39, 40] The sulfated polysaccharides appeared to impede metastasis by inhibiting tumor-induced heparan sulfate degradation in the basement membrane. The mechanism is uncertain, but perhaps they act as a decoy for GAG-degrading enzymes. Alternatively, they may induce signals in cancer cells that limit enzyme production.

Sulfated polysaccharides capable of inhibiting heparanase include dextran sulfate and xylan sulfate (components of the ECM), the common anticoagulant drug heparin, and fucoidan, a sulfated polysaccharide obtained from seaweed (*Sargassum kjellmanianum*). Additional work is needed to identify other natural compounds that inhibit heparanases.

Collagenases and Their Inhibitors

Collagenases are a family of enzymes that digest collagen, the fibrous protein found in connective tissue. Collagen is derived from the Greek words *kolla* (glue), and *gennan* (to produce), reflecting its role in "gluing" cells together. Collagen accounts for approximately 30 percent of the body's total protein store. Each type of collagenase degrades a specific type of collagen. For example, the basement membrane around capillaries contains type IV collagen, and therefore type IV collagenase is a particularly important enzyme in tumor invasion and metastasis. One specific group of collagenases

TABLE 9.2 NATURAL COMPOUNDS THAT AFFECT COLLAGEN			
COMPOUND	**STABILIZE COLLAGEN**	**INCREASE COLLAGEN SYNTHESIS**	**INHIBIT COLLAGENASE**
Anthocyanidins and proanthocyanidins	x	x	x
Centella asiatica		x	x
EGCG	x	x	x
EPA			x
Leukotriene inhibitors (see Table 8.2)			x
Curcumin			x
Emodin			x
Genistein			x
Luteolin and quercetin			x
PSK and other mushroom polysaccharides			x
Vitamin A (ATRA)			x
Vitamin C		x	
Note: See Table G.2 in Appendix G for details and references.			

of interest are matrix metalloproteinases (MMPs), a family of at least 15 zinc-dependent enzymes that collectively can degrade all components of the ECM. MMPs are inhibited by tissue inhibitors of metalloproteinases (TIMPs). TIMPs are being studied for their ability to inhibit tumor invasion and angiogenesis, although their use as chemotherapeutic agents is hampered by their rapid degradation in vivo.[41, 42, 43] Compounds that stimulate TIMP production in vivo may be more suitable than administration of TIMPs themselves.

Natural compounds that affect collagen or collagenase are listed in Table 9.2. Some of these also stimulate TIMP production (see Table G.2 for details). In addition, the table lists natural compounds that stabilize collagen or increase its production. These compounds may inhibit invasion by making collagen more resistant to destruction or by producing fresh collagen to replace degraded material. Some compounds that increase the stability of collagen do so by facilitating the cross-linking of collagen fibers. This approach has received little research but seems promising, especially when used as one part of a more complex anticancer strategy.

There is some concern that compounds that stimulate collagen synthesis might also increase angiogenesis in vivo. For example, vitamin C, which increases collagen production, was reported to increase angiogenesis in vitro; it is uncertain, however, whether this effect would occur in vivo. At least in some animal studies, vitamin C produced an anti- rather than a protumor effect (discussed in Chapter 15). Moreover, the other compounds listed that increase collagen synthesis also inhibit collagenases, an effect that may limit their ability to facilitate

tumor angiogenesis in vivo. Additional in-vivo studies are warranted on vitamin C and other compounds that increase collagen synthesis.

Note that many of the compounds discussed in Table 9.2 are antioxidants. Free radicals by themselves may degrade collagen or otherwise stimulate invasion. Oxygen radicals increased the invasive potential of mouse liver cancer cells, possibly by altering their plasma membrane or by altering signal transduction or both.[44]

The pathology of varicose veins bears some resemblance to cancer invasion, and in considering the resemblance, we find suggestions for compounds that may be useful in cancer treatment. In both cases, intermittent blood stasis causes tissue hypoxia and reperfusion, which leads to free radical generation. The free radicals then degrade collagen in the ECM and basement membrane. In addition, collagenases are produced, which further degrade collagen. At the same time, a dysregulation of normal matrix production occurs in both diseases, and GAG synthesis, primarily of hyaluronic acid, is excessively stimulated.[45, 46] This leads to a maldeveloped ECM and basement membrane that is collagen-poor and GAG-rich.

Proanthocyanidins and other compounds such as *Centella* and boswellic acid inhibit GAG synthesis and collagen degradation, and/or stimulate collagen production in vitro. In fact, proanthocyanidins are reportedly useful in vivo for increasing capillary resistance in diseases such as varicose veins (see Table F.1 in Appendix F). This suggests they might also be useful in cancer treatment.

TABLE 9.3 EFFECTS OF NATURAL COMPOUNDS ON CELL MIGRATION		
COMPOUND	**INHIBIT CANCER CELL MIGRATION**	**INHIBIT IMMUNE CELL MIGRATION**
1,25-D₃ (vitamin D₃)	x	x
Apigenin, luteolin, quercetin		x
Bromelain and other proteolytic enzymes		x
EPA/DHA	x	x
Boswellic acid		x
Genistein	x	x
Hyaluronidase inhibitors (see Table 9.1)	x	x
Melatonin	x	
Panax ginseng	x	
PKC inhibitors (see Table 4.3)	x	
PSK	x	
PTK inhibitors (see Table 4.2)	x	x
Note: See Table G.3 in Appendix G for details and references.		

ADHESION PROTEINS AND CANCER CELL MIGRATION

From the above, it should be clear that production of hyaluronidase or collagenase by tumor cells or other adjacent cells can lead to matrix digestion, which subsequently allows tumor cell invasion. One more aspect of this process is the mechanism by which tumor cells "walk" during invasion. It is useful to consider the close analogy between the migration of immune cells toward an infection site and the movement of cancer cells away from the central tumor. In both cases, the cells rely on the attraction of their surface adhesion proteins to other proteins in the extracellular matrix. Immune cells and cancer cells "walk" to their intended targets by gripping and then internalizing proteins of the ECM.[47, 48]

The "legs" of immune cells, fibroblasts, and some cancer cells appear to be RHAMM proteins (RHAMM = receptor for hyaluronic acid mediated motility) and variants of the CD44 family of proteins. CD44 proteins are surface receptors for both hyaluronic acid and collagen, and they mediate attachment, cellular uptake, and degradation of these proteins. RHAMM proteins are receptors for hyaluronic acid. CD44 and RHAMM proteins facilitate the uptake of hyaluronic acid and collagen into the cell, which are then degraded by enzymes.

In a number of human breast cancer cell lines, high CD44 expression has been associated with high invasive capacity.[49] One human study reported that elevated levels of soluble CD44 occurred in a high percentage of patients with metastatic disease, and removal of the primary tumor reduced these levels.[47] Accordingly, other human studies have reported that levels of soluble CD44

variants may act as an indicator of tumor burden and metastasis.[50, 51]

Resting immune cells produce normal CD44 proteins, which do not facilitate movement, whereas stimulated cells produce CD44 variants that do. Cancer cells appear to mimic stimulated immune cells by also expressing CD44 variants, thereby allowing increased migration.[51] The expression of CD44 variants may also play a role in metastasis. The basement membrane surrounding capillaries contains hyaluronic acid, and CD44 variants on blood-borne tumor cells help the cells attach to the vasculature.[52] In one study, intravenous injection of CD44 inhibitors (CD44 antibodies) reduced the proliferation and metastatic potential of CD44-expressing melanoma cells in mice.[53]

In addition to CD44 activity, cell migration is dependent on a number of other events, such as the presence of chemoattractant compounds (such as leukotrienes), growth factor signaling, and the interactions of other cell adhesion molecules (CAMs) with matrix components. These other adhesion molecules include integrins, selectins, cadherins, and the immunoglobulin superfamily of adhesion proteins (see Chapter 6).

A number of natural compounds inhibit cancer cell migration. Many of these also inhibit immune cell migration, since the mechanisms that govern both can be similar. However, at least some natural compounds, such as PSK, appear to inhibit cancer cell migration preferentially. Ginseng may do the same. The reason some natural compounds inhibit cancer cell migration but not that of immune cells is probably because cancer cells rely on such abnormal signals for activity that their activity is more easily inhibited.

Table 9.3 summarizes the effects of natural compounds on cancer cell and immune cell migration. Inhibitors of immune cell migration are included because these compounds are also likely to inhibit cancer cell migration. Note that as with Table 9.1, the data in Table 9.3 are probably incomplete. Future studies will identify additional compounds that affect cell migration and likely show that most of these compounds inhibit migration in both cell types (with cancer cells generally being more sensitive).

CONCLUSION

Cancer cells produce three types of compounds that facilitate invasion: abnormal matrix components or an abnormal mix of them that fails to bind growth factors and is easily invaded; enzymes such as collagenases and hyaluronidases that digest matrix components to allow room for invasion; and variant CD44 surface proteins that help them migrate. Natural compounds can be used to inhibit the production or action of all three, and it is reasonable to suppose natural compounds will have the greatest effect on invasion when all three are inhibited together. Active natural compounds are likely to include inhibitors of signal transduction, collagenase and hyaluronidase inhibitors, and compounds that stabilize ECM components and prevent their digestion.

REFERENCES

[1] Malik RK, Parsons JT. Integrin-mediated signaling in normal and malignant cells: A role of protein tyrosine kinases. Biochim Biophys Acta 1996 Jun 7; 1287(2–3):73–6.

[2] Robinson J, Viti M, Hook M. Structure and properties of an under-sulfated heparan sulfate proteoglycan synthesized by a rat hepatoma cell line. J Cell Biol 1984 March; 98:946–953.

[3] David G, van den Berghe H. Transformed mouse mammary epithelial cells synthesize undersulfated basement membrane proteoglycan. J Biol Chemistry 1983 June 25; 258(12):7338–7344.

[4] Nakamura N, Kojima J. Changes in charge density of heparan sulfate isolated from cancerous human liver tissue. Cancer Research 1981 January; 41:278–283.

[5] Winterbourne DJ, Mora PT. Cells selected for high tumorigenicity or transformed by simian virus 40 synthesize heparan sulfate with reduced degree of sulfation. The Journal of Biological Chemistry 1981 May 10; 256(9):4310–4320.

[6] Ida M, Kamada A. Changes in glycosaminoglycan characteristics during progression of a human gingival carcinoma xenograft line in nude mice. J Osaka Dent Univ 1995 Oct; 29(2):39–50.

[7] Tsara ME, Papageorgacopoulou N, Karavias DD, Theocharis DA. Distribution and changes of glycosaminoglycans in neoplasias of rectum. Anticancer Res 1995 Sep–Oct; 15(5B):2107–12.

[8] Wang C, Tammi M, Guo H, Tammi R. Hyaluronan distribution in the normal epithelium of esophagus, stomach, and colon and their cancers. Am J Pathol 1996 Jun; 148(6):1861–9.

[9] Fries H, Elsasser HP, Mahlbacher V, et al. Localisation of hyaluronate (HA) in primary tumors and nude mouse xenografts of human pancreatic carcinomas using a biotinylated HA-binding protein. Virchows Arch 1994; 424(1):7–12.

[10] Tamakoshi K, Kikkawa F, Maeda O, et al. Hyaluronidase activity in gynaecological cancer tissues with different metastatic forms. Br J Cancer 1997; 75(12):1807–11.

[11] Knudson W, Biswas C, Li XQ, et al. The role and regulation of tumor-associated hyaluronan. Ciba Foundation Symposium 1989; 143:150–169.

[12] Tzanakakis GN, Karamanos NK, Syrokou A, Hjerpe A. Effect of insulin and epidermal growth factors on the synthesis of glycosaminoglycans/proteoglycans in cultured human malignant mesothelioma cells of different phenotypic morphology. APMIS 1996 Oct; 104(10):718–28.

[13] Hasselbalch H, Hovgaard D, Nissen N, Junker P. Serum hyaluronan is increased in malignant lymphoma. Am J Hematol 1995 Dec; 50(4):231–3.

[14] Hernandez Hernandez JR; Garcia Garcia JM, Martinez Muniz MA, et al. Clinical utility of hyaluronic acid values in serum and bronchoalveolar lavage fluid as tumor marker for bronchogenic carcinoma. Int J Biol Markers 1995 Jul–Sep; 10(3):149–55.

[15] Kolarova M. Host-tumor relationship. XXXIV. Hyaluronidase activity and hyaluronidase inhibitor in the serum of patients with malignant tumors. Neoplasma 1977; 24(3):285–90.

[16] Kolarova M. Host-tumor relationship XXXIII. Inhibitor of hyaluronidase in blood serum of cancer patients. Neoplasma 1975; 22(4):435–9.

[17] Nakagawa T, Kubota T, Kabuto M, Kodera T. Hyaluronic acid facilitates glioma cell invasion in vitro. Anticancer Res 1996 Sep–Oct; 16(5A):2917–22.

[18] Rooney P, Kumar S, Ponting J, Wang M. The role of hyaluronan in tumour neovascularization (review). Int J Cancer 1995 Mar 3; 60(5):632–6.

[19] Lokeshwar VB, Öbek C, Soloway MS, Block NL. Tumor-associated hyaluronic acid: A new sensitive and specific urine marker for bladder cancer. Cancer Research 1997 Feb 15; 57:773–777.

[20] West DC, Kumar S. Hyaluronan and angiogenesis. Ciba Foundation Symposium 1989; 143:187–207.

[21] Honda A, Noguchi N, Takehara H, et al. Cooperative enhancement of hyaluronic acid synthesis by combined use of IGF-I and EGF, and inhibition by tyrosine kinase inhibitor genistein, in cultured mesothelial cells from rabbit pericardial cavity. J Cell Sci 1991 Jan; 98(Pt 1):91–8.

[22] Hall CL, Wang C, Lange LA, Turley EA. Hyaluronan and the hyaluronan receptor RHAMM promote focal adhesion turnover and transient tyrosine kinase activity. J Cell Biol 1994 Jul; 126(2):575–88.

[23] Syrokou A, Tzanakakis GN, Hjerpe A, et al. Proteoglycans in human malignant mesothelioma. Stimulation of their synthesis induced by epidermal, insulin and platelet-derived growth

factors involves receptors with tyrosine kinase activity. Biochimie 1999 Jul; 81(7):733–44.

24 Slevin M, Krupinski J, Kumar S, Gaffney J. Angiogenic oligosaccharides of hyaluronan induce protein tyrosine kinase activity in endothelial cells and activate a cytoplasmic signal transduction pathway resulting in proliferation. Lab Invest 1998 Aug; 78(8):987–1003.

25 Reddy GK, Chandrakasan G, Dhar SC. Studies on the metabolism of glycosaminoglycans under the influence of new herbal anti-inflammatory agents. Biochem Pharmacol 1989 Oct 15; 38(20):3527–34.

26 Fischer S, Slaga T. Arachidonic acid metabolism and tumor promotion. Boston: Martinus Nijhoff Publishing, 1985, p. 219.

27 Belman S, Garte SJ. Proteases and cyclic nucleotides. In *Arachidonic acid metabolism and tumor promotion*. Fischer SM, Slaga TJ, eds. Boston: Martinus Nijhoff Publishing, 1985.

28 Spruss T, Bernhardt G, Schonenberger H, Schiess W. Hyaluronidase significantly enhances the efficacy of regional vinblastine chemotherapy of malignant melanoma. J Cancer Res Clin Oncol 1995; 121(4):193–202.

29 Smith KJ, Skelton HG, Turiansky G, Wagner KF. Hyaluronidase enhances the therapeutic effect of vinblastine in intralesional treatment of Kaposi's sarcoma. J Am Acad Dermatol 1997 Feb; 36(2 Pt 1):239–42.

30 Muckenschnabel I, Bernhardt G, Spruss T, Buschauer A. Hyaluronidase pretreatment produces selective melphalan enrichment in malignant melanoma implanted in nude mice. Cancer Chemother Pharmacol 1996; 38(1):88–94.

31 Severini G, Aliberti LM. Serum N-acetyl-beta-glucosaminidase activity in breast cancer. Cancer Biochem Biophys 1994 Sep; 14(2):87–92.

32 Severini G, Diana L, Di Giovannandrea R, Tirelli C. A study of serum glycosidases in cancer. J Cancer Res Clin Oncol 1995; 121(1):61–3.

33 Niedbala MJ, Madiyalakan R, Matta K, et al. Role of glycosidases in human ovarian carcinoma cell mediated degradation of subendothelial extracellular matrix. Cancer Res 1987 Sep 1; 47(17):4634–41.

34 Woynarowska B, Wikiel H, Sharma M, et al. Inhibition of human ovarian carcinoma cell- and hexosaminidase- mediated degradation of extracellular matrix by sugar analogs. Anticancer Res 1992 Jan–Feb; 12(1):161–6.

35 Ho KJ, Kuo SH. Urinary beta-glucuronidase activity as an initial screening test for urinary tract malignancy in high risk patients. Comparison with conventional urine cytologic evaluation. Cancer 1995 Aug 1; 76(3):473–8.

36 Ho KJ. Urinary beta-glucuronidase in screening and followup of primary urinary tract malignancy [see comments]. J Urol 1995 Oct; 154(4):1335–8.

37 Szary A, Kowalczyk-Bronisz SH, Gieldanowski J. Indomethacin as inhibitor of hyaluronidase. Arch Immunol Ther Exp (Warsz) 1975; 23(1):131–4.

38 Parish CR, Coombe DR, Jakobsen KB, et al. Evidence that sulphated polysaccharides inhibit tumour metstasis by blocking tumour-cell-derived heparanases. Int J Cancer 1987; 40:511–518.

39 Coombe DR, Parish CR, Ramshaw IA, Snowden JM. Analysis of the inhibition of tumour metastasis by sulphated polysaccharides. Int J Cancer 1987; 39:82–88.

40 Kobayashi M, Yamashita T, Tsubura E. Inhibition of blood-borne pulmonary metastasis by sulfated polysaccharides. Tokushima J Exp Med 1979; 26:41–45.

41 Banda MJ, Howard EW, Herron GS, et al. Secreted inhibitors of metalloproteinases (IMPs) that are distinct from TIMP. Matrix Suppl 1992; 1:294–8.

42 Anand-Apte B, Bao L, Smith R, et al. A review of tissue inhibitor of metalloproteinases-3 (TIMP-3) and experimental analysis of its effect on primary tumor growth. Biochem Cell Biol 1996; 74(6):853–62.

43 Yu AE, Hewitt RE, Kleiner DE, Stetler-Stevenson WG. Molecular regulation of cellular invasion—role of gelatinase A and TIMP-2. Biochem Cell Biol 1996; 74(6):823–31.

44 Shinkai K, Mukai M, Akedo H. Superoxide radical potentiates invasive capacity of rat ascites hapatoma cells in vitro. Cancer Letters 1986; 32:7–13.

45 Drubaix I, Viljanen-Tarifa E, Robert AM, Robert L. [Role of glycosoaminoglycans in venous disease. Mode of action of some flavonoid drugs.] Pathol Biol (Paris) 1995 May; 43(5):461–70.

46 Drubaix I, Maraval M, Robert L, Robert AM. [Hyaluronic acid (hyaluronan) levels in pathological human saphenous veins. Effects of procyanidol oligomers.] Pathol Biol (Paris) 1997 Jan; 45(1):86–91.

47 Sherman L, Sleeman J, Herrlich P, Ponta H. Hyaluronate receptors: Key players in growth, differentiation, migration and tumor progression. Curr Opin Cell Biol 1994 Oct; 6(5):726–33.

48 Sy MS, Liu D, Schiavone R, et al. Interactions between CD44 and hyaluronic acid: Their role in tumor growth and metastasis. Curr Top Microbiol Immunol 1996; 213 (Pt 3):129–53.

49 Culty M, Shizari M, Thompson EW, Underhill CB. Binding and degradation of hyaluronan by human breast cancer cell lines expressing different forms of CD44: Correlation with invasive potential. J Cell Physiol 1994 Aug; 160(2):275–86.

50 Guo YJ, Liu G, Wang X, et al. Potential use of soluble CD44 in serum as indicator of tumor burden and metastasis in patients with gastric or colon cancer. Cancer Res 1994 Jan 15; 54(2):422–6.

51 Braumuller H, Gansauge S, Ramadani M, Gansauge F. CD44v6 cell surface expression is a common feature of macrophages and macrophage-like cells. Implication for a natural macrophage extravasation mechanism mimicked by tumor cells. FEBS Lett 2000 Jul 7; 476(3):240–7.

52 Sleeman JP, Arming S, Moll JF, et al. Hyaluronate-independent metastatic behavior of CD44 variant-expressing pancreatic carcinoma cells. Cancer Res 1996 Jul 1; 56(13):3134–41.

53 Guo Y, Ma J, Wang J, et al. Inhibition of human melanoma growth and metastasis in vivo by anti-CD44 monoclonal antibody. Cancer Res 1994 Mar 15; 54(6):1561–5.

Metastasis is the movement of malignant cells from a primary tumor site to a distant location where they form a new tumor. As discussed in the last chapter, invasion and metastasis are related—tumor cells must generally invade the basement membrane for metastasis to be successful. In this chapter we examine the role that invasion plays in metastasis, as well as a number of other events needed for metastasis. Natural compounds will be discussed that may be useful in inhibiting these events.

Most cancers do metastasize. Metastatic cells travel through the blood and lymphatic circulation systems, and the metastatic colonies they form are often more life threatening than the primary tumor. In fact, the growth of a tumor at its primary location is generally not a cause of death, except in a limited number of cancers such as those of the brain, liver, and lungs. (Brain cancer, for example, is one of the few cancers that rarely metastasize.) Since metastasis is what makes so many cancers life threatening, its inhibition is an important clinical goal.

STEPS OF METASTASIS

The metastatic process is inherently inefficient. In a study of patients with kidney cancer, between 10 million and 1 billion cancer cells were released from their tumors into the bloodstream per day. In spite of this enormous release, 20 percent of the patients showed no evidence of new tumor development, even after 30 months.[1] In animal tumors, only 0.001 percent of the released tumor cells develop into metastatic colonies.[2, 3] The reasons for the inefficiency of the metastatic process are uncertain, but since at least five different sequential steps are required for its success, interruption of any one of them could derail the whole process. The last step in this process seems particularly sensitive to inhibition.

A metastatic colony develops according to the steps listed below and illustrated in Figure 10.1. Like many aspects of cancer, metastasis is a complicated process, and numerous factors can affect each step.

1. Cells detach from the primary tumor and invade the basement membrane surrounding blood vessels to gain access to the bloodstream, a process called intravasation.

2. Once they are circulating in the bloodstream, the migrating cells evade attack by the immune system and survive other adverse conditions.

3. The migrating cells adhere to the wall of a blood vessel at the metastatic site—the process of cell arrest.

4. The arrested cells exit the blood vessel and, by invading through the basement membrane, enter the tissues. This process is called extravasation.

5. The tumor cells proliferate and the new tumor induces angiogenesis.

Studies with small video cameras suggest that at least in some cases, the majority of traveling metastatic cells come to rest in a target capillary bed and that most of these successfully exit the circulation (step four above). After this point, however, only a small fraction begins to proliferate and form a new tumor. The majority remains dormant, neither proliferating nor undergoing apoptosis.[4] Since the cells that do undergo proliferation likely do so in response to signals from growth factors, interactions with the extracellular matrix, and/or other signals such as free radicals or hypoxia, all the natural compounds mentioned in previous chapters that affect these signals may inhibit metastasis.

Each of the five steps is discussed individually below. Although they refer primarily to metastasis via the blood circulation, metastasis through the lymphatic system can occur by similar processes.

CELL DETACHMENT AND MOVEMENT INTO A VESSEL

The initial step in metastasis is detachment of cells from the primary tumor. Once detached, cancer cells contact a blood vessel (usually within the tumor) and secrete or induce the secretion of proteolytic enzymes, which digest the basement membrane. Tumor cells then slip between the cells of the vascular lining to enter the circulation. This process of intravasation is facilitated by the poorly developed basement membranes and fragile capillaries produced within the tumor during angiogenesis. An intact basement membrane is a barrier that inhibits metastasis. In some cases, broken capillaries may allow instant access to the circulation.

Cell detachment rates tend to increase as a tumor enlarges and as it undergoes central necrosis. Other fac-

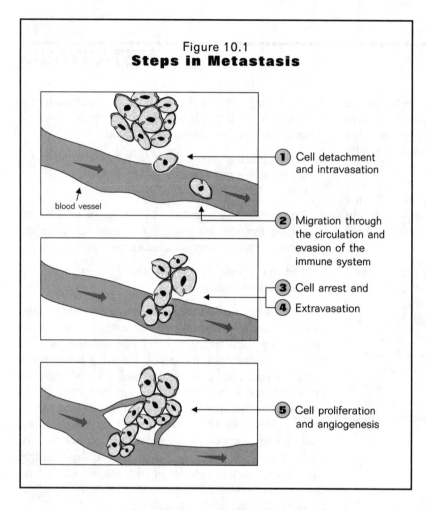

Figure 10.1
Steps in Metastasis

blood vessel

1 Cell detachment and intravasation

2 Migration through the circulation and evasion of the immune system

3 Cell arrest and
4 Extravasation

5 Cell proliferation and angiogenesis

limiting metastasis. The immune cells that appear to be most active in attacking migrating cancer cells are natural killer (NK) cells and macrophages. Studies suggest that

- metastasis is more frequent in animals with immune cell deficits, including deficits caused by immunosuppressive drugs;

- when animals are injected with tumor tissue, metastasis is more frequent if the macrophages within the tumor tissue are extracted before injection;

- metastasis is less frequent in mice that have high levels of NK cells.[5]

These observations suggest that natural compounds that stimulate the immune system may inhibit metastasis. This may be particularly true for those compounds that stimulate NK cell activity. For example, the mushroom polysaccharide PSK, an immune stimulant that enhances NK cell activity, has been reported to inhibit metastasis in tumor-bearing animals.[6, 7] Chapters 11 and 12 discuss the immune system in detail, along with natural compounds that affect it.

tors that may stimulate detachment include mechanical stress, increased hydrostatic pressure within tumors, increased activity by various proteolytic enzymes, and decreased expression of cell adhesion molecules on the cell's surface. Of these, CAMs and proteolytic enzymes are of particular importance in this book (see Chapters 6 and 9).

MIGRATION THROUGH THE CIRCULATION

Once cells detach from the tumor and enter the blood, the second step in metastasis is the migration of tumor cells through the circulation. A significant percentage of migrating tumor cells die in this step due to forces present in the circulation.

The most important of these forces may be the immune system. Although there is considerable evidence that the immune system plays a prominent role in inhibiting metastasis, the issue is complex, and no simple correlation between immune status and metastatic spread has been found. Nevertheless, numerous animal experiments do support a role for the immune system in

In addition to the immune system, other forces may destroy migrating tumor cells. These include mechanical stress as cells move through the small vessels, and toxicity caused by high oxygen levels in the blood.[8] It is difficult to affect these forces, and they are not discussed here other than to say that some investigators have studied the possibility of administering oxygen-rich air to cancer patients. There is also evidence that metastasizing cells are protected from apoptosis by high intracellular levels of the antioxidant glutathione.[9, 10] Thus antioxidants could potentially produce a prometastatic effect. Indeed, at least two studies have reported that antioxidants could increase metastasis in rodents (see Chapter 15).[11, 12] For this reason and others discussed there, I do not recommend the use of antioxidants as sole treatment agents. They may still be useful, however, as one part of a more complex anticancer strategy.

CELL ARREST AT A NEW LOCATION

The third step in metastasis is cell arrest. Because the environment within blood vessels is inhospitable to migrating tumor cells, the cells must leave the blood vessels in order to survive. This exit is initiated by attaching to the capillary wall, referred to as cell arrest. Several factors promote cell arrest at a given location, including CAM activity, vessel damage or thinning of the basement membrane, platelet aggregation, and fibrin formation. CAM activity was discussed in Chapter 6; the other factors are discussed below.

Damage to the Basement Membrane

Tumor cells adhere more efficiently to the exposed collagen of a damaged blood vessel than to normal vessel walls, and so damaged areas provide prime targets for cell arrest. Vessels can be damaged by trauma or inflammation; in fact, evidence is mounting that surgical removal of some tumors can promote tumor metastasis to existing wounds.[13, 14] This effect may also be facilitated by the growth factors present in wound fluid. Therefore, natural compounds that protect the vasculature or reduce inflammation may limit cell arrest. A host of anti-inflammatory and anticollagenase compounds have already been discussed (see Chapters 8 and 9). Some natural compounds like proanthocyanidins appear to have a specific affinity for vascular tissue and may be particularly useful.

Platelet Aggregation and Fibrin Production

Platelet aggregation and fibrin production can play an important role in metastasis. Three mechanisms by which they can promote metastasis are:[2, 3]

- Activated platelets are sticky and can act as a glue to enhance adhesion of tumor cells to the blood vessel lining.

- Platelet-secreted growth factors like platelet-derived growth factor (PDGF) can stimulate the proliferation of tumor cells and contribute to their survival within the blood circulation.

- The excessive fibrin production surrounding tumor cells enhances their stickiness and facilitates their arrest at metastatic sites. Fibrin helps tumor cells to aggregate with each other while migrating in the blood, thereby forming a larger clump that may more easily lodge in a capillary bed. In experimental studies on mice, the efficiency of metastasis was increased when either large numbers of tumor cells or clumps of tumor cells were injected.[15]

Regarding the last item, animal experiments have reported that oral administration of fibrinolytic enzymes such as bromelain and WOBE-MUGOS (a proprietary mixture of enzymes) inhibits tumor metastasis.[16, 17, 18] However, this effect could also be due to factors other than fibrinolysis, such as enzyme-induced digestion of CD44 surface proteins or immune stimulation.[a]

Experimental studies have reported that migrating cells from some cancers induce platelet aggregation by modifying the prostanoid balance.[8] Prostanoids were introduced in Chapter 7, and two additional ones are discussed here. Platelet aggregation depends on the relative balance of prostaglandin I (PGI, or prostacyclin) and thromboxane (see Figure 7.3). PGI is produced by vascular cells and inhibits platelet aggregation, whereas thromboxane is produced by platelets and enhances aggregation. Tumors promote platelet aggregation by inhibiting production of PGI or by stimulating production of thromboxane or both.

Platelet aggregation can readily be manipulated; however, numerous studies designed to test the antimetastatic effects of anticoagulants and platelet inhibitors have in general been inconclusive.[19, 20] One common drug that inhibits platelet aggregation is aspirin, which does so by preventing the formation of thromboxane. A single dose of aspirin can suppress platelet aggregation for 48 hours and longer. In one study on cancer-bearing mice, aspirin significantly reduced the number of lung metastases.[5] COX-2 inhibitors (see Tables 8.2 and F.2) might also have this effect, but again, the antimetastatic effect of platelet aggregation inhibitors is still in question. It is reasonable to speculate that the mixed results of the studies are due to the limited ability of platelet aggregation inhibitors to prevent metastasis when used alone, but that when used as one part of a larger combination therapy, they may be more effective.

Some cancer patients may be at risk for bleeding, and in fact, unexpected bleeding can be the initial symptom of cancers of the lung, colon, kidney, and uterus. In addition, patients can bleed after surgery. The indiscriminate use of fibrinolytic agents or agents that inhibit platelet aggregation in these patients could be disastrous. Not all cancer patients are at high risk for bleeding, however. Because of the potential danger in some patients and because studies on the use of anticoagulants and platelet inhibitors have been inconclusive, no new anticoagulant compounds are introduced in this chapter. In Table 10.1 the list of natural compounds that produce an anticoagulant effect through fibrinolysis or inhibition of platelet aggregation contains only those compounds otherwise mentioned in this book. Table 10.1 alerts the reader that these compounds should be used with cau-

---

[a] *In contrast, intravenous administration of fibrinolytic enzymes, which produces much higher plasma levels, may have either a positive or negative effect on metastasis. Intravenous doses of fibrinolytic compounds can also promote tumor growth and angiogenesis (see Chapter 8).*

TABLE 10.1 NATURAL ANTICOAGULANT COMPOUNDS	
COMPOUND	**REFERENCES**
Anthocyanidins	21
Astragalus membranaceus	22, 23, 24
Bromelain (fibrinolytic)	25, 26, 27
Curcumin	28, 29
Emodin	30
EPA	31, 32, 33
Feverfew	34
Flavonoids (including quercetin, apigenin and luteolin)	35–38
Ganoderma lucidum	39, 40
Garlic (fibrinolytic)	25, 41–43
Genistein and other PTK inhibitors	44, 45, 46
Panax ginseng	22, 23
PSK	47
Resveratrol	48, 49
Vitamin E	50, 51

tion in patients who may have a bleeding problem. Although no studies have compared their relative strengths, some of these compounds, such as bromelain, EPA, feverfew, garlic, PTK inhibitors, resveratrol, and vitamin E, might produce a relatively strong anticoagulant effect, while the others might produce a weaker one.

MOVEMENT OUT OF THE VESSEL

The fourth step in metastasis is extravasation, the movement of the metastatic colony out of the blood vessel. This is mediated by proteases and other factors in a process similar to movement into the blood vessel (step one). In both cases, the basement membrane provides an obstacle to the movement of tumor cells through the vessel wall.

One of the factors that mediates extravasation is local trauma (damaged capillaries). Just as trauma may facilitate intravasation (step one) and cell arrest (step three), it may also facilitate movement out of the vessel. One study reported that when cancer cells were injected into rabbits with traumatized tissues, metastasis to the trauma site was increased 20-fold over nontraumatized tissues.[5] Therefore, we again see that compounds that stabilize the vasculature or basement membrane may inhibit metastasis. These compounds were discussed in Chapter 8 (see Table 8.1) and Chapter 9 (see Tables 9.1 and 9.2).

INDUCTION OF ANGIOGENESIS

The fifth and final step in tumor metastasis is cell proliferation and induction of angiogenesis. Without angiogenesis, a tumor is unable to grow larger than a few millimeters in diameter. Once angiogenesis is established, the tumor can seed itself in a new cycle of metastasis. In fact, tumors generally do not metastasize until angiogenesis is initiated. The leaky vessels produced during angiogenesis allow tumor cells greater access to the circulation. Thus compounds that inhibit angiogenesis may inhibit metastasis (see Chapter 8). Similarly, any compounds discussed thus far that inhibit cell proliferation may also inhibit this last step in metastasis.

CONCLUSION

Metastasis is a five-step process consisting of cell detachment and intravasation, migration through the circulation, arrest at a new location, extravasation, and cell proliferation and angiogenesis. Successful metastasis is the deadly culmination of nearly every process we have discussed so far. At every step it seems likely that natural compounds might play a significant role in slowing down or even stopping its course.

REFERENCES

[1] Glaves D, Huben RP, Weiss L. Haematogenous dissemination of cells from human renal adenocarcinomas. Br J Cancer 1988; 57:32–35.

[2] Honn KV, Menter DG, Steinert BW, et al. Analysis of platelet, tumor cell, and endothelial cell interactions in vivo and in vitro. In *Prostaglandins in cancer research*. Garaci E, Paoletti R, Santoro MG, eds. New York: Springer-Verlag, 1987.

[3] Honn KV, Steinert BW, Onoda JM, et al. The role of platelets in metastasis. Biorheology 1987; 24(2):127–137.

[4] Morris VL, Schmidt EE, MacDonald IC, et al. Sequential steps in hematogenous metastasis of cancer cells studied by in vivo videomicroscopy. Invasion Metastasis 1997; 17(6):281–96.

[5] Calabresi P, Schein P. Medical oncology. 2nd ed. New York: McGraw-Hill, 1993, pp. 69–71.

[6] Nakamura K, Matsunaga K. Susceptibility of natural killer (NK) cells to reactive oxygen species (ROS) and their restoration by the mimics of superoxide dismutase (SOD). Cancer Biother Radiopharm 1998 Aug; 13(4):275–90.

[7] Suo J, Tanaka N, Hizuta A, Yunoki S, Orita K. Suppression of hepatic natural killer activity by liver metastasis of cancer and restoration of killer activity by oral administration of a Basidomycetes-derived polysaccharide, PSK. Acta Med Okayama 1994 Oct; 48(5):237–42.

[8] Tannock IF, Hill RP, eds. The basic science of oncology. 2nd ed. New York: McGraw-Hill, 1992, pp. 181–2.

9 Anasagasti MJ, Martin JJ, Mendoza L, et al. Glutathione protects metastatic melanoma cells against oxidative stress in the murine hepatic microvasculature. Hepatology 1998 May; 27(5):1249–56.

10 Eskenazi AE, Pinkas J, Whitin JC, et al. Role of antioxidant enzymes in the induction of increased experimental metastasis by hydroxyurea. J Natl Cancer Inst 1993 May 5; 85(9):711–21.

11 Evangelou A, Kalpouzos G, Karkabounas S, et al. Dose-related preventive and therapeutic effects of antioxidants-anticarcinogens on experimentally induced malignant tumors in Wistar rats. Cancer Lett 1997 May 1; 115(1):105–11.

12 Kanclerz A, Zbytniewski Z, Boeryd B. Influence of some synthetic antioxidants on the growth and metastases formation of Lewis lung carcinoma and amelanotic B16 melanoma in C57BL mice. Arch Geschwulstforsch 1981; 51(5):379–85.

13 Neuhaus SJ, Ellis T, Jamieson GG, Watson DI. Experimental study of the effect of intraperitoneal heparin on tumour implantation following laparoscopy. Br J Surg 1999 Mar; 86(3):400–4.

14 Abramovitch R, Marikovsky M, Meir G, Neeman M. Stimulation of tumour growth by wound-derived growth factors. Br J Cancer 1999 Mar; 79(9–10):1392–8.

15 Hill RP, Young SD, Cillo C, Ling V. Metastatic cell phenotypes: Quantitative studies using the experimental metastasis assay. Cancer Rev 1986; 5:118–151.

16 Klaschka, F. Oral enzymes in oncology: Clinical studies on Wobe-MuGos. MUCOS Pharma GmbH, 1997. http://www.mucos.de

17 Batkin S, Taussig S, Szekerczes J. Modulation of pulmonary metastasis (Lewis lung carcinoma) by bromelain, an extract of the pineapple stem (Ananas comosus) [letter]. Cancer Invest 1988; 6(2):241–2.

18 Batkin S, Taussig SJ, Szekerezes J. Antimetastatic effect of bromelain with or without its proteolytic and anticoagulant activity. J Cancer Res Clin Oncol 1988; 114(5):507–8.

19 Gasic GJ. Role of plasma, platelets, and endothelial cells in tumor metastasis. Cancer Metastasis Rev 1984; 3(2):99–114.

20 Al-Mondhiry H. Tumor interaction with hemostasis: The rationale for the use of platelet inhibitors and anticoagulants in the treatment of cancer. Am J Hematol 1984 Feb; 16(2):193–202.

21 Zaragoza F, Iglesias I, Benedi J. [Comparative study of the anti-aggregation effects of anthocyanosides and other agents.] Arch Farmacol Toxicol 1985 Dec; 11(3):183–8.

22 Wang SR, Guo ZQ, Liao JZ. Experimental study on the effects of 18 kinds of Chinese herbal medicine for synthesis of thromboxane A2 and PGI2. Chung Kuo Chung Hsi I Chieh Ho Tsa Chih 1993; 13(3):167–70.

23 Liao J, et al. Clinical and experimental studies of coronary heart disease treated with Yi-Qi Huo-Xue injection. J Trad Chin Med 1989; 9(3):193–8.

24 Li W, et al. Effects of Codonopsis pilosula-astralagus injection on platelet aggregation and activity of PGI2-like substance. J of Tradit Chinese Med 1986; 6(1):9–12.

25 Petry JJ. Surgically significant nutritional supplements. Plas Reconstr Surg 1996 Jan; 97(1):233–40.

26 Felton GE. Fibrinolytic and antithrombotic action of bromelain may eliminate thrombosis in heart patients. Med Hypothesis 1980; 6:1123–33.

27 Kelly GS. Bromelain: A literature review and discussion of its therapeutic applications. Alt Med Rev 1996; 1(4):243–257.

28 Srivastava KC. Extracts from two frequently consumed spices—cumin (Cuminum cyminum) and turmeric (Curcuma longa)—inhibit platelet aggregation and alter eicosanoid biosynthesis in human blood platelets. Prostaglandins Leukot Essent Fatty Acids 1989 Jul; 37(1):57–64.

29 Srivastava KC, Bordia A, Verma SK. Curcumin, a major component of food spice turmeric (Curcuma longa) inhibits aggregation and alters eicosanoid metabolism in human blood platelets. Prostaglandins Leukot Essent Fatty Acids 1995 Apr; 52(4):223–7.

30 Chung MI, Gan KH, Lin CN, et al. Antiplatelet effects and vasorelaxing action of some constituents of Formosan plants. J Nat Prod 1993 Jun; 56(6):929–34.

31 Yamada N, Takita T, Wada M, et al. Effects of dietary n-3/n-6 and polyunsaturated fatty acid/saturated fatty acid ratios on platelet aggregation and lipid metabolism in rats. J Nutr Sci Vitaminol (Tokyo) 1996 Oct; 42(5):423–34.

32 Mori TA, Beilin LJ, Burke V, et al. Interactions between dietary fat, fish, and fish oils and their effects on platelet function in men at risk of cardiovascular disease. Arterioscler Thromb Vasc Biol 1997 Feb; 17(2):279–86.

33 Mutanen M, Freese R. Polyunsaturated fatty acids and platelet aggregation. Curr Opin Lipidol 1996 Feb; 7(1):14–9.

34 Loesche W, Mazurov AV, Voyno-Yasenetskaya TA, et al. Feverfew—an antithrombotic drug? Folia Haematol Int Mag Klin Morphol Blutforsch 1988; 115(1–2):181–4.

35 Landolfi R, Mower RL, Steiner M. Modification of platelet function and arachidonic acid metabolism by bioflavonoids. Structure-activity relations. Biochem Pharmacol 1984 May 1; 33(9):1525–30.

36 Teng CM, Ko FN, Wang JP, et al. Antihaemostatic and antithrombotic effect of some antiplatelet agents isolated from Chinese herbs. J Pharm Pharmacol 1991 Sep; 43(9):667–9.

37 Gryglewski RJ, Korbut R, Robak R, Swies J. On the mechanism of antithrombotic action of flavonoids. Biochemical Pharmacology 1987; 36(3):317–322.

38 Tzeng SH, Ko WC, Ko FN, Teng CM. Inhibition of platelet aggregation by some flavonoids. Thromb Res 1991 Oct 1; 64(1):91–100.

39 Lin JM, Lin CC, Chin HF, et al. Evaluation of the anti-inflammatory and liver-protective effects of anoectochilus formosanus, Ganoderma lucidum and Gynostemma pentaphyllum in rats. American Journal of Chinese Medicine 1993; XXI(1):56–69.

40 Wang CN, Chen JC, Shiao MS, Wang CT. The inhibition of human platelet function by ganodermic acids. Biochem J 1991 Jul 1; 277 (Pt 1):189–97.

41 Katiyar SK, Agarwal R, Mukhtar H. Inhibition of tumor promotion in SENCAR mouse skin by ethanol extract of Zingiber officinale rhizome. Cancer Res 1996 Mar 1; 56(5):1023–30.

[42] Srivastava KC. Aqueous extracts of onion, garlic and ginger inhibit platelet aggregation and alter arachidonic acid metabolism. Biomed Biochim Acta 1984; 43(8–9):S335–46.

[43] Srivastava KC, Mustafa T. Spices: Antiplatelet activity and prostanoid metabolism. Prostaglandins Leukot Essent Fatty Acids 1989 Dec; 38(4):255–66.

[44] Wang X, Yanagi S, Yang C, et al. Tyrosine phosphorylation and Syk activation are involved in thrombin-induced aggregation of epinephrine-potentiated platelets. J Biochem (Tokyo) 1997 Feb; 121(2):325–30.

[45] Kubota Y, Arai T, Tanaka T, et al. Thrombopoietin modulates platelet activation in vitro through protein-tyrosine phosphorylation. Stem Cells 1996 Jul; 14(4):439–44.

[46] Furman MI Grigoryev D, Bray PF, et al. Platelet tyrosine kinases and fibrinogen receptor activation. Circ Res 1994 Jul; 75(1):172–80.

[47] Takahata K, Yamanaka M, Oka H. [Effect of PSK on prostaglandin metabolism.] Gan To Kagaku Ryoho 1985 May; 12(5):1131–6.

[48] Bertelli AA, Giovannini L, Giannessi D, et al. Antiplatelet activity of cis-resveratrol. Drugs Exp Clin Res 1996; 22(2):61–3.

[49] Bertelli AA, Giovannini L, Giannessi D, et al. Antiplatelet activity of synthetic and natural resveratrol in red wine. Int J Tissue React 1995; 17(1):1–3.

[50] Williams JC, Forster LA, Tull SP, et al. Dietary vitamin E supplementation inhibits thrombin-induced platelet aggregation, but not monocyte adhesiveness, in patients with hypercholesterolaemia. Int J Exp Pathol 1997 Aug; 78(4):259–66.

[51] Chan AC. Vitamin E and atherosclerosis. J Nutr 1998 Oct; 128(10):1593–6.

The immune system is a complex organization of white blood cells, antibodies, and blood factors that protects the body from foreign invaders. Many investigators believe the immune system plays a key role both in preventing the establishment of new cancers, a process known as "immune surveillance," and in limiting the progression of established tumors. As we will see in Chapter 12, natural compounds can be used to both support and stimulate immune function. It is too simplistic, however, to expect that using these kinds of immunoactive compounds alone will profoundly affect the course of an established cancer. Indeed, there is now much evidence that even powerful immune stimulants, such as the cytokine interleukin-2, have only moderate effects on established cancers, and then only on a few select types.

There are two reasons why immune stimulants have not been found highly effective against established cancers. The first, more theoretical reason is that the immune system acts as a kind of last-chance net for catching and ensuring the destruction of cancer cells. Just as excessive criminal activity in a city can overwhelm a police force, too many cancer cells can overwhelm the immune system. Thus to reduce the number of cancer cells, and thereby maximize the ability of the immune system to destroy them, cancer cells must be cut at their root; the aberrant signals that sustain their lives must be normalized. We have discussed in previous chapters how this might be accomplished.

The second, more mechanical reason immune stimulants have not been effective against established cancers is that cancer cells have devised numerous ways to evade immune recognition and attack. Thus even a well-functioning immune system will generally not destroy an established cancer.

In spite of its difficulties in destroying cancer, a healthy immune system is still important and immune stimulation does have a role in cancer treatment, particularly as one part of a multifaceted strategy. Such a strategy must, however, include compounds that prevent immune evasion, or immune stimulation will not play its role successfully.

The immune system is a complex world unto itself, and large books have been written attempting to describe how it works. Here I provide only a rudimentary overview as a background for understanding the relationship between it and cancer. We look at how it functions in general, and how it affects and is affected by cancer. We also look at ways immune stimulants have been used in conventional medicine to treat cancer, which provides context for using natural compounds to do the same (see Chapter 12).

INNATE AND ADAPTIVE IMMUNITY

Without an immune system we would quickly fall prey to the plethora of viruses, bacteria, and parasites that live within and around us. The immune system is a multilayered defense system. In its broadest sense, it includes physical barriers, such as the skin and the lining of the gastrointestinal tract; chemical barriers, such as stomach acid; microbial barriers, such as beneficial intestinal microflora; and the immune system proper (immune cells, antibodies, and so forth). This chapter focuses on the immune system proper.

The cells of the immune system are called white blood cells (leukocytes) that, like red blood cells (erythrocytes), are derived from stem cells in the bone marrow. The production of the different types of cells from the bone marrow is shown in Figure 11.1 (adapted from reference 1). Other cells important in the immune response but not shown in the figure (e.g., natural killer cells and dendritic cells) are discussed below.

As Figure 11.1 shows, leukocytes can be classified into two categories: those that derive from myeloid stem cells (macrophages and granulocytes) and those from lymphoid stem cells (the lymphocytes). Macrophages and granulocytes are involved with innate immunity, and lymphocytes are involved with adaptive immunity. Innate immunity provides the first line of defense against newly encountered pathogens.[a] It limits the initial progression of the pathogens and activates the adaptive immune system. Unlike the innate system, the adaptive system has the ability to remember previous pathogens and thereby mount a fast attack if the pathogen is encountered more than once.

The two systems function together to keep out foreign organisms, which are recognized as such by their foreign proteins or their lack of "self-proteins." In a simple analogy, the two systems can be likened to the security system at an international airport. A small group of se-

---

[a] *The immune system protects against four classes of pathogens: extracellular bacteria, parasites, and fungi; intracellular bacteria and parasites; intracellular viruses; and extracellular parasitic worms.*

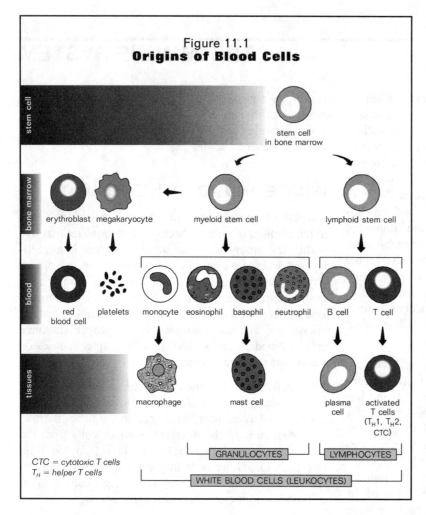

Figure 11.1
Origins of Blood Cells

stem cell

stem cell
in bone marrow

bone marrow

erythroblast   megakaryocyte   myeloid stem cell   lymphoid stem cell

blood

red   platelets   monocyte eosinophil basophil neutrophil   B cell   T cell
blood cell

tissues

macrophage   mast cell   plasma   activated
                                                      cell   T cells
                                                                 (T_H1, T_H2,
                                                                    CTC)

CTC = cytotoxic T cells
T_H = helper T cells

GRANULOCYTES   LYMPHOCYTES

WHITE BLOOD CELLS (LEUKOCYTES)

gregate formed by the MHC and antigen then rests at the surface of the innate immune cell, waiting for a cell from the adaptive system to come sample it. Cells of the adaptive system could not recognize the antigen as foreign if it were not presented to them in an MHC-antigen aggregate.

As the analogy illustrates, cells of the innate immune system handle the initial response to a pathogen. They attempt to clear the pathogen from the body, and if they are successful, the immune response ends. If unsuccessful and the amount of antigen reaches a threshold concentration, the adaptive immune system is stimulated. The cells of the adaptive immune system then help those of the innate system to destroy the pathogen. Furthermore, some of the B cells of the adaptive system form memory B cells that remember the specific antigen if it is encountered again. Other B cells differentiate to form plasma cells, which produce antibodies specific to the new foreign antigens. On reinfection with the same pathogen, the memory B cells quickly produce antibodies and engage the adaptive immune system.

curity guards—the cells of the innate system—are on guard at the security checkpoint to screen all incoming passengers, looking for "undesirable foreign elements." These guards have a rather nonspecific way of identifying suspects. Possibly they look for an absence of ordinary characteristics (a lack of self-proteins), or they look for generalized suspicious characteristics. If they spot suspects, they obtain their ID and call nearby guards—also cells of the innate system—for assistance. If there is trouble these guards can't handle, they call the state police—the adaptive immune system—who might take some time to arrive. Once they do, the guards present the suspect's IDs and the police take the suspects into custody. Importantly, the police also remember the suspect's IDs so that next time they come through the airport they can quickly be recognized.

The method that cells of the innate immune system use to "obtain" the IDs of foreign organisms and "present" them to the cells of the adaptive system is fascinating. Cells of the innate system ingest the foreign pathogens and, after digesting them a bit, "burp up" their protein fragments (called antigens) in a carrier molecule, called the major histocompatibility complex (MHC). The ag-

The different cell types of the innate and adaptive immune system are listed in Table 11.1, along with a description of what activates them, what their function is, and what cells assist them (accessory cells). Two cell types, natural killer (NK) cells and dendritic cells, not shown in Figure 11.1, are also listed. NK cells are a type of specialized lymphocyte that destroy foreign cells. The main function of dendritic cells is to present antigens to T cells. Each of these cell types are described later in this chapter.

In Table 11.1, T cells are categorized by their CD (cluster of differentiation) number. T_H1 and T_H2 cells are CD4 cells, and cytotoxic T cells are CD8 cells. The CD number is simply a way to identify cells by their prominent surface proteins. Recall from Chapter 9 that the CD44 protein is a cell adhesion molecule that binds to components of the extracellular matrix. Similarly, both CD4 and CD8 are proteins that assist T cells in the final phase of docking with antigen-presenting cells. The first phase is accomplished by ICAMs, which are surface proteins that allow cells to stick together (see Chapter 6).

The primary molecule that allows a CD4 or a CD8 T cell to dock with antigen-presenting cells is called the T-

TABLE 11.1 LEUKOCYTES IN INNATE AND ADAPTIVE IMMUNITY		
NONGRANULOCYTES IN INNATE IMMUNITY		
Name	**Activated by**	**Activated function**
Macrophages	general microbial constituents (but not antigens)	Eat (phagocytose) pathogens and tumor cells. Macrophages are the primary phagocytic cells of tissues outside the blood vessels; their name literally means "big eaters." They also present antigens from the pathogens they ingest to T cells.
Natural killer (NK) cells	uncertain, but may recognize a lack of MHC molecules on the surface of foreign cells	Release compounds that destroy some virus-infected cells; they can also kill tumor cells.

GRANULOCYTES IN INNATE IMMUNITY	
Name	**Activated function**
Neutrophils, eosinophils, basophils, and mast cells	Granulocytes are so named because of their densely staining intracellular granules. Neutrophils phagocytose pathogens and are the primary phagocytic cells of the blood. Eosinophils destroy antibody-coated parasites. Basophils release granules containing histamine and other inflammatory agents (see Chapter 8); those that reside in tissues are called mast cells. Granulocytes do not play as large a role in destroying cancer cells as macrophages and NK cells.

LEUKOCYTES IN ADAPTIVE IMMUNITY			
Name	**Description**	**Activated by**	**Activated Function**
CD4 T Cells	T_H1 cells: (helper T cells): a T lymphocyte that expresses the CD4 surface protein	antigen-MHC class II aggregate on infected macrophage	Activate macrophages to kill bacteria that lie within them. Release cytokines that attract macrophages.
	T_H2 cells (helper T cells): a T lymphocyte that expresses the CD4 surface protein	antigen-MHC class II aggregate on B cells	stimulate B cells to produce antibodies
CD8 T Cells	cytotoxic T cells: a T lymphocyte that expresses the CD8 surface protein	antigen-MHC class I aggregate on infected cell	destroy infected cells
B Cells	B lymphocytes	contact with antigen	present antigens to T cells and produce antibodies
Accessory Cells	**Name**	**Activated By**	**Activated Function**
Antigen-presenting cells (APCs)	dendritic cells, macrophages, and B cells	contact with antigen or by viral infection	Present antigens to T cells. Dendritic cells are the most important of the three types of antigen-presenting cells.

cell receptor. The T-cell receptor actually docks directly to the antigen-MHC aggregate, and in this way the antigen is presented to the T cell. CD4 and D8 proteins are called co-receptor molecules, since they assist the T-cell receptor molecule to dock.

ANTIGENS AND ANTIBODIES

The antibodies produced by the B cells of the adaptive system are a key element in the adaptive response. They are tiny Y-shaped proteins belonging to the immunoglobulin family of proteins; some CAMs are also related to this family (see Chapter 6). After being produced by B cells, antigens travel in the blood circulation and can reside in tissues.

Antibodies perform three important tasks. First, they neutralize antigens like bacterial toxins by surrounding them and preventing them from causing harm. Second, they coat (opsonize) pathogens in a way that makes the pathogens more attractive to immune cells, such as macrophages and natural killer cells. Lastly, antibodies activate the complement system; so-called because it "complements" the antibodies, helping them in their work of defense.

The complement system involves production of a series of plasma proteins that, when stimulated, bind to an antigen-antibody complex (this is called the classical complement pathway). The primary purpose of these proteins, like that of antibodies, is to make pathogens more recognizable and attractive to phagocytic immune cells like macrophages. Complement proteins can also bind to sugars on the pathogen surface or bind directly

TABLE 11.2 MACROPHAGE DESTRUCTION OF PATHOGENS AND THE ROLE OF T CELLS			
EVENTS	**PATHOGEN IN CYTOSOL**	**PATHOGEN IN VESICLES**	
Pathogen degraded in:	cytosol	acidified vesicles	acidified vesicles
Antigens bind to:	MHC class I	MHC class II	MHC class II
Antigens presented to:	CD8 T cells	CD4 T_H1 cells	CD4 T_H2 cells
Effect of antigen presentation:	CD8 T cells destroy macrophages and other cells displaying the antigen	CD4 T_H1 cells activate macrophage to kill pathogens in vesicles	CD4 T_H2 cells activate B cells to produce antibodies

Source: Reference 2.

to the pathogen and destroy it by rupturing its cell membrane (these are called the lectin and alternative pathways, respectively).

MHC MOLECULE

As mentioned, cells of the innate system, such as macrophages and dendritic cells, present antigens to cells of the adaptive system in the form of antigen-MHC (major histocompatibility) aggregates. Pathogens enter antigen-presenting cells in one of two ways: either the pathogen is ingested, as when a macrophage ingests bacteria, or the pathogen enters the cell by its own means, as occurs with a virus. Accordingly, there are two forms of the MHC, one for carrying antigens from ingested pathogens and one for carrying them from viruses. MHC class I molecules carry antigens from virally infected cells (the antigens being picked up in the cytosol), and class II molecules carry ones picked up from bacteria or other pathogens that were degraded in intracellular vesicles (see Figure 2.1 for the cytosol and intracellular vesicles). Intracellular vesicles function somewhat like the intestines in animals. Phagocytic immune cells eat pathogens and digest them with acids in vesicles.

T-helper cells of the adaptive system are designed to recognize antigen-MHC class II aggregates (again, which contain antigens obtained from vesicles). Upon recognition, the T-helper cells do one of two things: T-helper 1 (T_H1) cells stimulate macrophages so they can better digest the pathogens in their vesicles, and T-helper 2 (T_H2) cells stimulate B cells to make antibodies to the antigen.

In contrast, cytotoxic T cells of the adaptive system are designed to recognize antigen-MHC class I aggregates (containing antigens from the virally infected cytosol). Upon recognition, cytotoxic T cells destroy any cells that display the virus's antigen.

In order to pick up and deliver antigens to T cells, antigen-presenting cells circulate between the tissues, blood, and lymph organs. Although mature dendritic cells are found exclusively in the lymph organs, the precursors of these cells migrate in the blood and lymph to infection sites where they pick up antigens.

B and T cells also circulate between the bloodstream and the lymph organs. The most common location where antigen-presenting cells meet T cells is the lymph organs (spleen, tonsils, and other lymph nodes). The lymph organs are so designed that a high concentration of T and B cells come in contact with a high concentration of antigen-presenting cells. T and B cells that have not yet encountered antigens are called "naïve" cells. Upon contact with antigens, these naïve cells temporarily remain in the lymph node to proliferate, and their offspring differentiate into activated or "effector" lymphocytes capable of combating the infection. This is the reason people develop swollen glands during an infection. Eventually, these primed effector cells travel in the lymph and blood to the infection site.

The destruction of different pathogens by macrophages is summarized in Table 11.2. Although the table is specific to macrophages, the events occurring in other antigen-presenting cells are similar.

ROLE OF CYTOKINES IN IMMUNITY

Cytokines are a varied group of soluble proteins secreted by mammalian cells that affect the behavior of the secreting cell or that of nearby cells via specific cytokine receptors. Growth factors are also cytokines and can be produced by many cell types, but we use the term *cytokine* here to refer to soluble proteins produced by immune cells. Note that some proteins are referred to as both cytokines and growth factors, since they are produced by both immune cells and other cells. Cytokines, like the growth factors listed in Table 4.1, control a wide range of cellular behavior besides proliferation. Some cytokines like TGF-beta even inhibit cell proliferation. In this way cytokines play a significant role in the control of hematopoiesis (the production of red and white blood cells), the inflammatory response, and the immune response.

Cytokines and Immune Cell Activation

In the following sections we discuss how cytokines activate CD8 T cells (cytotoxic T cells), macrophages, B cells and CD4 T cells. The important points to remember here are simply that many cytokines are involved, and their moment-to-moment mix determines the effect on immune cell activation.

Cytokine Activation of CD8 T Cells

The primary cytokine that instructs CD8 T cells to proliferate after antigen presentation is IL-2; some of which comes from the T cell itself. When stimulated by contact with the appropriate antigen on the surface of a pathogen, the primed CD8 T cell secretes destructive proteases and cytotoxins such as perforin and granzymes. Stimulated CD8 cells also secrete other cytokines, including interferon-gamma (IFN-gamma) and tumor necrosis factor (TNF-alpha and TNF-beta), which can help destroy viruses and pathogens and stimulate other immune cells.

Cytokine Activation of Macrophages

The primary cytokine that activates macrophages is IFN-gamma. T_H1 cells activate macrophages by secreting IFN-gamma and other cytokines that assist IFN-gamma, including TNF and granulocyte macrophage-colony stimulating factor (GM-CSF). The activated macrophage then produces a wide variety of cytokine and noncytokine compounds, including free radicals, proteases, TNF, IL-1, and IL-6. Some of these stimulate other immune cells, and some destroy pathogens.

Cytokine Activation of B Cells

T_H2 cells activate B cells by secreting cytokines such as IL-4 and IL-5. Other cytokines produced by T_H2 cells include IL-3, IL-10, GM-CSF, and TGF-beta. After activation, some B cells become memory B cells, which remember antigens, and some become plasma cells, which produce antibodies for the encountered antigen.

Cytokine Activation of CD4 T Cells

Cytokines also control proliferation and activity of CD4 T cells. The first response of CD4 T cells to antigen presentation is IL-2 production, which leads to self-proliferation. The presence of other cytokines, including IL-12 and IFN-gamma, causes them to differentiate into T_H1 cells, and the presence of other cytokines, including IL-4, causes them to differentiate into T_H2 cells. Thus either T_H1 or T_H2 cells, but not both, are produced.

ROLE OF IMMUNE CELLS IN CANCER

Immune cells can destroy cancer cells within a tumor and also cancer cells that are metastasizing. T cells appear to play the largest role in the destruction of tumor cells, and macrophages and NK cells do the same in the destruction of metastasizing cells.

T Cells and Cancer

Although T cells are important in destroying cancer cells within a tumor, to be effective they require adequate antigen presentation. For this reason, T cells rely on antigen-presenting cells such as macrophages and dendritic cells. Since tumor cells often disrupt the mechanics of antigen presentation, they are able to evade T-cell recognition. Evasion of the immune response is discussed in more detail below.

NK Cells and Cancer

Natural killer (NK) cells are large, specialized, non-T, non-B lymphocytes. NK cells were discovered in the mid-1970s and constitute up to 15 percent of the total lymphocyte population in healthy subjects. They are capable of killing a broad range of human solid tumor, leukemic, and virus-infected cells. Depressed NK cell activity and depressed NK cell populations appear to be associated with the development and progression of cancer, as well as AIDS, chronic fatigue syndrome, psychiatric depression, various immunodeficiency syndromes, and certain autoimmune diseases.

NK cells may present the first line of defense against metastatic spread of tumors. In animal experiments, low

NK cell populations have been associated with greater survival of injected cancer cells and increased development of lung metastasis. Correction of the NK cell population restored resistance.[3–6] In human studies, patients with solid tumors commonly have diminished NK cell activity, but the association between low NK cell activity and metastatic spread is not so strong as in animals. This lack of correlation, however, may be due in part to the fact that most clinical studies of immunostimulants that affect NK cell activity were conducted in patients with advanced cancers. Patients with early stage cancers might be most likely to benefit from such therapies.[7]

NK cell activity appears to be a well-regulated system, subject to both inhibitory and excitatory controls. Some cytokines (interferons and IL-2) stimulate activity, while prostaglandins such as PGE_2 inhibit NK cell activity.[8] Although the exact mechanisms that regulate NK cell activity are still uncertain, recent research suggests that newly identified receptors on NK cells may recognize proteins similar to MHC class-I proteins on some tumor cells.[9] NK cells may also be activated by cells lacking MHC class I molecules.

Macrophages and Cancer

Like NK cells, macrophages do not recognize foreign antigens. In addition, they do not recognize self-proteins. Their activation mechanisms are poorly understood but may involve receptors for certain carbohydrates, complement, and other proteins. Although bacterial products are among the most potent activators, macrophages can also be activated by contact with tumor cells. Macrophages destroy foreign substances by phagocytosis (ingestion); by secretion of proteases, hydrogen peroxide, or other enzymes or radical species; or by secretion of certain cytokines, such as tumor necrosis factor, as discussed above.

Macrophages may play an important role in the immune response to cancer. A good bit of evidence supports this hypothesis:[10]

- Macrophages accumulate in considerable numbers within a variety of tumors, and they destroy a wide variety of cancer cells in vitro.

- Treatments that suppress the function of macrophages have been associated with increased tumor incidence and increased metastasis.

- Injection of activated macrophages into tumor-bearing animals inhibits metastatic spread of some tumor cell lines.

- Stimulation of macrophage activity has been associated with decreased tumor growth or decreased tumor incidence in animals.

Tumor-associated macrophages, however, have also been reported to promote angiogenesis and tumor growth (see Chapter 8). Since this negative effect may be mediated in large part by immunosuppressive compounds secreted by tumor cells, it is reasonable to suppose that the most effective strategies for increasing the antitumor effects of macrophages are those that include both immunostimulants and agents that prevent immunosuppression.

ROLE OF THE IMMUNE SYSTEM IN CANCER PREVENTION

Some researchers believe the immune system plays a critical role in preventing tumor development by searching out and destroying newly transformed cells. This process, known as immune surveillance, was first proposed by Ehrlich in 1909, and is supported by the following observations that associate immune depression with increased cancer risk:[11, 12]

- Children with immunodeficiency diseases have increased rates of lymphoma, leukemia, and Hodgkin's disease.

- Approximately 40 percent of patients with immunosuppression caused by the human immunodeficiency virus (HIV) are likely to develop cancer. Common cancers include Kaposi's sarcoma, non-Hodgkin's lymphoma, cervical cancer, and Hodgkin's disease.

- In organ transplant patients who receive immunosuppressive drugs, the incidence of malignancies is increased about 3-fold. In some studies on kidney transplant patients, the incidence of cancer has been observed to be 7-fold higher than in the general population. Commonly, these malignancies include Kaposi's sarcoma, non-Hodgkin's lymphoma, sarcoma, and cancers of the skin, kidney, cervix, and liver.

- Cancer risk increases with the duration of immunosuppressive treatment. In a study of heart transplant patients, cancer incidence increased 3-fold after one year of immunosuppressive treatment and 26-fold after five years. In some patients, regression of Kaposi's sarcoma and lymphoma was observed after immunosuppressive therapy ceased.

- Patients with autoimmune diseases treated with immunosuppressive therapy show increased incidence of acute leukemia, lymphoma, liver cancer, bladder cancer, and skin cancer.

Immunosuppressed patients appear to have a disproportionately high incidence of certain malignancies, such as skin cancers, Kaposi's sarcoma, lymphoma, and acute leukemia. Relatively few of the more common malignancies like breast and lung cancer are seen. This difference may be due to the longer latency period (15 to 20 years or more) of those tumors less apt to develop. Immunosuppressed patients may simply succumb to faster-developing tumors, or infections, before other slow-growing tumors can develop.

An alternate and more likely explanation for this disproportion is that cancers commonly associated with immunosuppressed states are virally induced, or they originate in the immune system itself. Accordingly, the problem is that the immune system fails to destroy viruses that cause or assist the development of cancer rather than that it fails to destroy tumor cells. In some cases, viruses can interfere with the *p53* tumor suppressor gene or can activate oncogenes. A number of human viruses are associated with increased risk of cancer. These include the Epstein-Barr virus (EBV), which has been associated with nasopharyngeal cancer and various lymphomas and leukemias. They also include human T-cell leukemia virus type I (HTLV-I), hepatitis B virus (HBV), human papilloma virus (HPV), and several herpes viruses (herpes virus 2, 6, 8, and 16), which have been associated with adult T-cell leukemia, liver cancer, cervical cancer, oral squamous cell carcinoma, nasopharyngeal cancer, Kaposi's sarcoma, multiple myeloma, lymphoma, Hodgkin's disease, oral squamous cell carcinoma, or penile cancer.[13–19]

Tumors of viral origin are sometimes referred to as "opportunistic" tumors, in reference to the "opportunistic infections" of immunosuppressed individuals. For example, the short induction time of Kaposi's sarcoma and lymphoma in immunosuppressed patients may reflect a virally induced opportunistic tumor. In organ transplant patients, whose immune systems are purposefully suppressed by drugs to avoid organ rejection, Kaposi's sarcoma appears, on average, within 20 months of transplant, and lymphoma appears, on average, within 34 months. This is in contrast to the 10- to 20-year period during which most solid tumors develop.

The immune system, then, may play a role in cancer prevention by destroying cancer cells soon after they arise or by destroying viruses that lead to cancer or both. It stands to reason that maintaining a healthy immune system will help prevent cancer.

IMMUNE SYSTEM IN CANCER TREATMENT

The immune system's postulated role in preventing cancer by destroying cancer cells, along with other evidence, tells us it can also help destroy cells of established cancers. Its ability to do so, referred to as antitumor immunity, involves both the innate and adaptive immune systems. For example, recent evidence suggests the immune system may be capable of detecting the protein products of oncogenes on the cell surface; immune responses to the HER-2/neu protein and mutated *ras* and *p53* gene products have been reported.[20, 21] In addition, antibodies against the patient's own tumor have been identified in the sera of some patients with soft-tissue sarcoma, malignant melanoma, ovarian carcinoma, and lung cancer.[22]

The degree to which the immune system can destroy established cancers, however, has not been established. In general, the immune system may be more effective against small tumors and metastatic spread than against established solid tumors. What is clear is that the success of the immune system is severely hampered by the ability of tumors to evade immunologic reactions, a problem now discussed in more detail.

Immune Evasion by Tumors

The immune system must recognize a cancer cell as foreign before it can be destroyed. If the immune system is able to recognize a substance as foreign, that substance is referred to as being antigenic. One might expect the immune system to have trouble recognizing tumors as foreign, but in fact most tumor cells appear to be strongly antigenic. Unfortunately, recognition of a foreign substance does not necessarily ensure that an immune reaction will take place. Although most human tumor cells are apparently strongly antigenic, they are only weakly immunogenic. (The ability of a foreign substance to evoke an immunologic reaction in a host is called its immunogenicity.) Therefore, rejection of the tumor is difficult, even with a fully functioning immune system. Recent investigations have reported that a few cancers, such as melanoma and kidney cancer, are more strongly immunogenic, but even these often escape destruction by the immune system. The low immunogenicity of most tumors may be due to their ability to successfully evade immune attack.

Immune evasion can occur through one or more of the following mechanisms:[23, 24, 25]

- *Modulation of surface proteins.* Tumor cells can evade immune cell recognition by reducing their expression of MHC molecules, adhesion molecules, or co-stimulatory molecules.

- *Antigenic modulation.* Antigenic modulation occurs when the tumor cell loses its surface antigens upon exposure to specific antibodies. In addition, contact between surface antigen and antibody may induce some cancer cells to absorb and degrade the antigen-antibody complex, leaving fewer ways for immune cells to recognize the cancer cell as foreign.

- *Induced immunosuppression.* Cancer patients are frequently immunosuppressed, a condition that can sometimes be corrected by removing the bulk of the tumor. There are a variety of ways tumor cells can induce local or systemic immunosuppression. One method is through the excessive production and shedding of antigens; the shed antigens combine with antibodies to form antigen-antibody complexes. This initially stimulates the immune system but in excess eventually overwhelms and suppresses it. Circulating immune complexes are elevated in many forms of cancer and have been suggested as potential tumor markers.[26] Tumors, or the immune cells they attract, can also locally produce immunosuppressive substances such as PGE_2, TGF-beta, IL-10, and others.[12, 27] In addition, unspecified substances produced by tumors can impair the function of the T-cell receptor complex.[11, 28]

- *Shedding of surface receptors.* Some tumor cells shed their receptors for TNF. As a result, TNF is unable to bind to the cell and destroy it. The shed receptors can also bind with TNF, thus preventing it from reaching other tumor cells.

Whatever the exact cause, patients with advanced cancers of any type frequently exhibit nonspecific defects in both innate and adaptive immunity. According to a recent study, they may also experience specific defects in immunity, such as lack of responsiveness of CD8 T cells to the tumor antigens present.[29] This finding supports the hypothesis that the immune system is able to recognize and respond to cancer cell antigens, even though this ability can be undermined.

Use of Immunotherapy in Conventional Cancer Medicine

We now look at how immunotherapy has been used in conventional cancer medicine. From this discussion, we obtain ideas on how natural compounds might be used to produce some of the same effects on the immune system, and we also see how the use of natural compounds differs from that of most conventional immunotherapy agents. The primary distinction between conventional immunotherapy agents and natural immunostimulant compounds is that the former tend to be cells or cytokines activated or generated outside the body, then injected into it, whereas the natural compounds cause the body to produce its own activated cells and cytokines. Still, the research showing that externally administered cells or cytokines can have an effect on cancer implies that natural compounds have the potential to produce the same effect.

The majority of human cancers exhibit low immunogenicity, probably due to one or more of the immune-evading mechanisms described earlier. This does not mean, however, that immunotherapy is necessarily ineffective against them. Conventional immunotherapy can be divided into two categories, active and passive, each discussed below. In general, conventional immunotherapy in humans is most effective in patients with a relatively healthy immune system and a low tumor burden (i.e., at an early stage of malignancy).

Active Immunotherapy

The term *active immunotherapy* refers to methods that directly stimulate an immune response by the body. In conventional medicine, this is often accomplished through immunization with damaged (nonviable) tumor cells or by injection of bacterial antigens, such as microbial agents. Examples of this type of therapy are the administration of Coley's toxins and the BCG bacterial product. (Recall that macrophages are activated by bacterial antigens.)

The clinical role of active immunotherapy as a sole agent may be limited, since prior to therapy the patient's immune system has had ample time to recognize and react to tumor antigens. Nonetheless, the use of various active immunotherapy agents has had some limited success in treating patients with osteosarcoma, leukemia, lymphoma, melanoma, and lung, kidney, bladder, ovarian, colon, and breast cancer.[30–33] Kidney cancer and melanoma exhibit the greatest immunogenicity and may respond better to active immunotherapy than other cancers. Also, transitional cell carcinoma of the bladder responds well to BCG bacterial products.[34] (In this case, the bacterial products are applied directly to the tumor.) In general, however, tumor-induced immunosuppression must be removed or reduced for active immunization to be successful.

Passive Immunotherapy

Passive immunotherapy refers to administration of agents that passively increase immune activity. Passive immunotherapy includes administration of serum or immune cells from immunized animals; administration of cloned antibodies; and administration of cloned immune cells and cytokines. Of these, passive immunotherapy with cloned immune cells or cytokines or both seems the most promising.

Two types of cloned cells have been investigated: tumor-infiltrating lymphocytes (TIL) and lymphokine-activated killer (LAK) cells. TIL therapy involves removing the T lymphocytes that migrate into solid tumors, cloning and activating them with IL-2, and then re-injecting them into the patient. The idea is that the T cells taken from inside the tumor, and their subsequent clones, are already sensitized to the tumor. TIL therapy has had some success against melanoma. LAK cell therapy is similar to TIL therapy, except that NK cells are used and the cells are obtained from the general circulation rather than from inside the tumor. LAK cells act similar to but are more active than NK cells. The cloning and activation of LAK cells in culture is made possible by the administration of IL-2.

Generating TIL and LAK cells and then injecting them into the body has relevance to the use of natural immunostimulant compounds, since both involve using cytokines to activate immune cells (one outside the body and one inside). As discussed in Chapter 12, a number of natural compounds increase production of IL-2, interferons, and other cytokines. Administration of these cytokines in their pure form can modestly affect some cancers (see below), and it seems reasonable that increasing their internal production using natural compounds will also modestly affect some cancers. It is also reasonable to suppose that the anticancer effects will be greater when these compounds are combined with ones that inhibit immune evasion and those that deter cancer by other means, such as inhibition of signal transduction.

Treatment with IL-2

A number of clinical trials have administered IL-2 alone or in combination with LAK cells.[35–39] Although IL-2 immune stimulation holds promise, so far the results have been modest. In past studies, the average total response rate has been roughly 20 to 30 percent, with the majority of these partial responses. For example, IL-2, with or without LAK cells, produced a response in up to 30 percent of patients with kidney cancer, but only 5 to 10 percent achieved long-lasting complete responses.[41] The clinical gains were modest in spite of the fact that immune function, as measured by NK cell activity, was successfully stimulated in the majority of patients.[36, 38] This again suggests that to obtain optimal clinical results, it may be necessary to combine immunotherapy with other anticancer therapies, including therapies that limit immune evasion.

Although IL-2 is a naturally occurring substance in the body, its use at high concentration produces serious, sometimes life-threatening, adverse effects. These effects are apparently due partly to increases in capillary permeability caused by IL-2. However, newer approaches, employing lower doses of IL-2 given intravenously or subcutaneously, may circumvent some of these problems. These newer approaches more closely mimic the increase in IL-2 concentrations that would be produced by the use of natural compounds (i.e., more gradual increases and lower peak concentrations).

Treatment with Interferons

Interferons (IFNs) have been the most extensively studied cytokines in cancer treatment. As a group, interferons affect a wide array of immunological functions. They mediate antiviral and antimicrobial activity, stimulate or inhibit leukocyte proliferation, suppress oncogenes, enhance tumor antigen expression, suppress angiogenesis, and augment the activity of NK cells, T lymphocytes, and macrophages. Interferons and tumor necrosis factor (TNF) also increase the burning of body fat stores, possibly to release energy reserves from fat cells for the immune system to use. In this capacity, they play a role in the development of cachexia (tissue wasting disease). Although this is a drawback to their use, interferons still produce an anticancer effect at tolerable doses.

Interferons have been effective against some nonsolid tumors such as hairy cell leukemia (85 percent response rate), chronic myelogenous leukemia (75 percent), and nodular lymphoma (45 percent).[40] Injections are usually administered daily for prolonged periods. Interferons are ineffective against chronic lymphocytic leukemia and multiple myeloma, but in the latter, administration of interferons may prolong the duration of chemotherapy-induced remission. Solid tumors respond less favorably to interferon therapy. Responses have been observed in Kaposi's sarcoma (33 percent response rate), brain cancer (40 percent), gastrointestinal cancers (20 percent), melanoma (15 percent), and kidney cancers (20 percent). As with IL-2, most of these responses were partial. In the case of kidney cancer, only about 3 to 5 percent of patients achieve long-lasting complete responses.[41] Local injection, as opposed to systemic therapy, has been used with some success against basal cell carcinoma (75 percent response rate), bladder cancer (40 percent), and ovarian cancer (45 percent).

Although life-threatening complications are rare from interferon administration, quality of life is commonly impaired because of fever, chills, headache, fatigue, anorexia, nausea, and other side effects. Some of these side effects may be due to increased secretion of tumor necrosis factor by stimulated macrophages.

Treatment with Multiple Cytokines

The results of clinical trials using individual cytokines such as IL-2 have been modest. Recent studies, however, have employed cocktails of cytokines and chemotherapy agents and the results of these trials are more promising. For example, studies have reported that the combination of chemotherapy with IL-2 and IFN-alpha produced responses in more than 50 percent of patients with metastatic melanoma, and approximately 10 percent achieved long-lasting complete responses.[42, 43] This again supports the concept that combinations of natural compounds that both stimulate the immune system and inhibit cancer by other means may be most effective. Importantly, natural immunostimulant compounds tend to stimulate a broad-based increase in cytokine production (see Chapter 12). Production of interleukins, interferons, and colony-stimulating factors may all be increased. In this way, such immunostimulants may naturally produce their own cocktail of cancer-fighting compounds.

CONCLUSION

The immune response to cancer consists of two arms: the innate immune response, which does not depend on tumor antigens, and the adaptive immune response, which does. Cells of the immune system communicate with and stimulate one another by transient docking and secretion of cytokines. Some of these cytokines have been produced in the laboratory and tested for their anti-cancer effects. Results with individual cytokines have been moderate, due partly to the ability of cancer cells to evade an immune response. It is likely the best results from immunotherapy will occur when immunostimulants are used in combination with compounds that prevent immune evasion, as well as in combination with those that inhibit cancer by other means. Natural compounds can, when used together, increase cytokine production, stimulate immune activity, and reduce the production or activity of compounds that allow immune evasion.

REFERENCES

[1] Janeway CA, Travers P. Immunobiology: The immune system in health and disease. New York: Garland Publishing, 1997, p. 1:4.

[2] Janeway CA, Travers P. Immunobiology: The immune system in health and disease. New York: Garland Publishing, 1997, pp. 4:3, 9:6.

[3] Kobayashi T. [Role of NK cells in lung metastasis immunosurveillance.] Gan To Kagaku Ryoho 1989 Apr; 16(4 Pt 2–1):1233–45.

[4] Woodruff MF. The cytolytic and regulatory role of natural killer cells in experimental neoplasia. Biochim Biophys Acta 1986 Aug 5; 865(1):43–57.

[5] Kim S, Iizuka K, Aguila HL, et al. In vivo natural killer cell activities revealed by natural killer cell-deficient mice. Proc Natl Acad Sci USA 2000 Mar 14; 97(6):2731–6.

[6] Dithmar SA, Rusciano DA, Armstrong CA, et al. Depletion of NK cell activity results in growth of hepatic micrometastases in a murine ocular melanoma model. Curr Eye Res 1999 Nov; 19(5):426–31.

[7] Whiteside TL, Vujanovic NL, Herberman RB. Natural killer cells and tumor therapy. Curr Top Microbiol Immunol 1998; 230:221–44.

[8] Herberman R, Santoni A. Regulation of NK-cell activity. In *Biological responses in cancer: Progress toward potential applications.* Vol 1. Mihich E, ed. New York: Plenum Press, 1982.

[9] Diefenbach A, Raulet DH. Natural killer cells: Stress out, turn on, tune in. Curr Biol 1999 Nov 18; 9(22):R851–3.

[10] Holleb AI, Fink DJ, Murphy GP. American Cancer Society textbook of clinical onocology. Atlanta: American Cancer Society, 1991.

[11] Penn I. Principles of tumor immunity: Immunocompetence and cancer. In *Biologic therapy of cancer.* DeVita V, Hellman S, Rosenberg S, eds. Philadelphia: JB Lippincott, 1991.

[12] Wojtowicz-Praga S. Reversal of tumor-induced immunosuppression: A new approach to cancer therapy [see comments]. J Immunother 1997 May; 20(3):165–77.

[13] Tung YC, Lin KH, Chu PY, et al. Detection of human papilloma virus and Epstein-Barr virus DNA in nasopharyngeal carcinoma by polymerase chain reaction. Kao Hsiung I Hsueh Ko Hsueh Tsa Chih 1999 May; 15(5):256–62

[14] Ohtsubo H, Arima N, Tei C. Epstein-Barr virus involvement in T-cell malignancy: Significance in adult T-cell leukemia. Leuk Lymphoma 1999 May; 33(5–6):451–8.

[15] Flaitz CM, Hicks MJ. Molecular piracy: The viral link to carcinogenesis. Oral Oncol 1998 Nov; 34(6):448–53.

[16] McCance DJ, Kalache A, Ashdown K, et al. Human papillomavirus types 16 and 18 in carcinomas of the penis from Brazil. Int J Cancer 1986 Jan 15; 37(1):55–9.

[17] Levi JE, Rahal P, Sarkis AS, Villa L. Human papillomavirus DNA and p53 status in penile carcinomas. Int J Cancer 1998 Jun 10; 76(6):779–83.

[18] Ylitalo N, Sorensen P, Josefsson AM, et al. Consistent high viral load of human papillomavirus 16 and risk of cervical carcinoma in situ: A nested case-control study. Lancet 2000 Jun 24; 355(9222):2194–8.

[19] Josefsson AM, Magnusson PK, Ylitalo N, et al. Viral load of human papilloma virus 16 as a determinant for development of cervical carcinoma in situ: A nested case-control study. Lancet 2000 Jun 24; 355(9222):2189–93.

[20] Tuttle TM. Oncogene products represent potential targets of tumor vaccines. Cancer Immunol Immunother 1996 Nov; 43(3):135–41.

[21] Chen HL, Carbone DP. p53 as a target for anti-cancer immunotherapy. Mol Med Today 1997 Apr; 3(4):160–7.

[22] Calabresi P, Schein P. Medical oncology. 2nd ed. New York: McGraw-Hill, 1993, pp. 325–6.

[23] Holland JF, Frei E, Bast R, et al. Cancer medicine. 3rd ed. Philadelphia: Lea & Febiger, 1993, p. 187.

[24] Calabresi P, Schein P. Medical oncology. 2nd ed. New York: McGraw-Hill, 1993, p. 331.

[25] Becker JC, Dummer R, Hartmann AA, et al. Shedding of ICAM-1 from human melanoma cell lines induced by IFN-gamma and tumor necrosis factor-alpha. Functional consequences on cell-mediated cytotoxicity. J Immunol 1991 Dec 15; 147(12):4398–401.

[26] Aziz M, Dass TK, Rattan A. Role of circulating immune-complexes as prognostic indicators of lympho-reticular and mesenchymal malignancies in children. J Trop Pediatr 1992 Aug; 38(4):185–8.

[27] Wahl LM, Kleinman HK. Tumor-associated macrophages as targets for cancer therapy. J Natl Cancer Inst 1998; 90(21):1583–4.

[28] Kiessling R, Kono K, Petersson M, Wasserman K. Immunosuppression in human tumor-host interaction: Role of cytokines and alterations in signal-transducing molecules. Springer Semin Immunopathol 1996; 18(2):227–42.

[29] Lee PP, Yee C, Savage PA, et al. Characterization of circulating T cells specific for tumor-associated antigens in melanoma patients. Nature Medicine 1999; 5(6):677–685.

[30] Hoover HC, Hanna, MG. Immunotherapy by active specific immunization: Clinical applications. In Biologic therapy of cancer. DeVita VT, Hellman S, Rosenberg S, eds. Philadelphia: JB Lippincott, 1991.

[31] Hersh EM, Taylor CW. Immunotherapy by active immunization of the host using nonspecific stimulants and immunomodulators. In Biologic therapy of cancer. DeVita VT, Hellman S, Rosenberg S, eds. Philadelphia: JB Lippincott, 1991.

[32] Tannock IF, Hill RP, eds. The basic science of oncology. 2nd ed. New York: McGraw-Hill, 1992, p. 245.

[33] Calabresi P, Schein P. Medical oncology. 2nd ed. New York: McGraw-Hill, 1993, p. 334.

[34] Nseyo UO, Lamm DL. Immunotherapy of bladder cancer. Semin Surg Oncol 1997 Sep–Oct; 13(5):342–9.

[35] Lotze MT, Rosenberg SA. Interleukin-2: Clinical applications. In Biologic therapy of cancer. DeVita VT, Hellman S, Rosenberg SA, eds. Philadelphia: JB Lippincott, 1991.

[36] Koretz MJ, Lawson DH, York RM, et al. Randomized study of interleukin 2 (IL-2) alone vs IL-2 plus lymphokine-activated killer cells for treatment of melanoma and renal cell cancer. Arch Surg 1991 Jul; 126(7):898–903.

[37] Rosenberg SA. Adoptive cellular therapy: Graft-versus-tumor responses after bone-marrow transplantation. In Biologic therapy of cancer. DeVita VT, Hellman S, Rosenberg SA, eds. Philadelphia: JB Lippincott, 1991.

[38] Weiss GR, Margolin KA, Aronson FR, et al. A randomized phase II trial of continuous infusion interleukin-2 or bolus injection interleukin-2 plus lymphokine-activated killer cells for advanced renal cell carcinoma. J Clin Oncol 1992 Feb; 10(2):275–81.

[39] Kruit WH, Stoter G. The role of adoptive immunotherapy in solid cancers. Neth J Med 1997 Feb; 50(2):47–68.

[40] Holland JF, Frei E, Bast R, et al. Cancer medicine. 3rd ed. Philadelphia: Lea & Febiger, 1993, p. 190.

[41] Canobbio L, Miglietta L, Boccardo F. Medical treatment of advanced renal cell carcinoma: Present options and future directions. Cancer Treat Rev 1996 Mar; 22(2):85–104.

[42] Atkins MB. The treatment of metastatic melanoma with chemotherapy and biologics. Curr Opin Oncol 1997 Mar; 9(2):205–13.

[43] Legha SS. Durable complete responses in metastatic melanoma treated with interleukin-2 in combination with interferon alpha and chemotherapy. Semin Oncol 1997 Feb; 24(1 Suppl 4):S39–43.

NATURAL COMPOUNDS THAT AFFECT THE IMMUNE SYSTEM

We have looked at how the immune system functions, how it may affect or be affected by cancer, and how its ability to find and destroy cancer cells is hindered by their evasion techniques. We saw also that regulation of immune cells happens largely through the release of various cytokines and that cytokines, especially interleukin-2 (IL-2) and interferons, have some value as anticancer agents. In this chapter, we examine natural compounds that can support or stimulate the immune system, and in this way may be useful in cancer treatment.

Compounds that support the immune system do so by providing proper nutrition to immune cells or by acting as antioxidants or both. (Immune cells such as macrophages require large amounts of antioxidants for protection from the free radicals they generate.) Some natural compounds also help the immune system by providing a regulatory influence, thereby normalizing the extremes in activity found in diseases like cancer. Compounds that stimulate the immune system often do so by increasing the production of cytokines, including IL-2 and interferons, but may act in other ways as well. These natural compounds tend to increase production of a broad range of cytokines

We also look at natural compounds that can cause immunosuppression. It is important to consider compounds with this characteristic because they could conceivably interfere with immunotherapy and, paradoxically, because many also produce anti-inflammatory or other effects that may inhibit cancer. For example, natural compounds that inhibit NF-κB activity can reduce the production of tumor necrosis factor. These compounds are potentially detrimental in that they could reduce the ability of immune cells to produce TNF, thereby interfering with an immune response. On the other hand, they are potentially beneficial in that they could reduce TNF-induced inflammation and angiogenesis, as well as NF-κB-mediated cell proliferation. Moreover, most natural compounds that inhibit NF-κB activity also inhibit PGE_2 production (compare Tables 5.2 and 8.2). Since PGE_2 is an immunosuppressive compound that helps cancer cells evade immune attack, these compounds could actually help the immune system attack cancer and thus work with immune stimulants to inhibit it.

This book does not resolve all the possible conflicts between using natural compounds that inhibit aspects of

the immune system and those that stimulate it. The effects of and interactions between both types of compounds are complex, and their final effect when used together will depend on many factors, not the least of which is the final mix of cytokines produced. Although additional research is needed to determine the optimal ways these types of compounds could be used in combination, it seems likely their concurrent use would be beneficial in most cases, as is discussed later.

NATURAL COMPOUNDS THAT STIMULATE AND/OR SUPPORT THE IMMUNE SYSTEM

A large number of natural compounds can stimulate or support the immune system or do both. A selected list of some of the major compounds is provided in Table 12.1. Note that many other natural compounds discussed in this book (and many not included) could act as immunostimulants or supportive agents. For example, CAPE has been reported to increase the susceptibility of tumor cells to NK cell attack and induce expression of tumor-associated antigens on human melanoma and brain cancer cells lines in vitro.[1, 2] As another example, oral administration of proanthocyanidins to mice has increased NK cell cytotoxicity and enhanced ex-vivo IL-2 production by immune cells.[3] Even though not comprehensive, Table 12.1 does include many of the well-known natural immunostimulants and supportive compounds. Reference books that discuss additional natural compounds with these effects are cited in Chapter 16.

In addition to stimulating the immune system, we must also inhibit immune evasion. One primary way cancer cells evade immune attack is by producing excessive amounts of immunosuppressive substances like PGE_2 and immunosuppressive cytokines, such as transforming growth factor-beta and IL-10. Natural compounds that reduce production of TGF-beta and/or IL-10 include PSK and other polysaccharides, proanthocyanidins, omega-3 fatty acids, monoterpenes, and vitamin E [3–11] In addition, protein kinase inhibitors like genistein can reduce the signaling effects of IL-10.[12] Natural compounds that inhibit PGE_2 production include omega-3 fatty acids and other compounds discussed in Chapter 8 (see Table 8.2). Lastly, compounds that reduce vascular endothelial growth factor production (see Chapter 8)

TABLE 12.1   NATURAL COMPOUNDS THAT ASSIST THE IMMUNE SYSTEM
HERBAL IMMUNOSTIMULANT COMPOUNDS
Astragalus membranaceus
Eleutherococcus senticosus
Ganoderma lucidum
Panax ginseng
Shiitake (*Lentinus edodes*), PSK, and other mushroom polysaccharides
ANTIOXIDANTS AND NUTRITIONAL COMPOUNDS
Glutamine
Glutathione-enhancing compounds (i.e., most antioxidants)
Selenium
Vitamin C
Vitamin E
OTHER COMPOUNDS
Bromelain and other enzymes
Melatonin
Note: See Table H.1 in Appendix H for details and references.

may limit immune evasion by cancer cells. In addition to its role in increasing vascular permeability, VEGF may also impede maturation of dendritic cells and thereby reduce the presentation of tumor antigens to lymphocytes.[13] Thus, between compounds that stimulate and/or support the immune system and those that limit immune evasion, we see that a large number, if not the majority of compounds discussed in this book, could affect tumor progression via immune-mediated mechanisms.

The compounds listed in Table 12.1 are divided into three categories: herbal immunostimulant compounds, antioxidants and nutritional compounds, and others. After discussing them, we look at some Chinese studies that have used herbal immunostimulants in cancer treatment.

Herbal Immunostimulant Compounds

The (probable) active ingredients of the herbal compounds in Table 12.1 tend to fall into a limited number of chemical families; one of these is high-molecular-weight polysaccharides, which are large sugar molecules. Natural compounds containing them include *Astragalus, Ganoderma, Eleutherococcus*, and PSK. A second family of immunostimulating compounds is the saponins. Natural compounds with these are *Eleutherococcus* and ginseng. It is tempting to speculate that the most effective combinations of herbal immune stimulants will contain compounds from both families, and in fact, most multiherb, immunostimulating formulas used in Chinese herbal medicine do have both. Some herbs

themselves also include compounds from both families, as is the case with *Eleutherococcus* and ginseng.

The mechanisms by which herbal compounds exert their immunostimulant effects are not well understood, but often they include the production of immunostimulating cytokines or modulation of cytokine effects. For example, *Astragalus* polysaccharides have been reported to potentiate the in-vitro antitumor cytotoxicity of lymphokine-activated killer cells generated with low-dose IL-2. The exact mechanism was uncertain but could have been due to *Astragalus*-induced increases in IL-2 receptor expression on the LAK cells, or some other form of increased IL-2 binding.[14] As another example, one study reported that *Ganoderma* polysaccharides increased production of cytokines by macrophages and T cells and increased the cytotoxic effect of macrophages against leukemia cells in vitro. The cytokines that were increased included IL-1, IL-6, TNF, and interferon-gamma.[15] Lastly, these compounds may work synergistically with IL-2 itself or possibly other natural compounds that increase IL-2 production. For example, a synergistic antimetastatic effect was seen when IL-2 was combined with the mushroom polysaccharide lentinan in mice. Little effect on metastasis occurred with either agent alone, but an 85 percent reduction was observed when the compounds were combined.[16]

Regardless of their exact modes of action, the final result of these herbal compounds is stimulation of both the innate and adaptive immune responses. As would be expected, these compounds produce antitumor effects in rodents. In humans, PSK has been the most extensively studied, and results suggest it may be useful in preventing recurrence after surgical removal of some tumors (see Chapter 16).

Antioxidants and Nutritional Support

The second category in Table 12.1 is compounds that are antioxidants or provide nutritional support. All cells need proper nutrition to function optimally, and immune cells are no exception. Although these require a variety of micro- and macronutrients, we focus here on a select few nutrients that have been extensively studied. In particular, several antioxidant vitamins appear to support immune function; when their levels are low, immune function can be hampered. Animal and human studies have reported that vitamins C and E support immune function through a number of mechanisms. For example, immune cells produce various noxious compounds, including reactive oxygen species (ROS) and reactive nitrogen species; antioxidants may help protect immune cells from self-destruction caused by the release of these compounds.

Antioxidants may also support immune function via their effects on intracellular glutathione levels. Glutathione plays an important role in immune function for three reasons. First, as a primary intracellular antioxidant, adequate glutathione is needed to protect the cell. Second, adequate glutathione levels are necessary for optimal T-cell activation by IL-2.[17] Third, high glutathione levels inhibit cellular production of PGE_2, an immunosuppressive substance.[18] Glutamine, listed in the table, induces glutathione synthesis and in addition can support immune function by acting as a fuel for immune cells. Antioxidants can also increase glutathione concentrations.

Lastly, selenium can support immune function. Selenium is not an antioxidant itself, but it is a crucial component of the antioxidant enzyme glutathione peroxidase. It therefore assists in the antioxidant effects of glutathione (see Figure 5.2). Moreover, either because of its influence on glutathione or through other means, selenium can enhance the expression of IL-2 receptors on immune cells.[19, 20, 21]

Other Compounds

Bromelain and melatonin act by somewhat different means than the other compounds listed. Bromelain's action is especially intriguing, since it appears to have a regulatory effect on the immune system that is mediated by a number of contradictory mechanisms.

Bromelain and Other Proteolytic Enzymes

Bromelain and other proteolytic (protein degrading) enzymes such as papain (from papaya) and trypsin and chymotrypsin (produced in the digestive tract) have been proposed as potential anticancer agents. These enzymes may affect cancer by a number of mechanisms, but one of the most important is through immune modification. Rather than being immune stimulants, proteolytic enzymes are considered immune regulators. They tend to bolster aspects of the immune system that are underactive and hinder aspects that are overactive.[22] For example, one study reported that oral administration of six bromelain tablets per day for 10 days corrected deficient macrophage activity in patients with breast cancer. In contrast, less of an effect on macrophage activity was seen in healthy subjects.[23] These enzymes have also produced anti-inflammatory and anti-edema effects, especially in acute conditions.[24–31]

This regulatory function is very useful, since either insufficient or excessive immune activity can reduce the body's ability to fight cancer. Immune dysregulation can lead to other adverse effects. For example, overproduction of TNF can lead to cachexia (tissue wasting), a potentially fatal condition associated with some types of cancer. Seven mechanisms by which proteolytic enzymes regulate the immune system are discussed below.

Digestion of Surface Proteins

Proteolytic enzymes like bromelain and trypsin can digest cell surface proteins, including CD4, CD8, and CD44, all of which are important regulators of immune response.[32–35] Recall that CD44 binds to components of the extracellular matrix (specifically, hyaluronic acid) and facilitates the invasion of tumor cells and the migration of immune cells (see Chapter 9). CD44, CD4, and CD8 also are involved in T-cell stimulation and IL-2 release (discussed in Chapter 11). Although this may help explain some of bromelain's anti-inflammatory effects, bromelain can also enhance T-cell activation, by up to 325 percent in some cases, an event that appears to be mediated through CD2-induced T-cell stimulation.[33, 35, 36] CD2, a cell adhesion molecule that helps T cells dock with antigen-presenting cells, is not digested by bromelain.

Increased Alpha$_2$-Macroglobulin Production

Alpha$_2$-macroglobulin is a large protein present in human serum; it is produced in the liver in response to high blood levels of proteolytic enzymes, which are found after administration of bromelain or other enzymes. It is also produced by macrophages in response to high tissues levels of proteolytic enzymes, like those found at inflammation sites. It has four actions that may affect the immune system and cancer.

First, it reduces tissue destruction by binding to endogenous proteases, such as plasmin, collagenase, elastase, and trypsin, and hastening their removal from the body.[37] Macroglobulin-protease complexes in the blood are removed by the liver, and complexes in inflamed tissues are removed by local macrophages. In regard to cancer, the binding and removal of plasmin and other proteases in inflamed areas by alpha$_2$-macroglobulin may inhibit cancer by limiting protease-dependent tumor cell invasion. Moreover, removal of proteases can also reduce protease destruction of cytokines, resulting in a greater concentration of cytokines and greater immune activity.

Second, alpha$_2$-macroglobulin transports and in some cases facilitates the removal of cytokines and growth factors.[38, 39] In this way, alpha$_2$-macroglobulin may regulate cytokine activity and the immune response. The alpha$_2$-macroglobulin molecule actually has two binding sites. Binding by a protease to the first site activates the molecule for fast removal from the body. The second site can then bind either another protease or a cytokine or growth factor. For example, IL-2 appears to compete effectively with trypsin for binding to the second site, and removal of IL-2 by trypsin-stimulated alpha$_2$-macroglobulin may explain the immunosuppressive effects of this complex.[40–43]

The third action of alpha$_2$-macroglobulin that may affect the immune system or cancer is that it binds other proteins besides proteinases, cytokines, and growth factors. In particular, it binds antigens. The removal of alpha$_2$-macroglobulin and associated antigens by local macrophages can increase by more than 100-fold the ability of macrophages to present antigens to T cells. In this way, alpha$_2$-macroglobulin may stimulate T-cell activity.

Lastly, alpha$_2$-macroglobulin directly stimulates macrophage activity. It appears there may be two distinct receptor sites on macrophages for alpha$_2$-macroglobulin; binding to the first controls alpha$_2$-macroglobulin uptake, and binding to the second stimulates macrophage activity.[44]

To sum up, orally administered enzymes increase production of alpha$_2$-macroglobulin. This may result in increased removal of proteases and cytokines, decreased destruction of cytokines by free proteases, increased antigen presentation to T cells, and increased macrophage stimulation. The final result of alpha$_2$-macroglobulin induction by orally administered enzymes appears to be immunoregulatory, either stimulating or inhibiting aspects of the immune system as needed.

Cytokine Production

In addition to affecting cytokine concentrations via alpha$_2$-macroglobulin production, a variety of proteolytic enzymes also stimulate cytokine production. The mechanisms involved are uncertain, but one possible explanation is that many cytokines, including TGF-beta and IL-1, are secreted from immune cells as inactive precursor molecules. Activation of these precursors is accomplished by proteolytic enzymes.[38, 45] In-vitro studies have reported that bromelain, papain, and a polyenzyme preparation (Wobenzym) all increased production of TNF, IL-1, and IL-6 by immune cells.[46–49] Of the three, bromelain was the most effective at increasing TNF production. Similar effects were seen after oral administration of the enzymes. Other studies have also reported that proteolytic enzymes can increase cytokine production in vitro and in vivo.[22, 50, 51]

Digestion of Immune Complexes

One way that cancer cells evade immune attack is through excessive shedding of surface antigens (see Chapter 11). When antibodies contact these antigens, they combine to form antigen-antibody complexes. Excessive formation of these complexes can induce immunosuppression by hindering macrophage-mediated immunity, by causing cells to secrete immunosuppressive substances (for example, PGE$_2$), and by other means.[52, 53] In addition to cancer, excessive production of immune complexes is also common in viral infections and autoimmune disorders.[22] Enzymes can digest immune complexes in vivo and may prevent immunosuppression. For example, intraperitoneal administration of the enzyme chymopapain has been reported to reduce immune complex concentrations in rodents.[54, 55]

Digestion of Fibrin

Tumors consist of cancer cells and immune cells embedded in a fibrin stroma; this stroma coats cancer cells and can inhibit immune cell recognition. Accordingly, proteolytic enzymes that increase fibrinolysis may improve immune cell destruction. Although the fibrinolytic effect of enzymes is diminished by binding with alpha$_2$-macroglobulin, some enzymes like bromelain contain components that induce plasmin production and therefore still produce a small fibrinolytic effect in vivo.[28, 56–59] Other investigators report a fibrinolytic effect by bromelain in vitro but not in vivo.[60]

Shedding of TNF Receptors

Cytokines such as TNF can induce production of their matching receptors in cells they contact. Although this is healthy in a normal immune response, in an excessive one it can lead to further tissue destruction and inflammation. Proteolytic enzymes counteract this process by inducing cells to shed cytokine receptors.[22]

Signal Transduction

Recently it has been reported that bromelain and other proteolytic enzymes can affect signal transduction in T cells. For example, bromelain can block the activation of kinases such as ERK-2, which are involved in the transduction of signals originating from T-cell receptors on the surface of T cells.[61]

Summary of Regulatory Function

We have seen that bromelain and other proteolytic enzymes may produce both immunostimulatory and immunosuppressive effects. The overall effect of enzyme therapy on the immune system tends to be regulatory rather than strictly stimulatory or suppressive, as summarized in Table 12.2. Although their effects are com-

TABLE 12.2 SUMMARY OF THE EFFECTS OF ENZYME THERAPY ON THE IMMUNE SYSTEM

ACTION	COMMENT	EFFECT
Digestion of surface proteins such as CD44	reduces immune cell migration and raises the stimulation threshold of T cells	immunosuppressive
Increased shedding of TNF receptors	cells become less sensitive to TNF	immunosuppressive
Increased alpha$_2$-macroglobulin production	numerous effects	immunosuppressive and immunostimulatory
Increased antigen presentation by macrophages	increases T-cell activity	immunostimulatory
Direct stimulation of macrophage activity	stimulation could occur via specific receptors	immunostimulatory
Increased cytokine production	stimulates immune cells	immunostimulatory
Digestion of immune complexes	allows macrophages to function properly	immunostimulatory
Increased fibrinolysis	increases circulation in inflamed areas and may expose tumor cells to immune attack	immunostimulatory

plex, there is growing evidence suggesting they can be helpful in cancer treatment, as well as in treatment of other conditions involving inflammation and immune suppression. Preliminary evidence indicates that enzymes can produce antitumor effects in vivo after oral administration (see Chapter 18).

Melatonin

Melatonin inhibits proliferation of breast cancer and some other cell lines in vitro. It also inhibits a number of cancer lines in animals, and human studies suggest it may be beneficial in cancer treatment (see Chapter 22). Although the exact mechanisms of action remain uncertain, a potential one is augmenting the anticancer effects of IL-2. For example, one study reported that in 90 patients with advanced solid neoplasms, the combination of low-dose IL-2 and melatonin (orally at 40 mg/day) significantly increased proliferation of immune cells as compared to IL-2 alone.[62] High-dose IL-2 is associated with significant adverse effects, and combining it with melatonin may allow lower, less toxic doses of IL-2 to be used without compromising its immunologic effects. Melatonin alone has no effect on the number of immune cells and requires the presence of IL-2 to produce an immune effect. The targets of melatonin activity appear to be helper T lymphocytes and macrophages, both of which are affected by IL-2.[63]

The relationship between melatonin and IL-2 is complex.[64] Both compounds are produced more abundantly at night, may affect one another, and are often abnormal in cancer patients.[65, 66, 67] For example, in a study on seven patients with advanced small-cell lung cancer, no patients had normal light-dark rhythms of melatonin secretion; however, administering IL-2 produced a normal melatonin rhythm in four of them.

Although the combination has not been investigated in human trials, it may be possible to combine melatonin with *Astragalus* or other natural compounds that induce IL-2 production to produce clinical benefits.

CLINICAL STUDIES WITH CHINESE HERBAL FORMULAS

No discussion on using natural immunostimulant compounds in cancer therapy would be complete without some consideration of the many clinical studies that have been done in China. Studies have been conducted on the combined use of chemotherapy and Chinese herbal medicine, as well as on the anticancer use of Chinese herbal medicine alone. The majority of herbal formulas used in the Chinese studies were composed primarily of immunostimulant herbs such as those in Table 12.1 (for example, most formulas included *Astragalus* or ginseng or both). In Chinese herbal medicine, most of these herbs are considered tonics for the *qi*, or vital energy.[a] (For contents of the herbal formulas mentioned below, see Table H.2 in Appendix H; for more information on the theory of using Chinese herbs in cancer treatment, see reference 68).

Unfortunately, the majority of the Chinese studies suffered design or reporting problems. None discussed here was double-blinded. In some cases, results were compared against historic controls rather than a randomized control group. If controls were provided, they often were not chosen to match the extent of disease, performance status of the patient, or the type of conventional treatment given. In many cases, the information published on the study agent, protocol, or results was inadequate to allow sufficient review. Therefore, the validity of most of these results is questionable. Although I omitted studies with particularly gross inadequacies, the

---

[a] *Herbs that in Chinese herbal medicine terms "clear heat," "regulate the blood," "supplement the blood," "supplement the yin," or "supplement the yang" are represented less frequently.*

studies taken together do suggest some beneficial effect may be occurring, warranting additional investigation.

Colon Cancer

In a study of 176 patients with cancer of the digestive tract who were undergoing chemotherapy, one group received injections of *Astragalus* and *Panax ginseng* extracts. The injections lessened the reduction in white blood cell count and macrophage activity caused by the chemotherapy and increased the patient's body weight, as compared to patients in the control group.[69]

Nasopharyngeal Cancer

In a study of 272 patients with nasopharyngeal cancer, half were treated with radiation therapy and half with radiation combined with the formula *Yi Qi Yang Yin Tang*. The five-year relapse rate was 68 percent lower for patients who received the combined therapy (12 percent versus 38 percent). Three- and five-year survival rates also significantly improved in the group that had the combined treatment (87 percent versus 66 percent at three years, and 67 percent versus 48 percent at five years).[70]

In a study on 197 patients with stage III and IV naso-pharyngeal cancer, approximately half had radiotherapy in combination with Formula #1, and half received radiotherapy alone. After one year, survival was 91 percent in the combined treatment group and 80 percent in the one receiving only radiotherapy. After three years, the survival rates were 67 percent and 33 percent respectively, and after five years, they were 52 percent and 24 percent.[71, 72] Although Formula #1 contains *Astragalus*, most of the others in the formula are ones that, in Chinese herbal medicine terms, "reduce blood stagnation."

Liver Cancer

In a study on 124 medium-stage liver cancer patients treated with radiotherapy in combination with the herbal formula *Si Jun Zi Tang*, the five-year observed survival rate was 43 percent.[73] For purposes of rough (and not statistically valid) comparison, the five-year relative survival rate for liver cancer patients in the United States is approximately 6 percent.

Lung Cancer

In a study of 40 patients with terminal lung cancer, administration of the formula *Fei Liu Ping* resulted in mean survival of 7.5 months, as compared to 6 months in control patients treated with cytotoxic chemotherapy. Body weight and immunologic indices were more normal in the group treated with the formula and gastrointestinal and other toxicity reactions were reduced.[74] The formula is comprised of immunostimulant herbs and herbs that, in the Chinese terms, "clear heat toxins."

Stomach Cancer

In one study, 158 patients with late-stage, postoperative stomach cancer received both chemotherapy and Formula #2. Some patients took the formula for more than four years. The observed 5-year survival rate was 30 percent, with seven patients living longer than 11 years. The 10-year survival rate was 12 percent. Immunological studies of the survivors revealed an enhancement of both innate and adaptive immunity, including an increase in NK cell function.[75, 76] The formula contains primarily immunostimulant herbs and ones that "clear heat toxins."

Some of the better-designed Chinese studies were conducted on the formula *Pishen Fang*, which contains a number of herbs that have immunostimulant effects. In a study of 81 patients with stage III stomach cancer who received chemotherapy, those who also took the formula experienced increased 5-year observed survival, as compared to controls (46 percent versus 20 percent). Digestive and bone marrow functions also improved.[77]

Pishen Fang was also investigated in 669 patients taking chemotherapy for late-stage stomach cancer. Of these, 365 had radical surgical operations. The patients were randomly divided into the treatment group (414 patients) that received the formula and the controls (255 patients). Improvements in body weight and appetite, as well as reductions in nausea and vomiting, were observed in the group that took the formula. The white blood cell count was depressed in 7 percent of the treatment group and in 33 percent of the controls. Macrophage activity increased 21 percent in the treatment group over that of controls. Five-year observed survival among 303 stage III and 63 stage IV patients who received followup were 53 percent and 10 percent respectively. After 10 years, 47 percent of the stage III patients were still alive.[78]

One study on postoperative stomach cancer patients followed 216 stage III and 110 stage IV patients who received chemotherapy treatment. Approximately half used the formula *Pishen Fang*. In the control group, 75 percent were able to finish the complete course of chemotherapy, as compared to 95 percent in the treatment group. In addition, more patients in the treatment group gained weight (23 percent versus 8 percent), fewer lost weight (6 percent versus 14 percent), fewer lost their appetites (10 percent versus 32 percent), and fewer suffered from vomiting (4 percent versus 12 percent).[79, 80]

TABLE 12.3 OBSERVED SURVIVAL RATES FOR PATIENTS WITH STOMACH CANCER TREATED WITH *LI WEI HUA JIE TANG*			
PATIENT CLASS	**3-YEAR SURVIVAL RATE (%)**	**5-YEAR SURVIVAL RATE (%)**	**10-YEAR SURVIVAL RATE (%)**
Radical operation (N=76)	61	47[*]	18
Palliative operation (N=177)	44	23	5

[*] *The observed five-year survival rate for patients with radical operations treated with conventional therapy in China is reported to be 11% to 22%.*

In a study of 81 stage III and IV stomach cancer patients treated with chemotherapy, approximately 75 percent received the formula *Shen Xue Tang*. After six weeks of treatment, none of the patients taking the formula suffered from diarrhea, as compared to 33 percent in the control group. Only 19 percent suffered from vomiting as compared to 33 percent in the control group, and 14 percent reported loss of appetite as compared with 22 percent in the control group.[81]

In a study of 320 patients with stomach cancer treated with both conventional medicine and the formula *Li Wei Hua Jie Tang*, the observed survival rates were as listed in Table 12.3.[82]

Lastly, one study on 39 patients with postsurgical gastrointestinal cancer who used the formula *Shi Quan Da Bu Tang* reported that NK cell activity was markedly elevated as compared to pretreatment levels.[83]

Other Studies

A study on 62 patients undergoing chemotherapy for various cancers investigated the effects of the formula *Ye Qi Sheng Xue Tang* on white blood cell count. Each patient received two daily doses of the formula. During the six-week trial, the patients who received the formula before breakfast and lunch experienced a less drastic decrease in white blood cell count than those who took the formula before lunch and supper (11 percent versus 26 percent). The incidence of low white blood cell count was also less frequent in the group that received the formula before breakfast and lunch (13 percent versus 48 percent). The authors suggested the difference in response between the two groups was due to the natural circadian rhythm of DNA synthesis in bone marrow. DNA synthesis is at a maximum in the morning, and apparently, agents that stimulate the bone marrow may be more effective if administered early in the day.[84] NK cell activity is also highest in the morning or early afternoon.[85]

In a study of 242 patients with a variety of cancers and a Chinese medicine diagnosis of "qi vacuity" (low vital energy), treatment with the formula *Shen Xue Tang* significantly improved a number of immune indices.

Macrophage activity improved 16 percent, helper T-lymphocyte populations increased 50 percent, and NK-cell function increased 81 percent.[86]

In a study of 40 patients with various types of cancers and depressed immune systems, administration of either *Astragalus* or a saponin-containing immunostimulant herb, *Gynostemma pentaphyllum*, increased lymphocyte activity by 46 percent and 26 percent respectively, as compared to pretreatment levels.[87]

NATURAL COMPOUNDS THAT SUPPRESS THE IMMUNE SYSTEM

Many natural compounds I discuss have the potential to inhibit aspects of the immune system. Although none of these is generally considered a primary immunosuppressive agent, each can produce immunosuppression as a secondary effect, at least under some circumstances. Natural compounds can induce immunosuppression in many ways, such as by reducing signal transduction (immune cells need signal transduction to function), reducing NF-κB activity, histamine release, vascular permeability, and immune cell migration, as well as by causing anti-inflammatory effects. The most potent anti-inflammatory compounds tend to be those that reduce production of PGE_2 or other inflammatory prostaglandins or leukotrienes. Taking all of these actions into account, we can see that most compounds included in this book have the potential to contribute to an immunosuppressive effect; however, earlier in this chapter we also saw that most could also contribute to a stimulatory effect. What is the overall effect of combinations on the immune system and are some compounds are incompatible with others? Based on the information below, it would seem that the compounds discussed in this book are compatible and that combinations of them will generally facilitate an immune response and are desirable to use.

Any immunosuppressive effects these compounds may produce do not appear to interfere with their ability to inhibit cancer progression in vivo, as attested to by the many successful animal antitumor studies cited in Part III. It is likely, in fact, that most of these compounds, at concentrations applicable to humans, produce relatively mild effects on the immune system in comparison to their effects on cancer. Because cancer cells rely on such abnormal and excessive signals to function, they are probably more susceptible than immune or other normal cells to compounds that inhibit signal transduction and other events that rely on signal transduction (for example, NF-κB activity and cell migration). As an analogy, aspirin has a marked effect on body temperature when the temperature is abnormally high (in fever), but relatively little effect when it is normal. In the same way, it is reasonable to suppose that these natural compounds will generally have more effect on the abnormal cellular activities found in cancer cells than they do on the normal activities found in immune or other healthy cells.

Concurrent use of immune stimulants and potential immunosuppressive compounds also seems compatible in that some of the latter actually increase the immune response. For example, although inflammation is part of the immune response, it can hinder the response when it is excessive. This immunosuppressive effect is largely due to excessive production of PGE_2, although other factors may play a role. Since most anti-inflammatory compounds act by reducing PGE_2 production, they have the potential to increase immune cell activity. Indeed, a recent review on impediments to successful immunotherapy emphasized that immunotherapy is unlikely to be effective unless methods of immune escape by cancer cells, such as the production of PGE_2 and other immunosuppressive compounds, are addressed.[88] Furthermore, one mouse study reported that a combination of IL-2 and ibuprofen, an inhibitor of prostaglandin synthesis, was more effective in inhibiting metastasis of transplanted breast cancer cells than either agent alone.[89]

Note that non-steroidal anti-inflammatory drugs (NSAIDs) such as aspirin and ibuprofen, which inhibit prostaglandin synthesis and reduce inflammation, are not necessarily contraindicated in patients with infections, even though these patients require an effective immune system. Indeed, some NSAIDs can assist rodents to overcome some types of bacterial infections, especially chronic ones.[90–93, a] Moreover, the beneficial effect produced by NSAIDs against infection can be increased by administering immune-stimulating cytokines like interferons.[94]

Turning again to natural inhibitors of NF-κB, these compounds reduce inflammation and TNF production and in so doing may cause immunosuppression, but they also tend to inhibit PGE_2 production and thus may in-

crease immune activity. Consider too the parallels between cancer treatment and treatment of patients with the HIV virus. Both diseases are driven by excessive NF-κB activity (although one could argue this is more true for HIV). Also, both diseases are associated with excessive ROS production, inflammation, and immunosuppression.[95] What is interesting is that inhibitors of NF-κB activity show promise in HIV treatment, in spite of the fact these patients are immunosuppressed.[96, 97] (In this case, NF-κB inhibitors serve to reduce rather than cause immunosuppression.) It seems possible that inhibitors of NF-κB could also be used in cancer patients without causing significant immunosuppression.

We can now identify some of the natural compounds with potential to cause immunosuppression. Inhibitors of signal transduction were discussed in Chapter 4; inhibitors of NF-κB activity were listed in Tables 5.1 and 5.2; those of PGE_2 production, histamine release, and increased vascular permeability in Chapter 8; and inhibitors of cell motility were listed in Table 9.3. Of these, we discuss flavonoids and EPA in more detail, since their use is important to this book and their immunosuppressive effects have received more study.

Flavonoids and Immune Function

The effects of flavonoids on the immune system are complex and poorly understood. Depending on the conditions, flavonoids may inhibit, assist, or have no effect on immune function. Their effects on immune function are due to their ability to inhibit eicosanoid-mediated inflammation, histamine-induced inflammation, PTK or PKC activity, cell motility, or several of these.

Many flavonoids can impede leukocyte proliferation and function in vitro. For example, genistein can inhibit T-cell and NK-cell activity in vitro at IC_{50} concentrations similar to that of cancer cell inhibition (about 1 to 100 μM).[98–102] This effect appears to be due partly to inhibition of PTK activity. Similarly, studies have reported that apigenin and quercetin can lower the generation and function of CD8 cytotoxic T cells in vitro (at about 5 to 20 μM).[103, 104, 105]

The above-cited studies tested pure flavonoids in vitro; flavonoids are present as glucuronide conjugates in vivo, however, and the conjugate forms appear to be much less inhibitory than the pure forms. For example, glucuronide conjugates of genistein inhibited NK cell activity at about 50-fold higher concentrations than that of free genistein.[99] In fact, genistein conjugates enhanced NK cell activity at concentrations that are relevant for therapy (0.1 to 10 μM). Moreover, quercetin enhanced natural killer cell activity in rats at oral doses relevant for therapy (at about 1.6 grams per day, as scaled to hu-

---

a In some cases, acute bacterial infections can be made worse by NSAIDs, since these drugs do reduce the initial immune response.

mans).[106] Similarly, oral administration of quercetin (at about 380 milligrams per day, as scaled to humans) increased macrophage-mediated antiviral effects in mice. Lastly, even in-vitro studies have reported that at low concentrations flavonoids can act as immunostimulants.[107, 108, 109]

Clearly, additional work remains to understand the effects of flavonoids on immune function and to determine how these effects may influence tumor progression. It does seem, however, that at doses relevant to humans, immunostimulation or no effect on the immune system is more likely to occur than an immunosuppressive effect.

EPA/DHA and Immune Function

Numerous in-vitro, animal, and human studies have reported that omega-3 fatty acids, in particular EPA and DHA, can suppress immune cell activity.[110–122] Omega-3 fatty acids are therefore potent anti-inflammatory agents, and for this reason EPA and fish oil (which contains EPA) have been reported useful in reducing the symptoms of autoimmune-related diseases such as lupus, rheumatoid arthritis, psoriasis, and colitis.[114, 123–125]

Although the exact mechanism of immune suppression is not well understood, it appears to involve the following:[115, 126–128]

- Reduced production of 2-series prostanoids (e.g., PGE$_2$) and 4-series leukotrienes.

- Reduced production of proinflammatory cytokines such as IL-1, IL-6, and TNF.

- Modification of gene expression, leading to reduced expression of T-cell stimulatory molecules.

- Increased production of transforming growth factor (TGF-beta) and Fas membrane receptors. (Fas is a membrane receptor in the same family as the TNF receptor.) Fas molecules can induce apoptosis in immune cells.

- Inhibition of PKC.

- Increased plasma membrane fluidity.

Regardless of the exact cause, the effects are predominantly a reduced ability of immune cells to present antigens to T cells and reduced T-cell activity. For example, fish oil inhibited the expression of foreign antigens/MHC aggregates on human monocytes in vitro and in vivo.[121, 129, 130] Macrophage and natural killer cell activity can also be affected.

In spite of these demonstrations of immunosuppressive activity, omega-3 fatty acids do not exert immunosuppressive effects under all experimental systems and, in some cases, have been found to improve immune function in humans. For example, EPA can augment macrophage activity, and fish oil (at 18 grams per day) has been reported to reduce immunosuppression in patients with solid tumors.[131, 132] Orally administered EPA (at 1.8 grams per day) improved lymphocyte proliferation and natural killer cell activity in patients after stressful surgery for esophageal cancer.[133] EPA also improved immune function in patients receiving chemoradiation therapy.[134] Furthermore, omega-3 fatty acids can increase the susceptibility of some leukemia cell lines to destruction by T lymphocytes.[135, 136]

The reasons for these apparent discrepancies are not entirely clear. Although many factors may determine the exact impact of omega-3 fatty acids on immune function, one of the more controllable ones may be antioxidant status.[114] EPA and DHA are more easily oxidized than other fatty acids, and when administered to animals and humans, they can cause lipid peroxidation and diminish vitamin E levels. Vitamin E is one of the most important antioxidants in preventing lipid peroxidation, and immune cells need adequate vitamin E. Free radicals generated during lipid peroxidation may contribute to the suppressive effects of omega-3 fatty acids on T-cell function. Therefore, it seems likely that some of the immunosuppressive effects reported were partly due to excessive free radical production. Vitamin E supplementation can ameliorate some of the immunosuppressive effects of omega-3 fatty acids, apparently without decreasing its anti-inflammatory effect. In humans, 300 I.U. of vitamin E reversed depressed T-cell activity that was induced by 15 grams per day of fish oil.[137] In a randomized control study of 60 patients with advanced solid tumors, 18 grams per day of fish oil with vitamin E increased TNF production and T cell function in a malnourished subgroup of patients. The survival of all patients was prolonged by EPA treatment.[138]

Clearly, the effects of omega-3 fatty acids on immune function are complex. While co-administration with vitamin E is likely to minimize any adverse effects and might even lead to immune stimulation, immunosuppression may occur in more limited instances. Even with vitamin E administration, however, omega-3 fatty acids may still produce an anti-inflammatory effect (due to reduced PGE$_2$ production, for example), and as we have discussed, this type of anti-inflammatory effect should be useful in cancer treatment. Regardless of the exact mechanisms affected, the overall effect of omega-3 fatty acids is generally one of cancer inhibition.

CONCLUSION

The methods by which natural compounds stimulate the immune system vary, but often they involve production of cytokines or modulation of cytokine activity. In this regard, combinations of natural compounds may be particularly effective, since combinations tend to increase production of a broad range of cytokines, including IL-2 and interferons. Indeed, mixtures of immunostimulant compounds have been used for centuries in herbal medicine traditions. More recently, they have been studied in China, where they appear to improve the survival of cancer patients receiving chemotherapy, while reducing its adverse effects. These studies and other human and animal studies on natural immunostimulant compounds, both alone and in combination, suggest they could play an important role in cancer treatment.

Cancer cells have developed ways to evade immune attack, one being the production of immunosuppressive compounds such as PGE_2. Therefore, the best results may be seen when immunostimulant, immune supportive, and immunoregulatory compounds are used in combination with natural compounds that inhibit production of PGE_2 and other immunosuppressive compounds. At the same time, it would be counterproductive to rely on treating the immune system alone. The underlying abnormalities in signal transduction, gene expression, and other processes that drive cancer cell proliferation and spread must be addressed.

REFERENCES

[1] Ghoneum M, Mermel O, Williams L, et al. Susceptibility of propolis-treated tumor cells to human natural killer cell activity in vitro. Cancer Detect Prevent 1995; 19(1):106.

[2] Guarini L, Su ZZ, Zucker S, et al. Growth inhibition and modulation of antigenic phenotype in human melanoma and glioblastoma multiforme cells by caffeic acid phenethyl ester (CAPE). Cellular and Molecular Biology 1992; 38(5):513–527.

[3] Cheshier JE, Ardestani-Kaboudanian S, Liang B, et al. Immunomodulation by pycnogenol in retrovirus-infected or ethanol-fed mice. Life Sci 1996; 58(5):PL 87–96.

[4] Nakajima N, Utsunomiya T, Kobayashi M, et al. In vitro induction of anti-type 2 T cells by glycyrrhizin. Burns 1996 Dec; 22(8):612–7.

[5] Yamashiki M, Nishimura A, Suzuki H, et al. Effects of the Japanese herbal medicine "Sho-saiko-to" (TJ-9) on in vitro interleukin-10 production by peripheral blood mononuclear cells of patients with chronic hepatitis C. Hepatology 1997 Jun; 25(6):1390–7.

[6] Schulz S, Reinhold D, Schmidt H, et al. Perillic acid inhibits Ras/MAP kinase-driven IL-2 production in human T lymphocytes. Biochem Biophys Res Commun 1997 Dec 29; 241(3):720–5.

[7] Hayashi N, Tashiro T, Yamamori H, et al. Effects of intravenous omega-3 and omega-6 fat emulsion on cytokine production and delayed type hypersensitivity in burned rats receiving total parenteral nutrition. JPEN J Parenter Enteral Nutr 1998 Nov–Dec; 22(6):363–7.

[8] Chavali SR, Weeks CE, Zhong WW, Forse RA. Increased production of TNF-alpha and decreased levels of dienoic eicosanoids, IL-6 and IL-10 in mice fed menhaden oil and juniper oil diets in response to an intraperitoneal lethal dose of LPS. Prostaglandins Leukot Essent Fatty Acids 1998 Aug; 59(2):89–93.

[9] Matsunaga K, Hosokawa A, Oohara M, et al. Direct action of a protein-bound polysaccharide, PSK, on transforming growth factor-beta. Immunopharmacology 1998 Nov; 40(3):219–30.

[10] Strickland FM, Darvill A, Albersheim P, et al. Inhibition of UV-induced immune suppression and interleukin-10 production by plant oligosaccharides and polysaccharides. Photochem Photobiol 1999 Feb; 69(2):141–7.

[11] Wang Y, Huang DS, Wood S, et al. Modulation of immune function and cytokine production by various levels of vitamin E supplementation during murine AIDS. Immunopharmacology 1995 Apr; 29(3):225–33.

[12] Bonig H, Korholz D, Pafferath B, et al. Interleukin 10 induced c-fos expression in human B cells by activation of divergent protein kinases. Immunol Invest 1996 Jan–Mar; 25(1–2):115–28.

[13] Gabrilovich DI, Ishida T, Nadaf S, et al. Antibodies to vascular endothelial growth factor enhance the efficacy of cancer immunotherapy by improving endogenous dendritic cell function. Clin Cancer Res 1999 Oct; 5(10):2963–70.

[14] Chu DT, Lepe-Zuniga J, Wong WL, et al. Fractionated extract of Astragalus membranaceus, a Chinese medicinal herb, potentiates LAK cell cytotoxicity generated by a low dose of recombinant interleukin-2. J Clin Lab Immunol 1988 Aug; 26(4):183–7.

[15] Wang SY, Hsu ML, Hsu HC, et al. The anti-tumor effect of Ganoderma lucidum is mediated by cytokines released from activated macrophages and T lymphocytes. Int J Cancer 1997 Mar 17; 70(6):699–705.

[16] Hamuro J, Takatsuki F, Suga T, et al. Synergistic antimetastatic effects of lentinan and interleukin 2 with pre- and post-operative treatments. Jpn J Cancer Res 1994 Dec; 85(12):1288–97.

[17] Liang CM, Lee N, Cattell D, Liang SM. Glutathione regulates interleukin-2 activity on cytotoxic T-cells. J Biol Chem 1989; 264(23):13519–523.

[18] Margalit A, Hauser SD, Zweifel BS, et al. Regulation of prostaglandin biosynthesis in vivo by glutathione. Am J Physiol 1998 Feb; 274(2 Pt 2):R294–302.

[19] Kiremidjian-Schumacher L, Roy M, et al. Regulation of cellular immune responses by selenium. Biol Trace Elem Res 1992 Apr–Jun; 33:23–35.

[20] Kiremidjian-Schumacher L, Roy M, Wishe HI, et al. Supplementation with selenium and human immune cell functions. II. Effect on cytotoxic lymphocytes and natural killer cells. Biol Trace Elem Res 1994 Apr–May; 41(1–2):115–27.

[21] Roy M, Kiremidjian-Schumacher L, Wishe HI, et al. Supplementation with selenium and human immune cell functions. I. Effect on lymphocyte proliferation and interleukin 2 receptor expression. Biol Trace Elem Res 1994 Apr–May; 41(1–2):103–14.

22 Klaschka, F. Oral enzymes in oncology. MUCOS Pharma GmbH, 1997. http://www.mucos.de

23 Eckert K, Grabowska E, Stange R, et al. Effects of oral bromelain administration on the impaired immunocytotoxicity of mononuclear cells from mammary tumor patients. Oncol Rep 1999 Nov–Dec; 6(6):1191–9.

24 Miller JM, Ginsberg M, McElfatrick GC, Zoll DR. The administration of bromelain orally in the treatment of inflammation and edema. Exp Med Surg 1964; 22:293–299.

25 Masson M. [Bromelain in blunt injuries of the locomotor system. A study of observed applications in general practice.] Fortschr Med 1995 Jul 10; 113(19):303–6.

26 Tsomides J, Goldberg RI. Controlled evaluation of oral chymotrypsin-trypsin treatment of injuries to the head and face. Clin Med 1969 Nov; 40–45.

27 Shaw PC. The use of trypsin-chymotrypsin formulation in fractures of the hand. Br J Clin Pract 1969; 23(1):25–26.

28 Bogner RL, Snyder CC. High dose oral chymotrypsin as an adjunct in plastic surgery. Plastic and Reconstructive Surgery 1962; 37(3):289–295.

29 Pirotta F, De Giuli-Morghen C. Bromelain: A deeper pharmacological study. Drugs Exptl Clin Res 1978; 4(1):1–20.

30 Netti C, Bandi GL, Pecile A. Anti-inflammatory action of proteolytic enzymes of animal vegetable or bacterial origin administered orally compared with that of known anti-phlogistic compounds. Farmaco [Prat] 1972 Aug; 27(8):453–66.

31 Gupta MK, Khanna JN, Khera SS. Evaluation of trypsin & chymotrypsin in the management of post-operative oedema. J Indian Dent Assoc 1985 Mar; 57(3):101–5.

32 Lehmann PV. Immunomodulation by proteolytic enzymes [editorial]. Nephrol Dial Transplant 1996 Jun; 11(6):952–5.

33 Hale LP, Haynes BF. Bromelain treatment of human T cells removes CD44, CD45RA, E2/MIC2, CD6, CD7, CD8, and Leu 8/LAM1 surface molecules and markedly enhances CD2-mediated T cell activation. J Immunol 1992 Dec 15; 149(12):3809–16.

34 Targoni OS, Tary-Lehmann M, Lehmann PV. Prevention of murine EAE by oral hydrolytic enzyme treatment. J Autoimmun 1999 May; 12(3):191–8.

35 Kleef R, Delohery TM, Bovbjerg DH. Selective modulation of cell adhesion molecules on lymphocytes by bromelain protease 5. Pathobiology 1996; 64(6):339–46.

36 Munzig E, Eckert K, Harrach T, et al. Bromelain protease F9 reduces the CD44 mediated adhesion of human peripheral blood lymphocytes to human umbilical vein endothelial cells. FEBS Lett 1994 Sep 5; 351(2):215–8.

37 de Wit CA, Westrom BR. Further studies of plasma protease inhibitors in the hedgehog, Erinaceus europaeus; collagenase, papain and plasmin inhibitors. Comp Biochem Physiol A 1987; 86(1):1–5.

38 LaMarre J, Wollenberg GK, Gonias SL, Hayes MA. Cytokine binding and clearance properties of proteinase-activated alpha 2-macroglobulins. Lab Invest 1991 Jul; 65(1):3–14.

39 Wollenberg GK, LaMarre J, Rosendal S, et al. Binding of tumor necrosis factor alpha to activated forms of human plasma alpha 2 macroglobulin. Am J Pathol 1991 Feb; 138(2):265–72.

40 Borth W, Teodorescu M. Inactivation of human interleukin-2 (IL-2) by alpha 2-macroglobulin-trypsin complexes. Immunology 1986 Mar; 57(3):367–71.

41 Mannhalter JW, Borth W, Eibl MM. Modulation of antigen-induced T cell proliferation by alpha 2M-trypsin complexes. J Immunol 1986 Apr 15; 136(8):2792–9.

42 Heumann D, Vischer TL. Immunomodulation by alpha 2-macroglobulin and alpha 2-macroglobulin-proteinase complexes: The effect on the human T lymphocyte response. Eur J Immunol 1988 May; 18(5):755–60.

43 Gravagna P, Gianazza E, Arnaud P, et al. Modulation of the immune response by plasma protease inhibitors. II. Alpha 2-macroglobulin subunits inhibit natural killer cell cytotoxicity and antibody-dependent cell-mediated cytotoxicity. Scand J Immunol 1982 Jan; 15(1):115–8.

44 Chu CT, Howard GC, Misra UK, Pizzo SV. α_2-Macroglobulin: A sensor for proteolysis. Ann New York Acad Sci 1994; 737:291–307.

45 Matsushima K, Taguchi M, Kovacs EJ, et al. Intracellular localization of human monocyte associated interleukin 1 (IL 1) activity and release of biologically active IL 1 from monocytes by trypsin and plasmin. J Immunol 1986 Apr 15; 136(8):2883–91.

46 Desser L, Rehberger A. Induction of tumor necrosis factor in human peripheral-blood mononuclear cells by proteolytic enzymes. Oncology 1990; 47:475–77.

47 Desser L, Kokron E, Rehberger A. Tumor necrosis factor (TNF), interleukin-1 (IL-1), and interleukin-6 (IL-6) synthesis in human peripheral blood mononuclear cells (PBMNC) induced by proteolytic enzymes and amylase in vitro and in vivo. J Cancer Res Clin Oncol 1992; 118(suppl):R81.

48 Desser L, Rehberger A, Paukovits W. Proteolytic enzymes and amylase induce cytokine production in human peripheral blood mononuclear cells in vitro. Cancer Biother 1994 Fall; 9(3):253–63.

49 Desser L, Rehberger A, Kokron E, et al. Cytokine synthesis in human peripheral blood mononuclear cells after oral administration of polyenzyme preparations. Oncology 1993; 50:403–7.

50 Zavadova E, Desser L, Mohr T. Stimulation of reactive oxygen species production and cytotoxicity in human neutrophils in vitro and after oral administration of a polyenzyme preparation. Cancer Biother 1995 Summer; 10(2):147–52.

51 Wrba H, Pecher O. Enzymes: A drug of the future. Strengthening the immunological system with enzyme therapy. MUCOS Pharma GmbH, 1996. http://www.mucos.de

52 Virgin HW 4th, Unanue ER. Immune complexes suppress cellular immunity. Ann N Y Acad Sci 1984; 437:16–27.

53 Esparza I, Green R, Schreiber RD. Inhibition of macrophage tumoricidal activity by immune complexes and altered erythrocytes. J Immunol 1983 Nov; 131(5):2117–21.

54 Nakazawa M, Emancipator SN, Lamm ME. Removal of glomerular immune complexes in passive serum sickness nephritis by treatment in vivo with proteolytic enzymes. Lab Invest 1986 Nov; 55(5):551–6.

55 Nakazawa M, Emancipator SN, Lamm ME. Proteolytic enzyme treatment reduces glomerular immune deposits and

proteinuria in passive Heymann nephritis. J Exp Med 1986 Dec 1; 164(6):1973–87.

56 Kelly GS. Bromelain: A literature review and discussion of its therapeutic applications. Alt Med Rev 1996; 1(4):243–257.

57 Felton GE. Fibrinolytic and antithrombotic action of bromelain may eliminate thrombosis in heart patients. Med Hypotheses 1980 Nov; 6(11):1123–33.

58 Ako H, Cheung AH, Matsuura PK. Isolation of a fibrinolysis enzyme activator from commercial bromelain. Arch Int Pharmacodyn Ther 1981 Nov; 254(1):157–67.

59 Taussig SJ, Batkin S. Bromelain, the enzyme complex of pineapple (Ananas comosus) and its clinical application. An update. J of Ethnopharmacol 1988; 22:191–203.

60 Alban S, Franz ME, Franz G. Influence of the therapeutically used enzymes bromelain, papain and trypsin on the blood coagulation in vitro. Pharm Pharmacol Lett 1997; 2/3:59–62.

61 Mynott TL, Ladhams A, Scarmato P, et al. Bromelain, from pineapple stems, proteolytically blocks activation of extracellular regulated kinase-2 in T cells. J Immunol 1999 Sep 1; 163(5):2568–75.

62 Lissoni P, Barni S, Tancini G, et al. Pineal-opioid system interactions in the control of immunioinflammatory responses. Ann NY Acad Sci 1994 Nov 25; 741:191–196.

63 Lissoni P, Barni S, Tancini G, Rovelli F, et al. A study of the mechanisms involved in the immunostimulatory action of the pineal hormone in cancer patients. Oncology. 1993; 50(6):399–402.

64 Blask DE. Neuroendocrine aspects of circadian pharmacodynamics. In *Circadian cancer therapy*. Hrushesky WJ, ed., Ann Arbor: CRC Press, 1994, pp. 43–59.

65 Maestroni GJ, Conti A. Melatonin in human breast cancer tissue: Association with nuclear grade and estrogen receptor status. Lab Invest 1996 Oct; 75(4):557–61.

66 Bartsch C, Bartsch H, Lippert TH. Rationales to consider the use of melatonin as a chrono-oncotherapeutic drug. in vivo 1995; 9:305–310.

67 Lissoni P, Rovelli F, Brivio F, et al. Circadian secretions of IL-2, IL-12, IL-6 and IL-10 in relation to the light/dark rhythm of the pineal hormone melatonin in healthy humans. Nat Immun 1998; 16(1):1–5.

68 Boik J. Cancer and natural medicine: A textbook of basic science and clinical research. Princeton, MN: Oregon Medical Press, 1996.

69 Li NQ. Clinical and experimental study on shen-qi injection with chemotherapy in the treatment of malignant tumor of digestive tract. Chung Kuo Chung Hsi I Chieh Ho Tsa Chih 1992; 12(10):588–92, 579.

70 Li L, Chen X, Li J. Observations on the long-term effects of "yi qi yang yin decoction" combined with radiotherapy in the treatment of nasopharyngeal carcinoma. J Tradit Chin Med 1992; 12(4):263–6.

71 Li PP. Treatment of tumors and their progress by improving blood circulation to remove stasis. Chung Kuo Chung Hsi I Chieh Ho Tsa Chih 1992; 12(10):634–6, 623.

72 Sun Y. The role of traditional Chinese medicine in supportive care of cancer patients. Recent Results in Cancer Research 1988; 108:327–334.

73 Zhang DZ. Prevention and cure by traditional Chinese medicine, of the side effects caused by radio-chemotherapy of cancer patients. Chung Hsi I Chieh Ho Tsa Chih 1988 Feb; 8(2):114–6.

74 Cheng JH, Zhang SL, Zhao DH, et al. Treatment of 20 patients with terminal primary bronchogenic carcinoma using feiliuping. Jiangxi Journal of Traditional Chinese Medicine 1991; 22(6):344–47.

75 Wang GT, Xu JY, Zheng A, et al. Treatment of operated late gastric carcinoma with prescription of strengthening the patient's resistance and dispelling the invading evil in combination with chemotherapy: Followup study of 158 patients and experimental study in animals. (meeting abstract) First Shanghai international symposium on gastrointestinal cancers. November 14–16, 1988, p. 244.

76 Wang GT. Treatment of operated late gastric carcinoma with prescription of strengthening the patient's resistance and dispelling the invading evil in combination with chemotherapy: Followup study of 158 patients and experimental study in animals. Chung Hsi I Chieh Ho Tsa Chih 1990; 10(12):712–6, 707.

77 Pan M. Cancer treatment with fu zheng pei ben principle. Fuijian: Fujian Science and Technology Publishing House, 1992, p. 34.

78 Yu G, Ren D, Sun G, et al. Clinical and experimental studies of JPYS in reducing side effects of chemotherapy in late-stage gastric cancer. J Tradit Chin Med 1993; 13(1):31–7.

79 Zhang DZ. Effects of traditional Chinese medicine and pharmacology on increasing sensitivity and reducing toxicity in tumor patients undergoing radio-chemical therapy Chung Kuo Chung Hsi I Chieh Ho Tsa Chih 1992; 12(3):135–8.

80 Ning CH, Wang GM, Zhao TY, et al. Therapeutical effects of jian pi yi shen prescription on the toxicity reactions of postoperative chemotherapy in patients with advanced gastric carcinoma. J Tradit Chin Med 1988; 8(2):113–6.

81 Rao XQ. Clinical and experimental studies of shengxue tang combined with chemotherapy in the treatment of late-stage gastric cancer. Chung Hsi I Chieh Ho Tsa Chih 1987; 7(12):715–7, 707.

82 Pan MJ, Li YH, Chen LF. Treatment of 320 cases of gastric cancer with liwei huajie decoction combined with surgery and chemotherapy. Chinese Journal of Combined Traditional and Western Medicine 1986; 6(5):268–70.

83 Okamoto T, Motohasi H, Takemiya S, et al. Clinical effects of Juzendaiho-to on immunologic and fatty metabolic states in postoperative patients with gastrointestinal cancer. Gan To Kagaku Ryoho 1989; 16(4 Pt 2–2):1533–7.

84 Li Y, Yu G. A comparative clinical study on prevention and treatment with selected chronomedication of leukopenia induced by chemotherapy. J of Trad Chin Med 1993; 13(4):257–261.

85 Whiteside T, Herberman R. The role of natural killer cells in human disease. Clinical Immunology and Immunotherapy 1989; 53:1–23.

86 Rao XQ, Yu RC, Zhang JH. Sheng xue tang on immunological functions of cancer patients with spleen deficiency syndrome. Chung Hsi I Chieh Ho Tsa Chih 1991; 11(4):218–9, 197.

87 Hou J, Liu S, Ma Z, et al. Effects of Gynostemma pentaphyllum makino on the immunological function of cancer patients. J Tradit Chin Med 1991; 11(1):47–52.

88 Hersey P. Impediments to successful immunotherapy. Pharmacol Ther 1999 Feb; 81(2):111–9.

89 Khoo NK, Chan FP, Saarloos MN, Lala PK. Immunotherapy of mammary adenocarcinoma metastases in C3H/HeN mice with chronic administration of cyclo-oxygenase inhibitors alone or in combination with IL-2. Clin Exp Metastasis 1992 Jul; 10(4):239–52.

90 Hockertz S, Heckenberger R, Emmendorffer A, Muller M. Influence of ibuprofen on the infection with Listeria monocytogenes. Arzneimittelforschung 1995 Jan; 45(1):104–7.

91 Hockertz S, Paulini I, Rogalla K, Schettler T. Influence of acetylsalicylic acid on a Listeria monocytogenes infection. Agents Actions 1993 Sep; 40(1–2):119–23.

92 Short BL, Gardiner M, Walker RI, et al. Indomethacin improves survival in gram-negative sepsis. Adv Shock Res 1981; 6:27–36.

93 Edwards CK 3d, Hedegaard HB, Zlotnik A, et al. Chronic infection due to Mycobacterium intracellulare in mice: Association with macrophage release of prostaglandin E2 and reversal by injection of indomethacin, muramyl dipeptide, or interferon-gamma. J Immunol 1986 Mar 1; 136(5):1820–7.

94 Hockertz S, Heckenberger R. Treatment of an acute bacterial infection with a combination of acetylsalicylic acid/ibuprofen and interferon gamma. Arzneimittelforschung 1996 Oct; 46(10):1012–5.

95 Israel N, Gougerot-Pocidalo MA. Oxidative stress in human immunodeficiency virus infection. Cell Mol Life Sci 1997 Dec; 53(11–12):864–70.

96 Dezube BJ. Pentoxifylline for the treatment of infection with human immunodeficiency virus. Clin Infect Dis 1994 Mar; 18(3):285–7.

97 Dezube BJ, Lederman MM. Pentoxifylline for the treatment of HIV infection and its complications. J Cardiovasc Pharmacol 1995; 25 Suppl 2:S139–42.

98 Dong Z, O'Brian CA, Fidler IJ. Activation of tumoricidal properties in macrophages by lipopolysaccharide requires protein-tyrosine kinase activity. J Leukoc Biol 1993 Jan; 53(1):53–60.

99 Zhang Y, Song TT, Cunnick JE, et al. Daidzein and genistein glucuronides in vitro are weakly estrogenic and activate human natural killer cells at nutritionally relevant concentrations. J Nutr 1999 Feb; 129(2):399–405.

100 Ting CC, Hargrove ME, Wang J, Patel AD. Differential requirement of protein tyrosine kinase and protein kinase C in the generation of IL-2-induced LAK cell and alpha CD3-induced CD3-AK cell responses. Cell Immunol 1995 Feb; 160(2):286–96.

101 Wang J, Hargrove ME, Ting CC. IL-2 and IL-4 mediate through two distinct kinase pathways for the activation of alphaCD3-induced activated killer cells. Cell Immunol 1996 Dec 15; 174(2):138–46.

102 Rosato A, Zambon A, Mandruzzato S, et al. Inhibition of protein tyrosine phosphorylation prevents T-cell-mediated cytotoxicity. Cell Immunol 1994 Dec; 159(2):294–305.

103 Schwartz A, Middleton E Jr. Comparison of the effects of quercetin with those of other flavonoids on the generation and effector function of cytotoxic T lymphocytes. Immunopharmacology 1984 Apr; 7(2):115–26.

104 Mookerjee BK, Lee TP, Logue GP, et al. The effects of flavonoids on human lymphocyte proliferative responses. Prog Clin Biol Res 1986; 213:511–20.

105 Schwartz A, Sutton SL, Middleton E Jr. Quercetin inhibition of the induction and function of cytotoxic T lymphocytes. Immunopharmacology 1982 Apr; 4(2):125–38.

106 Exon JH, Magnuson BA, South EH, Hendrix K. Dietary quercetin, immune functions and colonic carcinogenesis in rats. Immunopharmacol Immunotoxicol 1998 Feb; 20(1):173–90.

107 Welton AF, Hurley J, Will P. Flavonoids and arachidonic Acid Metabolism. In Plant flavonoids in biology and medicine II. New York: Alan R. Liss, Inc., 1988, pp. 301–02.

108 Del Rio M, Ruedas G, Medina S, et al. Improvement by several antioxidants of macrophage function in vitro. Life Sci 1998; 63(10):871–81.

109 Berg P, Daniel PT. Effects of flavonoid compounds on the immune response. In Plant flavonoids in biology and medicine II. New York: Alan R. Liss, Inc., 1988, pp. 157–171.

110 Linder MC, ed. Nutritional biochemistry and metabolism. 2nd ed. New York: Elsevier Science, 1991, p. 77.

111 Barone J, Hebert JR. Dietary fat and natural killer cell activity. Med Hypotheses 1988; 25:223–26.

112 Lu CY, Dustin LB, Vazquez MA. Macrophage tumoricidal activity is inhibited by docosahexaenoic acid (DHA), an omega-3 fatty acid. In Exercise, calories, fat, and cancer. Jacobs MM, ed. New York: Plenum Press, 1992.

113 Dyerberg J. Conference summary and future directions. In Health effects of w-3 polyunsaturated fatty acids in seafoods. World Rev Nutr Diet Simopoulos AP, et al., eds. Basel: Karger, 1991, pp. 66:16–9.

114 Meydani SN. Effect of (n-3) polyunsaturated fatty acids on cytokine production and their biologic function. Nutrition 1996 Jan; 12(1 Suppl):S8–14.

115 Erickson KL, Hubbard NE. Dietary fish oil modulation of macrophage tumoricidal activity. Nutrition 1996 Jan; 12(1 Suppl):S34–8.

116 Purasiri P, Murray A, Richardson S, et al. Modulation of cytokine production in vivo by dietary essential fatty acids in patients with colorectal cancer. Clinical Science 1994; 87:711–717.

117 Wu D, Meydani SN, Meydani M, et al. Immunologic effects of marine- and plant-derived n-3 polyunsaturated fatty acids in nonhuman primates. Am J Clin Nutr 1996 Feb; 63(2):273–80.

118 Endres S, von Schacky C. n-3 polyunsaturated fatty acids and human cytokine synthesis. Curr Opin Lipidol 1996 Feb; 7(1):48–52.

119 Endres S. n-3 polyunsaturated fatty acids and human cytokine synthesis. Lipids 1996 Mar; 31 Suppl:S239–42.

120 Hughes DA, Southon S, Pinder AC. (n-3) Polyunsaturated fatty acids modulate the expression of functionality associated molecules on human monocytes in vitro. J Nutr 1996 Mar; 126(3):603–10.

[121] Hughes DA, Pinder AC, Piper Z, et al. Fish oil supplementation inhibits the expression of major histocompatibility complex class II molecules and adhesion molecules on human monocytes. Am J Clin Nutr 1996 Feb; 63(2):267–72.

[122] Jolly CA, Jiang YH, Chapkin RS, McMurray DN. Dietary (n-3) polyunsaturated fatty acids suppress murine lymphoproliferation, interleukin-2 secretion, and the formation of diacylglycerol and ceramide. J Nutr 1997 Jan; 127(1):37–43.

[123] Blok WL, Katan MB, van der Meer JW. Modulation of inflammation and cytokine production by dietary (n-3) fatty acids. J Nutr 1996 Jun; 126(6):1515–33.

[124] Fortin PR, Lew RA, Liang MH, et al. Validation of a meta-analysis: The effects of fish oil in rheumatoid arthritis. J Clin Epidemiol 1995 Nov; 48(11):1379–90.

[125] Kremer JM. Effects of modulation of inflammatory and immune parameters in patients with rheumatic and inflammatory disease receiving dietary supplementation of n-3 and n-6 fatty acids. Lipids 1996 (Suppl.); 31:S-243-S-247.

[126] Fernandes G, Troyer DA, Jolly CA. The effects of dietary lipids on gene expression and apoptosis. Proc Nutr Soc 1998 Nov; 57(4):543–50.

[127] Robinson DR, Urakaze M, Huang R, et al. Dietary marine lipids suppress continuous expression of interleukin-1 beta gene transcription. Lipids 1996 Mar; 31 Suppl:S23–31.

[128] Karmali RA. Historical perspective and potential use of n-3 fatty acids in therapy of cancer cachexia. Nutrition 1996 Jan; 12(1 Suppl):S2–4.

[129] Hughes DA, Pinder AC. N-3 polyunsaturated fatty acids inhibit the antigen-presenting function of human monocytes. Am J Clin Nutr 2000 Jan; 71(1 Suppl):357S–60S.

[130] Hughes DA, Pinder AC. N-3 polyunsaturated fatty acids modulate the expression of functionally associated molecules on human monocytes and inhibit antigen-presentation in vitro. Clin Exp Immunol 1997 Dec; 110(3):516–23.

[131] Das UN. Gamma-linolenic acid, aracidonic acid, and eicosapentaenoic acid as potential anticancer drugs. Nutrition 1990; 6(6):429–34.

[132] Gogos CA, Ginopoulos P, Zoumbos NC, et al. The effect of dietary w-3 polyunsaturated fatty acids on T-lymphocyte subsets of patients with solid tumors. Cancer Det and Prev 1995; 19(5):415–417.

[133] Furukawa K, Tashiro T, Yamamori H, et al. Effects of soybean oil emulsion and eicosapentaenoic acid on stress response and immune function after a severely stressful operation. Ann Surg 1999 Feb; 229(2):255–61.

[134] Tashiro T, Yamamori H, Takagi K, et al. n-3 versus n-6 polyunsaturated fatty acids in critical illness. Nutrition. 1998; 14(6):551–3.

[135] Jenski LJ, Sturdevant LK, Ehringer WD, Stillwell W. Omega-3 fatty acid modification of membrane structure and function. I: Dietary manipulation of tumor cell susceptibility to cell- and complement-mediated lysis. Nutr Cancer 1993; (19):135–146.

[136] Pascale AW, Ehringer WD, Stillwell W, et al. Omega-3 fatty acid modification of membrane structure and function. II. Alteration by docosahexaenoic acid of tumor cell sensitivity to immune cytolysis. Nutr Cancer 1993; 19:147–157.

[137] Kremer JR, Schoene N, Douglass LW, et al. Increased vitamin E intake restores fish oil-induced suppressed blastogenesis of mitogenic-stimulated T-lymphocytes. Am J Clin Nutr 1991; 54:896.

[138] Gogos CA, Ginopoulos P, Salsa B, et al. Dietary omega-3 polyunsaturated fatty acids plus vitamin E restore immunodeficiency and prolong survival for severely ill patients with generalized malignancy: A randomized control trial. Cancer 1998; 82(2):395–402.

PART III
CLINICAL CONSIDERATIONS

In Parts I and II we explored how natural compounds may inhibit cancer. We looked at the many events that occur in cancer progression, both at the cellular level and at the level of the organism, and we also looked at natural compounds that could impede these events and thereby inhibit cancer. In Part III we shift our focus to the clinical aspects of using natural compounds.

Although actual clinical experience is lacking for most natural compounds, we can still explore clinical issues based on preclinical work that has been done. We do this in four primary ways for each compound. First, we examine work done on inhibiting cancer cell proliferation in-vitro and inhibiting cancer progression in animals and humans. Second, we examine ways the compound has been used, and at what doses, in the treatment of other, noncancerous diseases. Third, we review the material in Parts I and II to determine the procancer events the compound may inhibit. This review is primarily in table form. (For a full explanation of the tables, see Chapter 14.) Fourth, we estimate an effective dose and a maximum safe dose based on in-vitro and in-vivo data and results of computer modeling. Through these examinations, we begin to see how and when these compounds might be best used clinically. For convenience, the discussions for each compound in Chapters 14 to 22 begin with a brief summary of the results of the anticancer studies conducted, along with the conclusions that can be drawn from them.

Chapter 13 covers some important issues regarding synergism, the methods used to estimate doses, and strategies for designing combinations; the chapters that follow (14 to 22) focus on the natural compounds themselves. Each chapter discusses a group of compounds, with the groups loosely based on chemical family. For example, Chapter 14 covers the trace metals selenium, iron, and copper. The final chapter, Chapter 23, explores the use of natural compounds with chemotherapy or radiotherapy.

We discuss here what synergism is and why it is essential, as well as reasons to believe it may be practical, then summarize the methods for calculating doses and estimating toxicity of the individual compounds. Lastly, we outline strategies for designing effective combinations. Other issues discussed include the preferred forms of natural compounds for clinical use.

SYNERGISM

Thus far we have implied that synergism will occur in combinations that contain compounds from all three primary categories—direct acting, indirect acting, and immune stimulants. While this is likely the case and is still our clinical intention, when it comes to calculating doses we will act as if synergism occurs only between direct-acting compounds. This shift is needed because most studies on synergism have used only direct-acting compounds, few data are available on the others. Research has focused on direct-acting compounds because their anticancer effects are easier to study in vitro than those of other types of compounds, and when testing new therapies, in-vitro studies are usually done first. The in-vitro anticancer effects of indirect-acting compounds and immune stimulants are more difficult to study because these studies require multiple cell types and necessarily involve more complex interactions.

To provide hard evidence that compounds from all three categories interact synergistically to inhibit cancer, large combinations will need to be tested in vivo. My colleagues and I hope to start such studies soon.[a] Already, a recent study on rats has reported that apoptotic therapies work synergistically with therapies that stimulate the immune system.[b] In this study, a combination of an apoptosis inducer and IL-2 resulted in remissions of established colorectal cancers, whereas treatment with either therapy alone produced no remissions.[1] For the present, however, the possibility of synergism, and the associated reductions in dose that it allows, will be considered only for direct-acting compounds.

The Meaning of Synergism

Webster's defines synergism as the "interaction of discrete agencies or agents such that the total effect is greater than the sum of the individual effects." Although this concept is simple enough, measurement of synergism is complex, and researchers have yet to define a universally accepted formula for its determination. A number of formulas have been employed, but since each formula is somewhat different, the results depend on the particular formula used. Unless otherwise specified, we use the word *synergism* here in its general sense to refer to interactions that are either additive or synergistic.[c] One reason is that no universally accepted definition exists and a synergistic interaction to one researcher may be an additive one to another. Another reason is the awkwardness of repeating the phrase "additive or synergistic" throughout the text. There is some justification for using the term loosely, since either additive or synergistic interactions are sufficient to increase the potency of most natural compounds to the point their use becomes practical.

How Synergism Works

Synergism is still a rather mysterious process. Perhaps a dozen or more mechanisms come into play when two compounds interact synergistically, and one or several of these could be active in any given situation. Thus it is difficult to predict the exact mechanisms by which two compounds will interact, and even more difficult to predict those by which three or more compounds will interact. Nonetheless, synergistic interactions do occur between natural compounds, and it is likely the beneficial effects of combinations will be adequately demonstrated long before we understand completely how they occur. At this point, our knowledge of interactions is more theoretical than practical, and so we do not need to discuss potential interactions in detail. To show some

---

[a] *The reader is encouraged to regularly check the Oregon Medical Press web site at www.ompress.com for progress updates on antitumor and toxicity studies conducted by our group, which consists of Robert Newman, Ph.D., from M. D. Anderson Cancer Center, David Bailey, Ph.D., from Hauser Inc., and myself. All opinions, calculations, and conclusions presented in this book, however, are solely my own.*

[b] *The synergism produced in this study was apparently due to the following chain of events: The cytotoxic agent induced apoptosis, and the affected cells were ingested by macrophages. The macrophages then presented the cancer's antigens to T-lymphocytes, and in this way, the T cells became primed for attacking the cancer. The addition of an immune stimulant (IL-2) assisted the priming process. The overall effect then was one of increased immune response.*

---

[c] *Interactions between compounds can be inhibitive (where $1+1<2$), additive (where $1+1=2$), or supra-additive (where $1+1>2$).*

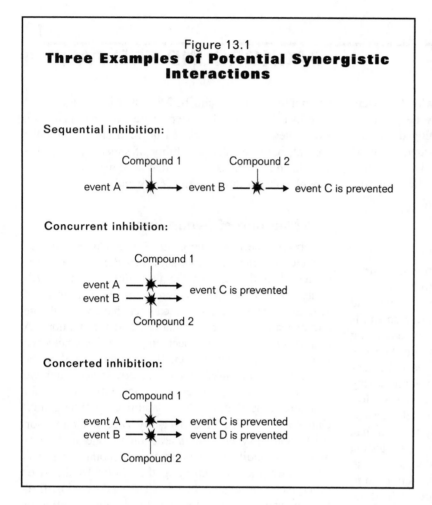

Figure 13.1

Three Examples of Potential Synergistic Interactions

Sequential inhibition:

Concurrent inhibition:

Concerted inhibition:

The concepts proposed here for using synergistic combinations are somewhat different from those historically used in cancer chemotherapy. For one thing, combinations discussed in this book have more targets, and thus their actions are broader in scope. As discussed in Chapter 1, the proposed strategy is to redundantly target all seven clusters of procancer events using combinations that include direct- and indirect-acting compounds and immune stimulants. In contrast, most combinations of chemotherapy drugs in current use focus primarily on one specific anticancer target: the disruption of DNA within cancer cells (see Chapter 2). Furthermore, the combinations proposed here are larger than those used with chemotherapy drugs. I suggest that optimal combinations might contain 15 to 18 natural compounds, whereas combinations of chemotherapy drugs tend to be smaller (usually 5 compounds or fewer). Lastly, my intention is for combinations to be used at doses that do not cause severe adverse effects. With chemotherapy, such effects are often accepted as part of the treatment.

possibilities, however, Figure 13.1 illustrates three common types (based on reference 2).

The first example shown is sequential inhibition. Here, two compounds inhibit a linear sequence of events, the result being the inhibition of a third event (event C) that is necessary for cancer cell proliferation. The second example is of concurrent inhibition; two compounds inhibit two parallel events, which inhibits a third event necessary for cancer cell proliferation. The third example is concerted inhibition, where two compounds inhibit two parallel events, resulting in inhibition of a third and fourth event, that are both necessary for cancer cell proliferation.

How Synergism Is Used

The concept of using combinations of drugs in cancer therapy is not new; chemotherapy regimes consisting of multiple drugs have been used since the 1960s. The idea of using combinations in cancer treatment was generated by the success of combination therapy with antibiotic drugs.[2]

Need for Synergism

According to the dose estimates made in Part III, about 65 percent of the direct-acting natural compounds will require synergism if they are to be effective against cancer. Their mild nature requires large doses relative to those of chemotherapy drugs. Although large doses of relatively nontoxic natural compounds would not seem to be a problem, in fact the required doses are so large in many cases that either they exceed doses likely to be safe or ones likely to be physically absorbed. Therefore, if these compounds are to demonstrate a high degree of safety, they must be used at lower doses. Synergistic combinations allow lower, safer doses to be utilized without sacrificing efficacy.

Safety of Synergistic Combinations

If synergistic combinations are potent in damaging cancer cells, it might seem they could also damage normal cells. The potential for such cannot be fully known until toxicity studies are done; however, there is reason to think that combinations like those proposed here would be safe. For one thing, a sizable percentage of the compounds discussed show some selectivity to cancer cells in vitro, harming cancer cells more than normal ones. One can reasonably suppose this same selectivity would occur using combinations.

There is also a precedent for safely using large combinations of natural compounds, including combinations that contain some of the compounds in this book. Both Chinese herbal medicine and Ayurvedic medicine, the ancient healing system of India, have been using large combinations of natural compounds for centuries, if not thousands of years. For example, in Chinese herbal medicine, single herbs are rarely prescribed, but combinations of 4 to 12 herbs are commonly employed. Considering that each herb may contain multiple active compounds, this is a large mix of compounds. The efficacy and safety of many of these formulas have been borne out by modern Chinese investigations.

There is one other precedent for the use of large combinations of natural compounds, and that is one set by cancer patients themselves. As mentioned in the preface, anywhere from 10 to 80 percent of cancer patients use some form of complementary medicine, and perhaps 40 to 60 percent of these use herbs, vitamins, antioxidants, or all three. It is probably safe to assume that a good number of these patients are ingesting large quantities of natural compounds in the mixtures they use. Moreover, patients with other diseases are probably doing the same. During the last decade, the sale of vitamins, herbs, and related food supplements in the United States has grown into a multimillion dollar business. Nevertheless, reports of adverse effects from combinations of supplements are rare.

Lastly, all the compounds I discuss have some history of use in herbal or other forms of medicine or in food. In some cases, they have been ingested in concentrated form, and in others as one among many components of a whole herb or food. For all compounds, their toxicity is negligible at commonly prescribed doses. Tentative dose recommendations for further research are made in Part III, and in all cases, the maximum recommended dose is at or below the maximum dose expected to be safe.

Of course, the above arguments do not prove the combinations discussed here are safe; nonetheless, they do support the likelihood that they are. This is not to say that mild adverse effects are unlikely. Gastrointestinal irritation or other forms of mild adverse effects can occur with any compound, especially in sensitive individuals, even at relatively low doses. It is also not possible to say that severe adverse effects cannot happen. Clearly, additional study on the toxicity of combinations of natural compounds is necessary.

Evidence for Synergism Against Cancer Cells

Research already provides evidence that synergistic interactions can occur within combinations of direct-acting natural compounds. Such interactions have been clearly documented by in-vitro studies. In addition, a small number of animal studies have also reported synergistic effects. For example, in three studies in mice, combinations of ATRA and 1,25-D_3 synergistically inhibited proliferation of transplanted human breast cancer cells or inhibited angiogenesis induced by cancer cells.[3, 4, 5] These three studies, in combination with many in-vitro and in-vivo studies showing synergistic interactions between groups of chemotherapy drugs, make the potential for inducing synergism seem high.

Evidence from Small Combinations

We first consider evidence from studies on small combinations in vitro; many such studies have been published, most of which used two or three compounds in combination. The studies presented here are not exhaustive but do provide a sampling of those available.

Combinations That Include Vitamin D_3 and/or ATRA

Numerous studies were conducted using 1,25-D_3 and/or ATRA in combination with other compounds. One study on 1,25-D_3 reported that when it was combined with curcumin, vitamin E, other antioxidants, or a variety of non-steroidal anti-inflammatory compounds, the differentiation of human leukemia cells was enhanced.[6] Another reported that curcumin (at 10 μM) enhanced the differentiation of human leukemia cells induced by 1,25-D_3 (at 5 nM).[7]

Curcumin has also been reported to act synergistically with ATRA. In one study, 10 nM of ATRA induced differentiation in only 10 percent of human leukemia cells, and 10 μM of curcumin induced differentiation in only 16 percent of cells, whereas a combination of the two induced differentiation in 65 percent of cells.[8] In this study, the effects on growth inhibition tended to be additive. Other investigators have reported similar results with these compounds.[9]

Other studies involving vitamin D_3 or ATRA or both are summarized below:

- 1,25-D_3 (at 24 nM) and ATRA (at 4 nM) markedly enhanced differentiation of human leukemia cells induced by genistein (at 19 μM).[10]

- Genistein (at 37 μM) enhanced differentiation of human leukemia cells induced by 1,25-D_3 (at 50

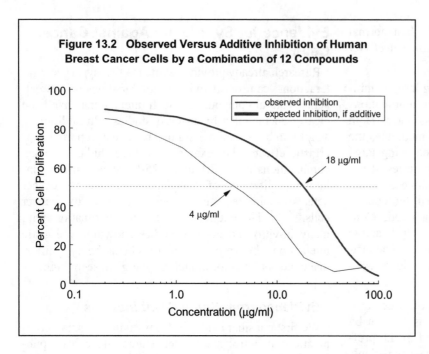

Figure 13.2   Observed Versus Additive Inhibition of Human Breast Cancer Cells by a Combination of 12 Compounds

nM).   Differentiation was increased threefold as compared to 1,25-D_3 alone.[11]

- Differentiation of human leukemia cells induced by both ATRA (at 0.1 μM) and 1,25-D_3 (150 nM) was enhanced by the addition of daidzein (40 μM).[12] Differentiation increased by about 55 percent when daidzein was added.

- The omega-3 fatty acid DHA (at 10 μM) markedly increased differentiation of human leukemic cells induced by ATRA (at 1 μM).[13]

Other Combinations

Additional studies tested compounds other than vitamin D_3 or ATRA, as summarized below:

- Curcumin and genistein synergistically inhibited proliferation of human breast cancer cells stimulated by estrogen and/or estrogenic pesticides. (Various pesticides, such as DDT and endosulfane, act as weak estrogens and stimulate proliferation of breast cancer cells in vitro.[14]) In these studies, combinations of genistein (at 25 μM) and curcumin (10 μM) almost completely inhibited the ability of these estrogenic compounds to stimulate proliferation.[15, 16, 17]

- Combinations of EGCG and curcumin were synergistic against human oral cancer cells. The combination allowed an eightfold reduction in EGCG concentration (from 18 to 2.1 μM) and a twofold reduction in curcumin concentration (from 5.2 to 2.1 μM), without loss of efficacy.[18]

- When used singularly, daidzein (at about 40 μM) and boswellic acid (about 11 μM) slightly induced dif-

ferentiation in human leukemia cells. When the two were used in combination, 80 percent of cells were induced to differentiate, and cell proliferation was markedly reduced.[19]

In summary, these studies provide good reason to be optimistic that additive or synergistic effects could occur between a variety of natural compounds.

Evidence from Large Combinations

The synergism studies mentioned above were conducted with no more than two or three natural compounds in combination. Our research group is attempting to demonstrate that synergism occurs in combinations containing many more compounds, and our preliminary data indicate that additive or synergistic effects do indeed occur in large combinations.[20]   Although much more work is needed to verify synergism both in vitro and in vivo, these data indicate it is possible to create highly effective combinations with a large number of compounds.

Briefly, we have tested 12 natural compounds, both individually and in a variety of combinations, for their ability to inhibit proliferation of human breast and prostate cancer cells in vitro. These compounds were CAPE, arctigenin, curcumin, apigenin, genistein, luteolin, EGCG, emodin, resveratrol, boswellic acid, parthenolide, and ATRA. Some of these were tested as pure substances and some as concentrated plant extracts. In all cases, the combinations were designed to have equal amounts of each compound in them; the concentration used for each was adjusted to take into account the compound's purity.

Our preliminary findings can be summarized in two graphs. The first, Figure 13.2, shows data for a combination containing all 12 compounds that was tested against human breast cancer cells. The thick line represents the mathematically expected inhibition of cell proliferation if all compounds interacted additively (the curve is based on their individual abilities to inhibit cell proliferation and their percentage in the combination). The thin line is the observed inhibition.

Simply put, the graph shows it would have taken 18 μg/ml of the combined compounds to inhibit cancer cell proliferation by 50 percent if they had interacted additively, but in fact the observed result was that it took only 4 µg/ml.[a] The remarkable 4.5-fold difference between the expected IC_{50} value based on additive interactions and the observed value suggests that supra-additive, or true synergistic effects were occurring.

The data in Figure 13.2 are for one combination tested against one cell line. Other combinations were also tested, and two cell lines were used (breast cancer and prostate cancer). Results from these tests also implied that supra-additive effects were occurring. Based on Figure 13.2, the ratio of the IC_{50} for the additive curve and the observed curve is 4.5. Similar ratios can be calculated for all the different combinations tested. Figure 13.3 shows a graph of such IC_{50} ratios (additive versus observed) plotted for different combinations for both cell lines. As can be seen, in all cases there was evidence of supra-additive effects. If purely additive effects had occurred, the curves for both cell lines would be horizontal lines at an IC_{50} ratio of 1.0. This is not the case, and in the breast cancer cell line, the greater the number of compounds used in the combination, the greater the supra-additive effect.

One other combination of natural compounds deserves mention here. PC-SPES, a mixture of extracts from eight herbs, has been tested in several animal and human trials. It was designed to treat prostate cancer and appears to act partly through an estrogenic action. Results suggest that it reduces plasma concentrations of PSA (prostate specific antigen), a tumor marker for prostate cancer, and in some cases reduces tumor burden.[21–24] Side effects are minimal, other than estrogenic reactions, which can be significant. Although promising, PC-SPES is not discussed in detail because its specific makeup is a trade secret and thus it does not meet the criteria for inclusion in this book (see Chapter 1). Note, however, that a recent paper explained that the effectiveness of PC SPES is due to its "complex composition which may target many signal transduction and metabolic pathways simultaneously, thereby eliminating the back-up or redundant mechanisms that otherwise promote cell survival when single-target agents are used."[21]

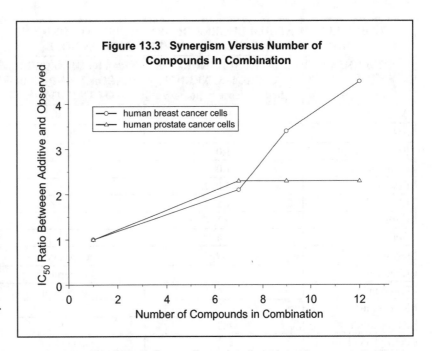

Figure 13.3 Synergism Versus Number of Compounds In Combination

This explanation supports the hypotheses proposed in this book.

Estimating Allowable Dose Reductions Due to Synergism

A primary reason we are so interested in synergistic interactions is that they will allow lower doses of each compound to be used. As stated, the calculations in Part III suggest that dose reductions due to synergistic interactions are required for most direct-acting compounds, if they are to be useful. A method for estimating allowable dose reductions follows; but keep in mind that it is based on results from our research, which was conducted in vitro. Translation of in-vitro data to in-vivo conditions is always full of uncertainties. Nonetheless, the method provides some logical basis for making an initial estimate of allowable dose reductions.

In spite of the promising preliminary results presented in Figure 13.3, our group still cannot statistically show that supra-additive effects were occurring. The data were obtained from three replicate samples for each individual test. Because of variations in the replicate samples, additional replicates are still needed to provide solid support for supra-additive effects. Although true synergism appears to be occurring, at this point it is safe to assume that, at the very least, additive effects were produced. Still, even additive effects are noteworthy and are sufficient to make the use of natural compounds seem practical.

Assuming additive interactions, allowable dose reductions can now be estimated. The estimating process is straightforward. For example, if 10 compounds were

---

[a] *Concentrations are reported in units of µg/ml, since many of the tested compounds were not pure compounds but concentrated extracts. Purities ranged from 22 to 100 percent. These IC_{50} values are higher than would be expected with pure compounds. Since the average molecular weight of these compounds is about 310 grams/mole, 1 µg/ml is roughly equal to 3.2 µM.*

TABLE 13.1 MINIMUM DEGREE OF SYNERGISM NEEDED AND MAXIMUM DOSE INCREASE OVER COMMON DOSE		
COMPOUND	MINIMUM DEGREE OF SYNERGISM NEEDED (fold increase in potency)	RATIO OF MAXIMUM RECOMMENDED DOSE TO COMMON DOSE
Apigenin	1.0[*]	180
Arctigenin	2.3	1.0[*]
Boswellic acid	1.0	2.8
Centella	1.0	19
Emodin	3.0	41
EPA/DHA	1.1	1.1
Garlic	6.1	1.0
Genistein	1.4	22
Geraniol	1.0	uncertain[†]
Limonene	7.9	uncertain
Luteolin	1.4	uncertain
Melatonin	1.0	6.7
Parthenolide	4.3	2.9
Perillyl alcohol	2.1	uncertain
Quercetin	2.1	1.8
Selenium	3.4	5.5
Vitamin E	1.0	1.0
Average	**2.5 (all values)** **3.0 (values greater than 1)**	**5.2[‡]**

[*] *A value of 1.0 means no increase or decrease is required.*

[†] *Uncertain means that no common dose is available.*

[‡] *Geometric average.*

used in combination at equal concentrations, then due to additive effects, the concentration of each compound within the combination could be reduced by a factor of 10. If 15 compounds were used, the concentration of each could be reduced by a factor of 15, and so on. To translate this to in-vivo conditions, we will simply assume that dose reductions will parallel the reductions in concentration seen in-vitro. Thus, if 15 compounds are used, the dose of each can be reduced by a factor of 15. As an example, suppose that to produce an anticancer effect, the target dose for a compound is 5 grams per day. If we use 10 compounds in combination, the target dose could theoretically be reduced 10-fold, and a 0.5-gram dose would be effective.

This does not necessarily mean, however, that a 0.5-gram dose should be used; the highest safe dose would generally be most appropriate because it would minimize the need for synergism and maximize the effect. Let's say that adverse reactions for this compound begin to appear at a dose of 1 gram per day. Then a 1-gram, rather than 0.5-gram, dose could be taken. Although synergism would still be needed, less would be needed than with a 0.5-gram dose. Because the 1-gram dose is

5-fold lower than the target dose of 5 grams (the target when the compound is used alone), synergistic interactions generated from using the compound in combination would need to compensate for the 5-fold dose reduction to maintain the same effectiveness. This should be possible, since according to our estimates, the use of 10 compounds in combination would allow a 10-fold maximum reduction.

This method assumes each compound appears in the plasma at an equal concentration. Although this is not exactly the case based on the dose estimates contained in Part III, it is often not far off. Similar plasma concentrations should be produced for most direct-acting compounds, since the dose estimates for most compounds used the same target plasma concentration (15 µM, as discussed later). For many direct-acting compounds, the calculated target dose is too high to be taken and the 15-µM plasma concentration will not be achieved, but plasma concentrations for most compounds still should not be much below 15 µM. (As we see below, the average dose reduction needed is about 3-fold; therefore, most compounds should occur in the plasma at concentrations between about 5 and 15 µM.)

For simplicity in analyzing dose requirements, we will assume that a maximum of 15 direct-acting compounds will be used in combination. Therefore, the maximum allowable dose reduction for each is 15-fold. As indicated in Table 13.1, a 15-fold dose reduction is more than enough to make essentially all direct-acting compounds seem practical. The first column of numbers in the table indicates how much the target dose would need to be reduced to make each direct-acting compound safe and practical (values taken from discussions in Part III). As shown at the bottom of the column, only a 2.5- to 3-fold dose reduction is required on the average. Some direct-acting compounds are not listed in the table because the target dose for these compounds was too uncertain to use as a base for calculations. Also, melatonin is listed, even though it is not categorized as a direct-acting compound, because it can still produce direct effects.

The 2.5- to 3-fold reduction in dose required by most compounds is well below the allowable 15-fold dose reduction estimated above, making it possible that all these compounds could be effective at safe and practical doses when used in combinations. The two compounds with the highest dose reduction requirements, garlic and limonene, are not as likely to be included in combinations, since other compounds may be more potent.[a] Removing these two compounds would lower the average required dose reduction even further (to 1.8).

Because the average required dose reduction due to synergism is 3-fold or lower does not mean that only three compounds should be used in combination. The values discussed here are only rough approximations that represent the minimum degree of synergism required, which means that for some compounds, a greater degree of synergism may be needed. This can be produced by using a larger number of compounds in combination. Equally important, larger combinations are necessary to target all seven primary clusters of procancer events (see Chapter 1).

The second column of numbers in Table 13.1 lists ratios of the maximum recommended dose and the commonly prescribed dose for noncancerous conditions; as shown, the maximum recommended doses are generally well above those normally prescribed. The average ratio is 5.2 (geometric average), but the range is rather large. (The high dose requirements are one reason concentrated extracts will be required for most compounds.) This average ratio would be a bit lower if we included indirect-acting and immune stimulant compounds in the calculation, since these compounds are used near their commonly prescribed dose. Although the tentative recommended doses are relatively large, in all cases they are at or below the dose estimated to be safe when used as single compounds.

ESTIMATING EFFECTIVE AND SAFE DOSES

Before a compound can be clinically used in cancer treatment, two crucial doses must be known: the effective dose and the safe dose. Unfortunately, for many of the natural compounds discussed, these values are still uncertain. Although some human data are available, very few of these compounds have been thoroughly

studied in humans; in-vitro and animal data are more prevalent. The best we can do at this point is to gather available data and make reasonable estimates. This effort is no small task, which may be why this book is among the first to attempt it for a broad range of compounds. Some readers will want a complete explanation of how doses were estimated, and Appendices B, I, and J provide this information. They discuss the general approach and models used and explain how specific estimates for each compound were reached. The discussions of each compound in Part III end with a summary of the results of these calculations. To clarify the dose summaries for each compound, as well as the tentative nature of the dose recommendations, an overview of the methods used is given below.

Estimating Effective Doses

There are three available data types on which to base estimates for an effective dose: human anticancer data; animal antitumor data; and a combination of pharmacokinetic and in-vitro data. Each type has advantages and disadvantages, but all can provide helpful information. In Part III, we estimate a target dose by using as many of these types as available data allow, then we compare the doses estimated with each to corroborate their values. For most compounds, human data are not available and doses can be estimated using only the last two data types.

If the dose estimate made from each available data type is in general agreement with the others (considered here as within a factor of two), we assume the target dose is relatively well known. In these cases, our target dose is generally chosen as an average of the available estimates. In actuality, a range of target doses may be more fitting, but for simplicity of calculations, we generally choose only one value. Note that the dose estimates we make are for the most part crude approximations based on numerous assumptions. They are useful as a starting point to conceptualize target doses but are still only an initial attempt based on limited data. They provide only ballpark approximations, and much more study is needed.

Use of the third data type, a combination of pharmacokinetic and in-vitro data, requires additional explanation. Briefly, we assume that a concentration effective in vitro will also be effective when produced in the plasma in vivo. This is not necessarily the case, as is discussed in Appendix B, but this assumption will work for our approximations. After identifying the effective plasma concentration from in-vitro data, we use pharmacokinetic data to determine how large a dose is needed to produce that concentration. (Pharmacokinetic data tell us how a given dose affects the plasma

---

[a] *Although limonene and garlic are listed as the weakest direct-acting compounds, vitamins A and D₃ are potentially weaker than both, based on worst-case scenarios. The strength of these vitamins is difficult to assess, however, since their target doses and/or safe doses are uncertain or variable and can be estimated only within a range of values.*

concentration.) The crucial pharmacokinetic parameter in these calculations is called the oral clearance. Simply put, the oral clearance value represents the amount of drug removed from the body per unit of time after oral administration.

Details of the method used to estimate a required dose based on pharmacokinetic and in-vitro data are provided in Appendix J, but a few points are highlighted here. First, oral clearance values can come from three sources: human studies, animal studies, and mathematical models. Values obtained from human studies are the most accurate, but again, few human studies are available. Values from animal data are next in accuracy and to be useful must be scaled to their human equivalent (see Appendix B). For some compounds, even animal values are unavailable. For this reason and as a way to corroborate animal and human values where they exist, the oral clearance can be predicted based on the chemical structure of the compound. I have developed a model to make these predictions; its details and limitations are presented in Appendix I.

The second point about this method is that the effective in-vitro concentration must be known. Although in-vitro data are available for most compounds, the effective concentrations generally vary over a wide range in different studies. Thus it is difficult to choose the most appropriate target concentration. Most of the compounds discussed in this book are effective within the same general range (1 to 50 µM, commonly 5 to 30 µM). To simplify the task of estimating doses, I chose a target concentration of 15 µM for most compounds, a value roughly the average for all the in-vitro studies.

For the phenolic compounds discussed in Chapters 19 and 20, the 15-µM target concentration is modified because these compounds tend to occur in the plasma in the form of conjugates, which are generally less potent than the free, unchanged compound. Conjugates are produced during phase II metabolism (a form of detoxification). Conjugation takes place in the liver as well as in other tissues like the intestinal lining. It is the body's attempt to make a foreign compound more water-soluble and thus more easily excreted in the urine. The conjugates produced during detoxification are comprised of the parent molecule or its metabolites linked to a second, more water-soluble molecule. This second molecule is either glucuronic acid (which is related to glucose), glutathione, or sulfate. For the phenolic compounds discussed, glucuronide conjugates predominate in the plasma. We assume here that these conjugates are essentially half as potent as the free parent compound (see Appendix J). Since most phenolic compounds appear in the plasma primarily in their conjugate form, we assume the target concentration of most phenolic compounds is

30 µM, or twice as high as the target of 15 µM used for most other compounds.

A final point is that the magnitude of the dose can affect both the absorption (since absorption is apt to be limited at high doses) and the type and concentration of active metabolites. Thus in addition to limits from safety issues, a human dose can also be limited by its ability to be absorbed or beneficially metabolized. Dose-dependent issues are likely to occur mostly for the phenolic compounds, which generally require the largest doses. In this book we conservatively assume that doses in excess of 1.8 grams per day (600 milligrams three times per day) of any single compound will produce limited gains in plasma concentration and/or will produce a different and less effective mix of metabolites in the plasma. We refer to this 1.8-gram limit as the general linear bioavailability limit (the reasoning behind this is presented in Appendix J). Some exceptions are noted in the text. To illustrate how this limit is used, imagine that the target dose of a compound is 18 grams and the safe dose is 20 grams. For this compound, the maximum recommended dose would be 1.8 grams; it would then need a 10-fold increase in potency due to synergism to make it as effective as an 18-gram dose.

Estimating Safe Doses

The best results will likely be obtained when the largest safe dose of each compound is used, as long as it is not above the 1.8-gram linear bioavailability limit. We view the largest safe dose as the one at which adverse effects just begin to be produced. This is referred to as the lowest-observable-adverse-effects level (LOAEL) dose and is generally determined from short-term toxicity studies. In these studies, animals are given a compound daily for several weeks (as opposed to a single administration given in acute toxicity studies).

The actual value of the human oral LOAEL dose is unknown for the majority of natural compounds, let alone for combinations of compounds, and must be estimated. LOAEL doses determined from animal studies are available for many compounds, and such doses can be scaled to their human equivalents. For some compounds, only lethal dose (LD_{50}) data are available. (The LD_{50} is the dose causing death in 50 percent of the test animals after a single administration.) As discussed in Appendix I, an approximate LOAEL dose can be estimated from the LD_{50}. For still other compounds, neither LOAEL dose nor LD_{50} animal data are available. Fortunately, LOAEL doses for almost all compounds can be estimated from the chemical structure, much as oral clearance values can be. These estimates, made by the TOPKAT model, along with data from animal and human studies, are used in Part III to estimate the human

TABLE 13.2 CATEGORIES OF DIRECT-ACTING NATURAL COMPOUNDS BASED ON A COMPARISON OF THE TARGET DOSE AND MAXIMUM RECOMMENDED DOSE (MRD)	
CATEGORY	**COMPOUNDS**
The target dose is relatively certain (a single target dose is used), and it is within 15-fold of the MRD. Synergism should allow the MRD to be effective	apigenin, arctigenin, boswellic acid, *Centella,* emodin, garlic, genistein, geraniol, EPA/DHA, limonene, luteolin, melatonin, parthenolide, perillyl alcohol, quercetin, selenium, vitamin E
The target dose is relatively uncertain (a range of target doses is used), and the maximum target dose is within 15-fold of the MRD. Synergism should allow the MRD to be effective.	CAPE (propolis), curcumin, ginseng, resveratrol, vitamin A, vitamin D_3
The target dose is relatively uncertain (a range of target doses is used), and the maximum target dose is not within 15-fold of the MRD. Synergism may be insufficient to allow the MRD to be effective. These compounds require more study than others before their potential for clinical use can be assessed.	EGCG, flaxseed, hypericin

LOAEL dose.[a] Of course, the human data are the most accurate; animal studies and TOPKAT predictions provide only rough estimates.

For some compounds, the maximum tolerated dose (MTD), rather than the LOAEL dose, is available; the MTD is generally larger than the LOAEL dose and is likely to cause at least mild adverse effects. Such a dose may need to be lowered slightly for clinical use.

Integrating Dose Estimates and Dose Limits

From the above, we have the necessary information—target doses, LOAEL doses, and the 1.8-gram bioavailability limit—to estimate maximum recommended doses for further research. (Minimum recommended doses are based on a slightly different set of values.) With these three values and the 15-fold dose reduction allowable through synergism, we can evaluate, at least in theory, whether the natural compounds discussed will be potent enough to produce an anticancer effect.

Target doses are estimated based on human and animal studies and a combination of pharmacokinetic and in-vitro data. If values from these studies agree with one another, the target dose is a single (average) value. If they do not agree, the target dose is more uncertain and a range of values is used. If the target dose is below both the 1.8-gram linear bioavailability limit and the LOAEL dose, we will set the maximum recommended dose (MRD) equal to the (maximum) target dose. If the target dose is higher than the 1.8-gram and LOAEL doses, we will set the maximum recommended dose

equal to the 1.8-gram limit or the LOAEL dose, whichever is lower.

In comparing the target dose to the MRD, we can group direct-acting natural compounds into the three categories listed in Table 13.2. Although not categorized here as direct-acting compounds, ginseng and melatonin are included in the table because they can have a direct inhibitory effect on cancer cells.

In the first category, the dose estimates agree, a single (average) target dose is used, and the difference between the target and MRD is less than 15-fold. For these compounds, synergism, if it is needed, should allow each to be effective at the MRD. Most of the direct-acting compounds fall into this category.

In the second category, the dose estimates do not agree, and a range of target doses is used. Even looking at a worst-case scenario, the difference between the maximum target dose and the MRD is still less than 15-fold. Again for these compounds, synergism, if needed, should allow each to be effective at the MRD. Although their target doses are somewhat uncertain and can be estimated only within a range, these compounds should still be useful.

In the third category, the dose estimates do not agree, and again a range of target doses is used. Looking at a worst-case scenario, the difference between the maximum target dose and the maximum recommended dose is greater than 15-fold. Synergism may not be sufficient to allow these compounds to be effective at the maximum recommended dose. Although all natural compounds require additional study, compounds in this last category require more study than others. Still, the three compounds in this category are discussed in Part III. Each provides an example of why a compound requires much additional study, and other reasons for their inclusion are provided in later chapters.

---

[a] *Oxford Molecular Group, creator of the TOPKAT toxicity assessment software program, which uses this method, has contributed estimates for rat oral LOAEL dose and LD$_{50}$ for many of the compounds discussed in this book. Information on the TOPKAT model and a listing of its predictions are presented in Appendix I.*

AVAILABLE FORMULATIONS

Natural compounds can be obtained in a variety of formulations, and for cancer treatment, some may be more preferable. Formulations include:

- *Decoctions.* Decoctions are teas made by boiling botanicals for an extended period in water, usually an hour or two. These are normally unavailable commercially and are made at home; they are commonly prescribed in Chinese herbal medicine. Infusions are similar to decoctions, but the botanicals are steeped in hot water or boiled for only a short time.

- *Powdered botanicals.* Powdered botanicals are available commercially in pill or capsule form. They are made from ground whole botanicals.

- *Extracts.* Extracts come in many forms. Solid extracts are made by extracting a botanical with a solvent (commonly water and/or alcohol), then removing the solvent under reduced pressure. Fluid extracts are prepared by soaking whole botanicals or highly concentrated solid extracts in a solvent (usually a water-alcohol mixture). Another type of extract, a tincture, is similar to a fluid extract only more dilute.

The strengths of these formulations vary. Powdered botanicals contain herbs in their natural dried state, and no attempt is made to concentrate the plant's active compounds. Decoctions are extractions representing about 1 part botanical to 30 parts water, depending on the amount of water used in the cooking process; their relative weakness is compensated for by the large doses given (about one to two cups per day). The strength of a fluid extracts is 1 part botanical in 1 part solvent, and that of a tincture is generally 1 part botanical in 4 to 10 parts solvent.

The strength of some solid and liquid extracts is expressed in terms of a known concentration of active ingredients. These are referred to as standardized extracts. For example, some *Eleutherococcus* pills on the market are standardized to contain 0.8 percent eleutheroside E and B, which are thought to be its primary active saponins. Another example is a standardized curcumin product that contains 97 percent curcumin.

As mentioned previously, relatively high doses of most compounds may be required to produce an anticancer effect. For this reason, concentrated extracts will usually be required to provide an adequate dose of active compound in a reasonable volume and at a reasonable cost. Since it is highly desirable to know exactly how much of a given active ingredient is being ingested, the preferred formulation in most cases is a standardized concentrated extract. Standardized extracts are becoming increasingly popular, and many of the natural compounds we discuss are now or soon will be available in this form.

Formulations other than concentrated extracts can be useful in limited circumstances. In the case of polysaccharide-rich herbs like *Astragalus*, decoctions are practical. Polysaccharides are easily extracted in hot water, and they occur at relatively high concentrations in the crude plant material. The same may be true of lignans, such as arctigenin. In contrast to concentrated extracts and decoctions, powdered whole botanicals and tinctures will likely play a lessor role in cancer treatment, due to their relatively low strength. One exception may be ginseng root, which has a relatively high concentration of active ingredients; it is sweet and can be sucked on in its whole form like candy.

In general, I subscribe to the theory that the best extracts for treating disease are those concentrated no more than necessary. Although there are exceptions, for cancer treatment this often means extracts containing at least 20 to 50 percent of the active compound. This approach is, of course, in opposition to the prevailing medical view that only pure substances should be investigated and developed into drugs. Although the benefits of using minimally concentrated extracts rather than pure compounds remain to be proven in cancer treatment, the philosophy is compelling. Minimally concentrated extracts provide the patient with a host of other compounds that could increase the effectiveness of treatment. For example, crude green tea extract contains not only the active compound EGCG but also other catechins that may be active. These catechins add to the inhibitory effect of EGCG against cancer cells in vitro (see Chapter 19). A similar argument could be made for crude propolis extract, which contains other active caffeic acid derivatives besides CAPE, the propolis compound we focus on.

Note that for a given herb, extracts made by different manufacturers might contain differing ratios and amounts of active ingredients, and thus their medicinal potency might vary. For example, one *Boswellia* extract could be weaker than another or even produce a slightly different effect. Therefore, we must use caution in generalizing results from studies on any particular extract. Nonetheless, this book tends to generalize, when such generalizations are likely to be reasonable; this tendency is in the spirit of making rough, not refined, dose estimates.

Let us briefly digress to talk about formulations used in animal studies. Animals may be given whole dried herb material, crude extracts of dried herbs, or more concentrated extracts. Unfortunately, some animal studies do not report the dose in terms of whole plant material equivalents. For example, a study may state that a crude extract of *Astragalus* was given at 300 mg/kg. This information is of limited value because we do not know how concentrated the extract was. This frustrating oversight is common, and I strongly encourage researchers to report dose information thoroughly. We can salvage some data by using common yield values. Although yields can vary depending on the plant, crude extracts generally yield about 30 percent of material, weight for weight.[25, 26] For example, if a study reported that a rat received an oral dose of 300 mg/kg of crude *Astragalus* root extract per day, we can assume that at a 30 percent yield this is roughly equivalent to about 1,000 mg/kg of whole root per day. Similar calculations were required in a few instances in Part III, mostly for polysaccharides.

COMBINATION DESIGN

As discussed in Chapter 1, the most practical method of designing combinations may be through a process of elimination. To do this, we can use the following five constraints, already listed there:

- Using a large number of compounds to assure redundancy, facilitate synergism, and target all seven clusters of procancer events. An ideal number of compounds might be 15 to 18, which means only about half the compounds we discuss in the book would be used.

- Choosing compounds so that all three categories of compounds (direct acting, indirect acting, and immune stimulants) are represented. Since each compound tends to inhibit multiple procancer events, by using a large combination and compounds from all three categories, it is likely that all seven clusters of procancer events will be inhibited.

- To assure diversity, if a pair or group of compounds appear to act very similarly, using only one of the pair or a few of the group.

- Eliminating compounds that are not practical for whatever reason. For example, some compounds discussed may not be commercially available at present.

- Eliminating compounds that do not appear to have strong anticancer effects relative to the other natural

TABLE 13.3 PRELIMINARY ARRANGEMENT FOR DESIGNING COMBINATIONS	
NUMBER TO CHOOSE	**COMPOUNDS**
Direct-Acting Compounds	
2 of 4	apigenin, luteolin, genistein, and quercetin
1	arctigenin
1 of 2	boswellic acid and *Centella*
1	CAPE
1	curcumin
1	emodin
1	EPA/DHA
0 or 1	garlic*
1 of 3	limonene,* perillyl alcohol, and geraniol
1	parthenolide
1	resveratrol
1	selenium
1	vitamin A
1	vitamin D$_3$
1 of 2	vitamin E* and vitamin E succinate
subtotal = 15 or 16	
Indirect-Acting Compounds	
1 of 2	anthocyanidins and proanthocyanidins
1 of 2	butcher's broom and horse chestnut
0 or 1	vitamin C*
subtotal = 2 or 3	
Immune Stimulants	
1	*Astragalus*
1	bromelain or polyenzyme mixture
1 of 2	*Eleutherococcus* and ginseng
1 of 3	*Ganoderma*, PSP/PSK, shiitake
1	melatonin
0 or 1	glutamine*
subtotal = 5 or 6	
Compounds for Which the Required Dose is Relatively Uncertain†	
0	EGCG, flaxseed, hypericin
Total: 22 to 25	

* *Compounds that may not produce as strong effects as others or may best be used in specific circumstances. For example, the best use of glutamine may be to help prevent gastrointestinal injury during chemotherapy.*
† *Obtained from the third category of Table 13.2.*

compounds. These include compounds in the third category of Table 13.2 and possibly those (limonene and garlic) in Table 13.1 that seem to have the highest need for synergism. It could also include antioxidant vitamins like vitamins C and E, which would not be expected to produce a strong effect.

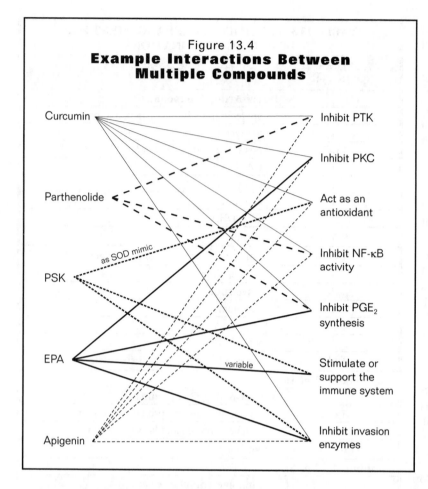

Figure 13.4
Example Interactions Between Multiple Compounds

only as affecting signal transduction. The terms used in the second column of Table 13.4 are similar to those used in Part III in tables that summarize the potential anticancer actions of each compound.

From Table 13.3, we have a general idea of how to create a combination. Although the process of elimination is relatively simple, refining the combination to optimize beneficial effects and meet the specific needs of a patient is more difficult. To spur the research needed to determine exactly which natural compounds would be most effective for a given patient and at what schedule and dose, I offer these preliminary suggestions:

Base choices on the characteristics of the cancer. To some degree, compounds can be chosen based on their appropriateness to the cancer's characteristics. Two examples follow:

- Brain cancer cells tend to have abnormally high levels of PKC, and focusing on PKC inhibition may be useful in their treatment. In comparison to healthy brain cells, PKC activity in cancer cells is at least one if not three orders of magnitude higher.[27] Furthermore, the level of PKC activity in brain cancer cells correlates with their proliferation rate, and PKC inhibitors can reduce proliferation rates up to 90 percent in vitro. PKC inhibitors also reduce the invasion of brain cancer cells in vitro.[28]

- Many oncogenes are overexpressed in breast cancer, including *H-ras, c-myc, erb13,* and *HER-2/neu.* Compounds that specifically inhibit expression or activity of these oncogenes could be useful. For example, emodin appears to be particularly effective against breast cancer cells that overexpress the *HER-2/neu* gene. *HER-2/neu* can also be overexpressed in other types of human cancers, including ovarian, lung, stomach, and oral cancers.[29]

Base choices on the results of appropriate assays. An individual patient's need for some compounds and response to treatment could be determined by appropriate assays. For example, assays are available to determine tissue levels of selenium and EPA. As another example, assays that measure capillary resistance could be useful to determine if compounds like proanthocyanidins are having their intended effect on vascular permeability.

Although this scheme is only one possible way to conceptualize the design process, it appears to be a useful one. To see how it works, the choices for compounds are laid out in Table 13.3.

As indicated in the table, a total of 22 to 25 compounds could be chosen. Some of these, however, are not yet on the market, may not be available in a standardized form, or for some other practical or personal reason may not be suitable. Excluding some then, the final total would likely be about 15 to 18 compounds. A combination this size seems reasonable based on the discussions in this book; it would contain enough compounds acting by enough means so that all seven clusters of procancer events would be targeted, each through diverse mechanisms. As an example, Figure 13.4 illustrates the procancer events that could be jointly affected with a group of only five compounds.

The generic actions of natural compounds and their effects on the seven clusters of procancer events are listed in Table 13.4. Note that some actions could affect more than one cluster of events. For example, antioxidants could affect almost every cluster of events but are listed only as affecting genetic instability. Likewise, PTK inhibitors could affect almost every cluster, but are listed

Similarly, assays that measure immune function could be useful in determining whether immune stimulants are needed or whether they are working. Lastly, new assays are becoming available to measure intermediate aspects of tumor progression, and these may be useful in guiding treatment. Under investigation are assays for measuring bFGF, VEGF, and other growth factors, as well as hyaluronidase, soluble CD44, adhesion molecules, motility factors, and immune-response-related molecules. Assays are also being developed for tumor-associated proteases and tumor vascularization. Established assays are already available for prostate-specific antigen (PSA) and other diagnostic markers that may have some use in guiding treatment. Currently though, the clinical relevance of the assays mentioned is still a matter of debate. As their clinical relevance becomes better defined, these assays could play an important role in determining which compounds may be needed and how they are working.

TABLE 13.4 ACTIONS THAT INHIBIT THE SEVEN CLUSTERS OF PROCANCER EVENTS	
CLUSTERS OF PROCANCER EVENTS	**INHIBITED BY NATURAL COMPOUNDS THAT:**
1. Reduce genetic instability	• Act as an antioxidant. • Assist in glutathione synthesis.
2. Inhibit abnormal transcription factor activity	• Inhibit NF-κB and/or AP-1 activity. • Support the function of p53 protein.
3. Inhibit abnormal signal transduction	• Inhibit PTK or PKC activity. • Normalize TGF-beta signaling. • Inhibit isoprene synthesis or otherwise inhibit the ras cascade
4. Encourage normal cell-to-cell communication	• Normalize CAM activity. • Improve gap junction communication.
5. Inhibit abnormal angiogenesis	• Degrade fibrin. • Normalize vascular permeability. • Inhibit the abnormal production or activity of bFGF, eicosanoids, histamine, TNF, VEGF, lactic acid, or insulin.
6. Inhibit invasion and metastasis	• Inhibit the abnormal production or activity of invasion enzymes. • Inhibit GAG synthesis. • Inhibit cell migration. • Inhibit platelet aggregation.
7. Increase or support the immune response	• Stimulate IL-2 production or otherwise stimulate, support, or regulate the immune system. • Inhibit the abnormal production or activity of eicosanoids, normalize TGF-beta signaling, or otherwise inhibit tumor-induced immunosuppression.

Focus on the most applicable procancer events. Not all procancer events discussed are active in all cancers, and compounds can be designed to focus on those events most applicable to a given situation. For example, brain cancers rarely metastasize, so an emphasis on antimetastatic compounds for these cancers is likely to be inappropriate. As another example, immune stimulants might play a larger role in treating immunogenic cancers like melanoma than they would in less immunogenic cancers. (Immunogenic cancers are those that are most able to evoke an immune reaction.)

Use rest periods. A resting period is advocated in many forms of therapy because it gives the body time to normalize its functions. For example, some immune stimulants may be more effective when administration includes a resting period. As discussed in Chapter 18 (for bromelain), 15 days of treatment followed by a 5-day rest period may be appropriate for some compounds.

Administer compounds at the most appropriate time of the day. A number of animal and human studies have demonstrated that side effects of chemotherapy or immunotherapy can be reduced and their efficacy increased by administration at the most appropriate times of the day.[30–33] These findings are related to the fact that many bodily functions follow a 24-hour cycle. For example, hormonal production and the absorption, transport, metabolism, and elimination of drugs follow 24-hour (chronobiologic) rhythms in animals and humans. Even in-vitro cell cultures show some 24-hour rhythms. These rhythms can likely be used to increase the efficacy and safety of natural compounds. For example, the effects of some herbal immunostimulants and melatonin may be optimized by administration at the appropriate time of day. Studies have indicated immunostimulants are best given in the morning and melatonin in the evening (see Chapters 12 and 22).

CONCLUSION

The information contained in this chapter is intended to place the discussions in remaining chapters in context and to illustrate how and why individual compounds should be used in combination. This chapter provides several reasons why synergism is both possible and essential and explains why only additive interactions and not true synergistic ones are likely needed to make direct-acting compounds effective at safe doses. The required additive interactions should be easily achieved in large combinations, opening the door to the potential use of combinations in cancer treatment.

REFERENCES

[1] Henry F, Bretaudeau L, Barbieux I, et al. Induction of antigen presentation by macrophages after phagocytosis of tumour apoptotic cells. Res Immunol 1998 Sep–Oct; 149(7–8):673–9.

[2] Mihich E, Grindey GB. Multiple basis of combination chemotherapy. Cancer 1977; 40:534–543.

[3] Koshizuka K, Kubota T, Said J, et al. Combination therapy of a vitamin D3 analog and all-*trans* retinoic acid: Effect on human breast cancer in nude mice. Anticancer Res 1999 Jan–Feb; 19(1A):519–24.

[4] Majewski S, Marczak M, Szmurlo A, et al. Retinoids, interferon alpha, 1,25-dihydroxyvitamin D3 and their combination inhibit angiogenesis induced by non-HPV-harboring tumor cell lines. RAR alpha mediates the antiangiogenic effect of retinoids. Cancer Lett 1995 Feb 10; 89(1):117–24.

[5] Majewski S, Skopinska M, Marczak M, et al. Vitamin D3 is a potent inhibitor of tumor cell-induced angiogenesis. J Investig Dermatol Symp Proc 1996; 1(1):97–101.

[6] Sokoloski JA, Sartorelli AC. Induction of the differentiation of HL-60 promyelocytic leukemia cells by nonsteroidal anti-inflammatory agents in combination with low levels of vitamin D3. Leuk Res 1998 Feb; 22(2):153–161.

[7] Sokoloski JA, Shyam K, Sartorelli AC. Induction of the differentiation of HL-60 promyelocytic leukemia cells by curcumin in combination with low levels of vitamin D3. Oncol Res 1997; 9(1):31–9.

[8] Liu Y, Chang RL, Cui XX, et al. Synergistic effects of curcumin on all-*trans* retinoic acid- and 1α,25-dihydroxyvitamin D3-induced differentiation in human promyelocytic leukemia HL-60 cells. Oncology Research 1997; 9:19–29.

[9] Conney AH, Lou YR, Xie JG, et al. Some perspectives on dietary inhibition of carcinogenesis: Studies with curcumin and tea. Proc Soc Exp Biol Med 1997 Nov; 216(2):234–45.

[10] Makishima M, Honma Y, Hozumi M, et al. Effects of inhibitors of protein tyrosine kinase activity and/or phosphatidylinositol turnover on differentiation of some leukemia myelomonocytic leukemia cells. Leukemia Res 1991; 15(8):701–708.

[11] Katagiri K, Katagiri T, Kajiyama K, et al. Modulation of monocytic differentiation of HL-60 cells by inhibitors of protein tyrosine kinases. Cell Immunol 1992 Apr; 140(2):282–94.

[12] Jing Y, Nakaya K, Han R. Differentiation of promyeloctic leukemia cells HL-60 induced by daidzen in vitro and in vivo. Anticancer Res 1993; 13(4):1049–54.

[13] Burns CP, Petersen ES, North JA, et al. Effect of docosahexaenoic acid on rate of differentiation of HL-60 human leukemia. Cancer Res 1989 Jun 15; 49(12):3252–8.

[14] Klotz DM, Beckman BS, Hill SM, et al. Identification of environmental chemicals with estrogenic activity using a combination of in vitro assays. Environ Health Perspect 1996 Oct; 104(10):1084–9.

[15] Verma SP, Salamone E, Goldin B. Curcumin and genistein, plant natural products, show synergistic inhibitory effects on the growth of human breast cancer MCF-7 cells induced by estrogenic pesticides. Biochem Biophys Res Commun 1997; 233:692–696.

[16] Verma SP, Goldin BR. Effect of soy-derived isoflavonoids on the induced growth of MCF-7 cells by estrogenic environmental chemicals. Nutr Cancer 1998; 30(3):232–9.

[17] Verma SP, Goldin BR, Lin PS. The inhibition of the estrogenic effects of pesticides and environmental chemicals by curcumin and isoflavonoids. Environ Health Perspect 1998 Dec; 106(12):807–812.

[18] Khafif A, Schantz SP, Chou TC, et al. Quantitation of chemopreventive synergism between (-)-epigallocatechin-3-gallate and curcumin in normal, premalignant and malignant human oral epithelial cells. Carcinogenesis 1998 Mar; 19(3):419–24.

[19] Jing YK, Han R. [Combination induction of cell differentiation of HL-60 cells by daidzein (S86019) and BC-4 or Ara-C.] Yao Hsueh Hsueh Pao 1993; 28(1):11–6.

[20] Boik J, Newman R, Bailey D. Unpublished observations. 1999.

[21] Darzynkiewicz Z, Traganos F, Wu JM, Chen S. Chinese herbal mixture PC SPES in treatment of prostate cancer. Int J Oncol 2000 Oct; 17(4):729–36.

[22] de la Taille A, Hayek OR, Burchardt M, et al. Role of herbal compounds (PC-SPES) in hormone-refractory prostate cancer: Two case reports. J Altern Complement Med 2000 Oct; 6(5):449–51.

[23] Small EJ, Frohlich MW, Bok R, et al. Prospective trial of the herbal supplement PC-SPES in patients with progressive prostate cancer. J Clin Oncol 2000 Nov 1; 18(21):3595–603.

[24] de la Taille A, Buttyan R, Hayek O, et al. Herbal therapy PC-SPES: In-vitro effects and evaluation of its efficacy in 69 patients with prostate cancer. J Urol 2000 Oct; 164(4):1229–34.

[25] Kimura M, Kimura I, Luo B, Kobayashi S. Antiinflammatory effect of Japanese-Sino medicine "keishi-ka-jutsubu-to" and its component drugs on adjuvant air pouch granuloma of mice. Phytotherapy Research 1991; 5:195–200.

[26] You JS, Hau DM, Chen KT, Huang HF. Combined effects of chuling (Polyporus umbellatus) extract and mitomycin C on experimental liver cancer. Am J Chinese Med 1994; 22(1):19–28.

[27] Baltuch GH, Yong VW. Signal transduction for proliferation of glioma cells in vitro occurs predominantly through a protein kinase C-mediated pathway. Brain Res 1996 Feb 26; 710(1–2):143–9.

[28] Baltuch GH, Dooley NP, Villemure JG, Yong VW. Protein kinase C and growth regulation of malignant gliomas. Can J Neurol Sci 1995 Nov; 22(4):264–71.

[29] Hung MC, Lau YK. Basic science of HER-2/neu: A review. Semin Oncol 1999 Aug; 26(4 Suppl 12):51–9.

[30] Levi F. Therapeutic implications of circadian rhythms in cancer patients. Novartis Found Symp 2000; 227:119–36; discussion 136–42.

[31] Levi F. Cancer chronotherapy. J Pharm Pharmacol 1999 Aug; 51(8):891–8.

[32] Cornelissen G, Gubin D, Halberg F, et al. Chronomedical aspects of oncology and geriatrics. In Vivo 1999 Jan–Feb; 13(1):77–82.

[33] Focan C. Marker rhythms for cancer chronotherapy. From laboratory animals to human beings. In Vivo 1995 Jul–Aug; 9(4):283–98.

Trace metals can play a number of roles in cancer initiation and progression, as well as in prevention and treatment. Although many trace metals can affect cancer, in this chapter we focus on three—selenium, iron, and copper—whose potential to affect disease outcome seems particularly high. The biochemistry of these trace metals is complex, and some of this complexity is related to their participation in redox reactions, which are themselves complex and poorly understood in vivo. Nonetheless, the information currently available strongly suggests that each could be manipulated in the clinical setting to prolong the survival of cancer patients.

All three metals participate easily in redox reactions and are components of enzymes and other proteins necessary for life, but their effects on cancer differ. Whereas selenium appears to protect against cancer and inhibit cancer progression, iron and copper have the opposite effect, and excessive concentrations of these are associated with increased cancer risk and progression. Therefore, we will discuss the potential benefits of administering selenium and lowering iron and copper concentrations.

SELENIUM

Summary of Research and Conclusions[a]

At least 35 in-vitro studies have reported that selenium produces cytotoxic effects on a variety of cancer cell lines.[1–5, b] At least 20 studies have reported that selenium produced antitumor effects in animals.[6–11, c] Hu-

man anticancer trials have not yet been conducted, other than one in which selenium was used in the symptomatic treatment of brain tumor patients.[12] In that trial, selenium, in combination with several other therapeutic agents, produced general improvements such as reductions in nausea and headaches. Still other studies have reported that selenium reduced the side effects of chemotherapy drugs; these are discussed in Chapter 23.

Apart from cancer treatment studies, a number of human trials have reported that selenium supplementation could reduce the risk of developing cancer.[13–17] Other large human cancer prevention trials are now in progress. Many animal studies also have reported that selenium may reduce cancer risk.[18–22] In addition to the above studies on supplementation, some epidemiological studies have reported that low dietary intake of selenium is associated with increased risk of several cancers, although the results of the epidemiologic studies as a whole are inconsistent.[23, 24]

In total, the studies on selenium suggest that supplementation may be useful in both cancer prevention and treatment. Although most human studies thus far have looked at its preventive effects, numerous animal studies have suggested selenium may be useful in treating established cancers. The results from in-vitro studies support its potential as an anticancer compound.

Introduction

Selenium is a trace metal well known for its incorporation into the antioxidant enzyme glutathione peroxidase (see Figure 5.2). As part of this important enzyme, selenium assists in converting hydrogen peroxide to water. One might initially guess that the cytotoxic and antitumor effects of selenium are due to this antioxidant role, but the situation is actually more complex. In fact, only small amounts of selenium are needed to produce maximal concentrations of glutathione peroxidase. Cancer prevention effects only begin at doses about 10-fold higher.[25] Thus other aspects of selenium biochemistry must be responsible for the cytotoxic and cancer preventive effects. Selenium compounds easily participate in redox reactions, and current research suggests that their effects on cancer may be due largely to redox activity.[26]

---

[a] *As in all sections of Part III with this heading, the information summarized was obtained primarily from the MEDLINE database; papers not indexed in MEDLINE are generally not included. The summaries are only for studies conducted with cancer cells; mechanistic studies not involving cancer cells (such as those on PTK inhibition, for example) are not summarized. Lastly, these summaries focus on studies pertinent to cancer treatment, not prevention.*

[b] *In all of Part III, if more than about seven studies demonstrated a particular effect, usually only about five will be listed as references; to list more would be too cumbersome. Those listed serve as examples that support the point.*

[c] *Technically, the term* antitumor *refers to a reduction in tumor volume in animals, whereas* anticancer *refers to the same in humans. To avoid awkward sentences, I use the two phrases interchangeably, and use both phrases in their broadest sense to refer not only to tumor regression but also to antiangiogenesis, anti-*

---

metastasis, anti-invasion, and other forms of cancer inhibition, prolongation of life span, or both.

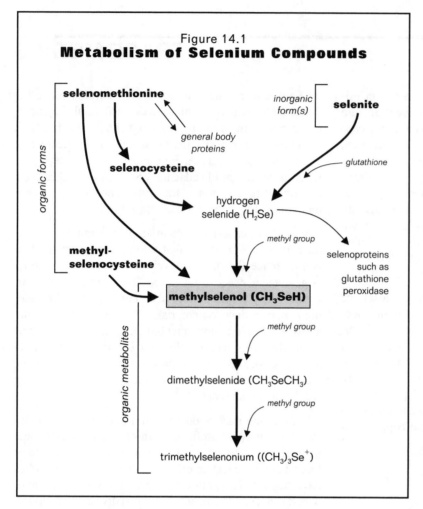

Figure 14.1
Metabolism of Selenium Compounds

Once in the body, most selenium, regardless of its starting form, is eventually metabolized to methylselenol, then to methylselenol derivatives. Methylselenol is of prime importance to us, since this form seems to be responsible for selenium's anticancer effects in vivo.[27, 28] The metabolism (or detoxification) of inorganic and organic forms to methylselenol and its derivatives is illustrated in Figure 14.1 (dietary compounds are in bold; figure adapted from references 29 and 30).

As shown on the right side, inorganic forms require the greatest metabolism on their way to becoming methylselenol. First they must be reduced (via glutathione) and then methylated (i.e., a methyl group, CH_3, must be added to the molecule). In contrast, as shown on the left, organic forms do not require reduction by glutathione in becoming methylselenol and often do not require methylation. Subsequent metabolism of methylselenol to its derivatives does entail additional methyl groups, but in total, organic forms require less than inorganic ones.

The principal methyl donor in the body is SAM, and selenium, especially the inorganic form, is toxic to the body at elevated doses because it depletes SAM reserves. Low SAM levels are associated with increased risk of a variety of diseases, including cancer (see Chapter 2). Accordingly, of the two forms, inorganic selenium causes the most adverse effects at high doses; it requires both extra methyl donors and extra antioxidants during its metabolism. Of the organic forms, methylselenocysteine, and to a lesser extent selenomethionine, are among those causing the least adverse effects at high doses, since they can be converted directly to methylselenol without methyl donors.

Methylselenocysteine occurs in selenium-enriched garlic and in some *Astragalus* species.[31, 32] Nevertheless, it is not widely used as a supplement because it occurs in very small concentrations in plants, and other selenium compounds such as selenomethionine are more abundant and economical.[30] For these reasons, selenomethionine is the most practical form of selenium for therapy. Another advantage of using selenomethionine is that it is readily stored in numerous body proteins. Consequently, animals previously supplemented with selenomethionine have shown higher activities of

To start, consider the basic question of what form of selenium is preferable in treatment. Fundamentally, there are only two types of selenium molecules: inorganic, which do not contain carbon, and organic, which do. Organic forms are preferable in treatment, since they are more easily metabolized to the active form in vivo.

Inorganic selenium occurs naturally in the earth's crust. A common example of it is selenite, a combination of selenium and sodium. In contrast, organic forms occur within living beings, including various plants and yeast; a common example is selenocysteine, a combination of selenium and the amino acid cysteine. Selenium supplements can contain inorganic forms (usually selenite) or organic ones (usually selenocysteine, selenomethionine, or methylselenocysteine). The structures for these four forms are illustrated in Figures A.11 to A.16 of Appendix A, along with the amino acids cysteine and methionine for comparison.[a]

---

[a] *Selenium can substitute for sulfur atoms, and as seen in the figures in Appendix A, it combines with cysteine and methionine molecules through this substitution.*

selenium-dependent enzymes for a longer period during selenium depletion than seen after previous administration of selenite.[30]

In-vitro Studies

Both inorganic and organic forms of selenium are cytotoxic to cancer cells in vitro. We do not, however, rely on the many in-vitro studies of inorganic selenium to explain why selenium should be useful, because these studies are based on conditions that do not occur in vivo. Inorganic selenium does not generally reach cancer tissues—it is metabolized first to organic selenium, as discussed, with most metabolism occurring in the liver. In vitro, cells exposed to inorganic selenium attempt to detoxify it to its organic forms, just as liver cells do in vivo. Since in-vitro concentrations usually overwhelm the ability of cells to detoxify selenium, cells are killed in large part because of depletion of SAM and antioxidant reserves.

TABLE 14.1 POTENTIAL ANTICANCER ACTIONS OF SELENIUM		
ACTIVITY	KNOWN EFFECTS	AS A PKC INHIBITOR, MAY:
Chapter 3: Results of Therapy at the Cellular Level		
Induce apoptosis	x	
Chapter 4: Growth Factors and Signal Transduction		
Inhibit PKC	x	—
Chapter 5: Transcription Factors and Redox Signaling		
Inhibit NF-κB/AP-1 activity	x	x
Chapter 6: Cell-to-Cell Communication		
Improve gap junction communication	x	x
Chapters 7 and 8: Angiogenesis		
Inhibit angiogenesis	x	x
Inhibit histamine effects		x
Inhibit TNF effects		x
Inhibit VEGF effects	x	x
Inhibit insulin resistance		x
Chapters 9 and 10: Invasion and Metastasis		
Inhibit invasion		x
Inhibit collagenase effects		x
Inhibit cell migration		x
Inhibit metastasis		x
Chapters 11 and 12: Immune System		
Support the immune system	x	

Understandably, selenite (inorganic selenium) has been reported to cause DNA strand breaks in cancer cells in vitro, probably via free radicals and/or SAM deficiency, and to induce p53-dependent apoptosis.[33] In contrast, methylselenocysteine and related organic forms act through a different means: they appear to induce apoptosis independent of DNA damage and p53 activity.[3]

The exact way that organic forms induce apoptosis in cancer cells is still uncertain, but it appears that organic selenium acts in a redox-mediated manner to switch protein activity on and off. There are a number of ways this can occur, and all are similar to the formation and destruction of disulfide bonds discussed in Chapter 5. For example, selenium compounds may react with cysteine residues in proteins to form sulfur-selenium-sulfur bonds. Selenium compounds may also catalyze the creation or dissolution of disulfide bonds between cysteine residues (see Figure 5.3). Whatever the exact reaction, oxidized selenium tends to turn proteins off, and reduced selenium tends to turn them on.

One protein selenium compounds are especially adept at turning off is PKC. Interestingly, selenium can inhibit PKC through a redox-sensitive mechanism despite the presence of adequate intracellular glutathione concentrations. Apparently, this is due to a shielding of the cysteine-rich regions of PKC caused by their close proximity to the plasma membrane.[34] In addition, selenium compounds may interact directly with transcription factors to switch them on or off.[25]

A summary of the potential anticancer actions of selenium is provided in Table 14.1. Similar tables are used throughout Part III for most compounds discussed. They summarize the material presented in Parts I and II and include inferred as well as known effects. The inferred effects have not yet been proven but are suggested by the general characteristics of the compound. For example, antioxidants in general tend to inhibit NF-κB activity, but not all antioxidants are the same in this respect. Therefore, the inferred effects may or may not occur, but they are included to provide suggestions for future research. Through these known (and inferred) effects, natural compounds have the potential to affect cancer progression in a multitude of ways. For convenience, activities for each compound are listed according to the chapter in which the activity was discussed. The dashes in the tables signify identical actions. For example, selenium inhibits PKC, so a dash appears in the line "Inhibit PKC" under the column heading "As a PKC inhibitor, may." In other words, any known PKC inhibitor obviously inhibits PKC.

Selenium compounds inhibit PKC and AP-1 activity at roughly 2 to 50 µM in vitro, with inorganic forms being slightly more potent than organic forms.[34, 35, 36] Within this same concentration range, selenium has been reported to inhibit neoplastic transformation and/or proliferation in a number of cell lines.[37–41] The low end of the active concentration range is similar to normal plasma concentrations; accordingly, such concentrations may be adequate to inhibit some cancer cell lines. Normal plasma concentrations of selenium range from about 1.3 to 5.2 µM, with the LOAEL (lowest-observable-adverse-effects level) concentration being about 13 µM.[35, 42, 57] Administration of selenium supplements (at 200 micrograms per day) can produce plasma concentrations at the high end of the normal range (roughly 5 µM). Normal plasma concentrations may be adequate to inhibit other aspects of cancer progression besides cancer cell proliferation. For example, at least one in-vitro study has reported that concentrations of 2 µM or less can partially inhibit proliferation of vascular cells during angiogenesis.[43]

In-vivo Studies

Many studies have reported that selenium produces anticancer effects in animals. Twelve of these are summarized below. Both inorganic and organic forms were reported to be effective, as expected, since the inorganic forms are metabolized to the organic forms in vivo. (The advantage of using organic selenium, as discussed above, has more to do with a reduced risk of adverse effects at high doses than an improved anticancer effect.) The typical oral doses used in the following studies were 2.3 to 5.8 milligrams per day, as scaled to humans. The geometric average of all oral doses used is 3.7 milligrams, as scaled to humans. Since this is an excessive dose even for organic forms, selenium will probably require synergism to be effective.

- Administration of about 480 µg/kg of selenium as selenite in the diet inhibited metastasis of melanoma cells and growth of metastatic lung tumors in mice.[7]

- Administration of 300 and 600 µg/kg of selenium as selenite in the diet inhibited the growth of Ehrlich ascites cells in mice. Intraperitoneal injection was more effective than oral.[44]

- Administration of 38 and 150 µg/kg of selenium as selenite in the diet increased the survival of rats injected with brain cancer cells.[11]

- Administration of 4 mg/kg of selenium as selenite in the diet had no effect on the growth of human breast cancer cells transplanted into nude mice. This high dose was also toxic to the mice.[45]

- Intraperitoneal injection of about 1.6 mg/kg of selenium as selenite inhibited some but not all types of leukemic cells injected into mice.[9]

- Intraperitoneal administration of 250 µg/kg of selenium as selenite inhibited the growth of Ehrlich ascites cells in mice.[46]

- Subcutaneous administration of 0.8 mg/kg of selenium as selenite inhibited the growth of transplanted breast cancer cells in mice.[47]

- Administration of about 600 µg/kg of selenium as selenomethionine in the diet inhibited metastasis of melanoma cells and growth of metastatic lung tumors in mice.[7]

- Administration of 240 µg/kg of selenium as selenium yeast in the diet inhibited metastasis of lung cancer cells in mice.[8]

- Administration of 150 µg/kg of selenium as selenium yeast in the diet inhibited the growth of breast cancer cells in rats.[48]

- Oral administration of about 230 µg/kg of various forms of selenium for seven weeks inhibited angiogenesis in rats with chemically induced breast cancer.[43]

- Intraperitoneal injection of 2 mg/kg of various forms of selenium inhibited Ehrlich ascites tumor growth in mice.[10]

Estimated Therapeutic and LOAEL Doses of Selenium

As stated above, the geometric average dose as scaled from animal studies is roughly 3.7 milligrams per day. We will use this as a target human dose, although it is much larger than the commonly prescribed selenium dose of 200 micrograms for noncancerous conditions. A 200-microgram dose was also used in most human risk reduction studies, as discussed below.

Doses higher than 200 micrograms per day could be safely used by most patients, especially for short to moderate periods. The LOAEL dose for selenium in humans is estimated to be about 2 milligrams (28 µg/kg) per day, and the NOAEL (no-observable-adverse-effects level) dose is estimated to be 1.1 milligrams (15 µg/kg).[49] Higher doses might be possible if methylselenocysteine or other methylated forms of selenium are used, but this remains to be confirmed. At high doses, signs of toxicity include depression, nervousness, nausea, vomiting, and a garlic odor of the breath and sweat. Ingestion of very high doses can cause hair and fingernail loss and fatigue, as seen in one woman who inadvertently ingested about 26 milligrams per day for three months.[50]

The therapeutic dose estimates are summarized in Table 14.2. The tentative dose recommendation is listed as 250 to 1,100 micrograms per day. The 250-microgram value is based on the assumption of a full 15-fold increase in potency by synergistic interactions, while the 1,100-microgram (or 1.1 milligram) value is based on the NOAEL dose.

It appears that synergistic interactions will be required for selenium to produce an anticancer effect in humans. In comparing the 3.7-milligram target dose to the 1.1-milligram maximum recommended dose, synergistic interactions will be needed to produce a minimum 3.4-fold increase in potency. This should be possible, since a 3.4-fold increase is well below the allowable 15-fold increase discussed in Chapter 13.

For chronic doses above 200 micrograms (11 µg/kg) per day, it would be especially important to use an organic form of selenium because, as noted, inorganic forms are more apt to produce adverse effects at high doses.[30] Doses as high as 4,000 micrograms of organic selenium (as kappa-selenocarrageenan) have been given safely to cancer patients over the short term (for eight days).[51] Nonetheless, it may be prudent to monitor patients receiving selenium at doses approaching the LOAEL for toxic effects, even if treatment is short or organic forms are used.

Cancer Prevention Studies

Some readers may be interested in the potential of selenium in cancer prevention as well as treatment. A number of studies have reported that low selenium levels are associated with increased cancer risk in humans.[52, 53, 54] Low levels have also been associated with increased risk of heart disease and reduced immune function.[55] Associations with cancer risk appear to be particularly strong for breast, colon, and prostate cancers. Some examples follow, along with studies that suggest selenium supplementation can reduce cancer risk:

- In a study on 321 subjects, 111 of whom later developed cancer, those with the lowest selenium levels were twice as likely to develop cancer as those with the highest levels. The association was strongest for cancers of the gastrointestinal tract and prostate.[23]

TABLE 14.2 ESTIMATED THERAPEUTIC AND LOAEL DOSES FOR SELENIUM	
DESCRIPTION	**SELENIUM DOSE (µg/day)**
Required dose as scaled from animal antitumor studies	2,300 to 5,800 (geometric average of 3,700)
Target dose based on animal antitumor studies	3,700
Minimum required antitumor dose assuming 15-fold synergistic benefits	250
Commonly prescribed human dose in noncancerous conditions	200
Estimated LOAEL dose	2,000
Estimated NOAEL dose	1,100
Tentative dose recommendation for further research	**250 to 1,100**
Minimum degree of synergism required	**3.4-fold potency increase**

- A cohort study of 33,700 men reported that prostate cancer risk was reduced in men who had higher dietary selenium intake.[24]

- In a study on women over 50, high blood levels of selenium were associated with a reduced risk of breast cancer.[56]

- In a seven-year study on 1,312 human subjects, 200 micrograms of selenium supplement per day (from yeast) reduced the incidence of prostate cancer by 63 percent, colon cancer by 58 percent, overall cancer incidence by 35 percent, and cancer mortality, 49 percent.[57] The incidence of skin cancer was not significantly affected.

- In a study on 974 men with a history of basal cell or squamous cell carcinoma, oral administration of 200 micrograms of selenium (from yeast) for 4.5 years reduced the risk of secondary prostate cancer by 63 percent. In addition, selenium supplementation reduced the risk of total cancer mortality, as well as the incidence of lung cancer, colorectal cancer, and total cancers.[16]

- Plasma selenium levels were lower in patients with malignant oral cavity lesions as compared to healthy controls and to patients with premalignant lesions. Twenty-two patients with premalignant lesions were treated with 300 micrograms per day of selenium supplements (selenite or organic selenium). After 12 weeks, lesions improved in 39 percent of the subjects.[58]

- Selenium supplementation of 200 micrograms (as selenite) significantly reduced the incidence of liver cancer in an area of China where selenium levels are low.[59]

In contrast to these studies, a few studies have reported no association between selenium deficiency and cancer

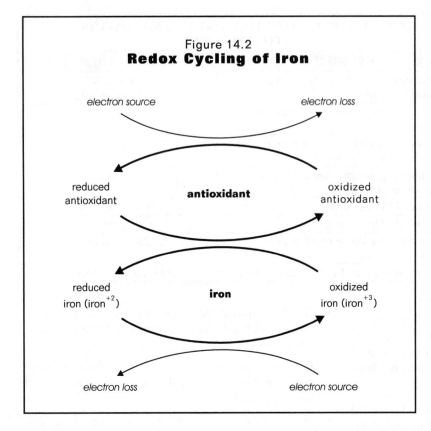

Figure 14.2
Redox Cycling of Iron

electron source   electron loss

reduced   **antioxidant**   oxidized
antioxidant   antioxidant

reduced   **iron**   oxidized
iron (iron^{+2})   iron (iron^{+3})

electron loss   electron source

been associated with increased risk of fungal or other infections.[69, 70, 71] The potential mechanisms for these detrimental effects include increased generation of ROS (reactive oxygen species), increased iron for DNA synthesis, and immune suppression induced by high iron levels.[66, 72] Therefore, anti-iron therapies may be useful in reducing cell transformation, cancer progression, and secondary effects of cancer like infection. However, since human life also requires iron, there is a limit to how far iron concentrations can be reduced. Thus there may be an optimal low level of tissue iron to strive for in cancer patients.

Iron and Redox Reactions[b]

As stated, excess iron can assist cancer through increased generation of ROS. We know that mild ROS concentrations can increase cell proliferation, angiogenesis, and invasion, as well as assist in other malignant behavior. In addition, ROS generation can be detrimental because it can damage healthy cells. Here we look more closely at the role iron plays in redox reactions and the kinds of ROS that can be produced.

Iron, like copper, is a reactive metal, which is why, for example, it is hard to keep it from rusting (oxidizing). We know iron gains or loses electrons during redox reactions, and in doing so, it cycles from reduced to oxidized forms and back, much like the antioxidants discussed in Chapter 5. In fact, the cycling of antioxidants and the cycling of iron are intertwined, since antioxidants can provide the electron source for cycling iron from oxidized to reduced states. The redox cycling of iron is illustrated in Figure 14.2.

As shown in the figure, the reduced form of iron is iron^{+2} (also called ferrous iron). Upon oxidation, it loses a negatively charged electron to become iron^{+3} (also called ferric iron). Many different antioxidants, including vitamin C and flavonoids, can participate in iron reduction. The iron redox cycle is important because the cycling of iron can lead to the formation of both hydrogen peroxide and the damaging hydroxyl radical, via the following reactions:

or have reported that selenium increases cancer risk.[60, 61] Based on the majority of studies, however, it appears that selenium is generally protective against cancer.

IRON

Iron is required for life by humans and many other organisms, including cancer cells and most bacteria. By virtue of its incorporation into hemoglobin, it plays a central role in oxygen and carbon dioxide transport by red blood cells. Iron is also a part of several key enzymes, including the antioxidant enzyme catalase and enzymes active in energy production, metabolism, and DNA synthesis. Furthermore, iron plays an important role in many redox reactions. Through these means, iron, essential as it is in human health, when present in excess can also play a role in cancer initiation and progression.

A large number of animal and human studies have reported that elevated iron levels are associated with increased risk of developing cancer.[62, 63, 64] Furthermore, increased iron loading may assist cancer progression and is associated with poor prognosis in some cancers.[65–68, a] Lastly, increased iron loading in cancer patients has

---

[a] *Increased iron loading can be judged by serum ferritin and transferrin levels and transferrin saturation.*

[b] *A summary of research and conclusions is not included for iron or copper because they are not intended to be used as therapeutic agents; instead, lowering their concentrations may be useful.*

$$antioxidant + iron^{+3} \rightarrow$$
$$oxidized\ antioxidant + iron^{+2}$$

$$iron^{+2} + O_2 \rightarrow iron^{+3} + H_2O_2$$

$$iron^{+2} + H_2O_2 \rightarrow iron^{+3} + OH^{\bullet} + OH^{-}$$

The first reaction is illustrated in Figure 14.2. In the second reaction, reduced iron reacts with molecular oxygen to produce oxidized iron and hydrogen peroxide (H_2O_2). In the third reaction, iron reacts with hydrogen peroxide to produce oxidized iron and the hydroxyl radical ($OH^{\bullet}$). This third reaction, which can also occur with copper and some other metal ions, is called the Fenton reaction. In addition to its role in producing the hydroxyl radical through the Fenton reaction, iron can also participate in the production of the hydroxyl radical by catalyzing the steps in the Haber-Weiss reaction:

$$O_2^{\bullet -} + H_2O_2 \rightarrow O_2 + OH^{\bullet} + OH^{-}$$

In this reaction, iron catalyzes the production of the hydroxyl radical from the superoxide radical and hydrogen peroxide. Although we are certain that the Fenton and Haber-Weiss reactions occur in vitro, it is likely that some variations on these themes occur in vivo.[73]

To limit the chance of unwanted redox reactions, most iron in the body is stored in the oxidized (ferric) form, sequestered to metal-binding proteins. For nonhemoglobin iron, the storage proteins are primarily ferritin inside the cell and transferrin in the blood. Inside the cell, iron can be picked up by other binding proteins, which vary in their ability to allow reactions. Most important to us is that in some situations, such as inflammation and tissue damage, a small amount of iron may be freed from its binding proteins. Iron may also be released during tumor invasion, where enzymes damage local tissues. Once free, iron is able to participate in redox reactions. This situation can also occur after cell damage caused by chemotherapy drugs and radiotherapy.[74] Thus free iron released after treatment with doxorubicin is believed to contribute to the adverse effects of this drug (for example, free iron can cause oxidative damage in heart tissue). In addition, chemotherapy drugs like doxorubicin can directly bind iron in a way that produces ROS, which is one way this drug kills cancer cells and also causes adverse reactions.[75]

Iron, Cell Proliferation, and Iron Withholding

In addition to its ability to increase oxidative damage, excess iron is detrimental because iron is needed for proliferation of bacteria and many other organisms, including most if not all cancer cells. In particular, iron is

needed for the enzyme ribonucleotide reductase, which plays an essential role in DNA synthesis. In fact, iron availability is commonly growth-limiting for many organisms. Since bacteria need iron, the body has developed ways to withhold iron when faced with infection. A large body of evidence demonstrates that one of the first responses to infection in animals is iron withholding.[76] The iron-withholding system can thus be considered part of the natural immune system. Many studies have reported that iron withholding reduces the severity of infection and that high iron levels favor more severe and more frequent infections.

Not surprisingly, the body responds to cancer in the same way it responds to infection—by withholding iron. Because of this response and the relationship between cancer, the immune system, and iron, it is useful to explore how iron withholding works, how excess iron affects the immune system, and how cancer cells strive to obtain iron.

There are at least three ways the body withholds iron. First, iron is sequestered in macrophages. In response to infection, immune cells secrete nitric oxide (NO) and other compounds that cause pathogens to export iron; the iron they release, along with that released from damaged cells, is picked up by iron-binding proteins secreted from neutrophils. One such protein is the multipurpose protein lactoferrin.[a] The iron-loaded lactoferrin is eventually ingested by macrophages. If iron levels are not too high, macrophages safely store the excess iron they ingest. In fact, in moderate amounts this iron can assist macrophages to produce ROS.[77] Ingestion of excessive amounts of iron, however, reduces their effectiveness and their ability to sequester additional iron. Thus very high iron levels can overwhelm storage capacity and have detrimental consequences for the immune system.

Second, the body controls iron availability during infection by reducing iron absorption in the intestines and by synthesizing immunoglobulins that attack the receptors for iron-binding proteins located on the surface of microbe cells.[78]

Lastly, the body regulates iron availability through synthesis of the iron-binding protein transferrin. Although transferrin also serves as an iron-supplying protein, it does play a role in removing iron from use.

Assays that measure the iron saturation level of transferrin are useful in determining the amount of available iron. The normal iron saturation level is about 30 percent, and levels at or below this point are helpful in fighting infection. In response to infection, iron-

---

[a] *Mother's milk has a high concentration of lactoferrin, which may help reduce the risk of infection in a child.*

withholding systems can lower transferrin saturation levels to about 15 percent, and serum iron can drop from a normal of about 18 μM down to about 5.3 μM.[76] In chronic infection, however, this self-induced drop in iron is prolonged and is responsible for the well-known anemic condition called the "anemia of chronic disease."

Iron withholding limits the ability of microbes to obtain needed iron; it also limits the same ability in cancer cells. Some cancer cells, however, have adapted to this limitation by producing iron-binding peptides that deliver iron to the cancer cell.[79, a] Still, in many cancer cell lines, proliferation is inhibited by iron withholding.

It is tempting to speculate that the spontaneous regressions seen in some cancer patients after severe infection and/or fever could be related at least in part to reductions in iron availability.[80–83] Not only does infection increase iron withholding, as discussed above, but fever, among its many effects, reduces the ability of pathogens and cancer cells to synthesize iron-binding proteins and their receptors.[84] Increased iron withholding, possibly in association with fever, may also be partly responsible for the antitumor effects of some bacterial injections.[76]

Iron-Withholding Strategies in Therapy

Because iron withholding assists in the treatment of cancer and infection, several strategies have been investigated that facilitate it:

- The simplest method to lower iron stores is bloodletting.[85, 86] It is interesting to note that bloodletting has been used since antiquity by a variety of cultures to treat infections and other diseases.[87] Modern research also indicates that bloodletting can have beneficial effects. For example, therapeutic bloodletting has been reported to reduce oxidation of serum cholesterol in smokers.[88] (Iron-withholding therapies can be expected to produce antioxidant effects.[89]) One common form of bloodletting is donating blood; this is associated with reduced cancer risk and reduced risk of heart attacks.[90, 91]

- Iron availability can be reduced by eating an iron-deficient diet. In one mouse study, an iron-deficient diet reduced the growth rate of spontaneous tumors by about 45 percent compared to mice on a normal diet.[92] Tumors in mice on low-iron diets also were smaller and grew more slowly than those in mice fed high-iron diets.[65] Although results of some studies

do conflict, other investigators have also reported that iron-deficient diets inhibit tumor growth in rodents without otherwise causing harm.[93] Note that vitamin C is able to increase iron uptake, since vitamin C reduces iron, and reduced iron is more easily assimilated. In Chapter 15, we discuss how vitamin C increased tumor growth in some animal studies. It is conceivable that some of the effects of vitamin C on tumor growth may have been related to increased iron absorption from the diet.

- Iron-chelating compounds (those that bind to iron and keep it from participating in reactions) have been tested for anticancer effects. Iron chelators can inhibit proliferation of many types of cancer cells in vitro.[94–98] The same is true for copper chelators.[99] Animal and human studies have also demonstrated that iron chelators can produce anticancer effects.[100, 101, 102] Some studies, however, reported that chelators were not effective, probably due to the ability of some tumors to synthesize iron-binding proteins and/or transferrin receptors and successfully compete for body iron stores.[79, 103] Iron chelators may also be beneficial in reducing adverse effects of chemotherapy drugs that generate ROS.[104] Since natural compounds that chelate copper also tend to chelate iron, the copper-chelating compounds discussed in Chapter 8 might be useful for iron chelation.

- It may be possible to reduce iron availability by administering the milk protein lactoferrin. In addition to its iron-binding effects discussed above, lactoferrin also acts as an immunostimulant; this has been reported after oral administration in rodents, cats, and humans.[105, 106] Immune effects have also been seen in vitro. For example, one study reported that lactoferrin increased the ability of natural killer cells to kill cancer cells.[107] Lactoferrin may also deter cancer in other ways, including inhibition of cyclin-dependent kinases.[108, 109] Regardless of the mechanism, lactoferrin can inhibit tumor growth and metastasis in vivo. For example, human and/or bovine lactoferrin impeded the growth or metastasis or both of *ras*-transformed fibroblasts, melanoma cells, colon cancer cells, and lymphoma cells in mice.[110, 111, 112] Nonetheless, bovine lactoferrin, which is commercially available, may not be effective against human cancer cells in some cases.[113] In spite of these positive results, administering bovine or human lactoferrin could also be harmful, since some tumor cells appear to produce lactoferrin and/or use it to supply themselves with iron.[87, 114–116] Therefore, although lactoferrin is potentially a useful compound in cancer therapy, it may be prudent to await further study before using it.

---

a Some tumor cells secrete an altered form of the iron-binding protein ferritin that is effective at picking up and bringing iron to them. The high serum ferritin levels seen in some cancer patients may originate from the tumor itself.

In summary, because excessive iron can facilitate cancer progression in several ways, we would like to lower high iron concentrations, if present. The degree that iron levels can be lowered, however, is limited by the need for iron by red blood cells and immune cells, as well as other normal cells. Moreover, excessively low iron levels can stimulate production of VEGF, as reported after high doses of iron chelators in vitro.[117] Since VEGF is an angiogenic factor, excessive iron withholding (including chelation) should be used with caution. The connection between low iron levels and VEGF is not surprising. Low iron conditions are associated with low oxygen conditions, which stimulate angiogeneses during wound healing. For these reasons, it is desirable to maintain an optimal low level of iron but not to drop below it.

A reasonable approach would be to monitor the level of iron in the system and, if it is excessive, lower its concentration through one or both of the first two strategies listed above, as appropriate to the situation. If a combination of natural compounds is already being used in treatment, it is likely that iron chelation (step three above) is already occurring to some degree.

COPPER

In many ways, copper is similar to iron; for one thing, both are needed for synthesis of important enzymes. Copper is necessary in the antioxidant enzyme copper/zinc superoxide dismutate, for example (see Figure 5.2). For another, both iron and copper are transition metals that can participate in redox reactions. Copper can participate in all the reactions discussed above for iron, including the Fenton and Haber-Weiss reactions. (In these, the reduced and oxidized forms of copper are copper^{+1} and copper^{+2}, respectively.) Like iron, copper is sequestered by proteins, thus preventing unwanted redox reactions. The storage protein for copper in the blood is ceruloplasmin, although albumin may also play a role. The storage proteins inside the cell are still uncertain, but metallothionein is thought to be one of them. As with iron, cell necrosis and tissue damage can release free copper, while oxidative stress alone can release free copper from metallothionein.[118]

Anticopper therapies may be useful in cancer treatment because cancer cells require copper for survival. For example, copper-deficient diets inhibited the growth of brain cancer cells in rats.[119, 120] Copper is also needed for angiogenesis, and copper-deficient diets, copper-chelating agents, or other forms of anticopper therapy can inhibit angiogenesis in rats, rabbits, and humans (see Chapter 8). As with iron, however, a certain level of copper is necessary to sustain life. Thus an optimum low level may exist that inhibits cancer but allows normal processes to continue.

Anticopper therapies could have the added benefit of increasing iron withholding, although the degree and conditions of this are still uncertain. It is clear that copper and iron metabolism are intertwined. Animals fed copper-deficient diets exhibit iron deficiency anemia and increased iron storage in organs such as the liver and brain.[121] In one study on mice, transferrin saturation was reduced by 50 percent after four weeks on a copper-deficient diet.[122] Conversely, iron deficiency can lead to increased copper levels in tissues.[123] The relationship between iron and copper is still not completely understood, but it appears copper may play a role in both iron influx into cells and iron efflux out of cells. Its effects on iron efflux are the most clearly documented.[124]

Anticopper therapies are likely to alter the iron status of tumor cells, but the form this alteration will take is not known exactly. Most tissues, except the brain and liver, show lowered iron content during copper deficiency. Tumor cells will possibly also show lowered iron content, which would be a beneficial effect. Conceivably, however, the reverse could occur. At this point, it seems that anticopper therapy might best be used in conjunction with anti-iron therapy; this may prevent unwanted increases in tissue levels of either metal. For example, if iron levels are high and anticopper therapy is used, excessive iron deposition may occur in some tissues.[125, 126] The same is true for copper deposition after anti-iron therapies.[127] Indeed, iron depletion has increased oxidative damage in rats, an effect thought to be due partly to increased copper deposition in the liver.[128]

Anticopper Strategies

Although copper-chelating compounds could be useful in lowering copper availability, the safest and most effective natural compounds known to do so are molybdenum and its relatives. Diets deficient in copper may also be of some use.

In the human study mentioned in Chapter 8, administration of the molybdenum compound tetrathiomolybdate appeared to stop the growth of advanced cancers in five of six patients, apparently by inhibiting angiogenesis. Tumor growth inhibition occurred when plasma ceruloplasmin concentrations were reduced to about 20 percent of baseline for 90 days or more. Side effects of the treatment were minimal as long as anemia was prevented by maintaining the hematocrit above 80 percent of baseline.[129] The dose of tetrathiomolybdate used was 120 milligrams per day in six divided doses.

(The findings in this phase I study must be verified by controlled studies.)

Tetrathiomolybdate, $(NH_4)_2MoS_4$, is an experimental drug used to treat Wilson's disease, which is marked by high concentrations of unbound copper and low plasma copper-binding proteins (ceruloplasmin).[130] The use of tetrathiomolybdate was pioneered by Dr. George Brewer. The idea for its use came from reports that copper deficiency symptoms appeared in livestock grazing on molybdenum-rich soils. Of the molybdenum compounds, tetrathiomolybdate is probably the most effective at lowering copper concentrations; because it is experimental, however, it is not yet available commercially.

Conceivably, it may be possible to use molybdenum compounds already available. The anticopper effect of molybdenum is greatly increased if sulfur is co-administered (sulfur occurs in tetrathiomolybdate). Thus sodium molybdate, Na_2MoO_4, could be combined with calcium sulfide, CaS, as an anticopper therapy. The dose of tetrathiomolybdate used in the human trials contained 44 milligrams of molybdenum per day. In animal experiments, the combination of sodium molybdate and calcium sulfide was roughly 10-fold less potent than tetrathiomolybdate in reducing copper levels.[131] Accordingly, doses as high as 440 milligrams of molybdenum in sodium molybdenum may be required when used in conjunction with calcium sulfide. This is an excessive molybdenum dose, however. Still, based on the ability of various molybdenum compounds to produce toxic effects in animals (via copper depletion), it may be possible that doses closer to 44 milligrams could still be effective. Clearly, many uncertainties remain about the required dose and effectiveness of sodium molybdate and calcium sulfide combinations. The use of such combinations is only mentioned here as an interesting possibility that requires further study.

The toxic molybdenum dose in humans is uncertain, but it appears that the LOAEL dose is about 1.6 mg/kg and the NOAEL dose about 0.9 mg/kg in rats. The human equivalent of these is about 26 and 15 milligrams per day, respectively. A dose of 26 milligrams per day is much higher than the 0.2 to 0.5 milligram per day dose commonly prescribed in noncancerous conditions. At high doses, side effects of molybdenum can include aching joints resembling gout, headache, anemia, and adverse effects on fetal development. Anemia and fetal impacts, which were seen in rodents, may be largely caused by low plasma copper concentrations: low copper concentrations can produce iron deficiency and inhibit the angiogenesis needed for fetal development.

The risks of adverse effects of long-term copper depletion remain to be fully characterized. Based on the human anticancer study mentioned above, copper depletion therapies do, however, promise few adverse effects. Copper does play crucial roles in the body, and a minimal amount is required to maintain normal functions. For example, since copper is a component of the antioxidant enzyme copper/zinc superoxide dismutase, copper deficiency can reduce antioxidant capability. Therefore, caution must be used in anticopper therapies, especially if they part of long-term treatment. It may be prudent to monitor iron, hematocrit, and ceruloplasmin in patients receiving high-dose molybdenum treatment.

We end by noting that although zinc is commonly used as an anticopper agent in the treatment of Wilson's disease, it may not be the best choice for lowering copper levels in cancer patients. Zinc, like copper, plays a role in many enzymes required for cell function, including immune cell function. The effects of zinc are thus complex, and studies on the metal have produced mixed results. On one hand, cancer patients are commonly deficient in zinc, zinc supplementation may improve immune response, zinc deficiency is associated with increased tumor load and stage of some cancers, and zinc supplementation may improve the efficacy of some chemotherapy drugs.[132–137] On the other, zinc chelators reduce cancer invasion in vitro, zinc enhances telomerase activity in vitro, zinc administration can promote metastasis and tumor growth in animals, high zinc levels are associated with increased metastasis of some cancers in humans, zinc deficiency inhibits tumor growth in animals, and animal tumors sequester zinc under zinc-deficient conditions.[138–148] Therefore, until the effects of zinc administration in human cancer patients become clear, anticopper therapies other than zinc administration may be preferable.

CONCLUSION

The trace metals selenium, iron, and copper can affect cancer initiation and progression in diverse ways. Whereas selenium appears to reduce cancer risk and may be useful in cancer treatment, iron and copper are associated with increased cancer risk, and high levels may negatively affect the survival of cancer patients. Therefore, selenium supplementation may be beneficial, as may iron and copper depletion.

Because of their interrelated biochemistries, it is prudent to consider both iron and copper if a depletion therapy is used. This may allow the greatest benefit with the least harm. Since both iron and copper are needed at low levels for health, any depletion therapy must be guided by adequate patient monitoring.

REFERENCES

1 Sinha R, Said TK, Medina D. Organic and inorganic selenium compounds inhibit mouse mammary cell growth in vitro by different cellular pathways. Cancer Lett 1996 Oct 22; 107(2):277–84.

2 Abdullaev FI, MacVicar C, Frenkel GD. Inhibition by selenium of DNA and RNA synthesis in normal and malignant human cells in vitro. Cancer Lett 1992 Jul 31; 65(1):43–9.

3 Lu J, Jiang C, Kaeck M, et al. Dissociation of the genotoxic and growth inhibitory effects of selenium. Biochem Pharmacol 1995 Jul 17; 50(2):213–9.

4 Zhu Z, Kimura M, Itokawa Y, et al. Effect of selenium on malignant tumor cells of brain. Biol Trace Elem Res 1995 Jul; 49(1):1–7.

5 Siwek B, Bahbouth E, Serra MA, et al. Effect of selenium compounds on murine B16 melanoma cells and pigmented cloned pB16 cells. Arch Toxicol 1994; 68(4):246–54.

6 Yan L, Yee JA, Li D, et al. Dietary supplementation of selenomethionine reduces metastasis of melanoma cells in mice. Anticancer Res 1999 Mar–Apr; 19(2A):1337–42.

7 Yan L, Yee JA, McGuire MH, Graef GL. Effect of dietary supplementation of selenite on pulmonary metastasis of melanoma cells in mice. Nutr Cancer 1997; 28(2):165–9.

8 Liu YH, Tian HS, Wang DX. Inhibitory effect of selenium yeast on the metastasis of Lewis lung carcinoma in C57BL mice. Studies with reference of histochemistry and ultrastructure. Chin Med J (Engl) 1987 Jul; 100(7):549–54.

9 Jiang XR, Macey MG, Lin HX, Newland AC. The anti-leukaemic effects and the mechanism of sodium selenite. Leuk Res 1992; 16(4):347–52.

10 Greeder GA, Milner JA. Factors influencing the inhibitory effect of selenium on mice inoculated with Ehrlich ascites tumor cells. Science 1980 Aug 15; 209(4458):825–7.

11 Zhang ZH, Kimura M, Itokawa Y. Inhibitory effect of selenium and change of glutathione peroxidase activity on rat glioma. Biol Trace Elem Res 1996 Oct–Nov; 55(1–2):31–8.

12 Pakdaman A. Symptomatic treatment of brain tumor patients with sodium selenite, oxygen, and other supportive measures. Biol Trace Elem Res 1998 Apr–May; 62(1–2):1–6.

13 Clark LC, Combs GF Jr, Turnbull BW, et al. Effects of selenium supplementation for cancer prevention in patients with carcinoma of the skin. A randomized controlled trial. JAMA 1996 Dec 25; 276(24):1957–63.

14 Yu SY, Zhu YJ, Li WG. Protective role of selenium against hepatitis B virus and primary liver cancer in Qidong. Biol Trace Elem Res 1997 Jan; 56(1):117–24.

15 Combs GF Jr, Clark LC, Turnbull BW. Reduction of cancer mortality and incidence by selenium supplementation. Med Klin 1997 Sep 15; 92 Suppl 3:42–5.

16 Clark LC, Dalkin B, Krongrad A, et al. Decreased incidence of prostate cancer with selenium supplementation: Results of a double-blind cancer prevention trial. Br J Urol 1998 May; 81(5):730–4.

17 Toma S, Micheletti A, Giacchero A, et al. Selenium therapy in patients with precancerous and malignant oral cavity lesions: Preliminary results. Cancer Detect Prev 1991; 15(6):491–4.

18 Ip C, Zhu Z, Thompson HJ, et al. Chemoprevention of mammary cancer with Se-allylselenocysteine and other selenoamino acids in the rat. Anticancer Res 1999 Jul–Aug; 19(4B):2875–80.

19 Reddy BS, Rivenson A, El-Bayoumy K, et al. Chemoprevention of colon cancer by organoselenium compounds and impact of high- or low-fat diets. J Natl Cancer Inst 1997 Apr 2; 89(7):506–12.

20 el-Bayoumy K, Chae YH, Upadhyaya P, Ip C. Chemoprevention of mammary cancer by diallyl selenide, a novel organoselenium compound. Anticancer Res 1996 Sep–Oct; 16(5A):2911–5.

21 Ip C, el-Bayoumy K, Upadhyaya P, et al. Comparative effect of inorganic and organic selenocyanate derivatives in mammary cancer chemoprevention. Carcinogenesis 1994 Feb; 15(2):187–92.

22 Ip C, Lisk DJ. Bioactivity of selenium from Brazil nut for cancer prevention and selenoenzyme maintenance. Nutr Cancer 1994; 21(3):203–12.

23 Willett WC, Polk BF, Morris JS, et al. Prediagnostic serum selenium and risk of cancer. Lancet 1983 Jul 16; 2(8342):130–134.

24 Yoshizawa K, Willett WC, Morris SJ, et al. Study of prediagnostic selenium level in toenails and the risk of advanced prostate cancer. J Natl Cancer Inst 1998 Aug 19; 90(16):1219–24.

25 Ganther HE. Selenium metabolism, selenoproteins and mechanisms of cancer prevention: Complexities with thioredoxin reductase. Carcinogenesis 1999 Sep; 20(9):1657–66.

26 Hasegawa T, Mihara M, Nakamuro K, Sayato Y. Mechanisms of selenium methylation and toxicity in mice treated with selenocystine. Arch Toxicol 1996; 71(1–2):31–8.

27 Ip C, Thompson HJ, Zhu Z, Ganther HE. In vitro and in vivo studies of methylseleninic acid: Evidence that a monomethylated selenium metabolite is critical for cancer chemoprevention. Cancer Res 2000 Jun 1; 60(11):2882–6.

28 Ip C, Hayes C, Budnick RM, Ganther HE. Chemical form of selenium, critical metabolites, and cancer prevention. Cancer Res 1991 Jan 15; 51(2):595–600.

29 Thompson HJ, Ip C, Ganther HE. Changes in ornithine decarboxylase activity and polyamine levels in response to eight different forms of selenium. J Inorg Biochem 1991 Dec; 44(4):283–92.

30 Schrauzer GN. Selenomethionine: A review of its nutritional significance, metabolism and toxicity. J Nutr 2000 Jul; 130(7):1653–1656.

31 Lu J, Pei H, Ip C, et al. Effect on an aqueous extract of selenium-enriched garlic on in vitro markers and in vivo efficacy in cancer prevention. Carcinogenesis 1996 Sep; 17(9):1903–7.

32 Neuhierl B, Thanbichler M, Lottspeich F, et al. A family of S-methylmethionine-dependent thiol/selenol methyltransferases. Role in selenium tolerance and evolutionary relation. J Biol Chem 1999 Feb 26; 274(9):5407–14.

33 Lu J, Kaeck M, Jiang C, et al. Selenite induction of DNA strand breaks and apoptosis in mouse leukemic L1210 cells. Biochem Pharmacol 1994 Apr 29; 47(9):1531–5.

[34] Gopalakrishna R, Chen ZH, Gundimeda U. Selenocompounds induce a redox modulation of protein kinase C in the cell, compartmentally independent from cytosolic glutathione: Its role in inhibition of tumor promotion. Arch Biochem Biophys 1997 Dec 1; 348(1):37–48.

[35] Su HD, Shoji M, Mazzei GJ, et al. Effects of selenium compounds on phospholipid/Ca2+-dependent protein kinase (protein kinase C) system from human leukemic cells. Cancer Res 1986 Jul; 46(7):3684–7.

[36] Sinha R, Kiley SC, Lu JX, et al. Effects of methylselenocysteine on PKC activity, cdk2 phosphorylation and gadd gene expression in synchronized mouse mammary epithelial tumor cells. Cancer Lett 1999 Nov 15; 146(2):135–45.

[37] Kuchan MJ, Milner JA. Influence of intracellular glutathione on selenite-mediated growth inhibition of canine mammary tumor cells. Cancer Res 1992 Mar 1; 52(5):1091–5.

[38] Shallom J, Juvekar A, Chitnis M. Selenium (Se) cytotoxicity in drug sensitive and drug resistant murine tumour. Cancer Biother 1995 Fall; 10(3):243–8.

[39] Yan L, Yee JA, Boylan LM, Spallholz JE. Effect of selenium compounds and thiols on human mammary tumor cells. Biol Trace Elem Res. 1991 Aug; 30(2):145-62.

[40] McGarrity TJ, Peiffer LP, Hartle RJ. Effect of selenium on growth, S-adenosylmethionine and polyamine biosynthesis in human colon cancer cells. Anticancer Res 1993 May–Jun; 13(3):811–5.

[41] Caffrey PB, Frenkel GD. Selenite cytotoxicity in drug resistant and nonresistant human ovarian tumor cells. Cancer Res 1992 Sep 1; 52(17):4812–6.

[42] Yang G, Zhou R. Further observations on the human maximum safe dietary selenium intake in a seleniferous area of China. J Trace Elem Electrolytes Health Dis 1994 Dec; 8(3–4):159–65.

[43] Jiang C, Jiang W, Ip C, et al. Selenium-induced inhibition of angiogenesis in mammary cancer at chemopreventive levels of intake. Mol Carcinog 1999 Dec; 26(4):213–225.

[44] Poirier KA, Milner JA. Factors influencing the antitumorigenic properties of selenium in mice. J Nutr 1983 Nov; 113(11):2147–54.

[45] Yan L, Boylan LM, Spallholz JE. Effect of dietary selenium and magnesium on human mammary tumor growth in athymic nude mice. Nutr Cancer 1991; 16(3–4):239–48.

[46] Milner JA. Effect of selenium on virally induced and transplantable tumor models. Fed Proc 1985 Jun; 44(9):2568–72.

[47] Watrach AM, Milner JA, Watrach MA, Poirier KA. Inhibition of human breast cancer cells by selenium. Cancer Lett 1984 Nov; 25(1):41–7.

[48] Ip C, Ip MM, Kim U. Dietary selenium intake and growth of the MT-W9B transplantable rat mammary tumor. Cancer Lett 1981 Oct; 14(1):101–7.

[49] Whanger P, Vendeland S, Park YC, Xia Y. Metabolism of subtoxic levels of selenium in animals and humans. Ann Clin Lab Sci 1996 Mar–Apr; 26(2):99–113.

[50] Murray MT. Encyclopedia of nutritional supplements. Rocklin, CA: Prima Publishing, 1996, p. 227.

[51] Hu YJ, Chen Y, Zhang YQ, et al. The protective role of selenium on the toxicity of cisplatin-contained chemotherapy regimen in cancer patients. Biol Trace Elem Res 1997 Mar; 56(3):331–41.

[52] Hocman G. Chemoprevention of cancer: Selenium. Int J Biochem 1988; 20(2):123–32.

[53] Willett WC, Stampfer MJ. Selenium and human cancer. Acta Pharmacol Toxicol 1986; 59 Suppl 7:240–7.

[54] Milner JA. Effect of selenium on virally induced and transplanted tumor models. Fed Proc 1985; 44(9):2568–72.

[55] Murray MT. Encyclopedia of nutritional supplements. Rocklin, CA: Prima Publishing, 1996, p. 223.

[56] Hardell L, Danell M, Angqvist CA, et al. Levels of selenium in plasma and glutathione peroxidase in erythrocytes and the risk of breast cancer. A case-control study. Biol Trace Res 1993 Feb; 36(2):99–108.

[57] Clark LC, Combs GF Jr, Turnbull BW, et al. Effects of selenium supplementation for cancer prevention in patients with carcinoma of the skin. A randomized controlled trial. JAMA 1996 Dec 25, 276(24):1957–63.

[58] Toma S, Micheletti A, Giachero A, et al. Selenium therapy in patients with precancerous and malignant oral cavity lesions: Preliminary results. Cancer Detection and Prevention 1991; 15(6):491–94.

[59] Yu SY, Zhu YJ, Li WG, et al. A preliminary report on the intervention trials of primary liver cancer in high-risk populations with nutritional supplementation of selenium in China. Biol Trace Elem Res 1991; 29(3):289–94.

[60] Neve J, Vertongen F, Molle L. Selenium deficiency. Clin Endocrinol Metab 1985; 14(3):629–56.

[61] Yan L, Boylan LM, Spallholz JE. Effect of dietary selenium and magnesium on human mammary tumor growth in athymic nude mice. Nutr Cancer 1991; 16(3–4):239–248.

[62] Weinberg ED. Roles of iron in neoplasia. Promotion, prevention, and therapy. Biol Trace Elem Res 1992 Aug; 34(2):123–40.

[63] Ullen H, Augustsson K, Gustavsson C, Steineck G. Supplementary iron intake and risk of cancer: Reversed causality? Cancer Lett 1997 Mar 19; 114(1–2):215–6.

[64] Herbert V, Shaw S, Jayatilleke E, Stopler-Kasdan T. Most free-radical injury is iron-related: It is promoted by iron, hemin, holoferritin and vitamin C, and inhibited by desferoxamine and apoferritin. Stem Cells 1994 May; 12(3):289–303.

[65] Hann HW, Stahlhut MW, Blumberg BS. Iron nutrition and tumor growth: Decreased tumor growth in iron-deficient mice. Cancer Res 1988 Aug 1; 48(15):4168–70.

[66] Toyokuni S. Iron-induced carcinogenesis: The role of redox regulation. Free Radic Biol Med 1996; 20(4):553–66.

[67] Milman N, Sengelov H, Dombernowsky P. Iron status markers in patients with small cell carcinoma of the lung. Relation to survival. Br J Cancer 1991 Nov; 64(5):895–8.

[68] Wu CW, Wei YY, Chi CW, et al. Tissue potassium, selenium, and iron levels associated with gastric cancer progression. Dig Dis Sci 1996 Jan; 41(1):119–25.

[69] Iglesias-Osma C, Gonzalez-Villaron L, San Miguel JF, et al. Iron metabolism and fungal infections in patients with haematological malignancies. J Clin Pathol 1995 Mar; 48(3):223–5.

[70] Gordeuk VR, Brittenham GM, McLaren GD, Spagnuolo PJ. Hyperferremia in immunosuppressed patients with acute nonlymphocytic leukemia and the risk of infection. J Lab Clin Med 1986 Nov; 108(5):466–72.

[71] Hunter RL, Bennett B, Towns M, Vogler WR. Transferrin in disease II: Defects in the regulation of transferrin saturation with iron contribute to susceptibility to infection. Am J Clin Pathol 1984 Jun; 81(6):748–53.

[72] Weinberg ED. Iron therapy and cancer. Kidney Int Suppl 1999 Mar; 69:S131–4.

[73] Liochev SL. The role of iron-sulfur clusters in in vivo hydroxyl radical production. Free Radic Res 1996 Nov; 25(5):369–84.

[74] Gordon LI, Brown SG, Tallman MS, et al. Sequential changes in serum iron and ferritin in patients undergoing high-dose chemotherapy and radiation with autologous bone marrow transplantation: Possible implications for treatment related toxicity. Free Radic Biol Med 1995 Mar; 18(3):383–9.

[75] Beare S, Steward WP. Plasma free iron and chemotherapy toxicity. Lancet 1996 Feb 10; 347(8998):342–3.

[76] Weinberg ED. Iron withholding: A defense against infection and neoplasia. Physiol Rev 1984 Jan; 64(1):65–102.

[77] Weinberg ED. Iron, infection, and neoplasia. Clin Physiol Biochem 1986; 4(1):50–60.

[78] Weinberg ED. Iron depletion: A defense against intracellular infection and neoplasia. Life Sci 1992; 50(18):1289–97.

[79] Selig RA, White L, Gramacho C, et al. Failure of iron chelators to reduce tumor growth in human neuroblastoma xenografts. Cancer Res 1998 Feb 1; 58(3):473–8.

[80] Nover L. 125 years of experimental heat shock research: Historical roots of a discipline. Genome 1989; 31(2):668–70.

[81] Wiernik PH. Spontaneous regression of hematologic cancers. Natl Cancer Inst Monogr 1976 Nov; 44:35–8.

[82] Cole WH. Spontaneous regression of cancer and the importance of finding its cause. Natl Cancer Inst Monogr 1976 Nov; 44:5–9.

[83] Muckle DS, Dickson JA, Johnston ID. High fever and cancer. Lancet 1971 May 8; 1(7706):972.

[84] Green MH, Vermeulen CW. Fever and the control of gram-negative bacteria. Res Microbiol 1994 May; 145(4):269–72.

[85] Weinberg F. Bloodletting. Can Fam Physician 1994 Jan; 40:131–4.

[86] Weinberg RJ, Ell SR, Weinberg ED. Blood-letting, iron homeostasis, and human health. Med Hypotheses 1986 Dec; 21(4):441–3.

[87] Weinberg ED. Development of clinical methods of iron deprivation for suppression of neoplastic and infectious diseases. Cancer Invest 1999; 17(7):507–13.

[88] Salonen JT, Korpela H, Nyyssonen K, et al. Lowering of body iron stores by blood letting and oxidation resistance of serum lipoproteins: A randomized cross-over trial in male smokers. J Intern Med 1995 Feb; 237(2):161–8.

[89] Polla BS. Therapy by taking away: The case of iron. Biochem Pharmacol 1999 Jun 15; 57(12):1345–9.

[90] Merk K, Mattsson B, Mattsson A, et al. The incidence of cancer among blood donors. Int J Epidemiol 1990 Sep; 19(3):505–9.

[91] Salonen JT, Tuomainen TP, Salonen R, et al. Donation of blood is associated with reduced risk of myocardial infarction. Am J Epidemiol 1998 Sep 1; 148(5):445–51.

[92] Hann HW, Stahlhut MW, Menduke H. Iron enhances tumor growth. Observation on spontaneous mammary tumors in mice. Cancer 1991 Dec 1; 68(11):2407–10.

[93] Wang F, Elliott RL, Head JF. Inhibitory effect of deferoxamine mesylate and low iron diet on the 13762NF rat mammary adenocarcinoma. Anticancer Res 1999 Jan–Feb; 19(1A):445–50.

[94] Renton FJ, Jeitner TM. Cell cycle-dependent inhibition of the proliferation of human neural tumor cell lines by iron chelators. Biochem Pharmacol 1996 Jun 14; 51(11):1553–61.

[95] Tanaka T, Muto N, Ido Y, et al. Induction of embryonal carcinoma cell differentiation by deferoxamine, a potent therapeutic iron chelator. Biochim Biophys Acta 1997 Jun 5; 1357(1):91–7.

[96] Simonart T, Noel JC, Andrei G, et al. Iron as a potential co-factor in the pathogenesis of Kaposi's sarcoma? Int J Cancer 1998 Dec 9; 78(6):720–6.

[97] Tanaka T, Muto N, Itoh N, et al. Induction of differentiation of embryonal carcinoma F9 cells by iron chelators. Res Commun Mol Pathol Pharmacol 1995 Nov; 90(2):211–20.

[98] Richardson DR. Potential of iron chelators as effective antiproliferative agents. Can J Physiol Pharmacol 1997 Oct–Nov; 75(10–11):1164–80.

[99] Oblender M, Carpentieri U. Control of the growth of leukemic cells (L1210) through manipulation of trace metals. Anticancer Res 1991 Jul–Aug; 11(4):1561–4.

[100] Hann HW, Stahlhut MW, Rubin R, Maddrey WC. Antitumor effect of deferoxamine on human hepatocellular carcinoma growing in athymic nude mice. Cancer 1992 Oct 15; 70(8):2051–6.

[101] Head JF, Wang F, Elliott RL. Antineoplastic drugs that interfere with iron metabolism in cancer cells. Adv Enzyme Regul 1997; 37:147–69.

[102] Donfrancesco A, Deb G, Dominici C, et al. Effects of a single course of deferoxamine in neuroblastoma patients. Cancer Res 1990 Aug 15; 50(16):4929–30.

[103] Blatt J. Deferoxamine in children with recurrent neuroblastoma. Anticancer Res 1994 Sep–Oct; 14(5B):2109–12.

[104] Satyamoorthy K, Chitnis MP, Advani SH. In vitro cytotoxicity of caracemide alone and in combination with hydroxyurea or iron-chelating agents in human chronic myeloid leukemia cells and murine tumors. Neoplasma 1988; 35(1):27–35.

[105] Yamauchi K, Wakabayashi H, Hashimoto S, et al. Effects of orally administered bovine lactoferrin on the immune system of healthy volunteers. Adv Exp Med Biol 1998; 443:261–5.

[106] Tomita M, Yamauchi K, Teraguchi S, Hayasawa H. Host defensive effects of orally administered bovine lactoferrin. Adv Exp Med Biol 1998; 443:189–97.

[107] Damiens E, Mazurier J, el Yazidi I, et al. Effects of human lactoferrin on NK cell cytotoxicity against haematopoietic and epithelial tumour cells. Biochim Biophys Acta 1998 Apr 24; 1402(3):277–87.

[108] Damiens E, El Yazidi I, Mazurier J, et al. Lactoferrin inhibits G1 cyclin-dependent kinases during growth arrest of human breast carcinoma cells. J Cell Biochem 1999 Sep 1; 74(3):486–98.

[109] Yoo YC, Watanabe R, Koike Y, et al. Apoptosis in human leukemic cells induced by lactoferricin, a bovine milk protein-derived peptide: Involvement of reactive oxygen species. Biochem Biophys Res Commun 1997 Aug 28; 237(3):624–8.

[110] Yoo YC, Watanabe S, Watanabe R, et al. Bovine lactoferrin and lactoferricin inhibit tumor metastasis in mice. Adv Exp Med Biol 1998; 443:285–91.

[111] Bezault J, Bhimani R, Wiprovnick J, Furmanski P. Human lactoferrin inhibits growth of solid tumors and development of experimental metastases in mice. Cancer Res 1994 May 1; 54(9):2310–2.

[112] Iigo M, Kuhara T, Ushida Y, et al. Inhibitory effects of bovine lactoferrin on colon carcinoma 26 lung metastasis in mice. Clin Exp Metastasis 1999 Feb; 17(1):35–40.

[113] Hurley WL, Hegarty HM, Metzler JT. In vitro inhibition of mammary cell growth by lactoferrin: A comparative study. Life Sci 1994; 55(24):1955–63.

[114] Campbell T, Skilton RA, Coombes RC, et al. Isolation of a lactoferrin cDNA clone and its expression in human breast cancer. Br J Cancer 1992 Jan; 65(1):19–26.

[115] Tuccari G, Giuffre G, Crisafulli C, Barresi G. Immunohistochemical demonstration of lactoferrin in human neoplastic tissues. Adv Exp Med Biol 1998; 443:337–40.

[116] Tuccari G, Giuffre G, Crisafulli C, Barresi G. Immunohistochemical detection of lactoferrin in human astrocytomas and multiforme glioblastomas. Eur J Histochem 1999; 43(4):317–22.

[117] Beerepoot LV, Shima DT, Kuroki M, et al. Up-regulation of vascular endothelial growth factor production by iron chelators. Cancer Res 1996 Aug 15; 56(16):3747–51.

[118] Fabisiak JP, Tyurin VA, Tyurina YY, et al. Redox regulation of copper-metallothionein. Arch Biochem Biophys 1999 Mar 1; 363(1):171–81.

[119] Yoshida D, Ikeda Y, Nakazawa S. Suppression of 9L gliosarcoma growth by copper depletion with copper-deficient diet and D-penicillamine. J Neurooncol 1993 Aug; 17(2):91–7.

[120] Yoshida D, Ikeda Y, Nakazawa S. Suppression of tumor growth in experimental 9L gliosarcoma model by copper depletion. Neurol Med Chir (Tokyo) 1995 Mar; 35(3):133–5.

[121] Chang A, Fink GR. Metal ion metabolism. The copper-iron connection. Curr Biol 1994 Jun 1; 4(6):532–3.

[122] Letendre ED, Holbein BE. Ceruloplasmin and regulation of transferrin iron during Neisseria meningitidis infection in mice. Infect Immun 1984 Jul; 45(1):133–8.

[123] Ward RJ, Scarino ML, Leone A, et al. Copper and iron homeostasis in mammalian cells and cell lines. Biochem Soc Trans 1998 May; 26(2):S191.

[124] Askwith C, Kaplan J. Iron and copper transport in yeast and its relevance to human disease. Trends Biochem Sci 1998 Apr; 23(4):135–8.

[125] Fields M, Lewis CG, Lure MD, et al. Low dietary iron prevents free radical formation and heart pathology of copper-deficient rats fed fructose. Proc Soc Exp Biol Med 1993 Feb; 202(2):225–32.

[126] Fields M, Lewis CG, Lure MD, et al. The severity of copper deficiency can be ameliorated by deferoxamine. Metabolism 1991 Jan; 40(1):105–9.

[127] Sugawara N, Sugawara C. An iron-deficient diet stimulates the onset of the hepatitis due to hepatic copper deposition in the Long-Evans Cinnamon (LEC) rat. Arch Toxicol 1999 Sep; 73(7):353–8.

[128] Knutson MD, Walter PB, Ames BN, Viteri FE. Both iron deficiency and daily iron supplements increase lipid peroxidation in rats. J Nutr 2000 Mar; 130(3):621–8.

[129] Brewer GJ, Dick RD, Grover DK, et al. Treatment of metastatic cancer with tetrathiomolybdate, an anticopper, antiangiogenic agent: Phase I study. Clin Cancer Res 2000; 6:1–10.

[130] Ogihara H, Ogihara T, Miki M, et al. Plasma copper and antioxidant status in Wilson's disease. Pediatr Res 1995 Feb; 37(2):219–26.

[131] Mills CF, El-Gallad TT, Bremner I. Effects of molybdate, sulfide, and tetrathiomolybdate on copper metabolism in rats. J Inorg Biochem 1981 Jun; 14(3):189–207.

[132] Prasad AS, Beck FW, Doerr TD, et al. Nutritional and zinc status of head and neck cancer patients: An interpretive review. J Am Coll Nutr 1998 Oct; 17(5):409–18.

[133] Doerr TD, Prasad AS, Marks SC, et al. Zinc deficiency in head and neck cancer patients. J Am Coll Nutr 1997 Oct; 16(5):418–22.

[134] Roosen N, Doz F, Yeomans KL, et al. Effect of pharmacologic doses of zinc on the therapeutic index of brain tumor chemotherapy with carmustine. Cancer Chemother Pharmacol 1994; 34(5):385–92.

[135] Doz F, Berens ME, Deschepper CF, et al. Experimental basis for increasing the therapeutic index of cis-diamminedicarboxylatocyclobutaneplatinum(II) in brain tumor therapy by a high-zinc diet. Cancer Chemother Pharmacol 1992; 29(3):219–26.

[136] Mathe G, Misset JL, Gil-Delgado M, et al. A phase II trial of immunorestoration with zinc gluconate in immunodepressed cancer patients. Biomed Pharmacother 1986; 40(10):383–5.

[137] Mei W, Dong ZM, Liao BL, Xu HB. Study of immune function of cancer patients influenced by supplemental zinc or selenium-zinc combination. Biol Trace Elem Res 1991 Jan; 28(1):11–9.

[138] Ferry G, Boutin JA, Hennig P, et al. A zinc chelator inhibiting gelatinases exerts potent in vitro anti-invasive effects. Eur J Pharmacol 1998 Jun 19; 351(2):225–33.

[139] Nemoto K, Kondo Y, Himeno S, et al. Modulation of telomerase activity by zinc in human prostatic and renal cancer cells. Biochem Pharmacol 2000 Feb 15; 59(4):401–5.

[140] Rath FW, Kortge R, Haase P, Bismarck M. The influence of zinc administration on the development of experimental lung metastases after an injection of tumour cells into the tail vein of rats. Exp Pathol 1991; 41(4):215–7.

[141] Gorodetsky R, Fuks Z, Sulkes A, et al. Correlation of erythrocyte and plasma levels of zinc, copper, and iron with evidence of metastatic spread in cancer patients. Cancer 1985 Feb 15; 55(4):779–87.

[142] Murray MJ, Erickson KL, Fisher GL. Effects of dietary zinc on melanoma growth and experimental metastasis. Cancer Lett 1983 Dec; 21(2):183–94.

[143] Minkel DT, Dolhun PJ, Calhoun BL, et al. Zinc deficiency and growth of Ehrlich ascites tumor. Cancer Res 1979 Jul; 39(7 Pt 1):2451–6.

[144] Mills BJ, Broghamer WL, Higgins PJ, Lindeman RD. Inhibition of tumor growth by zinc depletion of rats. J Nutr 1984 Apr; 114(4):746–52.

[145] Song MK, Adham NF, Costea NV. Effect of different levels of dietary zinc on longevity of BALB/c mice inoculated with plasmacytoma MOPC 104E. J Natl Cancer Inst 1984 Mar; 72(3):647–52.

[146] Takeda A, Goto K, Okada S. Zinc depletion suppresses tumor growth in mice. Biol Trace Elem Res 1997 Winter; 59(1–3):23–9.

[147] Wolters U, Muller JM, Wolfelschneider K, Iffland H. [Does varied parenteral zinc administration modify interaction between tumor and host? Studies based on an animal model.] Infusionstherapie 1991 Jun; 18(3):123–8.

[148] Murray MJ, Erickson KL, Fisher GL. Effects of supplemental zinc on melanoma metastasis in mice. Cancer Lett 1983 Apr; 18(3):339–47.

We now look at compounds that derive from saccharides, or sugars. Saccharides are the closest relatives to glucose, the starting material for all botanical compounds; in fact, glucose itself is a saccharide. The term saccharide refers to any carbohydrate, but is especially applied to the simple sugars—monosaccharides, disaccharides, oligosaccharides, and polysaccharides.[a]

This chapter discusses vitamin C, which is a monosaccharide derivative structurally similar to glucose (compare Figures A.17 and A.18 in Appendix A). It is the only monosaccharide derivative discussed in this book. Chapter 16 covers high-molecular-weight polysaccharides, which are large sugar molecules found in many immunostimulant herbs. The discussions on saccharides are split between chapters for two reasons. First, because their mechanisms of action are different, vitamin C and high-molecular-weight polysaccharides are likely to play greatly different roles in cancer treatment. Second, since vitamin C is one of the body's primary antioxidant compounds, our discussions on it serve as a springboard for an examination of antioxidants in general.

This book does not regard vitamin C or other antioxidants as essential elements in cancer therapy (this assessment does not apply to antioxidant compounds like flavonoids that inhibit cancer through nonantioxidant means). Nevertheless, vitamin C and antioxidants are explored in depth for several reasons. For one thing, antioxidants may be useful as supportive compounds, either within a large combination of natural compounds or in conjunction with chemotherapy or radiotherapy. For another, they are so popular that many people think of them first when they consider using natural compounds in cancer therapy. Popularity aside, a heated debate is currently under way in the research community on how and when antioxidants could be useful, or whether in fact they may be detrimental in some circumstances. This controversy is the third and most important reason why the discussions here are so extensive. Since the conclusions I present are by no means universally accepted, thorough explanations for their basis are provided.

As we examine ways antioxidants may affect cancer, we primarily look at studies that used antioxidants alone. In Chapter 23 we review studies conducted in combination with chemotherapy or radiotherapy. Here we see that the controversy surrounding antioxidants is not surprising, since antioxidants can produce contradictory results under different in-vitro and in-vivo conditions. For example, oral vitamin C has been reported to both increase and decrease tumor growth in animals. With such contradictions, additional studies are needed before we fully understand what takes place.

Still, based on the limited information available, we can draw some preliminary conclusions about the oral use of primary antioxidants in cancer treatment. The term *primary antioxidant* is used here to refer to vitamin C, vitamin E, alpha-lipoic acid, *N*-acetylcysteine, and any other related compound whose primary therapeutic effect is to increase intracellular antioxidant stores. Of course, other natural compounds discussed can also function as antioxidants, but the greatest effect of these compounds on cancer is not likely to be mediated through an antioxidant mechanism. For example, quercetin functions as an antioxidant, but its most powerful effects on cancer are probably mediated through kinase inhibition or other nonantioxidant actions. For convenience, we refer to these compounds as *secondary antioxidants*.

Our first conclusion is that primary antioxidants are not suitable as single treatment agents, and their use as such is best avoided. The same holds true for combinations of primary antioxidants. Results from such antioxidant therapies would be unpredictable and possibly detrimental under some conditions.

Second, to help assure a marked inhibitory effect on cancer, the best use of primary antioxidants is likely to be in combination both with one another and with other anticancer compounds, such as those discussed elsewhere in this book. My central hypothesis is that the most effective treatments will be those that strongly and redundantly address all seven clusters of procancer events. Using a combination of primary antioxidants alone would obviously not follow this strategy.

Our third conclusion is that even in the context of large and diverse combinations, primary antioxidants should probably not be viewed as the key players; their role is more of a supportive one. If constraints dictate that only a limited number of compounds can be used in therapy, compounds other than primary antioxidants could be

---

[a] *Carbohydrates are those compounds that fit the general formula $C_x(H_2O)_n$; they include these saccharides, their derivatives, and other smaller groups of compounds like the inositols. The prefixes* mono, di, oligo, *and* poly *refer to one, two, a few, and many linked saccharide units, respectively.*

chosen that are more potent against cancer. This conclusion does not ignore the antioxidant needs of the cancer patient: any needs not met through diet could be filled by secondary antioxidant compounds. For example, most of the phenolic compounds in Chapters 19 and 20 are secondary antioxidant compounds; the example of quercetin was given above. As another example, while vitamin E itself may have only a moderate effect on most cancers, secondary antioxidants like vitamin E succinate may have a more profound effect. (Most of the inhibitory effects of vitamin E succinate are unrelated to its antioxidant action.) Many more examples of secondary antioxidants could be cited, including melatonin.

VITAMIN C

Summary of Research and Conclusions

The results of in-vitro cancer studies on vitamin C have been conflicting. Over 37 in-vitro cytotoxicity studies have been conducted on the vitamin as a single agent. The majority of these have reported that vitamin C, especially at high concentrations (1 to 10 mM), can inhibit cancer cell proliferation by a free-radical-mediated mechanism while causing little harm to normal cells.[1-5] At least six studies have reported, however, that lower concentrations (10 to 300 µM) of vitamin C can stimulate proliferation of some cancer lines in vitro.[6-11]

Animal studies have likewise been contradictory. At least eight animal studies reported that vitamin C used alone or with copper can produce an antitumor effect (copper increases free radical generation).[12-19] On the other hand, at least four animal studies reported that vitamin C used alone did not produce such an effect.[20-23] Moreover, at least five animal studies reported an increase in growth or metastasis of some tumors when vitamin C was used alone.[22, 24-27]

Human studies have also been conflicting. Two series of case studies have been published suggesting that vitamin C may prolong the survival of terminally ill patients.[28, 29] Three retrospective trials and one prospective trial (all nonrandomized) were also published; the retrospective trials suggested an anticancer effect in a majority of terminal cancer patients, but the prospective trial reported no increase in life span for early-stage breast cancer patients.[30-33] In fact, the latter study inferred harm in a subset of patients, but this was not statistically analyzed and may have been due to chance.[34] In addition to these studies, two randomized, double-blind, placebo-controlled trials reported no benefit for terminal colon cancer patients.[35, 36] In one of

these, survival time was slightly lower in patients receiving vitamin C in comparison to placebo, although this negative effect was not statistically analyzed and may again have been due to chance.

Lastly, vitamin C has been tested in combination with other antioxidants, again with conflicting results.[37-41] For example, one animal study reported that a combination of antioxidants increase metastasis without affecting the growth of the primary tumor. On the other hand, one human study reported that a combination of antioxidants reduced the risk of recurrence after treatment for bladder cancer.[40, 42]

These inconsistencies are certainly perplexing, and to some degree, they probably reflect the complex biochemistries of antioxidants/oxidants found in vivo. In addition, some inconsistencies found in in-vitro, animal, and human studies may be attributed to differences in the experimental procedures used.

Overall, the studies suggest vitamin C can inhibit cancer proliferation in vitro and in vivo through a free-radical-mediated process, if the free radical concentration is sufficiency high. But if the free radical concentration is mild, vitamin C can have variable effects, stimulating proliferation in some cases. The exact mechanisms behind these actions are still poorly understood. Based on available information, if vitamin C is found useful as a single agent, it will probably be when it is administered intravenously at high doses, in which case it would inhibit cancer through a prooxidant effect. Since I do not advocate the use of prooxidant therapies, and since a prooxidant effect cannot be assured after oral administration even if we wanted one, the use of oral vitamin C as a single agent is not recommend.

Introduction to Vitamin C

Vitamin C can affect cancer in a multitude of ways, but the mechanisms are still poorly understood in spite of the relatively large number of studies conducted. As we have seen, various studies have reported that vitamin C inhibits cancer, has no effect on cancer, or it facilitates cancer progression.

A primary reason for the slow progress and conflicting results in vitamin C research is that its effects on cancer are largely mediated through redox reactions, and the study of these in biological systems is a complex undertaking. Like all antioxidants, vitamin C can act as both an antioxidant and prooxidant. Its prooxidant effects are mediated through the vitamin C free radical, which in high concentrations inhibits tumor growth but in low concentrations may stimulate it. Unfortunately, much of our understanding of the effects of free radicals in health and disease has come only recently, and the role the vitamin C free radical plays in the vitamin's anticancer effects was not fully appreciated in early studies. Consequently, early studies were not always careful to account for its production and involvement, making the results of different investigations difficult to interpret. The study of vitamin C also is difficult and results are conflicting because in addition to redox-mediated effects, vitamin C may affect cancer through a number of indirect means, such as through immune enhancement.

Mechanisms of Action

As an antioxidant, vitamin C may inhibit cancer progression through a variety of actions, listed in Table 15.1. Its ability to stimulate apoptosis is mediated by its prooxidant effect.

Any of the actions listed may contribute to tumor inhibition in vivo, but some actions will likely be more active than others. Nearly all mechanistic studies conducted so far have focused on vitamin C's ability to directly inhibit cancer cells by acting as a prooxidant, thereby inducing apoptosis. Much less is known about its ability to inhibit cancer through the indirect means listed, such as inhibition of invasion. Additional study is required to determine the role each of these indirect mechanisms may play, but we now use the available evidence to make preliminary conclusions about both direct and indirect effects, with the latter discussion necessarily more brief.

Indirect Effects of Vitamin C

Most of the activities listed in Table 15.1 are those that would indirectly inhibit cancer, including actions that inhibit angiogenesis, invasion, and metastasis and those that support the immune system. Although data are scarce, it appears that indirect means will likely play a lesser role in tumor inhibition in vivo than direct means. Furthermore, we can estimate that the inferred actions listed are less likely to be involved than the known actions. Indeed, inhibition of metastasis is listed as an inferred activity, yet vitamin C increased metastasis in

TABLE 15.1 POTENTIAL ANTICANCER ACTIONS OF VITAMIN C			
ACTIVITY	**KNOWN EFFECTS**	**AS AN ANTIOXIDANT, MAY:**	**AS A HYALURONIDASE INHIBITOR, MAY:**
Chapter 2: Mutations, Gene Expression, and Proliferation			
Act as an antioxidant	x	—	
Chapter 3: Results of Therapy at the Cellular Level			
Induce apoptosis	x		
Chapter 5: Transcription Factors and Redox Signaling			
Inhibit NF-κB activity	weak	x	
Chapters 7 and 8: Angiogenesis			
Inhibit angiogenesis		x	x
Inhibit bFGF effects			x
Inhibit histamine effects	x		
Inhibit TNF effects		x	
Inhibit VEGF effects		x	
Chapters 9 and 10: Invasion and Metastasis			
Inhibit invasion			x
Inhibit hyaluronidase and beta-glucuronidase	x		—
Inhibit collagenase effects	stimulates collagen synthesis	x	
Inhibit cell migration			x
Inhibit metastasis			x
Chapters 11 and 12: Immune System			
Support the immune system	x		

some animal studies when used alone or in combinations with other vitamins.[22, 43]

The known indirect activities listed in Table 15.1 are inhibition of histamine, support of the immune system, and support of ECM integrity (via inhibition of hyaluronidase and beta-glucuronidase and stimulation of collagen synthesis).[a] Although the ability of vitamin C to inhibit histamine and improve immune response has been demonstrated in healthy humans, it is unlikely these effects alone would be sufficient to produce the antitumor effects observed in some animal studies. Histamine is one of many secondary mediators of angiogenesis, and its reduction alone would not be expected to influence angiogenesis dramatically.

---

[a] *The effects of vitamin C on the ECM and immune system are apparent in scurvy, or vitamin C deficiency. Symptoms of scurvy are bleeding gums, poor wound healing, extensive bruising, and susceptibility to infection.*

Likewise, Vitamin C can support the immune system through a number of mechanisms, but it is not an immune stimulant per se; its role is supportive in nature, so effects on the immune system are not likely responsible by themselves for the observed antitumor effects. Indeed, the antitumor effects in some animal studies were seen within a short enough time period to exclude major immune involvement.[13] Interestingly, one way vitamin C supports the immune system is by inhibiting histamine production.[44] Excess histamine can have a suppressive effect on the immune system.

Lastly, the effects of vitamin C on the ECM are also unlikely to account for observed antitumor effects. The effects of vitamin C on the ECM have been studied in cancer-bearing animals and humans, but results have varied. One study on tumor-bearing mice reported that orally administered vitamin C affected the architecture of implanted ascites tumors; in a human study, however, the authors reported as a minor observation that no correlations were evident between plasma vitamin C concentrations and the architectural changes of skin cancers.[45, 46] Furthermore, two in-vitro studies reported that vitamin C does not reduce collagenase production by tumor cells or make the ECM more resistant to tumor degradation.[47, 48]

In summary, while the above-mentioned indirect effects may add to an anticancer action, their contribution is likely to be relatively minor, except possibly in cases of overt vitamin C deficiency.

Direct Effects of Vitamin C

In contrast to indirect effects, it seems probable that vitamin C can produce antitumor effects solely through direct effects on cancer cells. A large body of evidence suggests that the direct effects of vitamin C are mediated by its free radical. As stated earlier, however, prooxidant therapies have their drawbacks and are not advocated in this book. Nonetheless, the prooxidant effects of vitamin C are discussed below, to explain how vitamin C can kill cancer cells and to provide background for later discussions on other antioxidants. Moreover, at lower concentrations, the vitamin C free radical can stimulate proliferation of some tumors, and for that reason needs to be discussed.

Ascorbate Free Radical

Vitamin C occurs in four forms. Dry vitamin C is called ascorbic acid. When placed in solution, it ionizes to form ascorbate.[a] Ascorbate can donate an electron

(hydrogen atom) to neutralize a free radical, and in the process it becomes a free radical itself, called the ascorbate free radical or AFR. AFR can then donate another electron, and in doing so, it becomes oxidized vitamin C or dehydroascorbate (DHAsc).[b] Vitamin C cycles in vivo between its reduced form (ascorbate), its free radical form (AFR), and its oxidized form (DHAsc). These forms, along with ascorbic acid itself, are illustrated in Figures A.18 through A.21 in Appendix A. In this chapter, we use the terms *ascorbate* and *vitamin C* (ascorbic acid) interchangeably.

The vitamin C cycle is intimately involved with the cycle of at least two other major intracellular antioxidants, glutathione and vitamin E. Their relationships are illustrated (in simplified form) in Figure 15.1 (adapted from reference 49).

Three important ideas are illustrated in the figure. First, each of these antioxidants cycles between a reduced (antioxidant) form and an oxidized form. Thus the figure shows three cycles, one for glutathione, one for vitamin C, and one for vitamin E.

Second, the reduced forms of each antioxidant can recycle other antioxidants. For example, reduced glutathione can cycle oxidized vitamin C to its reduced form, producing oxidized glutathione in the process. Likewise, ascorbate can cycle oxidized vitamin E to its reduced form, producing oxidized vitamin C. These interactions are important in vivo, as they allow antioxidants to keep each other in their reduced forms.[50, 51, 52]

Third, the figure illustrates that the ascorbate free radical is produced as an intermediary between the reduced and oxidized forms of the vitamin. Like DHAsc, oxidized glutathione is also produced through a two-step electron loss process, with the glutathione free radical (GFR) produced in the first step.

Also of interest in the figure is that the source of electrons for reducing glutathione (and through glutathione, other antioxidants) is NADH, which is obtained from the burning of glucose (see Chapter 5). Thus in addition to providing energy for other cellular functions, glucose provides the fundamental energy to maintain antioxidants in their reduced states.

As shown, some of the AFR produced can be cycled directly back to ascorbate (reduced vitamin C). A larger portion, however, is converted to DHAsc. Since DHAsc

---

[a] *Ionization is a common event. For example, salt (NaCl) ionizes (splits apart) in water to form sodium (Na^+) and chloride (Cl^-)*

ions. When vitamin C is mixed with water, a hydrogen ion dissociates from the rest of the molecule to produce ascorbate and H^+.

[b] *Ascorbate free radical is also referred to as semidehydroascorbate, signifying its midpoint existence between ascorbate and dehydroascorbate.*

is quite unstable and quickly degrades in vitro and in vivo to other inactive compounds, this represents a significant form of vitamin C loss.[53] (Only minor amounts of DHAsc can be cycled back to ascorbate.) Thus antioxidant recycling is not complete, and regular dietary replenishment of vitamin C, as well as vitamin E, is needed, along with synthesis of additional glutathione.

Almost all of the body's extracellular and intracellular vitamin C is in its reduced form. DHAsc accounts for only about 8 percent of the total vitamin C plasma concentration.[54]   Although DHAsc is produced in significant quantities during conditions of oxidative stress, its low plasma concentration is due to its rapid degradation and to the uptake of DHAsc into cells, where it is converted to the reduced form. Cells maintain very high concentrations of ascorbate relative to plasma levels, and immune cells have especially high intracellular ascorbate concentrations. Intracellular concentrations of immune cells can be as high as 6 mM, whereas plasma concentrations are usually below 70 μM.[55]

AFR is a relatively long-lived and mild-acting free radical. Because it is long-lived, it can readily be measured in the blood and other fluids. In comparison to highly reactive oxygen free radicals, like the hydroxyl radical, it is not as likely to directly produce DNA or protein damage. Because of this and because of antioxidant recycling, the overall effect of vitamin C in vivo at normal dietary intake is as an antioxidant.[56] Nonetheless, AFR or AFR-generated free radicals can stimulate or inhibit cancer and other cells in vitro and in vivo. Whether proliferation is stimulated, inhibited, or unaffected depends on a number of factors, including the concentration of ascorbate and free radicals present, the characteristics of the cell, and the availability of metal ions, as discussed below.

Inhibition of Cell Proliferation

In order to better understand the direct effects of vitamin C on cancer in vivo, we review the way AFR is produced and how it may lead to cell death. The three main points are relatively simple: vitamin C can scav-

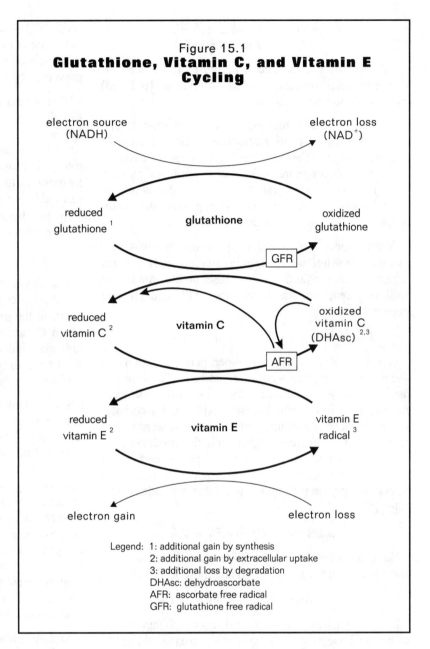

Figure 15.1
Glutathione, Vitamin C, and Vitamin E Cycling

electron source (NADH) → electron loss (NAD⁺)

reduced glutathione [1]   glutathione   oxidized glutathione

GFR

reduced vitamin C [2]   vitamin C   oxidized vitamin C (DHAsc) [2,3]

AFR

reduced vitamin E [2]   vitamin E   vitamin E radical [3]

electron gain   electron loss

Legend: 1: additional gain by synthesis
         2: additional gain by extracellular uptake
         3: additional loss by degradation
         DHAsc: dehydroascorbate
         AFR: ascorbate free radical
         GFR: glutathione free radical

enge free radicals, but in the process AFR is produced; vitamin C can react with oxygen to produce hydrogen peroxide; and copper and iron ions can react with hydrogen peroxide to produce harmful hydroxyl radicals, DNA damage, and cell death. These concepts were introduced earlier and are discussed here in more detail to provide a more complete understanding of how vitamin C works against cancer.

Production and Effects of AFR

Ascorbate free radical (AFR) is produced when ascorbate reduces (donates an electron or hydrogen atom), to another compound. For example, vitamin C can reduce the vitamin E radical to produce AFR and reduced vitamin E:

ascorbate + vitamin E radical →
AFR + reduced vitamin E

This reaction is illustrated in Figure 15.1. Thus ascorbate can keep vitamin E in its antioxidant (reduced) state, ready to protect the cell.

Another important reaction in which vitamin C and some other antioxidants participate is the reduction of iron and copper. This reaction is important for two reasons: it produces more AFR, and it produces reduced iron and copper, which can then react in other ways. In the following discussions, we use copper as the example, but similar reactions occur with iron.

When copper^{+2} (oxidized copper) and ascorbate are available in solution, copper gains an electron (i.e., gains a negative charge) and ascorbate loses an electron by the following reaction, which produces AFR and reduced copper:[57]

$$ascorbate + copper^{+2} \rightarrow AFR + copper^{+1}$$

In some animal antitumor experiments, solutions of ascorbate and copper were administered. Thus we can assume AFR was produced in these solutions. Although not particularly harmful by itself, AFR (and ascorbate) can participate in producing other, more dangerous free radicals. This process begins with the production of hydrogen peroxide, usually in two steps. Ascorbate, in the presence of a catalyst such as copper, can react with molecular oxygen (O_2) to produce the superoxide radical ($O_2^{\bullet -}$):[58]

$$ascorbate + O_2 \rightarrow AFR + O_2^{\bullet -}$$

Next, ascorbate and superoxide radical can react to form hydrogen peroxide (H_2O_2) and more AFR:[59, a]

$$ascorbate + O_2^{\bullet -} \rightarrow AFR + H_2O_2$$

In a similar way, AFR can also react with superoxide to produce ascorbate and hydrogen peroxide. In either case, the result is hydrogen peroxide.

The ability of vitamin C to make hydrogen peroxide in vitro is well documented.[60] Furthermore, its production after intravenous administration of vitamin C analogs has been demonstrated in cancer-bearing rats.[61] In this study, hydrogen peroxide generation was particularly strong at cancer sties. This was most likely caused by an availability of copper ions at the sites due to inflammation and tissue destruction and also low catalase production by tumors; the latter is an enzyme that degrades hydrogen peroxide to form water and oxygen (see Fig-

ure 5.2). In-vitro studies confirm that the cytotoxicity of ascorbate is greatly increased in the presence of copper, is associated with hydrogen peroxide generation, and is prevented by catalase.[3, 62, 63]

We now explore ways that hydrogen peroxide can lead to cell death. Hydrogen peroxide is not a free radical but is considered a reactive oxygen species (ROS) because it is easily converted to free radicals. Furthermore, hydrogen peroxide can easily pass through membranes to reach any intracellular compartment.[64] It can oxidize copper^{+1} (return it to copper^{+2}) and thereby form the damaging hydroxyl radical (OH $^\bullet$); this is the Fenton reaction first discussed in Chapter 14:[65]

$$copper^{+1} + H_2O_2 \rightarrow copper^{+2} + OH^\bullet + OH^-$$

In addition to the Fenton reaction, superoxide can also react with copper^{+2} to produce the hydroxyl radical. Thus, in the presence of oxygen and copper or iron, vitamin C can produce hydrogen peroxide and hydroxyl radicals. Indeed, mixtures of iron and vitamin C have been used for decades as a source of hydroxyl radicals for laboratory experiments.

Since vitamin C can assist in producing hydroxyl radicals, why is it not dangerous in living systems? First, the body limits vitamin C plasma concentrations, thereby limiting the potential for damage. Second, copper and iron are not freely available in most situations to act as catalysts. Third, other antioxidant enzymes work in conjunction with vitamin C to reduce any reactive oxygen species produced. As noted above, catalase is able to degrade hydrogen peroxide, producing water and oxygen. When these safety checks are overridden, for instance, when vitamin C is administered intravenously at high doses or with copper or iron, it can be dangerous, especially to cancer cells, which tend to produce low amounts of catalase.

Although hydroxyl radicals are probably involved in vitamin C's antitumor effect, they are not the whole story. The exact mechanisms of cytotoxicity in vivo are still under investigation.[66, 67] For example, scavengers of hydroxyl radicals do not reduce the cytotoxicity of vitamin C in in-vitro studies.[68] One theory is that through a series of steps involving the formation of complexes between copper ions and DNA, the hydroxyl radical is eventually produced directly at the DNA site in the presence of vitamin C.[69] In this way, the hydroxyl radical can act swiftly, leaving insufficient time for hydroxyl scavengers to stop the process.

Note that vitamin C is not the only reducing agent that can cause the above reactions to occur. A number of other antioxidants, including glutathione, *N*-acetylcysteine, and NADH, are capable of doing so.[69, 70] Of

---

[a] *Hydrogen peroxide can also form from the action of the antioxidant enzyme superoxide dismutase (SOD), which converts superoxide to hydrogen peroxide.*

these, ascorbic acid is the most effective; it causes the greatest DNA damage and is active at physiologic concentrations of 10 to 100 µM in vitro.

Like copper, iron can also induce DNA damage in the presence of antioxidants, but it is less effective than copper and appears to act through a slightly different pathway, one more dominated by hydroxyl radical formation. Iron-mediated DNA damage can be inhibited by hydroxyl radical scavengers.[71]

Results of Studies Dependent on Experimental Procedures Used

Understanding how vitamin C directly inhibits cancer, we can consider how differences in experimental procedure could account for some of the inconsistencies reported in the animal and human studies. Several of the human studies that tested vitamin C and found it ineffective did so in a way that failed to produce a prooxidant effect, thereby eliminating its direct-acting properties and causing it to be ineffective.

Several forms of vitamin C were given in different animal and human studies, and the choice of form may have greatly affected the results. These forms include dry oral, oral in solution, oral in solution with copper, and intravenous solution. From the above discussions, it is clear these forms of administration are not equivalent, either in their redox activity or their ability to increase plasma concentrations. Therefore, they would be expected to produce different results. Of all the forms, dry vitamin C given orally could be expected to produce the least AFR and the smallest anticancer effect. Indeed, two animal studies reported that vitamin C was ineffective when given in food as the dry form (at 1.9 to 9.6 grams per day, as scaled to humans) but was effective at this dose when given in drinking water, especially if copper was added.[72, 73] (AFR is produced in solution, especially if copper is added.)

It may not be a coincidence then that all the human case studies and clinical trials reporting anticancer effects used intravenous or oral solutions of vitamin C.[28–32] We could expect AFR or other radicals to be present in such solutions, and expect intravenous administration to produce the relatively high plasma concentrations necessary for a prooxidant effect. In contrast, the two randomized, double-blind clinical trials that reported no anticancer effect used oral administration of dry vitamin C, as did the nonrandomized prospective trial that reported no effect.[34, 35, 36] We would expect AFR or other radicals to be missing in these forms and oral administration to produce a relatively low plasma concentration. We can say, therefore, that the studies reporting no anticancer effect used a form of vitamin C (dry oral) least likely to be effective.

Stimulation of Cell Proliferation

We have reviewed ways that vitamin C can cause a direct inhibitory effect on cancer cells; however, it can have a direct stimulatory effect too. A major reason for using caution with vitamin C is that in some studies it has stimulated cancer cell proliferation, not only in vitro but also in animals. Although the human studies have reported no clear signs that vitamin C is detrimental, several do raise the possibility it could be harmful in a small subset of patients.

Before considering its effects in humans, let us examine how vitamin C could stimulate cancer. The fact that free radicals can stimulate cell proliferation is not a new concept to us; the stimulating properties of radicals on growth factor receptors, PKC activity, and NF-κB activity were discussed in Chapter 5.[74, 75] In addition, AFR and other radicals may stimulate proliferation through a process called transmembrane electron transport, where cells reduce extracellular AFR to ascorbate by sending electrons through their plasma membrane. The reasons why transmembrane electron transport stimulates cell proliferation are still uncertain, but may be due partly to a subsequent increase in the intracellular pH, which favors cell proliferation.[76, 77] Considering the above, it is not surprising that cancer cell proliferation can be stimulated by AFR under the right conditions, as well as by other radicals such as hydrogen peroxide and nitric oxide.[77, 78, 79]

In addition, there are a number of indirect ways vitamin C may facilitate cancer progression. For example, it could facilitate the synthesis of collagen, which is needed during angiogenesis, or its antioxidant properties could protect cancer cells from oxidative damage.[80] The latter is consistent with the ability of tumors to sequester high amounts of vitamin C.[81, 82] (The ability of antioxidants to protect cancer cells is discussed below.)

The method cancer and immune cells use to increase vitamin C concentrations is quite interesting. These cells efficiently take up extracellular dehydroascorbate (DHAsc) through their glucose transporters.[83, 84, 85] (Recall that vitamin C is a glucose derivative.) Indeed, glucose transporters are overexpressed on both cancer cells and activated immune cells. Primarily through DHAsc uptake, cancer cells can amass more than twofold higher vitamin C concentrations than can surrounding tissues.[86] In both immune and cancer cells, the uptake of the reduced form of vitamin C from extracellular fluids is much less efficient than the uptake of DHAsc. Thus, the kind of oxidizing conditions seen in inflammation and at cancer sites causes or allows immune and cancer cells to take up additional vitamin C.

Whether vitamin C stimulates cancer cell proliferation in humans by one or more of these means is still unknown. If detrimental effects occur in humans, they likely do so only in a subset of patients, as suggested by an in-vitro study where vitamin C stimulated proliferation of fresh leukemic stem cells obtained from 35 percent of 151 patients and suppressed proliferation of stem cells from 15 percent.[8] This selectivity probably involves the relative ability of cancers from different patients to produce catalase (which neutralizes hydrogen peroxide), the relative abundance of free metal ions present, and the relative sensitivity of growth factor receptors and PKC to free radical modification. Clinical studies too have implied that detrimental effects could have occurred in some patients, but these studies were not looking for harm and did not statistically analyze the results based on harm.[34, 87] In the second study cited, which was double-blind and placebo-controlled, the mean survival of terminal colorectal cancer was 4.1 months for controls and 2.9 months for patients taking 10 grams of vitamin C orally per day. It is reasonable to suppose that any detrimental effects vitamin C might have on cancer patients could be reduced or eliminated if it is used in combination with nonantioxidant anticancer compounds (i.e., it is used as a supportive compound for other therapies). When moderate doses are used in conjunction with other anticancer compounds, vitamin C could be safe and even useful.

In-vitro and In-vivo Studies

With some understanding of the basic mechanisms, we can review some highlights of the in-vitro and in-vivo studies. First we briefly discuss the pharmacokinetics of the vitamin to help understand the effects of different routes of administration.

Normal plasma levels of vitamin C are about 40 to 70 μM.[88, 89, 90] Humans eating a diet deficient in vitamin C (less than 5 milligrams of vitamin C per day) may have plasma levels of 10 μM or less.[91] A recent analysis of previously published data suggests that gastrointestinal absorption occurs in a saturable process, and renal excretion rises sharply with increasing plasma concentrations.[92] Both events serve to limit plasma concentrations. The authors of the analysis suggest that single doses of 250 to 500 milligrams will produce plasma concentrations of 70 to 100 μM, but that doses higher than this produce minor increases. They speculate that absorption could be improved by frequent small doses, especially taken with food, but even with these efforts, plasma concentrations would still be limited by concentration-dependent renal excretion.[92]

In-vitro studies suggest that high concentrations of vitamin C are needed to inhibit cancer cell proliferation. Although some cells are more sensitive than others, common IC_{50} concentrations are about 1 to 7 mM.[93, 94, 95] This is far above the normal plasma levels and those attainable with oral administration. For cells that are stimulated by vitamin C in vitro, stimulation occurs at lower concentrations, usually between 10 and 100 μM.[96, 97] These levels are within the normal range.

In spite of the fact that high concentrations normally are needed to inhibit cancer cell proliferation, some animal studies reported that oral vitamin C can inhibit tumor growth. That relatively low concentrations from oral administration can produce antitumor effects in vivo suggests the situation is complex. As mentioned, one factor may be the availability of copper ions, which would facilitate free radical production and DNA damage. Indeed, copper ions can reduce the IC_{50} of vitamin C by nearly two orders of magnitude in vitro.[63] Another factor discussed previously may be the concentration of AFR or other radicals in the vitamin C dose given, solutions containing more AFR than dry forms. A third factor may be the ability of the particular tumor cells to produce catalase. Cells with low catalase concentrations are more likely to be inhibited by low concentrations of vitamin C. Lastly, tumor grade may play a role. Well-differentiated cancer cells may be more easily inhibited, and undifferentiated cancer cells may be more easily stimulated.[98]

Many of the early studies on vitamin C in cancer patients were conducted by Linus Pauling, Ewan Cameron, and associates. In the successful human studies, vitamin C was administered in solution either orally or intravenously.[28, 31] In these and later studies by Cameron and Pauling, vitamin C was typically administered intravenously for the first 10 days at doses of 5 to 40 grams per day and orally afterward at doses of 10 to 30 grams per day; the doses most often were 10 grams per day, either by intravenous or oral administration. Based on the pharmacokinetics of vitamin C, we can assume that the high oral doses did not produce high plasma concentrations. Still, the fact they were in solution and may have contained AFR or other radicals suggests they could have contributed to an anticancer effect, if such an effect was indeed produced. Although the retrospective studies by Cameron and Pauling suggested it was, they were not randomized and blinded studies.[31, 33, 99] The evidence from these studies is not as strong as it would have been in randomized, blinded ones.

To give an idea of the benefits reported by Cameron and Pauling, survival data are presented in Figure 15.2 from a study of 100 terminal patients with various cancers (data from reference 31). Vitamin C was administered as discussed above. Survival was compared to the average of 10 matched historical pairs treated in the same hospital without vitamin C. The dotted vertical line at a 1-fold change signifies no effect. Although about 20 percent of the patients actually had lower survival than matched pairs, the negative effect does not appear to be statistically significant. The axis of the figure is broken at a value of 11—the highest increase for a patient was about a 43-fold increase. Overall, the geometric average survival was about 2.2-fold greater than matched pairs (96 versus 45 days). A Japanese retrospective trial on 130 cancer patients using similar methods reported similar gains in survival.[100]

In contrast to these positive studies, note that in a prospective nonblinded trial with 25 early-stage breast cancer patients, oral administration of dry vitamin C (at 3 grams per day) to 13 patients did not affect five-year survival in comparison to controls.[34] Moreover, the study implied that a subset of patients who took vitamin C might actually have died faster than controls but that those in the vitamin C group who lived suffered fewer recurrences. This negative effect was not statistically analyzed and may have been an artifact of the small study population.

Estimated Therapeutic and LOAEL Doses of Vitamin C

As stated earlier, I do not view orally administered vitamin C as an essential element in cancer therapy but rather as a supportive compound to be used only with other anticancer compounds. In this regard, it may have some benefit.

If used alone, its efficacy could be improved by combining it with copper or giving it in solution (especially intravenously at high doses); these would induce a prooxidant effect. While a prooxidant therapy may have benefits in the short term, it may have adverse effects in the long term. For one thing, prooxidant therapies are unlikely to destroy every cancer cell in the body, and those that survive the oxidative conditions could be primed for an increased rate of gene mutations, leading to a more aggressive cancer. Although this possibility is still a matter of debate, it may have been suggested by some human studies on vitamin C. According to Cameron, advanced cancer patients treated with vitamin C solutions (often intravenously) typically experienced an initial plateau of comparative well-being lasting for

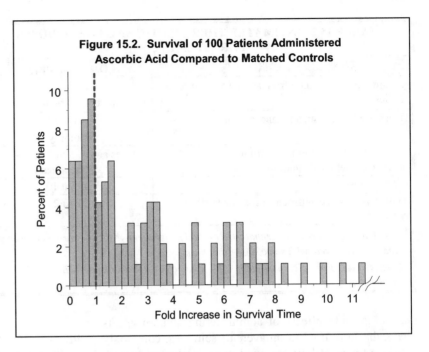

Figure 15.2. Survival of 100 Patients Administered Ascorbic Acid Compared to Matched Controls

months or even years, then entered an abrupt downhill phase with explosive metastasis.[101] It is reasonable to suppose that the oxidative conditions produced by the vitamin C solutions could have led to an increased mutation rate, eventually creating a more aggressive and better-adapted cancer.

In addition, a prooxidant therapy could induce cancers in healthy tissue. Many anticancer drugs, such as doxorubicin, mitomycin, and bleomycin, as well as radiotherapy, induce apoptosis or necrosis through a prooxidant mechanism.[102, 103] The risk of secondary cancers induced by chemotherapy or radiotherapy is substantial.[104]

In light of the above, this book does not advocate the use of vitamin C as a prooxidant, and again considers vitamin C as a supportive compound to be used within a larger combination of natural compounds.

Human studies have employed oral doses between about 3 and 30 grams per day, while animal studies have used a somewhat larger range of doses, as scaled to humans. Based on the pharmacokinetics of vitamin C and considering our purposes, a dose of about 1 to 2 grams per day divided into three administrations may be sufficient. The estimated therapeutic doses are summarized in Table 15.2.

To be complete, we also look at the use of higher doses. In human studies, the primary side effect of high doses was diarrhea, which occurred at oral doses near or above 10 grams per day. Other than such gastrointestinal effects, oral vitamin C is generally considered free of adverse reactions, but the potential for these is greatly increased by intravenous administration. According to

TABLE 15.2 ESTIMATED THERAPEUTIC AND LOAEL DOSES FOR VITAMIN C

DESCRIPTION	DOSE (g/day)
Required dose as scaled from animal antitumor studies	0.2 to 60 (average about 20)[*]
Doses used in human anticancer studies	3 to 30[†] (commonly 10)
Required dose as determined from pharmacokinetic calculations	doses above 1 to 2 grams are not necessary
LOAEL dose	about 10
Tentative dose recommendation for further research	**1 to 2**

[*] *Based on nine animal studies that used oral administration. Note that results of these studies were mixed, with some suggesting harm.*

[†] *Some studies, especially those using higher range doses, administered vitamin C intravenously.*

Cameron, side effects of administering sodium ascorbate, the form used in intravenous solutions, commonly include transient fluid retention due to sodium overload, which may be dangerous in patients with cardiac impairment. Side effects may rarely include life-threatening septicemic shock caused by sudden necrosis of the tumor load.[105] Because sensitivities are possible, Cameron advised low initial test doses. Contraindications include renal insufficiency, hemodialysis patients, and unusual iron overload.[106] The danger of oxalate stone formation suggested by some early investigators does not appear to be well founded.[107, 108] Before intravenous dosing, screening for red blood cell dehydrogenase deficiency is recommended. An intravenous dose as high as 150 grams over a 24-hour period appears to be safe.[106] Slow drip (eight-hour) intravenous infusion of 60 to 115 grams is capable of maintaining a plasma concentration of 5,700 μM without causing short-term adverse effects.

Synergism and Vitamin C

A number of natural compounds appear to act synergistically with vitamin C to produce cytotoxic effects via stimulation of free radicals. These include vitamin K_3 and high-molecular-weight compounds such as PSK and lignans. Each is described briefly below. Since their clinical use would involve prooxidant mechanisms, as well as intravenous administration, such synergistic combinations are not advocated; they are mentioned only because some readers may find references to them in the literature.

Vitamin K is used medicinally as a procoagulant agent in hemorrhagic (bleeding) diseases and as an antidote to anticoagulant overdose. Vitamin K_3 potentiates the cytotoxic effects of vitamin C in vitro, the optimum ratio being approximately 1:100. This combination may be 4- to 61-fold more potent than vitamin C alone, depending on the cell line and exposure times.[109, 110] Vitamin K_3 by itself also displays cytotoxic activity in a variety of cell lines. In addition, it augments the antitumor effect of the anticoagulant drug warfarin and the antitumor activity of a number of cytotoxic drugs when used with vitamin C.[111–117] Possible mechanisms of vitamin K_3 antitumor activity include induction of free radical damage, inhibition of DNA synthesis, induction of apoptosis, modulation of coagulation, and inhibition of growth factor binding. The antitumor effects of a combination of vitamins C and K_3 are completely prevented by the addition of catalase, suggesting that free radical production is a necessary component.[118]

High-molecular-weight substances such as the mushroom extract PSK and lignans from pine cones increase vitamin C oxidation and synergistically enhance the cytotoxicity of vitamin C against human leukemia and brain cancer cells in vitro.[119, 120, 121] Again, a prooxidant mechanism is at work. Optimal results in vitro are obtained when a sodium solution is used to dissolve vitamin C, the mixture is freshly made before testing, the vitamin C concentration is 300 μM or greater, and the lignin to vitamin C ratio is roughly 20 to 1 (weight to weight).

Combining vitamin K_3 or high-molecular-weight substances with vitamin C is not practical for our purposes. To provide optimal results, high concentrations of vitamin C are still required, which would require intravenous administration. To achieve sufficient plasma concentrations, vitamin K_3 would also need to be administered intravenously. Lastly, the required dose of PSK or other lignans would be excessive. Both vitamin K_3 and PSK can, of course, be used in combination with vitamin C, but it is unlikely that using these compounds alone at oral doses applicable to humans would produce significant synergistic effects or high cell kill.

ANTIOXIDANTS

In the following sections, we explore the effects of antioxidants in general. Many issues that applied to vitamin C apply to other antioxidants as well, and our preliminary conclusions regarding their use are the same as those for vitamin C. In short, most antioxidants have the capacity to increase, decrease, or not effect cancer cell proliferation. To help assure an anticancer effect, they are best used as supportive agents within a larger combination of natural compounds and/or drugs.

In-vitro Redox Effects of Antioxidants

We begin by looking at the potential of antioxidants to act as prooxidants. Since we are not seeking a prooxidant effect, it is important to know when such an effect may be produced; it becomes more likely when single antioxidants are used and doses are large. Conversely, an antioxidant effect is more likely with combinations of antioxidants used at moderate oral doses.

As with vitamin C, most antioxidants exhibit both antioxidant and prooxidant effects in vitro, depending on conditions that include the concentration of the antioxidant, the presence of other antioxidants, and the presence of iron and copper ions. Table 15.3 summarizes some studies on the prooxidant capabilities of compounds normally considered antioxidants. Note that other compounds discussed in this book can also produce prooxidant effects. For example, omega-3 fatty acids, at high doses, can inhibit tumor growth in vivo through a prooxidant mechanism.[122, 123] These doses are larger than those recommended in this book, however (see Chapter 17).

In contrast to the studies listed in the table, a large number have also documented the antioxidant capabilities for each of these compounds in vitro. Thus, the data in Table 15.3 show only half the story; nonetheless, they clearly reveal that antioxidant compounds can produce prooxidant effects under the right circumstances. In light of the discussion on vitamin C, this is not surprising.

The fact that antioxidants can produce prooxidant effects in vitro complicates interpretation of some in-vitro studies on cancer cells. For example, in the studies

TABLE 15.3 PROOXIDANT EFFECTS OF ANTIOXIDANTS IN VITRO	
COMPOUND	COMMENT
Apigenin and luteolin	• In tests on a series of flavonoids, apigenin produced the greatest prooxidant effect independent of metal ions. Apparently, apigenin oxidized intracellular glutathione, and the oxidized glutathione then participated in the generation of additional free radicals.[124, 125] • Apigenin and luteolin acted as antioxidants at low iron concentrations but as prooxidants at high iron concentrations.[126]
Beta-carotene	• Induced DNA damage in cancer cells via a prooxidant mechanism.[127]
Curcumin	• Induced DNA damage in the presence of copper.[128, 129] • Induced apoptosis in cancer cells through a prooxidant mechanism, and antioxidants prevented curcumin-induced apoptosis.[130, 131]
EGCG	• Induced apoptosis in human lung cancer cells through a prooxidant mechanism.[132]
Glutathione	• Glutathione (and NADH) induced DNA damage in the presence of copper through a prooxidant mechanism.[69, 133, 134]
N-acetylcysteine (NAC)	• Induced DNA damage in the presence of copper via a prooxidant mechanism.[70]
Quercetin	• Mutagenic in vitro due to its ability to induce DNA damage through a prooxidant mechanism. • Induced DNA damage in the presence of copper via a prooxidant mechanism.[135] • Produced dose-dependent cytotoxic effects due to a prooxidant mechanism.[136]
Vitamin A	• Retinol induced DNA damage in whole cells and in isolated DNA in the presence of copper via a prooxidant mechanism.[137]
Vitamin E	• Induced DNA damage in the presence of copper via a prooxidant mechanism.[138]

summarized in the table, curcumin induced apoptosis in cancer cells in vitro through a prooxidant mechanism. Under normal in-vivo conditions, however, curcumin is more likely to produce an antioxidant effect. Consequently, the relevance of the curcumin studies listed, as well as those for other compounds, to in-vivo conditions is uncertain. In other words, these in-vitro studies cannot be construed as suggesting these compounds will be useful in cancer therapy. Fortunately, however, other in-vitro studies reviewed in this book do suggest their usefulness, only not as prooxidants. Indeed, their ability to act as antioxidants in most situations may support their other anticancer actions, such as inhibition of signal transduction, for example.

In-vivo Redox Effects of Antioxidants

As with in-vitro studies, the effects an antioxidant produces in vivo are likely to be dependent on its concentration, the presence of metal ions, and the amount of other antioxidants and ROS present. In addition, the metabolism of the compound can greatly affect its redox reactivity. For example, quercetin, which shows both antioxidant and prooxidant effects in vitro, occurs in the plasma mainly in its conjugate forms (i.e., quercetin combined with glucuronic acid, a derivative of glucose). The conjugate form is less reactive than free quercetin in vitro and generally acts as a mild antioxidant in vivo.[139–143]

Similar to vitamin C, normal dietary doses of most antioxidants will probably have antioxidant effects in most in-vivo conditions, and one is more assured if combinations of antioxidants are used.[144] For example, oral administration of a diverse group and high quantity of antioxidants produced greater protection from oxidative damage in rodents than fewer antioxidants and lower quantities.[145, 146, 147] In another study, combinations of antioxidants were more effective in reducing cancer initiation in hamsters than single antioxidants.[148] Like vitamin C, however, all antioxidants are capable of acting as prooxidants under limited circumstances. As the dose increases beyond a crucial point, the chances of producing a prooxidant effect also increase, especially when used alone or given intravenously.

One antioxidant that has received quite a bit of attention is beta-carotene. In a large trial on smokers (the Beta-Carotene and Retinol Efficiency Trial), researchers found that 30 milligrams of beta-carotene per day actually increased lung cancer rates.[149–154] Reasons for this unexpected effect are still uncertain but are probably due to oxidation of beta-carotene in the free-radical-rich environment of a smoker's lungs and/or the altered metabolism of beta carotene caused by changed detoxification enzymes in the smoker's lungs.[155] One other factor may have been the high plasma concentration of beta-carotene produced, relative to that provided by normal dietary intake. For example, one in-vitro study reported that at concentrations created by normal dietary intake (1 to 3 μM), beta-carotene provided protection from oxidative DNA damage. However, at concentrations just above this level (4 to 10 μM, as can be produced during supplementation), the protection was lost and beta-carotene (and lycopene) facilitated DNA damage.[156]

Other human studies on in-vivo effects of beta-carotene are mixed. Some reported that supplementation of beta-carotene had no effect on oxidative DNA damage in lymphocytes, while others found that beta-carotene supplementation (at 25 milligrams per day) was protective.[157–160] Still others reported that beta-carotene (at 60 milligrams per day) increased oxidative damage in the lymphocytes of smokers but was protective in nonsmokers.[161]

The effect of vitamin E on DNA damage has also been studied in vivo. Again, studies suggest vitamin E can produce antioxidant or prooxidant effects, depending on conditions. Vitamin E supplementation (at 280 milligrams per day) produced both DNA protection in human lymphocytes and, under the right conditions, carcinogenic effects in animals.[138, 158, 162] One study reported that susceptibility of red blood cells to oxidative damage was increased by high and prolonged doses of vitamin E (1600 I.U. per day for 20 weeks) in nonsmokers, but not at lower doses, for shorter time periods, or in smokers.[163] Supplementation with normal therapeutic doses of vitamin E (400 to 800 I.U. per day) probably produces antioxidant effects under most in-vivo conditions.[164]

The effect of other antioxidants on oxidative DNA damage has been studied in vivo as well. From earlier discussions, we know that high doses of vitamin C (especially given intravenously) can produce prooxidant effects in vivo. In other studies, oral supplementation with small doses of vitamin C (100 to 250 milligrams per day) protected DNA from oxidative damage in humans, while in still others, oral vitamin C showed no protective effect.[158, 160, 161, 162] Neutral results were seen in one of these studies even though plasma concentration of vitamin C increased during supplementation.

Even studies on multivitamin supplements have produced surprising results. One reported that multivitamin supplements increased mortality from cancer in male smokers but decreased it in nonsmokers or quitters.[165] Some subjects took additional vitamin A, C, or E with their multivitamins, and the results were the same.

The inconsistencies in these experiments again point to the dynamic nature of redox reactions in vivo and the likelihood that various factors, such as antioxidant dose, the presence of other antioxidants, the presence of metal ions, and the degree of oxidative stress, may determine the effect seen. It is hoped that future studies on antioxidants will consider these factors in their design. For example, we may one day find that doses of antioxidants are best determined based on the results of patient monitoring. Along these lines, one recent study on the use of *N*-acetylcysteine (NAC) to treat cancer cachexia (tissue wasting) based the dose on the plasma cystine to thiol ratio (this ratio is an indicator of oxidative stress).[166] In this type of design, an excess amount of antioxidants would not be given, and any prooxidant effects produced would be quickly discovered.

Implications for Cancer Therapy

From the above discussions, we see that high doses of antioxidant compounds can produce prooxidant effects in vivo, especially when single antioxidants are given. This, of course, is a drawback to using high doses in cancer therapy. An antioxidant effect is likely, however, if moderate to low doses of antioxidants are used, and they are used in combination.

If antioxidants are used to produce an antioxidant rather than prooxidant effect, the antioxidant effect produced will generally be beneficial to the body. For example, immune cells may function better when they contain adequate antioxidants. Cancer cells may also benefit, however. Using antioxidants in cancer treatment is currently a matter of much debate, and it is especially heated regarding use of antioxidants in combination with chemotherapy. In theory, because many chemotherapy drugs act by generating ROS, antioxidants could reduce ROS-induced apoptosis in cancer cells. Indeed, several in-vitro studies have reported that antioxidants can protect cancer cells from ROS-induced apoptosis.[167–173] Moreover, in-vitro and in-vivo studies have reported that low levels of glutathione within cancer cells can increase apoptosis induced by both immune cells and chemotherapy.[174–177] Lastly, antioxidants are known to protect tumors under some therapeutic circumstances; for example, vitamin E can markedly reduce the anticancer effects of large doses of fish oil in animals.[122]

In spite of the above, many of the animal studies have reported that antioxidants do not increase tumor growth and do not reduce the effectiveness of chemotherapy. Some have actually found that the effectiveness of chemotherapy increases with antioxidant use (see Chapter 23). Still, the antioxidant issue is complex, and some animal studies have reported that antioxidants (vitamin C) can increase tumor growth. Fortunately, a number of animal and human studies are in the planning stages or will soon be completed. Their results should help clarify the conditions in which antioxidants may be beneficial or detrimental.

Even if antioxidants like vitamins C or E are found to be detrimental on their own or to decrease the efficacy of chemotherapy, these findings will not necessarily negate possible benefits from using natural compounds. We consider antioxidants as supportive compounds, rather than as primary anticancer agents. Therefore, if it became necessary, primary antioxidants like vitamin C could be omitted from therapy. To test the theories of this book, large combinations of natural compounds, rather than groups of antioxidant vitamins, will need to be studied in vivo.

A Theory on Antioxidant Effects

If we bring together what is known, it is possible to construct a theory that makes sense of the conflicting data and goes beyond the simplistic argument of whether antioxidants are good or bad. Instead, we focus attention on how different conditions within various patients might alter the effects of antioxidants on cancer cell proliferation.

The conclusions from this theory were summarized in Chapter 2, where we stated that depending on the circumstances, antioxidants used alone could produce beneficial, detrimental, or insignificant effects in cancer patients. When used in combination with other anticancer compounds (i.e., natural compounds or chemotherapy drugs), however, their effects are more likely to be beneficial, or at least not harmful. Lastly, we concluded that even when beneficial, the effects will probably be mild for many patients. For these reasons, we see antioxidants as supportive agents, best used in larger combinations of cancer-inhibiting compounds.

The graphs presented here pull together our knowledge about the relationship between changes in oxidative stress and changes in cancer cell proliferation. They illustrate a plausible answer to the question, why do antioxidants have different effects in different situations? The graphs are not meant to represent exact numerical values but simply to put the general results of research in graphic form.

Figure 15.3 illustrates the approximate relationship between oxidative stress at the tumor site and cancer cell proliferation. We see that at levels of oxidative stress normal for healthy tissue (point A on the curve), cancer cell proliferation is low; at stress levels that are mildly elevated for healthy tissue (point D), cancer cell proliferation is high; and at levels high for healthy tissue (point H), cancer cells are killed.

We know from previous chapters that mild oxidative stress can assist cancer cell proliferation in many ways, so proliferation will be high at sites that experience mild stress. For example, oxidative stress can increase sensitivity of growth factor receptors and PKC, decrease the function of the p53 protein, and increase NF-κB activity, angiogenesis, and invasion. We also know that high oxidative stress will kill cancer cells, as it does other kinds of cells. Moreover, we can assume that normal (or nominal) oxidative stress will effect proliferation somewhere between that of mild and high stress. Note that this figure takes into account only the component of cancer cell proliferation related to oxidative stress. To determine actual tumor growth or inhibition, other factors, such as inhibition of proliferation due to drugs or immune activity, would need to be factored in.

Figure 15.3 does not reveal the role antioxidants play in oxidative stress and cancer cell proliferation. Intracellular antioxidants certainly do affect the level of oxi-

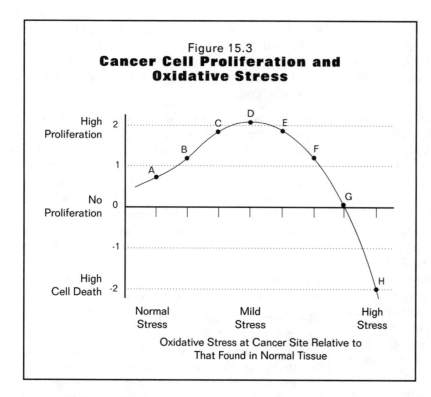

Figure 15.3
Cancer Cell Proliferation and Oxidative Stress

Oxidative Stress at Cancer Site Relative to That Found in Normal Tissue

dant intake cannot keep up with the rate of antioxidant depletion.

Second, the figure indicates there is a limit to the total amount of antioxidants that can be taken up by cancer cells, if they are still to act as antioxidants (high concentrations could act as prooxidants). This is indicated by the horizontal line at the top of the graph.

Third, cancer cells tend to have a higher antioxidant reserve than the body as a whole. Tumors exist in an oxidative environment, and to cope with their environment, they tend to trap antioxidants. For example, cancer cells are known to sequester high concentrations of vitamins C and E in vivo.[81, 178–182] High concentrations of glutathione have also been found in cancer cells relative to surrounding cells.[180, 183, 184] Looking at an example in the figure, point B on the bottom curve represents a condition of normal extracellular ROS concentration at a tumor site in a patient with low body reserves of antioxidants. In this situation, the cancer cells would tend to have moderate antioxidant reserves (as shown on the vertical axis) as opposed to the low levels in other body tissues.

dative stress, but they are not the only factor; an equally important one is the magnitude of ROS concentrations around the cell. Since three factors are involved (antioxidant reserves, ROS concentrations, and cell proliferation), a three-dimensional graph is needed to show their relationships. Figure 15.4 is the equivalent of such a graph. The vertical axis shows the level of antioxidant reserves in the cancer cells and the horizontal axis shows the level of ROS at the tumor site. Points A through H, which refer back to Figure 15.3, show the degree of proliferation (point D is the highest, point H is the lowest, and so on). Figure 15.4 also adds a missing element—the patient, who has a certain level of antioxidant reserves in his body. The three curved lines represent patients with relatively low, moderate, or high body antioxidant reserves. Note that antioxidant reserves in the body are generally not the same as those in cancer cells, which can sequester antioxidants.

What happens to cell proliferation when the patient's level of antioxidant reserves is changed by giving antioxidants? Several examples are given below, using Figures 15.3 and 15.4 as a basis. First, however, some fundamental relationships illustrated in the latter figure need to be highlighted.

Figure 15.4 shows that as ROS concentrations at the cancer site increase, antioxidant reserves in the cancer cells decrease for all three types of patients, and they decrease most dramatically for each at high ROS concentrations; at high levels of ROS, the rate of antioxi-

Lastly, the figure illustrates that cancer cells in patients with low antioxidant reserves are more susceptible to oxidative stress than cancer cells in patients with high antioxidant reserves, as would be expected. For example, point D from Figure 15.3 represents a condition of mild oxidative stress where cancer cell proliferation is at a maximum. In Figure 15.4, this same point D is marked on each of the three curves representing patients with different body antioxidant reserves. As expected, when ROS concentrations increase, point D occurs first in patients with low antioxidant reserves and last in ones with high reserves. A similar statement can be made for any of the other points marked in Figure 15.3. For example, point H represents a point of high oxidative stress; in Figure 15.4, as ROS concentrations increase, point H is reached first in patients with low antioxidant reserves and last in those with high reserves.

Now we look at four examples of how antioxidant supplementation may affect cancer cell proliferation under different circumstances. We examine the circumstances in which we would expect supplementation to greatly increase cancer cell proliferation, moderately decrease proliferation, have little effect either way, and finally, to moderately increase proliferation. These discussions refer to what happens in an average cancer cell; any given cell in a tumor may experience a greater or lesser amount of oxidative stress and may react accordingly. When reading these examples, keep in mind that Figures 15.3 and 15.4 take into account only the component of cancer cell proliferation related to oxidative stress. Actual tumor growth or inhibition also depends on additional factors like the actions of drugs, other natural compounds, or immune cells.

Conditions That May Greatly Increase Cancer Cell Proliferation

We can see that antioxidant supplementation could greatly increase cancer cell proliferation by looking, for example, at the point marked H on the bottom curve of Figure 15.4. Here we have the situation of high oxidant stress (fairly high extracellular ROS concentrations in a patient with low antioxidant reserves). If this patient is given a sizable dose of antioxidants, enough to create high reserves, we can follow an imaginary vertical line going up through this point H to the top curve (since we now have a patient with high antioxidant reserves), where we arrive at point F. Looking at Figure 15.3, we see that a movement from point H to point F represents a dramatic increase in proliferation of about 3 units (from –2 to 1). (Again, the units of proliferation are arbitrary and are only intended to allow statements on general trends.)

Such an increase would be expected. In highly oxidizing conditions, cancer cell proliferation is likely to be limited both by oxidative damage and by the generation of lipid peroxides, which can act as negative regulators of proliferation in most cell lines.[185–188] Giving antioxidants in this situation would greatly decrease oxidative stress and the formation of lipid peroxides, and thereby increase cancer cell proliferation. This is not necessarily bad, however. Such high levels of oxidative stress would most likely occur in patients undergoing conventional chemotherapy, and for these, an increase in cancer cell proliferation is actually beneficial. Since most chemotherapy drugs currently in use will not kill cells unless they are actively proliferating, such an increase should enhance the effectiveness of chemotherapy.[189]

In addition, in conditions of high oxidant stress, antioxidants can induce cancer cells to die of apoptosis rather than necrosis. Apoptosis is the preferred form of cell death. As discussed in Chapter 3, cells dying of

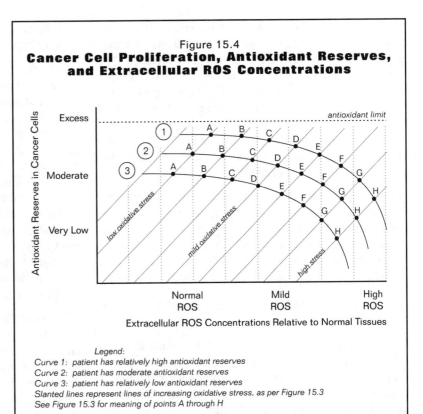

Figure 15.4
Cancer Cell Proliferation, Antioxidant Reserves, and Extracellular ROS Concentrations

antioxidant limit

Antioxidant Reserves in Cancer Cells

Excess

Moderate

Very Low

① ② ③

A B C D E
A B C D E F
A B C D E F G
      F G H
         G H
            H

low oxidative stress

mild oxidative stress

high stress

Normal ROS   Mild ROS   High ROS

Extracellular ROS Concentrations Relative to Normal Tissues

Legend:
Curve 1: patient has relatively high antioxidant reserves
Curve 2: patient has moderate antioxidant reserves
Curve 3: patient has relatively low antioxidant reserves
Slanted lines represent lines of increasing oxidative stress, as per Figure 15.3
See Figure 15.3 for meaning of points A through H

apoptosis are engulfed by macrophages before they can rupture and spill their contents, but necrotic cells discharge their contents into the extracellular space before they are devoured. Necrosis and the resulting spillage have a number of disadvantages. For one thing, spillage produces inflammation, which is associated with ROS production and increased cancer progression. Moreover, it reduces the ability of macrophages to present the tumor's antigens to T cells, which need antigen presentation to target other cancer cells. The ingestion of tumor antigens by macrophages, and hence antigen presentation, is more efficient when whole apoptotic cells rather than bits and pieces of necrotic cells are ingested. The oxidative stress caused by chemotherapy drugs, coupled with the preexisting oxidative stress at the tumor site, appears to favor necrosis, and so inhibits the effectiveness of chemotherapy drugs.[190] Antioxidants, by decreasing oxidative stress and favoring apoptosis, could increase the effectiveness of conventional chemotherapy.

Conditions That May Decrease Cancer Cell Proliferation

A situation in which antioxidant supplementation could moderately decrease cancer cell proliferation is seen at the point marked D on the bottom curve of Figure 15.4. Here we have the situation of mild oxidant stress (normal to mild extracellular ROS concentrations in a patient with low antioxidant reserves). If this patient is given a sizable dose of antioxidants to create high reserves, we can follow an imaginary vertical line going up through this point D to the top curve, arriving midway between points B and C. Looking at Figure 15.3, we see that a movement from point D to midway between points B and C represents a decrease in proliferation of about one half-unit (from 2 to 1.5), which is a moderate decrease relative to the increase of 3 units discussed in the previous example.

This scenario would probably develop in patients who have not undergone chemotherapy, since ROS concentrations here are only moderately elevated. In these conditions, antioxidants could inhibit cell proliferation by several means, such as normalizing the activity of growth factor receptors, PKC, and transcription factors.

Conditions That May Have Little Effect on Cancer Cell Proliferation

Antioxidant supplementation could have only minimal effects on cancer cell proliferation. In the previous examples, giving antioxidants to patients with low reserves produced high reserves. Now, we consider the more common example of a patient with normal antioxidant reserves and with extracellular ROS concentrations a bit stronger than mild; this might be the case of a patient with early- to mid-stage cancer who has not undergone chemotherapy. This situation is represented by point E both in Figure 15.3 and on the middle curve of Figure 15.4. In other words, tumors in most patients not receiving chemotherapy probably exist in an oxidative environment on the verge of causing extensive cell kill if oxidative stress increases. If this patient is given enough antioxidants to create high reserves, we can follow an imaginary vertical line up through point E to the top curve, just to the right of point D. In Figure 15.3, we see that moving from point E to the right of point D represents almost no change in proliferation.

Based on animal studies, this may be a common scenario. A recent study on mice looked at the effects of antioxidant depletion and supplementation on the growth of de novo brain tumors.[191] The authors reported that severe depletion of dietary antioxidants (vitamins E and A) inhibited tumor growth via a prooxidant mechanism. Administration of moderate amounts of antioxidants (170 I.U. vitamin E and 9,200 I.U. vitamin A as scaled to humans), however, did not appreciably affect tumor growth compared to controls receiving half this amount (normal dietary amounts). In addition, several other animal studies reported that antioxidant administration did not greatly affect tumor growth one way or the other (see below and Chapter 23).

Conditions That May Moderately Increase Cancer Cell Proliferation

Consider the case of a terminal cancer patient who is not going through chemotherapy. Antioxidant reserves may be depleted and oxidative stress may be relatively high, but not as high as if chemotherapy were given. The proliferation of the patient's cancer cells would fall, on average, around point F on Figure 15.3, somewhere between maximal and no proliferation. In Figure 15.4, this situation corresponds to point F on the bottom curve. If the patient receives enough antioxidants to create high reserves, we can follow an imaginary vertical line up through point F to the top curve, just to the right of point D. Looking at Figure 15.3, we see that a movement from point H to the right of point D represents an increase in proliferation of about 3/4 units, which is a moderate increase.

It is possible this type of scenario occurred in some of the vitamin C animal studies where tumor growth increased. In fact, since dietary vitamin C tends to increase iron absorption, and iron tends to increase ROS production, it may be that a more extreme situation was happening (i.e., starting closer to point G on the bottom curve of Figure 15.4). Because of the potential for antioxidants to increase tumor growth by this means, we again conclude that antioxidants are best not used alone.

We look now at how other natural compounds could turn a detrimental result of antioxidant use into a beneficial one. It seems reasonable to suppose that combinations of compounds that act primarily by nonantioxidant mechanisms to inhibit signal transduction and the other clusters of procancer events (see Chapter 1) could produce an anticancer effect regardless of whether primary antioxidants were also used. In fact, since primary antioxidants could put more cells in the cell cycle, they might increase an anticancer effect, just as they may do with chemotherapy.

There is one other way primary antioxidants could work with other natural compounds to maximize an anticancer effect. Looking again at Figure 15.3, the most beneficial point on the curve from the patient's perspective is point A. (Point H is more desirable in terms of cell death but is less so in terms of oxidative stress.) In Figure 15.4, if cancer cells in the average patient might be at point E (on any curve), we see that the greatest opportunity to reach point A for all three types of patients is by decreasing ROS generation, not increasing antioxidant reserves. In other words, antioxidant supplementation can play a supportive role in reaching point A, but the main therapeutic emphasis is better placed on decreasing ROS production. Such a decrease can be accomplished by using anti-inflammatory compounds, compounds that reduce iron and copper levels, and compounds that prevent tissue damage, such as enzyme inhibitors and ECM protectors. Anti-inflammatory compounds include those that inhibit PGE_2 production, NF-κB activity, vascular permeability, and histamine release. To some degree, the use of antioxidants alone will also reduce extracellular ROS levels, but they would not necessarily reduce ROS generation.

Still, in Figure 15.3 we see that reaching point A is not enough to kill tumor cells, only to reduce their proliferation. It follows that antioxidants and compounds that reduce ROS generation must be combined with other compounds that inhibit cancer through other means.

In summary, we can theorize that antioxidant supplementation will increase, decrease, or have only mild effects on cancer cell proliferation, depending on the antioxidant reserves of the patient and the concentration of extracellular ROS. To avoid detrimental effects, they should probably not be used alone. In those cases where they are used with other anticancer compounds or chemotherapy drugs, and proliferation is increased, this could be beneficial because it may help to increase cell kill. When antioxidants are used with other natural compounds, their anticancer effects could be maximized by including compounds that reduce ROS generation, such as anti-inflammatory compounds.

Antioxidants may have other beneficial effects; for example, they can protect normal tissues from adverse effects of chemotherapy, at least in some cases (see Chapter 23). In addition, they may reduce the mutation rate and, over time, result in less aggressive cancers, ones less able to adapt to changing conditions. Although this effect remains to be proven in vivo, it is a reasonable supposition. Lastly, antioxidants can help normal tissues function correctly. Because immune cells need a certain amount of antioxidants to function, taking antioxidants can produce healthier immune cells, which are more likely to inhibit cancer than unhealthy ones.

Effects of Antioxidants on Metastasis

There are concerns that antioxidants may facilitate metastasis. That they may have this effect in some situations should not be surprising, given the above discussions. In one of the few animal studies that tested combined antioxidants, metastasis increased.[192] In this study, high and very high doses of antioxidants were given in drinking water to rats with established, carcinogen-induced tumors. The high doses were about 2.4 grams of vitamin C and 1,200 I.U. of vitamin E per day (as scaled to humans). The very high doses were 10-fold greater. Both groups received selenium (at 2 μg/kg) and a thiol antioxidant compound (2-MPG, at 15

mg/kg). The high-dose therapy was not effective in increasing life span nor was tumor size greater, but secondary metastases increased. Life span was increased 1.4-fold in the very high dose group, but again secondary metastases increased equal to the high-dose group. The results suggest the antioxidants may have protected metastasizing cells from apoptosis. Perhaps metastasizing cells are under greater oxidative stress than tumor cells and require additional antioxidants. They are certainly under great oxidative stress while they travel through the lungs during circulation. Another study also reported that synthetic antioxidants increased metastasis of lung cancer cells injected into mice but did not affect growth of the primary tumor that formed.[193] Moreover, other studies have reported metastasizing cells are protected from apoptosis by high intracellular glutathione levels in vivo.[194, 195] As we will see in Chapter 18, some antioxidants, including vitamins C and E, increase intracellular glutathione concentrations.[196, 197]

The above discussions indicate that primary antioxidants have the potential to promote metastasis, another reason to avoid their sole use. If they are used in combination with other cancer inhibitors, any assistance antioxidants may give to metastatic cells should, in theory, be negated by the effects of the other active compounds. Along these lines, secondary antioxidants could be expected to inhibit cancer more potently than primary ones.

Antioxidants may be more useful in preventing cancer than treating established cancers. A recent large clinical trial reported that prostate cancer rates were lowered in smokers who took vitamin E supplements.[198] A mixture of natural compounds is likely to be even more effective. Even mixtures of primary antioxidants may be more useful than single ones, as reported recently for a combination of vitamin C and N-acetylcysteine (NAC) in mice.[199]

Antioxidant supplements also seem to be useful in preventing recurrence after treatment. For example, they were a prominent part of a protocol used in a randomized, double-blind study of 65 postsurgical patients with bladder cancer.[40] All patients were treated with the immunostimulating bacterial compound BCG. Those who received RDA doses of multivitamins plus 40,000 I.U. vitamin A, 100 milligrams vitamin B6, 2 grams vitamin C, 400 I.U. vitamin E, and 90 milligrams zinc per day had a 41 percent recurrence rate after five years. In comparison, those receiving only BCG plus RDA multivitamins had 91 percent recurrence.

CONCLUSION

The in-vitro, animal, and human cancer studies on vitamin C have produced inconsistent results, probably due in part to vitamin C prooxidant effects. These effects appear to be mediated by a number of conditions, including the concentration of the antioxidant, the presence of metal ions, the concentration of ROS present, and the tumor's ability to produce antioxidant enzymes. Based on available evidence, it appears that vitamin C could inhibit or facilitate tumor progression, or have no effect, depending on the above conditions.

Although other antioxidant compounds have not received as much study as vitamin C, it is likely they will behave similarly. When used alone at high doses, especially, high intravenous ones or orally in copper solutions, they may also have a prooxidant effect and kill cancer cells. On the other hand, when used orally at moderate doses, vitamin C and other antioxidants are likely to create an antioxidant effect, especially when used in combination.

Based on the limited data available, our preliminary conclusions are that antioxidants can produce variable results on cancer cell proliferation. Depending on oxidative stress at the cancer site, they could increase or decrease cancer cell proliferation, or have only nominal effects on it. The same may also be true of their effects on metastasis. For these reasons, antioxidants are not considered here as sole treatment agents, but they are viewed as potentially useful in a supportive role, in combination with other compounds or drugs. (We refer here to antioxidant supplementation; normal dietary intake is likely safe under any circumstances.) Antioxidants may be most beneficial when combined with compounds that inhibit ROS generation, since together these groups of compounds can reduce oxidative stress at cancer sites, leading to minimal proliferation. To induce apoptosis in cancer cells, however, antioxidants and anti-ROS compounds are best combined with other natural compounds that inhibit cancer by other means.

REFERENCES

[1] Maramag C, Menon M, Balaji KC, et al. Effect of vitamin C on prostate cancer cells in vitro: Effect on cell number, viability, and DNA synthesis. Prostate 1997 Aug 1; 32(3):188–95.

[2] Leung PY, Miyashita K, Young M, Tsao CS. Cytotoxic effect of ascorbate and its derivatives on cultured malignant and nonmalignant cell lines. Anticancer Res 1993 Mar–Apr; 13(2):475–80.

[3] Sakagami H, Satoh K, Ohata H, et al. Relationship between ascorbyl radical intensity and apoptosis-inducing activity. Anticancer Res 1996 Sep–Oct; 16(5A):2635–44.

[4] Bishun N, Basu TK, Metcalfe S, Williams DC. The effect of ascorbic acid (vitamin C) on two tumor cell lines in culture. Oncology 1978; 35(4):160–2.

[5] Park CH, Amare M, Savin MA, Hoogstraten B. Growth suppression of human leukemic cells in vitro by L-ascorbic acid. Cancer Res 1980 Apr; 40(4):1062–5.

[6] Park CH, Bergsagel DE, McCulloch EA. Ascorbic acid: A culture requirement for colony formation by mouse plasmacytoma cells. Science 1971 Nov; 174(10):720–2.

[7] Liotti FS, Menghini AR, Guerrieri P, et al. Effects of ascorbic and dehydroascorbic acid on the multiplication of tumor ascites cells in vitro. J Cancer Res Clin Oncol 1984; 108(2):230–2.

[8] Park CH, Kimler BF. Growth modulation of human leukemic, preleukemic, and myeloma progenitor cells by L-ascorbic acid. Am J Clin Nutr 1991 Dec; 54(6 Suppl):1241S-1246S.

[9] Alcain FJ, Buron MI, Rodriguez-Aguilera JC, et al. Ascorbate free radical stimulates the growth of a human promyelocytic leukemia cell line. Cancer Res 1990 Sep 15; 50(18):5887–91.

[10] Liotti FS, Bodo M, Talesa V. Stimulating effect of ascorbic acid on ascites tumor cell multiplication in vitro. J Cancer Res Clin Oncol 1983; 106(1):69–70.

[11] Park CH. Vitamin C in leukemia and preleukemia cell growth. Prog Clin Biol Res 1988; 259:321–30.

[12] Meadows GG, Pierson HF, Abdallah RM. Ascorbate in the treatment of experimental transplanted melanoma. Am J Clin Nutr 1991 Dec; 54(6 Suppl):1284S-1291S.

[13] Tsao CS. Inhibiting effect of ascorbic acid on the growth of human mammary tumor xenografts. Am J Clin Nutr 1991 Dec; 54(6 Suppl):1274S-1280S.

[14] Tsao CS, Dunham WB, Leung PY. In vivo antineoplastic activity of ascorbic acid for human mammary tumor. In Vivo 1988 Mar–Apr; 2(2):147–50.

[15] Pavelic K, Kos Z, Spaventi S. Antimetabolic activity of L-ascorbic acid in human and animal tumors. Int J Biochem 1989; 21(8):931–5.

[16] Gardiner NS, Duncan JR. Inhibition of murine melanoma growth by sodium ascorbate. J Nutr 1989 Apr; 119(4):586–90.

[17] Chakraborty A, Chatterjee R. Prevention of growth of transplanted sarcoma in mice by vitamin C. Indian J Exp Biol 1985 Aug; 23(8):472–3.

[18] Leung PY, Dunham WB, Tsao CS. Ascorbic acid with cupric ions as a chemotherapy for human lung tumor xenografts implanted beneath the renal capsule of immunocompetent mice. In Vivo 1992 Jan–Feb; 6(1):33–40.

[19] Kimoto E, Tanaka H, Gyotoku J, et al. Enhancement of antitumor activity of ascorbate against Ehrlich ascites tumor cells by the copper: glycylglycylhistidine complex. Cancer Res 1983 Feb; 43(2):824–8.

[20] Stratton JA, Rettenmaier MA, DiSaia PJ. In vivo antineoplastic activity of various biological response modifiers for tumors of the ovary and breast. J Clin Lab Immunol 1983 Aug; 11(4):181–7.

[21] Abul-Hajj YJ, Kelliher M. Failure of ascorbic acid to inhibit growth of transplantable and dimethylbenzanthracene induced rat mammary tumors. Cancer Lett 1982 Oct; 17(1):67–73.

22. Silverman J, Rivenson A, Reddy B. Effect of sodium ascorbate on transplantable murine tumors. Nutr Cancer 1983; 4(3):192–7.

23. Hubert DD, Holiat SM, Smith WE, Baylouny RA. Inhibition of transplanted carcinomas in mice by retinoids but not by vitamin C. Cancer Treat Rep 1983 Dec; 67(12):1061–5.

24. Migliozzi JA. Effect of ascorbic acid on tumour growth. Br J Cancer 1977 Apr; 35(4):448–53.

25. Kallistratos GI, Fasske EE, Karkabounas S, Charalambopoulos K. Prolongation of the survival time of tumor bearing Wistar rats through a simultaneous oral administration of vitamins C + E and selenium with glutathione. Prog Clin Biol Res 1988; 259:377–89.

26. Schwartz J, Shklar G, Trickler D. Vitamin C enhances the development of carcinomas in the hamster buccal pouch experimental model. Oral Surg Oral Med Oral Pathol 1993 Dec; 76(6):718–22.

27. Pierson HF, Meadows GG. Sodium ascorbate enhancement of carbidopa-levodopa methyl ester antitumor activity against pigmented B16 melanoma. Cancer Res 1983 May; 43(5):2047–51.

28. Cameron E, Campbell A. The orthomolecular treatment of cancer. II. Clinical trial of high-dose ascorbic acid supplements in advanced human cancer. Chem Biol Interact 1974 Oct; 9(4):285–315.

29. Cameron E, Campbell A, Jack T. The orthomolecular treatment of cancer. III. Reticulum cell sarcoma: Double complete regression induced by high-dose ascorbic acid therapy. Chem Biol Interact 1975 Nov; 11(5):387–93.

30. Cameron E, Pauling L. Supplemental ascorbate in the supportive treatment of cancer: Reevaluation of prolongation of survival times in terminal human cancer. Proc Natl Acad Sci USA 1978 Sep; 75(9):4538–42.

31. Cameron E, Pauling L. Supplemental ascorbate in the supportive treatment of cancer: Prolongation of survival times in terminal human cancer. Proc Natl Acad Sci USA 1976 Oct; 73(10):3685–9.

32. Murata A, Morishige F, Yamaguchi H. Prolongation of survival times of terminal cancer patients by administration of large doses of ascorbate. Int J Vitam Nutr Res Suppl 1982; 23:103–13.

33. Cameron E, Campbell A. Innovation vs. quality control: An "unpublishable" clinical trial of supplemental ascorbate in incurable cancer. Med Hypotheses 1991 Nov; 36(3):185–9.

34. Poulter JM, White WF, Dickerson JW. Ascorbic acid supplementation and five year survival rates in women with early breast cancer. Acta Vitaminol Enzymol 1984; 6(3):175–82.

35. Creagan ET, Moertel CG, O'Fallon JR, et al. Failure of high-dose vitamin C (ascorbic acid) therapy to benefit patients with advanced cancer. A controlled trial. N Engl J Med 1979 Sep 27; 301(13):687–90.

36. Moertel CG, Fleming TR, Creagan ET, et al. High-dose vitamin C versus placebo in the treatment of patients with advanced cancer who have had no prior chemotherapy. A randomized double-blind comparison. N Engl J Med 1985 Jan 17; 312(3):137–41.

37. Kallistratos GI, Fasske EE, Karkabounas S, Charalambopoulos K. Prolongation of the survival time of tumor bearing Wistar rats through a simultaneous oral administration of vitamins C + E and selenium with glutathione. Prog Clin Biol Res 1988; 259:377–89.

38. Evangelou A, Kalpouzos G, Karkabounas S, et al. Dose-related preventive and therapeutic effects of antioxidants-anticarcinogens on experimentally induced malignant tumors in Wistar rats. Cancer Lett 1997 May 1; 115(1):105–11.

39. Prasad KN, Kumar A, Kochupillai V, Cole WC. High doses of multiple antioxidant vitamins: Essential ingredients in improving the efficacy of standard cancer therapy. J Am Coll Nutr 1999 Feb; 18(1):13–25.

40. Lamm DL, Riggs DR, Shriver JS, et al. Megadose vitamins in bladder cancer: A double-blind clinical trial. J Urol 1994 Jan; 151(1):21–6.

41. Satoh K, Ida Y, Hosaka M, et al. Induction of apoptosis by cooperative action of vitamins C and E. Anticancer Res 1998 Nov–Dec; 18(6A):4371–5.

42. Evangelou A, Kalpouzos G, Karkabounas S, et al. Dose-related preventive and therapeutic effects of antioxidants-anticarcinogens on experimentally induced malignant tumors in Wistar rats. Cancer Lett 1997 May 1; 115(1):105–11.

43. Evangelou A, Kalpouzos G, Karkabounas S, et al. Dose-related preventive and therapeutic effects of antioxidants-anticarcinogens on experimentally induced malignant tumors in Wistar rats. Cancer Lett 1997 May 1; 115(1):105–11.

44. Johnston CS. The antihistamine action of ascorbic acid. Subcell Biochem 1996; 25:189–207.

45. Gruber HE, Tewfik HH, Tewfik FA. Cytoarchitecture of Ehrlich ascites carcinoma implanted in the hind limb of ascorbic acid-supplemented mice. Eur J Cancer 1980 Apr; 16(4):441–8.

46. Moriarty MJ, Mulgrew S, Malone JR, O'Connor MK. Results and analysis of tumour levels of ascorbic acid. Ir J Med Sci 1977 Mar; 146(3):74–8.

47. DeClerck YA, Jones PA. Effect of ascorbic acid on the resistance of the extracellular matrix to hydrolysis by tumor cells. Cancer Res 1980 Sep; 40(9):3228–31.

48. Boggust WA, McGauley H. Ascorbic acid and dehydroascorbic acid in HeLa cells: Their effect on the collagen-peptidase activity of glucose-deficient cultures. Br J Cancer 1978 Jul; 38(1):100–105.

49. Winkler BS, Orselli SM, Rex TS. The redox couple between glutathione and ascorbic acid: A chemical and physiological perspective. Free Radic Biol Med 1994 Oct; 17(4):333–49.

50. Tanaka K, Hashimoto T, Tokumaru S, et al. Interactions between vitamin C and vitamin E are observed in tissues of inherently scorbutic rats. J Nutr 1997 Oct; 127(10):2060–4.

51. Johnston CS, Meyer CG, Srilakshmi JC. Vitamin C elevates red blood cell glutathione in healthy adults. Am J Clin Nutr 1993 Jul; 58(1):103–5.

52. Igarashi O, Yonekawa Y, Fujiyama-Fujihara Y. Synergistic action of vitamin E and vitamin C in vivo using a new mutant of Wistar-strain rats, ODS, unable to synthesize vitamin C. J Nutr Sci Vitaminol (Tokyo) 1991 Aug; 37(4):359–69.

[53] Koshiishi I, Mamura Y, Liu J, Imanari T. Degradation of dehydroascorbate to 2,3-diketogulonate in blood circulation. Biochim Biophys Acta 1998 Sep 16; 1425(1):209–14.

[54] Koshiishi I, Imanari T. Measurement of ascorbate and dehydroascorbate contents in biological fluids. Anal Chem 1997 Jan 15; 69(2):216–20.

[55] May JM, Mendiratta S, Qu ZC, Loggins E. Vitamin C recycling and function in human monocytic U-937 cells. Free Radic Biol Med 1999 Jun; 26(11–12):1513–23.

[56] Halliwell B. Vitamin C: Antioxidant or pro-oxidant in vivo? Free Radic Res 1996 Nov; 25(5):439–54.

[57] Ozawa T, Hanaki A, Onodera K, Kasai M. Reactions of copper(II)-N-polycarboxylate complexes with hydrogen peroxide in the presence of biological reductants: ESR evidence for the formation of hydroxyl radical. Biochem Int 1992 Mar; 26(3):477–83.

[58] Scarpa M, Stevanato R, Viglino P, Rigo A. Superoxide ion as active intermediate in the autoxidation of ascorbate by molecular oxygen. Effect of superoxide dismutase. J Biol Chem 1983 Jun 10; 258(11):6695–7.

[59] Scarpa M, Stevanato R, Viglino P, Rigo A. Superoxide ion as active intermediate in the autoxidation of ascorbate by molecular oxygen. Effect of superoxide dismutase. J Biol Chem 1983 Jun 10; 258(11):6695–7.

[60] Sestili P, Brandi G, Brambilla L, et al. Hydrogen peroxide mediates the killing of U937 tumor cells elicited by pharmacologically attainable concentrations of ascorbic acid: Cell death prevention by extracellular catalase or catalase from cocultured erythrocytes or fibroblasts. J Pharmacol Exp Ther 1996 Jun; 277(3):1719–25.

[61] Asano K, Satoh K, Hosaka M, et al. Production of hydrogen peroxide in cancerous tissue by intravenous administration of sodium 5,6-benzylidene-L-ascorbate. Anticancer Res 1999 Jan–Feb; 19(1A):229–36.

[62] Sestili P, Brandi G, Brambilla L, et al. Hydrogen peroxide mediates the killing of U937 tumor cells elicited by pharmacologically attainable concentrations of ascorbic acid: Cell death prevention by extracellular catalase or catalase from cocultured erythrocytes or fibroblasts. J Pharmacol Exp Ther 1996 Jun; 277(3):1719–25.

[63] Satoh K, Kadofuku T, Sakagami H. Copper, but not iron, enhances apoptosis-inducing activity of antioxidants. Anticancer Res 1997; 17:2487–2490.

[64] Toyokuni S, Okamoto K, Yodoi J, Hiai H. Persistent oxidative stress in cancer. FEBS Lett 1995 Jan 16; 358(1):1–3.

[65] Ozawa T, Hanaki A, Onodera K, Kasai M. Reactions of copper(II)-N-polycarboxylate complexes with hydrogen peroxide in the presence of biological reductants: ESR evidence for the formation of hydroxyl radical. Biochem Int 1992 Mar; 26(3):477–83.

[66] Amano Y, Sakagami H, Tanaka T, et al. Uncoupling of incorporation of ascorbic acid and apoptosis induction. Anticancer Res 1998 Jul–Aug; 18(4A):2503–6.

[67] Sakagami H, Kuribayashi N, Iida M, et al. The requirement for and mobilization of calcium during induction by sodium ascorbate and by hydrogen peroxide of cell death. Life Sci 1996; 58(14):1131–8.

[68] Menon M, Maramag C, Malhotra RK, Seethalakshmi L. Effect of vitamin C on androgen independent prostate cancer cells (PC3 and Mat-Ly-Lu) in vitro: Involvement of reactive oxygen species-effect on cell number, viability and DNA synthesis. Cancer Biochem Biophys 1998 Jun; 16(1–2):17–30.

[69] Oikawa S, Kawanishi S. Site-specific DNA damage induced by NADH in the presence of copper(II): Role of active oxygen species. Biochemistry 1996 Apr 9; 35(14):4584–90.

[70] Oikawa S, Yamada K, Yamashita N, et al. N-acetylcysteine, a cancer chemopreventive agent, causes oxidative damage to cellular and isolated DNA. Carcinogenesis 1999 Aug; 20(8):1485–90.

[71] Oikawa S, Kawanishi S. Distinct mechanisms of site-specific DNA damage induced by endogenous reductants in the presence of iron(III) and copper(II). Biochim Biophys Acta 1998 Jul 30; 1399(1):19–30.

[72] Tsao CS, Dunham WB, Leung PY. In vivo antineoplastic activity of ascorbic acid for human mammary tumor. In Vivo 1988 Mar–Apr; 2(2):147–50.

[73] Tsao CS. Inhibiting effect of ascorbic acid on the growth of human mammary tumor xenografts. Am J Clin Nutr 1991; 54:1274S-80S.

[74] Monteiro HP, Stern A. Redox modulation of tyrosine phosphorylation-dependent signal transduction pathways. Free Radic Biol Med 1996; 21(3):323–33.

[75] Peranovich TM, da Silva AM, Fries DM, et al. Nitric oxide stimulates tyrosine phosphorylation in murine fibroblasts in the absence and presence of epidermal growth factor. Biochem J 1995 Jan 15; 305 (Pt 2):613–9.

[76] Brigelius-Flohe R, Flohe L. Ascorbic acid, cell proliferation, and cell differentiation in culture. Subcell Biochem 1996; 25:83–107.

[77] Villalba JM, Cordoba F, Navas P. Ascorbate and the plasma membrane. A new view of cell growth control. Subcell Biochem 1996; 25:57–8.

[78] Burdon RH, Gill V, Rice-Evans C. Oxidative stress and tumour cell proliferation. Free Radic Res Commun 1990; 11(1–3):65–76.

[79] Peranovich TM, da Silva AM, Fries DM, et al. Nitric oxide stimulates tyrosine phosphorylation in murine fibroblasts in the absence and presence of epidermal growth factor. Biochem J 1995 Jan 15; 305 (Pt 2):613–9.

[80] Nicosia RF, Belser P, Bonanno E, Diven J. Regulation of angiogenesis in vitro by collagen metabolism. In Vitro Cell Dev Biol 1991 Dec; 27 A(12):961–6.

[81] Agus DB, Vera JC, Golde DW. Stromal cell oxidation: A mechanism by which tumors obtain vitamin C. Cancer Res 1999 Sep 15; 59(18):4555–8.

[82] Piyathilake CJ, Bell WC, Johanning GL, et al. The accumulation of ascorbic acid by squamous cell carcinomas of the lung and larynx is associated with global methylation of DNA. Cancer 2000 Jul 1; 89(1):171–6.

[83] Vera JC, Rivas CI, Velasquez FV, et al. Resolution of the facilitated transport of dehydroascorbic acid from its intracellular accumulation as ascorbic acid. J Biol Chem 1995 Oct 6; 270(40):23706–12.

[84] Vera JC, Rivas CI, Zhang RH, et al. Human HL-60 myeloid leukemia cells transport dehydroascorbic acid via the glucose

transporters and accumulate reduced ascorbic acid. Blood 1994 Sep 1; 84(5):1628–34.

85 Laggner H, Goldenberg H. Interaction of respiratory burst and uptake of dehydroascorbic acid in differentiated HL-60 cells. Biochem J 2000 Jan 15; 345 Pt 2:195–200.

86 Moriarty M, Mulgrew S, Mothersill C, et al. Some effects of administration of large doses of vitamin C in patients with skin carcinoma. Ir J Med Sci 1978 May; 147(5):166–70.

87 Moertel CG, Fleming TR, Creagan ET, et al. High-dose vitamin C versus placebo in the treatment of patients with advanced cancer who have had no prior chemotherapy. A randomized double-blind comparison. N Engl J Med 1985 Jan 17; 312(3):137–41.

88 Lykkesfeldt J, Loft S, Nielsen JB, Poulsen HE. Ascorbic acid and dehydroascorbic acid as biomarkers of oxidative stress caused by smoking. Am J Clin Nutr 1997 Apr; 65(4):959–63.

89 Hultqvist M, Hegbrant J, Nilsson-Thorell C, et al. Plasma concentrations of vitamin C, vitamin E and/or malondialdehyde as markers of oxygen free radical production during hemodialysis. Clin Nephrol 1997 Jan; 47(1):37–46.

90 Herrick AL, Rieley F, Schofield D, et al. Micronutrient antioxidant status in patients with primary Raynaud's phenomenon and systemic sclerosis. J Rheumatol 1994 Aug; 21(8):1477–83.

91 Levine M, Conry-Cantilena C, Wang Y, et al. Vitamin C pharmacokinetics in healthy volunteers: Evidence for a recommended dietary allowance. Proc Natl Acad Sci USA 1996 Apr 16; 93(8):3704–9.

92 Blanchard J, Tozer TN, Rowland M. Pharmacokinetic perspectives on megadoses of ascorbic acid. Am J Clin Nutr 1997 Nov; 66(5):1165–71.

93 Iwasaka K, Koyama N, Nogaki A, et al. Role of hydrogen peroxide in cytotoxicity induction by ascorbates and other redox compounds. Anticancer Res 1998 Nov–Dec; 18(6A):4333–7.

94 Sakagami H, Satoh K, Ohata H, et al. Relationship between ascorbyl radical intensity and apoptosis-inducing activity. Anticancer Res 1996 Sep–Oct; 16(5A):2635–44.

95 Bram S, Froussard P, Guichard M, et al. Vitamin C preferential toxicity for malignant melanoma cells. Nature 1980 Apr 17; 284(5757):629–31.

96 Nemoto S, Otsuka M, Arakawa N. Inhibitory effect of ascorbate on cell growth: Relation to catalase activity. J Nutr Sci Vitaminol (Tokyo) 1996 Apr; 42(2):77–85.

97 Menon M, Maramag C, Malhotra RK, Seethalakshmi L. Effect of vitamin C on androgen independent prostate cancer cells (PC3 and Mat-Ly-Lu) in vitro: Involvement of reactive oxygen species-effect on cell number, viability and DNA synthesis. Cancer Biochem Biophys 1998 Jun; 16(1–2):17–30.

98 Evangelou A, Kalpouzos G, Karkabounas S, et al. Dose-related preventive and therapeutic effects of antioxidants-anticarcinogens on experimentally induced malignant tumors in Wistar rats. Cancer Lett 1997 May 1; 115(1):105–11.

99 Cameron E, Pauling L. Supplemental ascorbate in the supportive treatment of cancer: Reevaluation of prolongation of survival times in terminal human cancer. Proc Natl Acad Sci USA 1978 Sep; 75(9):4538–42.

100 Murata A, Morishige F, Yamaguchi H. Prolongation of survival times of terminal cancer patients by administration of large doses of ascorbate. Int J Vitam Nutr Res Suppl 1982; 23:103–13.

101 Cameron E. Protocol for the use of vitamin C in the treatment of cancer. Med Hypotheses 1991 Nov; 36(3):190–4.

102 Doroshow JH. Role of hydrogen peroxide and hydroxyl radical formation in the killing of Ehrlich tumor cells by anticancer quinones. Proc Natl Acad Sci USA 1986 Jun; 83(12):4514–8.

103 Doroshow JH. Prevention of doxorubicin-induced killing of MCF-7 human breast cancer cells by oxygen radical scavengers and iron chelating agents. Biochem Biophys Res Commun 1986 Feb 26; 135(1):330–5.

104 Green DM, Hyland A, Barcos MP, et al. Second malignant neoplasms after treatment for Hodgkin's disease in childhood or adolescence. J Clin Oncol 2000 Apr; 18(7):1492–9.

105 Cameron E. Protocol for the use of vitamin C in the treatment of cancer. Med Hypothesis 1991; 36:190–94.

106 Riordan NH, Riordan HD, Meng X, et al. Intravenous ascorbate as a tumor cytotoxic chemotherapeutic agent. Medical Hypotheses 1995; 44:207–213.

107 Diplock AT. Safety of antioxidant vitamins and β-carotene. Am J Clin Nutr 1995; 62(suppl):1510S-6S.

108 Auer BL, Auer D, Rodgers AL. the effect of ascorbic acid ingestion on the biochemical and physiochemical risk factors associated with calcium oxalate kidney stone formation. Clin Chem Lab Med 1998; 36(3):143–147.

109 Venugopal M, Jamison JM, Gilloteaux J, et al. Synergistic antitumor activity of vitamins C and K3 on human urologic tumor cell lines. Life Sci 1996; 59(17):1389–400.

110 Noto V, Taper HS, Yi-Hua, J, et al. Effects of sodium ascorbate (vitamin C) and 2-methyl-1,4-naphthoquinone (vitamin K_3) treatment on human tumor cell growth in vitro. Cancer 1989 Mar 1; 63:901–906.

111 Lupulescu AP. Hormones, vitamins, and growth factors in cancer treatment and prevention. A critical appraisal. Cancer 1996 Dec 1; 78(11):2264–80.

112 Lupulescu A. The role of hormones, growth factors and vitamins in carcinogenesis. Crit Rev Oncol Hematol 1996 Jun; 23(2):95–130.

113 Wang Z, Wang M, Finn F, Carr BI. The growth inhibitory effects of vitamins K and their actions on gene expression. Hepatology 1995 Sep; 22(3):876–82.

114 Taper HS, deGerlache J, Lans M, Roberfroid M. Non-toxic potentiation of cancer chemotherapy by combined C and K_3 vitamin pre-treatment. Int J Cancer 1987; 40:575–579.

115 Taper HS, Roberfroid M. Non-toxic sensitization of cancer chemotherapy by combined vitamin C and K3 pretreatment in a mouse tumor resistant to oncovin. Anticancer Res 1992 Sep–Oct; 12(5):1651–4.

116 De Loecker W, Janssens J, Bonte J, Taper HS. Effects of sodium ascorbate (vitamin C) and 2-methyl-1,4-naphthoquinone (vitamin K3) treatment on human tumor cell growth in vitro. II. Synergism with combined chemotherapy action. Anticancer Res 1993 Jan–Feb; 13(1):103–6.

117 Chlebowski RT, Akman SA, Block JB. Vitamin K in the treatment of cancer. 1985; 12:49–63.

[118] Noto V, Taper HS, Yi-Hua, J, et al. Effects of sodium ascorbate (vitamin C) and 2-methyl-1,4-naphthoquinone (vitamin K_3) treatment on human tumor cell growth in vitro. Cancer 1989 Mar 1; 63:901–906.

[119] Sakagami H, Satoh K. Stimulation of two step degradation of sodium ascorbate by lignins. Anticancer Res 1996 Sep–Oct; 16(5A):2849–51.

[120] Satoh K, Sakagami H, Nakamura K. Enhancement of radical intensity and cytotoxic activity of ascorbate by PSK and lignins. Anticancer Res 1996 Sep–Oct; 16(5A):2981–6.

[121] Satoh K, Sakagami H. Ascorbyl radical scavenging activity of polyphenols. Anticancer Res 1996 Sep–Oct; 16(5A):2885–90.

[122] Maehle L, Lystad E, Eilertsen E, et al. Growth of human lung adenocarcinoma in nude mice is influenced by various types of dietary fat and vitamin E. Anticancer Res 1999 May–Jun; 19(3A):1649–55.

[123] Gonzalez MJ. Fish oil, lipid peroxidation and mammary tumor growth. J Am Coll Nutr 1995 Aug; 14(4):325–35.

[124] Chan T, Galati G, O'Brien PJ. Oxygen activation during peroxidase catalysed metabolism of flavones or flavanones. Chem Biol Interact 1999 Aug 30; 122(1):15–25.

[125] Galati G, Chan T, Wu B, O'Brien PJ. Glutathione-dependent generation of reactive oxygen species by the peroxidase-catalyzed redox cycling of flavonoids. Chem Res Toxicol 1999 Jun; 12(6):521–5.

[126] Sugihara N, Arakawa T, Ohnishi M, Furuno K. Anti- and pro-oxidative effects of flavonoids on metal-induced lipid hydroperoxide-dependent lipid peroxidation in cultured hepatocytes loaded with alpha-linolenic acid. Free Radic Biol Med 1999 Dec; 27(11–12):1313–23.

[127] Woods JA, Bilton RF, Young AJ. Beta-carotene enhances hydrogen peroxide-induced DNA damage in human hepatocellular HepG2 cells. FEBS Lett 1999 Apr 23; 449(2–3):255–8.

[128] Ahsan H, Parveen N, Khan NU, Hadi SM. Pro-oxidant, anti-oxidant and cleavage activities on DNA of curcumin and its derivatives demethoxycurcumin and bisdemethoxycurcumin. Chem Biol Interact 1999 Jul 1; 121(2):161–75.

[129] Ahsan H, Hadi SM. Strand scission in DNA induced by curcumin in the presence of Cu(II). Cancer Lett 1998 Feb 13; 124(1):23–30.

[130] Kuo ML, Huang TS, Lin JK. Curcumin, an antioxidant and anti-tumor promoter, induces apoptosis in human leukemia cells. Biochim Biophys Acta 1996 Nov 15; 1317(2):95–100.

[131] Bhaumik S, Anjum R, Rangaraj N, et al. Curcumin mediated apoptosis in AK-5 tumor cells involves the production of reactive oxygen intermediates. FEBS Lett 1999 Aug 6; 456(2):311–4.

[132] Yang GY, Liao J, Kim K, et al. Inhibition of growth and induction of apoptosis in human cancer cell lines by tea polyphenols. Carcinogenesis 1998 Apr; 19(4):611–6.

[133] Oikawa S, Kawanishi S. Distinct mechanisms of site-specific DNA damage induced by endogenous reductants in the presence of iron(III) and copper(II). Biochim Biophys Acta 1998 Jul 30; 1399(1):19–30.

[134] Milne L, Nicotera P, Orrenius S, Burkitt MJ. Effects of glutathione and chelating agents on copper-mediated DNA oxidation: Pro-oxidant and antioxidant properties of glutathione. Arch Biochem Biophys 1993 Jul; 304(1):102–9.

[135] Yamashita N, Tanemura H, Kawanishi S. Mechanism of oxidative DNA damage induced by quercetin in the presence of Cu(II). Mutat Res 1999 Mar 10; 425(1):107–15.

[136] Metodiewa D, Jaiswal AK, Cenas N, et al. Quercetin may act as a cytotoxic prooxidant after its metabolic activation to semiquinone and quinoidal product. Free Radic Biol Med 1999 Jan; 26(1–2):107–16.

[137] Murata M, Kawanishi S. Oxidative DNA damage by vitamin A and its derivative via superoxide generation. J Biol Chem 2000 Jan 21; 275(3):2003–8.

[138] Yamashita N, Murata M, Inoue S, et al. Alpha-tocopherol induces oxidative damage to DNA in the presence of copper(II) ions. Chem Res Toxicol 1998 Aug; 11(8):855–62.

[139] Noroozi M, Angerson WJ, Lean ME. Effects of flavonoids and vitamin C on oxidative DNA damage to human lymphocytes. Am J Clin Nutr 1998 Jun; 67(6):1210–8.

[140] da Silva EL, Piskula MK, Yamamoto N, et al. Quercetin metabolites inhibit copper ion-induced lipid peroxidation in rat plasma. FEBS Lett 1998 Jul 3; 430(3):405–8.

[141] Terao J. Dietary flavonoids as antioxidants in vivo: Conjugated metabolites of (-)-epicatechin and quercetin participate in antioxidative defense in blood plasma. J Med Invest 1999 Aug; 46(3–4):159–68.

[142] Lean ME, Noroozi M, Kelly I, et al. Dietary flavonols protect diabetic human lymphocytes against oxidative damage to DNA. Diabetes 1999 Jan; 48(1):176–81.

[143] Manach C, Morand C, Crespy V, et al. Quercetin is recovered in human plasma as conjugated derivatives which retain antioxidant properties. FEBS Lett 1998 Apr 24; 426(3):331–6.

[144] Dickancaite E, Nemeikaite A, Kalvelyte A, Cenas N. Prooxidant character of flavonoid cytotoxicity: Structure-activity relationships. Biochem Mol Biol Int 1998 Aug; 45(5):923–30.

[145] Chen H, Tappel AL. Protection of vitamin E, selenium, trolox C, ascorbic acid palmitate, acetylcysteine, coenzyme Q0, coenzyme Q10, beta-carotene, canthaxanthin, and (+)-catechin against oxidative damage to rat blood and tissues in vivo. Free Radic Biol Med 1995 May; 18(5):949–53.

[146] Chen H, Tappel AL. Vitamin E, selenium, trolox C, ascorbic acid palmitate, acetylcysteine, coenzyme Q, beta-carotene, canthaxanthin, and (+)-catechin protect against oxidative damage to kidney, heart, lung and spleen. Free Radic Res 1995 Feb; 22(2):177–86.

[147] Chen H, Tappel AL. Protection by vitamin E selenium, trolox C, ascorbic acid palmitate, acetylcysteine, coenzyme Q, beta-carotene, canthaxanthin, and (+)-catechin against oxidative damage to liver slices measured by oxidized heme proteins. Free Radic Biol Med 1994 Apr; 16(4):437–44.

[148] Shklar G, Schwartz J, Trickler D, Cheverie SR. The effectiveness of a mixture of beta-carotene, alpha-tocopherol, glutathione, and ascorbic acid for cancer prevention. Nutr Cancer 1993; 20(2):145–51.

[149] Omenn GS, Goodman GE, Thornquist MD, et al. Risk factors for lung cancer and for intervention effects in CARET, the Beta-Carotene and Retinol Efficacy Trial [see comments]. J Natl Cancer Inst 1996 Nov 6; 88(21):1550–9.

150 Albanes D, Heinonen OP, Taylor PR, et al. Alpha-Tocopherol and beta-carotene supplements and lung cancer incidence in the alpha-tocopherol, beta-carotene cancer prevention study: Effects of base-line characteristics and study compliance [see comments]. J Natl Cancer Inst 1996 Nov 6; 88(21):1560–70.

151 Omenn GS, Goodman G, Thornquist M, et al. The beta-carotene and retinol efficacy trial (CARET) for chemoprevention of lung cancer in high risk populations: Smokers and asbestos-exposed workers. Cancer Res 1994 Apr 1; 54(7 Suppl):2038s-2043s.

152 Omenn GS, Goodman GE, Thornquist M, Brunzell JD. Long-term vitamin A does not produce clinically significant hypertriglyceridemia: Results from CARET, the beta-carotene and retinol efficacy trial. Cancer Epidemiol Biomarkers Prev 1994 Dec; 3(8):711–3.

153 Goodman GE, Omenn GS, Thornquist MD, et al. The Carotene and Retinol Efficacy Trial (CARET) to prevent lung cancer in high-risk populations: Pilot study with cigarette smokers. Cancer Epidemiol Biomarkers Prev 1993 Jul–Aug; 2(4):389–96.

154 Omenn GS, Goodman GE, Thornquist MD, et al. The Carotene and Retinol Efficacy Trial (CARET) to prevent lung cancer in high-risk populations: Pilot study with asbestos-exposed workers. Cancer Epidemiol Biomarkers Prev 1993 Jul–Aug; 2(4):381–7.

155 Wang XD, Russell RM. Procarcinogenic and anticarcinogenic effects of beta-carotene. Nutr Rev 1999 Sep; 57(9 Pt 1):263–72.

156 Lowe GM, Booth LA, Young AJ, Bilton RF. Lycopene and beta-carotene protect against oxidative damage in HT29 cells at low concentrations but rapidly lose this capacity at higher doses. Free Radic Res 1999 Feb; 30(2):141–51.

157 Collins AR, Olmedilla B, Southon S, et al. Serum carotenoids and oxidative DNA damage in human lymphocytes. Carcinogenesis 1998 Dec; 19(12):2159–62.

158 Duthie SJ, Ma A, Ross MA, Collins AR. Antioxidant supplementation decreases oxidative DNA damage in human lymphocytes. Cancer Res 1996 Mar 15; 56(6):1291–5.

159 Collins AR, Gedik CM, Olmedilla B, et al. Oxidative DNA damage measured in human lymphocytes: Large differences between sexes and between countries, and correlations with heart disease mortality rates. FASEB J 1998 Oct; 12(13):1397–400.

160 Collins AR. Oxidative DNA damage, antioxidants, and cancer. Bioessays 1999 Mar; 21(3):238–46.

161 Welch RW, Turley E, Sweetman SF, et al. Dietary antioxidant supplementation and DNA damage in smokers and nonsmokers. Nutr Cancer 1999; 34(2):167–72.

162 McCall MR, Frei B. Can antioxidant vitamins materially reduce oxidative damage in humans? Free Radic Biol Med 1999 Apr; 26(7–8):1034–53.

163 Brown KM, Morrice PC, Duthie GG. Erythrocyte vitamin E and plasma ascorbate concentrations in relation to erythrocyte peroxidation in smokers and nonsmokers: Dose response to vitamin E supplementation. Am J Clin Nutr 1997 Feb; 65(2):496–502.

164 Kontush A, Finckh B, Karten B, et al. Antioxidant and prooxidant activity of alpha-tocopherol in human plasma and low density lipoprotein. J Lipid Res 1996 Jul; 37(7):1436–48.

165 Watkins ML, Erickson JD, Thun MJ, et al. Multivitamin use and mortality in a large prospective study. Am J Epidemiol 2000 Jul 15; 152(2):149–62.

166 Hack V, Breitkreutz R, Kinscherf R, et al. The redox state as a correlate of senescence and wasting and as a target for therapeutic intervention. Blood 1998 Jul 1; 92(1):59–67.

167 Witenberg B, Kletter Y, Kalir HH, et al. Ascorbic acid inhibits apoptosis induced by X irradiation in HL60 myeloid leukemia cells. Radiat Res 1999 Nov; 152(5):468–78.

168 Witenberg B, Kalir HH, Raviv Z, et al. Inhibition by ascorbic acid of apoptosis induced by oxidative stress in HL-60 myeloid leukemia cells. Biochem Pharmacol 1999 Apr 1; 57(7):823–32.

169 Hawkins RA, Sangster K, Arends MJ. Apoptotic death of pancreatic cancer cells induced by polyunsaturated fatty acids varies with double bond number and involves an oxidative mechanism. J Pathol 1998 May; 185(1):61–70.

170 Zhang D, Okada S, Yu Y, et al. Vitamin E inhibits apoptosis, DNA modification, and cancer incidence induced by iron-mediated peroxidation in Wistar rat kidney. Cancer Res 1997 Jun 15; 57(12):2410–4.

171 Lotem J, Peled-Kamar M, Groner Y, Sachs L. Cellular oxidative stress and the control of apoptosis by wild-type p53, cytotoxic compounds, and cytokines. Proc Natl Acad Sci USA 1996 Aug 20; 93(17):9166–71.

172 Cossarizza A, Franceschi C, Monti D, et al. Protective effect of N-acetylcysteine in tumor necrosis factor-alpha-induced apoptosis in U937 cells: The role of mitochondria. Exp Cell Res 1995 Sep; 220(1):232–40.

173 Satoh K, Sakagami H. Effect of cysteine, N-acetyl-L-cysteine and glutathione on cytotoxic activity of antioxidants. Anticancer Res 1997 May–Jun; 17(3C):2175–9.

174 Obrador E, Navarro J, Mompo J, et al. Regulation of tumour cell sensitivity to TNF-induced oxidative stress and cytotoxicity: Role of glutathione. Biofactors 1998; 8(1–2):23–6.

175 Obrador E, Navarro J, Mompo J, et al. Glutathione and the rate of cellular proliferation determine tumour cell sensitivity to tumour necrosis factor in vivo. Biochem J 1997 Jul 1; 325 (Pt 1):183–9.

176 Chen MF, Chen LT, Boyce HW Jr. 5-Fluorouracil cytotoxicity in human colon HT-29 cells with moderately increased or decreased cellular glutathione level. Anticancer Res 1995 Jan–Feb; 15(1):163–7.

177 Yellin SA, Davidson BJ, Pinto JT, et al. Relationship of glutathione and glutathione-S-transferase to cisplatin sensitivity in human head and neck squamous carcinoma cell lines. Cancer Lett 1994 Oct 14; 85(2):223–32.

178 Cheeseman KH, Collins M, Proudfoot K, et al. Studies on lipid peroxidation in normal and tumour tissues. The Novikoff rat liver tumour. Biochem J 1986 Apr 15; 235(2):507–14.

179 Cheeseman KH, Burton GW, Ingold KU, Slater TF. Lipid peroxidation and lipid antioxidants in normal and tumor cells. Toxicol Pathol 1984; 12(3):235–9.

180 Ray S, Chakrabarti P. Altered lipid peroxidation and antioxidant potential in human uterine tumors. Indian J Exp Biol 1999 May; 37(5):439–43.

[181] Gerber M, Richardson S, Favier F, et al. Vitamin E and tumor growth. Adv Exp Med Biol 1990; 264:129–32.

[182] Piyathilake CJ, Bell WC, Johanning GL, et al. The accumulation of ascorbic acid by squamous cell carcinomas of the lung and larynx is associated with global methylation of DNA. Cancer 2000 Jul 1; 89(1):171–6.

[183] Allalunis-Turner MJ, Lee FY, Siemann DW. Comparison of glutathione levels in rodent and human tumor cells grown in vitro and in vivo. Cancer Res 1988 Jul 1; 48(13):3657–60.

[184] Russo A, DeGraff W, Friedman N, Mitchell JB. Selective modulation of glutathione levels in human normal versus tumor cells and subsequent differential response to chemotherapy drugs. Cancer Res 1986 Jun; 46(6):2845–8.

[185] Bartoli GM, Galeotti T. Growth-related lipid peroxidation in tumour microsomal membranes and mitochondria. Biochim Biophys Acta 1979 Sep 28; 574(3):537–41.

[186] Chajes V, Sattler W, Stranzl A, Kostner GM. Influence of n-3 fatty acids on the growth of human breast cancer cells in vitro: Relationship to peroxides and vitamin-E. Breast Cancer Res Treat 1995 Jun; 34(3):199–212.

[187] Morisaki N, Lindsey JA, Stitts JM, et al. Fatty acid metabolism and cell proliferation. V. Evaluation of pathways for the generation of lipid peroxides. Lipids 1984 Jun; 19(6):381–94.

[188] Muzio G, Salvo RA, Trombetta A, et al. Dose-dependent inhibition of cell proliferation induced by lipid peroxidation products in rat hepatoma cells after enrichment with arachidonic acid. Lipids 1999 Jul; 34(7):705–11.

[189] Conklin KA. Dietary antioxidants during cancer chemotherapy: Impact on chemotherapeutic effectiveness and development of side effects. Nutr Cancer 2000; 37(1):1–18.

[190] Shacter E, Williams JA, Hinson RM, et al. Oxidative stress interferes with cancer chemotherapy: Inhibition of lymphoma cell apoptosis and phagocytosis. Blood 2000 Jul 1; 96(1):307–313.

[191] Salganik RI, Albright CD, Rodgers J, et al. Dietary antioxidant depletion: Enhancement of tumor apoptosis and inhibition of brain tumor growth in transgenic mice. Carcinogenesis 2000 May; 21(5):909–914.

[192] Evangelou A, Kalpouzos G, Karkabounas S, et al. Dose-related preventive and therapeutic effects of antioxidants-anticarcinogens on experimentally induced malignant tumors in Wistar rats. Cancer Lett 1997 May 1; 115(1):105–11.

[193] Kanclerz A, Zbytniewski Z, Boeryd B. Influence of some synthetic antioxidants on the growth and metastases formation of Lewis lung carcinoma and amelanotic B16 melanoma in C57BL mice. Arch Geschwulstforsch 1981; 51(5):379–85.

[194] Anasagasti MJ, Martin JJ, Mendoza L, et al. Glutathione protects metastatic melanoma cells against oxidative stress in the murine hepatic microvasculature. Hepatology 1998 May; 27(5):1249–56.

[195] Eskenazi AE, Pinkas J, Whitin JC, et al. Role of antioxidant enzymes in the induction of increased experimental metastasis by hydroxyurea. J Natl Cancer Inst 1993 May 5; 85(9):711–21.

[196] Hu JJ, Roush GC, Berwick M, et al. Effects of dietary supplementation of α-tocopherol on plasma glutathione and DNA repair activities. Cancer Epidem Biomarkers Prev 1996; 5:263–270.

[197] Johnston CS, Meyer CG, Srilakshmi JC. Vitamin C elevates red blood cell glutathione in healthy adults. Am J Clin Nutr 1993; 58:103–5.

[198] Heinonen OP, Albanes D, Virtamo J, et al. Prostate cancer and supplementation with alpha-tocopherol and beta-carotene: Incidence and mortality in a controlled trial. J Natl Cancer Inst 1998 Mar 18; 90(6):440–6.

[199] D'Agostini F, Balansky RM, Camoirano A, De Flora S. Interactions between N-acetylcysteine and ascorbic acid in modulating mutagenesis and carcinogenesis. Int J Cancer 2000 Dec 1; 88(5):702–7.

Having looked at vitamin C, a monosaccharide derivative, we now examine polysaccharides. As the name implies, polysaccharides consist of multiple monosaccharides (simple sugars) linked together. Although many important compounds are polysaccharides (starch, hyaluronic acid, and cellulose, for example), in this chapter we are concerned with high-molecular-weight (large) polysaccharides with immunostimulating properties. Quite a few medicinal plants contain these high-molecular-weight polysaccharides (hereafter referred to simply as polysaccharides).

Polysaccharide-rich plants have a long history of use in traditional medicines such as Chinese herbal medicine, where they are commonly employed to increase the vital energy of a patient. Modern medicine has also investigated their properties. All the polysaccharide-rich plants discussed here increase production of immune-stimulating cytokines, generating a cytokine cocktail that stimulates immune activity. As discussed in Chapter 11, cocktail mixes are believed to be among the most effective ways to use cytokines in cancer treatment. In addition, several polysaccharides appear to inhibit production or activity of immunosuppressive cytokines and in this way may also have an anticancer effect. Not surprisingly then, studies like the Chinese clinical trials discussed in Chapter 12 suggest that polysaccharides may be useful in cancer treatment. Also, a large number of Japanese clinical trials have reported that polysaccharide-rich mushroom products, such as PSK, have some benefit in conjunction with chemotherapy. Some of these studies, along with additional animal and human studies on polysaccharides, are reported in this chapter. Keep in mind that although some studies report polysaccharides can be beneficial alone, our position is that polysaccharides, and all other natural compounds discussed, are most beneficial within a larger combination of compounds.

INTRODUCTION TO POLYSACCHARIDES

Although many natural compounds can stimulate the immune system, natural immunostimulants often fall into one of two chemical families: high-molecular-weight polysaccharides and saponins.[1, a] In Chinese herbal medicine, plants containing these compounds are often classified as vital energy (*qi*) tonics; for example, *Astragalus membranaceus* contains high-molecular-weight polysaccharides and *Panax ginseng* contains saponins. Both are considered qi tonics. Actually, many herbs that stimulate the immune system include compounds from both chemical families. *Eleutherococcus senticosus* is an example. Ginseng also contains both saponins and polysaccharides, although the former are more prominent. In this chapter we focus on a few of the most common polysaccharide-rich herbs and extracts, and in Chapter 21 we discuss a few saponin-rich herbs. The reader is referred to herbal medicine guidebooks for information regarding additional herbs that act as immunostimulants.[2–10]

Polysaccharides have been studied both in crude form (the entire polysaccharide fraction of a plant) and semipurified and purified forms (various levels of purification for specific polysaccharides). Purified polysaccharides that have received research attention include lentinan, from the edible mushroom *Lentinus edodes* (shiitake), schizophyllan, from the fungus *Schizophyllum commune*, and pachyman, from the fungus *Poria cocos*. Semipurified polysaccharides include PSK and PSP, from the mushroom *Coriolus versicolor*, and KS-2, from *Lentinus edodes*. All three—crude, semipurified, and purified polysaccharides—can produce antitumor effects in animals, and some beneficial effects have been reported in human patients.[11, 12]

INDIVIDUAL COMPOUNDS

Six polysaccharide-rich plants or extracts are examined in this chapter: *Astragalus, Eleutherococcus, Ganoderma*, shiitake, PSK, and PSP. These plants and extracts act in part by increasing production of immunostimulating cytokines (such as IL-1, IL-2, IL-6, interferons, TNF, and colony-stimulating factors); by increasing the responsiveness of cytokine receptors; and/or by decreasing the production or reducing the action of cytokines that inhibit the immune system, such as TGF-beta and IL-10.[13–21] The resulting effect is, in gen-

---

[a] *As a reference point, high-molecular-weight polysaccharides have a molecular weight between about 10,000 and 800,000 grams/mole. The average molecular weight of the polysaccha-rides discussed here is roughly 200,000 grams/mole. This is in comparison with glucose, a monosaccharide with a molecular weight of 180 grams/mole, as well as with most other natural compounds discussed in this book, which have an average molecular weight of about 360 grams/mole.*

eral, increased proliferation and heightened function of natural killer cells, macrophages, and T cells.

In the following, only brief discussions are provided for most compounds, since much of the information on immune stimulation is included in Chapter 12 and Table H.1. A more in-depth discussion is provided for the mushroom polysaccharides PSK and PSP, however, because they have been researched extensively.

Although not all polysaccharide-rich plants have received the same amount of research, this does not mean some are more beneficial than others. In fact, many likely share similar qualities and so may be somewhat interchangeable in clinical practice. Also, as we will see, their active dosages are quite similar. To assure the greatest benefits though, it may be prudent to use a mixture of polysaccharide-rich plants, and, as always, to combine this mixture with compounds that inhibit cancer by other means. The concept of using mixtures of polysaccharide-rich plants has a long history in Chinese and other herbal traditions.

Astragalus membranaceus

Summary of Research and Conclusions

Although *Astragalus* is one of the most commonly used Chinese herbs and is used extensively in Chinese hospitals for treating cancer patients (in combination with chemotherapy), relatively few studies on *Astragalus* are indexed in the MEDLINE database. Presumably, many more are available in Chinese journals. Because of the custom of using combinations in Chinese herbal medicine, most of the indexed studies of *Astragalus* are ones on herbal combinations.

Some 13 in-vitro studies relate to cancer or immune function.[22–26] In general, these reported that *Astragalus*, alone or in combination with other Chinese herbs, stimulated IL-2 production, immune cell activity, and immune cell killing of cancer cells.

Thirteen animal studies are indexed.[27–31] These support the in-vitro data by reporting that herbal combinations with *Astragalus* can stimulate the immune system, inhibit tumor growth, and prevent chemotherapy- or radiotherapy-induced immunosuppression. A few animal studies presented conflicting results, however; at least one reported that an *Astragalus* combination was unable to prevent cyclophosphamide-induced immunosuppression, whereas another reported *Astragalus* polysaccharides to be effective in this regard.[28, 32]

Five human studies, one of which is a review, also reported that *Astragalus* combinations stimulated the immune system and inhibited chemotherapy-induced immunosuppression in cancer patients.[33–37] Overall, these in-vitro, animal, and human studies suggest *Astragalus* could have beneficial effects. Much of this would come from immune stimulation but *Astragalus* may also inhibit metastasis by inhibiting platelet aggregation (see Table 10.1).

General Information

The root of the legume *Astragalus membranaceus* (milk vetch or yellow vetch) is one of the most common tonic herbs in Chinese herbal medicine. *Astragalus* is a very large genus; in North America there are nearly 400 *Astragalus* species, located mainly in the western United States. Some of these, such as the infamous "locoweed," are poisonous to livestock due to their high selenium content. Other species of *Astragalus*, like *membranaceus*, are nontoxic. The common food and cosmetic ingredient, gum tragacanth, is obtained from several nontoxic *Astragalus* species.[38] The medicinal use of *Astragalus membranaceus* was discussed in the 2,000-year-old Chinese text, *Shen Nong Ben Cao Jing (Divine Husbandman's Classic of the Materia Medica)*.

In Chinese medicine, *Astragalus* is prescribed for various forms of insufficient qi. It has a marked effect on the immune system of humans and rodents and has been clinically studied in China as an adjuvant for chemotherapy. The common daily dose in noncancer conditions is 9 to 30 grams of dried herb in decoction. In exceptional cases, up to 60 grams per day may be given.[39] When treating cancer patients in China, clinicians commonly prescribe a dose of roughly 30 to 60 grams per day.

The toxicity of *Astragalus membranaceus* is very low; oral doses of 75 to 100 g/kg did not cause acute toxicity in mice.[40] Although side effects are minimal at normal doses, higher doses of *Astragalus* (and many of the other herbal immunostimulants discussed here) may cause insomnia, increased heart rate, palpitations, hypertension, a general feeling of overstimulation, or all of these.

Eleutherococcus senticosus

Summary of Research and Conclusions

At least four papers have been published on the in-vitro effects of *Eleutherococcus* that relate to immune stimulation or cancer. One reported that extracts of *Eleutherococcus* inhibited T-cell and B-cell activity while enhancing macrophage activity, and interestingly, the other three found that *Eleutherococcus* could inhibit cancer cells directly, without affecting immune cell activity.[41–44]

Seven out of eight published animal studies, in contrast to the in-vitro ones, reported that *Eleutherococcus* stimulated immune activity and inhibited tumor growth primarily through an immune-mediated mechanism.[45–51] The eighth study reported that *Eleutherococcus* protected mice from adverse effects of radiotherapy.[52]

At least three human studies are indexed, the first reporting that *Eleutherococcus* stimulated the immune system, including T-cell activity, of healthy volunteers.[53] The second study found that *Eleutherococcus* stimulated the immune system of breast cancer patients, and the third reported it could prevent infection or other postoperative complications of surgery in elderly cancer patients.[54, 55] Based on these limited studies, it seems likely *Eleutherococcus* may have an immunostimulating effect in humans and could be useful in cancer treatment.

General Information

Eleutherococcus senticosus is a shrubby member of the ginseng family. Like *Astragalus*, it is a common Chinese herb and is mentioned in the *Shen Nong Ben Cao Jing*. A complex taxonomic controversy exists regarding similarities between the *Eleutherococcus* and *Acanthopanax* species, however, and it is not certain that the *Shen Nong Ben Cao Jing* was actually referring to *Eleutherococcus senticosus*. Some scholars have combined *Eleutherococcus* and *Acanthopanax* into the same (*Eleutherococcus*) genus, while others have recognized *Eleutherococcus* as a distinct genus. Today, most of the world's scientists refer to the plant as *Eleutherococcus senticosus*, while Chinese scientists refer to it as *Acanthopanax senticosus*. Not until the 1970s, when the plant was imported into the United States as an herbal "adaptogen," was it given the common name Siberian ginseng.[a] Extensive clinical research on the plant has been conducted in Russia since the 1950s.[56]

In Chinese herbal medicine, *Eleutherococcus* (or *Acanthopanax*) is used as a qi tonic and as an anti-inflammatory agent in arthritic conditions. The dose is commonly 6 to 15 grams per day of the dried herb in decoction.[57] The Russian studies commonly used a 33 percent (1:3) alcohol extract, of which 2 to 16 milliliters were taken 1 to 3 times per day; this dose is roughly equivalent to 1 to 16 grams per day of the dried herb. Treatment was commonly continued for up to 60 days, followed by a rest period of 2 to 3 weeks.[56] As noted earlier, some type of treatment-rest schedule may help

---

[a] *The Russian scientist N.V. Lazarev coined the term* adaptogen *in 1947 to refer to agents that help increase "nonspecific resistance of an organism to adverse influence."*

all compounds we discuss to perform at their best (see Chapter 13). Side effects of *Eleutherococcus* appear to be minimal at low to moderate doses.

Eleutherococcus may inhibit cancer through several mechanisms. In addition to its affects on the immune system, it may inhibit angiogenesis by reducing histamine availability (see Table 8.3) and may block cancer cell proliferation by inhibiting cyclin-dependent kinases (see Chapter 4). It may also alter the plasma membrane or its components, as suggested by some of the in-vitro studies.

Ganoderma lucidum and Shiitake

Summary of Research and Conclusions

The immunostimulating and antitumor properties of *Ganoderma* and shiitake mushrooms have been discussed in at least five reviews.[58–62] In addition to these, two in-vitro studies have reported they can increase cytokine production, stimulate immune cells, and induce differentiation of cancer cells via cytokine activity.[63, 64] Nine studies have reported antitumor effects in animals.[65–73] A large number of additional animal and human cancer studies have been published on the purified polysaccharide lentinan, isolated from shiitake.[74–77]

Based on the extensive anticancer data of lentinan, it would seem reasonable that crude shiitake extracts could also produce an immunostimulating effect and be useful in cancer treatment. The few studies on crude shiitake and *Ganoderma* extracts suggest both may indeed be helpful.

General Information

Ganoderma lucidum, also called reishi mushroom, is a common Chinese fungus mentioned in the *Shen Nong Ben Cao Jing*. Like a variety of other mushrooms, including the edible shiitake mushroom (*Lentinus edodes*), *Ganoderma* acts as an immunostimulant in both animals and humans. In addition to its potential to inhibit cancer through immune stimulation, *Ganoderma* may impede metastasis by inhibiting platelet aggregation (see Table 10.1).

Intraperitoneal administration (400 mg/kg every other day) of crude *Ganoderma* extract, with and without chemotherapy treatment, increased the life span of mice with lung cancer.[69] The equivalent human intraperitoneal dose is about 1.9 grams per day of crude *Ganoderma* extract. If we assume this crude extract provided a 30 percent yield of material (as explained in Chapter 13), then the equivalent human oral dose is about 32 grams of whole dried *Ganoderma*. The normal dose of the whole herb in Chinese herbal medicine is about 9 grams per day in decoction.[78] Since the polysaccharide content of many polysaccharide-rich herbs is roughly 7 percent (commonly 5 to 10 percent), a 32-gram dose of *Ganoderma* provides about 2.2 grams per day of polysaccharides.[79–83]

The antitumor effects of the purified polysaccharide lentinan, which is obtained from *Lentinus edodes* (the shiitake mushroom), have been extensively studied in mice. The results have been very encouraging; an antitumor effect has been reported against many types of cancers.[11] Lentinan has also been studied in humans with promising results. Human clinical trials have reported increased survival when used in combination with chemotherapy.[12, 75] In rodent studies, the dose generally given (1 mg/kg intraperitoneal) is low relative to doses of other polysaccharides discussed here. Low intravenous doses were also used in the human studies. The beneficial effects seen at low doses are due to the purified nature of lentinan and the route of administration. Clearly, the successes of lentinan demonstrate that shiitake mushrooms contain potent immunomodulating substances.

The whole shiitake mushroom also produces an antitumor effect. An oral dose of 12 g/kg per day of raw shiitake inhibited the growth of sarcoma tumors in mice by 40 percent. Doses two- and threefold greater produced additional inhibition. The growth of five other tumor types was also reduced, although generally to a lesser degree.[84, 85] The human equivalent of a 12-g/kg dose in mice is roughly 120 grams per day. This dose is prohibitively large but provides only about 8 grams of polysaccharides per day (assuming a 7 percent polysaccharide content), which is similar to the polysaccharide doses used in other studies discussed in this chapter.

PSK and PSP

Summary of Research and Conclusions

PSK (also called Krestin) and PSP (polysaccharide peptide) are semipurified polysaccharides obtained from the mushroom *Coriolus versicolor*. Of the two, PSK has received the most research attention, primarily in Japan, where PSK is now used clinically in cancer treatment in some situations.[86, 87] A relatively large number of papers have been published documenting the effects of PSK or PSP. More than 16 examined their ability to stimulate immune cells or inhibit cancer cell proliferation in-vitro.[88–92] Thirty-nine looked at their ability to inhibit metastasis, angiogenesis, and/or tumor growth in animals.[93–97] Of these, 13 focused on their interactions with chemotherapy drugs or radiotherapy or their ability

to decrease the immunosuppression caused by these therapies.[98–102] Fifty-four focused on their ability to inhibit cancer progression in humans.[103–107] The great majority of these studies were on PSK combined with chemotherapy, radiotherapy, other immune stimulants, or a combination of these. As a whole, these studies strongly suggest that PSK and/or PSP inhibit cancer progression in animals and improve postoperative survival in humans. These effects are probably due to a combination of immune stimulation and inhibition of immunosuppressive cytokines, although other factors like inhibition of invasion may also play a role.

In-vitro Studies

Most of the in-vitro studies on PSK/PSP have focused on their ability to stimulate immune cells. In one study, PSK (at about 1.1 µM) increased proliferation of lymphocytes obtained from patients with stomach and colorectal cancer by 1- to 3-fold (average 1.4-fold).[88] In another study, the same concentration of PSK stimulated the cytotoxic effect of tumor-infiltrating lymphocytes obtained from gastrointestinal patients.[89] The same beneficial effect was reported with lymphocytes taken from other types of cancers.[91] Other studies reported that the cytotoxicity of natural killer cells against cancer cells was increased by PSK concentrations of 1.1 µM in vitro.[108] A PSK plasma concentration of roughly 1.1 µM is achieved after oral administration of about 3 grams per day. Markedly higher doses are not recommended, since in-vitro studies have reported that 10-fold higher PSK concentrations actually reduced immune cell activity.[108]

A smaller number of in-vitro studies reported on other effects of PSK/PSP. For example, two studies reported that PSK inhibited the invasion of leukemia cells in vitro; at about 1.1 µM, PSK reduced the number of invading cells by half. The effect was thought to be due to inhibition of enzymes that digest the extracellular matrix.[109, 110] One study reported an inhibition of melanoma invasion in vitro by PSK. Part of this inhibition was attributed to decreased tumor cell binding to the basement membrane.[94]

In-vitro studies have reported PSK can inhibit TGF-beta activity, a desirable characteristic since it allows PSK to interrupt TGF-beta-mediated immune evasion by cancer cells (cancer cells can produce TGF-beta, and high concentrations of TGF-beta are immunosuppressive).[111] Moreover, since TGF-beta lowers production of the antioxidant enzyme SOD (superoxide dismutase), PSK can increase SOD production.[112, 113] The result is an antioxidant effect (see Figure 5.2).

At the end of Chapter 5, I mentioned a study in which stimulation of an immune response by implanting a gelatin sponge next to weakly tumorigenic cancer cells caused the cells to form aggressive tumors.[114] This response was associated with a decline in intracellular antioxidant enzymes. Administration of PSK to animals increased the antioxidant capacity at such tumor sites and inhibited transformation into aggressive tumors.[112, 113]

At higher PSK concentrations (about 5.5 to 11 μM), PSK can increase the SOD capacity of cancer cells through another means, apparently by acting as an electron donor. In-vitro studies have reported that at these PSK concentrations, cancer cells were directly inhibited by PSK treatment, presumably due to the hydrogen peroxide produced when SOD activity is increased (see Figure 5.2).[115, 116, 117, a] Increased production of SOD and hydrogen peroxide may also be responsible for reports of PSK-induced enhancement of cisplatin activity against cancer cells in vitro.[118] The ability of PSK to kill cancer cells by producing hydrogen peroxide is probably limited to in-vitro studies, since the required PSK concentrations could not easily be reached in vivo. This is not of concern here though, since we are not interested in producing a prooxidant effect.

Animal Studies

Animal studies have corroborated the results observed in in-vitro studies. Some 39 studies reported that PSK stimulates the immune system of tumor-bearing rodents, prevents metastasis or angiogenesis, and increases survival. Thirteen of these were conducted in conjunction with chemotherapy or radiotherapy, but three examples where PSK was used alone are as follows:

- Oral administration of PSK reduced the growth of colon cancer cells transplanted into mice. Optimal effects were seen at about 360 to 720 mg/kg.[119] The equivalent human dose is about 3.4 to 6.8 grams per day. The effects were associated with improved immune function, suppression of TGF-beta activity, and restoration of interferon-gamma production. Higher doses had no effect on tumor growth.

- Oral administration of 1,000 mg/kg inhibited the growth of two types of tumors in mice (of three types tested). The effect was due to a reduction of tumor-induced immunosuppression.[120]

- Oral administration of 500 mg/kg increased NK cell activity and inhibited metastasis of liver cancer cells in rats.[121]

In addition to these oral studies, other studies reported antitumor effects after intraperitoneal, intratumoral, or intratumoral and oral administration.[96, 97, 122, 123] Some of these studies reported that a combination of preoperative intratumoral treatment and postoperative oral treatment was highly effective at eradicating metastatic tumors. In general, the effects of PSK were greater on small tumors and were specific to certain tumor types.[93, 124] One factor in tumor sensitivity appeared to be tumor susceptibility to NK cell activity.[125]

A small number of studies have reported that PSK inhibited angiogenesis in tumor-bearing rodents.[126] For example, intraperitoneal administration of 50 mg/kg inhibited angiogenesis induced by liver cancer cells in mice. The mechanism of action was uncertain but may have involved inhibition of bFGF activity.[95]

Summarizing the above discussions and those from previous chapters, Table 16.1 lists the potential antitumor activities of PSK and PSP.

Human Studies

As listed in Table 1.3, the 54 human studies conducted on PSK/PSP are more than that for any other compound discussed. All of these studies used PSK/PSP—with or without other immunostimulants—in conjunction with chemotherapy or radiotherapy. Although the effects of natural compounds on chemotherapy or radiotherapy generally are covered in Chapter 23, we discuss those for PSK/PSP here because all human studies conducted used them in combination with chemotherapy or radiotherapy.

Five of the 54 studies were review articles, and most of the studies these reviewed were trials on stomach cancer patients in Japan.[127–131] In general, they suggested that combinations of chemotherapy and PSK resulted in greater increases in life span than chemotherapy alone.

Twenty-four randomized control trials have been conducted, many of which were large, multicenter trials. The general finding was that adding PSK to treatment regimes improved patient survival. In some studies, the effect of PSK administration was not statistically significant, but many revealed a trend for increased survival.[132–135] Some examples of the randomized controlled trials are summarized below (the dose of PSK used was 3 grams per day orally unless noted):

- Two hundred sixty-two postoperative stomach cancer patients were randomized to receive chemotherapy or chemotherapy plus PSK. The addition of PSK increased the five-year disease-free rate (from

---

[a] *If SOD activity is increased relative to catalase and/or glutathione peroxidase activity, hydrogen peroxide will be produced.*

TABLE 16.1 POTENTIAL ANTICANCER ACTIONS OF PSK AND PSP		
ACTIVITY	**KNOWN EFFECTS**	**AS A COLLAGENASE INHIBITOR, MAY:**
Chapter 3: Results of Therapy at the Cellular Level		
Inhibit TGF-beta	x	
Chapters 7 and 8: Angiogenesis		
Inhibit angiogenesis	x	x
Inhibit bFGF effects	x	x
Inhibit VEGF effects	via PDGF and TGF-beta binding	
Chapters 9 and 10: Invasion and Metastasis		
Inhibit invasion	x	x
Inhibit collagenase effects	x	—
Inhibit cell migration	x	
Inhibit metastasis	x	x
Inhibit platelet aggregation	x	
Chapters 11 and 12: Immune System		
Stimulate the immune system	x	
Inhibit tumor-induced immunosuppression	x	
Chapters 16: Polysaccharides		
Act as an SOD mimic	x	

59 to 71 percent) and the five-year survival rate (from 60 to 73 percent).[104]

- Four hundred sixty-two patients with curatively re-sected colorectal cancer were randomized to receive chemotherapy or chemotherapy plus PSK. PSK administration increased the three-year disease-free rate (from 68 to 77 percent) and the three-year survival rate (from 79 to 86 percent).[105]

- One hundred eleven patients with curatively resected colorectal cancer were randomized to receive chemotherapy or chemotherapy plus PSK. PSK administration increased the eight-year disease-free rate (from about 7.8 to 28 percent) and the 10-year survival rate (from about 19 to 36 percent).[136]

- Two hundred seventy-eight patients with stage IIA T2N1 estrogen-dependent and node-negative breast cancer were randomized to receive chemotherapy or chemotherapy plus PSK. PSK administration increased the five-year survival rate (from 81 to 96 percent). Disease-free survival also increased, but the increase was not statistically significant. Node-negative breast cancer patients with some other classifications were also helped by PSK treatment, but the improvements were not statistically significant.[137]

- Thirty-eight patients with nasopharynx cancer who were treated with radiotherapy, with or without chemotherapy, were randomized to receive PSK or no

PSK. PSK administration increased the five-year survival rate (from 15 to 28 percent). The survival time was also increased (from 25 to 35 months). The PSK dose was 1 gram per day orally.[106]

- Seventy-three patients in remission from acute nonlymphocytic leukemia were randomized to receive either maintenance chemotherapy or maintenance chemotherapy plus PSK. Although there were no statistical differences in duration of remission or survival between the two groups on the whole, when a smaller subset of patients was looked at, PSK administration increased the remission period by 418 days (from 467 to 885 days); this subset was made of patients maintaining a remission period for more than 270 days.[138] In other words, those patients who were doing well did even better with PSK.

ESTIMATED THERAPEUTIC AND LOAEL DOSES OF POLYSACCHARIDES

The estimated required dose of crude polysaccharides from different sources as scaled from animal studies reasonably agrees with doses used in human studies. Based on these values, the human polysaccharide dose required for cancer treatment is likely to be 2 to 9 grams per day.

In studies on mice, optimal antitumor effects of poly-saccharides from a variety of plants were observed at daily intraperitoneal doses of 25 to 250 mg/kg per day.[139–145] The midrange (140 mg/kg) corresponds to a human oral dose of about 6.6 grams per day; a dose similar to the commonly prescribed polysaccharide dose for cancer patients in China (based on decoctions of polysaccharide-rich herbs). These decoctions often contain 30 to 90 grams per day of herbs. Assuming the herbs contain about 7 percent polysaccharides, the poly-saccharide dose would be 2 to 6 grams per day. This dose is also similar to the commonly prescribed PSK dose of 3 grams per day.

In addition, the above doses are similar to the required dose as calculated from in-vitro and pharmacokinetic data (see Appendix J). Using a target concentration of 2.2 μM (for stimulation of immune cells), the required polysaccharide dose is 9.3 grams per day.

The LOAEL dose for polysaccharides has not been established but is likely to be much greater than the polysaccharide dose of 2 to 9 grams recommended here.

TABLE 16.2 ESTIMATED THERAPEUTIC AND LOAEL DOSES FOR POLYSACCHARIDES*	
DESCRIPTION	DOSE (g/day)
Required dose as scaled from animal antitumor studies	6.6 (midrange)
Common human dose in cancer treatment	2 to 6
Required dose as determined from pharmacokinetic calculations	9.3
Estimated LOAEL dose	much greater than 6
Tentative dose recommendation for further research	**2 to 9**

See Appendix J for details.

For all practical purposes, these compounds are nontoxic, although a general feeling of overstimulation can occur at high doses or in sensitive individuals.

Dose calculations for polysaccharides are summarized in Table 16.2. Note that synergism is not mentioned in the table, since polysaccharides are not classified as direct-acting compounds. Nevertheless, as discussed in Chapter 13, synergistic interactions could still be expected between immune stimulants and other indirect- and direct-acting compounds, and the best clinical effects may occur when all three groups are used together.

USING COMBINATIONS OF POLYSACCHARIDES

The dose required for a variety of polysaccharides may range from 2 to 9 grams per day. To achieve this without using excessive amounts of any single herb, combinations of herbs can be used. For example, a decoction comprised of 30 grams of *Astragalus* and 15 grams of *Eleutherococcus* contains a polysaccharide dose of roughly 3 grams, assuming that each herb contains about 7 percent polysaccharides. Herbs can also be combined with semi-purified polysaccharides like PSK to achieve the desired dose.

Combinations of herbs are of course used in Chinese herbal medicine, and most Chinese formulas intended for immune stimulation (or qi stimulation) contain polysaccharide-rich herbs. For the interested reader, we mention two historic Chinese herbal formulas as examples. These formulas, *Shi Quan Da Bu Tang* and *Bu Zhong Yi Qi Tang*, contain combinations of both polysaccharide- and saponin-rich herbs (see Table H.2 in Appendix H for ingredients). Each formula is put to a slightly different use in Chinese herbal medicine, but both produce effects on the immune system.

Shi Quan Da Bu Tang contains twelve common Chinese herbs, including *Astragalus* and ginseng. The formula inhibited tumor growth and increased the survival rate of mice with chemically induced bladder tumors treated with the chemotherapy drug cisplatin. It also protected mice against kidney and liver toxicity and bone marrow suppression caused by cisplatin. The formula increased the survival of leukemia-bearing mice treated with mitomycin, as compared to those treated only with mitomycin. It also helped prevent the low blood count and weight loss associated with mitomycin treatment and helped delay death caused by a lethal dose of mitomycin. Injection of the extract suppressed the growth of ascites cancer in mice, and oral administration prolonged survival of the mice. Of 116 traditional formulas tested, this formula was most effective as a biological response modifier.[16, 33, 146–151]

Bu Zhong Yi Qi Tang contains eight common Chinese herbs, including *Astragalus* and ginseng. Administration of this formula stimulated the immune system and suppressed the growth of cancer in mice.[152, 153]

CONCLUSION

High-molecular-weight polysaccharides can increase production of immune-stimulating cytokines, decrease production or activity of immunosuppressive cytokines, and act in other ways to inhibit cancer. They have been reported to stimulate the immune system in animals and humans, inhibit cancer progression in animals, and improve survival in humans when used with conventional therapies. Based on earlier discussions (see Chapter 11), immune stimulants are not likely to produce profound anticancer effects in humans unless combined with compounds that prevent immune evasion and those that address some of the fundamental abnormalities in cancer cells that allow them to proliferate and spread. Thus, although animal studies report that polysaccharides can inhibit cancer on their own, the best effects are most likely to be seen when they are used in combination with other anticancer compounds.

REFERENCES

[1] Wagner H. Immunostimulants from medicinal plants. In *Advances in Chinese medicinal materials research*. Chang HM, Yeung W, Tso W, Koo A, eds. Singapore: World Scientific, 1985.

[2] Bensky D, Gamble A. Chinese herbal medicine materia medica. Seattle: Eastland Press, 1993.

[3] Bensky D, Barolet R. Chinese herbal medicine formulas & strategies. Seattle: Eastland Press, 1990.

[4] Foster S, Yue C. Herbal emissaries: Bringing Chinese herbs to the West. Rochester, VT: Healing Arts Press, 1992.

[5] Hsu HY, Chen YP, Shen SJ, et al. Oriental materia medica: A concise guide. Long Beach, CA: Oriental Healing Arts Institute, 1986.

[6] Duke J. The green pharmacy. Emmaus, PA: Rodale Press, 1997.

[7] Tierra M. Planetary herbology. Twin Lakes, WI: Lotus Press, 1988.

[8] Tyler V. Herbs of choice: The therapeutic use of phytomedicines. Binghamton, NY: Pharmaceutical Products Press, 1994.

[9] Weiss RF. Herbal medicine. Gothenburg, Sweden: AB Arcanum, 1988.

[10] Murray MT. The healing power of herbs. Rocklin, CA: Prima Publishing, 1995.

[11] Chihara G, Hamuro J, Maeda YY, et al. Antitumor and metastasis-inhibitory activities of lentinan as an immunomodulator: An overview. Cancer Detection and Prevention Supplement 1987; 1:423–443.

[12] Taguchi T. Clinical efficacy of lentinan on patients with stomach cancer: End point results of a four-year follow-up survey. Cancer Detection and Prevention Supplement 1987; 1:333–349.

[13] Matsunaga K, Hosokawa A, Oohara M, et al. Direct action of a protein-bound polysaccharide, PSK, on transforming growth factor-beta. Immunopharmacology 1998 Nov; 40(3):219–30.

[14] Yang YZ, Jin PY, Guo Q, et al. Effect of Astralagus membranaceus on natural killer cell activity and induction of alpha- and gamma-interferon in patients with coxsackie B viral myocarditis. Chin Med J (Engl) 1990; 103(4):304–7.

[15] Zhao KW, Kong HY. Effect of astragalan on secretion of tumor necrosis factors in human peripheral blood mononuclear cells. Chung Kuo Chung Hsi I Chieh Ho Tsa Chih 1993; 13(5):263–5.

[16] Jin R, Kurashige S. Effect of shi-ka-ron on cytokine production of lymphocytes in mice treated with cyclophosphamide. Am J Chin Med 1996; 24(1):37–44.

[17] Strickland FM, Darvill A, Albersheim P, et al. Inhibition of UV-induced immune suppression and interleukin-10 production by plant oligosaccharides and polysaccharides. Photochem Photobiol 1999 Feb; 69(2):141–7.

[18] Kitani H, Tsuru S, Oguchi M, et al. Effect of PSK on interferon production in tumor-bearing mice. J Clin Lab Immunol 1984 Dec; 15(4):211–4.

[19] Kobayashi H, Matsunaga K, Oguchi Y. Antimetastatic effects of PKS (Krestin), a protein-bound polysaccharide obtained from Basidiomycetes: An overview. Cancer Epidem Biomarkers Prev 1995; 4:275–281.

[20] Adachi Y, Okazaki M, Ohno N, et al. Enhancement of cytokine production by macrophages stimulated with (1-->3)-beta-D-glucan, grifolan (GRN), isolated from Grifola frondosa. Biol Pharm Bull 1994 Dec; 17(12):1554–60.

[21] Wang SY, Hsu ML, Hsu HC, et al. The anti-tumor effect of Ganoderma lucidum is mediated by cytokines released from activated macrophages and T lymphocytes. Int J Cancer 1997 Mar 17; 70(6):699–705.

[22] Chu DT, Lepe-Zuniga J, Wong WL, et al. Fractionated extract of Astragalus membranaceus, a Chinese medicinal herb, potentiates LAK cell cytotoxicity generated by a low dose of recombinant interleukin-2. J Clin Lab Immunol 1988 Aug; 26(4):183–7.

[23] Chu DT, Wong WL, Mavligit GM. Immunotherapy with Chinese medicinal herbs. I. Immune restoration of local xenogeneic graft-versus-host reaction in cancer patients by fractionated Astragalus membranaceus in vitro. J Clin Lab Immunol 1988 Mar; 25(3):119–23.

[24] Sun Y, Hersh EM, Lee SL, et al. Preliminary observations on the effects of the Chinese medicinal herbs Astragalus membranaceus and Ligustrum lucidum on lymphocyte blastogenic responses. J Biol Response Mod 1983; 2(3):227–37.

[25] Rittenhouse JR, Lui PD, Lau BH. Chinese medicinal herbs reverse macrophage suppression induced by urological tumors. J Urol 1991 Aug; 146(2):486–90.

[26] Wang Y, Qian XJ, Hadley HR, Lau BH. Phytochemicals potentiate interleukin-2 generated lymphokine-activated killer cell cytotoxicity against murine renal cell carcinoma. Mol Biother 1992 Sep; 4(3):143–6.

[27] Lau BH, Ruckle HC, Botolazzo T, Lui PD. Chinese medicinal herbs inhibit growth of murine renal cell carcinoma. Cancer Biother 1994 Summer; 9(2):153–61.

[28] Chu DT, Wong WL, Mavligit GM. Immunotherapy with Chinese medicinal herbs. II. Reversal of cyclophosphamide-induced immune suppression by administration of fractionated Astragalus membranaceus in vivo. J Clin Lab Immunol 1988 Mar; 25(3):125–9.

[29] Zhao KS, Mancini C, Doria G. Enhancement of the immune response in mice by Astragalus membranaceus extracts. Immunopharmacology 1990 Nov–Dec; 20(3):225–33.

[30] Hsu HY, Hau DM, Lin CC. Effects of kuei-pi-tang on cellular immunocompetence of gamma-irradiated mice. Am J Chin Med 1993; 21(2):151–8.

[31] Hsu HY, Ho YH, Lian SL, Lin CC. Preliminary study on antiradiation effect of kuei-pi-tang. Am J Chin Med 1991; 19(3–4):275–84.

[32] Khoo KS, Ang PT. Extract of Astragalus membranaceus and Ligustrum lucidum does not prevent cyclophosphamide-induced myelosuppression. Singapore Med J 1995 Aug; 36(4):387–90.

[33] Zee-Cheng RK. Shi-quan-da-bu-tang (ten significant tonic decoction), SQT. A potent Chinese biological response modifier in cancer immunotherapy, potentiation and detoxification of anticancer drugs. Methods Find Exp Clin Pharmacol 1992 Nov; 14(9):725–36.

[34] Zhang R, Qian J, Yang G, et al. Medicinal protection with Chinese herb-compound against radiation. Aviat Space Environ Med 1990; 61:729–31.

[35] Cha RJ, Zeng DW, Chang QS. [Non-surgical treatment of small cell lung cancer with chemo-radio-immunotherapy and traditional Chinese medicine.] Chung Hua Nei Ko Tsa Chih 1994 Jul; 33(7):462–6.

[36] Li NQ. [Clinical and experimental study on shen-qi injection with chemotherapy in the treatment of malignant tumor of digestive tract.] Chung Kuo Chung Hsi I Chieh Ho Tsa Chih 1992 Oct; 12(10):588–92, 579.

[37] Hou J, Liu S, Ma Z, et al. Effects of Gynostemma pentaphyllum makino on the immunological function of cancer patients. J Tradit Chin Med 1991; 11(1):47–52.

[38] Foster S, Yue C. Herbal emissaries: Bringing Chinese herbs to the West. Rochester, VT: Healing Arts Press, 1992, pp. 27–8.

[39] Bensky D, Gamble A. Chinese herbal medicine materia medica. Seattle: Eastland Press, 1993, pp. 319–320.

[40] Lueng AY, Foster S. Encyclopedia of common natural ingredients. New York: John Wiley & Sons, 1996, p. 52.

[41] Shan BE, Yoshita Y, Sugiura T, Yamashita U. Suppressive effect of Chinese medicinal herb, Acanthopanax gracilistylus, extract on human lymphocytes in vitro. Clin Exp Immunol 1999 Oct; 118(1):41–8.

[42] Shan BE, Zeki K, Sugiura T, et al. Chinese medicinal herb, Acanthopanax gracilistylus, extract induces cell cycle arrest of human tumor cells in vitro. Jpn J Cancer Res 2000 Apr; 91(4):383–389.

[43] Hacker B, Medon PJ. Cytotoxic effects of Eleutherococcus senticosus aqueous extracts in combination with N6-(delta 2-isopentenyl)-adenosine and 1-beta-D-arabinofuranosylcytosine against L1210 leukemia cells. J Pharm Sci 1984 Feb; 73(2):270–2.

[44] Tong L, Huang TY, Li JL. [Effects of plant polysaccharides on cell proliferation and cell membrane contents of sialic acid, phospholipid and cholesterol in S 180 and K 562 cells.] Chung Kuo Chung Hsi I Chieh Ho Tsa Chih 1994 Aug; 14(8):482–4.

[45] Shen ML, Zhai SK, Chen HL, et al. Immunomopharmacological effects of polysaccharides from Acanthopanax senticosus on experimental animals. Int J Immunopharmacol 1991; 13(5):549–54.

[46] Wagner H, Proksch A, Riess-Maurer I, et al. [Immunostimulating action of polysaccharides (heteroglycans) from higher plants.] Arzneimittelforschung 1985; 35(7):1069–75.

[47] Wagner H, Proksch A, Riess-Maurer I, et al. [Immunostimulant action of polysaccharides (heteroglycans) from higher plants. Preliminary communication.] Arzneimittelforschung 1984; 34(6):659–61.

[48] Wang JZ, Tsumura H, Shimura K, Ito H. Antitumor activity of polysaccharide from a Chinese medicinal herb, Acanthopanax giraldii Harms. Cancer Lett 1992 Jul 31; 65(1):79–84.

[49] Wang JZ, Tsumura H, Ma N, et al. Biochemical and morphological alterations of macrophages and spleen cells produced by antitumor polysaccharide from Acanthopanax obovatus roots. Planta Med 1993 Feb; 59(1):54–8.

[50] Xie SS. [Immunoregulatory effect of polysaccharide of Acanthopanax senticosus (PAS). I. Immunological mechanism of PAS against cancer.] Chung Hua Chung Liu Tsa Chih 1989 Sep; 11(5):338–40.

[51] Wang JZ, Mao XJ, Ito H, Shimura K. Immunomodulatory activity of polysaccharide from Acanthopanax obovatus roots. Planta Med 1991 Aug; 57(4):335–6.

[52] Miyanomae T, Frindel E. Radioprotection of hemopoiesis conferred by Acanthopanax senticosus Harms (Shigoka) administered before or after irradiation. Exp Hematol 1988 Oct; 16(9):801–6.

[53] Bohn B, Nebe CT, Birr C. Flow-cytometric studies with Eleutherococcus senticosus extract as an immunomodulatory agent. Arzneimittelforschung 1987 Oct; 37(10):1193–6.

[54] Kupin VI, Polevaia EB. [Stimulation of the immunological reactivity of cancer patients by Eleutherococcus extract.] Vopr Onkol 1986; 32(7):21–6.

[55] Starosel'skii IV, Lisetskii VA, Kaban AP, et al. [Prevention of postoperative complications in the surgical treatment of cancer of the lung, esophagus, stomach, large intestine and the rectum in patients over 60 years old.] Vopr Onkol 1991; 37(7–8):873–7.

[56] Foster S, Yue C. Herbal emissaries: Bringing Chinese herbs to the West. Rochester, VT: Healing Arts Press, 1992, pp. 73–6.

[57] Hsu HY, Chen YP, Shen SJ, et al. Oriental materia medica: A concise guide. Long beach, CA: Oriental Healing Arts Institute, 1986, p. 318.

[58] Wasser SP, Weis AL. Therapeutic effects of substances occurring in higher Basidiomycetes mushrooms: A modern perspective. Crit Rev Immunol 1999; 19(1):65–96.

[59] Jong SC, Birmingham JM. Medicinal benefits of the mushroom Ganoderma. Adv Appl Microbiol 1992; 37:101–34.

[60] Borchers AT, Stern JS, Hackman RM, et al. Mushrooms, tumors, and immunity. Proc Soc Exp Biol Med 1999 Sep; 221(4):281–93.

[61] Chang R. Functional properties of edible mushrooms. Nutr Rev 1996 Nov; 54(11 Pt 2):S91–3.

[62] Jong SC, Birmingham JM. Medicinal and therapeutic value of the shiitake mushroom. Adv Appl Microbiol 1993; 39:153–84.

[63] Lieu CW, Lee SS, Wang SY. The effect of Ganoderma lucidum on induction of differentiation in leukemic U937 cells. Anticancer Res 1992 Jul–Aug; 12(4):1211–5.

[64] Wang SY, Hsu ML, Hsu HC, et al. The anti-tumor effect of Ganoderma lucidum is mediated by cytokines released from activated macrophages and T lymphocytes. Int J Cancer 1997 Mar 17; 70(6):699–705.

[65] Maruyama H, Yamazaki K, Murofushi S, et al. Antitumor activity of Sarcodon aspratus (Berk.) S. Ito and Ganoderma lucidum (Fr.) Karst. J Pharmacobiodyn 1989 Feb; 12(2):118–23.

[66] Sasaki T, Arai Y, Ikekawa T, et al. Antitumor polysaccharides from some polyporaceae, Ganoderma applanatum (Pers.) Pat and Phellinus linteus (Berk. et Curt) Aoshima. Chem Pharm Bull (Tokyo) 1971 Apr; 19(4):821–6.

[67] Zhang J, Wang G, Li H, et al. Antitumor active protein-containing glycans from the Chinese mushroom songshan lingzhi, Ganoderma tsugae mycelium. Biosci Biotechnol Biochem 1994 Jul; 58(7):1202–5.

[68] Wang G, Zhang J, Mizuno T, et al. Antitumor active polysaccharides from the Chinese mushroom Songshan lingzhi, the fruiting body of Ganoderma tsugae. Biosci Biotechnol Biochem 1993 Jun; 57(6):894–900.

[69] Furusawa E, Chou SC, Furusawa A, et al. Antitumor activity of Ganoderma lucidum, an edible mushroom, on intraperitoneally implanted Lewis lung carcinoma in synergenic mice. Phytotherapy Research 1992; 6:300–304.

[70] Nanba H, Kuroda H. Antitumor mechanisms of orally administered shiitake fruit bodies. Chem Pharm Bull (Tokyo) 1987 Jun; 35(6):2459–64.

[71] Nanba H, Mori K, Toyomasu T, Kuroda H. Antitumor action of shiitake (Lentinus edodes) fruit bodies orally administered to mice. Chem Pharm Bull (Tokyo) 1987 Jun; 35(6):2453–8.

[72] Fujii T, Maeda H, Suzuki F, Ishida N. Isolation and characterization of a new antitumor polysaccharide, KS-2, extracted from culture mycelia of Lentinus edodes. J Antibiot (Tokyo) 1978 Nov; 31(11):1079–90.

[73] Chihara G, Maeda Y, Hamuro J, et al. Inhibition of mouse sarcoma 180 by polysaccharides from Lentinus edodes (Berk.) sing. Nature 1969 May 17; 222(194):687–8.

[74] Chihara G, Hamuro J, Maeda YY, et al. Antitumor and metastasis-inhibitory activities of lentinan as an immunomodulator: An overview. Cancer Detect Prev Suppl 1987; 1:423–43.

[75] Nakano H, Namatame K, Nemoto H, et al. A multi-institutional prospective study of lentinan in advanced gastric cancer patients with unresectable and recurrent diseases: Effect on prolongation of survival and improvement of quality of life. Kanagawa Lentinan Research Group. Hepatogastroenterology 1999 Jul–Aug; 46(28):2662–8.

[76] Matsuoka H, Seo Y, Wakasugi H, et al. Lentinan potentiates immunity and prolongs the survival time of some patients. Anticancer Res 1997 Jul–Aug; 17(4A):2751–5.

[77] Hamuro J, Takatsuki F, Suga T, et al. Synergistic antimetastatic effects of lentinan and interleukin 2 with pre- and post-operative treatments. Jpn J Cancer Res 1994 Dec; 85(12):1288–97.

[78] Hsu HY, Chen YP, Shen SJ, et al. Oriental materia medica: A concise guide. Long beach, CA: Oriental Healing Arts Institute, 1986, pp. 640–1.

[79] Wang Q, Chen SQ, Zhang ZH. Determiniation of polysaccharide contents in fructus Lycii. Chinese Traditional and Herbal Drugs 1991; 22(2):67–8.

[80] Zhang J, Wang G, Li H, et al. Antitumor polysaccharides from a Chinese mushroom, "Yuhuangmo," the fruiting body of Pleurotus citrinnopileatus. Biosci Biotech Biochem 1994; 58(7):1195–1201.

[81] Nanba H, Hamaguchi A, Kuroda H. The chemical structure of an antitumor polsaccharide in fruit bodies of Grifola frondosa (Maitake). Chem Pharm Bull 1987; 35(3):1162–1168.

[82] You JS, Hau DM, Chen KT, Huang HF. Combined effects of chuling (Polyporus umbellatus) extract and mitomycin C on experimental liver cancer. Am J Chinese Med 1994; 22(1):19–28.

[83] Choy YM, Leung KN, Cho CS, et al. Immunopharmacological studies of low molecular weight polysaccharide from Angelica sinensis. American Journal of Chinese Medicine 1994; 22(2):137–145.

[84] Nanba H, Mori K, Toyomasu T, Kuroda H. Antitumor action of shiitake (Lentinus edodes) fruit bodies orally administered to mice. Chem Pharm Bull (Tokyo) 1987 Jun; 35(6):2453–8.

[85] Nanba H, Kuroda H. Antitumor mechanisms of orally administered shiitake fruit bodies. Chem Pharm Bull (Tokyo) 1987 Jun; 35(6):2459–64.

[86] Ng TB. A review of research on the protein-bound polysaccharide (polysaccharopeptide, PSP) from the mushroom Coriolus versicolor (Basidiomycetes: Polyporaceae). Gen Pharmacol 1998 Jan; 30(1):1–4.

[87] Ooi VE, Liu F. Immunomodulation and anti-cancer activity of polysaccharide-protein complexes. Curr Med Chem 2000 Jul 1; 7(7):715–729.

[88] Sugimachi K, Maehara Y, Kusumoto T, et al. In vitro reactivity to a protein-bound polysaccharide PSK of peripheral blood lymphocytes from patients with gastrointestinal cancer. Anticancer Res 1995 Sep–Oct; 15(5B):2175–9.

[89] Noguchi K, Tanimura H, Yamaue H, et al. Polysaccharide preparation PSK augments the proliferation and cytotoxicity of tumor-infiltrating lymphocytes in vitro. Anticancer Res 1995 Mar–Apr; 15(2):255–8.

[90] Aoyagi H, Iino Y, Takeo T, et al. Effects of OK-432 (picibanil) on the estrogen receptors of MCF-7 cells and potentiation of antiproliferative effects of tamoxifen in combination with OK-432. Oncology 1997 Sep–Oct; 54(5):414–23.

[91] Kariya Y, Okamoto N, Fujimoto T, et al. Lysis of fresh human tumor cells by autologous peripheral blood lymphocytes and tumor-infiltrating lymphocytes activated by PSK. Jpn J Cancer Res 1991 Sep; 82(9):1044–50.

[92] Kariya Y, Inoue N, Kihara T, et al. Activation of human natural killer cells by the protein-bound polysaccharide PSK independently of interferon and interleukin 2. Immunol Lett 1992 Feb 15; 31(3):241–5.

[93] Algarra I, Collado A, Garcia Lora A, Garrido F. Differential effect of protein-bound polysaccharide (PSK) on survival of experimental murine tumors. J Exp Clin Cancer Res 1999 Mar; 18(1):39–46.

[94] Matsunaga K, Ohhara M, Oguchi Y, et al. Antimetastatic effect of PSK, a protein-bound polysaccharide, against the B16-BL6 mouse melanoma. Invasion Metastasis 1996; 16(1):27–38.

[95] Kanoh T, Matsunaga K, Saito K, Fujii T. Suppression of in vivo tumor-induced angiogenesis by the protein-bound polysaccharide PSK. In Vivo 1994 Mar–Apr; 8(2):247–50.

[96] Matsunaga K, Aota M, Nyunoya Y, et al. Antitumor effect of biological response modifier, PSK, on C57BL/6 mice with syngeneic melanoma B16 and its mode of action. Oncology 1994 Jul–Aug; 51(4):303–8.

[97] Ebina T, Kohya H, Ishikawa K. Antitumor effect of PSK: Role of regional lymph nodes and enhancement of concomitant and sinecomitant immunity in the mouse. Jpn J Cancer Res 1989 Feb; 80(2):158–66.

[98] Qian ZM, Xu MF, Tang PL. Polysaccharide peptide (PSP) restores immunosuppression induced by cyclophosphamide in rats. Am J Chin Med 1997; 25(1):27–35.

[99] Ebina T, Murata K. Antitumor effect of PSK at a distant site: Tumor-specific immunity and combination with other

chemotherapeutic agents. Jpn J Cancer Res 1992 Jul; 83(7):775–82.

100 Takenoshita S, Hashizume T, Asao T, et al. Inhibitory effects of combined administration of 5-FU and Krestin on liver cancer KDH-8 in WKA/H rats. J Invest Surg 1995 Jan–Feb; 8(1):1–5.

101 Mickey DD, Carvalho L, Foulkes K. Combined therapeutic effects of conventional agents and an immunomodulator, PSK, on rat prostatic adenocarcinoma. J Urol 1989 Dec; 142(6):1594–8.

102 Mickey DD. Combined therapeutic effects of an immunomodulator, PSK, and chemotherapy with carboquone on rat bladder carcinoma. Cancer Chemother Pharmacol 1985; 15(1):54–8.

103 Niimoto M, Hattori T, Tamada R, et al. Postoperative adjuvant immunochemotherapy with mitomycin C, futraful and PSK for gastric cancer. An analysis of data on 579 patients followed for five years. Jpn J Surg 1988 Nov; 18(6):681–6.

104 Nakazato H, Koike A, Saji S, et al. Efficacy of immunochemotherapy as adjuvant treatment after curative resection of gastric cancer. Lancet 1994 May 7; 343(8906):1122–6.

105 Mitomi T, Tsuchiya S, Iijima N, et al. Randomized, controlled study on adjuvant immunochemotherapy with PSK in curatively resected colorectal cancer. Dis Colon Rectum 1992 Feb; 35(2):123–30.

106 Go P, Chung CH. Adjuvant PSK immunotherapy in patients with carcinoma of the nasopharynx. J Int Med Res 1989 Mar–Apr; 17(2):141–9.

107 Hayakawa K, Mitsuhashi N, Saito Y, et al. Effect of Krestin as adjuvant treatment following radical radiotherapy in non-small cell lung cancer patients. Cancer Detect Prev 1997; 21(1):71–7.

108 Pedrinaci S, Algarra I, Garrido F. Protein-bound polysaccharide (PSK) induces cytotoxic activity in the NKL human natural killer cell line. Int J Clin Lab Res 1999; 29(4):135–40.

109 Ebina T, Murata K. [Antitumor effect of intratumoral administration of BRM: Inhibition of tumor cell invasion in vitro.] Gan To Kagaku Ryoho 1995 Sep; 22(11):1626–8.

110 Ebina T, Murata K. [Antitumor effect of intratumoral administration of a Coriolus preparation, PSK: Inhibition of tumor invasion in vitro.] Gan To Kagaku Ryoho 1994 Sep; 21(13):2241–3.

111 Matsunaga K, Hosokawa A, Oohara M, et al. Direct action of a protein-bound polysaccharide, PSK, on transforming growth factor-beta. Immunopharmacology 1998 Nov; 40(3):219–30.

112 Habelhah H. [Induction of manganese superoxide dismutase by an immunopotentiator as a mechanism of inhibiting of malignant progression of murine tumor cells.] Hokkaido Igaku Zasshi 1998 Sep; 73(5):519–29.

113 Habelhah H, Okada F, Nakai K, et al. Polysaccharide K induces Mn superoxide dismutase (Mn-SOD) in tumor tissues and inhibits malignant progression of QR-32 tumor cells: Possible roles of interferon alpha, tumor necrosis factor alpha and transforming growth factor beta in Mn-SOD induction by polysaccharide K. Cancer Immunol Immunother 1998 Aug; 46(6):338–44.

114 Okada F, Nakai K, Kobayashi T, et al. Inflammatory cell-mediated tumour progression and minisatellite mutation correlate with the decrease of antioxidative enzymes in murine fibrosarcoma cells. Br J Cancer 1999 Feb; 79(3–4):377–85.

115 Kobayashi Y, Kariya K, Saigenji K, Nakamura K. Suppressive effects on cancer cell proliferation of the enhancement of superoxide dismutase (SOD) activity associated with the protein-bound polysaccharide of Coriolus versicolor QUEL. Cancer Biother 1994 Summer; 9(2):171–8.

116 Kobayashi Y, Kariya K, Saigenji K, Nakamura K. Suppression of cancer cell growth in vitro by the protein-bound polysaccharide of Coriolus versicolor QUEL (PS-K) with SOD mimicking activity. Cancer Biother 1994 Spring; 9(1):63–9.

117 Kariya K, Nakamura K, Nomoto K, et al. Mimicking of superoxide dismutase activity by protein-bound polysaccharide of Coriolus versicolor QUEL, and oxidative stress relief for cancer patients. Mol Biother 1992 Mar; 4(1):40–6.

118 Kobayashi Y, Kariya K, Saigenji K, Nakamura K. Enhancement of anti-cancer activity of cisdiaminedichloroplatinum by the protein-bound polysaccharide of Coriolus versicolor QUEL (PS-K) in vitro. Cancer Biother 1994 Winter; 9(4):351–8.

119 Harada M, Matsunaga K, Oguchi Y, et al. Oral administration of PSK can improve the impaired anti-tumor CD4+ T-cell response in gut-associated lymphoid tissue (GALT) of specific-pathogen-free mice. Int J Cancer 1997 Jan 27; 70(3):362–72.

120 Matsunaga K, Morita I, Iijima H, et al. Competitive action of a biological response modifier, PSK, on a humoral immunosuppressive factor produced in tumor-bearing hosts. J Clin Lab Immunol 1990 Mar; 31(3):127–36.

121 Suo J, Tanaka N, Hizuta A, Yunoki S, Orita K. Suppression of hepatic natural killer activity by liver metastasis of cancer and restoration of killer activity by oral administration of a Basidomycetes-derived polysaccharide, PSK. Acta Med Okayama 1994 Oct; 48(5):237–42.

122 Ebina T, Murata K. Antitumor effect of PSK at a distant site: Inductions of interleukin-8-like factor and macrophage chemotactic factor in murine tumor. Jpn J Cancer Res 1990 Dec; 81(12):1307–13.

123 Ebina T, Murata K, Tamura K. Antitumor effect of intratumoral administration of biological response modifiers: Induction of immunosuppressive acidic protein, a type of alpha 1-acid glycoprotein, in mice. Jpn J Cancer Res 1994 Jan; 85(1):93–100.

124 Mickey DD, Bencuya PS, Foulkes K. Effects of the immunomodulator PSK on growth of human prostate adenocarcinoma in immunodeficient mice. Int J Immunopharmacol 1989; 11(7):829–38.

125 Algarra I, Collado A, Garrido F. Protein bound polysaccharide PSK abrogates more efficiently experimental metastases derived from H-2 negative than from H-2 positive fibrosarcoma tumor clones. J Exp Clin Cancer Res 1997 Dec; 16(4):373–80.

126 Kumar S, Saitoh K, Kumar P. Antiangiogenesis strategies in cancer therapy with special reference to Krestin. EXS 1992; 61:463–70.

[127] Saji S, Sugiyama Y, Kunieda K, Umemoto T. [Recent progress in biological therapies for cancer.] Gan To Kagaku Ryoho 1999 Jun; 26 Suppl 1:32–41.

[128] Torisu M, Uchiyama A, Goya T, et al. [Eighteen-year experience of cancer immunotherapies—evaluation of their therapeutic benefits and future.] Nippon Geka Gakkai Zasshi 1991 Sep; 92(9):1212–6.

[129] Saji S, Tanemura H, Kunieda K, Sugiyama Y. [Recent advance and its problem of postoperative immunotherapy on gastric cancer—with references to effects and host dependent factors.] Nippon Geka Gakkai Zasshi 1991 Sep; 92(9):1221–4.

[130] Sakamoto J, Nakazato H. [Evaluation of adjuvant immunochemotherapy in advanced gastric cancer.] Gan To Kagaku Ryoho 1993 Dec; 20(16):2525–30.

[131] Fukushima M. Adjuvant therapy of gastric cancer: The Japanese experience. Semin Oncol 1996 Jun; 23(3):369–78.

[132] Morimoto T, Ogawa M, Orita K, et al. Postoperative adjuvant randomised trial comparing chemoendocrine therapy, chemotherapy and immunotherapy for patients with stage II breast cancer: 5-year results from the Nishinihon cooperative study group of adjuvant chemoendocrine therapy for breast cancer (ACETBC) of Japan. Eur J Cancer 1996 Feb; 32A(2):235–42.

[133] Iino Y, Yokoe T, Maemura M, et al. Immunochemotherapies versus chemotherapy as adjuvant treatment after curative resection of operable breast cancer. Anticancer Res 1995 Nov–Dec; 15(6B):2907–11.

[134] Ogoshi K, Satou H, Isono K, et al. Immunotherapy for esophageal cancer. A randomized trial in combination with radiotherapy and radiochemotherapy. Am J Clin Oncol 1995 Jun; 18(3):216–22.

[135] Suto T, Fukuda S, Moriya N, et al. Clinical study of biological response modifiers as maintenance therapy for hepatocellular carcinoma. Cancer Chemother Pharmacol 1994; 33 Suppl:S145–8.

[136] Torisu M, Hayashi Y, Ishimitsu T, et al. Significant prolongation of disease-free period gained by oral polysaccharide K (PSK) administration after curative surgical operation of colorectal cancer. Cancer Immunol Immunother 1990; 31(5):261–8.

[137] Toi M, Hattori T, Akagi M, et al. Randomized adjuvant trial to evaluate the addition of tamoxifen and PSK to chemotherapy in patients with primary breast cancer. 5-Year results from the Nishi-Nippon group of the adjuvant chemoendocrine therapy for breast cancer organization. Cancer 1992 Nov 15; 70(10):2475–83.

[138] Ohno R, Yamada K, Masaoka T, et al. A randomized trial of chemoimmunotherapy of acute nonlymphocytic leukemia in adults using a protein-bound polysaccharide preparation. Cancer Immunol Immunother 1984; 18(3):149–54.

[139] Wang G, Li Y, Wang B, et al. [Anti-tumor effect of Cetraria laevigata Rassad. polysaccharides.] Chung Kuo Chung Yao Tsa Chih 1991 Apr; 16(4):242–4, 256.

[140] Lin PF. [Antitumor effect of actinidia chinensis polysaccharide on murine tumor.] Chung Hua Chung Liu Tsa Chih 1988 Nov; 10(6):441–4.

[141] Wang JZ, Tsumura H, Shimura K, et al. Antitumor activity of polysaccharide from a Chinese medicinal herb, Acanthopanax giraldii Harms. Cancer Lett 1992; 65(1):79–84.

[142] Yamada H, Komiyama K, Kiyohara H, et al. Structural characterization and antitumor activity of a pectic polysaccharide from the roots of Angelica acutiloba. Planta Medica 1990; 56:182–186.

[143] Wang JZ, Tsumura H, Ma N, et al. Biochemical and morphological alterations of macrophages and spleen cells produced by antitumor polysaccharide from Acanthopanax obovatus roots. Planta Med 1993; 59(1):54–8.

[144] Wang JZ, Mao XJ, Ito H, Shimura K. Immunomodulatory activity of polysaccharide from Acanthopanax obovatus roots. Planta Med 1991 Aug; 57(4):335–6.

[145] Xiang DB, Li XY. Antitumor activity and immuno-potentiating actions of Achyranthes bidentata polysaccharides. Chung Kuo Yao Li Hsueh Pao 1993 Nov; 14(6):556–61.

[146] Sun Y, Hersh EM, Talpaz M, et al. Immune restoration and/or augmentation of local graft versus host reaction by traditional Chinese medicinal herbs. Cancer 1983; 52(1):70–3.

[147] He J, Li Y, Wei S, et al. Effects Of mixture Of Astragalus membranaceus, fructus Ligustri And Eclipta prostrata On immune function In mice. Hua Hsi I Ko Ta Hsueh Pao 1992; 23(4):408–11.

[148] Jin R, Wan LL, Mitsuishi T, et al. Effect of shi-ka-ron and Chinese herbs on cytokine production of macrophage in immunocompromised mice. American Journal of Chinese Medicine 1994; XXII(3–4). 255–266.

[149] Ebisuno S, Hirano A, Kyoku I, et al. Basal studies on combination of Chinese medicine in cancer chemotherapy: Protective effects on the toxic side effects of CDDP and antitumor effects with CDDP on murine bladder tumor (MBT-2). Nippon Gan Chiryo Gakkai Shi 1989; 24(6):1305–12.

[150] Yamada H. Chemical characterization and biological activity of the immunologically active substances in Juzen-taiho-to (Japanese kampo prescription). Gan To Kagaku Ryoho 1989 Apr; 16(4 Pt 2–2):1500–5.

[151] Aburada M, Takeda S, Ito E, et al. Protective effects of juzentaihoto, dried decoctum of 10 Chinese herbs mixture, upon the adverse effects of mitomycin C in mice. J Pharmacobiodyn 1983; 6(12):1000–4.

[152] Ito H, Shimura K. Studies on the antitumor activity of traditional Chinese medicines. II. The antitumor mechanism of traditional Chinese medicines. Gan To Kagaku Ryoho 1985; 12(11):2149–54.

[153] Ito H, Shimura K. Studies on the antitumor activity of traditional Chinese medicines. I. Gan To Kagaku Ryoho 1985; 12(11):2145–8.

Everyone knows that a high-fat-diet can lead to obesity and that obesity is associated with increased health risks. What is less commonly understood is that, depending on the amount and type of fat consumed, dietary fats may also stimulate or inhibit the progression of an established cancer. This chapter focuses on two types of dietary fat, omega-6 and omega-3 fatty acids. Research suggests that, in general, omega-6 fatty acids tend to promote cancer progression and omega-3 fatty acids tend to inhibit it.

After reviewing the possible role of omega-6 fatty acids (and saturated fats) in cancer progression, we turn to the role of omega-3 fatty acids in inhibiting cancer progression, concluding with comments on the clinical use of fish oil. These discussions should clarify the potential benefits of reducing intake of omega-6 fatty acids and increasing intake of fish oil, a natural source of omega-3 fatty acids.

TYPES OF DIETARY FAT AND THEIR SOURCES

Fatty acids are long, straight-chain molecules of 4 to 24 carbon atoms that can be categorized as saturated, monounsaturated, or polyunsaturated. The differences between these are based on the chemistry of the molecule. Saturated fats contain only single bonds between all carbon atoms; single bonds leave the maximum number of bonding sites open, which are then filled by hydrogen atoms. As a result, these compounds are said to be fully saturated with hydrogen. In contrast, monounsaturated fatty acids contain one double bond, and polyunsaturated fatty acids contain more than one double bond. The primary dietary source of saturated fats is animal fats, the primary source of monounsaturated fats is olive oil, and that of polyunsaturated fats is vegetable oils like corn oil.

Among other things, the number of double bonds predicts how solid the fatty acid will be at room temperature; saturated fat, with no double bonds, is solid. The number also predicts how susceptible the fatty acid is to free radical damage. Each double bond is a potential site of oxidative damage, and vegetable oils, with multiple double bonds, are more prone to lipid peroxidation and have a shorter shelf life than saturated fats.

Two groups of polyunsaturated fatty acids, omega-3 and omega-6, are of primary interest here. The omega-6 fatty acids of interest are primarily linoleic acid, ob-

tained from vegetable oils, and arachidonic acid, obtained directly from animal fats and indirectly through conversion of linoleic acid in vivo (see Figure 7.4). The omega-3 fatty acids of interest are primarily EPA (eicosapentaenoic acid) and DHA (docosahexaenoic acid), obtained from fish oil. The "3" and "6" designations refer to how many carbon atoms the location of the first double carbon bond is from the "omega" end, or tail, of the fatty acid chain. The locations of the omega-6 and omega-3 double carbon bonds for arachidonic acid, EPA, and DHA are readily apparent in Figures A.22 through A.24 of Appendix A.

Table 17.1 lists the fatty acid content of various common dietary oils. The table heading also gives the numerical nomenclature for the different fatty acids, which is useful to know because some articles use the nomenclature rather than the name of the fatty acid. The numbers simply specify how many carbon atoms and double bonds the fatty acid contains. For example, EPA is a 20:5 fatty acid, which means it contains 20 carbon molecules, 5 of which are double bonds.

Note in the table that in contrast to other oils, olive oil is a very rich source of omega-9 fatty acids. Therefore, discussions on omega-6 and omega-3 fatty acids in this chapter do not pertain to olive oil. Although data are still being gathered, it appears that omega-9 fatty acids are neutral in their effects on cancer, as compared to either omega-6 or omega-3 fatty acids.[1]

STIMULATION OF CANCER PROGRESSION BY SATURATED AND OMEGA-6 FATTY ACIDS

In 1982, the National Research Council identified fats (referring to saturated and omega-6 fatty acids) as the single dietary component most strongly related to cancer risk. One of their recommendations was that fat intake be reduced to no more than 30 percent of total dietary calories.[2] The average American now consumes approximately 33 percent of dietary calories as fat.[3, 4] This is down slightly from 36 to 40 percent in the late 1970s.

The Council report was based on early studies that suggested a strong correlation between fat consumption and incidence of gastrointestinal, prostate, and breast cancers. Correlations were also seen with cancers of the testis, ovary, and uterus.[5] More recent studies, however, suggest the link between fat intake and cancer risk may

TABLE 17.1 PERCENT FATTY ACID CONTENT OF VARIOUS OILS						
OIL		OMEGA-9	OMEGA-6		OMEGA-3	
	SATURATED	OLEIC (18:1)	LINOLEIC (18:2)	ARACHIDONIC (20:4)	ALPHA-LINOLENIC (18:3)	EPA AND DHA (20:5 AND 22:6)
Canola oil	>6	24	15	—	5.2	7.4
Coconut oil	88	7	1	—	—	—
Cod liver oil	19	23	2	0.7	1	24
Corn oil	13	31	39	—	1	—
Flaxseed oil	13	17	13	—	55	—
Olive oil	14	72	8	—	1	—
Peanut oil	19	55	26	2.2	1	—
Safflower oil	9	11	74	—	0.5	—
Salmon oil	26	—	1	—	1	13
Sesame seed oil	>12	40	42	—	0.4	—
Soybean oil	15	22	53	—	8	—
Sunflower seed oil	10	22	55	—	0.5	—
Walnut oil	11	—	55	—	11	—
Wheat germ oil	>16	27	42	—	—	1

Source: References 12 and 13.

not be as clear as previously thought, at least not for breast, colon, and prostate cancer.[6, 7, 8] For example, a pooled analysis of cohort studies suggests that fat intake is not a risk factor for development of breast cancer.[9] Other recent studies have reported that a lower total fat intake (from about 33 percent to about 20 percent of calories) is not associated with decreased breast cancer risk.[3] Still other meta-analysis studies have reported conflicting results.[10] Importantly, some studies reported that a high omega-6 to omega-3 ratio in fat tissue, rather than total fat consumption, might be associated with increased breast cancer risk.[11]

Although the correlation between fat intake and cancer risk is not as clear as previously thought, research does suggest that a strong correlation exists between fat intake and disease progression. Many studies indicate that omega-6 fatty acids, and to some degree saturated fats, tend to facilitate progression of some cancers. For example, one study found that omega-6 fatty acids could enhance invasion and metastasis of breast and possibly prostate cancer.[14] In another study, increased intake of saturated fat was associated with increased frequency of lymph node involvement in newly diagnosed postmenopausal breast cancer patients.[15] Other studies have esti-

mated that the risk of death at any time in breast cancer patients increases 1.4-fold for each kilogram increase in monthly fat intake.[16, 17] In a five-year study of 384 men treated for prostate cancer, patients with the highest saturated-fat intake had a threefold higher risk of dying than patients with the lowest saturated-fat intake.[18]

In rodent studies, a low-fat diet (21 percent of calories or less as fat) markedly slowed the growth of established human prostate tumors.[19] Progressively lower fat levels produced better results. In one 10-week study on mice with transplanted human prostate cancer cells, the mean tumor weight of a group receiving a high-fat diet (20 percent fat by diet weight) was double that of a group receiving a 5 percent fat diet.[20] Note that a diet of 21 percent of calories by fat is far different from a diet of 20 percent fat by weight. The first contains roughly 50 grams of fat per day, while the second contains roughly 190 grams per day. A low-fat diet then might have about 5 percent of fat by weight, or roughly 20 percent of calories as fat.

A number of mechanisms exist by which dietary fats may promote development and growth of cancer. Omega-6 fatty acids can increase production of 2-series prostanoids and 4-series leukotrienes, increase estrogen bioavailability, impair the immune system, increase total calorie intake, and/or induce mild oxidative stress.[21] Each of these mechanisms is discussed below.

Increased Production of Prostanoids and Leukotrienes

Consumption of animal fats and omega-6 vegetable oils can increase the arachidonic acid content of cell membranes, especially membranes of some cancer cells.[22] For example, breast and lung cancer cells have an increased percentage of arachidonic acid compared to normal cells. In human lung cancer cells, up to 40 percent of the fatty acid composition of the cell wall has been reported to be arachidonic acid, a much larger percentage than found in normal cells.[23, 24, 25] The arachidonic acid, in turn, acts as a substrate for production of inflammatory eicosanoids like PGE_2 and the 4-series leukotrienes, such as leukotriene A_4 (see Figures 7.3 and 7.4). Increased production of eicosanoids has been implicated as the active mechanism in omega-6-induced invasion and metastasis of a number of cancers, including breast cancer.[26, 27, 28]

These inflammatory eicosanoids are produced in excessive quantities by many types of tumors. Production of PGE_2 has been linked both with tumor metastasis to bone and poor survival in breast cancer patients.[29] PGE_2 and leukotrienes may promote tumor development and progression by stimulating release of invasion-enhancing enzymes from tumor cells, inducing inflammation, increasing angiogenesis, stimulating migration of cancer cells, and helping migrating tumor cells adhere to capillary walls.[30] In addition, these eicosanoids can affect immune parameters. For example, PGE_2 can inhibit natural killer cell activity.[31] PGE_2 is not the only eicosanoid that assists cancer progression and recent evidence suggests that, depending on the type of cancer, leukotrienes can play an even more important role than prostaglandins.[32–35]

The relative roles of leukotrienes and prostaglandins in cancer progression will doubtless become more apparent with future research. What is already clear is that saturated fats and omega-6 fatty acids are direct and indirect sources of arachidonic acid and that arachidonic acid is converted to both inflammatory leukotrienes and prostanoids in vivo.

Increased Estrogen Availability

Intake of saturated and omega-6 fatty acids may promote cancer progression partly by increasing the production or availability of estrogen.[36, 37, 38] Estrogen is a growth factor for a number of cancers, including many breast cancers. High-fat diets and associated increases in fat tissue can increase estrogen availability in a number of ways:

- Fat tissue is a major source of estrogen production in postmenopausal women. Increased estrogen production by fat tissue may partially account for the association between high body weight and decreased survival in breast cancer patients.[39, 40]

- Obesity, and possibly insulin resistance, can decrease the levels of sex hormone binding globulin (SHBG) in men and women and increase breast cancer risk or cancer progression.[41–45] SHBG is a plasma protein that binds and transports sex hormones, including estrogen and testosterone. By binding with SHBG, hormones become less biologically available. Thus binding of estrogen to SHBG may deprive breast cancer cells of estrogen stimulation.[46] In addition, in estrogen-dependent human breast cancer cells, bind-

ing between estrogen, SHBG, and the SHBG receptor causes an antiproliferative, antiestrogenic effect.[47]

- Obesity can alter estrogen metabolism in the liver in favor of removal of byproducts with low estrogenic activity and retention of estrogen byproducts with high estrogenic activity.[48]

- High-fat diets may reduce the amount of estrogen excreted through the feces.

In contrast, low-fat (and high-fiber) diets can reduce circulating estrogen levels.[49] The Women's Health Trial Vanguard Group has studied 303 women at increased risk for breast cancer to determine the feasibility of reducing dietary fat to 20 percent of calories, since animal studies suggested that diets containing less than 20 percent of calories as fat reduced the incidence of breast cancer.[50, 51] Results indicated that patients can comply successfully with dietary fat restrictions and that serum estrogen levels can be decreased.[36, 52] Smaller studies have reported similar results. For example, one study reported that a 10 percent fat diet could reduce estrogen levels in postmenopausal women by 50 percent.[53]

In light of these results, some investigators have recommended a diet containing no more than 15 percent calories from fat as an adjuvant therapy for postmenopausal breast cancer patients, and prostate cancer patients as well.[54, 55, 56] Others have advised breast cancer patients to eat even lower levels, no more then 10 percent of calories as fat.[57] Although the benefits of low-fat diets are still under investigation, it would seem reasonable based on available evidence for some patients to consume significantly less than 30 percent of calories as fat. Low-fat diets alone, however, are probably not enough to produce optimal effects; a significant portion of the total fat consumed should be comprised of omega-3 fatty acids.

Decreased Immune Response

A diet high in saturated and omega-6 fatty acids may promote cancer partly by decreasing immune function. In a study of 17 men who reduced their fat intake to less than 30 percent of calories, natural killer (NK) cell activity was markedly increased compared to baseline levels. In this study, the lower the fat content, the greater the NK cell activity.[58] The exact mechanism of this inhibition was uncertain, but it may have been related to increased PGE_2 production, which has an immunosuppressive effect.

Increased Calorie Intake

Calorie intake by itself may stimulate cancer progression, and dietary fat is a major source of calories. In a study of 149 women treated for breast cancer, higher levels of total fat intake were associated with increased risks of recurrence and death. A large part of this risk increase appeared to be due to increased calorie intake.[59] In rats, a 30 percent reduction of calorie intake reduced growth of transplanted human prostate cancer cells, vascular endothelial growth factor (VEGF) production, and tumor angiogenesis.[60] Interestingly, exercise, which burns calories, reduced the growth of transplanted human breast cancer cells in mice fed a high-fat diet.[61]

Mild Oxidative Stress

As mentioned, polyunsaturated fatty acids are susceptible to free radical damage because of their high number of double carbon bonds. Therefore, moderate intake of polyunsaturated fatty acids may stimulate cancer progression by inducing mild oxidative stress within tumors. Recent studies have suggested that diets containing 15 percent of calories polyunsaturated fatty acids significantly increase DNA oxidative damage to lymphocytes and other indicators of oxidative stress in humans as compared to diets containing 5 percent polyunsaturated fatty acids.[62, 63] Not surprisingly, in these and other studies vitamin E reduced the negative effects of high-fat diets. In one study vitamin E (at about 170 I.U., as scaled to humans) inhibited the ability of high-fat diets to promote growth of transplanted human prostate cancer cells in mice.[64]

INHIBITION OF CANCER BY OMEGA-3 FATTY ACIDS

We have seen that intake of saturated and omega-6 fatty acids may promote tumor progression through a variety of mechanisms. Now we turn to the potential of omega-3 fatty acids, primarily EPA and DHA as found in fish oil, to inhibit tumor development and metastasis. Many of the successful animal studies used high doses of EPA or fish oil, which produced anticancer effects through a prooxidant mechanism. Although these results are not very relevant to our interests—the doses are excessive and we do not advocate a prooxidant strategy—a smaller number of studies have suggested that moderate doses, which do not act by prooxidant means, may still be beneficial. Also, negative effects were reported in a few high-dose animal studies; these could likely be reduced or eliminated by using lower doses of fish oil, which would not cause prooxidant effects and would be less likely to cause immunosuppression.

Summary of Research and Conclusions

A relatively large number of in-vitro and animal studies have been published regarding the ability of omega-3 fatty acids, and specifically EPA, DHA, or fish oil, to inhibit cancer proliferation and progression. At least 57 in-vitro studies have been published, and of these, 47 reported that omega-3 fatty acids could inhibit proliferation or invasion, or induce differentiation of cancer cells.[35, 65–68] Eleven studies directly correlated the antiproliferative effect with increased lipid peroxidation.[69–73] In addition to these, at least 11 reported that omega-3 fatty acids could increase the effectiveness of chemotherapy or radiotherapy against cancer cells.[74–78] This effect is likely due to increased lipid peroxidation and drug uptake.

Of the 66 animal studies on omega-3 fatty acids:

- Thirty-eight reported that omega-3 fatty acids could inhibit tumor growth and metastasis in rodents.[79–83] Five other studies were negative or reported increased metastasis.[84–88]

- Seven studies directly correlated the antiproliferative effect with increased lipid peroxidation.[89–92]

- Eleven studies focused on the ability of omega-3 fatty acids to inhibit cachexia.[93–97] All but one reported a beneficial effect.[98]

- Six studies reported that omega-3 fatty acids could inhibit tumor growth through other mechanisms such as inhibition of angiogenesis, ras protein activity, or invasion enzymes.[99–104]

- Five studies reported that omega-3 fatty acids increased the effectiveness of chemotherapy drugs.[105–109]

Of the 11 human studies conducted on the anticancer effects of omega-3 fatty acids, seven examined their potential anticachectic effects. As a whole, these suggested EPA could inhibit tumor-induced cachexia.[110–116] Four studies explored the effects of omega-3 fatty acids on the immune function of cancer patients, with three of these reporting positive effects and one, no effect.[117–120]

To sum up, in-vitro, animal, and human studies indicate omega-3 fatty acids can inhibit cell proliferation and tumor growth through a free-radical-mediated mechanism, which is probably the primary cause of cell kill seen at high EPA or fish oil doses. At more moderate doses, other mechanisms may be acting, including inhibition of inflammation, angiogenesis, ras protein activity, or invasion enzymes. Moderate doses may also inhibit tumor cachexia.

Discussion

A large number of animal studies have reported that omega-3 fatty acids, especially EPA found in fish oil, produce an antitumor effect.[29, 30, 91, 121–126] For example, EPA, or fish oil containing EPA, inhibited development and growth of colon, prostate, and pancreatic cancers and the growth and metastasis of breast cancer in rodents. The doses used in most studies were high—about 10 to 20 percent of diet, or the human equivalent of about 120 to 240 grams per day. At this excessive dose, the primary mechanism of tumor inhibition apparently was increased lipid peroxidation.[89, 90, 91] Not surprisingly then, the effect could be inhibited by vitamin E treatment.[92]

A prooxidant mechanism is also responsible for many of the cytotoxic results seen in vitro.[127] Both omega-3 and omega-6 fatty acids are cytotoxic to human breast, lung, and prostate cancer cells in vitro but not to normal cells.[128, 129] In fact, polyunsaturated fatty acids are cytotoxic in vitro to at least 16 different human cell lines derived from 11 different organs.[128] As mentioned, polyunsaturated fatty acids contain multiple carbon double bonds, and each double bond is a target for free radical damage. Some cancer cells have an increased content of arachidonic acid (four double bonds), which makes them more susceptible than normal cells to lipid peroxide damage.[25] Incorporation of EPA, which has five double bonds, and DHA, with six, further increases susceptibility to lipid peroxide damage. In one study, treatment of leukemia cells with DHA increased the number of unsaturated double bonds in the plasma membrane by 31 percent.[23, 25]

Since multiple antioxidant mechanisms are active in vivo, the moderate doses of EPA suitable for humans are not likely to produce enough lipid peroxidation to inhibit tumor growth by this means. Oral administration of EPA or DHA at 5.8 grams per day (as scaled to humans) did not affect red blood cell susceptibility to oxidative stress in rats, even though EPA and DHA tissue concentrations were increased.[130] Thus it appears that the results of the high-dose animal studies and the in-vitro studies, which relied on lipid peroxidation, are not directly applicable to treating human patients. Moreover, such a prooxidant effect, even if it could be achieved, may not be beneficial over the long run.

Fortunately, relatively moderate doses of EPA/DHA may still inhibit cancer through a number of nonoxidative mechanisms, although results may not be as dramatic as those seen at high doses; to assure effectiveness, moderate doses of EPA/DHA may best be used in combination with other anticancer compounds. Some animal studies reported that EPA inhibited tumor growth and/or reduced metastasis at doses of about 1 to 2 percent of diet.[22, 131, 132] The human equivalent is about 12 to 24 grams per day of EPA. DHA can also be effective at moderate doses; for example, at 2 percent of diet it inhibited metastasis of human breast cancer cells in mice.[131] In another study, DHA at 4 percent of diet inhibited growth of transplanted human breast cancer cells in mice and inhibited angiogenesis.[100] The human equivalents of a 2 and 4 percent diet are about 24 and 48 grams per day.

At moderate doses (12 to 48 grams per day) EPA and DHA may inhibit cancer progression through the actions listed in Table 17.2, all have been discussed previously except for increased membrane fluidity and decreased cachexia, reviewed below. The ability of EPA to affect eicosanoid synthesis is also discussed further.

EPA and Eicosanoids

A number of investigators have reported that omega-3 supplementation can inhibit production of 2-series prostanoids and 4-series leukotrienes by normal cells and cancer cells. These eicosanoids can assist angiogenesis and cancer progression (see Chapters 7 and 8). Even moderate doses of omega-3 fatty acids can change tissue fatty acid profiles and PGE_2 production. For example, a 3-gram dose of fish oil (containing 540 milligrams of EPA and 360 milligrams of DHA) increased the ratio of omega-3 to omega-6 fatty acids in breast tissue and plasma in patients with breast cancer, and an 11-gram dose (2.1 grams of EPA and 1.9 grams of DHA) reduced production of PGE_2 by intestinal cells in healthy subjects.[133, 134, a]

The ability of omega-3 fatty acids to inhibit eicosanoid production is dependent on the dietary omega-3 to omega-6 ratio. Ideal dietary ratios of total omega-3 to total omega-6 fatty acids for eicosanoid inhibition, health promotion, and disease treatment may be about 1:1 to 1:2.[35, 135–137] The ratio in the Western diet is far lower, at about 1:20 to 1:30.[138]

Increased Plasma Membrane Fluidity

Polyunsaturated fatty acids can increase fluidity of the plasma membrane of tumor cells. Membrane fluidity is a measure of the ability of lipid molecules (and the proteins they sandwich) to move about; fluidity thus affects

---

[a] In plasma, the omega-6 to omega-3 ratio changed from 0.9 to 0.41. To give an idea of plasma concentrations, the total omega-3 fatty acid concentration changed from 390 to 1,200 μM. EPA plasma concentrations changed from 34 to 690 μM and DHA plasma concentrations changed from 330 to 530 μM.

TABLE 17.2 POTENTIAL ANTICANCER ACTIONS OF EPA/DHA				
ACTIVITY	**KNOWN EFFECTS**	**AS A PKC INHIBITOR, MAY:**	**AS AN EICOSANOID INHIBITOR, MAY:**	**AS A COLLAGENASE INHIBITOR, MAY:**
Chapter 3: Results of Therapy at the Cellular Level				
Induce differentiation	x			
Induce apoptosis	x		x	
Chapter 4: Growth Factors and Signal Transduction				
Inhibit PKC	x	—		
Inhibit isoprene synthesis	x			
Chapter 5: Transcription Factors and Redox Signaling				
Inhibit NF-κB activity		x	x	
Chapter 6: Cell-to-Cell Communication				
Affect CAMs	x	x	x	
Chapters 7 and 8: Angiogenesis				
Inhibit angiogenesis	x	x	x	x
Inhibit bFGF effects				x
Inhibit histamine effects		x		
Inhibit eicosanoid effects	x		—	
Inhibit TNF effects		x		
Inhibit VEGF effects	x	x	x	
Inhibit insulin resistance	x	x		
Chapters 9 and 10: Invasion and Metastasis				
Inhibit invasion		x		x
Inhibit hyaluronidase, beta-glucuronidase, or elastase			x	
Inhibit collagenase effects	x	x	x	—
Inhibit cell migration	x	x		
Inhibit metastasis	x	x		x
Inhibit platelet aggregation	x			
Chapters 11 and 12: Immune System				
Stimulate the immune system	variable			
Inhibit tumor-induced immunosuppression	x			
Chapter 17: Lipids				
Increase membrane fluidity	x			
Decrease cachexia	x			

be more fluid than those of normal cells, possibly due to their relatively high arachidonic acid content.[139] In addition, the plasma membranes of highly metastatic tumor cell variants are commonly more fluid than their low metastatic counterparts.[140, 141]

While increased membrane fluidity can assist cancer cells in some respects and omega-3 fatty acids can increase membrane fluidity, the latter do not generally promote tumor progression. They do increase drug transport across the cell wall, however. For example, EPA increased the uptake of the chemotherapy drug mitomycin in colon cancer cells but not in normal cells.[142] Similar effects were seen in other cancer cell lines.[143] Furthermore, omega-3 fatty acids do not increase tumor cell's ability to deform and squeeze through passages. For example, in one study on leukemia cells, the higher the DHA content, the less the leukemic cells were able to deform.[144] Lastly, omega-3 fatty acids can alter antigen structures on tumor cells and make them more susceptible to immune attack. For example, leukemia cells from mice fed large doses of fish oil (58 to 120 grams per day, as scaled to humans) were more susceptible to destruction by cytotoxic T cells.[145] Another in-vitro study reported the same result.[146]

It would seem from these studies that EPA and DHA can increase membrane fluidity but in a way that inhibits rather than promotes tumor progression. Their ability to increase drug uptake may make them valuable during some forms of chemotherapy treatment (see Chapter 23).

Decreased Cachexia

Causes of Cachexia

Cachexia is a complex metabolic syndrome characterized by malnutrition and tissue wasting (greater than 10

the mobility of membrane proteins such as receptors, enzymes, antigens, and CAMs.

Moderate increases in fluidity are associated with greater freedom of molecular motion, greater drug transport across the cell wall, increased cell metabolism, a greater capacity for division, and a greater ability to deform and squeeze between vascular cells during migration. The effects of increased fluidity are complex, however, and not all of these events necessarily occur together. The plasma membranes of tumor cells tend to to 15 percent weight loss). Not all cancers are associated with cachexia; it is relatively rare in patients with breast cancer and sarcoma. Still, it is responsible for 4 to 23 percent of all cancer-related deaths.[147] There is evidence from animal and human studies that EPA may reduce cachexia.

Patients with tumors of the digestive tract are particularly vulnerable to cachexia, since these can interfere with digestive function. Systemic mechanisms of cachexia also exist, however, as evidenced by the relatively high rates of cachexia in patients with nongastrointestinal cancers, such as lung cancer. Regardless of the cause, patients without weight loss tend to survive substantially longer.

Systemic causes of cachexia are related to disruptions in the metabolism of carbohydrates, proteins, and fats. The cachectic patient is not able to gain weight, even with adequate nutrition. Changes in glucose metabolism are often central to cachexia. Tumors can produce factors that decrease sensitivity of normal cells to insulin, creating insulin resistance and resulting in hyperglycemia and the production of more insulin. Recall from Chapter 7 that insulin can act as a growth factor for cancer cells; their increased demand for glucose is aggravated by the fact that they metabolize glucose in an inherently inefficient anaerobic process. The high glucose demand is met in part by converting fat and muscle into glucose. It is also met by gluconeogenesis, a process by which the byproduct of anaerobic metabolism, lactic acid, circulates back to the liver and is metabolized into glucose. Gluconeogenesis itself is an energy-intensive process that further depletes energy stores and causes additional tissue wasting.

A second metabolic change that leads to tissue wasting is altered fat metabolism. The exact mechanism causing the change is unclear. Until recently, it was thought to be primarily due to increased production of cytokines like tumor necrosis factor (TNF) and interleukin-6 (which also induces anorexia). Because of its effect on cachexia, tumor necrosis factor was originally termed *cachectin*. TNF is secreted by macrophages and can both destroy cancer cells and facilitate angiogenesis; it has a secondary effect of mobilizing fat and protein energy stores, possibly for use as an energy source for im-

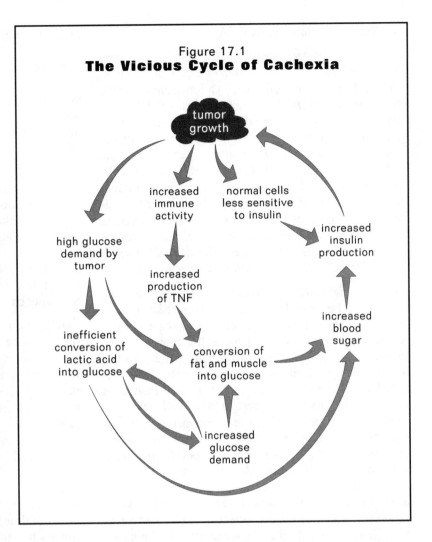

Figure 17.1
The Vicious Cycle of Cachexia

mune cells. In short-term conditions like infection, excessive fat metabolism does not lead to a critical loss in tissue mass, but in chronic diseases such as cancer, elevated fat metabolism eventually depletes fat and muscle stores. The vicious cycle leading to cachexia, as well as tumor growth, is illustrated in Figure 17.1.

In cancer patients, insulin resistance as well as cachexia is associated with increased production of TNF and IL-6.[148, 149] It has recently been suggested, however, that neither of these is the primary culprit in cancer cachexia; a newly described factor, proteolysis-inducing factor (PIF), may be involved.[93, 150] It appears that PIF induces cachexia as a result of increased production of the leukotriene 15-HETE.[151] Nevertheless, to the degree that TNF assists cachexia, natural agents that limit its production may help reduce cachectic effects. These agents were discussed in Chapters 5 and 8 (recall that NF-κB activation can lead to increased TNF production).

Inhibition of Cachexia by EPA

EPA effectively reverses cachexia induced by colon cancer in mice.[152, 153, 154] Other omega-3 or omega-6 fatty acids were not effective. Optimal anticachectic effects were observed at daily doses of 1.2 to 5 g/kg.[155, 156, 157] The lower range is equal to roughly 12 grams per day in humans. In EPA-treated mice, survival was approximately double that of controls, and no cachexia was apparent.[155] Oral administration of EPA (at 4.8 grams per day, as scaled to humans) also inhibited cachexia induced directly by PIF in mice.[150] Although a number of mechanisms may be involved in EPA-induced inhibition of cachexia, the primary mechanism appears to be a direct blocking of the sensitivity of fat cells to tumor-produced cachectic factors.[150]

Positive results with omega-3 fatty acids were reported in four uncontrolled clinical trials on weight-losing pancreatic cancer patients. Pancreatic cancer is a disease in which up to 90 percent of patients suffer from cachexia. In one study, administration of 12 grams per day of fish oil (containing 2.2 grams EPA and 1.4 grams DHA) resulted in an overall weight gain after three months of treatment.[158] The EPA content in blood cells increased from undetectable levels before supplementation to 5.3 percent after one month. DHA increased from 3.5 percent to 6.6 percent. A similar dose was effective in another study, in which oral administration of 2.2 grams EPA and 0.96 grams DHA per day in combination with a multivitamin supplement reversed weight loss in cachectic pancreatic cancer patients.[111] This same dose was effective in a third study without the multivitamin supplement.[115] In the fourth study, a dose of 6 grams per day of pure EPA reversed weight loss in pancreatic cancer patients.[116]

Tumor characteristics may determine the success of EPA treatment. For example, mice bearing a poorly differentiated, fast-growing cancer that induces cachexia did not respond to EPA treatment (at 14 grams per day, as scaled to humans). EPA may be most effective in well-differentiated, slower-growing tumors.[159] In support of this, moderately differentiated colon cancer cells appear to incorporate more omega-3 fatty acids into their plasma membrane than do poorly differentiated cells.[160]

Other Natural Agents That May Inhibit Cachexia

In addition to fatty acids, other natural compounds may be useful in treating cachexia. One such group of compounds are those that protect the gastrointestinal lining from physical trauma, such as that induced by chemotherapy. For example, plantain, a type of starchy banana, increases the thickness of the gastric mucosa and has shown significant promise as an anti-ulcer agent.[161, 162] In one study, a preparation of plantain sap prevented the acute toxic effects of chemotherapy on the intestines in tumor-bearing mice. Furthermore, the combined treatment was more effective in inhibiting tumor growth than chemotherapy alone.[163] The amino acid glutamine may also help protect the intestinal cells of patients undergoing chemotherapy. (Glutamine is discussed in Chapter 18.)

Vitamin E may also be useful. In mice, administration of a large dose of vitamin E (at approximately 640 mg/kg) markedly inhibited development of TNF-induced cachexia. The effect was not because TNF production was blocked but apparently because of inhibition of the TNF receptor or a post-receptor pathway in muscle tissue.[164] The human equivalent is about 6.1 grams per day, or about 9,200 I.U.

Melatonin may help treat cachexia also; in a study of 100 advanced patients, oral administration of melatonin (at 20 milligrams per day) reduced TNF production and the rate of weight loss.[165] It is possible this effect was due partly to inhibition of NF-κB activity. In another study, melatonin inhibited cachexia in patients receiving chemotherapy. In a randomized study of 70 patients with advanced non-small-cell lung cancer treated with cisplatin and etoposide, the addition of melatonin (at 20 milligrams per day, orally) increased the one-year survival rate as compared to those receiving only chemotherapy (from 19 to 44 percent). In addition, the adverse effects of drug treatment, particularly myelosuppression, neuropathy, and cachexia, diminished in the group receiving melatonin. In the group taking melatonin and chemotherapy, no cachexia was reported, but in the one taking chemotherapy only, 44 percent of patients experienced cachexia.[166]

The effects of vitamin E and melatonin may be common to antioxidants in general. Oral administration of N-acetylcysteine (at 0.6 to 4.2 grams per day) prevented loss of body mass in late-stage cancer patients treated with IL-2; the N-acetylcysteine dose given to each subject was based on the plasma cystine to thiol ratio, since this ratio indicates oxidative stress.[167]

Clinical Use of Fish Oil

The two primary commercial sources of omega-3 fatty acids are fish oil and flaxseed oil. Although most anti-cancer studies have been conducted with fish oil, or its components EPA and DHA, flaxseed oil presents a tempting alternative. It is far less expensive and contains a greater percentage of omega-3 fatty acids; its content of alpha-linolenic acid is approximately 58 percent of the total fat.[168] Flaxseed oil does not seem as promising in cancer treatment, however.

In vivo, alpha-linolenic acid is converted to EPA by a series of enzymes, including delta-6 desaturate (see Figure 7.4). In studies on healthy humans, flaxseed oil (at 1.5 tablespoons per day) was as effective in increasing tissue EPA levels as direct EPA supplementation, so long as the dietary content of omega-6 fatty acids was restricted.[169] Similarly, canola oil, also rich in linolenic acid, moderately increased tissue EPA levels in humans, but the degree of conversion appeared to be restricted and unreliable.[170, 171] The difficulty with flaxseed oil is that it may not be effectively converted to EPA in the tissue of some tumors, since many cancer lines are deficient in delta-6 desaturase, the enzyme needed for this conversion. In fact, *ras* overexpression may result in the loss of delta-6 desaturase activity.[172] One study in mice with transplanted human prostate cancer cells reported that an 18 percent flaxseed and 5 percent corn oil diet did not reduce the tumor burden or increase life span, whereas an 18 percent EPA/DHA and 5 percent corn oil diet did.[20] In addition, some studies have associated dietary intake of alpha-linolenic acid with increased risk of prostate cancer. Therefore, fish oil may be the better choice for treatment.

One important factor in the clinical use of EPA is the amount and type of other fatty acids in the diet, since the presence of saturated and omega-6 fatty acids may affect uptake and metabolism of EPA.[35] For example, omega-6 fatty acids compete with EPA for cellular uptake.[173, 174, 175] To be effective, then, EPA is best combined with a diet low in omega-6 fatty acids and saturated fats. As discussed previously, an ideal omega-3 to omega-6 ratio may be in the range of 1:1 to 1:2. These low ratios may be difficult to achieve, but ratios just above this range should be attainable. For example, a 1:3 ratio could be produced with a daily fish oil dose of about 15 grams (containing roughly 10 grams of EPA and DHA in total) and a daily omega-6 fatty acid intake of about 30 grams. (Since intake of omega-9 fatty acids like olive oil does not factor into this ratio, total fat intake could be larger than 40 grams.)

Estimated Therapeutic and Tolerated Doses of EPA/DHA

EPA has been studied as a treatment agent for a number of noncancerous conditions, including autoimmune

TABLE 17.3 ESTIMATED THERAPEUTIC AND MTD DOSES FOR FISH OIL AND/OR EPA/DHA	
DESCRIPTION	**DOSE (g/day)**
Required dose as scaled from animal antitumor studies (fish oil and/or EPA/DHA)	120 to 240 (high dose) 12 to 48 (moderate dose)
Human dose reported useful in inhibiting cachexia (pure EPA)	2 to 12 (about 6 to 36 as fish oil)
Target dose based on an average from animal and human studies (fish oil)	23
Minimum required cytotoxic dose assuming 15-fold synergistic benefits	1.5
Common human dose in noncancerous conditions (fish oil)	2 to 20
Maximum tolerated dose (MTD) of fish oil	21
Tentative dose recommendation for further research (fish oil)	**6 to 21**
Minimum degree of synergism required	**1.1-fold potency increase**

disorders and heart disease. Although effective dosages of fish oil are still uncertain, common doses range from 2 to 20 grams per day.[176, 177] The various effects become apparent within four weeks of administration.

The optimal dose of EPA/DHA and its efficacy in treating human cancer are still uncertain. The antitumor dose of EPA, DHA, or fish oil scaled from rodent experiments is 12 to 48 grams per day in studies using a moderate dose and 120 to 240 grams in those that used a high dose. Benefits in the high-dose studies were likely from a prooxidant effect, and we are more interested here in studies that used moderate doses. As mentioned, an estimated EPA dose for treating cachexia is 2 to 12 grams per day of pure EPA, based on animal and human studies. This might be equivalent to a fish oil dose of about 6 to 36 grams, assuming that commercial fish oil products contain about 33 percent pure EPA. Lastly, an 18-gram fish oil dose containing 3.1 grams of EPA and 2.1 grams of DHA (with 300 I.U. vitamin E) improved immune indices of severely ill cancer patients and significantly prolonged their survival (50 percent survival of about 400 days versus 180 days with placebo).[117] Thus an effective human dose of fish oil might be in the range of 6 to 48 grams per day. We use an average of all the above doses (excluding those from the high-dose animal studies) as a target, which is then 23 grams per day of fish oil.

A 23-gram dose is likely to cause mild adverse effects. In a recent phase I trial, the maximum tolerated dose of fish oil for cachectic patients was 21 grams daily (0.3 g/kg).[110] This dose contained about 15 grams of total omega-3 fatty acids. Dose-limiting side effects were reversible gastrointestinal upsets like diarrhea, nausea, and cramping. Moreover, note that moderate doses of fish oil are likely to inhibit platelet aggregation, and caution should be used in patients at risk for bleeding.

The estimated therapeutic doses for fish oil and/or EPA/DHA are summarized in Table 17.3. The tentative recommended dose is 6 to 21 grams per day of fish oil. The 6-gram value is approximate and assumes that the minimum effective dose of pure EPA may be about 2 grams (as per the studies on cachexia) and that commercial fish oil products contain about 33 percent pure EPA. The 21-gram value is equal to the maximum tolerated dose.

It appears that synergistic interactions may be required for fish oil to produce an anticancer effect in humans. In comparing the 23-gram target dose to the 21-gram maximum dose, synergistic interactions will be needed to produce a minimum 1.1-fold increase in potency. This should be possible, since a 1.1-fold increase is well below the allowable 15-fold increase discussed in Chapter 13. If a 15-fold increase in potency were produced, a dose as low as 1.5 grams per day could be effective.

Although EPA and DHA appear to have some of the same actions, there are differences, and EPA may be more effective, at least for treating cachexia. Diets with a high EPA/DHA ratio were also reported to be more effective at inhibiting arthritis-related inflammation in rats than diets with an equal ratio.[178] Fish oil products that contain a high ratio of EPA to DHA may be most appropriate for treating cachexia and possibly other aspects of cancer. Commercial products are available with an EPA to DHA ratio of at least 5:2.

It may be prudent to use vitamin E in conjunction with fish oil to prevent lipid peroxidation. While vitamin E may be useful in preventing immunosuppression induced by fish oil, it is not clear, however, if immunosuppression would occur at the fish oil doses recommended here. Other antioxidants that would be part of a large combination of natural compounds could be used instead of vitamin E to prevent lipid peroxidation; for example, oral administration of curcumin or quercetin inhibited lipid peroxidation in mice.[179, 180] Moreover, a combination of quercetin and catechin reduced lipid peroxidation in rats fed a diet high in polyunsaturated fatty acids.[181]

CONCLUSION

The available research strongly suggests that omega-6 fatty acids, which are contained in most vegetable oils, may promote cancer progression. Saturated fats may also do so, although the evidence is not as clear as for omega-6 fatty acids. Due to their effects and the fact that they comprise the bulk of dietary fats, some scientists have suggested that fat intake be reduced to 10 to 20 percent of total calories (roughly 25 to 50 grams per day). In contrast, fish oil, which contains EPA, may inhibit cancer progression through many mechanisms, including inhibition of angiogenesis, invasion, metastasis, and cachexia. Thus, during treatment, a significant portion of daily fat intake should come as omega-3 fatty acids.

While much of the information on omega-3 fatty acids comes from animal experiments, inhibition of cachexia has been observed in human patients. Although the research on fish oil is not yet conclusive, its multitude of effects, along with its safe use in noncancerous conditions, makes it very promising as a natural anticancer agent.

REFERENCES

[1] Lasekan JB, Clayton MK, Gendron-Fitzpatrick A. Dietary olive and safflower oils in the promotion of DMBA-induced mammary tumorgenesis in rats. Nutr Cancer 1990; 13:153–63.

[2] National Research Council. Diet, nutrition, and cancer. Cancer Res 1983; 43:3018–3023.

[3] Holmes MD, Hunter DJ, Colditz GA, et al. Association of dietary intake of fat and fatty acids with risk of breast cancer. JAMA 1999 Mar 10; 281(10):914–20.

[4] Krebs-Smith SM. Progress in improving diet to reduce cancer risk. Cancer 1998 Oct 1; 83(7):1425–32.

[5] Creasey W. Diet and cancer. Philadelphia: Lea & Febiger, 1985, pp. 86–102.

[6] Kolonel LN, Nomura AM, Cooney RV. Dietary fat and prostate cancer: Current status. J Natl Cancer Inst 1999 Mar 3; 91(5):414–28.

[7] Snyderwine EG. Diet and mammary gland carcinogenesis. Recent Results Cancer Res 1998; 152:3–10.

[8] Willett WC. Dietary fat intake and cancer risk: A controversial and instructive story. Semin Cancer Biol 1998 Aug; 8(4):245–53.

[9] Hunter DJ, Spiegelman D, Adami HO, et al. Cohort studies of fat intake and the risk of breast cancer—a pooled analysis. NEJM 1996; 334:356–61.

[10] Harrison RA, Waterbor JW. Understanding meta-analysis in cancer epidemiology: Dietary fat and breast cancer. Cancer Detect Prev 1999; 23(2):97–106.

[11] Simonsen N, van't Veer P, Strain JJ, et al. Adipose tissue omega-3 and omega-6 fatty acid content and breast cancer in the EURAMIC study. Am J Epidemiol 1998 Feb 15; 147(4):342–52.

[12] Linder MC, ed. Nutritional biochemistry and metabolism. 2nd ed. New York: Elsevier Science, 1991, p. 74.

[13] Murray M, Pizzorno J. Encyclopedia of natural medicine. Rocklin, CA: Prima Publishing, 1991, p. 163.

[14] Rose DP. Dietary fatty acids and cancer. Am J Clin Nutr 1997 Oct; 66(4 Suppl):998S-1003S.

[15] Verreault R, Brisson J, Deschenes L, et al. Dietary fat in relation to prognostic indicators in breast cancer. J National Cancer Institute 80(11):819–825.

[16] Gregorio DI, Emrich LJ, Graham S, et al. Dietary fat consumption and survival among women with breast cancer. J Natl Cancer Inst 1985; 75(1):37–41.

[17] Holm LE, Nordevang E, Hjalmar ML, et al. Treatment failure and dietary habits in women with breast cancer. J Natl Cancer Inst 1993; 85(1):32–36.

[18] Fradet Y, Meyer F, Bairati I, et al. Dietary fat and prostate cancer progression and survival. Eur Urol 1999; 35(5–6):388–91.

[19] Wang Y, Corr JG, Thaler HY, et al. Decreased growth of established human prostate LNCaP tumors in nude mice fed a low-fat diet. J Natl Cancer Inst 1995 October 4; 87(19):1456–62.

[20] Connolly JM, Coleman M, Rose DP. Effects of dietary fatty acids on DU145 human prostate cancer cell growth in athymic nude mice. Nutrition and Cancer 1997; 29(2):114–119.

[21] Broitman SA, Cannizzo, Jr F. A model system for studying nutritional interventions on colon tumor growth: Effects of marine oil. In Exercise, calories, fat and cancer. Jacobs MM, ed. New York: Plenum Press, 1992.

[22] Karmali RA, Marsh J, Fuchs C. Effect of omega-3 fatty acids on growth of a rat mammary tumor. JNCL 1984; 73(2):457.

[23] Bockman RS, Hickok N, Rapuano B. Prostaglandins and calcium metabolism in cancer. In Prostaglandins in cancer research. Garaci E, Paoletti R, Santoro MG, ed. Berlin: Springer-Verlag, 1987.

[24] Burns CP, Petersen ES, North JA, et al. Effect of docosahexaenoic acid on rate of differentiation of HL-60 human leukemia. Cancer Research 1989; 49:3252–58.

[25] Cullis P, Hope MJ. Physical properties and functional roles of lipids in membranes. In Biochemistry of lipids, lipoproteins and membranes. Vance DE, Vance JE, eds. Amsterdam: Elsevier, 1991.

[26] Rose DP, Hatala MA. Dietary fatty acids and breast cancer invasion and metastasis. Nutr Cancer 1994; 21:103–111.

[27] Bandyopadhyay GK, Hwang SI, Imagawa W, Nandi S. Role of polyunsaturated fatty acids as signal transducers: Amplification of signals from growth factor receptors by fatty acids in mammary epithelial cells. Prostaglandins Leuko Essent Fatty Acids 1993; 48:71–78.

[28] Rose DP, Connolly JM. Influence of dietary linoleic acid on experimental human breast cancer cell metastasis in athymic nude mice. Int J Oncol 1998 Dec; 13(6):1179–83.

[29] Carroll KK. Dietary fats and cancer 1–3. Am J Clin Nutr 1991; 53:1064s-67s.

[30] Cave WT Jr. Dietary omega-3 polyunsaturated fats and breast cancer. Nutrition 1996 Jan; 12(1Suppl):S39–42.

[31] Barone J, Hebert JR. Dietary fat and natural killer cell activity. Med Hypotheses 1988; 25:223–26.

[32] Connolly JM, Liu XH, Rose DP. Dietary linoleic acid-stimulated human breast cancer cell growth and metastasis in nude mice and their suppression by indomethacin, a cyclooxygenase inhibitor. Nutr Cancer 1996; 25(3):231–40.

[33] Rose DP, Connolly JM, Rayburn J, Coleman M. Influence of diets containing eicosapentaenoic or docosahexaenoic acid on growth and metastasis of breast cancer cells in nude mice. Journal of the National Cancer Institute 1995 Apr 19; 87(8):587–592.

[34] Noguchi M, Rose DP, Earashi M, Miyazaki I. The role of fatty acids and eicosanoid synthesis inhibitors in breast carcinoma. Oncology 1995; 52:265–271.

[35] Noguchi M, Earashi M, Minami M, et al. Effects of eicosapentaenoic and docosahexaenoic acid on cell growth and prostaglandin E and leukotriene B production by a human breast cancer cell line (MDA-MB-231). Oncology 1995; 52:458–464.

[36] Dwyer JT. Dietary fat and breast cancer: Testing interventions to reduce risks. In Exercise, calories, fat and cancer. Jacobs MM, ed. New York: Plenum Press, 1992.

[37] Fernandes G, Venkatraman JT. Possible mechanisms through which dietary lipids, calorie restriction and exercise modulate breast cancer. In Exercise, calories, fat and cancer. Jacobs MM, ed. New York: Plenum Press, 1992.

[38] Wu AH, Pike MC, Stram DO. Meta-analysis: Dietary fat intake, serum estrogen levels, and the risk of breast cancer. J Natl Cancer Inst 1999 Mar 17; 91(6):529–34.

[39] Albanes D. Energy balance, body size, and cancer. Crit Rev Oncol Hematol 1990; 10(3):283–303.

[40] Hebert JR, Hurley TG, Ma Y. The effect of dietary exposures on recurrence and mortality in early stage breast cancer. Breast Cancer Res Treat 1998 Sep; 51(1):17–28.

[41] Stoll BA. Western nutrition and the insulin resistance syndrome: A link to breast cancer. Eur J Clin Nutr 1999 Feb; 53(2):83–7.

[42] Stoll BA. Essential fatty acids, insulin resistance, and breast cancer risk. Nutr Cancer 1998; 31(1):72–7.

[43] Yoshikawa T, Noguchi Y, Doi C, et al. Insulin resistance was connected with the alterations of substrate utilization in patients with cancer. Cancer Lett 1999 Jul 1; 141(1–2):93–8.

[44] Tymchuk CN, Tessler SB, Aronson WJ, Barnard RJ. Effects of diet and exercise on insulin, sex hormone-binding globulin, and prostate-specific antigen. Nutr Cancer 1998; 31(2):127–31.

[45] Sherif K, Kushner H, Falkner BE. Sex hormone-binding globulin and insulin resistance in African-American women. Metabolism 1998 Jan; 47(1):70–4.

[46] Zeginiadou T, Kortsaris AH, Koliais S, et al. Sex hormone binding globulin inhibits strongly the uptake of estradiol by human breast carcinoma cells via a deprivative mechanism. Cancer Biochem Biophys 1998 Oct; 16(3):253–63.

[47] Fortunati N, Becchis M, Catalano MG, et al. Sex hormone-binding globulin, its membrane receptor, and breast cancer: A new approach to the modulation of estradiol action in neoplastic cells. J Steroid Biochem Mol Biol 1999 Apr–Jun; 69(1–6):473–9.

[48] Rose D. Diet, hormones, and cancer. Annu Rev Publ Health 1993; 14:1–17.

[49] Bagga D, Ashley JM, Geffrey SP, et al. Effects of a very low fat, high fiber diet on serum hormones and menstrual function. Cancer 1995; 76:2491–6.

50 Cohen LA, Thompson DO, Maeura Y, et al. Dietary fat and mammary cancer. Promoting effects of different dietary fats on N-nitrosomethylurea-induced mammary tumorigenesis. J Natl Cancer Inst. 1986; 77:33.

51 Cohen LA, Choi K, Weisburger JH, et al. Effect of varying proportions of dietary fat on the development of N-nitrosomethylurea-induced rat mammary tumors. Anticancer Res. 1986; 6:215.

52 Boyar AP, Rose JR, Loughridge A, et al. Response to a diet low in total fat in women with postmenopausal breast cancer: A pilot study. Cancer and Nutrition 1988; 11:93–99.

53 Heber D, Ashley JM, Leaf DA, et al. Reduction of serum estradiol in postmenopausal women given free access to low-fat high carbohydrate diet. Nutrition 1991; 7:137.

54 Wynder EL, Taioli E, Rose DP. Breast cancer—The optimal diet. In *Exercise, calories, fat and cancer*. Jacobs MM, ed. New York: Plenum Press, 1992.

55 Cohen LA, Rose DP, Wynder EL. A rationale for dietary intervention in postmenopausal breast cancer patients: An update. Nutr Cancer 1993; 19:1–10.

56 Wynder EL, Rose DP, Cohen LA. Nutrition and prostate cancer: A proposal for dietary intervention. Nutr Cancer 1994; 22:1–10.

57 Nicholson A. Diet and the prevention and treatment of breast cancer. Altern Ther Health Med 1996 Nov; 2(6):32–8.

58 Barone J, Hebert JR, Reddy MM. Dietary fat and natural-killer-cell activity. Am J Clin Nutr 1989 Oct; 50(4):861–867.

59 Saxe GA, Rock CL, Wisha MS, Schottenfeld D. Diet and risk for breast cancer recurrence and survival. Breast Cancer Res Treat 1999 Feb; 53(3):241–53.

60 Mukherjee P, Sotnikov AV, Mangian HJ. Energy intake and prostate tumor growth, angiogenesis, and vascular endothelial growth factor expression. J Natl Cancer Inst 1999 Mar 17; 91(6):512–23.

61 Welsch MA, Cohen LA, Welsch CW. Inhibition of growth of human breast carcinoma xenografts by energy expenditure via voluntary exercise in athymic mice fed a high-fat diet. Nutr Cancer 1995; 23(3):309–18.

62 Jenkinson AM, Collins AR, Duthie SJ, et al. The effect of increased intakes of polyunsaturated fatty acids and vitamin E on DNA damage in human lymphocytes. FASEB J 1999 Dec; 13(15):2138–42.

63 Jenkinson A, Franklin MF, Wahle K, Duthie GG. Dietary intakes of polyunsaturated fatty acids and indices of oxidative stress in human volunteers. Eur J Clin Nutr 1999 Jul; 53(7):523–8.

64 Fleshner N, Fair WR, Huryk R, Heston WD. Vitamin E inhibits the high-fat diet promoted growth of established human prostate LNCaP tumors in nude mice. J Urol 1999 May; 161(5):1651–4.

65 Burns CP, Petersen ES, North JA, Ingraham LM. Effect of docosahexaenoic acid on rate of differentiation of HL-60 human leukemia. Cancer Res 1989 Jun 15; 49(12):3252–8.

66 Connolly JM, Rose DP. Effects of fatty acids on invasion through reconstituted basement membrane ("Matrigel") by a human breast cancer cell line. Cancer Lett 1993 Dec 10; 75(2):137–42.

67 Maehle L, Eilertsen E, Mollerup S, et al. Effects of n-3 fatty acids during neoplastic progression and comparison of in vitro and in vivo sensitivity of two human tumour cell lines. Br J Cancer 1995 Apr; 71(4):691–6.

68 Lai PB, Ross JA, Fearon KC, et al. Cell cycle arrest and induction of apoptosis in pancreatic cancer cells exposed to eicosapentaenoic acid in vitro. Br J Cancer 1996 Nov; 74(9):1375–83.

69 Kumar GS, Das UN. Free radical-dependent suppression of growth of mouse myeloma cells by alpha-linolenic and eicosapentaenoic acids in vitro. Cancer Lett 1995 May 25; 92(1):27–38.

70 Das UN. Tumoricidal action of cis-unsaturated fatty acids and their relationship to free radicals and lipid peroxidation. Cancer Lett 1991 Mar; 56(3):235–43.

71 Das UN, Begin ME, Ells G, et al. Polyunsaturated fatty acids augment free radical generation in tumor cells in vitro. Biochem Biophys Res Commun 1987 May 29; 145(1):15–24.

72 Chajes V, Sattler W, Stranzl A, Kostner GM. Influence of n-3 fatty acids on the growth of human breast cancer cells in vitro: Relationship to peroxides and vitamin-E. Breast Cancer Res Treat 1995 Jun; 34(3):199–212.

73 Hawkins RA, Sangster K, Arends MJ. Apoptotic death of pancreatic cancer cells induced by polyunsaturated fatty acids varies with double bond number and involves an oxidative mechanism. J Pathol 1998 May; 185(1):61–70.

74 Tsai WS, Nagawa H, Muto T. Differential effects of polyunsaturated fatty acids on chemosensitivity of NIH3T3 cells and its transformants. Int J Cancer 1997 Jan 27; 70(3):357–61.

75 Vartak S, Robbins ME, Spector AA. Polyunsaturated fatty acids increase the sensitivity of 36B10 rat astrocytoma cells to radiation-induced cell kill. Lipids 1997 Mar; 32(3):283–92.

76 Zijlstra JG, de Vries EG, Muskiet FA, et al. Influence of docosahexaenoic acid in vitro on intracellular adriamycin concentration in lymphocytes and human adriamycin-sensitive and -resistant small-cell lung cancer cell lines, and on cytotoxicity in the tumor cell lines. Int J Cancer 1987 Dec 15; 40(6):850–6.

77 Plumb JA, Luo W, Kerr DJ. Effect of polyunsaturated fatty acids on the drug sensitivity of human tumour cell lines resistant to either cisplatin or doxorubicin. Br J Cancer 1993 Apr; 67(4):728–33.

78 Kinsella JE, Black JM. Effects of polyunsaturated fatty acids on the efficacy of antineoplastic agents toward L5178Y lymphoma cells. Biochem Pharmacol 1993 May 5; 45(9):1881–7.

79 Rose DP, Connolly JM. Effects of dietary omega-3 fatty acids on human breast cancer growth and metastases in nude mice. J Natl Cancer Inst 1993 Nov 3; 85(21):1743–7.

80 de Bravo MG, de Antueno RJ, Toledo J, et al. Effects of an eicosapentaenoic and docosahexaenoic acid concentrate on a human lung carcinoma grown in nude mice. Lipids 1991 Nov; 26(11):866–70.

81 Iwamoto S, Senzaki H, Kiyozuka Y, et al. Effects of fatty acids on liver metastasis of ACL-15 rat colon cancer cells. Nutr Cancer 1998; 31(2):143–50.

82 Iigo M, Nakagawa T, Ishikawa C, et al. Inhibitory effects of docosahexaenoic acid on colon carcinoma 26 metastasis to the lung. Br J Cancer 1997; 75(5):650–5.

83 Rose DP, Connolly JM, Rayburn J, Coleman M. Influence of diets containing eicosapentaenoic or docosahexaenoic acid on growth and metastasis of breast cancer cells in nude mice. J Natl Cancer Inst 1995 Apr 19; 87(8):587–92.

84 Adams LM, Trout JR, Karmali RA. Effect of n-3 fatty acids on spontaneous and experimental metastasis of rat mammary tumour 13762. Br J Cancer 1990 Feb; 61(2):290–1.

85 Coulombe J, Pelletier G, Tremblay P, et al. Influence of lipid diets on the number of metastases and ganglioside content of H59 variant tumors. Clin Exp Metastasis 1997 Jul; 15(4):410–7.

86 Fady C, Reisser D, Lagadec P, et al. In vivo and in vitro effects of fish-containing diets on colon tumour cells in rats. Anticancer Res 1988 Mar–Apr; 8(2):225–8.

87 Kort WJ, Weijma IM, Stehmann TE, et al. Diets rich in fish oil cannot control tumor cell metastasis. Ann Nutr Metab 1987; 31(6):342–8.

88 Griffini P, Fehres O, Klieverik L, et al. Dietary omega-3 polyunsaturated fatty acids promote colon carcinoma metastasis in rat liver. Cancer Res 1998 Aug 1; 58(15):3312–9.

89 Gonzalez MJ, Schemmel RA, Dugan L Jr, et al. Dietary fish oil inhibits human breast carcinoma growth: A function of increased lipid peroxidation. Lipids 1993 Sep; 28(9):827–32.

90 Gonzalez MJ. Fish oil, lipid peroxidation and mammary tumor growth. J Am Coll Nutr 1995 Aug; 14(4):325–35.

91 Gonzalez MJ, Schemmel RA, Gray JI, et al. Effect of dietary fat on growth of MCF-7 and MDA-MB231 human breast carcinomas in athymic nude mice: Relationship between carcinoma growth and lipid peroxidation product levels. Carcinogenesis 1991 Jul; 12(7):1231–5.

92 Maehle L, Lystad E, Eilertsen E, et al. Growth of human lung adenocarcinoma in nude mice is influenced by various types of dietary fat and vitamin E. Anticancer Res 1999 May–Jun; 19(3A):1649–55.

93 Hussey HJ, Tisdale MJ. Effect of a cachectic factor on carbohydrate metabolism and attenuation by eicosapentaenoic acid. Br J Cancer 1999 Jun; 80(8):1231–5.

94 Tisdale MJ, Beck SA. Inhibition of tumour-induced lipolysis in vitro and cachexia and tumour growth in vivo by eicosapentaenoic acid. Biochem Pharmacol 1991 Jan 1; 41(1):103–7.

95 Tisdale MJ, Dhesi JK. Inhibition of weight loss by omega-3 fatty acids in an experimental cachexia model. Cancer Res 1990 Aug 15; 50(16):5022–6.

96 Beck SA, Smith KL, Tisdale MJ. Anticachectic and antitumor effect of eicosapentaenoic acid and its effect on protein turnover. Cancer Res 1991 Nov 15; 51(22):6089–93.

97 Dagnelie PC, Bell JD, Williams SC, et al. Effect of fish oil on cancer cachexia and host liver metabolism in rats with prostate tumors. Lipids 1994 Mar; 29(3):195–203.

98 Costelli P, Llovera M, Lopez-Soriano J, et al. Lack of effect of eicosapentaenoic acid in preventing cancer cachexia and inhibiting tumor growth. Cancer Lett 1995 Oct 20; 97(1):25–32.

99 Skopinska-Rozewska E, Krotkiewski M, Sommer E, et al. Inhibitory effect of shark liver oil on cutaneous angiogenesis induced in Balb/c mice by syngeneic sarcoma L-1, human urinary bladder and human kidney tumour cells. Oncol Rep 1999 Nov–Dec; 6(6):1341–4.

100 Rose DP, Connolly JM. Antiangiogenicity of docosahexaenoic acid and its role in the suppression of breast cancer cell growth in nude mice. Int J Oncol 1999 Nov; 15(5):1011–5.

101 Singh J, Hamid R, Reddy BS. Dietary fat and colon cancer: Modulating effect of types and amount of dietary fat on ras-p21 function during promotion and progression stages of colon cancer. Cancer Res 1997 Jan 15; 57(2):253–8.

102 Liu XH, Rose DP. Suppression of type IV collagenase in MDA-MB-435 human breast cancer cells by eicosapentaenoic acid in vitro and in vivo. Cancer Lett 1995 May 25; 92(1):21–6.

103 Suzuki I, Iigo M, Ishikawa C, et al. Inhibitory effects of oleic and docosahexaenoic acids on lung metastasis by colon-carcinoma-26 cells are associated with reduced matrix metalloproteinase-2 and -9 activities. Int J Cancer 1997 Nov 14; 73(4):607–12.

104 Mukutmoni-Norris M, Hubbard NE, Erickson KL. Modulation of murine mammary tumor vasculature by dietary n-3 fatty acids in fish oil. Cancer Lett 2000 Mar 13; 150(1):101–9.

105 Horie T, Nakamaru M, Masubuchi Y. Docosahexaenoic acid exhibits a potent protection of small intestine from methotrexate-induced damage in mice. Life Sci 1998; 62(15):1333–8.

106 Shao Y, Pardini L, Pardini RS. Intervention of transplantable human mammary carcinoma MX-1 chemotherapy with dietary menhaden oil in athymic mice: Increased therapeutic effects and decreased toxicity of cyclophosphamide. Nutr Cancer 1997; 28(1):63–73.

107 Hardman WE, Moyer MP, Cameron IL. Fish oil supplementation enhanced CPT-11 (irinotecan) efficacy against MCF7 breast carcinoma xenografts and ameliorated intestinal side-effects. Br J Cancer 1999 Oct; 81(3):440–8.

108 Germain E, Lavandier F, Chajes V, et al. Dietary n-3 polyunsaturated fatty acids and oxidants increase rat mammary tumor sensitivity to epirubicin without change in cardiac toxicity. Lipids 1999; 34 Suppl:S203.

109 Shao Y, Pardini L, Pardini RS. Dietary menhaden oil enhances mitomycin C antitumor activity toward human mammary carcinoma MX-1. Lipids 1995 Nov; 30(11):1035–45.

110 Burns CP, Halabi S, Clamon GH, et al. Phase I clinical study of fish oil fatty acid capsules for patients with cancer cachexia: Cancer and leukemia group B study 9473. Clin Cancer Res 1999 Dec; 5(12):3942–7.

111 Barber MD, Ross JA, Voss AC, et al. The effect of an oral nutritional supplement enriched with fish oil on weight-loss in patients with pancreatic cancer. Br J Cancer 1999 Sep; 81(1):80–6.

112 Wigmore SJ, Ross JA, Falconer JS, et al. The effect of polyunsaturated fatty acids on the progress of cachexia in patients with pancreatic cancer. Nutrition 1996 Jan; 12(1 Suppl):S27–30.

[113] Wigmore SJ, Fearon KC, Maingay JP, Ross JA. Down-regulation of the acute-phase response in patients with pancreatic cancer cachexia receiving oral eicosapentaenoic acid is mediated via suppression of interleukin-6. Clin Sci (Colch) 1997 Feb; 92(2):215–21.

[114] Barber MD, Ross JA, Preston T, et al. Fish oil-enriched nutritional supplement attenuates progression of the acute-phase response in weight-losing patients with advanced pancreatic cancer. J Nutr 1999 Jun; 129(6):1120–5.

[115] Barber MD, McMillan DC, Preston T, et al. Metabolic response to feeding in weight-losing pancreatic cancer patients and its modulation by a fish-oil-enriched nutritional supplement. Clin Sci (Colch) 2000 Apr; 98(4):389–99.

[116] Wigmore SJ, Barber MD, Ross JA. Effect of oral eicosapentaenoic acid on weight loss in patients with pancreatic cancer. Nutr Cancer 2000; 36(2):177–84.

[117] Gogos CA, Ginopoulos P, Salsa B, et al. Dietary omega-3 polyunsaturated fatty acids plus vitamin E restore immunodeficiency and prolong survival for severely ill patients with generalized malignancy: A randomized control trial. Cancer 1998 Jan 15; 82(2):395–402.

[118] Gogos CA, Ginopoulos P, Zoumbos NC, et al. The effect of dietary omega-3 polyunsaturated fatty acids on T-lymphocyte subsets of patients with solid tumors. Cancer Detect Prev 1995; 19(5):415–7.

[119] Tashiro T, Yamamori H, Takagi K, et al. n-3 versus n-6 polyunsaturated fatty acids in critical illness. Nutrition 1998 Jun; 14(6):551–3.

[120] McCarter MD, Gentilini OD, Gomez ME, Daly JM. Preoperative oral supplement with immunonutrients in cancer patients. JPEN J Parenter Enteral Nutr 1998 Jul–Aug; 22(4):206–11.

[121] Cave WT Jr. Omega-3 polyunsaturated fatty acids in rodent models of breast cancer. Breast Cancer Res Treat 1997 Nov–Dec; 46(2–3):239–46.

[122] Rose DP. Dietary fatty acids and prevention of hormone-responsive cancer. Proc Soc Exp Biol Med 1997 Nov; 216(2):224–33.

[123] Butrum RR, Messina MJ. Cancer. In *Health effects of w-3 polyunsaturated fatty acids in seafoods*. World Rev Nutr Diet. Simopoulos AP, et al., eds. Basel: Karger, 1991, pp. 66:48–50.

[124] Karmali RA. Lipid nutrition, prostaglandins and cancer. In *Biochemistry of arachidonic acid metabolism*. Lands W, ed. Boston: Martinus Nijhoff Publishing, 1985.

[125] Istfan N, Wan J, Bistrian B. Nutrition and tumor promotion: In-vitro methods for measurement of cellular proliferation and protein metabolism. J of Parenteral and Enteral Nutrition 1992; 6(6) supp:76s-81s.

[126] Pritchard GA, Jones DL, Mansel RE. Lipids in breast carcinogenesis. Br J Surg 1989; 76:1069–73.

[127] Das UN. Gamma-linolenic acid, arachidonic acid, and eicosapentaenoic acid as potential anticancer drugs. Nutrition 1990; 6(6):429–34.

[128] Norman A, Bennett LR, Mead JF, et al. Antitumor activity of sodium linoleate. Nutrition and Cancer 1988; 11:107–15.

[129] Begin ME, Ells G, Das UN, et al. Differential killing of human cacinoma cells supplemented with n-3 and n-6 polyunsaturated fatty acids. JNCL 1986 Nov; 77(5):1053–60.

[130] Calviello G, Palozza P, Franceschelli P, Bartoli GM. Low-dose eicosapentaenoic or docosahexaenoic acid administration modifies fatty acid composition and does not affect susceptibility to oxidative stress in rat erythrocytes and tissues. Lipids 1997 Oct; 32(10):1075–83.

[131] Rose DP, Connolly JM, Coleman M. Effect of omega-3 fatty acids on the progression of metastases after the surgical excision of human breast cancer cell solid tumors growing in nude mice. Clin Cancer Res 1996 Oct; 2(10):1751–6.

[132] Calviello G, Palozza P, Piccioni E, et al. Dietary supplementation with eicosapentaenoic and docosahexaenoic acid inhibits growth of Morris hepatocarcinoma 3924A in rats: Effects on proliferation and apoptosis. Int J Cancer 1998 Mar 2; 75(5):699–705.

[133] Bagga D, Capone S, Wang HJ, et al. Dietary modulation of omega-3/omega-6 polyunsaturated fatty acid ratios in patients with breast cancer. J Natl Cancer Inst 1997 Aug 6; 89(15):1123–31.

[134] Bartram HP, Gostner A, Scheppach W, et al. Effects of fish oil on rectal cell proliferation, mucosal fatty acids, and prostaglandin E2 release in healthy subjects. Gastroenterology 1993 Nov; 105(5):1317–22.

[135] Simopoulos AP. Evolutionary aspects of omega-3 fatty acids in the food supply. Prostaglandins Leukot Essent Fatty Acids 1999 May–Jun; 60(5–6):421–9.

[136] Minami M, Noguchi M. Effects of low-dose eicosapentaenoic acid, docosahexaenoic acid and dietary fat on the incidence, growth and cell kinetics of mammary carcinomas in rats. Oncology 1996 Sep–Oct; 53(5):398–405.

[137] Karmali RA. Eicosanoids in neoplasia. Prev Med 1987 Jul; 16(4):493–502.

[138] Simopoulos AP. Essential fatty acids in health and chronic disease. Am J Clin Nutr 1999 Sep; 70(3 Suppl):560S-569S.

[139] Booyens J, Maguire L, Katzeff IE. Dietary fats and cancer. Med Hypotheses 1985 Aug; 17(4):351–62.

[140] Taraboletti G, Perin L, Bottazzi B, et al. Membrane fluidity affects tumor-cell motility, invasion and lung-colonizing potential. Int J Cancer 1989; 44:707–713.

[141] Kier AB, Franklin C. Membranes of high- and low-metastatic L tumor cell variants. Invasion and Metastasis 1991; 11:25–37.

[142] Tsai WS, Nagawa H, Muto T. Differential effects of polyunsaturated fatty acids on chemosensitivity of NIH3T3 cells and its transformants. Int J Cancer 1997 Jan 27; 70(3):357–61.

[143] Maehle L, Eilertsen E, Mollerup S, et al. Effects of n-3 fatty acids during neoplastic progression and comparison of in vitro and in vivo sensitivity of two human tumour cell lines. British Journal of Cancer 1995; 71:691–696.

[144] Zerouga M, Jenski LJ, Booster S, et al. Can docosahexaenoic acid inhibit metastasis by decreasing deformability of the tumor cell plasma membrane? Cancer Lett 1997 Nov 11; 119(2):163–8.

[145] Jenski LJ, Sturdevant LK, Ehringer WD, et al. Omega-3 fatty acid modification of membrane structure and function. I. Dietary manipulation of tumor cell susceptibility to cell- and complement-mediated lysis. Nutr Cancer 1993; 19(2):135–46.

146 Pascale AW, Ehringer WD, Stillwell W, et al. Omega-3 fatty acid modification of membrane structure and function. II. Alteration by docosahexaenoic acid of tumor cell sensitivity to immune cytolysis. Nutr Cancer 1993; 19(2):147–57.

147 Calabresi P, Schein P. Medical oncology. 2nd ed. New York: McGraw-Hill, 1993, p. 1149.

148 Noguchi Y, Yoshikawa T, Marat D, et al. Insulin resistance in cancer patients is associated with enhanced tumor necrosis factor-alpha expression in skeletal muscle. Biochem Biophys Res Commun 1998 Dec 30; 253(3):887–92.

149 Makino T, Noguchi Y, Yoshikawa T, et al. Circulating interleukin 6 concentrations and insulin resistance in patients with cancer. Br J Surg 1998 Dec; 85(12):1658–62.

150 Tisdale MJ. Inhibition of lipolysis and muscle protein degradation by EPA in cancer cachexia. Nutrition 1996 Jan; 12(1 Suppl):S31–3.

151 Smith HJ, Lorite MJ, Tisdale MJ. Effect of a cancer cachectic factor on protein synthesis/degradation in murine C2C12 myoblasts: Modulation by eicosapentaenoic acid. Cancer Res 1999 Nov 1; 59(21):5507–13.

152 Tisdale MJ. Mechanism of lipid mobilization associated with cancer cachexia: Interaction between the polyunsaturated fatty acid, eicosapentaenoic acid, and inhibitory guanine nucleotide-regulatory protein. Prostaglandins Leukot Essent Fatty Acids 1993; 48(1):105–9.

153 Hudson EA, Beck SA, Tisdale MJ. Kinetics of the inhibition of tumour growth in mice by eicosapentaenoic acid—reversal by linoleic acid. UK Biochem Pharmacol 1993; 45(11):2189–94.

154 Smith KL, Tisdale MJ. Mechamism of muscle protein degradation in cancer cachexia. Br J Cancer 1993; 68(2):314–8.

155 Beck SA, Smith KL, Tisdale MJ. Anticachectic and antitumor effect of eicosapentaenoic acid and its effect on protein turnover. Cancer Res 1991; 51(22):6089–93.

156 Tisdale MJ, Beck SA. Inhibition of tumour-induced lipolysis in vitro and cachexia and tumour growth in vivo by eicosapentaenoic acid. Biochemical Pharmacology 1991; 41(1):103–7.

157 Hudson EA, Tisdale MJ. Comparison of the effectiveness of eicosapentaenoic acid administered as either the free acid or ethyl ester as an anticachectic and antitumour agent. Prostaglandins Leukot Essent Fatty Acids 1994 Aug; 51(2):141–5.

158 Wigmore SJ, Ross JA, Falconer JS, et al. The effect of polyunsaturated fatty acids on the progress of cachexia in patients with pancreatic cancer. Nutrition 1996 Jan; 12(1 Suppl):S27–30.

159 Costelli P, Llovera M, Lopez-Soriano J, et al. Lack of effect of eicosapentaenoic acid in preventing cancer cachexia and inhibiting tumor growth. Cancer Letters 1995; 97:25–32.

160 Meterissian SH, Forse RA, Steele GD, Thomas P. Effect of membrane free fatty acid alterations on the adhesion of human colorectal carcinoma cells to liver macrophages and extracellular matrix proteins. Cancer Letters 1995; 89:145–152.

161 Best R, et al. The anti-ulcerogenic activity of the unripe plantian banana (Musa species). British Journal of Pharmacology 1984; 82:107–16.

162 Goel RK, et al. Anti-ulcerogenic effect of banana powder (Musa sapientum var. paradisiaca) and its effect on mucosal resistance. Journal of Ethno-Pharmacology 1986; 18:33–44.

163 Borovskaia TG, Udintsev SN, Zueva EP, et al. Dilution of the toxic action of 5-fluorouracil on the mucosa of the small intestine in mice using the sap of plantain. Vopr Onkol 1987; 33(7):60–64.

164 Buck M, Chojkier M. Muscle wasting and dedifferentiation induced by oxidative stress in a murine model of cachexia is prevented by inhibitors of nitric oxide synthesis and antioxidants. EMBO J 1996 Apr 15; 15(8):1753–65.

165 Lissoni P, Paolorossi F, Tancini G, et al. Is there a role for melatonin in the treatment of neoplastic cachexia? Eur J Cancer 1996; 32A(8):1340–3.

166 Lissoni P, Paolorossi F, Ardizzoia A, et al. A randomized study of chemotherapy with cisplatin plus etoposide versus chemoendocrine therapy with cisplatin, etoposide and the pineal hormone melatonin as a first-line treatment of advanced non-small cell lung cancer patients in a poor clinical state. J Pineal Res 1997 Aug; 23(1):15–9.

167 Hack V, Breitkreutz R, Kinscherf R, et al. The redox state as a correlate of senescence and wasting and as a target for therapeutic intervention. Blood 1998 Jul 1; 92(1):59–67.

168 Murray MT. Encyclopedia of nutritional supplements. Rocklin, CA: Prima Publishing, 1996, p. 243.

169 Mantzioris E, James MJ, Gibson RA, Cleland LG. Dietary substitution with α-linolenic acid-rich vegetable oil increases eicosapentaenoic acid concentrations in tissues. Am J Clin Nutr 1994; 59:1304–9.

170 Weaver BJ, Corner EJ, Bruce VM, et al. Dietary canola oil: Effect on the accumulation of eicosapentaenoic acid in the alkenylacyl fraction of human platelet ethanolamine phosphoglyceride. Am J Clin Nutr 1990 Apr; 51(4):594–8.

171 Gerster H. Can adults adequately convert alpha-linolenic acid (18:3n-3) to eicosapentaenoic acid (20:5n-3) and docosahexaenoic acid (22:6n-3)? Int J Vitam Nutr Res 1998; 68(3):159–173.

172 Bardon S, Le MT, Alessandri JM. Metabolic conversion and growth effects of n-6 and n-3 polyunsaturated fatty acids in the T47D breast cancer cell line. Cancer Lett 1996 Jan 19; 99(1):51–8.

173 Rubin D, Laposata M. Cellular interactions between n-6 and n-3 fatty acids: A mass analysis of fatty acid elongation/desturation, distribution among complex lipids, and conversion to eicosanoids. Journal of Lipid Research 1992; 33:1431–40.

174 Whelan J. Antagonistic effects of dietary arachidonic acid and n-3 polyunsaturated fatty acids. J Nutr 1996 Apr; 126(4 Suppl):1086S-91S.

175 Ling PR, Boyce P, Bistrian BR. Role of arachidonic acid in the regulation of the inflammatory response in TNF-alpha-treated rats. J Parenter Enteral Nutr 1998 Sep–Oct; 22(5):268–75.

176 Sanders TAB, Roshanai F. The influence of different types of w-3 polyunsaturated fatty acids on blood lipids and platelet

function in healthy volunteers. Clinical Science 1983; 64:91–99.

[177] Linder MC, ed. Nutritional biochemistry and metabolism. 2nd ed. New York: Elsevier Science, 1991, p. 78.

[178] Volker DH, FitzGerald PE, Garg ML. The eicosapentaenoic to docosahexaenoic acid ratio of diets affects the pathogenesis of arthritis in Lew/SSN rats. J Nutr 2000 Mar; 130(3):559–65.

[179] Soudamini KK, Unnikrishnan MC, Soni KB, Kuttan R. Inhibition of lipid peroxidation and cholesterol levels in mice

by curcumin. Indian J Physiol Pharmacol 1992 Oct; 36(4):239–43.

[180] Kawagoe M, Nakagawa K. Attenuation of luminol-amplified chemiluminescent intensity and lipid peroxidation in the livers of quercetin-fed mice. Toxicol Lett 2000 Apr 3; 114(1–3):189–96.

[181] Fremont L, Gozzelino MT, Franchi MP, Linard A. Dietary flavonoids reduce lipid peroxidation in rats fed polyunsaturated or monounsaturated fat diets. J Nutr 1998 Sep; 128(9):1495–502.

AMINO ACIDS AND RELATED COMPOUNDS

In this chapter, we look at two amino acids, glutathione and glutamine, that have a special significance in cancer treatment. Glutathione is one of the most important antioxidants within a cell, and glutamine, among its many effects, can increase glutathione concentrations. Two other compounds, garlic and bromelain, although not amino acids themselves, are loosely related to amino acids and are discussed also. Certain garlic compounds are similar to glutathione in that, like glutathione, they possess thiol (sulfur-hydrogen) groups that give them antioxidant capacity. Bromelain is included because as a protein it is composed of large numbers of amino acids.

AMINO ACIDS

Although we discuss glutathione and glutamine in this section, glutathione is not recommended as a treatment compound since its administration does not appear to effectively increase intracellular glutathione concentrations; administering vitamin C or other antioxidants or glutamine may be more effective than glutathione itself. If antioxidants are taken, the guidance in Chapter 15 applies: in brief, antioxidants are not considered suitable as sole treatment agents. Glutamine does not have the same potential as antioxidants to increase cancer cell proliferation, since it appears to produce an antioxidant effect only in normal, not in cancer cells. Nonetheless, glutamine too could be expected to produce a greater anticancer effect when combined with other natural compounds.

Glutathione

Functions of Glutathione

Glutathione plays an essential role in both normal and cancer cells, and on that basis, it is worth reviewing in detail. In addition, since glutathione is commercially available and has been recommended as an antioxidant by some authors, it seems important to explain why this book does not support its use.

Adequate glutathione concentrations are crucial to cells because glutathione is the most abundant low-molecular-weight thiol antioxidant they contain. In this regard, glutathione's role is twofold. First, it sacrifices electrons to free radicals to neutralize them, and second, it acts in conjunction with the selenium-dependent antioxidant enzyme glutathione reductase to transform hydrogen peroxide into water. In these two ways, it plays a crucial role in many different redox reactions, including those that control apoptosis.[1, 2, 3]

In addition to antioxidant effects, glutathione is also needed for the cellular detoxification of noxious compounds, particularly for electrophilic (positively charged) compounds. In this type of detoxification, noxious compounds are joined with glutathione molecules within the cell to form conjugates; these have a low reactivity and are easily and safely transported out of the cell. Although liver cells are particularly adept at performing this and other types of detoxification, all cells, including cancer cells, perform detoxification. For example, cancer cells use this detoxification system to export several types of chemotherapy drugs, thereby inducing drug resistance. The enzyme glutathione S-transferase, which catalyzes the conjugation process, is commonly overexpressed in drug-resistant cancer cells.[4, 5, 6]

The antioxidant and detoxification actions of glutathione are illustrated in Figure 18.1. Glutathione also serves other functions not shown in the figure. High concentrations inhibit eicosanoid production, particularly the production of PGE_2 (see Chapter 8).[7] It also is required for optimal IL-2 activity, and thus for T-cell function (see Chapter 12). Lastly, glutathione acts as a storage and transport vehicle for cysteine, an amino acid used in many cellular functions (cysteine is a component of glutathione).[8]

Because of its many functions, all cells need adequate glutathione. Interestingly, its levels decrease with age, and the aging process itself may be due partly to low levels of glutathione.[9–12] In animal studies, low levels are associated with reduced immune response, increased cancer risk, impaired detoxification of noxious substances, and many other detrimental events.[13–17]

Since glutathione is used in detoxifying several chemotherapy drugs, there is some concern that administering antioxidants, which increase intracellular glutathione concentrations, could strengthen cancer cell's resistance to therapy. Indeed, some animal and human studies have reported that high glutathione concentrations within cancer cells are associated with a decreased response to chemotherapy drugs.[18, 19, 20] Nevertheless, the majority of animal studies that tested antioxidants in combination with chemotherapy reported that they either assist or do not affect the ability of chemotherapy drugs to kill cancer cells (see Chapter 23). We can reason then

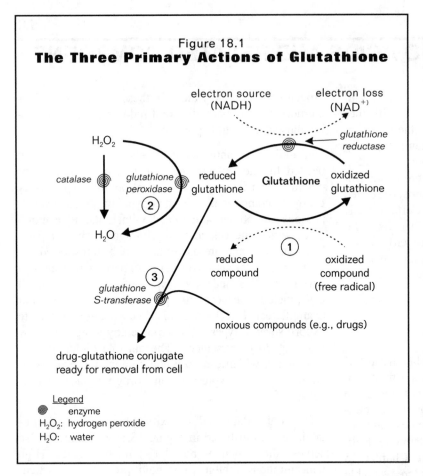

Figure 18.1
The Three Primary Actions of Glutathione

electron source
(NADH)

electron loss
(NAD$^{+)}$)

glutathione reductase

H$_2$O$_2$

catalase

glutathione peroxidase

②

reduced glutathione

Glutathione

oxidized glutathione

H$_2$O

①

reduced compound

oxidized compound (free radical)

③

glutathione S-transferase

noxious compounds (e.g., drugs)

drug-glutathione conjugate
ready for removal from cell

Legend
⊚   enzyme
H$_2$O$_2$: hydrogen peroxide
H$_2$O: water

that, whatever effects antioxidants may have on intracellular glutathione concentrations, their overall effect on chemotherapy is still either benign or supportive.

Effects of Antioxidants on Glutathione Concentrations

Although glutathione is essential to all cells, we do not place a high priority here on increasing intracellular glutathione concentrations. If producing such high concentrations were a goal, one of the most effective means to accomplish it would be by using antioxidants like vitamin C, not glutathione itself. As discussed in Chapter 15, however, antioxidants are viewed as supportive compounds, most helpful within larger combinations. It follows that any increases in intracellular glutathione concentrations from using antioxidants can also be seen as a supportive and not a priority goal. Glutamine, which appears to increase glutathione concentrations in normal but not cancer cells, is also viewed as supportive. While adequate glutathione will assist healthy cells to function and thus may add to an anticancer effect, other compounds are still necessary to produce a maximum one.

The basic reason glutathione appears to have limited clinical value has to do with the way it enters cells. Glutathione is a tripeptide amino acid composed of the amino acids cysteine, glycine, and glutamic acid. (The presence of the thiol group within cysteine gives glutathione its antioxidant activity.) Glutathione itself is poorly transported across the plasma membrane of cells, and so intracellular glutathione concentrations are not maintained by its direct transport into the cell, but by disassembly of glutathione at the outer plasma membrane, transport of the three individual amino acids into the cell, and then reassembly of the glutathione molecule within the cell.

Glutathione must also be broken down when passing through intestinal membranes, as it must after oral administration. This process of breakdown, transport, and restructuring is not highly efficient, and studies have reported that oral administration of glutathione does not effectively increase plasma or intracellular glutathione concentrations.[8, 32] For example, oral administration of 3 grams did not increase plasma glutathione or cysteine concentrations in seven healthy subjects.[21] This is not to say that orally administered glutathione cannot increase glutathione concentrations. A small number of studies have reported that oral doses do increase plasma glutathione levels in humans and rodents.[22, 23, 24] The majority of studies, however, suggested that its ability to do so is limited.

A more efficient way to increase intracellular glutathione concentrations is by taking antioxidants, glutamine, or certain other natural compounds discussed below. Antioxidants such as vitamins C and E and thiol antioxidants like alpha-lipoic acid and melatonin are all capable of increasing plasma and intracellular glutathione concentrations.[25–28] (Antioxidants appear to increase glutathione concentrations by sparing glutathione oxidation.) For example, one study reported that oral administration of 60 to 200 milligrams of vitamin E (90 to 300 I.U.) increased plasma glutathione concentrations after 31 days in healthy subjects.[29] In another study, repeated oral administration of high amounts of vitamin C (123 mg/kg) increased plasma glutathione levels in a 45-month old girl with hereditary glutathione deficiency.[30] Similarly, repeated oral doses of more moderate amounts of vitamin C (500 milligrams per day) increased red blood cell glutathione content by 50 percent in healthy adults.[31] In yet another study, vitamin C, but not glutathione, was able to prevent cellular oxidative damage caused by experimentally induced glutathione depletion in rodents.[32] Lastly, intraperitoneal injection of alpha-lipoic acid (at 4 to 16 mg/kg) in mice also increased intracellular glutathione concentrations.[33] The equivalent human oral dose is about 38 to 150 milligrams per day.

Glutathione as a Prooxidant

Disassembling the glutathione molecule at the plasma membrane (before it can enter the cell as individual amino acids) is accomplished by the enzyme GGT (gamma-glutamyl transpeptidase). Ironically, in the process of splitting glutathione, GGT produces a significant amount of hydrogen peroxide. Since cancer cells are generally under oxidative stress and therefore need additional glutathione, many cell lines overexpress GGT. When adequate extracellular glutathione is present, enough hydrogen peroxide can be generated to either stimulate cell proliferation in vitro (at low hydrogen peroxide concentrations) or inhibit it (at high concentrations).[34–39] In most conditions seen in vivo, however, extracellular concentrations of glutathione and overexpression of GGT are probably not high enough to produce so much hydrogen peroxide that cancer cells are killed. Rather, in in-vivo conditions, GGT overexpression tends to increase tumor growth and reduce the effectiveness of chemotherapy drugs like cisplatin (since the glutathione produced assists in drug detoxification).[40]

Although this mechanism may be one way cancer cells make low concentrations of hydrogen peroxide in vivo (and low concentrations of hydrogen peroxide can assist cancer cell progression), this is no reason to avoid using antioxidants. Antioxidants increase glutathione concentrations by sparing its destruction, and thus would not be expected to increase hydrogen peroxide production. Moreover, they can affect cancer in several different ways, and their overall effect is of greatest concern. Antioxidants are likely to be beneficial to the patient if they are used in combination with other anticancer compounds.

Glutathione as an Anticancer Compound

Even though glutathione administration is probably not the most effective means to increase intracellular glutathione concentrations, it still has shown some effects in animal antitumor studies. To the degree that administration can increase glutathione concentrations, we would expect that, like any antioxidant, it could have no

effect on cancer progression or could assist or inhibit it. Each of these results has been observed in animal studies. For example, in one study in rats, 5.3 grams per day, as scaled to humans, given orally caused partial or complete regression in 81 percent of established aflatoxin-induced liver tumors.[41] In another rat study, oral administration of 2 g/kg of glutathione inhibited growth of transplanted breast cancer cells; tumor inhibition was associated with a decrease in PGE_2 production, suggesting that intracellular concentrations of glutathione were increased.[42] At least one animal study reported detrimental effects: 500 mg/kg of glutathione in the drinking water increased the size of chemically induced tumors in rats.[43] In other animal studies, glutathione had no effect on tumor growth.[44]

The discrepancies among these studies are not surprising, for in addition to the complexities of glutathione synthesis and function, antioxidants in general yield complex results (see Chapter 15). Positive studies notwithstanding, glutathione administration cannot be counted on to increase glutathione concentrations, and its use is not recommended. Available evidence does suggest that a number of antioxidants, as well as glutamine, may be more effective than glutathione itself.

Glutamine

Summary of Research and Conclusions

At least 5 reviews have been published on glutamine as a therapeutic agent in cancer treatment.[45–49] Although the results reviewed are promising, the use of glutamine has been hampered by concern that cancer cells may use it as a fuel source. Well over 7 in-vitro studies have reported glutamine could be used as a fuel.[50–56] The situation in vivo appears to be different, however; at least 21 animal studies have reported that glutamine does not promote tumor growth in vivo and in fact inhibits it, inhibits cachexia, or reduces adverse effects of chemotherapy or radiotherapy.[57–62] Glutamine's beneficial effects are attributed largely to its ability to increase glutathione concentrations in, and act as a fuel for, immune, intestinal, and other normal cells, but not cancer cells.

At least 17 human studies have been conducted, all designed to determine if glutamine could reduce adverse effects of conventional therapy. Five of these were on patients undergoing bone marrow transplantation. Most but not all of the human studies reported a beneficial effect.[63–67] Although a minority found no effect, no studies reported a detrimental one.[68–71]

In total, the above studies suggest that glutamine may reduce adverse effects of some chemotherapy and radiotherapy regimes by increasing the glutathione content of normal cells, by acting as a fuel source for intestinal or immune cells, or all three.

Effect of Glutamine on Glutathione Concentrations

Glutamine increases the glutathione concentration of normal cells because they metabolize it to glutamate, the salt of glutamic acid, one of the three amino acids needed for glutathione synthesis. (The structures of glutathione and glutamine are illustrated in Figures A.25 and A.26 of Appendix A.) Glutamine-induced increases in glutathione synthesis have been reported in cells of the gut lining and in many other types of cells.[46] In fact, oral glutamine has increased intracellular glutathione synthesis up to threefold in some cell lines.[72, 100] Using glutamine-enriched intravenous nutrition to increase glutathione concentrations and reduce mortality in intensive care units is well documented.[73]

Although effective in normal cells, glutamine does not appear to increase glutathione concentrations in cancer cells. When administered with chemotherapy or radiotherapy, glutamine can actually lower the content of glutathione in cancer cells and increase the concentration of some chemotherapy drugs (since cells with low glutathione concentrations are less able to expel drugs).[46, 62, 74] In cancer-bearing animals treated with chemotherapy, glutamine enhanced the therapeutic effect, reduced adverse effects, and improved survival.[75, 76] These beneficial effects were due mostly to increased glutathione synthesis in normal cells. For example, oral glutamine (at 1 g/kg per day) protected rats against doxorubicin-induced cardiotoxicity, apparently by upregulating glutathione synthesis in the heart.[61]

The reasons why glutamine does not increase tumor growth or tumor glutathione content in vivo are still a matter of debate. One suggestion is that glutathione concentrations in cancer cells do not increase because of the acidic environment within them; such an environment decreases the efficiency of the enzyme 5-oxoprolinase (5-OP), which plays a role in glutathione synthesis.[76]

Glutamine as a Cellular Fuel

One of the dose-limiting adverse effects of cytotoxic chemotherapy and abdominal radiotherapy is intestinal injury. Therapy-induced intestinal damage affects a significant number of cancer patients, and in some cases, the damage is severe enough to require surgical intervention, intravenous nutrition, or both. Glutamine is the most abundant amino acid in the blood and is a major energy source for cells of the intestinal lining. Studies suggest that it may protect the gut lining against radiotherapy- and chemotherapy-induced injury.[77, 78, 79] In studies on rats receiving chemotherapy or abdominal radiation, glutamine at oral doses of up to 1 g/kg reduced bowel damage and bloody diarrhea and increased survival.[80–86]

In human studies, oral doses of 8 grams per day reduced the severity and duration of chemotherapy-induced mouth and throat inflammation (mucositis).[87, 88] An oral dose of 18 grams per day reduced the duration and severity of diarrhea in leukemia patients undergoing chemotherapy.[89] The same dose reduced diarrhea and improved gut integrity in patients with colorectal cancer treated with chemotherapy.[90] Twenty-one grams per day given orally increased tumor destruction and improved gut parameters in prostate cancer patients undergoing radiotherapy.[91] An intravenous dose of 14 to 22 grams per day reduced mucositis and ulceration of the gastrointestinal lining in patients with colorectal cancer receiving chemotherapy.[63] A 30-gram oral dose protected T cells and gut permeability in patients with advanced esophageal cancer undergoing chemotherapy and radiotherapy.[65] Adding glutamine to parenteral nutrition mixtures may also help patients recover from bone marrow transplantations. Although two studies reported no effect, several reported beneficial effects.[67, 70, 71, 92–95]

Glutamine's ability to provide energy to cells could in theory increase cancer cell proliferation, and in fact, in-vitro studies have reported glutamine can act as an energy source for cancer cells, as it does for immune and intestinal cells.[96] Furthermore, glutaminase, an enzyme that reduces plasma glutamine levels, can reduce angiogenesis in tumor-bearing mice.[97] Because of this, agents that lower glutamine levels have been tested as anticancer drugs against leukemia and other malignancies.[98, 99]

Although the in-vitro evidence that cancer cells use glutamine as a fuel might seem strong, in-vivo studies tell a different story. Neither oral nor intravenous glutamine administration has been reported to increase tumor growth in animal or humans. The reasons for the contrasting effects between normal cells and cancer cells in vivo are still unclear. In rodents, oral glutamine administration did not increase the growth of a variety of cancers, even at doses as high as 2 g/kg.[59, 100–104] Instead, tumor-induced weight loss was actually reduced in some of these studies; possibly due to a glutamine-induced increase in muscle protein synthesis (since glutamine is used by muscle cells).

Glutamine and the Immune System

Glutamine may inhibit tumor progression in part through its ability to increase immune activity; it can improve both natural killer cell and T-cell activity in vitro and in vivo.[46, 105] Glutamine may also reduce immuno-suppression caused by tumors. Because some enzymes involved in PGE_2 production are inhibited by glutathione, and because PGE_2 is an immunosuppressive compound, glutamine, as an inducer of glutathione synthesis, can reduce immunosuppression.[106] The ability of cancer cells to evade immune destruction is one of the main reasons conventional immunostimulant drugs have had only limited success (see Chapters 11 and 12). The potential anticancer effects of glutamine are summarized in Table 18.1.

Estimated Therapeutic and LOAEL Doses of Glutamine

The human studies conducted with glutamine have primarily been concerned with reducing side effects of chemotherapy, as discussed above. In these studies, oral glutamine was effective at doses of 8 to 30 grams per day. Similar doses have been used in animal experiments, often about 1 to 2 g/kg. The human equivalent of a 1-g/kg dose in rats is about 16 grams per day; a dose of 16 to 30 grams per day is considered safe in humans.[89, 107] Although this may sound like a large dose, normal dietary intake is about 5 to 10 grams per day.[45] The estimated therapeutic doses of glutamine are summarized in Table 18.2.

Other Compounds That Selectively Increase Intracellular Glutathione Concentrations

A number of other compounds have been investigated for their ability to increase glutathione concentrations in normal but not cancer cells. Most of these compounds act by delivering cysteine to the cell (cysteine being the component of glutathione that is usually in shortest supply). One of these cysteine-delivery agents, OTZ (1-2-oxothiazolidine-4-carboxylate), is split by the enzyme 5-OP to form a compound that is easily converted to cysteine in the cell. Since 5-OP is downregulated in many cancer cells, only normal cells can take advantage of OTZ for glutathione synthesis.[108, 109] In fact, as with glutamine, OTZ administration can lead to decreased glutathione levels in cancer cells.[110] The reasons are

TABLE 18.1 POTENTIAL ANTICANCER ACTIONS OF GLUTAMINE

ACTIVITY	KNOWN EFFECTS	AS AN EICOSANOID INHIBITOR, MAY:
Chapter 3: Results of Therapy at the Cellular Level		
Induce apoptosis		x
Chapter 5: Transcription Factors and Redox Signaling		
Inhibit NF-κB activity		x
Chapters 7 and 8: Angiogenesis		
Inhibit angiogenesis		x
Inhibit eicosanoid effects	x	—
Inhibit VEGF effects		x
Chapters 11 and 12: Immune System		
Stimulate/support the immune system	x	
Chapters 18: Amino Acids and Related Compounds		
Protect normal cells from chemotherapy/radiotherapy	x	

TABLE 18.2 ESTIMATED THERAPEUTIC AND LOAEL DOSES FOR GLUTAMINE

DESCRIPTION	DOSE (g/day)
Required dose as scaled from animal antitumor studies	up to 32
Doses used in human anticancer studies	8 to 30
LOAEL dose	30 or more
Tentative dose recommendation for further research	**8 to 30**

unclear, but perhaps OTZ drives some process, such as GGT activity, that requires glutathione, leading to lower glutathione concentrations. Although OTZ is not discussed here as a natural compound for treatment, it is of interest because of the similarities between OTZ and whey proteins.

Whey proteins from milk also increase glutathione concentrations in normal cells but not cancer cells. The mechanisms are still uncertain, but whey contains a number of cysteine-rich proteins. The whey proteins involved in its effects include albumin, alpha-lactalbumin, and lactoferrin. (As discussed in Chapter 14, lactoferrin is also involved in iron metabolism.) Apparently, these three proteins deliver cysteine to normal cells but not to cancer cells, the selectivity probably due to low 5-OP concentrations in cancer cells. Not surprisingly, whey products and/or their isolated proteins have been reported to inhibit carcinogenesis in animals and cancer cell proliferation in vitro, and to increase glutathione concentrations in immune and other normal cells in vivo.[111–116] Like glutamine and OTZ, whey proteins can also reduce tumor glutathione concentrations in animals.[117]

The amounts of whey used in these animal studies were generally large. Mouse studies commonly used about 24 g/kg, the human equivalent of about 230 grams per day. The few human studies conducted used lower doses of 20 to 40 grams per day, which still increased glutathione concentrations in immune cells.[118, 119] In one study, a daily dose of 30 grams given to six patients with metastatic cancer lowered the abnormally high glutathione concentrations in lymphocytes of some patients. Apparently, these concentrations reflected high tumor glutathione concentrations. Thus the authors of this study suggested that whey proteins could reduce excessive glutathione concentrations in human tumors. Two of the six patients showed signs of tumor regression.[120]

GARLIC

Summary of Research and Conclusions

At least seven in-vitro studies have reported that garlic or its primary constituent, diallyl disulfide (DADS), inhibited proliferation of a variety of cancer cell lines.[121–127] Seven animal studies and three reviews reported that garlic or DADS inhibited tumor progression in vivo.[128–137] In addition, a large number of studies have investigated the effects of garlic supplementation in cancer prevention, and a few have explored the in-vitro cytotoxicity of other minor garlic constituents.

The active garlic constituents contain sulfur-hydrogen (thiol) groups or easily react to form thiol groups, thus garlic compounds are redox active and this probably plays a large role in its cancer inhibitory effects. A number of studies reported that garlic compounds alter intracellular thiol proteins, including glutathione and glutathione enzymes.[138, 139] In fact, garlic compounds can increase the glutathione concentration of cancer cells in vitro.[140]

Because of their redox activity, garlic compounds may produce variable effects. While low doses of garlic compounds are likely to produce an antioxidant effect, it is possible a prooxidant effect could result from high doses. For example, garlic compounds are generally anticarcinogenic, but they can also act as tumor promoters in some circumstances.[141, 142, 143] High concentrations of garlic compounds can also produce lipid peroxidation in vitro.[144] Like all antioxidants then, garlic should probably not be used as a sole treatment agent, especially at high doses.

Relatively low doses of garlic (19 to 29 grams per day) may have moderate effects on cancer, primarily through antioxidant-, immune-, and eicosanoid-mediated mechanisms. Higher doses (40 to 150 grams per day) may

inhibit isoprene synthesis and ras protein activity and yield more dramatic anticancer effects. At high doses, garlic probably inhibits HMGR, the rate-limiting enzyme in isoprene synthesis, by a prooxidant mechanism. The doses required for this effect, however, appear to be higher than the maximum dose of 15 grams estimated as safe for chronic use in humans. If we assume that the target dose is high (91 grams per day), then a relatively high degree of synergism (a 6.1-fold potency increase) is required to make the allowable 15-gram dose effective. From this perspective, garlic is the second weakest direct-acting compound discussed in this book (see Table 13.1).

Introduction

Garlic (*Allium sativum*) is a member of the lily family and is cultivated worldwide for culinary and medicinal uses. In Chinese herbal medicine, it is used to treat parasitic conditions and infections, especially intestinal ones. In the West, it is more commonly used for reducing cholesterol and blood pressure. Animal, human, and in-vitro studies have confirmed that garlic exhibits antimicrobial, antibacterial, antifungal, antihelmintic (antiworm), antiviral, anti-inflammatory, antiatherosclerotic, and immune-enhancing effects. It also reduces platelet aggregation, stimulates fibrinolysis, inhibits eicosanoid synthesis, and reduces high blood pressure.[145–159]

Its active constituents are primarily found in the volatile oils, which comprise 0.1 to 0.5 percent by weight. They include allicin, diallyl disulfide (DADS), and diallyl trisulfide (DATS). Other garlic components include alliin, selenium, and the enzyme alliinase.[145, a]

Allinin is the principal starting material for production of the other organosulfur compounds. The metabolism of allinin is shown in Figure 18.2 (adapted from references 160 and 161). When garlic is crushed, the enzyme alliinase is released, which converts alliin to the biologically active (and pungent) compound allicin. Allicin is further metabolized as shown. After exposure to alliinase, the essential oil of garlic yields approximately 60 percent allicin. At moderate doses in the isolated rat liver, allicin is completely metabolized after the first pass. The primary metabolite is DADS, and to a much lesser extent, a degradation product of DADS, allyl mercaptan.[160] Alliinase is inactivated by heat, so cooked garlic is less pungent and less biologically active than raw garlic.

In addition to the lipid-soluble compounds mentioned, alliinase-activated garlic also contains water-soluble

---

[a] *The structures of allicin and DADS are shown in Figures A.27 and A.28 of Appendix A, respectively.*

compounds such as S-allylcysteine (SAC) and S-allylmercaptocysteine (SAMC). These and the other organosulfur compounds are more or less unstable.

In-vitro and Animal Studies

A number of organosulfur compounds can produce anticancer effects in animals and inhibit proliferation of a variety of cancer cell lines in vitro. These include allicin, DADS, DATS, SAC, and SAMC.[162] The mechanism of growth inhibition is uncertain but is probably due to the formation of redox-active sulfur metabolites that affect intracellular proteins.[163] A variety of other mechanisms may be involved, however. The potential anticancer actions of garlic are listed in Table 18.3.

Of the compounds mentioned above, DATS and DADS have the strongest effects in vitro. DATS is active in vitro at concentrations of about 10 μM, and DADS is active at concentrations of about 100 μM.[136, 164–167] In contrast, SAMC is active at 100 to 500 μM and SAC is active at 1 to 10 mM.[165, 168–172] Results differ, however, depending on the cell lines and experimental conditions. Because it is a primary metabolite, DADS may be the most reasonable therapeutic garlic compound.

At least three rodent studies have reported antitumor effects for DADS:

- Oral administration (at 190 mg/kg three times per week, or 81 mg/kg per day) delayed tumor growth and decreased tumor volume in nude mice injected with *ras*-transformed cells. The effect appeared to be related to inhibition of isoprene synthesis.[132] The equivalent human dose is approximately 780 milligrams of DADS per day, which, when translated to an equivalent dose of whole garlic, is roughly 150 grams, which is prohibitive.

- Intraperitoneal and oral administration of 50 mg/kg DADS three times a week inhibited colon cancer cells in nude mice with no adverse effects.[173] (Intraperitoneal administration reduced tumor growth by 63 percent, whereas oral doses reduced it by 29 percent.) The equivalent human oral doses are about 290 and 210 milligrams of DADS, respectively (roughly 40 to 55 grams of whole garlic).

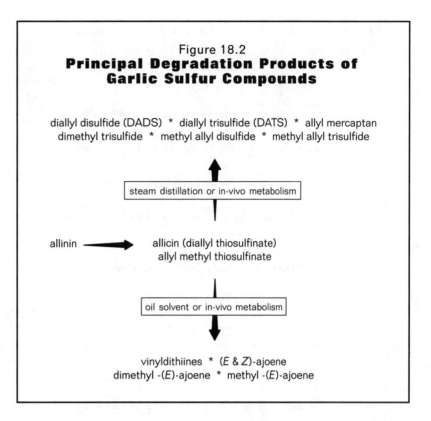

Figure 18.2
Principal Degradation Products of Garlic Sulfur Compounds

diallyl disulfide (DADS) * diallyl trisulfide (DATS) * allyl mercaptan
dimethyl trisulfide * methyl allyl disulfide * methyl allyl trisulfide

↑

steam distillation or in-vivo metabolism

allinin → allicin (diallyl thiosulfinate)
allyl methyl thiosulfinate

oil solvent or in-vivo metabolism

↓

vinyldithiines * (*E* & *Z*)-ajoene
dimethyl -(*E*)-ajoene * methyl -(*E*)-ajoene

- Higher intraperitoneal doses of DADS (400 mg/kg) produced significant anticancer effects but were toxic to rodents.[166]

Whole garlic has also been studied in rodents. Administration of 3 g/kg per day of garlic in the diet prolonged survival of nude mice with transplanted colon cancer cells.[137] The equivalent human dose is about 29 grams per day. Doses of 3.8 g/kg per day of garlic in the diet reduced the growth of transplanted liver cancer in rats.[136] The human equivalent is about 62 grams per day. An oral dose of 2 g/kg increased survival of mice with transplanted Dalton's lymphoma cells.[134] The human equivalent is about 19 grams per day.

Two primary effects may have occurred in the above rodent studies on DADS and whole garlic. Some of these studies used nude mice, which have an impaired immune system. The antitumor effects of garlic in these mice were clearly not mediated by the immune system and were probably due in part to inhibition of isoprene and/or eicosanoid synthesis. The immune system may have played a role in the other rodent studies, however. Garlic is known to improve immune cell response, probably in part by its ability to increase glutathione concentrations.[174, 175, 176] Isoprene synthesis is inhibited at relatively high DADS concentrations in vitro (about 500 μM), whereas immunostimulation and modulation of eicosanoid production may occur at lower concentrations.[177, 178] Thus, based on data scaled from rodent studies, garlic may inhibit tumor growth in humans at

TABLE 18.3 POTENTIAL ANTICANCER ACTIONS OF GARLIC			
ACTIVITY	**KNOWN EFFECTS**	**AS AN ANTIOXIDANT, MAY:**	**AS AN EICOSANOID INHIBITOR, MAY:**
Chapter 2: Mutations, Gene Expression, and Proliferation			
Act as an antioxidant	x	—	
Chapter 3: Results of Therapy at the Cellular Level			
Induce apoptosis	x		x
Chapter 4: Growth Factors and Signal Transduction			
Inhibit isoprene synthesis	x		
Chapter 5: Transcription Factors and Redox Signaling			
Support p53 function		x	
Inhibit NF-κB activity		x	x
Chapter 6: Cell-to-Cell Communication			
Affect CAMs			x
Chapters 7 and 8: Angiogenesis			
Inhibit angiogenesis		x	x
Degrade fibrin	x		
Inhibit eicosanoid effects	x		—
Inhibit TNF effects		x	
Inhibit VEGF effects		x	x
Chapters 9 and 10: Invasion and Metastasis			
Inhibit hyaluronidase, beta-glucuronidase, or elastase			x
Inhibit collagenase effects		x	x
Inhibit platelet aggregation	x		
Chapter 18: Amino Acids and Related Compounds			
Increase glutathione concentrations	x	x	
Support/stimulate the immune system	x	x	

doses of 19 to 150 grams per day. Effects at the lower side of this dose range are probably mediated by the immune system and disruptions in eicosanoid production, and effects at the higher side probably by isoprenoid inhibition.[a]

Estimated Therapeutic and LOAEL Doses of Garlic

The estimated required dose as scaled from animal antitumor studies is in reasonable agreement with the required dose as calculated from pharmacokinetic and in-

vitro data; the former is from 19 to 150 grams per day and the latter is similar. Using a target in-vivo concentration of 100 μM of DADS, the required garlic dose is about 110 grams per day. Based on an average of 110 grams and the higher end of the dose range scaled from animals, the target human dose is estimated to be about 91 grams per day. Such a dose could act by inhibiting isoprene synthesis and ras activity, and the effects would be more dramatic than those expected at lower doses.

The LOAEL dose for garlic is estimated to be about 15 grams per day (see Appendix J). Side effects are likely to be mild near the LOAEL dose and may include heartburn, flatulence, and related gastrointestinal problems.[179]

Dose calculations for garlic are summarized in Table 18.4. The tentative recommended dose range is 6 to 15 grams per day, with the 6-gram value based on assuming a full 15-fold increase in potency by synergistic interactions. The 15-gram value is based on the estimated LOAEL dose.

It appears that synergistic interactions will be required for garlic to produce an anticancer effect in humans. In comparing the 91-gram target dose to the 15-gram maximum dose, synergistic interactions will be needed to cause about a 6.1-fold increase in potency. This should be possible, since such an increase is well below the allowable 15-fold increase discussed in Chapter 13. We note again, however, that at the relatively low recommended dose, certain antitumor effects of garlic, specifically, inhibition of isoprene synthesis and ras activity, may not happen and its usefulness at these low doses may be limited. Additional studies are needed to shed more light on the effects of low garlic doses in combination with other natural compounds.

---

[a] *One may wonder why relatively high doses of DADS are required when oral garlic can reduce cholesterol production in humans at moderate doses. The difference is probably because allicin concentrations in the liver are high after oral administration of garlic, and the liver is the major producer of cholesterol in the body. Allicin is about 10-fold more effective at inhibiting isoprene synthesis than DADS.*

BROMELAIN AND OTHER PROTEOLYTIC ENZYMES

This section covers bromelain, a proteolytic enzyme from pineapple, as well as polyenzyme mixtures, which may or may not contain bromelain. We focus on bromelain since it is commonly used as a supplement and many in-vitro and animal studies have suggested it may affect a variety of procancer events. The comments on bromelain, however, also pertain to other proteolytic enzymes, in particular, trypsin, chymotrypsin, and papain. If enzymes are used in therapy, they may be most effective as part of a polyenzyme combination. Polyenzyme mixtures without bromelain may also be effective and in fact have been studied as anticancer agents.

TABLE 18.4 ESTIMATED THERAPEUTIC AND LOAEL DOSES FOR GARLIC[*]	
DESCRIPTION	DOSE (g/day)
Required dose as scaled from animal antitumor studies	19 to 150
Required dose as determined from pharmacokinetic calculations	110
Target dose based on an average from animal antitumor studies (higher dose range) and pharmacokinetic calculations	91
Minimum required antitumor dose assuming 15-fold synergistic benefits	6.1
Commonly prescribed human dose in noncancerous conditions	4 to 15
Estimated LOAEL dose	15
Tentative dose recommendation for further research	**6 to 15**
Minimum degree of synergism required	**6.1-fold potency increase**

[*] *See Appendix J for details.*

Summary of Research and Conclusions

Six reviews have been published on the general effects of enzymes and/or their potential in cancer treatment.[180–185] In addition, at least 14 in-vitro studies have been published, 11 of which looked at immune effects. These studies reported that enzyme treatment in vitro or ex vivo (after oral administration) produced cleavage of immune complexes and CD44 cell adhesion molecules, induced TNF, IL-1, and IL-6 production, increased the cytotoxicity of macrophages and neutrophils against cancer cells, and inhibited *ras* signaling in T cells.[186–196] Three of the in-vitro studies looked at the effect of enzymes on cancer cells. One of these reported that bromelain induced differentiation, one that it inhibited proliferation, and one that it stimulated proliferation.[197, 198, 199]

At least 11 studies have investigated the effects of enzymes in animals. Seven reported that enzymes inhibited inflammation or alleviated the signs and symptoms of autoimmune diseases.[200–206] Four found that enzymes inhibited tumor growth and metastasis in rodents.[207–210]

Six studies on the effects of enzymes in cancer patients reported that enzymes prolonged survival time when used in combination with other conventional or alternative therapies, reduced chemotherapy-induced adverse effects, improved tumor boundaries prior to radiotherapy, or reduced fluid escape in the lungs due to metastasis.[211–216]

In total, the in-vitro, animal, and human studies suggested that polyenzyme combinations could beneficially regulate the immune system and also inhibit cancer through other means. The normalizing effects of these enzymes on the immune system may make them an essential part of larger immune strategies.

Introduction

Enzymes are protein molecules composed of very long chains of amino acids, whose function is to catalyze specific biochemical reactions in the body.[a] Their molecular weight can range from 20,000 to 40,000 grams per mole or more, as compared to an average of 360 grams per mole for most other natural compounds discussed in this book. They have highly defined surface structures and internal cavities, and like a lock and key, only specific molecules fit into these cavities. In this way, enzymes interact only with specific targets. By convention, enzymes are given the suffix *–ase*, although in the past, some were given the suffix *-in*, as in trypsin.

There are six broad classes of enzymes. Together they account for more than 50,000 different enzymes active in the human body. Two classes, isomerases and hydrolases, are discussed in this book. Isomerases (i.e., topoisomerases), discussed in Chapter 2, catalyze the rearrangement of chemical groups in a molecule. In contrast, hydrolases cleave chemical bonds in the presence of water, thereby breaking molecules apart. Hydrolases are important in many internal processes, for

---

[a] *A catalyst is a compound that increases the rate of a chemical reaction but is itself unchanged by the process.*

TABLE 18.5 POTENTIAL ANTICANCER ACTIONS OF BROMELAIN	
ACTIVITY	**KNOWN EFFECTS**
Chapter 3: Results of Therapy at the Cellular Level	
Induce differentiation	x
Chapters 7 and 8: Angiogenesis	
Degrade fibrin	x
Chapters 9 and 10: Invasion and Metastasis	
Inhibit metastasis	x
Inhibit cell migration	x
Inhibit platelet aggregation	x
Chapters 11 and 12: Immune System	
Stimulate or regulate the immune system	x
Chapter 18: Amino Acids	
Increase drug absorption	x

example in digestion. Two subclasses of hydrolases, glycosidases and proteases, were first introduced in Chapter 9. Glycosidases split sugar bonds, and proteases split protein bonds. The enzymes discussed in this chapter are all proteases and include bromelain, trypsin, chymotrypsin, and papain. Bromelain itself contains a mixture of proteases and lesser amounts of a peroxidase, protease inhibitors, and other compounds.

The proteases used in therapy vary in their ability to degrade different molecules, and hence they have different effects in humans.[217] Due to its effects on various proteins, bromelain is especially efficient in reducing edema. Papain is especially efficient at cleaving antigen-antibody complexes, and trypsin and chymotrypsin at cleaving fibrin. That enzymes differ in their efficiencies is one reason why polyenzyme preparations may be more effective than single enzymes.[185] At least one study has reported that a mixture of enzymes had a more potent anti-inflammatory effect than single enzymes.[218]

In-vitro and Animal Studies

Most of the in-vitro and animal studies conducted on bromelain and polyenzyme therapies focused on their effects on immune function and/or inflammation; these were discussed in Chapter 12. The evidence indicates that immune modulation and anti-inflammatory effects may account for a large part of any anticancer effects seen in animals or humans.

Only three in-vitro studies have investigated the direct effects of bromelain on cancer cells. One study reported that bromelain (at 5 to 8 μM) inhibited the proliferation of mouse lymphoma, lung, and ascites tumor cells.[219] The effects appeared due to the peroxidase activity of bromelain. (Peroxidases are enzymes that catalyze the conversion of hydrogen peroxide to water.) The second study reported bromelain induced differentiation in leu-

kemic cells, probably due to its ability to alter cytokine synthesis, which again points to the role of bromelain in immune modulation.[197] In the third, a combination of bromelain and trypsin stimulated the proliferation of Ehrlich ascites tumor cells.[220] This finding may not be relevant to in-vivo conditions during enzyme therapy, however.

Four animal studies examined the antitumor effects of bromelain or polyenzymes. In two of the studies, oral administration of 140 to 400 mg/kg bromelain (about 1.3 to 3.8 grams per day, as scaled to humans) inhibited metastasis of lung cancer cells in mice.[207, 208] In the other two, rectal administration of 45 mg/kg two times per day of a polyenzyme formula (WOBE-MUGOS) reduced metastasis and increased survival of mice with transplanted melanoma and lung cancer cells.[210, 221] Doses were rectally given to improve absorption. The equivalent human dose is roughly 870 milligrams per day.

Oral enzyme therapy may inhibit cancer progression or improve the effects of chemotherapy drugs through a number of mechanisms. The potential anticancer activities of bromelain are listed in Table 18.5. Although the focus is on bromelain, other proteolytic enzymes are likely to share similar characteristics. All activities except for the ability of proteolytic enzymes to increase drug absorption have been discussed in previous chapters.

Increased Drug Absorption

Orally administered proteolytic enzymes can increase absorption and tissue diffusion of some drugs, including some antibiotics and chemotherapy drugs.[222] In part, this may be due to the moderate fibrinolytic effects produced by enzymes that assist the free flow of therapeutic drugs to inflamed sites. It may also come from the ability of proteolytic enzymes, especially mixed ones, to open tight junctions in the intestinal lining and allow the passage of large drug molecules.[223] Enzymes like chymotrypsin have increased the concentration of chemotherapy drugs within tumor cells in vitro and potentiated the effects of antibiotics.[224] Combinations of enzyme therapy and chemotherapy have been used in Germany in preliminary experiments with good results, including more rapid remissions, reduced side effects, and reductions in therapy costs.[185, 212, 217, 225, 226] Reduced side effects appear partly the result of inhibiting chemotherapy-induced production of inflammatory substances.

Human Studies

Human studies on enzymes have been published in journal articles and books, as well as in literature from manufacturers. We start with the six human studies published in journals. Unfortunately, five of these were only available in abstract form (three articles were not in English and two were published only as abstracts); all five were uncontrolled. Briefly, one study reported that Wobenzym, a polyenzyme product, in combination with hyperthermia, immunostimulants, and hormone therapy, improved survival of patients with advanced pancreatic cancer.[211] The second reported that unspecified proteolytic enzymes degraded plasma proteins and reduced hyperviscosity symptoms in patients with hematological cancers.[227] Hyperviscosity syndrome is a collective term for the multitude of clinical manifestations that result from impaired blood flow due to abnormal blood thickness; one cause in cancer patients is an abnormally high amount of plasma proteins, such as antibodies. The three other studies reported that polyenzymes could reduce bleomycin-induced lung toxicity, improve the boundaries of lymphoma masses for subsequent radiotherapy, and reduce fluid escape in the lungs due to metastasis.[213, 215, 228]

The sixth study was a two-year, unblinded, uncontrolled, pilot study on 10 patients with inoperable pancreatic cancer.[216] This study by Nicholas Gonzalez, M.D., and Linda Isaacs, M.D., was a continuation of work originally started by Dr. John Beard and others in the early 1900s and later carried on by William Kelly, a dentist from Texas.[229, 230, 231] Dr. Gonzalez became interested in the effects of proteolytic enzymes and other modalities after reviewing the work of Dr. Kelly. In this study, patients were treated with an intensive program of diet, oral supplementation of nutrients and enzymes, and routines such as coffee enemas (for the purpose of liver detoxification). The proteolytic enzymes are the proposed anticancer element in the program, while the other components are considered supportive in nature. The daily dose of pancreas enzymes (derived from pigs) was 25 to 40 grams, which was spread out over multiple doses throughout the day and night. Although the exact protocol has not been published, based on public comments by Dr. Gonzalez it would appear the enzymes were ingested about every four hours on an empty stomach and treatments were given for 15 consecutive days, followed by a 5-day rest period.

The results are intriguing: 81 percent of the patients survived one year, 45 percent survived two years, and 36 percent survived three years. This is far above the average survival rates of 25 percent at one year and 10 percent at two years as reported in the National Cancer Data Base from 1995. Because of this success, Dr.

Gonzalez was awarded a large grant in June 2000 to conduct a larger clinical trial using his protocol.

Other human studies using enzymes have been published in books or appeared in articles published by the MUCOS pharmaceutical company, or they were articles not indexed in MEDLINE.[a] These studies are discussed below.

Max Wolf, M.D., treated over 1,000 cancer patients in Germany using a multiple-enzyme product named WOBE-MUGOS, or similar multienzyme products.[232, b] Dr. Wolf began treating patients about 1949 with a variety of enzyme formulations, and after its introduction in 1959, WOBE-MUGOS was used exclusively. The original formula for WOBE-MUGOS contained chymotrypsin, trypsin, papain, and calf thymus extract. It was reformulated in 1991, and the thymus extract was removed. Early treatment protocols used oral doses of 200 milligrams per day, and protocols in later years used 2 to 4 grams per day. Enzyme treatments were often combined with surgery, vitamins, heparin, or other agents. Where possible, treatment included intratumoral injection or topical application of the enzymes. With colon cancer, retention enemas were employed. Although it is difficult to evaluate the success of this early work based on available data, especially since the studies were not controlled and randomized, the following conclusions were suggested by Wolf:

- Enzyme therapy was generally not curative but appeared to inhibit metastasis and moderately prolong survival. For example, breast cancer was the most common cancer treated. Of 107 postmastectomy patients, the five-year observed survival rate was 84 percent. The authors reported that observed survival rates for conventional therapy at the time were 43 to 48 percent. The benefits gained with other types of cancers were less clear, although the authors asserted that patients generally benefited.

- Systemic treatment was less successful than localized treatment using intratumoral injections, topical salves, bladder infusions, or other treatments.

- The best results in inhibiting metastasis were seen in patients who were on long-term therapy.

- High doses and mixed plant and animal enzymes provided better results than low doses and single enzymes.

---

[a] *The German company MUCOS Pharma GmbH is a leader in the production and testing of polyenzyme products.*

[b] *The name WOBE-MUGOS derives from the two early principal investigators, Max Wolf (WO) and Helen Benitez (BE) and from the MUCOS pharmaceutical company that later took over the production and investigative work.*

This early work was continued by the MUCOS company. According to preliminary studies cited in the manufacturer's literature, initial clinical trials yielded promising results in patients with malignancies of the breast, colon, head, neck, and multiple myeloma. In multiple myeloma, retrospective cohort studies reported life span prolongation. Prospective studies are under way on patients with multiple myeloma, breast, and colon cancer to verify these results. In the completed studies, enzyme therapy commonly resulted in weight gain, reductions in fatigue and depression, and improved quality of life. A slowing of tumor progression was also suggested in some cases.[226]

Other doctors have used multienzyme formulas to treat cancer patients. For example, in the 1960s Frank Shively, M.D., treated more than 96 advanced cancer patients using a combination of chymotrypsin, trypsin, amylase, and other agents. The enzymes were administered intravenously, with more than 3,000 infusions given to these patients in total. Case studies of some of these and cautions and contraindications of the treatment are available.[233] According to Dr. Shively, many patients responded favorably to the enzyme treatment. In many cases, the tumors apparently became necrotic, detached from their surrounding tissue, and were easily removed by surgery. The most commonly treated tumors were carcinomas of the breast, gastrointestinal tract, and genitals.

Other investigators have suggested that bromelain alone may be useful in treating cancer patients. Gerard was one of the first.[234] In a case series on 12 patients with various tumors who were given bromelain, resolution of masses was reported in patients with ovarian and breast cancers. Nieper experimented with higher doses of bromelain in combination with standard chemotherapy and also reported some success.[235] These physicians have suggested that the optimum dose of bromelain may be 1 to 2.4 grams daily.

Estimated Therapeutic and LOAEL Doses of Enzymes

Since they are such large molecules, the intestinal absorption of enzymes has been questioned, but ample evidence now demonstrates that enzymes are indeed absorbed in their active forms in humans and animals. This has been reported for bromelain, trypsin, papain, and chymotrypsin in a number of studies, including animal studies using radiolabeled enzymes and antibody studies in humans.[236, 237] Approximately 6 percent of papain and 38 percent of orally administered bromelain are found in plasma and lymph fluids, still in their active form.[185, 217, 238] The highest concentration is usually seen between two and four hours after administration. The capacity of the intestines to absorb enzymes may be limited, however. For example, in a series of human studies, single doses of a polyenzyme product (bromelain and trypsin) above about 200 milligrams did not further increase plasma proteolytic activity.[239, 240, 241]

Orally administered enzymes are very safe. In Germany in 1992, over 1.4 million prescriptions were made for enzyme preparations with no reports of any grave adverse effects.[217] No lethal dose for orally administered polyenzyme preparations could be determined in animal models, even at a daily dose of 15 g/kg. This was also true for individual enzymes (trypsin, chymotrypsin, papain, and bromelain). At high doses mild effects may be seen, such as stool modifications, sedation, appetite reduction, and weight loss.[185]

Contraindications to bromelain or polyenzyme therapy include the following:

- Enzymes should be used with caution in individuals who suffer from protein allergies, since they may be allergic to the enzymes.

- Enzymes should not be used within 24 hours of any surgery because they may reduce platelet stickiness and increase fibrinolysis, and therefore inhibit blood coagulation. For the same reason, enzymes should not be used in patients with blood coagulation disturbances or in conjunction with anticoagulants.

- As with all compounds in this book, enzymes should be used carefully by pregnant women, if used at all.

- Bromelain may increase heart rate and thus are best used cautiously by patients with heart palpitations or tachycardia.

The estimated therapeutic doses of bromelain and polyenzyme mixtures are summarized in Table 18.6. Enzymes are usually taken on an empty stomach with plenty of water. If they are taken with food, some of their activity may go toward digesting food proteins rather than the intended therapeutic use. Although this has yet to be verified, the assumption is reasonable.[242] To improve absorption, daily doses can be divided into three or more equal portions, and treatment should be intermittent, an example being 15 days of treatment followed by a 5-day rest period.

Note that the maximum recommend dose in the table is 4 grams, which is considerably lower than the 25 to 40 grams used by Dr. Gonzalez. The 4-gram limit is based on the general linear bioavailability limit of 600 milligrams per administration (with six administrations per day). It would seem that even the 4-gram limit might be excessive, since doses much greater than 200 milligrams (per administration) may not further increase plasma concentrations. More research is needed to determine the optimal maximum daily dose.

CONCLUSION

I have characterized both glutamine and bromelain as immune stimulants. Glutamine supports immune function by increasing glutathione concentrations in immune cells and by acting as fuel for immune cells. The mechanisms by which bromelain and other enzymes affect immune function are less understood, but their actions appear regulatory in nature. Both glutamine and enzymes have other characteristics that make them useful; for example, glutamine can protect intestinal cells from injury induced by chemotherapy or radiotherapy, and bromelain can produce anti-inflammatory effects.

Based on current research, garlic does not seem quite as promising as many other compounds discussed, since it may require a relatively high degree of synergism to be effective at allowable doses. Nonetheless, it may still be useful; garlic compounds such as DADS do inhibit cancer through a variety of mechanisms, depending on the dose. At high doses, DADS is likely to act through inhibition of isoprene synthesis and ras protein activity. It is unlikely such high doses could be used safely in humans, however. Lower doses may inhibit cancer through other mechanisms, such as inhibiting eicosanoid production, but such effects at lower doses are likely to be more moderate than those seen at higher doses.

TABLE 18.6 ESTIMATED THERAPEUTIC AND LOAEL DOSES FOR BROMELAIN AND POLYENZYME MIXTURES

DESCRIPTION	DOSE (g/day)
Required dose as scaled from animal antitumor studies	1.3 to 3.8
Human doses used in anticancer studies	1 to 40
LOAEL dose	high
Tentative dose recommendation for further research	**1 to 4**

REFERENCES

[1] Hall AG. Review: The role of glutathione in the regulation of apoptosis. Eur J Clin Invest 1999 Mar; 29(3):238–45.

[2] Voehringer DW. BCL-2 and glutathione: Alterations in cellular redox state that regulate apoptosis sensitivity. Free Radic Biol Med 1999 Nov; 27(9–10):945–50.

[3] Obrador E, Navarro J, Mompo J, et al. Regulation of tumour cell sensitivity to TNF-induced oxidative stress and cytotoxicity: Role of glutathione. Biofactors 1998; 8(1–2):23–6.

[4] Nakanishi Y, Kawasaki M, Bai F, et al. Expression of p53 and glutathione S-transferase-pi relates to clinical drug resistance in non-small cell lung cancer. Oncology 1999 Nov; 57(4):318–23.

[5] Wang K, Ramji S, Bhathena A, et al. Glutathione S-transferases in wild-type and doxorubicin-resistant MCF-7 human breast cancer cell lines. Xenobiotica 1999 Feb; 29(2):155–70.

[6] Morrow CS, Smitherman PK, Townsend AJ. Combined expression of multidrug resistance protein (MRP) and glutathione S-transferase P1-1 (GSTP1-1) in MCF7 cells and high level resistance to the cytotoxicities of ethacrynic acid but not oxazaphosphorines or cisplatin. Biochem Pharmacol 1998 Oct 15; 56(8):1013–21.

[7] Margalit A, Hauser SD, Zweifel BS, et al. Regulation of prostaglandin biosynthesis in vivo by glutathione. Am J Physiol 1998 Feb; 274(2 Pt 2):R294–302.

[8] Meister A. Glutathione deficiency produced by inhibition of its synthesis, and its reversal: Applications in research and therapy. Pharmacol Ther 1991; 51(2):155–94.

[9] Ames BN, Shigenaga MK, Hagen TM. Oxidants, antioxidants and the degenerative diseases of aging. Proc Natl Acad Sci USA 1993 Sep; 90:7915–22.

[10] Richie JP Jr, Leutzinger Y, Parthasarathy S, et al. Methionine restriction increases blood glutathione and longevity in F344 rats. FASEB J 1994 Dec; 8(15):1302–7.

[11] Fletcher RH, Fletcher SW. Glutathione and ageing: Ideas and evidence. Lancet 1994 Nov 19; 344(8934):1379–80.

[12] Stio M, Iantomasi T, Favilli F, et al. Glutathione metabolism in heart and liver of the aging rat. Biochem Cell Biol 1994 Jan–Feb; 72(1–2):58–61.

[13] Robinson MK, Rodrick ML, Jacobs DO, et al. Glutathione depletion in rats impairs T-cell and macrophage immune function. Arch Surg 1993 Jan; 128(1):29–34; discussion 34–5.

[14] Mizutani T, Nakahori Y, Yamamoto K. p-Dichlorobenzene-induced hepatotoxicity in mice depleted of glutathione by

treatment with buthionine sulfoximine. Toxicology 1994 Nov–Dec; 94(1–3):57–67.

[15] Mizutani T, Satoh K, Nomura H, Nakanishi K. Hepatotoxicity of eugenol in mice depleted of glutathione by treatment with DL-buthionine sulfoximine. Res Commun Chem Pathol Pharmacol 1991 Feb; 71(2):219–30.

[16] Hirano T, Yamaguchi Y, Kasai H. Inhibition of 8-hydroxyguanine repair in testes after administration of cadmium chloride to GSH-depleted rats. Toxicol Appl Pharmacol 1997 Nov; 147(1):9–14.

[17] Rotstein JB, Slaga TJ. Effect of exogenous glutathione on tumor progression in the murine skin multistage carcinogenesis model. Carcinogenesis 1988 Sep; 9(9):1547–51.

[18] Sargent JM, Williamson C, Hall AG, et al. Evidence for the involvement of the glutathione pathway in drug resistance in AML. Adv Exp Med Biol 1999; 457:205–9.

[19] van der Kolk DM, Vellenga E, Muller M, de Vries EG. Multidrug resistance protein MRP1, glutathione, and related enzymes. Their importance in acute myeloid leukemia. Adv Exp Med Biol 1999; 457:187–98.

[20] Kigawa J, Minagawa Y, Cheng X, Terakawa N. Gamma-glutamyl cysteine synthetase up-regulates glutathione and multidrug resistance-associated protein in patients with chemoresistant epithelial ovarian cancer. Clin Cancer Res 1998 Jul; 4(7):1737–41.

[21] Witschi a, Reddy S, Stofer B, et al. The systemic availability of oral glutathione. Eur J Clin Pharmacol 1992; 43(6):667–9.

[22] Jones DP, Coates RJ, Flagg EW, et al. Glutathione in foods listed in the National Cancer Institute's health habits and history food frequency questionnaire. Nutr Cancer 1992; 17:57–75.

[23] Jones DP, Hagen TM, Weber R. Oral administration of glutathione (GSH) increases plasma GSH concentration in humans. FASEBJ 1989; 3:1250A.

[24] Hagen TM, Grazyna T, et al. Bioavailability of dietary glutathione: Effect on plasma concentration. Am Physiol Soc 1990; G524-G529.

[25] Packer L, Witt EH, Tritschler HJ. Alpha-lipoic acid as a biological antioxidant. Free Radic Biol Med 1995; 19(2):227–250.

[26] Han D, Tritschler HJ, Packer L. Alpha-lipoic acid increases intracellular gluathione in a human T-lymphocyte Jurkat cell line. Biochem Biophys Res Commun 1995 Feb 6; 207(1):258–64.

[27] Wahab MH, Akoul ES, Abdel-Aziz AA. Modulatory effects of melatonin and vitamin E on doxorubicin-induced cardiotoxicity in Ehrlich ascites carcinoma-bearing mice. Tumori 2000 Mar–Apr; 86(2):157–62.

[28] Lopez PM, Finana IT, De Agueda MC, et al. Protective effect of melatonin against oxidative stress induced by ligature of extra-hepatic biliary duct in rats: Comparison with the effect of S-adenosyl-L-methionine. J Pineal Res 2000 Apr; 28(3):143–9.

[29] Hu JJ, Roush GC, Berwick M, et al. Effects of dietary supplementation of α-tocopherol on plasma glutathione and DNA repair activities. Cancer Epidem Biomarkers Prev 1996; 5:263–270.

[30] Jain A, Buist NRM, Kennaway NG, et al. Effect of ascorbate or N-acetylcysteine treatment in a patient with hereditary glutathione synthetase deficiency. J Pediatr 1994; 124:229–33.

[31] Johnston CS, Meyer CG, Srilakshmi JC. Vitamin C elevates red blood cell glutathione in healthy adults. Am J Clin Nutr 1993; 58:103–5.

[32] Anderson, ME. Glutathione and glutathione delivery compounds. Advances in Pharmacology 1997; 38:65–78.

[33] Busse E, Zimmer G, Schopohl B, Kornhuber B. Influence of alpha-lipoic acid on intracellular glutathione in vitro and in vivo. Arzneimittelforschung 1992 Jun; 42(6):829–31.

[34] Lewis AD, Hayes JD, Wolf CR. Glutathione and glutathione-dependent enzymes in ovarian adenocarcinoma cell lines derived from a patient before and after the onset of drug resistance: Intrinsic differences and cell cycle effects. Carcinogenesis 1988 Jul; 9(7):1283–7.

[35] Hanigan MH. Gamma-glutamyl transpeptidase, a glutathionase: Its expression and function in carcinogenesis. Chem Biol Interact 1998 Apr 24; 111–112:333–42.

[36] Dominici S, Valentini M, Maellaro E, et al. Redox modulation of cell surface protein thiols in U937 lymphoma cells: The role of gamma-glutamyl transpeptidase-dependent H2O2 production and S-thiolation. Free Radic Biol Med 1999 Sep; 27(5–6):623–35.

[37] Perego P, Paolicchi A, Tongiani R, et al. The cell-specific anti-proliferative effect of reduced glutathione is mediated by gamma-glutamyl transpeptidase-dependent extracellular pro-oxidant reactions. Int J Cancer 1997 Apr 10; 71(2):246–50.

[38] del Bello B, Paolicchi A, Comporti M, et al. Hydrogen peroxide produced during gamma-glutamyl transpeptidase activity is involved in prevention of apoptosis and maintainance of proliferation in U937 cells. FASEB J 1999 Jan; 13(1):69–79.

[39] Drozdz R, Parmentier C, Hachad H, et al. Gamma-glutamyltransferase dependent generation of reactive oxygen species from a glutathione/transferrin system. Free Radic Biol Med 1998 Nov 1; 25(7):786–92.

[40] Hanigan MH, Gallagher BC, Townsend DM, Gabarra V. Gamma-glutamyl transpeptidase accelerates tumor growth and increases the resistance of tumors to cisplatin in vivo. Carcinogenesis 1999 Apr; 20(4):553–9.

[41] Novi AM. Regression of aflatoxin B1-induced hepatocellular carcinomas by reduced gluthione. Science 1981; 212(1):541–2.

[42] Karmali RA. Growth inhibition and prostaglandin metabolism in the R3230AC mammary adenocarcinoma by reduced glutathione. Cancer Biochem Biophys 1984 Jun; 7(2):147–54.

[43] Chen MF, Chen LT, Boyce HW Jr. Cruciferous vegetables and glutathione: Their effects on colon mucosal glutathione level and colon tumor development in rats induced by DMH. Nutr Cancer 1995; 23(1):77–83.

[44] Cook JR, Huang DP, Burkhardt AL, et al. Assessment of the anti-tumor potential of glutathione. Cancer Lett 1984 Jan; 21(3):277–83.

[45] Miller AL. Therapeutic considerations of L-glutamine: A review of the literature. Altern Med Rev 1999 Aug; 4(4):239–48.

46 Klimberg VS, McClellan JL. Claude H. Organ, Jr. honorary lectureship. Glutamine, cancer, and its therapy. Am J Surg 1996 Nov; 172(5):418–24.

47 Wilmore DW, Schloerb PR, Ziegler TR. Glutamine in the support of patients following bone marrow transplantation. Curr Opin Clin Nutr Metab Care 1999 Jul; 2(4):323–7.

48 Wilmore DW. Metabolic support of the gastrointestinal tract: Potential gut protection during intensive cytotoxic therapy. Cancer 1997 May 1; 79(9):1794–803.

49 Souba WW. Glutamine and cancer. Ann Surg 1993 Dec; 218(6):715–28.

50 Wasa M, Bode BP, Abcouwer SF, et al. Glutamine as a regulator of DNA and protein biosynthesis in human solid tumor cell lines. Ann Surg 1996 Aug; 224(2):189–97.

51 Kovacevic Z, McGivan JD. Mitochondrial metabolism of glutamine and glutamate and its physiological significance. Physiol Rev 1983 Apr; 63(2):547–605.

52 Kallinowski F, Runkel S, Fortmeyer HP, et al. L-glutamine: A major substrate for tumor cells in vivo? J Cancer Res Clin Oncol 1987; 113(3):209–15.

53 Turowski GA, Rashid Z, Hong F, et al. Glutamine modulates phenotype and stimulates proliferation in human colon cancer cell lines. Cancer Res 1994 Nov 15; 54(22):5974–80.

54 Santoso JT, Lucci JA 3rd, Coleman RL, et al. Does glutamine supplementation increase radioresistance in squamous cell carcinoma of the cervix? Gynecol Oncol 1998 Dec; 71(3):359–63.

55 Kovacevic Z, Brkljac O, Bajin K. Control and function of the transamination pathways of glutamine oxidation in tumour cells. Biochem J 1991 Jan 15; 273(Pt 2):271–5.

56 Collins CL, Wasa M, Souba WW, Abcouwer SF. Determinants of glutamine dependence and utilization by normal and tumor-derived breast cell lines. J Cell Physiol 1998 Jul; 176(1):166–78.

57 Holm E, Hagmuller E, Staedt U, et al. Substrate balances across colonic carcinomas in humans. Cancer Res 1995 Mar 15; 55(6):1373–8.

58 Shewchuk LD, Baracos VE, Field CJ. Dietary L-glutamine supplementation reduces the growth of the Morris Hepatoma 7777 in exercise-trained and sedentary rats. J Nutr 1997 Jan; 127(1):158–66.

59 Robinson LE, Bussiere FI, Le Boucher J, et al. Amino acid nutrition and immune function in tumour-bearing rats: A comparison of glutamine-, arginine- and ornithine 2-oxoglutarate-supplemented diets. Clin Sci (Colch) 1999 Dec; 97(6):657–69.

60 Yoshida S, Kaibara A, Yamasaki K, et al. Effect of glutamine supplementation on protein metabolism and glutathione in tumor-bearing rats. JPEN J Parenter Enteral Nutr 1995 Nov–Dec; 19(6):492–7.

61 Cao Y, Kennedy R, Klimberg VS. Glutamine protects against doxorubicin-induced cardiotoxicity. J Surg Res 1999 Jul; 85(1):178–82.

62 Rubio IT, Cao Y, Hutchins LF, et al. Effect of glutamine on methotrexate efficacy and toxicity. Ann Surg 1998 May; 227(5):772–8; discussion 778–80.

63 Decker-Baumann C, Buhl K, Frohmuller S, et al. Reduction of chemotherapy-induced side-effects by parenteral glutamine supplementation in patients with metastatic colorectal cancer. Eur J Cancer 1999 Feb; 35(2):202–7.

64 Anderson PM, Schroeder G, Skubitz KM. Oral glutamine reduces the duration and severity of stomatitis after cytotoxic cancer chemotherapy. Cancer 1998 Oct 1; 83(7):1433–9.

65 Yoshida S, Matsui M, Shirouzu Y, et al. Effects of glutamine supplements and radiochemotherapy on systemic immune and gut barrier function in patients with advanced esophageal cancer. Ann Surg 1998 Apr; 227(4):485–91.

66 Huang EY, Leung SW, Wang CJ, et al. Oral glutamine to alleviate radiation-induced oral mucositis: A pilot randomized trial. Int J Radiat Oncol Biol Phys 2000 Feb 1; 46(3):535–9.

67 Ziegler TR, Young LS, Benfell K, et al. Clinical and metabolic efficacy of glutamine-supplemented parenteral nutrition after bone marrow transplantation. A randomized, double-blind, controlled study. Ann Intern Med 1992 May 15; 116(10):821–8.

68 Bozzetti F, Biganzoli L, Gavazzi C, et al. Glutamine supplementation in cancer patients receiving chemotherapy: A double-blind randomized study. Nutrition 1997 Jul–Aug; 13(7–8):748–51.

69 Jebb SA, Osborne RJ, Maughan TS, et al. 5-fluorouracil and folinic acid-induced mucositis: No effect of oral glutamine supplementation. Br J Cancer 1994 Oct; 70(4):732–5.

70 Schloerb PR, Skikne BS. Oral and parenteral glutamine in bone marrow transplantation: A randomized, double-blind study. JPEN J Parenter Enteral Nutr 1999 May–Jun; 23(3):117–22.

71 Schloerb PR, Amare M. Total parenteral nutrition with glutamine in bone marrow transplantation and other clinical applications (a randomized, double-blind study). JPEN J Parenter Enteral Nutr 1993 Sep–Oct; 17(5):407–13.

72 Cao Y, Feng Z, Hoos A, Klimberg VS. Glutamine enhances gut glutathione production. JPEN J Parenter Enteral Nutr 1998 Jul–Aug; 22(4):224–7.

73 Amores-Sanchez MI, Medina MA. Glutamine, as a precursor of glutathione, and oxidative stress. Mol Genetics Metab 1999; 67:100–105.

74 Klimberg VS, Pappas AA, Nwokedi E, et al. Effect of supplemental dietary glutamine on methotrexate concentrations in tumors. Arch Surg 1992 Nov; 127(11):1317–20.

75 Klimberg VS, Nwokedi E, Hutchins LF, et al. Glutamine facilitates chemotherapy while reducing toxicity. JPEN J Parenter Enteral Nutr 1992 Nov–Dec; 16(6 Suppl):83S–87S.

76 Rouse K, Nwokedi E, Woodliff JE, et al. Glutamine enhances selectivity of chemotherapy through changes in glutathione metabolism. Annals of Surgery 1995; 221(4):420–426.

77 Cascinu S, Catalano G. Intensive weekly chemotherapy for elderly gastric cancer patients, using 5-fluorouracil, ciplatin, epi-doxorubicin, 6S-leucovorin and glutathione with the support of G-CSF. Tumori 1995 Jan–Feb; 81(1):32–5.

78 Gebbia V, Valenza R, Testa A, et al. Weekly 5-fluorouracil and folinic acid plus escalating doses of cisplatin with glutathione protection in patients with advanced head and neck cancer. Med Oncol Tumor Pharmacother 1992; 9(4):165–8.

79 Sumiyoshi Y, Hashine K, Kasahara K, Karashima T. [Glutathione chemoprotection therapy against CDDP-induced

neurotoxicity in patients with invasive bladder cancer.] Gan To Kagaku Ryoho 1996 Sep; 23(11):1506–8.

80 Klimberg VS, Salloum RM, Kasper M, et al. Oral glutamine accelerates healing of the small intestine and improves outcome after whole abdominal radiation. Arch Surg 1990; 125:1040–1045.

81 Fox AD, Kripke SA, Berman JR, et al. Reduction of the severity of enterocolitis by glutamine-supplemented enteral diets. Surg Forum 1987; 38:43.

82 Fox AD, DePaula JA, Kripke SA, et al. Glutamine-supplemented elemental diets reduce endotoxemia in a lethal model of enterocolitis. Surg Forum 1988; 39:46.

83 O'Dwyer ST, Scott T, Smith RJ, et al. 5-Fluorouracil toxicity on small intestinal mucosa but not white blood cells is decreased by glutamine. Clin Res 1987; 35:369A.

84 Jacobs DO, Evans A, O'Dwyer ST, et al. Disparate effects of 5-fluorouracil on the ileum and colon of enterally fed rats with protection by dietary glutamine. Surg Forum 1987; 38:45–49.

85 Jensen JC, Schaefer R, Nwokedi E, et al. Prevention of chronic radiation enteropathy by dietary glutamine. Annals Surgical Oncology 1994; 1(2):157–163.

86 Klimberg S. Prevention of radiogenic side effects using glutamine-enriched elemental diets. Recent Results Cancer Res 1991; 121:283–5.

87 Skubitz KM, Anderson PM. Oral glutamine to prevent chemotherapy induced stomatitis: A pilot study. J Lab Clin Med 1996 Feb; 127(2):223–8.

88 Anderson PM, Schroeder G, Skubitz KM. Oral glutamine reduces the duration and severity of stomatitis after cytotoxic cancer chemotherapy. Cancer 1998 Oct 1; 83(7):1433–9.

89 Muscaritoli M, Micozzi A, Conversano L, et al. Oral glutamine in the prevention of chemotherapy-induced gastrointestinal toxicity [letter]. Eur J Cancer 1997 Feb; 33(2):319–20.

90 Daniele B, Perrone F, Gallo C, et al. Oral glutamine in the prevention of fluorouracil induced intestinal toxicity: A double blind, placebo controlled, randomised trial. Gut 2001 Jan; 48(1):28-33.

91 Richards EW, Long CL, Pinkston JA, et al. The role of oral glutamine in the prevention of radiation-induced enterocolitis in prostate cancer patients. FASEB J 1992; 6(5):A1680.

92 Brown SA, Goringe A, Fegan C, et al. Parenteral glutamine protects hepatic function during bone marrow transplantation. Bone Marrow Transplant 1998 Aug; 22(3):281–4.

93 Goringe AP, Brown S, O'Callaghan U, et al. Glutamine and vitamin E in the treatment of hepatic veno-occlusive disease following high-dose chemotherapy. Bone Marrow Transplant 1998 Apr; 21(8):829–32.

94 MacBurney M, Young LS, Ziegler TR, Wilmore DW. A cost-evaluation of glutamine-supplemented parenteral nutrition in adult bone marrow transplant patients. J Am Diet Assoc 1994 Nov; 94(11):1263–6.

95 Ziegler TR, Bye RL, Persinger RL, et al. Effects of glutamine supplementation on circulating lymphocytes after bone marrow transplantation: A pilot study. Am J Med Sci 1998 Jan; 315(1):4–10.

96 Wasa M, Bode BP, Abcouwer SF, et al. Glutamine as a regulator of DNA and protein biosynthesis in human solid tumor cell lines. Ann Surg 1996 Aug; 224(2):189–97.

97 Maity P, Chakraborty S, Bhattacharya P. Angiogenesis a putative new approach in glutamine related therapy. Pathol Oncol Res 1999 Dec 1; 5(4):309–314.

98 Holcenberg JC, Kien CL. The effects of protein or amino acid intake on the nitrogen balance and antitumor activity of glutaminase treatment. Current Topics in Cellular Regulation 1985; 26:395–402.

99 Hidalgo M, Rodriguez G, Kuhn JG, et al. A phase I and pharmacological study of the glutamine antagonist acivicin with the amino acid solution aminosyn in patients with advanced solid malignancies. Clin Cancer Res 1998 Nov; 4(11):2763–70.

100 Klimberg VS, McClellan JL. Glutamine, cancer and its therapy. Am J Surg 1996 Nov; 172(5):418–24.

101 Shewchuk LD, Baracos VE, Field CJ. Dietary L-glutamine supplementation reduces the growth of the Morris Hepatoma 7777 in exercise-trained and sedentary rats. J Nutr 1997 Jan; 127(1):158–66.

102 Bartlett DL, Charland S, Torosian MH. Effect of glutamine on tumor and host growth. Ann Surg Oncol 1995 Jan; 2(1):71–6.

103 Klimberg VS, Souba WW, Salloum RM, et al. Glutamine-enriched diets support muscle glutamine metabolism without stimulating tumor growth. J Surg Res 1990; 48:319–323.

104 Yoshida S, Kaibara A, Yamasaki K, et al. Effect of glutamine supplementation on protein metabolism and glutathione in tumor-bearing rats. JPEN J Parenter Enteral Nutr 1995 Nov–Dec; 19(6):492–7.

105 Fahr MJ, Kornbluth J, Blossom S, et al. Harry M. Vars research award. Glutamine enhances immunoregulation of tumor growth. J Parenter Enteral Nutr 1994 Nov–Dec; 18(6):471–6.

106 Klimberg VS, Kornbluth J, Cao Y, et al. Glutamine suppresses PGE2 synthesis and breast cancer growth. J Surg Res 1996 Jun; 63(1):293–7.

107 Ziegler TR, Benfell K, Smith RJ, et al. Safety and metabolic effects of L-glutamine administration in humans. JPEN J Parenter Enteral Nutr 1990 Jul–Aug; 14(4 Suppl):137S-146S.

108 Wang T, Chen X, Schecter RL, et al. Modulation of glutathione by a cysteine pro-drug enhances in vivo tumor response. J Pharmacol Exp Ther 1996 Mar; 276(3):1169–73.

109 Chen X, Batist G. Sensitization effect of L-2-oxothiazolidine-4-carboxylate on tumor cells to melphalan and the role of 5-oxo-L-prolinase in glutathione modulation in tumor cells. Biochem Pharmacol 1998 Sep 15; 56(6):743–9.

110 Baruchel S, Wang T, Farah R, et al. In vivo selective modulation of tissue glutathione in a rat mammary carcinoma model. Biochem Pharmacol 1995 Oct 26; 50(9):1505–8.

111 Bounous G, Batist G, Gold P. Immunoenhancing property of dietary whey protein in mice: Role of glutathione. Clin Invest Med 1989 Jun; 12(3):154–61.

112 Bounous G, Gold P. The biological activity of undenatured dietary whey proteins: Role of glutathione. Clin Invest Med 1991 Aug; 14(4):296–309.

113 Bounous G, Batist G, Gold P. Whey proteins in cancer prevention. Cancer Lett 1991 May 1; 57(2):91–4.

114 Svensson M, Hakansson A, Mossberg A, et al. Conversion of alpha-lactalbumin to a protein inducing apoptosis. Proc Natl Acad Sci USA 2000 Apr 11; 97(8):4221–6.

[115] Hakkak R, Korourian S, Shelnutt SR, et al. Diets containing whey proteins or soy protein isolate protect against 7,12-dimethylbenz(a)anthracene-induced mammary tumors in female rats. Cancer Epidemiol Biomarkers Prev 2000 Jan; 9(1):113–7.

[116] Papenburg R, Bounous G, Fleiszer D, Gold P. Dietary milk proteins inhibit the development of dimethylhydrazine-induced malignancy. Tumour Biol 1990; 11(3):129–36.

[117] Baruchel S, Viau G. In vitro selective modulation of cellular glutathione by a humanized native milk protein isolate in normal cells and rat mammary carcinoma model. Anticancer Res 1996 May–Jun; 16(3A):1095–9.

[118] Bounous G, Baruchel S, Falutz J, Gold P. Whey proteins as a food supplement in HIV-seropositive individuals. Clin Invest Med 1993 Jun; 16(3):204–9.

[119] Lands LC, Grey VL, Smountas AA. Effect of supplementation with a cysteine donor on muscular performance. J Appl Physiol 1999 Oct; 87(4):1381–5.

[120] Kennedy RS, Konok GP, Bounous G, et al. The use of a whey protein concentrate in the treatment of patients with metastatic carcinoma: A phase I-II clinical study. Anticancer Res 1995 Nov–Dec; 15(6B):2643–9.

[121] Sakamoto K, Lawson LD, Milner JA. Allyl sulfides from garlic suppress the in vitro proliferation of human A549 lung tumor cells. Nutr Cancer 1997; 29(2):152–6.

[122] Sundaram SG, Milner JA. Diallyl disulfide inhibits the proliferation of human tumor cells in culture. Biochim Biophys Acta 1996 Jan 17; 1315(1):15–20.

[123] Siegers CP, Steffen B, Robke A, Pentz R. The effects of garlic preparations against human tumor cell proliferation. Phytomedicine 1999 Mar; 6(1):7–11.

[124] Knowles LM, Milner JA. Depressed p34cdc2 kinase activity and G2/M phase arrest induced by diallyl disulfide in HCT-15 cells. Nutr Cancer 1998; 30(3):169–74.

[125] Musk SR, Stephenson P, Smith TK, et al. Selective toxicity of compounds naturally present in food toward the transformed phenotype of human colorectal cell line HT29. Nutr Cancer 1995; 24(3):289–98.

[126] Sundaram SG, Milner JA. Impact of organosulfur compounds in garlic on canine mammary tumor cells in culture. Cancer Lett 1993 Oct 15; 74(1–2):85–90.

[127] Sundaram SG, Milner JA. Diallyl disulfide induces apoptosis of human colon tumor cells. Carcinogenesis 1996 Apr; 17(4):669–73.

[128] Riggs DR, DeHaven JI, Lamm DL. Allium sativum (garlic) treatment for murine transitional cell carcinoma. Cancer 1997 May 15; 79(10):1987–94.

[129] Lamm DL, Riggs DR. The potential application of Allium sativum (garlic) for the treatment of bladder cancer. Urol Clin North Am 2000 Feb; 27(1):157–62, xi.

[130] Milner JA. Garlic: Its anticarcinogenic and antitumorigenic properties. Nutr Rev 1996 Nov; 54(11 Pt 2):S82–6.

[131] Sundaram SG, Milner JA. Diallyl disulfide suppresses the growth of human colon tumor cell xenografts in athymic nude mice. J Nutr 1996 May; 126(5):1355–61.

[132] Singh SV, Mohan RR, Agarwal R, et al. Novel anti-carcinogenic activity of an organosulfide from garlic: Inhibition of H-RAS oncogene transformed tumor growth in vivo by diallyl disulfide is associated with inhibition of p21H-ras processing. Biochem Biophys Res Commun 1996 Aug 14; 225(2):660–5.

[133] Choy YM, Kwok TT, Fung KP, Lee CY. Effect of garlic, Chinese medicinal drugs and amino acids on growth of Erlich ascites tumor cells in mice. Am J Chin Med 1983; 11(1–4):69–73.

[134] Unnikrishnan MC, Kuttan R. Tumour reducing and anticarcinogenic activity of selected spices. Cancer Lett 1990 May 15; 51(1):85–9.

[135] Marsh CL, Torrey RR, Woolley JL, et al. Superiority of intravesical immunotherapy with Corynebacterium parvum and Allium sativum in control of murine bladder cancer. J Urol 1987 Feb; 137(2):359–62.

[136] Lea MA. Organosulfur compounds and cancer. In *Dietary phytochemicals in cancer prevention and treatment*. New York: Plenum Press, 1996, pp. 147–154.

[137] Cheng JY, Meng CL, Tzeng CC, Lin JC. Optimal dose of garlic to inhibit dimethylhydrazine-induced colon cancer. World J Surg 1995 Jul–Aug; 19(4):621–5; discussion 625–6.

[138] Sheen LY, Chen HW, Kung YL, et al. Effects of garlic oil and its organosulfur compounds on the activities of hepatic drug-metabolizing and antioxidant enzymes in rats fed high- and low-fat diets. Nutr Cancer 1999; 35(2):160–6.

[139] Rabinkov A, Miron T, Konstantinovski L, et al. The mode of action of allicin: Trapping of radicals and interaction with thiol containing proteins. Biochim Biophys Acta 1998 Feb 2; 1379(2):233–44.

[140] Pinto JT, Qiao C, Xing J, et al. Effects of garlic thioallyl derivatives on growth, glutathione concentration, and polyamine formation of human prostate carcinoma cells in culture. Am J Clin Nutr 1997 Aug; 66(2):398–405.

[141] Fukushima S, Takada N, Hori T, Wanibuchi H. Cancer prevention by organosulfur compounds from garlic and onion. J Cell Biochem Suppl 1997; 27:100–5.

[142] Takada N, Matsuda T, Otoshi T, et al. Enhancement by organosulfur compounds from garlic and onions of diethylnitrosamine-induced glutathione S-transferase positive foci in the rat liver. Cancer Res 1994 Jun 1; 54(11):2895–9.

[143] Delker DA, Papanikolaou A, Suhr YJ, Rosenberg DW. Diallyl sulfide enhances azoxymethane-induced preneoplasia in Fischer 344 rat colon. Chem Biol Interact 2000 Feb 1; 124(3):149–60.

[144] Sheen LY, Sheu SF, Tsai SJ, et al. Effect of garlic active principle, diallyl disulfide, on cell viability, lipid peroxidation, glutathione concentration and its related enzyme activities in primary rat hepatocytes. Am J Chin Med 1999; 27(1):95–105.

[145] Murray MT. The healing power of herbs. Rocklin, CA: Prima Publishing, 1995, pp. 121–131.

[146] Lau BH, Yamasaki T, Gridley DS. Garlic compounds modulate macrophage and T-lymphocyte functions. Mol Biother 1991 Jun; 3(2):103–7.

[147] CGEOG, Cooperative group for essential oil of garlic: The effect of essential oil of garlic on hyperlipidemia and platelet aggregation—an analysis of 308 cases. J of Tradit Chinese Med 1986; 6(2)-117–20.

[148] Yue Z, et al. Effect of allitridi on platelet aggregation, a preliminary study. J of Tradit Chinese Med 1984; 4(1):29–32.

[149] Kiesewetter H, Jung F, Pindur G, et al. Effect of garlic on thrombocyte aggregation, microcirculation, and other risk factors. Int J Clin Pharmacol Ther Toxicol 1991; 29(4):151–5.

[150] Srivastava KC. Aqueous extracts of onion, garlic and ginger inhibit platelet aggregation and alter arachidonic acid metabolism. Biomed Biochim Acta 1984; 43(8–9):S335–46.

[151] Mayeux PR, Agrawal KC, Tou JS, et al. The pharmacological effects of allicin, a constituent of garlic oil. Agents Actions 1988 Aug; 25(1–2):182–90.

[152] Srivastava KC, Mustafa T. Spices: Antiplatelet activity and prostanoid metabolism. Prostaglandins Leukot Essent Fatty Acids 1989 Dec; 38(4):255–66.

[153] Sendl A, Elbl G, Steinke B, et al. Comparative pharmacological investigations of Allium ursinum and Allium sativum. Planta Med 1992 Feb; 58(1):1–7.

[154] Ernst E. Garlic therapy? Theories of a folk remedy (author's translation). MMW Munch Med Wochenschr 1981; 123(41):1537–8.

[155] Arora RC, Arora S, Gupta RK. The long-term use of garlic in ischemic heart disease—an apraisal. Atherosclerosis 1981; 40(2):175–9.

[156] Chang HM, But PPH. Pharmacology and applications of Chinese materia medica. Vol. 1. Teaneck, NJ: World Scientific, 1986, p. 90.

[157] Katiyar SK, Agarwal R, Mukhtar H. Inhibition of tumor promotion in SENCAR mouse skin by ethanol extract of Zingiber officinale rhizome. Cancer Res 1996 Mar 1; 56(5):1023–30.

[158] Legnani C, Frascaro M, Guazzaloca G, et al. Effects of dried garlic preparations on fibrinolysis and platelet aggregation in healthy subjects. Arzneim Forsch 1993; 43(2):119–122.

[159] Kandil OM, Abdullah TH, Elkadi A. Garlic and the immune system in humans: Its effect on natural killer cells. Fed Proc 1987; 46:441.

[160] Egen-Schwind C, Eckard R, Kemper FH. Metabolism of garlic constituents in the isolated perfused rat liver. Planta Med 1992 Aug; 58(4):301–5.

[161] Lawson LD, Wang ZYJ, Hughes BG. Identification and HPLC quantification of the sulfides and dialk(en)yl thiosulfinates in commercial garlic products. Planta Medica 1991; 57:363–70.

[162] Block E. Recent results in the organosulfur and organoselenium chemistry of genius Allium and Brassica plants. In *Dietary phytochemicals in cancer prevention and treatment*. New York: Plenum Press, 1996, pp. 155–169.

[163] Lee ES, Steiner M, Lin R. Thioallyl compounds: Potent inhibitors of cell proliferation. Biochim Biophys Acta 1994 Mar 10; 1221(1):73–7.

[164] Sundaram SG, Milner JA. Diallyl disulfide induces apoptosis of human colon tumor cells. Carcinogenesis 1996 Apr; 17(4):669–73.

[165] Sundaram SG, Milner JA. Diallyl disulfide inhibits the proliferation of human tumor cells in culture. Biochim Biophys Acta 1996 Jan 17; 1315(1):15–20.

[166] Sundaram SG, Milner JA. Impact of organosulfur compounds in garlic on canine mammary tumor cells in culture. Cancer Lett 1993 Oct 15; 74(1–2):85–90.

[167] Sakamoto K, Lawson LD, Milner JA. Allyl sulfides from garlic suppress the in vitro proliferation of human A549 lung tumor cells. Nutrition and cancer 1997; 152–156.

[168] Pinto JT, Qiao C, Xing J, et al. Effects of garlic thioallyl derivatives on growth, glutathione concentration, and polyamine formation of human prostate carcinoma cells in culture [see comments]. Am J Clin Nutr 1997 Aug; 66(2):398–405.

[169] Sigounas G, Hooker J, Anagnostou A, Steiner M. S-allylmercaptocysteine inhibits cell proliferation and reduces the viability of erythroleukemia, breast, and prostate cancer cell lines. Nutr Cancer 1997; 27(2):186–91.

[170] Sigounas G, Hooker JL, Li W, et al. S-allylmercaptocysteine, a stable thioallyl compound, induces apoptosis in erythroleukemia cell lines. Nutr Cancer 1997; 28(2):153–9.

[171] Takeyama H, Hoon DS, Saxton RE, et al. Growth inhibition and modulation of cell markers of melanoma by S-allyl cysteine. Oncology 1993; 50(1):63–9.

[172] Welch C, Wuarin L, Sidell N. Antiproliferative effect of the garlic compound S-allyl cysteine on human neuroblastoma cells in vitro. Cancer Lett 1992 Apr 30; 63(3):211–9.

[173] Sundaram SG, Milner JA. Diallyl disulfide suppresses the growth of human colon tumor cell xenografts in athymic nude mice. J Nutr 1996 May; 126(5):1355–61.

[174] Colic M, Savic M. Garlic extracts stimulate proliferation of rat lymphocytes in vitro by increasing IL-2 and IL-4 production. Immunopharmacol Immunotoxicol 2000 Feb; 22(1):163–81.

[175] Salman H, Bergman M, Bessler H, et al. Effect of a garlic derivative (alliin) on peripheral blood cell immune responses. Int J Immunopharmacol 1999 Sep; 21(9):589–97.

[176] Lau BH, Yamasaki T, Gridley DS. Garlic compounds modulate macrophage and T-lymphocyte functions. Mol Biother 1991 Jun; 3(2):103–7.

[177] Kumar RV, Banerji A, Kurup CK, Ramasarma T. The nature of inhibition of 3-hydroxy-3-methylglutaryl CoA reductase by garlic-derived diallyl disulfide. Biochim Biophys Acta 1991 Jun 24; 1078(2):219–25.

[178] Omkumar RV, Kadam SM, Banerji A, Ramasarma T. On the involvement of intramolecular protein disulfide in the irreversible inactivation of 3-hydroxy-3-methylglutaryl-CoA reductase by diallyl disulfide. Biochim Biophys Acta 1993 Jun 24; 1164(1):108–12.

[179] Tyler V. Herbs of choice: The therapeutic use of phytomedicines. Binghamton, NY: Pharmaceutical Products Press, 1994, pp. 107–8.

[180] Taussig SJ, Batkin S. Bromelain, the enzyme complex of pineapple (Ananas comosus) and its clinical application. An update. J Ethnopharmacol 1988 Feb–Mar; 22(2):191–203.

[181] Richards BA. The enzyme knife—a renewed direction for cancer therapy? Discussion paper. J R Soc Med 1988 May; 81(5):284–5.

[182] [No authors listed]. Monograph: Bromelain. Altern Med Rev 1998 Aug; 3(4):302–5.

[183] Taussig SJ, Yokoyama MM, Chinen A, et al. Bromelain: A proteolytic enzyme and its clinical application. A review. Hiroshima J Med Sci 1975 Sep; 24(2–3):185–93.

[184] Taussig SJ. The mechanism of the physiological action of bromelain. Med Hypotheses 1980 Jan; 6(1):99–104.

185 Lotz-Winter H. On the pharmacology of bromelain: An update with special regard to animal studies on dose-dependent effects. Planta Med 1990; 56:249–53.

186 Mynott TL, Ladhams A, Scarmato P, Engwerda CR. Bromelain, from pineapple stems, proteolytically blocks activation of extracellular regulated kinase-2 in T cells. J Immunol 1999 Sep 1; 163(5):2568–75.

187 Boyle MD, Ohanian SH, Borsos T. Lysis of tumor cells by antibody and complement. VI. Enhanced killing of enzyme-pretreated tumor cells. J Immunol 1976 Mar; 116(3):661–8.

188 Zavadova E, Desser L, Mohr T. Stimulation of reactive oxygen species production and cytotoxicity in human neutrophils in vitro and after oral administration of a polyenzyme preparation. Cancer Biother 1995 Summer; 10(2):147–52.

189 Hale LP, Haynes BF. Bromelain treatment of human T cells removes CD44, CD45RA, E2/MIC2, CD6, CD7, CD8, and Leu 8/LAM1 surface molecules and markedly enhances CD2-mediated T cell activation. J Immunol 1992 Dec 15; 149(12):3809–16.

190 Desser L, Rehberger A, Kokron E, Paukovits W. Cytokine synthesis in human peripheral blood mononuclear cells after oral administration of polyenzyme preparations. Oncology 1993 Nov–Dec; 50(6):403–7.

191 Desser L, Rehberger A. Induction of tumor necrosis factor in human peripheral-blood mononuclear cells by proteolytic enzymes. Oncology 1990; 47(6):475–7.

192 Kleef R, Delohery TM, Bovbjerg DH. Selective modulation of cell adhesion molecules on lymphocytes by bromelain protease 5. Pathobiology 1996; 64(6):339–46.

193 Steffen C, Menzel J. [Basic studies on enzyme therapy of immune complex diseases.] Wien Klin Wochenschr 1985 Apr 12; 97(8):376–85.

194 Desser L, Rehberger A, Paukovits W. Proteolytic enzymes and amylase induce cytokine production in human peripheral blood mononuclear cells in vitro. Cancer Biother 1994 Fall; 9(3):253–63.

195 Sakalova A, Kunze R, Holomanova D, et al. [Density of adhesive proteins after oral administration of proteolytic enzymes in multiple myeloma.] Vnitr Lek 1995 Dec; 41(12):822–6.

196 Eckert K, Grabowska E, Stange R, et al. Effects of oral bromelain administration on the impaired immunocytotoxicity of mononuclear cells from mammary tumor patients. Oncol Rep 1999 Nov–Dec; 6(6):1191–9.

197 Maurer HR, Hozumi M, Honma Y, Okabe-Kado J. Bromelain induces the differentiation of leukemic cells in vitro: An explanation for its cytostatic effects? Planta Med 1988 Oct; 54(5):377–81.

198 Taussig SJ, Szekerczes J, Batkin S. Inhibition of tumour growth in vitro by bromelain, an extract of the pineapple plant (Ananas comosus). Planta Med 1985 Dec; (6):538–9.

199 Adamietz IA, Kurfurst F, Muller U, et al. Growth acceleration of Ehrlich ascites tumor cells treated by proteinase in vitro. Eur J Cancer Clin Oncol 1989 Dec; 25(12):1837–41.

200 Ito C, Yamaguchi K, Shibutani Y, et al. [Anti-inflammatory actions of proteases, bromelain, trypsin and their mixed preparation.] Nippon Yakurigaku Zasshi 1979 Apr 20; 75(3):227–37.

201 Rovenska E, Svik K, Stancikova M, Rovensky J. Enzyme and combination therapy with cyclosporin A in the rat developing adjuvant arthritis. Int J Tissue React 1999; 21(4):105–11.

202 Klein G, Kullich W. [Reducing pain by oral enzyme therapy in rheumatic diseases.] Wien Med Wochenschr 1999; 149(21–22):577–80.

203 Kumakura S, Yamashita M, Tsurufuji S. Effect of bromelain on kaolin-induced inflammation in rats. Eur J Pharmacol 1988 Jun 10; 150(3):295–301.

204 Vellini M, Desideri D, Milanese A, et al. Possible involvement of eicosanoids in the pharmacological action of bromelain. Arzneimittelforschung 1986; 36(1):110–2.

205 Targoni OS, Tary-Lehmann M, Lehmann PV. Prevention of murine EAE by oral hydrolytic enzyme treatment. J Autoimmun 1999 May; 12(3):191–8.

206 Pirotta F, de Giuli-Morghen C. Bromelain—A deeper pharmacological study. Note I—Antiinflammatory and serum fibrinolytic activity after oral administration in the rat. Drugs Exptl Res 1978; 4(1):1–20.

207 Batkin S, Taussig S, Szekerczes J. Modulation of pulmonary metastasis (Lewis lung carcinoma) by bromelain, an extract of the pineapple stem. Cancer Invest 1988; 6(2):241–2.

208 Batkin S, Taussig SJ, Szekerezes J. Antimetastatic effect of bromelain with or without its proteolytic and anticoagulant activity. J Cancer Res Clin Oncol 1988; 114(5):507–8.

209 Wald M, Zavadova E, Pouckova P, et al. Polyenzyme preparation WOBE-MUGOS inhibits growth of solid tumors and development of experimental metastases in mice. Life Sci 1998; 62(3):PL43–8.

210 Wald M, Olejar T, Pouckova P, Zadinova M. Proteinases reduce metastatic dissemination and increase survival time in C57Bl6 mice with the Lewis lung carcinoma. Life Sci 1998; 63(17):PL237–43.

211 Hager ED, Sube B, Strama H, Schrittwieser G. Multimodal treatment of patients with advanced pancreatic cancer in combination with locoregional hyperthermia. South Med J 1996; 89(10):S145.

212 Schedler M, Lind A, Schatzle W, Stauder G. Adjuvant therapy with hydrolytic enzymes in oncology—a hopeful effort to avoid bleomycinum induced pneumotoxicity? J Cancer Res Clin Oncol 1990; 116(Suppl I):697.

213 Gubareva AA. [The use of enzymes in treating patients with malignant lymphoma with a large tumor mass.] Lik Sprava 1998 Aug; (6):141–3.

214 Sakalova A, Mikulecky M, Holomanova D, et al. [The favorable effect of hydrolytic enzymes in the treatment of immunocytomas and plasmacytomas.] Vnitr Lek 1992 Sep; 38(9):921–9.

215 Kokron O. [Local therapy of metastatic pleural effusions with zusammenfassung proteolytic enzymes.] Osterr Kneipp Mag 1977 Dec 19; 4(4):82–5.

216 Gonzalez NJ, Isaacs LL. Evaluation of pancreatic proteolytic enzyme treatment of adenocarcinoma of the pancreas, with nutrition and detoxification support. Nutr Cancer 1999; 33(2):117–24.

[217] Wrba H, Pecher O. Enzymes: A drug of the future. Strengthening the immunological system with enzyme therapy. MUCOS Pharma GmbH, 1996. http://www.mucos.de

[218] Ito C, Yamaguchi K, Shibutani Y, et al. [Anti-inflammatory actions of proteases, bromelain, trypsin and their mixed preparation (author's transl).] Nippon Yakurigaku Zasshi 1979 Apr 20; 75(3):227–37.

[219] Taussig SJ, Szekerczes J, Batkin S. Inhibition of tumour growth in vitro by bromelain, an extract of the pineapple plant (ananas comosus). Planta Medica 1985; 538–9.

[220] Miyata S, Koshikawa N, Yasumitsu H, Miyazaki K. Trypsin stimulates integrin alpha(5)beta(1)-dependent adhesion to fibronectin and proliferation of human gastric carcinoma cells through activation of proteinase-activated receptor-2. J Biol Chem 2000 Feb 18; 275(7):4592–8.

[221] Wald M, Zavadova E, Pouckova P, et al. Polyenzyme preparation WOBE-MUGOS inhibits growth of solid tumors and development of experimental metastases in mice. Life Sciences 62(3):PL 43–48.

[222] Stankler L. Tetracycline and proteolytic enzymes combined compared with tetracycline alone in acne vulgaris. Br J Clin Pract 1976 Mar; 30(3):65–6.

[223] Bock U, Kolac C, Borchard G, et al. Transport of proteolytic enzymes across Caco-2 cell monolayers. Pharm Res 1998 Sep; 15(9):

[224] Maloman EN, Syrbu VT, Lupashku BK. [Effect of proteolytic enzymes on the antimicrobial activity of antibiotics.] Antibiotiki 1975 Jun; 20(7):613–7.

[225] Lahousen M. [Modification of liver parameters by adjuvant administration of proteolytic enzymes following chemotherapy in patients with ovarian carcinoma.] Wien Med Wochenschr 1995; 145(24):663–8.

[226] Klaschka, F. Oral Enzymes in Oncology: Clinical studies on Wobe-MuGos. MUCOS Pharma GmbH, 1997. http://www.mucos.de

[227] Sakalova A, Mikulecky M, Holomanova D, Langer D, et al. The favorable effect of hydrolytic enzymes in the treatment of immunocytomas and plasmacytomas. Vnitr Lek 1992; 38(9):921–9.

[228] Schedler M, Lind A, Schatzle W, Stauder G. Adjuvant therapy with hydrolytic enzymes in oncology—a hopeful effort to avoid bleomycinum induced pneumotoxicity? J Cancer Res Clin Oncol 1990; 116(Suppl I):697.

[229] Beard J. The action of trypsin upon the living cells of Jensen's mouse tumor. Br. Med J 1906; 4:140–141.

[230] Beard J. The enzyme treatment of cancer. Dayton, OH: Johnson-Watson, 1969.

[231] Kelley, WD. One answer to cancer: An ecological approach to the successful treatment of malignancy. Kelley Foundation, c1969, Rev. ed., 1974.

[232] Wolf M, Ransberger K. Enzyme therapy. New York: Vantage Press, 1972, pp. 184–204.

[233] Shively FL. Multiple proteolytic enzyme therapy of cancer. Dayton: Johnson-Watson Printing, 1969.

[234] Gerard G. Therapeutique anti-cancreuse et bromelaines. Agressologie 1972; 3:261–74.

[235] Nieper HA. Bromelain in der kontrolle malignen washstums. Krebsgeschehen 1976; 1:9–15.

[236] Kolac C, Streichhan P, Lehr CM. Oral bioavailability of proteolytic enzymes. European J Pharm Biopharm 1996; 42(4):222–232.

[237] Castell JV, Friedrich G, Kuhn CS, Poppe GE. Intestinal absorption of undegraded proteins in men: Presence of bromelain in plasma after oral intake. Am J Physiol 1997 Jul; 273(1 Pt 1):G139–46.

[238] Klaschka, F. Oral enzymes in oncology: Fundamentals of systemic enzyme therapy. MUCOS Pharma GmbH, 1997. http://www.mucos.de

[239] Kleine MW, Stauder GM, Gebauer F, et al. Kinetics of proteolytic enzyme activity of serum in a controlled randomized double blind study. 2nd International Congress on Biological Response Modifiers, San Diego, California, USA, Jan 29–31, 1993.

[240] Lehmann PV, et al. Beeinflussung der autoimmunen T-cell-antwort durch hydrolytische enzyme. In *Systemisch enzymtherapie. Aktueller stand und fortschritte*. Wrba H, Kleine MW, Miehlke K, et al. eds. München, Germany: MMW Medizin Verlag, 1996.

[241] Maehder K, Weigelt O. Die bestimmung der proteolytischen und fibrinolytischen aktivität auf blut- und hämoglobin-agarplatten. Arzneimittel-Forsch 1972; 22:116–117.

[242] Kelly GS. Bromelain: A literature review and discussion of its therapeutic applications. Alt Med Rev 1996; 1(4):243–257.

The next two chapters turn to the large family of phenolic compounds. In this one, flavonoids, the single largest group of phenolic compounds, are discussed, and Chapter 20 looks at nonflavonoid phenolics. The primary flavonoids covered here are apigenin, luteolin, quercetin, genistein, the green tea catechin EGCG, anthocyanidins, and proanthocyanidins, with others like daidzein mentioned more briefly.

Phenolic compounds, and flavonoids in particular, are capable of inhibiting cancer cells through multiple means. These include inhibition of PTK, PKC, and other enzymes involved in signal transduction, and inhibition of NF-κB, cyclooxygenase, and lipoxygenase. Questions remain as to the exact mode of action, but several likely contribute to an anticancer effect in any given situation. Questions also remain regarding the pharmacokinetic characteristics of flavonoids; for one thing, most if not all flavonoids are heavily metabolized in vivo, and a large amount of work remains to identify the active metabolites and their disposition (see Appendix J). Still, based on the many in-vitro studies and the few in-vivo studies available, flavonoids do have potential in cancer treatment, and additional study is warranted. As we will see, some flavonoids are better characterized than others, with data more consistent for some than others. Future research will identify those having the greatest potential and how they may best be used.

INTRODUCTION

Flavonoids, also called bioflavonoids, are a group of roughly 3,000 naturally occurring phenolic compounds sharing a similar chemical structure. They are found in every family and nearly every species of higher plants, and thus are in almost all fruits, vegetables, and medicinal herbs.[1] In many cases, they function as pigments or copigments and give plants their characteristic colors. In citrus fruit, they may represent up to 1 percent of fresh material. Beverages such as beer, wine, tea, and coffee also contain considerable amounts of flavonoids. The average daily dietary intake of flavonoids may be as high as 1 gram per day, mostly as quercetin, although some studies have suggested this value may be overestimated.[1, 2] Flavonoids seem to be active constituents in numerous medicinal plants, and plants containing them are widely used in herbal medicine traditions around the world. As a whole, flavonoids tend to improve capillary

resistance, inhibit inflammation, scavenge free radicals, and inhibit a variety of enzymes.

Flavonoids can be classified into six categories. (Some authors consider flavanols and isoflavones as separate categories, but it is also accepted to include these within flavonoids.) The categories are:

- *Flavanones.* Flavanones are viewed as minor flavonoids due to their limited natural distribution; they are found principally in citrus fruits.[3] Flavanones include tangeretin and naringin.

- *Flavones.* Flavones have much wider distribution. Although there are few primary flavones, these can combine with various sugar compounds in different ways to form thousands of different glycosides.[a] Primary flavones include luteolin and apigenin.

- *Isoflavones.* Isoflavones, or isoflavonoids, are found mostly in legumes, such as soy. Genistein and daidzein are common ones. Isoflavones also occur naturally as glycosides.

- *Flavonols.* As with flavones, there are only a few primary flavonols, but these are found as a variety of glycosides. Flavonols occur in most plant families and primary ones include quercetin and kaempferol.

- *Flavanols.* Flavanols are also seen as minor flavonoids because of their limited natural distribution. Flavanols (also called flavan-3-ols) are found in onions, kale, broccoli, apples, cherries and berries, tea, and red wine, and they include catechins such as EGCG.

- *Anthocyanidins and proanthocyanidins.* Anthocyanidins are red-blue pigments in plants, found mainly in their glycoside form, anthocyanins. They are highly concentrated in red and blue fruits like berries. Proanthocyanidins derive their name from the fact that under acidic conditions and high temperature they yield anthocyanidins. Proanthocyanidins are sometimes referred to by the trademark term *pycnogenols*, coined by the French researcher Jacques Masquelier, meaning "that which creates condensation"; it refers to the tendency of proantho-

---

[a] *A glycoside consists of the pure compound (called the aglycone), attached to a sugar molecule. Most phenolic compounds discussed in this book occur naturally as glycosides in the plant world. Glycosides are more useful to plants, one major reason being that they are more water-soluble than the aglycone.*

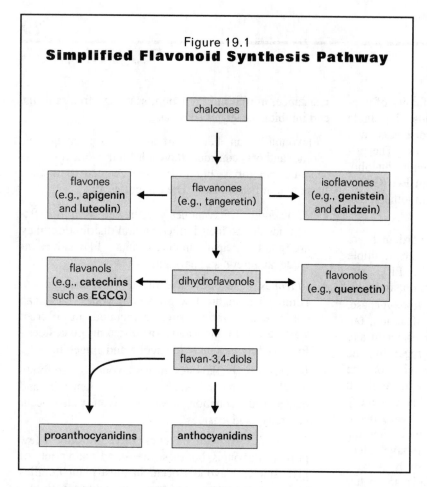

Figure 19.1
Simplified Flavonoid Synthesis Pathway

istein inhibited proliferation of a wide variety of cancer cell lines.[4–8] In these studies, genistein was generally active at about 1 to 50 µM.

Twenty-one animal antitumor studies have been conducted with genistein, or genistein-rich soy isoflavone mixtures, or both. Of these, 14 reported that genistein or soy isoflavonoid extracts inhibited tumor growth, metastasis, and/or angiogenesis in rodents.[9–13] In contrast, 5 studies reported that genistein either stimulated the growth of estrogen-dependent breast cancers or did not affect tumor growth in animals.[14–18] Thus while genistein shows promise, its use may not be appropriate against cancers that are estrogen-dependent. The two remaining studies were on genistein as a component of high-soy diets or its use as a pretreatment agent for cancer cells injected into animals.

Flavones

Over 26 in-vitro studies have been conducted on the cytotoxic effects of apigenin and/or luteolin (about half on each). Almost all noted that these flavones inhibited proliferation of a wide variety of cancer cell lines.[19–24] In these studies, apigenin and luteolin were generally active at about 1 to 50 µM.

Only two animal studies have been done on these flavones. In one, subcutaneously injected luteolin inhibited growth of breast cancer cells injected into mice.[25] In the other, intraperitoneal administration of apigenin inhibited growth and metastasis of melanoma cells in mice.[26]

cyanidins to occur as dimers (two similar compounds joined together).

All of these flavonoids primarily derive from the same (chalcone) precursor, as illustrated in Figure 19.1 (minor pathways are not shown). The figure gives a general idea of how interrelated the synthesis of these compounds is in the plant world. The flavonoids discussed in detail here are shown in bold type. The structures of all of these are of course similar, which can be seen by comparing Figures A.29 to A.40 in Appendix A.

ISOFLAVONES, FLAVONES, AND FLAVONOLS

Summary of Research and Conclusions

Isoflavones

Over 85 in-vitro studies have been conducted on the cytotoxic effects of genistein and/or daidzein, with most studies on the former. Although a few reported that very low concentrations stimulated proliferation of estrogen-dependent cancer cells, the vast majority found that gen-

Flavonols

Over 73 in-vitro studies have been examined the cytotoxic effects of quercetin, with almost all reporting that it inhibited proliferation of a wide variety of cancer cell lines.[27–31] Quercetin was generally active at about 1 to 50 µM in these studies.

Only four antitumor studies on quercetin have been done on animals. In one, a low oral dose did not affect metastasis of melanoma cells in mice.[32] In the second study, intraperitoneal administration slightly but not significantly increased the life span of mice injected with lympholeukemia ascites cancer cells.[33] In the third, intraperitoneal administration dramatically inhibited growth of human head and neck squamous cell carcinoma cells implanted into chambers in rats.[34] And the fourth reported that intraperitoneal administration of quercetin inhibited growth and metastasis of melanoma cells injected into mice.[26, a]

One human phase I study has also been completed using intravenously administered quercetin; the safe dose was established and evidence of tumor inhibition was seen in a few patients.[35]

In summary, these flavonoid have been the subject of a large number of in-vitro studies and a small number of in-vivo ones. They suggest these flavonoids are able to inhibit cancer cell proliferation in vitro and in vivo. At this point, it appears that genistein could also stimulate growth of estrogen-dependent cancers, and for this reason I believe it should not be used in trials against these types of cancers.

In addition to the above-mentioned studies, others have investigated the effects of these flavonoids on chemotherapy drugs. Research on their interactions will be discussed in Chapter 23.

The major commercial and dietary source of the isoflavones genistein and daidzein is soy products. Of the two, genistein is our primary interest here but daidzein is still important because almost any soy-based genistein product will contain approximately equal amounts of daidzein, and daidzein has some beneficial actions on its own. For practical reasons, genistein and daidzein would likely be used together, much as EPA and DHA from fish oil are (see Chapter 17). Note that soy is not the only source of genistein; some plants contain even higher concentrations, but soy is still the most common commercial source.[36]

Estrogenic and Antiestrogenic Effects of Isoflavones, Flavones, and Flavonols

Introduction

Estrogen acts as a growth factor for several types of cancer, especially several types of breast cancer. Since isoflavones, flavones, and flavonols can produce estrogenic effects, there is some concern they may stimulate growth of estrogen-dependent cancers. On the other hand, these same compounds can also produce antiestrogenic effects, which could inhibit growth of these cancers. Of the flavonoids discussed, genistein appears

most capable of producing an estrogenic effect and stimulating cancer growth.

Although studies are not so complete for flavonoids like apigenin, luteolin, and quercetin, or other phytoestrogens, it appears these compounds are much less likely to stimulate progression of estrogen-dependent cancers. For example, one in-vitro study reported that the estrogenic effects of luteolin, resveratrol, apigenin, and quercetin were 58, 22, 16, and 10 percent that of genistein.[37] Based on this and other in-vitro and in-vivo studies, it would seem these compounds are safe, but as a precaution, they are best used only within a larger combination of anticancer compounds.

Estrogenic and Antiestrogenic Effects

A number of natural compounds can produce estrogenic and antiestrogenic effects. These compounds, which include isoflavonoids, flavones, and flavonols, as well as stilbenes like resveratrol and mammalian lignans like those produced after flaxseed ingestion, are referred to as phytoestrogens. (Resveratrol and flaxseed are discussed in Chapter 20.)

The factors that dictate what response a phytoestrogen will produce are actually complex, but in general, phytoestrogens possess weak estrogenic activity as compared to estrogen, and they compete with estrogen for estrogen receptors in a cell's nucleus. In addition, they can occur at much higher plasma concentrations than estrogen. Therefore, when estrogen levels are low (as in postmenopausal women), they have the potential to produce estrogenic effects. At least one human study using moderate isoflavone doses (140 milligrams per day, from soy concentrate) noted a slight but significant estrogenic effect in postmenopausal women.[38]

Using the same reasoning, when estrogen levels are high (as in premenopausal women), we would expect genistein or other phytoestrogens to produce antiestrogenic effects. The effects of genistein on premenopausal women, however, are still uncertain. Mild estrogenic effects from genistein have been reported in some human studies, and two studies have noted that soy intake (at 38 to 60 grams per day) had a stimulatory effect on the breast tissue of healthy premenopausal women.[39–42] In another study, a high (60 gram) soy diet for two weeks produced estrogenic effects in the healthy breast tissue of premenopausal women, but these effects were weak.[43]

Based on the above, we conclude that genistein is likely to produce estrogenic effects in postmenopausal women and may or may not produce them in premenopausal women. Some readers aware of the epidemiologic studies may be surprised at this conclusion; such

---

[a] A fifth study was indexed in MEDLINE, but it was in Polish and had no abstract.

studies have reported, for example, that the risk of developing breast and endometrial cancers is reduced 5 to 10-fold in women who regularly consume soy.[44, 45, 46, a] On the surface, these results suggest that genistein does not produce estrogenic effects in women. The results are not consistent, however, and the role of isoflavonoids in risk reduction is still uncertain. Importantly, there is some recent evidence that a protective effect, at least for breast cancer, may be due to early-life exposure to genistein as opposed to current exposure.[47, 48, 49] Furthermore, other soy components besides isoflavones may be involved in any protective effects.

Effects of Phytoestrogens on Proliferation of Cancer Cells In Vitro

Ultimately, we are interested in the estrogenic effects of genistein on cancer cells. A number of in-vitro studies with estrogen-dependent cancer cells have been conducted, and indeed it appears that genistein and some other flavonoids can stimulate cell proliferation. Their ability to do so, however, seems to depend on the flavonoid concentration and the presence or absence of estrogen.

In-vitro studies have shown that low concentrations of genistein (1 nM to 1 μM) can stimulate proliferation of estrogen-dependent human breast cancer cells when estrogen is not present. At higher concentrations (10 to 100 μM), genistein strongly inhibits proliferation. Apparently, mechanisms active at higher concentrations override the stimulating effects at low ones. This biphasic effect was also seen with genistein in an estrogen-dependent pituitary cancer cell line.[50] A similar effect on estrogen-dependent breast cancer cells occurred with apigenin, luteolin, and enterolactone in some studies, where concentrations less than 10 μM increased proliferation and concentrations greater than 20 μM inhibited it.[51] (Enterolactone is discussed in Chapter 20.)

Any stimulatory effect from these compounds, however, may be attenuated by the presence of estrogen, as occurs in vivo. Most in-vitro studies suggest that apigenin, luteolin, genistein, and other flavonoids that can stimulate proliferation of estrogen-dependent breast cancer cells do not do so in the presence of estrogen.[17, 52, 53] For example, some studies found that genistein (at 5 μM) actually counteracted the growth-stimulatory effect of estrogen on human breast cancer cells in vitro.[54, 55] Still, not all studies reported a counteractive effect, and in some, genistein did not appreciably alter estrogen-induced proliferation.[56]

---

[a] *Epidemiologic studies also associate a reduced risk of prostate, stomach, colorectal, and lung cancer with soy consumption.*

Effects of Isoflavones in Estrogen-Dependent Tumors in Animals

If genistein and other phytoestrogens can, under some conditions, stimulate proliferation of estrogen-dependent cancer cells in vitro, we want to know whether this effect occurs in vivo. Unfortunately, very few in-vivo studies have been conducted with estrogen-dependent cancers. One, discussed in more detail later, reported that luteolin reduced growth of human breast cancer cells in mice.[25] In a study on soy, administration of a very large dose (20 percent of diet) to mice with transplanted human breast cancer cells did not affect growth of the primary tumor but did reduce proliferation of metastatic tumors in the lungs.[57] One study on genistein also reported anticancer effects, but these were surprising considering the low dose used (roughly 15 milligrams per day, as scaled to humans), and additional study is needed to verify these findings.[58]

In contrast to the above, three studies reported that genistein promoted the growth of breast cancer in vivo. In one study, soy extracts (at 90 mg/kg intraperitoneal) promoted growth and metastasis of breast cancer in rats.[16] The equivalent human dose is about 6.8 grams. In the second, genistein (at 90 mg/kg in diet) enhanced growth of estrogen-dependent human breast cancer cells in mice that had their ovaries removed.[17] These mice would have low estrogen levels, however, and would be particularly sensitive to the estrogenic effects of genistein. In the third study, both genistein and its glycoside (at 90 mg/kg in diet) increased growth of human estrogen-dependent breast cancer cells in mice; removing either from the diet resulted in tumor regression.[18] The human equivalent of 90 mg/kg in mice is about 870 milligrams per day of genistein.

In summary, it appears that genistein (or soy) is able to stimulate the growth of estrogen-dependent cancers under some in-vivo conditions. Therefore, again, the conservative recommendation given here is that genistein should not be administered to patients who have estrogen-dependent cancers. This recommendation pertains primarily to genistein supplementation. Normal dietary intake of soy and other foods that contain genistein should not pose a problem, especially if they are consumed only occasionally.

Type II Estrogen Receptors

One reason why phytoestrogens other than genistein may be less problematic is that they appear to inhibit cancer through additional estrogen-receptor-related means. Thus far we have discussed the effects of genistein and other phytoestrogens on what is called the classic estrogen receptor, or type I receptor. A second type has also been reported, the type II estrogen receptor; its existence is still somewhat controversial, since it has not yet been possible to purify its protein. Some researchers believe this will take place in the near future, however.[59] Type II receptors apparently exist at a higher concentration on the nuclear surface than type I and have a lower affinity for estrogen. Type II receptors do not induce a classic estrogen response after activation and appear to have a different function.

A number of in-vitro studies have indicated that flavones and flavonols could inhibit cancer cell proliferation by binding to type II estrogen receptors. Apparently, type II estrogen receptors are overexpressed in a wide range of human tumors, including breast, pancreatic, prostate, lymphatic, skin, ovarian, kidney, colon, and lung. Although type II receptors weakly bind estrogen, they more potently bind a compound identified as methyl-p-hydroxyphenyllactate (MeHPLA). Flavonoids and/or their metabolites mimic MeHPLA and bind to type II receptors, in competition with estrogen.[60, 61] Receptor binding with MeHPLA or flavonoids inhibits cell proliferation, whereas binding with estrogen stimulates it. For example, in some in-vitro studies luteolin and quercetin inhibited cancer cell proliferation by binding to type II receptors; in one, luteolin inhibited proliferation of human breast cancer cells at an IC_{50} of about 42 μM, reportedly by this mechanism.[60, 62] A number of other in-vitro studies have reported that quercetin (at about 10 μM) inhibited a wide variety of human tumor cell lines by affecting type II receptors.[60, 63–68]

In addition to inhibiting cell proliferation by binding to type II receptors, flavones have prevented the overexpression of MeHPLA esterase by cancer cells; this enzyme degrades MeHPLA, thereby decreasing its growth-inhibitory effects. Oral administration of luteolin (at 56 mg/kg) in drinking water for seven days blocked estrogen stimulation of MeHPLA esterase in rat uterine tissues.[61] The equivalent human dose is roughly 910 milligrams of luteolin per day. Similar results were seen after subcutaneous administration of luteolin in rats (at 5 mg/kg).[69] The equivalent human oral dose is about 540 milligrams per day.

Flavones and flavonols (i.e., apigenin, luteolin, and quercetin) may inhibit cancer in vivo through one or both of the above mechanisms (mimicking MeHPLA and preventing its destruction). One study reported that subcutaneous administration of luteolin (at about 23 to 91 mg/kg) inhibited growth of transplanted human breast cancer cells in mice.[25] The authors hypothesized that the results were related to type II binding or in-

TABLE 19.1 IN-VITRO ANTIOXIDANT ACTIVITY OF VARIOUS COMPOUNDS	
COMPOUND	ACTIVITY RELATIVE TO VITAMIN C[*]
Proanthocyanidins	about 5.0
Quercetin	4.7
Cyanidin	4.4
Epicatechin	2.5
Catechin	2.4
Resveratrol	2.0
Apigenin	1.5
Caffeic acid	1.3
Genistein	1.0
Vitamin C	1.0
Vitamin E	1.0
Glutathione	0.9

[*] Based on TEAC values. TEAC is Trolox equivalent antioxidant activity in aqueous phase.
Sources: References 70–73.

creased MeHPLA availability. The equivalent human oral dose is about 1.5 to 5.8 grams per day.

Antioxidant Effects of Isoflavones, Flavones, Flavonols, and other Phenols

Phenolic compounds, including isoflavones, flavones, and flavonols, can act as antioxidants due to the hydrogen-donating capacity of their phenolic groups and, in some cases, their metal-chelating potential. The latter may block the generation of copper- and iron-induced free radicals. Table 19.1 ranks various phenolics and other antioxidants in comparison to vitamin C in their ability to scavenge aqueous free radicals in vitro. As seen, most flavonoids are more active than vitamins C and E.

Some phenolic compounds that normally act as antioxidants can also act as prooxidants under the right circumstances (see Chapter 15). For example, some in-vitro conditions are adequate to auto-oxidize quercetin, and the prooxidant effect produced may account for some of quercetin's ability to cause gene mutations in vitro. In one study that tested 55 flavonoids, quercetin was the most mutagenic.[74] Other flavonoids in Table 19.1 do not appear to auto-oxidize as readily or tend to be mutagenic in vitro; apigenin may actually inhibit mutagenesis under some circumstances.[75–78] Even in the presence of copper, which is a catalyst for oxidation, apigenin was much less apt than quercetin to induce DNA damage.[79, 80] Still, at moderate doses in vivo, it is likely that quercetin and the other flavonoids produce an antioxidant, rather than prooxidant effect. For one thing, most of the flavonoids found in the plasma occur in the conjugate form, which is less reactive. Indeed, a recent study of men with chronic prostatitis suggested that even a high dose of quercetin produces an antioxidant effect in vivo.[81] In this study, a dose of 500 milligrams was given twice per day. Potential carcinogenic effects of quercetin are covered again later in this chapter.

In-vitro Cytotoxicity of Flavones, Flavonols, and Isoflavones

Apigenin, luteolin, quercetin, daidzein, and genistein produce cytotoxic effects in vitro at concentrations of 1 to 100 μM, although the IC$_{50}$ is often in the range of 10 to 30 μM. Data on their cytotoxicity against various cell lines is presented in Appendix K. Flavones, flavonols, and isoflavones can induce cell death through many possible means. Quite likely, the active means vary between cell lines. The potential anticancer actions of apigenin, luteolin, quercetin, and genistein are listed in Table 19.2.

In-vivo Antitumor Effects of Flavones, Flavonols, and Isoflavones

Unfortunately, very few animal antitumor studies have been conducted on flavones and flavonols. As discussed previously, one study on luteolin reported that it inhibited growth of human breast cancer cells in mice. Another mouse study found that intraperitoneal administration of 25 and 50 mg/kg apigenin inhibited growth and metastasis of transplanted melanoma cells.[26] The equivalent human oral dose is about 1.2 and 2.5 grams per

TABLE 19.2 POTENTIAL ANTICANCER ACTIONS OF APIGENIN (A), LUTEOLIN (L), QUERCETIN (Q), AND GENISTEIN (G)

ACTIVITY	KNOWN EFFECTS	AS ANTIOXIDANTS, MAY:	AS PTK INHIBITORS, MAY:	AS PKC INHIBITORS, MAY:	AS NF-κB INHIBITORS, MAY:	AS EICOSANOID INHIBITORS, MAY:	AS INVASION ENZYME INHIBITORS, MAY:
Chapter 2: Mutations, Gene Expression, and Proliferation							
Act as an antioxidant	x	—					
Inhibit topoisomerases	x						
Chapter 3: Results of Therapy at the Cellular Level							
Induce differentiation	x						
Induce apoptosis	x			x		x	
Chapter 4: Growth Factors and Signal Transduction							
Inhibit PTK	x		—				
Inhibit PKC	A,L,Q			—			
Induce *p21* or *p27* activity	A,G						
Inhibit *ras* cascade	A,Q,G		x	x			
Chapter 5: Transcription Factors and Redox Signaling							
Support p53 function	x	x					
Inhibit NF-κB/AP-1 activity	x	x	x	x	—	x	
Chapter 6: Cell-to-Cell Communication							
Affect CAMs	x		x	x	x	x	
Improve gap junction communication	A,G	x			x	x	
Chapters 7 and 8: Angiogenesis							
Inhibit angiogenesis	A,L,G	x	x	x	x	x	x
Inhibit bFGF effects							x
Reduce lactic acid	x						
Inhibit histamine effects	x		x	x	x		
Inhibit eicosanoid effects	x		x		x	—	
Inhibit TNF effects	G	x	x	x	x		
Inhibit VEGF effects	G	x	x	x		x	
Inhibit insulin resistance	G			x			
Chapters 9 and 10: Invasion and Metastasis							
Inhibit invasion				x			x
Inhibit hyaluronidase, collagenase, or elastase	A,L, G,Q	x		x		x	—
Inhibit GAG synthesis				x			
Inhibit cell migration	x		x	x			x
Inhibit metastasis				x			x
Inhibit platelet aggregation	x			x			
Chapters 11 and 12: Immune System							
Inhibit tumor-induced immunosuppression	G		x			x	
Chapter 19: Flavonoids							
Affect type II estrogen receptors	A,L,Q						

day. Moreover, apigenin inhibited the initiation and promotion phases of cancer in animal experiments.[76, 82]

Four animal studies examined the antitumor effects of quercetin:

- A low oral dose (the human equivalent of 290 milligrams) did not affect metastasis of melanoma cells in mice (the same dose of curcumin was inhibitory).[32]

- Intraperitoneal administration of 20 to 80 mg/kg slightly but not significantly increased the life span of mice injected with lympholeukemia ascites cancer cells.[33] The equivalent human oral dose is 1.2 to 4.9 grams.

- Intraperitoneal administration of 20 to 800 mg/kg dramatically inhibited growth of human head and neck squamous cell carcinoma implanted into chambers in rats.[34] The 800-mg/kg dose only moderately increased inhibition compared to the 20-mg/kg doses. The human oral equivalent of 20 mg/kg is about 2.1 grams.

- Intraperitoneal administration of 25 and 50 mg/kg inhibited growth and metastasis of transplanted melanoma cells in mice.[26] The equivalent human oral dose is about 1.5 and 3.1 grams per day.

In addition to these, one animal study examined the effects of quercetin chalcone, a proprietary, water-soluble form of quercetin. Given orally to mice at a daily dose of 310 and 620 milligrams it reduced the growth of transplanted colon cancer cells by 29 and 65 percent, respectively.[83]

One human phase I study has also been completed using intravenously administered quercetin. Although phase I trials are designed for determining safe doses rather than inducing an anticancer effect, evidence of tumor inhibition was seen in a few patients in the study.[35]

In contrast to flavones and flavonols, many more in-vivo studies have been conducted on isoflavones. As mentioned above, soy is a natural source of the isoflavones genistein and daidzein. Epidemiological studies indicate that soy consumption may be responsible for the decreased incidence of a number of cancers in Chinese and Japanese populations. Some of these studies were mentioned above in relation to the estrogenic effects of isoflavones. In another study, Japanese men consuming high quantities of soy products exhibited a low mortality rate from prostate cancer.[84]

Risk reduction is also seen in animals. In approximately 70 percent of the 30 or so animal studies conducted, soy administration in the diet produced a cancer preventive effect. The effect was generally an increase in latency, suggesting that soy delays the appearance and growth of new tumors.[85, 86, 87] However, soy components other than isoflavones could have been responsible for some of the cancer preventive effects.[88]

A number of rodent studies have suggested that soy or isolated isoflavones could also inhibit progression of established cancers in vivo. Again, in studies on soy, additional components may have been active. In one study, a large dose of a soybean protein isolate (10 to 20 percent of diet) inhibited metastasis formation and reduced tumor growth in mice injected with melanoma cells.[89] In a second one, large doses of soy (33 percent of diet) inhibited growth of transplanted prostate cells in rats.[90] In a third, a low-fat diet containing a soy isoflavone concentrate (about 220 mg/kg) and soy protein (about 24 g/kg) inhibited growth of human prostate cancer cells injected into mice.[91]

Several studies have been done on genistein, daidzein, or isoflavonoid-rich soy extracts. Based on those listed below, we can conclude that genistein and daidzein may inhibit growth or progression of many types of cancers in vivo, although not necessarily estrogen-dependent cancers. The average dose in all the successful oral, intraperitoneal, and subcutaneous studies on genistein discussed below is about 2.3 grams (range of 250 milligrams to 9.9 grams, all as scaled to human oral equivalents):

- Administration of about 1.2 g/kg of an isoflavone-rich soy concentrate in the diet inhibited the growth of transplanted human prostate cancer cells in mice by 30 percent, as well as angiogenesis. The actual isoflavone dose was about 200 mg/kg, approximately half of which was from genistein and half from daidzein.[12] The equivalent human isoflavone dose is about 1.9 grams per day.

- Genistein (at about 180 mg/kg in diet) inhibited the growth of human prostate cancer cells in mice. A soy isoflavone concentrate (at 600 mg/kg in diet) and a diet rich in soy protein but depleted of isoflavones also inhibited tumor growth.[13] The human equivalent of a 180-mg/kg dose is about 1.7 grams per day.

- Genistein (at about 40 mg/kg in diet) inhibited growth of transplanted melanoma cells in mice by about 50 percent.[11] The equivalent human dose is about 380 milligrams per day.

- Genistein (at about 120 and 240 mg/kg in diet) reduced metastasis of melanoma cells in mice and reduced tumor growth. A 30-mg/kg dose was not effective.[92] The equivalent human dose is about 1.2 and 2.4 grams per day.

- Oral administration of 54 mg/kg of genistein inhibited lung metastasis by 54 percent in mice with

TABLE 19.3   ESTIMATED THERAPEUTIC AND LOAEL DOSES FOR ISOFLAVONES, FLAVONES, AND FLAVONOLS[*]

DESCRIPTION	GENISTEIN DOSE (g/day)	APIGENIN DOSE (g/day)	LUTEOLIN DOSE (g/day)	QUERCETIN DOSE (g/day)
Required dose as scaled from animal antitumor studies	0.25 to 9.9 (average 2.3)	1.2 to 2.5	1.1 to 3.4	1.2 to 4.9
Required dose as scaled from animal anti-inflammatory studies	none	0.66 to 4.1	0.66 to 4.1	1 to 4
Required dose as estimated from pharmacokinetic calculations	0.72	0.93	2.9	5.2
Target dose based on an average from animal antitumor studies and pharmacokinetic calculations	1.5	1.5	2.5	3.8
Minimum required antitumor dose assuming 15-fold synergistic benefits	0.1	0.1	0.17	0.25
Commonly prescribed human dose in noncancerous conditions	0.05	0.01	uncertain	1
Estimated LOAEL dose	1.6	3.2	4.4	6.5
Tentative dose recommendation for further research	**0.1 to 1.1[†]**	**0.1 to 1.5**	**0.17 to 1.8[‡]**	**0.25 to 1.8[‡]**
Minimum degree of synergism required	**1.4-fold potency increase**	**none**	**1.4-fold potency increase**	**2.1-fold potency increase**

[*] *See Appendix J for details.*
[†] *Upper value based on daidzein LOAEL.*
[‡] *Upper value based on the general linear bioavailability limit of 1.8 grams per day.*

transplanted human melanoma cells, but daidzein was not effective.[93] The equivalent human dose is about 520 milligrams per day.

- Oral administration of 22 mg/kg of genistein per day to rats with transplanted prostate cancer reduced tumor-associated macrophage numbers, angiogenesis, and tumor volume.[94] The equivalent human dose is about 360 milligrams per day.

In addition to the oral studies, genistein also inhibited the growth, metastasis, and/or angiogenesis of a variety of tumors in mice and rats after intraperitoneal or subcutaneous administration.[9, 10, 95–98] Daidzein has also been reported effective. Intraperitoneal administration of 25 to 50 mg/kg daidzein reduced tumor volume by more than 50 percent and induced differentiation of leukemia cells held in chambers in mice.[99] The equivalent human oral dose is about 1.1 to 2.3 grams per day.

Lastly, at least two studies found that genistein was not effective; one of these, on rats, used very low doses in the drinking water (0.07 to 0.285 mg/kg). In this study, genistein did not inhibit the growth of transplanted human prostate cancer cells. The equivalent human dose is about 1.1 to 4.6 milligrams per day.[15] In the other study, oral administration of about 90 mg/kg of genistein in the diet did not inhibit growth of new or established estrogen-independent breast cancer cells transplanted into

mice.[14] The equivalent human dose is about 870 milligrams per day.

Estimated Therapeutic and LOAEL Doses of Isoflavones, Flavones, and Flavonols

The estimated required doses as scaled from animal antitumor studies (and anti-inflammatory studies) reasonably agree with estimated doses calculated from pharmacokinetic and in-vitro data. The required dose scaled from animal antitumor studies ranges from 250 milligrams to 9.9 grams, and that based on pharmacokinetic calculations is similar. Using a target in-vivo concentration of 15 μM for each compound (30 μM after adjustment for conjugates; see Appendix J), the required dose ranges from 720 milligrams to 5.2 grams. We can estimate target human doses by using an average of the doses scaled from animal studies and those calculated from pharmacokinetic and in-vitro data. For all compounds, the target doses are below the LOAEL doses.

The therapeutic dose estimates are summarized in Table 19.3. For all four flavonoids, the low end of the tentative recommended dose range is equal to the dose calculated by assuming a full 15-fold increase in potency by synergistic interactions. For genistein, the high end of the tentative recommended dose range is equal to the estimated LOAEL dose for daidzein; these two isoflavones normally occur in about 1 to 1 ratios in most soy-based genistein products, and the estimated LOAEL dose for daidzein is lower than for genistein. For apigenin, the high end of the tentative recommended dose range is equal to the target dose of 1.5 grams. For luteolin and quercetin, the high end of the tentative recommended dose range is equal to the assumed general linear bioavailability limit of 1.8 grams per day (see Appendix J). Higher doses, up to the estimated LOAEL dose, could be used, but it is uncertain whether they would be fully absorbed or would produce metabolites similar to those achieved by the lower doses.

It appears that synergistic interactions may be required for genistein, luteolin, and quercetin to produce an anticancer effect in humans. In comparing the target doses listed in Table 19.3 to the maximum tentative recommended doses, synergistic interactions will be needed to generate a minimum 1.4-fold, 1.4-fold, and 2.1-fold increase in potency, respectively. This should be possible, since these required increases are well below the allowable 15-fold increase discussed in Chapter 13.

The actual dose necessary to reach a desired plasma concentration (and its effect) will vary depending on many factors. These include the type of sugars that comprise the glycosides, the length of exposure to the flavonoid, and the individual's sex and particular gut microflora.[100–104] Nonetheless, the above dose calculations are useful in preliminary estimates. These estimates are for ingestion of the aglycone, and the doses of products containing glycosides would need to be increased about 1.6-fold (since the molecular weights of flavonoid glycosides are generally about 1.6-fold greater than that of the aglycones).

Potential Carcinogenic Effects of Flavonoids

Since flavonoids can produce a prooxidant effect invitro (see Table 15.3), their ability to induce cancer has been of concern. Quercetin has been of most concern due to its high redox activity; of all the flavonoids it produces the greatest mutagenetic effects in vitro, as discussed previously.

When quercetin is used with a carcinogen, it can increase carcinogen's effects (in this situation, quercetin acts as a *tumor-promoting* agent). For example, it enhanced the carcinogenic activity of 3-methylcholanthrene in mice and azoxymethane in rats.[105, 106] In the first study, quercetin was only active when it was co-injected subcutaneously with the carcinogen in the mice, and therefore these results have little relevance to oral administration. In the second, perhaps more relevant study, an oral dose of about 1.3 g/kg combined with the carcinogen decreased development of breast cancer in rats but increased that of colon cancer. It is reasonable to suppose that the very high concentration of the (reactive) aglycone in the intestines, in combination with the carcinogen, caused a local prooxidant effect that led to tumor development. The human equivalent of a 1.3-g/kg dose in rats is about 21 grams per day. Quercetin has also been reported to increase development of cancers outside the intestines; in one study, a dose of 12 g in the diet (as scaled to humans) increased the risk of pancreatic cancer in rats treated with a carcinogen.[107]

When quercetin was used alone, however, as it has been in many animal studies, results suggest the compound was not carcinogenic. In rats fed diets containing up to 5 percent quercetin (about 3.8 g/kg) for two years, no carcinogenic effects were observed, although benign kidney tumors did appear in some male rats.[108, 109] A lack of carcinogenic effects was also noted in hamsters and rats on a 10 percent quercetin diet for up to two years.[110, 111] In a review of a Japanese National Toxicology Program report concerning the long-term carcinogenic effect of quercetin in rats, the authors concluded that "therefore, although the data of [the program] do indicate possible carcinogenic activity, its risk potential for man on the basis of our present knowledge must be considered to be negligible."[112] In fact, some studies have reported that quercetin produces anticarcinogenic effects.[113] For example, oral administration of a high quercetin dose (about 1.5 to 3.8 g/kg in the diet) inhibited the incidence and number of palpable breast cancers in rats injected with the carcinogen N-nitrosomethylurea.[114]

The general lack of carcinogenic effects by quercetin is likely for two reasons. First, quercetin occurs as conjugates in the plasma. As discussed in Appendix J, these conjugates are less reactive than the free compound. Second, although the doses used were very high (the human equivalent of about 24 to 120 grams per day), it is unlikely such high doses were completely absorbed or metabolized in the same way lower doses would be. At doses above about 1.8 grams per day, many compounds are either poorly absorbed or are metabolized quite differently than lower doses (see Appendix J); in some cases, high doses are heavily methylated, which severely restricts their ability to undergo redox reactions. Thus, it seems the body has built-in mechanisms that help prevent systemic prooxidant effects caused by high doses of orally administered flavonoids.

FLAVANOLS—EGCG AND RELATED GREEN TEA CATECHINS

Summary of Research and Conclusions

At least 29 in-vitro studies have been conducted on the cytotoxic effects of green tea extract or EGCG against cancer cells.[115–119] As a whole, these studies suggest that green tea extract and/or EGCG can inhibit proliferation of many different cell lines, although a minority of lines do not appear to be affected. Although the active concentrations of EGCG are commonly high (50 to 80 μM), a few studies suggested that lower concentrations (roughly 15 μM) may be cytotoxic if exposure is prolonged.

In 6 animal studies, green tea extract or EGCG inhibited tumor growth, angiogenesis, or metastasis in mice.[120–125] A much larger number of animal studies reported that green tea extract or EGCG reduced cancer risk.

In addition, some studies observed that EGCG improved the effects of chemotherapy drugs; these are discussed in Chapter 23.

Although the in-vitro and animal studies are promising, important questions on EGCG remain unanswered. There are a number of inconstancies between the human, rat, and mouse pharmacokinetic and dosage data (see Appendix J). Due to the inconsistencies, the required target dose can be estimated only within a large range. In a worst-case scenario (a target dose at the high end of this range), it is possible EGCG would not be effective at the maximum safe human dose, even with synergism. The effective use of EGCG is also made difficult by its short half-life in humans (about one to four hours) and its chemical instability. A short half-life requires frequent dosing to maintain reasonably uniform plasma concentrations (therapeutic compounds are best dosed about once every half-life). For these reasons, a relatively large amount of study is needed before the required dose and clinical potential of EGCG can be fully assessed (see Table 13.2). Despite these shortcomings, green tea extract and EGCG are still discussed here because future studies may resolve the inconsistencies. Moreover, current studies suggest that EGCG and green tea may be useful in cancer prevention, and there is great interest in these compounds by the public.

Introduction

Green tea, *Camellia sinensis*, is one of the most popular beverages in the world and is a rich source of flavanols. It is made from tea leaves dried in a manner to avoid oxidation of the phenolic compounds. The principal flavanol compounds in tea are called catechins. Of the green tea catechins, the primary compounds include catechin, epicatechin, epicatechin gallate, epigallocatechin, and eipgallocatechin gallate (EGCG), the last two being most predominant.[126] EGCG is thought to be the primary anticancer agent in green tea.

In a clinical setting, the most practical form for EGCG administration is within decaffeinated, freeze-dried green tea solids, commonly referred to as green tea extract (GTE). Green tea extract standardized for EGCG is available commercially. Standardized green tea extract is more useful than green tea itself, since the EGCG dose can be precisely monitored and the extract allows greater doses without excessive intake of liquids or caffeine. The potential anticancer actions of EGCG are listed in Table 19.4.

In-vitro Activity of EGCG

EGCG has inhibited proliferation of many cancer cell lines in vitro. Some of these studies are summarized in Table 19.5. A density analysis of the data shown suggests that the IC_{50} for most cell lines is 50 to 80 μM and that a smaller number of cell lines have an IC_{50} of about 900 μM. The differences between cells lines may simply reflect that some cancer cell lines are more sensitive to EGCG than others. They may also reflect, at least in part, differences in experimental procedures, which can affect sensitivity. For example, EGCG is slowly transported across the plasma membrane, and relatively long treatment periods are required to ensure adequate EGCG uptake. Some in-vitro tests may have been too short to allow adequate uptake.

Combinations of green tea catechins appear to be more effective than EGCG or other single catechins alone. A combination of epicatechin and EGCG was about 2.6-fold more effective at reducing the proliferation of human lung cancer cells than EGCG.[127]

In-vivo Activity of EGCG

Both EGCG alone and green tea extract appear to have cancer preventive effects in vivo, largely due to inhibition of free radical damage and improved carcinogen metabolism. Dozens of studies have reported that topical, oral, or intravenous administration of EGCG or GTE inhibited development of rodent neoplasms in a variety of tissues (tongue, lung, stomach, skin, for example) by a variety of chemical inducers and promoters.[128–140, 160] In the mouse studies, the typical dose was a 1 to 2 percent tea (from tea leaf) as the sole source of drinking water.[141–145] This provided the equivalent of about 330 to 660 mg/kg of GTE. The equivalent human dose is about 3.2 to 6.4 grams per day of GTE, or about 380 to 760 grams per day of EGCG.

Epidemiologic studies sought to determine if tea drinkers have lower rates of cancer. Although a number have reported some reduction in risk for various cancers, in general green tea drinking does not seem to reduce cancer rates, except possibly for colorectal and pancreatic cancer.[146–149] One reason for lack of risk reduction may be that green tea drinkers do not usually ingest enough of it to be effective. Green tea may still be useful in some cases, however, for increased consumption prior to diagnosis has been correlated with improved prognosis of stage I and II breast cancer patients in Japan.[150] GTE is currently being investigated as a cancer preventive agent by the National Cancer Institute.[151]

Apart from any preventive effect, EGCG and GTE can inhibit cancer progression in vivo. This was seen in most but not all animal studies.[152, 153] Some successful studies are summarized below:

- Oral administration of GTE (about 110 mg/kg of EGCG) inhibited metastasis of transplanted lung cancer cells in mice, an effect possibly due to the extract's ability to inhibit invasion through the collagen-rich basement membrane.[120]

- Oral administration of approximately 100 mg/kg of EGCG in drinking water inhibited metastasis of transplanted melanoma cells in mice by about 72 percent.[121]

- Oral administration of 400 mg/kg of green tea extract (about 48 mg/kg EGCG) inhibited the growth of sarcoma cells transplanted into mice by 50 percent.[122]

- Oral administration of 500 mg/kg per day of green tea extract (about 60 mg/kg EGCG) inhibited the proliferation of Ehrlich carcinoma cells by 32 percent in mice.[123]

- Intraperitoneal administration of 40 mg/kg EGCG inhibited growth of androgen-sensitive and andro-

TABLE 19.4 POTENTIAL ANTICANCER ACTIONS OF EGCG

ACTIVITY	KNOWN EFFECTS	AS AN ANTI-OXIDANT, MAY:	AS A PTK INHIBITOR, MAY:	AS A PKC INHIBITOR, MAY:	AS AN EICOSANOID INHIBITOR, MAY:	AS A COLLAGENASE INHIBITOR, MAY:
Chapter 2: Mutations, Gene Expression, and Proliferation						
Act as an antioxidant	x	—				
Chapter 3: Results of Therapy at the Cellular Level						
Induce apoptosis	x		x		x	
Chapter 4: Growth Factors and Signal Transduction						
Inhibit PTK	x		—			
Inhibit PKC	x			—		
Induce *p21* or *p27* activity	x					
Chapter 5: Transcription Factors and Redox Signaling						
Support p53 function		x				
Inhibit NF-κB activity	varies	x	x	x	x	
Inhibit AP-1 activity	x		x			
Chapter 6: Cell-to-Cell Communication						
Affect CAMs			x	x	x	
Improve gap junction communication	x					
Chapters 7 and 8: Angiogenesis						
Inhibit angiogenesis		x	x	x	x	x
Inhibit bFGF effects						x
Inhibit histamine effects	x		x	x		
Inhibit eicosanoid effects	x		x		—	
Inhibit TNF effects		x	x	x		
Inhibit VEGF effects	x	x	x	x	x	
Inhibit insulin resistance				x		
Chapters 9 and 10: Invasion and Metastasis						
Inhibit invasion				x		x
Inhibit hyaluronidase, beta-glucuronidase, or elastase					x	
Inhibit collagenase effects	x	x		x	x	—
Inhibit GAG synthesis			x			
Inhibit cell migration			x	x		
Inhibit metastasis				x		x
Inhibit platelet aggregation			x			
Chapters 11 and 12: Immune System						
Inhibit tumor-induced immunosuppression			x			
Chapter 19: Flavonoids						
Inhibit telomerase activity	x					

TABLE 19.5   INHIBITION OF TUMOR CELLS BY EGCG IN VITRO

CELL LINE	EFFECT
Human acute leukemia blast cells	Inhibited proliferation at 50 µM and above. Complete inhibition at 500 µM.[154]
Human and mouse leukemia cell lines	IC_{50} = about 50 µM.[117]
Mouse erythroleukemia cells	82% inhibition at about 220 µM.[164]
Human lymphoid leukemia cells	Inhibited proliferation by 18% at 50 µM and 93% at 100 µM.[155, 156]
Human lung cancer cells	IC_{50} = 100 µM.[157, 158]
Two human lung cancer cell lines	IC_{50} = 22 µM. EGCG was two- to threefold less effective against another human lung cancer line and human colon cancer cells.[118]
Mouse lung cancer cells	Inhibited proliferation by 36% at 1,000 µM.[159]
Two mouse lung cancer lines	IC_{50} = 35 and 42 µM.[160]
Human melanoma and human breast, colon, and lung cancer cell lines	IC_{50} = about 100 to 150 µM.[161]
Human oral cancer cells	IC_{50} = 18 µM.[162]
Human epidermoid cancer cells	IC_{50} = about 130 µM.[163]
Rat liver cancer cells	IC_{50} = about 220 µM.[164]
Three human prostate cancer cell lines	IC_{50} between 1 and 25 µM.[165]
Two mouse breast cancer cell lines	IC_{50} = 770 and 925 µM.[160]
Virally transformed human fibroblast cells	IC_{50} = 10 µM for cancer cells and 120 µM for normal cells.[166]

gen-insensitive human prostate cancer cells and estrogen-dependent human breast cancer cells transplanted into mice.[125]

• Although not a study on tumors, 1.3 percent green tea as drinking water (about 140 mg/kg EGCG) inhibited VEGF-induced corneal angiogenesis in mice.[124]

The oral doses used in the mouse studies ranged from 48 to 140 mg/kg of EGCG. The equivalent human dose is about 0.46 to 1.3 grams per day. This range is somewhat higher than the dose range of 380 to 760 milligrams as scaled from the mouse cancer prevention studies above. This difference is expected, since for most compounds the doses required for antitumor effects are larger than those needed to prevent cancer.

As listed in Table 19.4, a number of mechanisms may be responsible for the in-vivo effects of EGCG. As mentioned, cytotoxic effects were generally seen at concentrations greater than 50 µM. In some cases, however, EGCG may impede cancer through indirect means at doses lower than those required for direct cytotoxic effects. EGCG inhibited collagenases produced from mouse lung cancer cells at an IC_{50} of about 9 µM.[167] Invasion of mouse lung cancer cells was inhibited at an IC_{50} of about 25 µM.[120] Also, EGCG inhibited leuko-

triene LTB$_4$ release from stimulated rat cells at concentrations of about 10 µM.[168]

EGCG may show other effects in vivo that it does not readily show in vitro. For example, its ability to reduce telomerase activity in cancer cells may be more apparent in vivo than in most in-vitro studies. Telomerase is an enzyme that preserves the tips of chromosomes during cell division and allows cells to maintain a high proliferative capacity. EGCG at 15 µM markedly reduced telomerase activity in human leukemia and adenocarcinoma cells. At this low concentration, however, the proliferation rate reached a plateau only after treatment for 40 to 60 days; in-vitro cytotoxicity tests are rarely carried out this long.[169] Furthermore, although EGCG inhibited chemically induced TNF production and NF-κB activity in vitro only at high concentrations (100 mM), oral administration of 500 mg/kg in mice, which produced a total EGCG plasma concentration of only about 22 µM, reduced TNF by more than 80 percent.[170]

Estimated Therapeutic and LOAEL Doses of EGCG

The estimated required dose of EGCG as scaled from animal antitumor studies is not in close agreement with that calculated from pharmacokinetic and in-vitro data. This discrepancy suggests the target human dose is still highly uncertain; it can be estimated only within a large range. The required dose as scaled from antitumor experiments in animals is about 460 milligrams to 1.3 grams per day, but the dose based on pharmacokinetic calculations is much higher. Using a target in-vivo concentration of 15 µM of EGCG (30 µM after adjustment for conjugates), the required EGCG dose is about 12 grams per day. The reasons for this large difference are not clear. As discussed in Appendix J, the difference in doses reflects a number of inconstancies between the human, rat, and mouse data, and further study is necessary. Lacking additional data, we can estimate a target human dose between 460 milligrams and 12 grams per day.

The LOAEL dose for EGCG also is not certain but is estimated to be between 210 and 550 milligrams per day (see Appendix J). The lower range of this dose is about equal to commonly prescribed doses; the dose of EGCG for noncancerous conditions recommended on some standardized green tea products is about 200 milligrams per day.

The therapeutic dose estimates are summarized in Table 19.6, with the tentative dose recommendation 460 to 550 milligrams per day. The 460-milligram value is based on the low end of the antitumor dose scaled from animals, and the 550-milligram on the estimated high end of the LOAEL dose range.

TABLE 19.6 ESTIMATED THERAPEUTIC AND LOAEL DOSES FOR EGCG*

DESCRIPTION	DOSE (g/day)
Required dose as scaled from animal antitumor studies	0.46 to 1.3
Required cytotoxic dose as determined from pharmacokinetic calculations	12
Target dose based on range from animal antitumor studies and pharmacokinetic calculations	0.46 to 12
Minimum required antitumor dose assuming 15-fold synergistic benefits	0.031 to 0.8
Commonly prescribed human dose in noncancerous conditions	0.2
Estimated LOAEL dose	0.21 to 0.55
Tentative dose recommendation for further research	**0.46 to 0.55**
Minimum degree of synergism required	uncertain

See Appendix J for details.

Since the target dose is uncertain, it is also not clear if synergistic interactions are required to produce an anticancer effect in humans, or if such effect could take place even with the benefits of synergism. Consider a worst-case scenario, where the target dose is 12 grams and the LOAEL dose is only 210 milligrams. The full 15-fold allowable increase in potency from synergism would lower the target dose to 800 milligrams, which is still above the LOAEL dose. Thus, a dose of 210 or even 550 milligrams may not produce an anticancer effect if the required dose is 12 grams.

Although the required dose is uncertain and EGCG may not be effective even with synergism, dose details are still given in the table for the sake of completeness and because the tentatively recommended dose is not expected to cause harm and a beneficial effect cannot be ruled out.

As with most natural compounds, the EGCG daily dose is best divided into at least three equally spaced administrations, if it is used. Since it has a relatively short half-life, a dose given more than three times a day may be desirable. Single EGCG doses greater than about 220 milligrams may not have their intended effect, since one study reported that doses above that (as part of GTE) begin to saturate uptake mechanisms, resulting in little additional gain in EGCG plasma concentrations.[171] Other investigators place the saturation dose closer to 380 milligrams of EGCG in GTE.[172]

A dose of 460 milligrams per day is equal to about 12 cups of green tea per day, or about 3.8 grams of GTE. Note that some manufacturers make a green tea polyphenol extract that is more concentrated than the aver-age GTE, and therefore lower doses of these products would suffice.

ANTHOCYANIDINS AND PROANTHOCYANIDINS

Summary of Research and Conclusions

At least six in-vitro studies have been conducted on the cytotoxic effects of anthocyanidins.[173–178] Overall, these studies suggested that anthocyanidins or their glycosides, anthocyanins, inhibited proliferation of cancer cell lines at concentrations between 5 and 100 μM, with anthocyanins being somewhat less potent than anthocyanidins. At least two animal studies have been performed, which reported that oral administration of anthocyanins inhibited growth of lymphoma cells transplanted into mice.[176, 179]

Some five in-vitro studies have been done on proanthocyanidins, suggesting they reduced cancer cell proliferation or induced differentiation at concentrations between 8 and 86 μM.[180–184]

Although in-vitro and in-vivo studies have been conducted on cyanidins and proanthocyanidins, most looked for direct cytotoxic effects, which were in fact seen in the in-vitro studies but only at relatively high concentrations. Because of the unfavorable pharmacokinetic characteristics of these compounds, such high concentrations could not be achieved in human plasma after oral dosing. This book is among the first to suggest anthocyanidins and proanthocyanidins may be useful in cancer treatment for their indirect and not their direct effects. Indirect effects such as protection of the vascu-

TABLE 19.7 ESTIMATED THERAPEUTIC AND LOAEL DOSES FOR ANTHOCYANINS*	
DESCRIPTION	**DOSE (g/day)**
Required dose as scaled from animal antitumor studies	0.12 to 0.28
Required dose as scaled from animal anti-edema studies	0.4 to 3
Required cytotoxic dose as determined from pharmacokinetic calculations	250
Commonly prescribed human dose in noncancerous conditions	0.06 to 0.12
Estimated LOAEL dose	2.2
Tentative dose recommendation for further research	**0.12 to 1.8 grams**[†]

* See Appendix J for details.

† Upper value based on the general linear bioavailability limit of 1.8 grams per day.

lature occur with reasonable oral doses. So, while the following discussions show that excessive doses are necessary to produce cytotoxic effects, this is not a problem since the compounds could still inhibit cancer through indirect effects at lower doses.

Anthocyanidins

Anthocyanidins are red-blue pigments in plants, and they are especially high in fruits such as blueberries, bilberries, and other berries. Like many other flavonoids, anthocyanidins exist in nature almost exclusively in their glycoside (anthocyanin) forms. Although the glycosides are found in many plants, the primary commercial source of anthocyanins is *Vaccinium myrtillus* (bilberry), in which they occur at about 3 percent.[185] Bilberries are eaten as food and have also been used medicinally to treat scurvy, urinary infections, diarrhea (due to their astringent characteristics), and varicose veins, as well to improve night vision and treat other eye disorders.[186]

Anthocyanins are available commercially as bilberry extract standardized for 25 percent anthocyanins and as standardized elderberry extracts. The common dose of standardized bilberry extract is 240 to 480 milligrams per day in divided doses, which provides an actual anthocyanin dose of 60 to 120 milligrams per day.[187]

Anthocyanins may have a protective effect on the vasculature due to their high affinity for connective tissue. This affinity has been demonstrated in a rat study, where concentrations were higher in connective tissue (skin) than in the plasma, and the half-life in connective tissue was prolonged. Four hours after administration, connective tissue concentrations were fivefold higher than

plasma concentrations.[188] In rabbits, the standardized bilberry extract at an oral dose of 200 to 400 mg/kg prevented chemically induced increases in skin capillary permeability.[189] The human equivalent of the 400 mg/kg dose is about 3 grams of anthocyanins. In rats, oral administration of 25 to 100 mg/kg was effective in inhibiting increased skin capillary permeability due to dietary deficiencies.[189] The human equivalent of 100 mg/kg of bilberry extract in rats is about 400 milligrams of anthocyanins. Oral administration of about 500 mg/kg of bilberry extract blocked increases in blood-brain barrier permeability caused by surgery in rats.[190] The equivalent human dose is about 2 grams per day of anthocyanins.

Anthocyanins and their aglycone have reduced cancer cell proliferation in vitro, as summarized below. Anthocyanidins (the aglycones) inhibited proliferation at concentrations between 5 and 100 µM, with glycosides being somewhat less potent:

The IC_{50} for a variety of mixed anthocyanins from different plants against human colon cancer and lymphoma cells averaged about 13 µM. This same concentration was cytotoxic to normal human fibroblast cells. The aglycones were about 1.5-fold more potent than the glycosides, and about 2 to 6 times more potent than genistein and other flavonoid aglycones.[191]

- Various anthocyanins (apparently the glycoside form) inhibited proliferation of human colon cancer cells at roughly 220 µM. Lower concentrations were not tested.[177]

- Anthocyanins from red wine inhibited proliferation of human stomach cancer cells at an IC_{50} of about 5 µM and human colon cancer cells at an IC_{50} between 5 and 28 µM.[175]

- Various anthocyanidins (apparently the aglycone form) inhibited the proliferation of human colon cancer cells at an IC_{50} between roughly 0.3 and 70 µM.[178]

- Anthocyanidins from grape rinds and red rice inhibited proliferation of human colon cancer cells at an IC_{50} between 70 and 100 µM. Anthocyanins (glycosides) were less potent.[174]

- Anthocyanidins from red soybeans and red beans inhibited proliferation of human colon cancer cells at an IC_{50} of roughly 87 µM.[176]

Two animal studies have reported that anthocyanins reduced tumor growth in vivo.[176, 179] At a dose of roughly 12 to 29 mg/kg (in drinking water), anthocyanins from red beans, red soybeans, *Camellia* species, or *Hibiscus* species increased the survival of mice with transplanted lymphoma cells. The percent of those surviving after 30 days was generally about double that of control mice. The equivalent human dose is about 120 to 280 milligrams per day.

Estimated Therapeutic and LOAEL Doses of Anthocyanidins

The estimated required doses based on animal studies and pharmacokinetic calculations are not in close agreement. The antitumor dose as scaled from mouse studies is 120 to 280 milligrams, but the dose based on pharmacokinetic calculations is higher. Using a target in-vivo concentration of 15 µM (30 µM after adjustment for conjugates) for anthocyanins, the required anthocyanin dose is about 250 grams per day, which is prohibitive. The large difference in doses is expected and not problematic, however; it merely reiterates that anthocyanidins would function as indirect-acting, not direct-acting cytotoxic compounds. Cytotoxic concentrations will not be produced in the plasma after oral dosing.

ACTIVITY	KNOWN EFFECTS, ANTHOCYANIDINS	KNOWN EFFECTS, PROANTHOCYANIDINS	AS ANTIOXIDANTS, MAY:	AS COLLAGENASE INHIBITORS, MAY:	AS HYALURONIDASE INHIBITORS, MAY:
Chapter 2: Mutations, Gene Expression, and Proliferation					
Act as an antioxidant	x	x	—		
Chapter 5: Transcription Factors and Redox Signaling					
Support p53 function			x		
Inhibit NF-κB activity		x	x		
Chapters 7 and 8: Angiogenesis					
Inhibit angiogenesis			x	x	x
Inhibit bFGF effects				x	x
Inhibit histamine effects		x			
Inhibit TNF effects			x		
Impede increased vascular permeability	x	x			
Inhibit VEGF effects			x		
Chapters 9 and 10: Invasion and Metastasis					
Inhibit invasion				x	x
Inhibit hyaluronidase, beta-glucuronidase, or elastase		x			—
Inhibit collagenase effects	x	x	x	—	
Inhibit cell migration					x
Inhibit metastasis				x	x
Inhibit platelet aggregation	x				
Chapters 11 and 12: Immune System					
Stimulate the immune system		x			
Inhibit tumor-induced immunosuppression		x			

TABLE 19.8 POTENTIAL ANTICANCER ACTIONS OF ANTHOCYANIDINS AND PROANTHOCYANIDINS

The estimated LOAEL dose for anthocyanins in humans is 2.2 grams per day (see Appendix J), which is just below the average LOAEL dose (2.9 grams) for all flavonoids discussed. The 2.2-gram value is much higher than the commonly prescribed daily dose of 120 milligrams.

Therapeutic dose estimates are summarized in Table 19.7, with the tentative recommended range at 120 milligrams to 1.8 grams per day. The 120-milligram value is based on the low end of the effective range in animal antitumor studies. The 1.8-gram value is equal to the general linear bioavailability limit of 1.8 grams per day (see Appendix J). Higher doses, up to the estimated LOAEL dose, could be used, but it is uncertain whether they would be fully absorbed or produce metabolites similar to those from lower doses.

One more advantage of anthocyanidins, though probably not a major one, appears when we look at their metabolism. Anthocyanidins appear to be unstable in vivo and quickly metabolized to protocatechuic acid.[192] The plasma concentration of protocatechuic acid may be about sevenfold greater than that of anthocyanins. Protocatechuic acid is a simple phenolic compound that appears as a metabolite of many different flavonoids. It is cytotoxic in vitro to human lung and stomach cancer cells, but only at high concentrations (approaching 650 µM).[193] Nevertheless, some studies have reported it

TABLE 19.9 ESTIMATED THERAPEUTIC AND LOAEL DOSES FOR PROANTHOCYANIDINS[*]	
DESCRIPTION	**DOSE (g/day)**
Required dose as scaled from animal anti-edema studies	0.49 to 6.5
Required cytotoxic dose as determined from pharmacokinetic calculations	87
Commonly prescribed human dose in noncancerous conditions	0.05 to 0.3
Estimated LOAEL dose	2.2
Tentative dose recommendation for further research	**0.49 to 1.8 grams**[†]

[*] *See Appendix J for details.*
[†] *Upper value based on the general linear bioavailability limit of 1.8 grams per day.*

could produce antioxidant and cancer preventive effects.[194, 195]

Proanthocyanidins

Proanthocyanidins are dimers composed of one flavanol compound joined with a flavan-3,4-diol compound (see Figure 19.1). They apparently share many qualities with anthocyanidins, including potential antitumor actions, as listed in Table 19.8. Note that most of these actions would inhibit cancer progression through indirect means rather than through direct cytotoxic effects.

Like anthocyanidins, proanthocyanidins are also active in vitro against cancer cells. Proanthocyanidins from barley induced differentiation in human leukemia cells at about 8 μM. The same study reported that proanthocyanidins potentiated the ability of retinoic acid to induce differentiation. In combination with low levels of retinoic acid, proanthocyanidins were about twice as potent as when used alone.[181] Proanthocyanidins from grape seed were cytotoxic to human breast, lung, and stomach cancer cells in vitro; the IC$_{50}$ was about 86 μM, although nearly similar effects (43 percent inhibition) were seen at 43 μM. In this study, no cytotoxicity was observed with leukemia cells, and the proliferation of normal human stomach cells and rat macrophage cells was actually enhanced.[196] It seems then that proanthocyanidins may have some selective inhibitory effects against certain cancer cells. In three other in-vitro studies, proanthocyanidins (at 75 to 86 μM) inhibited proliferation of human breast cancer cells and human prostate cancer cells. Again, selective effects against cancer cells were noted.

Estimated Therapeutic and LOAEL Doses of Proanthocyanidins

The estimated required doses based on animal studies and pharmacokinetic calculations are not in close agreement. As with anthocyanins, this difference in doses is not surprising or problematic. Proanthocyanidins are not considered cytotoxic compounds here. Like anthocyanins, proanthocyanidins inhibit edema, protect the vasculature, and are regarded as indirect-acting compounds.

Although proanthocyanidins have not been tested in antitumor experiments, they have been for vascular conditions as listed in Table 8.1 (see also Table F.1 of Appendix F). The required dose as scaled from animal experiments is 490 milligrams to 6.5 grams per day. Doses up to 300 milligrams per day have been used in human noncancer studies.

The anticancer dose based on pharmacokinetic calculations is higher, but again this is not problematic since proanthocyanidins are not viewed here as direct-acting cytotoxic compounds. Using a target in-vivo concentration of 15 μM (30 μM after adjustment for conjugates), the required proanthocyanidin dose is about 87 grams per day. This is probably a low estimate, since most in-vitro studies suggested that concentrations greater than 15 μM are required.

The estimated human LOAEL dose is 2.2 grams per day, similar to anthocyanidins (see Appendix J). This value is higher than the dose of 300 milligrams per day used in some human studies.

The therapeutic dose estimates are summarized in Table 19.9. The tentative recommended dose range is 490 milligrams to 1.8 grams per day, with the 490-milligram value based on the low end of the effective dose range in animal anti-edema studies. The 1.8-gram value is equal to the assumed general linear bioavailability limit of 1.8 grams per day (see Appendix J). Higher doses, up to the estimated LOAEL dose, could be taken, but whether they would be fully absorbed or produce similar metabolites to those from lower doses is unknown.

CONCLUSION

Phenolic compounds represent a diverse group of compounds with anticancer potential. As a whole, they may inhibit cancer progression through cytotoxic means, as well as a variety of indirect ones. Although a number of questions remain regarding their effects in vivo, their use in cancer treatment seems promising, especially when used in synergistic combinations. Even flavonoids such as anthocyanidins and proanthocyanidins, which are unlikely to inhibit cancer progression through direct cytotoxicity, may be more effective when used in combinations. Their use in combinations could increase the overall anticancer effect by increasing the number of procancer events targeted.

REFERENCES

[1] Kuhnau J. The flavonoids. A class of semi-essential food components: Their role in human nutrition. World Rev Nutr Diet 1976; 24:117–91.

[2] Hertog MG, Hollman PC, Katan MB, Kromhout D. Intake of potentially anticarcinogenic flavonoids and their determinants in adults in The Netherlands. Nutr Cancer 1993; 20(1):21–9.

[3] Hollman PCH. Bioavailability of flavonoids. European J of Clinical Nutrition 1997; 51(suppl 1):S66–69.

[4] Alhasan SA, Ensley JF, Sarkar FH. Genistein induced molecular changes in a squamous cell carcinoma of the head and neck cell line. Int J Oncol 2000 Feb; 16(2):333–8.

[5] Dixon-Shanies D, Shaikh N. Growth inhibition of human breast cancer cells by herbs and phytoestrogens. Oncol Rep 1999 Nov–Dec; 6(6):1383–7.

[6] Shen F, Xue X, Weber G. Tamoxifen and genistein synergistically down-regulate signal transduction and proliferation in estrogen receptor-negative human breast carcinoma MDA-MB-435 cells. Anticancer Res 1999 May–Jun; 19(3A):1657–62.

[7] Lyn-Cook BD, Stottman HL, Yan Y, et al. The effects of phytoestrogens on human pancreatic tumor cells in vitro. Cancer Lett 1999 Jul 19; 142(1):111–9.

[8] Balabhadrapathruni S, Thomas TJ, Yurkow EJ, et al. Effects of genistein and structurally related phytoestrogens on cell cycle kinetics and apoptosis in MDA-MB-468 human breast cancer cells. Oncol Rep 2000 Jan–Feb; 7(1):3–12.

[9] Wietrzyk J, Opolski A, Madej J, Radzikowski C. Antitumour and antimetastatic effect of genistein alone or combined with cyclophosphamide in mice transplanted with various tumours depends on the route of tumour transplantation. In Vivo 2000 Mar–Apr; 14(2):357–62.

[10] Iishi H, Tatsuta M, Baba M, et al. Genistein attenuates peritoneal metastasis of azoxymethane-induced intestinal adenocarcinomas in Wistar rats. Int J Cancer 2000 May 1; 86(3):416–20.

[11] Record IR, Broadbent JL, King RA, et al. Genistein inhibits growth of B16 melanoma cells in vitro and in vivo and promotes differentiation in vitro. Int J Cancer 1997; 72:860–864.

[12] Zhou JR, Gugger ET, Tanaka T, et al. Soybean phytochemicals inhibit the growth of transplantable human prostate carcinoma and tumor angiogenesis in mice. J Nutr 1999 Sep; 129(9):1628–35.

[13] Zhou JR, Zhong Y, Blackburn GL. Soybean components inhibit orthotropic growth of human prostate LNCaP cells in

SCID mice. Third international symposium on the role of soy in preventing and treating chronic disease. October 31-November 3, 1999. Washington, DC, USA.

[14] Santell RC, Kieu N, Helferich WG. Genistein inhibits growth of estrogen-independent human breast cancer cells in culture but not in athymic mice. J Nutr 2000 Jul; 130(7):1665–1669.

[15] Naik HR, Lehr JE, Pienta KJ. An in vitro and in vivo study of antitumor effects of genistein on hormone refractory prostate cancer. Anticancer Res 1994 Nov–Dec; 14(6B):2617–9.

[16] Charland SL, Hui JW, Torosian MH. The effects of a soybean extract on tumor growth and metastasis. Int J Mol Med 1998; 2(2):225–228.

[17] Hsieh CY, Santell RC, Haslam SZ, Helferich WG. Estrogenic effects of genistein on the growth of estrogen receptor-positive human breast cancer (MCF-7) cells in vitro and in vivo. Cancer Res 1998 Sep 1; 58(17):3833–8.

[18] Allred CD, Allred KF, Helferich WG. Genistin, the glycoside form of genistein, stimulates growth of estrogen-dependent human breast cancer cells in vivo. Third international symposium on the role of soy in preventing and treating chronic disease. October 31-November 3, 1999. Washington, DC, USA.

[19] Fotsis T, Pepper MS, Montesano R, et al. Phytoestrogens and inhibition of angiogenesis. Baillieres Clin Endocrinol Metab 1998 Dec; 12(4):649–66.

[20] Yin F, Giuliano AE, Van Herle AJ. Growth inhibitory effects of flavonoids in human thyroid cancer cell lines. Thyroid 1999 Apr; 9(4):369–76.

[21] Jing Y, Waxman S. Structural requirements for differentiation-induction and growth-inhibition of mouse erythroleukemia cells by isoflavones. Anticancer Res 1995 Jul–Aug; 15(4):1147–52.

[22] Yin F, Giuliano AE, Van Herle AJ. Signal pathways involved in apigenin inhibition of growth and induction of apoptosis of human anaplastic thyroid cancer cells. Anticancer Res 1999 Sep–Oct; 19(5B):4297–303.

[23] Huang YT, Hwang JJ, Lee PP, et al. Effects of luteolin and quercetin, inhibitors of tyrosine kinase, on cell growth and metastasis-associated properties in A431 cells overexpressing epidermal growth factor receptor. Br J Pharmacol 1999 Nov; 128(5):999–1010.

[24] Kawaii S, Tomono Y, Katase E, et al. Antiproliferative activity of flavonoids on several cancer cell lines. Biosci Biotechnol Biochem 1999 May; 63(5):896–9.

[25] Markaverich BM, Gregory RR, Alejandro M, et al. Methyl p-hydroxyphenyllactate and nuclear type II binding sites in malignant cells: Metabolic fate and mammary tumor growth. Cancer Res 1990 Mar 1; 50(5):1470–8.

[26] Caltagirone S, Rossi C, Poggi A, et al. Flavonoids apigenin and quercetin inhibit melanoma growth and metastatic potential. Int J Cancer 2000 Aug 15; 87(4):595–600.

[27] Yoshida M, Sakai T, Hosokawa N, et al. The effect of quercetin on cell cycle progression and growth of human gastric cancer cells. FEBS Lett 1990 Jan 15; 260(1):10–3.

[28] Larocca LM, Teofili L, Leone G, et al. Antiproliferative activity of quercetin on normal bone marrow and leukaemic progenitors. Br J Haematol 1991 Dec; 79(4):562–6.

[29] Kandaswami C, Perkins E, Soloniuk DS, et al. Antiproliferative effects of citrus flavonoids on a human squamous cell carcinoma in vitro. Cancer Lett 1991 Feb; 56(2):147–52.

[30] Huang YT, Hwang JJ, Lee PP, et al. Effects of luteolin and quercetin, inhibitors of tyrosine kinase, on cell growth and metastasis-associated properties in A431 cells overexpressing epidermal growth factor receptor. Br J Pharmacol 1999 Nov; 128(5):999–1010.

[31] Csokay B, Prajda N, Weber G, Olah E. Molecular mechanisms in the antiproliferative action of quercetin. Life Sci 1997; 60(24):2157–63.

[32] Menon LG, Kuttan R, Kuttan G. Inhibition of lung metastasis in mice induced by B16F10 melanoma cells by polyphenolic compounds. Cancer Lett 1995 Aug 16; 95(1–2):221–5.

[33] Molnar J, Beladi I, Domonkos K, et al. Antitumor activity of flavonoids on NK/Ly ascites tumor cells. Neoplasma 1981; 28(1):11–8.

[34] Castillo MH, Perkins E, Campbell JH, et al. The effects of the bioflavonoid quercetin on squamous cell carcinoma of head and neck origin. Am J Surg 1989 Oct; 158(4):351–5.

[35] Ferry DR, Smith A, Malkhandi J, et al. Phase I clinical trial of the flavonoid quercetin: Pharmacokinetics and evidence for in vivo tyrosine kinase inhibition. Clin Cancer Res 1996 Apr; 2(4):659–68.

[36] Kaufman PB, Duke JA, Brielmann H, et al. A comparative survey of leguminous plants as sources of the isoflavones, genistein and daidzein: Implications for human nutrition and health. J Altern Complement Med 1997 Spring; 3(1):7–12.

[37] Zand RS, Jenkins DJ, Diamandis EP. Steroid hormone activity of flavonoids and related compounds. Breast Cancer Res Treat 2000 Jul; 62(1):35–49.

[38] Duncan AM, Underhill KE, Xu X, et al. Modest hormonal effects of soy isoflavones in postmenopausal women. J Clin Endocrinol Metab 1999 Oct; 84(10):3479–84.

[39] Duncan AM, Merz BE, Xu X, et al. Soy isoflavones exert modest hormonal effects in premenopausal women. J Clin Endocrinol Metab 1999 Jan; 84(1):192–7.

[40] Nagata C, Takatsuka N, Inaba S, et al. Effect of soymilk consumption on serum estrogen concentrations in premenopausal Japanese women. J Natl Cancer Inst 1998 Dec 2; 90(23):1830–5.

[41] Petrakis NL, Barnes S, King EB, et al. Stimulatory influence of soy protein isolate on breast secretion in pre- and postmenopausal women. Cancer Epidemiol Biomarkers Prev 1996 Oct; 5(10):785–94.

[42] Bingham SA, Atkinson C, Liggins J, et al. Phyto-oestrogens: Where are we now? Br J Nutrition 1998; 79:393–406.

[43] Hargreaves DF, Potten CS, Harding C, et al. Two-week dietary soy supplementation has an estrogenic effect on normal premenopausal breast. J Clin Endocrinol Metab 1999 Nov; 84(11):4017–24.

[44] Wu AH, Ziegler RG, Nomura AM, et al. Soy intake and risk of breast cancer in Asians and Asian Americans. Am J Clin Nutr 1998 Dec; 68(6 Suppl):1437S–1443S.

[45] Fournier DB, Erdman JW, Gordon GB. Soy, its components, and cancer prevention: A review of the in vitro, animal, and human data. Cancer Epidemiol Biomarkers Prev 1998 Nov; 7(11):1055–65.

[46] Messina M, Barnes S. The role of soy products in reducing risk of cancer. Journal of the National Cancer Institute 1991; 83(8):541–6.

[47] Lamartiniere CA, Zhang JX, Cotroneo MS. Genistein studies in rats: Potential for breast cancer prevention and reproductive and developmental toxicity. Am J Clin Nutr 1998 Dec; 68(6 Suppl):1400S–1405S.

[48] Fritz WA, Coward L, Wang J, Lamartiniere CA. Dietary genistein: Perinatal mammary cancer prevention, bioavailability and toxicity testing in the rat. Carcinogenesis 1998 Dec; 19(12):2151–8.

[49] Lamartiniere CA. Protection against breast cancer with genistein: A component of soy. Am J Clin Nutr 2000 Jun; 71(6 Suppl):1705S-7S; discussion 1708S-9S.

[50] Stahl S, Chun TY, Gray WG. Phytoestrogens act as estrogen agonists in an estrogen-responsive pituitary cell line. Toxicol Appl Pharmacol 1998 Sep; 152(1):41–8.

[51] Wang C, Kurzer MS. Phytoestrogen concentration determines effects on DNA synthesis in human breast cancer cells. Nutr Cancer 1997; 28(3):236–47.

[52] Le Bail JC, Varnat F, Nicolas JC, Habrioux G. Estrogenic and antiproliferative activities on MCF-7 human breast cancer cells by flavonoids. Cancer Lett 1998 Aug 14; 130(1–2):209–16.

[53] Wang C, Kurzer MS. Effects of phytoestrogens on DNA synthesis in MCF-7 cells in the presence of estradiol or growth factors. Nutr Cancer 1998; 31(2):90–100.

[54] Fioravanti L, Cappelletti V, Miodini P, et al. Genistein in the control of breast cancer cell growth: Insights into the mechanism of action in vitro. Cancer Lett 1998 Aug 14; 130(1–2):143–52.

[55] Miodini P, Fioravanti L, Di Fronzo G, Cappelletti V. The two phyto-oestrogens genistein and quercetin exert different effects on oestrogen receptor function. Br J Cancer 1999 Jun; 80(8):1150–5.

[56] Zava DT, Duwe G. Estrogenic and antiproliferative properties of genistein and other flavonoids in human breast cancer cells in vitro. Nutr Cancer 1997; 27(1):31–40.

[57] Liu XH, Upadhyaya P, El-Bayoumy K, et al. The effect of dietary soy on human breast cancer metastasis in nude mice. Adv Exp Biol Med 1996; 401:283–4.

[58] Shao ZM, Wu J, Shen ZZ, Barsky SH. Genistein exerts multiple suppressive effects on human breast carcinoma cells. Cancer Res 1998 Nov 1; 58(21):4851–7.

[59] Markaverich BM. Personal communication. 2000.

[60] Piantelli M, Rinelli A, Macri E, Maggiano N, et al. Type II estrogen binding sites and antiproliferative activity of quercetin in human meningiomas. Cancer 1993; 71(1):193–8.

[61] Maybruck WM, Markaverich BM. Partial purification and characterization of methyl-p-hydroxyphenyllactate esterase in rat uterine cytosol. Steroids 1997; 62:321–330.

[62] Markaverich BM, Gregory RR. Preliminary assessment of luteolin as an affinity ligand for type II estrogen-binding sites in rat uterine nuclear extracts. Steroids 1993; 58:268–274.

[63] Larocca LM, Giustacchini M, Maggiano N, Ranelletti FO, et al. Growth-inhibitory effect of quercetin and presence of type II

estrogen binding sites in primary human transitional cell carcinomas. J Urol 1994; 152(3):1029–33.

[64] Scambia G, Ranelletti FO, Benedetti PP, Piantelli M, et al. Quercetin inhibits the growth of a multidrug-resistant estrogen-receptor-negative MCF-7 human breast-cancer cell line expressing type II estrogen-binding sites. Cancer Chemother Pharmacol 1991; 28(4):255–8.

[65] Scambia G, Ranelletti FO, Panici PB, et al. Inhibitory effect of quercetin on OVCA 433 cells and presence of type II oestrogen binding sites in primary ovarian tumours and cultured cells. Br J Cancer 1990 Dec; 62(6):942–946.

[66] Scambia G, Ranelletti FO, Panici PB, Piantelli M, et al. Quercetin induces type-II estrogen-binding sites in estrogen-receptor-negative (MDA-MB231) and estrogen-receptor-positive (MCF-7) human breast-cancer cell lines. Int J Cancer 1993; 54(3):462–6.

[67] Ranelletti FO, Ricci R, Larocca LM, Maggiano N, et al. Growth-inhibitory effect of quercetin and presence of type-II estrogen-binding sites in human colon-cancer cell lines and primary colorectal tumors. Int J Cancer 1992; 50(3):486–92.

[68] Larocca LM, Teofili L, Leone G, Sica S, et al. Antiproliferative activity of quercetin on normal bone marrow and leukaemic progenitors. Br J Haematol 1991; 79(4):562–6.

[69] Markaverich BM, Roberts RR, Alejandro MA, et al. Bioflavonoid interaction with rat uterine type II binding sites and cell growth inhibition. J Steroid Biochem 1988; 30:71–78.

[70] Rice-Evans CA, Miller NJ, Bolwell PG, et al. The relative antioxidant activities of plant-derived polyphenolic flavonoids. Free Radic Res 1995 Apr; 22(4):375–83.

[71] Schwitters B, Masquelier J. OPC in practice: Bioflavinoids and their application. Rome, Italy: Alfa Omega Publishers, 1993, pp. 28–35.

[72] Bagchi D, Garg A, Krohn RL, et al. Oxygen free radical scavenging abilities of vitamins C and E, and a grape seed proanthocyanidin extract in vitro. Res Commun Mol Pathol Pharmacol 1997 Feb; 95(2):179–89.

[73] Miller NJ, Rice-Evans CA. Antioxidant activity of resveratrol in red wine. Clin Chem 1995; 41(12):1789.

[74] Nagao M, Morita N, Yahagi T, et al. Mutagenicities of 61 flavonoids and 11 related compounds. Environ Mutagen 1981; 3(4):401–19.

[75] Kuo ML, Lee KC, Lin JK. Genotoxicities of nitropyrenes and their modulation by apigenin, tannic acid, ellagic acid and indole-3-carbinol in the Salmonella and CHO systems. Mutat Res 1992 Nov 16; 270(2):87–95.

[76] Birt DF, Walker B, Tibbels MG, Bresnick E. Anti-mutagenesis and anti-promotion by apigenin, robinetin and indole-3-carbinol. Carcinogenesis 1986 Jun; 7(6):959–63.

[77] Heo MY, Yu KS, Kim KH, et al. Anticlastogenic effect of flavonoids against mutagen-induced micronuclei in mice. Mutat Res 1992 Dec 16; 284(2):243–9.

[78] Wall ME, Wani MC, Hughes TJ, Taylor H. Plant antimutagens. Basic Life Sci 1990; 52:61–78.

[79] Rahman A, Shahabuddin, Hadi SM, et al. Strand scision in DNA induced by quercetin and Cu(II): Role of Cu(I) and oxygen free radicals. Carcinogenesis 1989; 10(10):1833–1839.

[80] Ahmad MS, Fazal F, Rahman A, et al. Activities of flavonoids for the cleavage of DNA in the presence of Cu(II): Correlation with generation of active oxygen species. Carcinogenesis 1992; 13(4):605–608.

[81] Shoskes DA, Zeitlin SI, Shahed A, Rajfer J. Quercetin in men with category III chronic prostatitis: A preliminary prospective, double-blind, placebo-controlled trial. Urology 1999 Dec; 54(6):960–3.

[82] Huang YT, Kuo ML, Liu JY, et al. Inhibitions of protein kinase C and proto-oncogene expressions in NIH 3T3 cells by apigenin. Eur J Cancer 1996 Jan; 32A(1):146–51.

[83] Hayashi A, Gillen AC, Lott JR. Effects of daily oral administration of quercetin chalcone and modified citrus pectin. Altern Med Rev 2000 Dec; 5(6):546–552.

[84] Adlercreutz H, Markkanen H, Watanabe S. Plasma concentrations of phyto-oestrogens in Japanese men. Lancet 1993 Nov 13; 342(8881):1209–10.

[85] Barnes S. Effect of genistein on in vitro and in vivo models of cancer. J Nutr 1995 Mar; 125(3 Suppl):777S-783S.

[86] Hawrylewicz EJ, Zapata JJ, Blair WH. Soy and experimental cancer: Animal studies. J Nutr 1995; 125:698S-708S.

[87] Messina MJ, Persky V, Barnes S, Setchell KD. Soy intake and cancer risk: A review of the in vitro and in vivo data. Nutr Cancer 1994; 21:113–131.

[88] Hawrylewicz EJ, Zapata JJ, Blair WH. Soy and experimental cancer: Animal studies. J Nutr 1995 Mar; 125(3 Suppl):698S-708S.

[89] Yan L, Yee JA, McGuire MH, Graef GL. Effect of dietary supplementation of soybeans on experimental metastasis of melanoma cells in mice. Nutrition and Cancer 1997; 29(1):1–6.

[90] Landstrom M, Zhang JX, Hallmans G, et al. Inhibitory effects of soy and rye diets on the development of Dunning R3327 prostate adenocarcinoma in rats. Prostate 1998 Aug 1; 36(3):151–61.

[91] Aronson WJ, Tymchuk CN, Elashoff RM, et al. Decreased growth of human prostate LNCaP tumors in SCID mice fed a low-fat, soy protein diet with isoflavones. Nutr Cancer 1999; 35(2):130–6.

[92] Li D, Yee JA, McGuire MH, et al. Soybean isoflavones reduce experimental metastasis in mice. J Nutr 1999 May; 129(5):1075–8.

[93] Menon LG, Kuttan R, Nair MG, et al. Effect of isoflavones genistein and daidzein in the inhibition of lung metastasis in mice induced by B16F-10 melanoma cells. Nutr Cancer 1998; 30(1):74–77.

[94] Joseph IB, Isaacs JT. Macrophage role in the anti-prostate cancer response to one class of antiangiogenic agents. J Natl Cancer Inst 1998 Nov 4; 90(21):1648–53.

[95] Zhou JR, Mukherjee P, Gugger ET, et al. Inhibition of murine bladder tumorigenesis by soy isoflavones via alterations in the cell cycle, apoptosis, and angiogenesis. Cancer Res 1998 Nov 15; 58(22):5231–8.

[96] Schleicher RL, Lamartiniere CA, Zheng M, Zhang M. The inhibitory effect of genistein on the growth and metastasis of a transplantable rat accessory sex gland carcinoma. Cancer Lett 1999 Mar 1; 136(2):195–201.

[97] Kakeji Y, Teicher BA. Preclinical studies of the combination of angiogenic inhibitors with cytotoxic agents. Invest New Drugs 1997; 15(1):39–48.

[98] Teicher BA, Holden SA, Ara G, et al. Comparison of several antiangiogenic regimens alone and with cytotoxic therapies in the Lewis lung carcinoma. Cancer Chemother Pharmacol 1996; 38(2):169–77.

[99] Jing Y, Nakaya K, Han R. Differentiation of promyeloctic leukemia cells HL-60 induced by daidzen in vitro and in vivo. Anticancer Res 1993; 13(4):1049–54.

[100] Hollman PCH, van Trijp JMP, Buysman MCNP. Relative bioavailability of the antioxidant flavonoid quercetin from various foods in man. FEBS Letters 1997; 418:152–156.

[101] Lu LJ, Lin SN, Grady JJ, et al. Altered kinetics and extent of urinary daidzein and genistein excretion in women during chronic soya exposure. Nutr Cancer 1996; 26(3):289–302.

[102] Lu LJ, Grady JJ, Marshall MV, et al. Altered time course of urinary daidzein and genistein excretion during chronic soya diet in healthy male subjects. Nutr Cancer 1995; 24(3):311–23.

[103] Xu X, Harris KS, Wang HJ, et al. Bioavailability of soybean isoflavones depends upon gut microflora in women. J Nutr 1995 Sep; 125(9):2307–15.

[104] Lu LJ, Anderson KE. Sex and long-term soy diets affect the metabolism and excretion of soy isoflavones in humans. Am J Clin Nutr 1998 Dec; 68(6 Suppl):1500S-1504S.

[105] Ishikawa M, Oikawa T, Hosokawa M, Hamada J, et al. Enhancing effect of quercetin on 3-methylcholanthrene carcinogenesis in C57B1/6 mice. Neoplasma 1985; 32(4):435–41.

[106] Pereira MA, Grubbs CJ, Barnes LH, et al. Effects of the phytochemicals, curcumin and quercetin, upon azoxymethane-induced colon cancer and 7,12-dimethylbenz[a]anthracene-induced mammary cancer in rats. Carcinogenesis 1996 Jun; 17(6):1305–11.

[107] Barotto NN, Lopez CB, Eynard AR, et al. Quercetin enhances pretumorous lesions in the NMU model of rat pancreatic carcinogenesis. Cancer Lett 1998 Jul 3; 129(1):1–6.

[108] Dunnick JK, Hailey JR. Toxicity and carcinogenicity studies of quercetin, a natural component of foods. Fundam Appl Toxicol 1992; 19(3):423–31.

[109] Ito N, Hagiwara A, Tamano S, Kagawa M, et al. Lack of carcinogenicity of quercetin in F344/DuCrj rats. Jpn J Cancer Res 1989; 80(4):317–25.

[110] Morino K, Matsukara N, Kawachi T, Ohgaki H, et al. Carcinogenicity test of quercetin and rutin in golden hamsters by oral administration. Carcinogenesis 1982; 3(1):93–7.

[111] Hirono I, Ueno I, Hosaka S, et al. Carcinogenicity examination of quercitin and rutin in ACI rats. Cancer Letters 1981; 13:15–21.

[112] Ito N. Is quercetin carcinogenic? Jpn J Cancer Res; Letter to the editor 1992; 83:312–14.

[113] Fujiki H, Takahiko H, Yamashita K, et al. Inhibition of tumor promotion by flavonoids. In *Plant flavonoids in biology and medicine II*. New York: Alan R. Liss, Inc., 1986, pp. 429–40.

[114] Verma AK, Johnson JA, Gould MN, et al. Inhibition of 7,12-dimethylbenz(a)antracene- and n-nitrosommethylurea-induced rat mammary cancer by dietary flavonol quercetin. Cancer Res 1988; 48:5754–58.

[115] Lyn-Cook BD, Rogers T, Yan Y, et al. Chemopreventive effects of tea extracts and various components on human pancreatic and prostate tumor cells in vitro. Nutr Cancer 1999; 35(1):80–6.

[116] Chung JY, Huang C, Meng X, et al. Inhibition of activator protein 1 activity and cell growth by purified green tea and black tea polyphenols in H-ras-transformed cells: Structure-activity relationship and mechanisms involved. Cancer Res 1999 Sep 15; 59(18):4610–7.

[117] Otsuka T, Ogo T, Eto T, et al. Growth inhibition of leukemic cells by (-)-epigallocatechin gallate, the main constituent of green tea. Life Sci 1998; 63(16):1397–403.

[118] Yang GY, Liao J, Kim K, et al. Inhibition of growth and induction of apoptosis in human cancer cell lines by tea polyphenols. Carcinogenesis 1998 Apr; 19(4):611–6.

[119] Kennedy DO, Nishimura S, Hasuma T, et al. Involvement of protein tyrosine phosphorylation in the effect of green tea polyphenols on Ehrlich ascites tumor cells in vitro. Chem Biol Interact 1998 Apr 3; 110(3):159–72.

[120] Sazuka M, Murakami S, Isemura M, et al. Inhibitory effects of green tea infusion on in vitro invasion and in vivo metastasis of mouse lung carcinoma cells. Cancer Lett 1995 Nov 27; 98(1):27–31.

[121] Taniguchi S, Fujiki H, Kobayashi H, et al. Effect of (-)-epigallocatechin gallate, the main constituent of green tea, on lung metastasis with mouse B16 melanoma cell lines. Cancer Letters 1992; 65:51–4.

[122] Oguni I, Nasu K, Yamamoto S, Nomura T. On the antitumor activity of fresh green tea leaf. Agric Biol Chem 1988; 52:1879–1880.

[123] Yan YS. Effect of Chinese tea extract on the immune function of mice bearing tumor and their antitumor activity. Chung Hua Yu Fang I Hsueh Tsa Chih 1992; 26(1):5–7.

[124] Cao Y, Cao R. Angiogenesis inhibited by drinking tea. Nature 1999 Apr 1; 398(6726):381.

[125] Liao S, Umekita Y, Guo J, et al. Growth inhibition and regression of human prostate and breast tumors in athymic mice by tea epigallocatechin gallate. Cancer Lett 1995 Sep 25; 96(2):239–43.

[126] Maiani G, Serafini M, Salucci M, et al. Application of a new high-performance liquid chromatographic method for measuring selected polyphenols in human plasma. J Chromatography B 1997; 692:311–317.

[127] Suganuma M, Okabe S, Kai Y, et al. Synergistic effects of (-)-epicatechin gallate with (-)-epicatechin, sulindac, or tamoxifen on cancer-preventive activity in the human lung cancer cell line PC-9. Cancer Res 1999; 59:44–7

[128] Katiyar SK, Agarwal R, Wang ZY, et al. (-)-Epigallocatechin-3-gallate in camellia sinensis leaves from himalayan region of sikkim: Inhibitory effects against biochemical events and tumor initiation in sencar mouse skin. Nutr Cancer 1992; 18(1):73–83.

[129] Katiyar SK, Agarwal R, Mukhtar H. Protective effects of green tea polyphenols administered by oral intubation against chemical carcinogen-induced forestomach and pulmonary neoplasia in A/J mice. Cancer Lett 1993; 73(2–3):167–72.

[130] Katiyar SK, Agarwal R, Mukhtar H. Inhibition of both stage I and stage II skin tumor promotion in SENCAR mice by a polyphenolic fraction isolated from green tea: Inhibition depends on the duration of polyphenol treatment. Carcinogenesis 1993; 14(12):2641–3.

[131] Katiyar SK, Agarwal R, Mukhtar H. Protection against malignant conversion of chemically induced benign skin papillomas to squamous cell carcinomas in SENCAR mice by a polyphenolic fraction isolated from green tea. Cancer Res 1993; 53(22):5409–12.

[132] Katiyar SK, Agarwal R, Mukhtar H. Inhibition of spontaneous and photo-enhanced lipid peroxidation in mouse epidermal microsomes by epicatechin derivatives from green tea. Cancer Lett 1994 Apr 29; 79(1):61–6.

[133] Tanaka T, Kojima T, Kawamori T, et al. Inhibition of 4-nitroquinoline-1-oxide-induced rat tongue carcinogenesis by the naturally occurring plant phenolics caffeic, ellagic, chlorogenic and ferulic acids. Carcinogenesis 1993; 14(7):1321–5.

[134] Luo D, Li Y. Preventive effect of green tea on MNNG-induced lung cancers and precancerous lesions in LACA mice. Hua Hsi I Ko Ta Hsueh Hsueh Pao 1992; 23(4):433–7.

[135] Heur YH, Zeng W, Stoner GD, et al. Synthesis of ellagic acid O-alkyl derivatives and isolation of ellagic acid as a tetrahexanoyl derivative from Fragaria ananassa. J Nat Prod 1992; 55(10):1402–7.

[136] Agarwal R, Katiyar SK, Zaidi SI, et al. Inhibition of skin tumor promoter-caused induction of epidermal ornithine decarboxylase in sencar mice by polyphenolic fraction isolated from green tea and its individual epicatechin derivatives. Cancer Res 1992; 52(13):3582–8.

[137] Fujita Y, Yamane T, Tanaka M, et al. Inhibitory effect of (-)-epigallocatechin gallate on carcinogenesis with N-ethyl-N'-nitro-N-nitroguanidine in moude duodenum. Jpn J Cancer Res 1989; 80(6):503–5.

[138] Agarwal R, Mukhtar H. Cancer chemoprevention by polyphenols in green tea and artichoke. Adv Exp Med Biol 1996; 401:35–50.

[139] Qin G, Gopalan-Kriczky P, Su J, et al. Inhibition of aflatoxin B1-induced initiation of hepatocarcinogenesis in the rat by green tea. Cancer Lett 1997 Jan 30; 112(2):149–54.

[140] Narisawa T, Fukaura Y. A very low dose of green tea polyphenols in drinking water prevents N-methyl-N-nitrosourea-induced colon carcinogenesis in F344 rats. Jpn J Cancer Res 1993 Oct; 84(10):1007–9.

[141] Wang ZY, Hong JY, Huang MT, et al. Inhibition of N-nitrosodiethylamine- and 4-(methylnitrosamino)-1-(3-pyridyl)-1-butanone-induced tumorigenesis in A/J mice by green tea and black tea. Cancer Res 1992 Apr 1; 52(7):1943–7.

[142] Wang ZY, Huang MT, Lou YR, et al. Inhibitory effects of black tea, green tea, decaffeinated black tea, and decaffeinated green tea on ultraviolet B light-induced skin carcinogenesis in 7,12-dimethylbenz[a]anthracene-initiated SKH-1 mice. Cancer Res 1994 Jul 1; 54(13):3428–35.

[143] Katiyar SK, Agarwal R, Zaim MT, Mukhtar H. Protection against N-nitrosodiethylamine and benzo[a]pyrene-induced forestomach and lung tumorigenesis in A/J mice by green tea. Carcinogenesis 1993 May; 14(5):849–55.

[144] Wang ZY, Huang MT, Ferraro T, et al. Inhibitory effect of green tea in the drinking water on tumorigenesis by ultraviolet light and 12-O-tetradecanoylphorbol-13-acetate in the skin of SKH-1 mice. Cancer Res 1992 Mar 1; 52(5):1162–70.

[145] Hu G, Han C, Chen J. Inhibition of oncogene expression by green tea and (-)-epigallocatechin gallate in mice. Nutr Cancer 1995; 24(2):203–9.

[146] Ji BT, Chow WH, Hsing AW, et al. Green tea consumption and the risk of pancreatic and colorectal cancers. Int J Cancer 1997 Jan 27; 70(3):255–8.

[147] Kohlmeier L, Weterings KG, Steck S, Kok FJ. Tea and cancer prevention: An evaluation of the epidemiologic literature. Nutr Cancer 1997; 27(1):1–13.

[148] Blot WJ, Chow WH, McLaughlin JK. Tea and cancer: A review of the epidemiological evidence. Eur J Cancer Prev 1996 Dec; 5(6):425–38.

[149] Kuroda Y, Hara Y. Antimutagenic and anticarcinogenic activity of tea polyphenols. Mutat Res 1999 Jan; 436(1):69–97.

[150] Nakachi K, Suemasu K, Suga K, et al. Influence of drinking green tea on breast cancer malignancy among Japanese patients. Jpn J Cancer Res 1998 Mar; 89(3):254–61.

[151] NCI/DCPC. Clinical development plan: Tea extracts. Green tea polyphenols. Epigallocatechin gallate. J Cell Biochem Suppl 1996; 26:236–57.

[152] Hirose M, Mizoguchi Y, Yaono M, et al. Effects of green tea catechins on the progression or late promotion stage of mammary gland carcinogenesis in female Sprague-Dawley rats pretreated with 7,12-dimethylbenz(a)anthracene. Cancer Lett 1997 Jan 30; 112(2):141–7.

[153] Tanaka H, Hirose M, Kawabe M, et al. Post-initiation inhibitory effects of green tea catechins on 7,12-dimethylbenz[a]anthracene-induced mammary gland carcinogenesis in female Sprague-Dawley rats. Cancer Lett 1997 Jun 3; 116(1):47–52.

[154] Asano Y, Okamura S, Ogo T, et al. Effect of (-)-epigallocatechin gallate on leukemic blast cells from patients with acute myeloblastic leukemia. Life Sci 1997; 60(2):135–42.

[155] Hibasami H, Achiwa Y, Fujikawa T, Komiya T. Induction of programmed cell death (apoptosis) in human lymphoid leukemia cells by catechin compounds. Anticancer Res 1996 Jul–Aug; 16(4A):1943–6.

[156] Achiwa Y, Hibasami H, Katsuzaki H, et al. Inhibitory effects of Persimmon (Diospyros kaki) extract and related polyphenol compounds on growth of human lymphoid leukemia cells. Biosci Biotech Biochem 1997; 61(7):1099–1101.

[157] Okabe S, Suganuma M, Hayashi M, et al. Mechanisms of growth inhibition of human lung cancer cell line, PC-9, by tea polyphenols. Jpn J Cancer Res 1997 Jul; 88(7):639–43.

[158] Fujiki H, Suganuma M, Okabe S, et al. Cancer inhibition by green tea. Mutat Res 1998 Jun 18; 402(1–2):307–10.

[159] Isemura M, Suzuki Y, Satoh K, et al. Effects of catechins on the mouse lung carcinoma cell adhesion to the endothelial cells. Cell Biol Int 1993; 17(6):559–64.

[160] Komori A, Yatsunami J, Okabe S, et al. Anticarcinogenic activity of green tea polyphenols. Jpn J Clin Oncol 1993; 23(3):186–90.

[161] Valcic S, Timmermann BN, Alberts DS, et al. Inhibitory effect of six green tea catechins and caffeine on the growth of four selected human tumor cell lines. Anticancer Drugs 1996 Jun; 7(4):461–8.

[162] Khafif A, Schantz SP, Chou TC, et al. Quantitation of chemopreventive synergism between (-)-epigallocatechin-3-gallate and curcumin in normal, premalignant and malignant human oral epithelial cells. Carcinogenesis 1998 Mar; 19(3):419–24.

[163] Ahmad N, Feyes DK, Nieminen AL, et al. Green tea constituent epigallocatechin-3-gallate and induction of apoptosis and cell cycle arrest in human carcinoma cells. J Natl Cancer Inst 1997 Dec 17; 89(24):1881–6.

[164] Lea MA, Xiao Q, Sadhukhan AK, Cottle S, et al. Inhibitory effects of tea extracts and (-)-epigallocatechin gallate on DNA synthesis and proliferation of hepatoma and erythrleukemia cells. Cancer Letters 1993; 68:231–36.

[165] Paschka AG, Butler R, Young CYF. Induction of apoptosis in prostate cancer cell lines by the green tea component, (-)-epigallocatechin-3-gallate. Cancer Lett 1998 Aug 14; 130(1–2):1–7.

[166] Chen ZP, Schell JB, Ho CT, Chen KY. Green tea epigallocatechin gallate shows a pronounced growth inhibitory effect on cancerous cells but not on their normal counterparts. Cancer Lett 1998 Jul 17; 129(2):173–9.

[167] Sazuka M, Imazawa H, Shoji Y, et al. Inhibition of collagenases from mouse lung carcinoma cells by green tea catechins and black tea theaflavins. Biosci Biotechnol Biochem 1997 Sep; 61(9):1504–6.

[168] Matsuo N, Yamada K, Yamashita K, et al. Inhibitory effect of tea polyphenols on histamine and leukotriene B4 release from rat peritoneal exudate cells. In Vitro Cell Dev Biol Anim 1996 Jun; 32(6):340–4.

[169] Naasani I, Seimiya H, Tsuruo Y. Telomerase inhibition, telomere shortening, and senescence of cancer cells by tea catechins. Biochem Biophys Res Commun 1998 Aug 19; 249(2):391–6.

[170] Yang F, De Villiers WJS, McClain CJ, Varilek GW. Green tea polyphenols block endotoxin-induced tumor necrosis factor-production and lethality in a murine model. J Nutr 1998 Dec; 128(12):2334–40.

[171] Yang CS, Chen L, Lee MJ, et al. Blood and urine levels of tea catechins after ingestion of different amounts of green tea by human volunteers. Cancer Epidemiol Biomarkers Prev 1998 Apr; 7(4):351–4.

[172] Nakagawa K, Okuda S, Miyazawa T. Dose-dependent incorporation of tea catechins, (-)-epigallocatechin-3-gallate and (-)-epigallocatechin, into human plasma. Biosci Biotechnol Biochem 1997 Dec; 61(12):1981–5.

[173] Kamei H, Kojima T, Hasegawa M, et al. Suppression of tumor cell growth by anthocyanins in vitro. Cancer Invest 1995; 13(6):590–4.

[174] Koide T, Kamei H, Hashimoto Y, et al. Antitumor effect of hydrolyzed anthocyanin from grape rinds and red rice. Cancer Biother Radiopharm 1996 Aug; 11(4):273–7.

[175] Kamei H, Hashimoto Y, Koide T, et al. Anti-tumor effect of methanol extracts from red and white wines. Cancer Biother Radiopharm 1998 Dec; 13(6):447–52.

[176] Koide T, Hashimoto Y, Kamei H, et al. Antitumor effect of anthocyanin fractions extracted from red soybeans and red beans in vitro and in vivo. Cancer Biother Radiopharm 1997 Aug; 12(4):277–80.

[177] Koide T, Kamei H, Hashimoto Y, et al. Influence of flavonoids on cell cycle phase as analyzed by flow-cytometry. Cancer Biother Radiopharm 1997 Apr; 12(2):111–5.

[178] Kamei H, Kojima T, Koide T, et al. Influence of OH group and sugar bonded to flavonoids on flavonoid-mediated suppression of tumor growth in vitro. Cancer Biother Radiopharm 1996 Aug; 11(4):247–9.

[179] Kamei H, Koide T, Kojimam T, et al. Flavonoid-mediated tumor growth suppression demonstrated by in vivo study. Cancer Biother Radiopharm 1996 Jun; 11(3):193–6.

[180] Ye X, Krohn RL, Liu W, et al. The cytotoxic effects of a novel IH636 grape seed proanthocyanidin extract on cultured human cancer cells. Mol Cell Biochem 1999 Jun; 196(1–2):99–108.

[181] Tamagawa K, Fukushima S, Kobori M, et al. Proanthocyanidins from barley bran potentiate retinoic acid-induced granulocytic and sodium butyrate-induced monocytic differentiation of HL60 cells. Biosci Biotechnol Biochem 1998 Aug; 62(8):1483–7.

[182] Huynh HT, Teel RW. Selective induction of apoptosis in human mammary cancer cells (MCF-7) by pycnogenol. Anticancer Res 2000 Jul–Aug; 20(4):2417–20.

[183] Agarwal C, Sharma Y, Zhao J, Agarwal R. A polyphenolic fraction from grape seeds causes irreversible growth inhibition of breast carcinoma MDA-MB468 cells by inhibiting mitogen-activated protein kinases activation and inducing G1 arrest and differentiation. Clin Cancer Res 2000 Jul; 6(7):2921–30.

[184] Agarwal C, Sharma Y, Agarwal R. Anticarcinogenic effect of a polyphenolic fraction isolated from grape seeds in human prostate carcinoma DU145 cells: Modulation of mitogenic signaling and cell-cycle regulators and induction of G1 arrest and apoptosis. Mol Carcinog 2000 Jul; 28(3):129–38.

[185] Lueng AY, Foster S. Encyclopedia of common natural ingredients. New York: John Wiley & Sons, 1996, p. 84.

[186] Murray MT. The healing power of herbs. Rocklin, CA: Prima Publishing, 1992, pp. 50–59.

[187] Pizzorno J, Murray M. Vaccinium myrtillus. In *A textbook of natural medicine*. Seattle, John Bastyr College Publications, 1987.

[188] Lietti A, Cristoni A, Picci M. Studies on Vaccinium myrtillus anthocyanosides. II. Aspects of anthocyanins pharmacokinetics in the rat. Arzneimittelforschung 1976; 26(5):832–5.

[189] Lietti A, Cristoni A, Picci M. Studies on Vaccinium myrtillus anthocyanosides. I. Vasoprotective and antiinflammatory activity. Arzneimittelforschung 1976; 26(5):829–32.

[190] Detre Z, Jellinek H, Miskulin M, Robert AM. Studies on vascular permeability in hypertension: Action of anthocyanosides. Clin Physiol Biochem 1986; 4(2):143–9.

[191] Kamei H, Kojima T, Hasegawa M, et al. Suppression of tumor cell growth by anthocyanins in vitro. Cancer Investigation 1995; 13(6):590–594.

[192] Tsuda T, Horio F, Osawa T. Absorption and metabolism of cyanidin 3-O-beta-D-glucoside in rats. FEBS Lett 1999 Apr 23; 449(2–3):179–82.

[193] Lee IR, Yang MY. Phenolic compounds from Duchesnea chrysantha and their cytotoxic activities in human cancer cell. Arch Pharm Res 1994; 17(6):476–479.

[194] Boulton DW, Walle UK, Walle T. Fate of the flavonoid quercetin in human cell lines: Chemical instability and metabolism. J Pharm Pharm 1999; 51:353–359.

[195] Tanaka T, Kojima T, Kawamori T, et al. Chemoprevention of diethylnitrosamine-induced hepatocarcinogenesis by a simple phenolic acid protocatechuic acid in rats. Cancer Res 1993; 53(12):2775–9.

[196] Ye X, Krohn RL, Liu W, et al. The cytotoxic effects of a novel IH636 grape seed proanthocyanidin extract on cultured human cancer cells. Mol Cell Biochem 1999 Jun; 196(1–2):99–108.

In this chapter we continue our discussions of phenolic compounds by examining several nonflavonoids: CAPE (from propolis), curcumin, lignans (from *Arctium* seed and flaxseed), the stilbene resveratrol, and the quinones emodin and hypericin. As with the flavonoids, questions remain regarding the metabolism and pharmacokinetics of these phenolics in vivo, as well as their in-vivo antitumor effects. Still, the in-vitro and limited in-vivo studies available suggest that most could play a role in cancer treatment, especially if used in synergistic combinations. For flaxseed and hypericin, however, the uncertainties are particularly strong, and they require more study than others. The structures of all compounds discussed here are illustrated in Figures A.41 to A.58 of Appendix A.

CAPE AND PROPOLIS

Summary of Research and Conclusions

At least 11 in-vitro studies have reported that propolis extract and/or CAPE inhibited proliferation of a variety of cancer cell lines.[1-5] In many cases, inhibition was more pronounced on cancer cells than normal cells. For cancer cells, the effective concentrations were generally between 1 and 35 µM (for CAPE itself). In addition to the in-vitro studies, propolis also produced antitumor effects in one animal study.[6]

Although relatively few in-vitro and in-vivo studies have been conducted on propolis or CAPE, the results look promising. In addition, the ability of propolis and CAPE to inhibit inflammation in animals also suggests they produce biological effects in vivo and could inhibit tumor progression. The metabolism and pharmacokinetics of CAPE are still uncertain, however. Based on the limited information available, there are inconsistencies between the dose found effective in animal studies and the dose estimated from in-vitro and pharmacokinetic data; because of these the required target dose can only be estimated within a large range. Nonetheless, even in a worst-case scenario (a target dose in the high end of this range), propolis could still be effective at the maximum safe human dose, with the benefits of synergism.

Introduction

Caffeic acid phenethyl ester (CAPE) is an active component of bee propolis. Propolis also contains several other related compounds that are cytotoxic to cancer

cells. For this reason, the most clinically useful source of CAPE is likely to be a propolis extract standardized for CAPE and containing additional caffeic acid esters. Crude propolis itself is not an ideal source because the concentration of CAPE in propolis can vary greatly. Such a standardized extract is not yet available commercially, however, and so crude propolis is discussed here as a source of CAPE. Aside from CAPE and related caffeic acid esters, propolis also has a number of flavonoids present at a total concentration of 10 to 30 percent or more.[7] In 15 different samples the most abundant flavonoid was apigenin (about 5 percent).[8] While apigenin may be useful in cancer treatment (see Chapter 19), we focus on CAPE and related compounds here.

Propolis, or "bee glue," is a complex resinous mixture gathered from plants and used by honeybees as a general-purpose sealer and antibiotic in their hives. In North and South America, Europe, and western Asia the dominant source for propolis is the bud exudate of the poplar tree (*Populus sp.*), although other species are frequently used.[8, 9] The name *propolis* comes from the Greek *pro* (for) and *polis* (city), referring to its function in the construction of hives.

Propolis has a long history of use in the herbal medicine traditions of many cultures and currently is utilized in dermatological products to treat burns, wounds, leg ulcers, herpes simplex, sprains, and other conditions, and in dentistry as an anesthetic and in toothpaste and mouthwash preparations. It is also marketed in tablets and capsules for internal use. Studies have reported that propolis extracts exhibit antibacterial, antiviral, antifungal, liver protective, anti-inflammatory, and other properties.[10-16]

CAPE and related caffeic acid esters are present in propolis at a total concentration of about 19 percent. In propolis, the major ester is caffeic acid benzyl ester, which accounts for about 14 percent of the ester fraction.[7] CAPE concentrations in propolis can vary greatly depending on the source of the propolis; it is commonly present at 1 to 5 percent, but some propolis samples appear to contain none.[17, 18]

The oral dose recommended by manufacturers of propolis products is generally from 200 milligrams to 3 grams per day. Animal studies suggest this range may be effective for inhibiting some types of inflammation. For example, oral administration of 100 to 150 mg/kg decreased acute and chronic inflammation in rats.[19] The equivalent human dose is about 1.6 to 2.4 grams per

TABLE 20.1 POTENTIAL ANTICANCER ACTIONS OF CAPE

ACTIVITY	KNOWN EFFECTS	AS AN ANTIOXIDANT, MAY:	AS A PTK INHIBITOR, MAY:	AS A PKC INHIBITOR, MAY:	AS AN EICOSANOID INHIBITOR, MAY:
Chapter 2: Mutations, Gene Expression, and Proliferation					
Act as an antioxidant	x	—			
Chapter 3: Results of Therapy at the Cellular Level					
Induce differentiation	x				
Induce apoptosis	x		x		x
Chapter 4: Growth Factors and Signal Transduction					
Inhibit PTK	x		—		
Inhibit PKC	x			—	
Chapter 5: Transcription Factors and Redox Signaling					
Support p53 function		x			
Inhibit NF-κB activity	weak	x	x	x	x
Inhibit AP-1 activity			x		
Chapter 6: Cell-to-Cell Communication					
Affect CAMs			x	x	x
Improve gap junction communication	x				
Chapters 7 and 8: Angiogenesis					
Inhibit angiogenesis		x	x	x	x
Inhibit histamine effects			x	x	
Inhibit eicosanoid effects	x		x		—
Inhibit TNF effects		x	x	x	
Inhibit VEGF effects		x	x	x	x
Inhibit insulin resistance				x	
Chapters 9 and 10: Invasion and Metastasis					
Inhibit invasion				x	
Inhibit hyaluronidase, beta-glucuronidase, or elastase					x
Inhibit collagenase effects		x		x	x
Inhibit GAG synthesis			x		
Inhibit cell migration			x	x	
Inhibit metastasis				x	
Inhibit platelet aggregation			x		
Chapters 11 and 12: Immune System					
Stimulate the immune system	x				
Inhibit tumor-induced immunosuppression			x		

day. Oral administration of 100 mg/kg per day decreased vascular permeability in mice.[19] The equivalent human dose is about 960 milligrams per day. Oral administration (about 650 mg/kg) of an aqueous propolis extract markedly reduced the inflammatory response in rats treated with radiation.[20] The equivalent human dose is about 11 grams daily.

In-vitro and In-vivo Anticancer Effects

Both propolis and CAPE inhibit cancer cell proliferation in vitro. In one study, crude extracts of propolis were cytotoxic to transformed mouse fibroblast cells. Proliferation was completely inhibited at about 220 μM, while CAPE alone was roughly six times more potent (90 percent inhibition at 35 μM).[21, a] In another study, the IC_{50} of a propolis extract against human nasopharyngeal and cervical cancer cells was about 13 to 33 μM.[2] CAPE alone inhibited a large number of rodent and human cell lines; the IC_{50} for most was 1 to 35 μM.[3–5, 21–24] The effects of CAPE seem to be specific to cancer cells. For example, it was selectively toxic to transformed fibroblast and melanocyte cells as compared to normal cells.[21]

At least one animal antitumor study has been conducted. In this study, intraperitoneal administration of an ethanol extract made from roughly 60 mg/kg of propolis markedly increased the survival of mice injected with Ehrlich carcinoma cells.[6] The equivalent human oral dose is about 1.3 grams per day of propolis.

CAPE may also have some cancer preventive effects. An oral dose of about 180 mg/kg inhibited tumor formation in mice genetically prone to cancer.[25] The equivalent human dose is about 1.7 grams. In addition, out of 25 natural compounds tested for cancer preventive activity, CAPE and genistein were the most effective in a series of in-vitro tests.[26]

---

[a] *This 220 μM value assumes that the average molecular weight of the active caffeic acid derivatives is about 300 grams/mole.*

The cytotoxic effects of CAPE may actually come from its metabolite, caffeic acid, which is also found in high quantity in a number of plants, including artichokes. Caffeic acid itself was not effective at inhibiting proliferation of various cell lines in vitro, probably because it is poorly transported across the cell membrane; however, esterification of caffeic acid with a lipophilic alcohol (i.e., CAPE) facilitates its uptake. Once inside the cell, CAPE may be hydrolyzed to caffeic acid, where it subsequently reduces cell proliferation.[21] In addition, although caffeic acid is not particularly cytotoxic, it can sensitize cancer cells to chemotherapy drugs and possibly natural cytotoxic compounds. Caffeic acid (at 10 μM) increased the sensitivity of human breast cancer cells to doxorubicin in vitro, and importantly, this effect was particularly pronounced in multi-drug-resistant cancer cell variants.[27]

Besides CAPE, other caffeic acid esters in propolis may have biological effects. Intraperitoneal administration of 10 mg/kg per day of methyl caffeate inhibited growth of injected sarcoma cells in mice by 21 percent.[28] In addition, oral administration of 45 mg/kg of methyl caffeate decreased chemically induced PTK membrane activity in the colon and liver of rats, as well as chemically induced leukotriene production in the liver of rats.[29] Another caffeic acid derivative, phenylethyl dimethylcaffeate (PEDMC), was more potent than CAPE in inhibiting proliferation of human colon cancer cells in vitro (IC_{50}s of 36 μM and 55 μM, respectively). PEDMC also decreased PTK activity in these cells.[30]

The potential anticancer actions of CAPE are listed in Table 20.1. In addition to these, at least one in-vitro study reported that the cytotoxic effects of CAPE were due to a prooxidant effect.[23] As discussed in Chapter 15, many antioxidant compounds can produce prooxidant effects in vitro but antioxidant effects in vivo.

Estimated Therapeutic and LOAEL Doses of Propolis

The estimated required dose of propolis scaled from animal antitumor studies is not in close agreement with that calculated from pharmacokinetic and in-vitro data. This discrepancy suggests an uncertain target human dose that can be estimated only within a large range. The required dose scaled from an animal antitumor ex-

TABLE 20.2 ESTIMATED THERAPEUTIC AND LOAEL DOSES FOR PROPOLIS*

DESCRIPTION	DOSE (g/day)
Required dose as scaled from an animal antitumor study	1.3
Required dose as scaled from animal anti-inflammatory study	0.96 to 11
Required cytotoxic dose as determined from pharmacokinetic calculations	72
Target dose based on range from animal antitumor studies and pharmacokinetic calculations	1.3 to 72
Minimum required antitumor dose assuming 15-fold synergistic benefits	0.087 to 4.8
Commonly prescribed human dose in noncancerous conditions	0.2 to 3
Estimated LOAEL dose	15
Tentative dose recommendation for further research	**3 to 15**
Minimum degree of synergism required	**uncertain**

* See Appendix J for details.

periment is about 1.3 grams daily, similar to the 0.96 to 11 grams scaled from animal anti-inflammatory experiments. The dose based on pharmacokinetic calculations is much higher, however. Using a target in-vivo concentration of 15 μM (30 μM after adjustment for conjugates), the required propolis dose is about 72 grams per day. The reasons for this large difference are not clear, but a number of questions exist regarding the metabolism and pharmacokinetics of CAPE and other active propolis compounds. It seems likely, however, that the 72-gram dose is overestimated. Lacking additional data, we can only estimate that the target human dose is between 1.3 and 72 grams per day. Since the target dose is uncertain, it is also unclear whether synergistic interactions will be required to produce an anticancer effect in humans. At the low end of this target range, synergism would not be needed, but it would be at the high end. The commonly prescribed human dose in noncancerous conditions is from 200 milligrams to 3 grams per day; the LOAEL dose is higher at about 15 grams per day (see Appendix J).

The therapeutic dose estimates of propolis are summarized in Table 20.2; the tentative dose recommendation is given as 3 to 15 grams per day. The 3-gram value is based on the high end of the commonly prescribed dose range, while the 15-gram value is based on the estimated LOAEL dose.

Although the target dose is uncertain, even in a worst-case scenario an anticancer effect may still be possible within the recommended dose range with the benefits of

TABLE 20.3   INHIBITION OF TUMOR CELLS BY CURCUMIN IN VITRO

CELL LINE	EFFECT
Breast cancer cells	Curcumin (at 3 µM) inhibited the proliferation of 7 different human breast cancer cell lines by 74% or more. These included multi-drug-resistant, TNF-resistant, estrogen-dependent, and estrogen-independent cell lines. Normal cells were relatively resistant to curcumin treatment.[31] Other studies on drug-resistant human breast cancer cells reported that normal cells are 3.5-fold less sensitive than cancer cells to curcumin treatment.[32]
Leukemia cells	IC$_{50}$ = about 20 µM for human chronic myeloid leukemia cells.[33]
Leukemia cells	Curcumin (at 6 to 50 µM) inhibited proliferation in 5 leukemia cell lines, but also inhibited proliferation in 3 normal lines.[34]
Leukemia and lymphoma cells	Curcumin caused 100 percent cell death in normal and leukemic lymphocytes at 22 µM, and in lymphoma cells at 11 µM.[47]
Ehrlich ascites and lymphoma cells	Curcumin inhibited the proliferation of Ehrlich ascites cells and mouse lymphoma cells at IC$_{50}$s of 27 and 16 µM.[42]
Oral cancer cells	IC$_{50}$ = 5.2 µM in human oral cancer cells.[38]

synergism. Consider a scenario where the target dose is 72 grams and the LOAEL dose is 15 grams. The full 15-fold allowable increase in potency due to synergism would lower the target dose to 4.8 grams, which is below the LOAEL dose. Thus a 15-gram dose could well produce an anticancer effect, even in the extreme case. (A 4.8-fold increase in potency would be required, which is similar to that for other direct-acting compounds, as listed in Table 13.1.)

Propolis can cause allergic dermatitis after topical contact in sensitive individuals, and oral administration may sensitize a person to this. Accordingly, it is contraindicated in persons with known allergies to bee products. There is also some concern about potential carcinogenic effects of caffeic acid, a metabolite of CAPE. The propolis doses considered here, however, are unlikely to produce such an effect (see Appendix J).

CURCUMIN

Summary of Research and Conclusions

Some 19 in-vitro studies have reported that curcumin inhibited proliferation of a variety of cancer cell lines.[35–39] In most cases, the active concentration was between 3 and 50 µM. Several of these also found that curcumin could decrease invasion and angiogenesis of cancer cells. In three animal antitumor studies, curcumin increased the life span of rodents with transplanted tumors, inhibited tumor growth, or inhibited metasta-

sis.[40, 41, 42] One human study reported that topical application of a curcumin ointment provided symptomatic relief for patients with external cancerous lesions.[43]

Other animal studies suggested that curcumin could reduce side effects or increase the antitumor action of some chemotherapy drugs (see Chapter 23). Lastly, a number of other animal studies indicated that curcumin has cancer preventive effects.[44, 45, 46]

Although relatively few animal or human antitumor studies have been conducted on curcumin, those that have look promising. In addition, curcumin's ability to decrease inflammation in animals also suggests it has biological effects in vivo and could inhibit tumor progression. As with its relatives caffeic acid and CAPE, however, the pharmacokinetics and metabolism of curcumin are poorly understood. Based on the limited information available, there are inconsistencies between the doses effective in animal studies and those estimated from in-vitro and pharmacokinetic studies. Due to the inconsistencies, the required target dose can be estimated only within a large range. Nevertheless, even considering a target dose in the high end of this range, with synergism curcumin could still be effective at the maximum safe human dose.

Introduction

Curcumin (from *Curcuma longa*) is the orange-yellow pigment that gives the spice turmeric its unique color. *Curcuma*, a perennial herb of the ginger family, is widely cultivated in tropical areas. Turmeric is the major component of curry powder and has been safely used for centuries as a spice; the curcumin content of turmeric is 1 to 5 percent.[47, 48, 49] *Curcuma* extracts are also used medicinally in both Chinese and Indian herbal medicine.

Curcumin has a number of biological effects. It is a potent antioxidant, stronger than vitamin E in preventing lipid peroxidation in vitro.[50, 51] It increases bile flow in dogs and rats and lowers plasma cholesterol levels in rats.[52, 55] Its ability to increase bile flow is reminiscent of caffeic acid, to which it has some structural similarities.

Curcumin also produces anti-inflammatory effects in vivo after oral administration. Approximately 50 and 100 mg/kg reduced acute inflammation by 50 percent in rats and mice, respectively, and acute inflammation in rats was decreased by an intraperitoneal dose of 2.1 mg/kg.[53] The human equivalent of a 100-mg/kg dose in mice is about 960 milligrams and the human oral equivalent of the intraperitoneal dose is about 230 milligrams. Chronic inflammation was reduced by 20 to 30 percent in rats after an oral dose of 160 mg/kg; the equivalent human dose is about 2.6 grams. In the acute inflammation tests, curcumin's effect was comparable to that of phenylbutazone, an anti-inflammatory drug.[54, 55] Human studies also reported an anti-inflammatory effect; oral administration of 1.2 grams daily produced a greater anti-inflammatory response than placebo in patients with postoperative inflammation.[56]

Curcumin also retains its antioxidant effects after oral administration; 74 mg/kg protected rats against free radical damage induced by whole body irradiation.[57] Curcumin at 200 mg/kg reduced inflammation and lipid peroxidation and increased antioxidant defense mechanisms in the lung tissue of rats treated with the chemotherapy agent cyclophosphamide.[58] The equivalent human dose is about 3.2 grams. Similar effects were observed in the lung tissue of bleomycin-treated rats after oral doses of 200 mg/kg of curcumin.[59] Furthermore, 200 mg/kg given orally reduced lipid peroxidation and protected against chemically induced myocardial infarction in rats.[60]

In-vitro and In-vivo Anticancer Studies

Curcumin's potential as a cancer preventive agent is supported by several studies.[61, 62] In addition to prevention, it may also be useful in cancer treatment. Many studies have noted that it decreased proliferation of cancer cells in vitro. Selected studies are summarized in Table 20.3; the IC_{50} for these typically ranged from 3 to 50 μM. Curcumin may inhibit cancer progression through a number of mechanisms, listed in Table 20.4.

A small number of animal antitumor studies have been conducted. In two of them, oral administration of 74 mg/kg on alternate days decreased lung metastasis of melanoma cells injected into mice and increased mouse

TABLE 20.4 POTENTIAL ANTICANCER ACTIONS OF CURCUMIN

ACTIVITY	KNOWN EFFECTS	AS AN ANTIOXIDANT, MAY:	AS A PTK INHIBITOR, MAY:	AS A PKC INHIBITOR, MAY:	AS A NF-κB INHIBITOR, MAY:	AS AN EICOSANOID INHIBITOR, MAY:	AS A COLLAGENASE INHIBITOR, MAY:
Chapter 2: Mutations, Gene Expression, and Proliferation							
Act as an antioxidant	x	—					
Chapter 3: Results of Therapy at the Cellular Level							
Induce apoptosis	x		x		x		
Increase TGF-beta	x						
Chapter 4: Growth Factors and Signal Transduction							
Inhibit PTK	x	—					
Inhibit PKC	x			—			
Chapter 5: Transcription Factors and Redox Signaling							
Support p53 function	x	x					
Inhibit NF-κB activity	x	x	x	x	—	x	
Inhibit AP-1 activity	x	x					
Chapter 6: Cell-to-Cell Communication							
Affect CAMs			x	x	x	x	
Chapters 7 and 8: Angiogenesis							
Inhibit angiogenesis		x	x	x	x	x	x
Inhibit bFGF effects							x
Inhibit histamine effects			x	x	x		
Inhibit eicosanoid effects	x		x		x	—	
Inhibit TNF effects		x	x	x	x		
Inhibit VEGF effects	x	x	x	x		x	
Inhibit insulin resistance				x			
Chapters 9 and 10: Invasion and Metastasis							
Inhibit invasion					x		x
Inhibit hyaluronidase, beta-glucuronidase, or elastase						x	
Inhibit collagenase effects	x	x			x	x	—
Inhibit GAG synthesis			x				
Inhibit cell migration			x	x			
Inhibit metastasis					x		x
Inhibit platelet aggregation	x	x					
Chapters 11 and 12: Immune System							
Inhibit tumor-induced immunosuppression			x				

TABLE 20.5 ESTIMATED THERAPEUTIC AND LOAEL DOSES FOR CURCUMIN*

DESCRIPTION	DOSE (g/day)
Required dose as scaled from animal antitumor studies	0.36 to 3.2
Required dose as scaled from animal anti-inflammatory studies	0.23 to 3.2
Required cytotoxic dose as determined from pharmacokinetic calculations	8.7
Target dose based on range from animal antitumor studies and pharmacokinetic calculations	0.36 to 8.7
Minimum required antitumor dose assuming 15-fold synergistic benefits	0.024 to 0.58
Commonly prescribed human dose in noncancerous conditions	0.75 to 1.5
Estimated LOAEL dose	greater than 43
Tentative dose recommendation for further research	**1.5 to 1.8†**
Minimum degree of synergism required	**uncertain**

* See Appendix J for details.

† Upper value based on the general linear bioavailability limit of 1.8 grams per day.

life span.[40, 41] The equivalent human dose is about 360 milligrams per day. Intraperitoneal administration of 50 mg/kg reduced tumor volume and increased the life span of mice injected with Ehrlich ascites cancer cells by 50 percent.[42] The equivalent human oral dose is about 3.2 grams daily. Curcumin has also demonstrated some antitumor activity in conjunction with cisplatin. Twenty-eight mg/kg per day given orally with cisplatin reduced the progression of fibrosarcoma in rats better than cisplatin alone.[63] The equivalent human dose is about 450 milligrams per day.

Estimated Therapeutic and LOAEL Doses of Curcumin

The estimated required dose of curcumin scaled from animal antitumor studies is different than the estimated dose as calculated from pharmacokinetic and in-vitro data, thus the target human dose is still uncertain and can be estimated only within a large range. The required dose as scaled from animal antitumor experiments is 360 milligrams to 3.2 grams per day; similar doses were effective in animal anti-inflammatory experiments. The anticancer dose based on pharmacokinetic calculations is larger. Using a target in-vivo concentration of 15 μM (30 μM after adjustment for conjugates), the required curcumin dose is about 8.7 grams daily. The reasons for this large difference are not clear, and lacking additional data, we can only estimate a target human dose of between 360 milligrams and 8.7 grams per day.

Curcumin is a very safe compound, the LOAEL dose likely being greater than 43 grams per day (see Appendix J). The commonly prescribed human dose in noncancerous conditions is 750 milligrams to 1.5 grams per day.

Therapeutic dose estimates for curcumin are summarized in Table 20.5; the tentative dose recommendation is 1.5 to 1.8 grams daily. The 1.5-gram value is based on the high end of the commonly prescribed dose range, while the 1.8-gram value is the general linear bioavailability limit (see Appendix J). Higher doses up to the estimated LOAEL dose could be used, but they may not be fully absorbed or produce metabolites similar to those generated by lower doses.

In looking at a worst-case scenario, even though the target dose is uncertain an anticancer effect may still be possible within the recommended dose range. Consider a target dose of 8.7 grams and a maximum allowable dose of 1.8 grams. The full 15-fold allowable increase in potency from synergism would lower the target dose to 580 milligrams, well below the 1.8-gram dose. Thus, the latter could produce an anticancer effect. A 4.8-fold increase in potency would be required, which is similar to that needed for other direct-acting compounds (see Table 13.1).

LIGNANS

Lignans are widely distributed in the plant kingdom, with several hundred lignan compounds isolated in about 70 different families.[64] Lignans may produce a number of medicinal effects. For example, many appear to have liver-protective properties, including silybin from milk thistle (*Silybum marianum*) and schizandrin from *Schizandra chinensis*, both of which are used in herbal medicine. Some lignans have caused cytotoxic effects in cancer cells, an example being podophyllotoxin, obtained from the mayapple plant (*Podophyllum peltatum*). In fact, the FDA has approved its semisynthetic derivatives teniposide and etoposide as anticancer drugs. In this section, we focus on two lignan-containing plants, *Arctium lappa* (burdock), which is used in Chinese herbal medicine, and flaxseed, which is used as a food and a bulking agent for treating constipation. *Arctium* seed contains the plant lignan arctigenin, and flaxseed contains secoisolariciresinol (SECO), a precursor for the production of mammalian lignans in vivo. See Appendix J for dose information on silybin from milk thistle, which also may have some anticancer properties.

Arctium Seed

Summary of Research and Conclusions

Relatively few in-vitro and no rodent or human studies have been conducted on *Arctium* seed or its lignan arctigenin. Six in-vitro studies reported that arctigenin induced differentiation in or inhibited the proliferation of various cancer cell lines.[65–69] In addition, cytotoxic effects against two cancer cell lines have been observed by our research group.[70] Since few studies have been done, the discussions on *Arctium* seed are necessarily brief; this does not mean it should be discounted, however. For one thing, results from in-vitro studies have been promising. In some studies, arctigenin was active at relatively low concentrations and was more potent than many other lignans tested. For another, lignans in general appear promising for cancer treatment. One advantage arctigenin has over other lignans is that its pharmacokinetic characteristics are relatively favorable, which should make it effective at oral doses lower than those needed for other lignans. In addition, arctigenin occurs in relatively high concentrations in *Arctium* seed, and the seed has a long history of safe use in Chinese herbal medicine.

Discussion

The seed of *Arctium lappa* is widely used in Chinese herbal medicine to treat colds, sore throats, coughs, and other conditions, usually in combination with other herbs. It contains a number of lignans, including arctigenin and its glycoside arctiin.

As discussed in Appendix D (Table D.1), arctigenin induced differentiation and inhibited proliferation of leukemia cells at concentrations less than 10 μM, and it was nontoxic to normal lymphocytes. In an additional study, arctigenin inhibited the proliferation of two human leukemia cell lines at IC_{50}s of 0.2 and 1.4 μM.[66] Arctigenin's cytotoxic effects are not limited to leukemia cell lines, however; in a study on five nonleukemic cancer cell lines, the average IC_{50} for arctigenin was 4.3 μM, and that for arctiin, its glycoside, was 8.9 μM.[65] In another study, the IC_{50} for human liver cancer cells was

TABLE 20.6 ESTIMATED THERAPEUTIC AND LOAEL DOSES FOR ARCTIGENIN AND *ARCTIUM* SEED[*]

DESCRIPTION	ARCTIGENIN DOSE (g/day)	*ARCTIUM* SEED DOSE (g/day)
Required cytotoxic dose as determined from pharmacokinetic calculations	1.4	27
Target dose based on pharmacokinetic calculations	1.4	27
Minimum required antitumor dose assuming 15-fold synergistic benefits	0.093	1.7
Commonly prescribed human dose in noncancerous conditions	0.5	9
Estimated LOAEL dose	0.65	12
Tentative dose recommendation for further research	**0.65**	**12**
Minimum degree of synergism required	2.3-fold potency increase	

* See Appendix J for details.

3.5 μM for arctigenin and 4.9 μM for arctiin.[67] In addition to producing cytotoxic effects and inducing differentiation, arctigenin has also regulated immune response in human lymphocytes in vitro, and it could act either as an immune stimulant (under some conditions) or as an inhibitor of TNF production.[71]

Estimated Therapeutic and LOAEL Doses of Arctigenin and Arctium Seed

Since animal antitumor data are lacking, the doses of arctigenin or *Arctium* seed needed to produce an anticancer effect can be estimated only by making calculations based on pharmacokinetic and in-vitro data. Therefore, the resulting estimates cannot be confirmed with an independent source of data. Using a target in-vivo concentration of 15 μM (30 μM after adjustment for conjugates), the required arctigenin dose is about 1.4 grams per day. The corresponding *Arctium* seed dose is about 27 grams per day. We will use these values as our target human doses. If animal studies were available, the doses scaled from them would likely be lower than the arctigenin dose of 1.4 grams, since for most natural compounds discussed the doses scaled from animal studies are lower than those based on pharmacokinetic and in-vitro data.

The commonly prescribed dose of *Arctium* seed for noncancerous conditions in Chinese herbal medicine is about 9 grams per day, which provides about 500 milligrams of arctigenin. The LOAEL dose for arctigenin is uncertain, but based on predictions for the LD_{50}, we will estimate it at 650 milligrams, or 12 grams of *Arctium* seed (see Appendix J); this is the tentative dose recommendation listed in Table 20.6.

It appears that synergistic interactions will be required for arctigenin to produce an anticancer effect in humans. In comparing the 27-gram target dose for *Arctium* seed to the 12-gram maximum dose, synergistic interactions will be needed to produce a minimum 2.3-fold increase in potency. This should be possible, since a 2.3-fold increase is well below the allowable 15-fold increase (see Chapter 13).

Flaxseed

Summary of Research and Conclusions

When ingested, the active flaxseed lignan SECO (secoisolariciresinol) and a variety of other plant lignans are acted on by gut bacteria to produce the mammalian lignans enterodiol and enterolactone, which then circulate in the plasma. Enterolactone appears to be more potent than enterodiol against cancer cells and it has been the subject of at least seven in-vitro studies.[66, 72–77] As a whole, these studies found that enterolactone inhibited proliferation of several cancer cells lines at concentrations of 10 to 50 µM.

Three animal antitumor studies and one review reported that flaxseed or SECO decreased metastasis of melanoma cells in mice and reduced the growth of chemically induced breast cancer at a late stage of carcinogenesis in mice.[78–81]

Like some of the flavonoids discussed in the previous chapter, enterolactone can act as a phytoestrogen in vitro; it has been reported to stimulate proliferation of estrogen-dependent cell lines at concentrations below about 10 µM and to inhibit proliferation at higher concentrations. Its estrogenic effect does not appear to be as great as that of genistein, and like some flavonoids it has antiestrogenic effects in the presence of estrogen. More work is needed to fully characterize its estrogenic potential, but for these reasons it does not seem that flaxseed would be contraindicated in patients with estrogen-dependent cancers, especially if used in combination with other anticancer compounds.

Although the few in-vitro and animal studies conducted on flaxseed look promising, questions remain about the pharmacokinetics and metabolism of enterolactone and enterodiol after flax administration. As discussed in Appendix J, there are inconsistencies between the flaxseed doses found effective in animal studies and the dose estimated from in-vitro and pharmacokinetic data, and so the required target dose of flaxseed can be estimated only within a large range. If the effective target dose is at the high end of this range, flaxseed would probably not be effective at the maximum safe human dose, even with synergism. For these reasons, a relatively large amount of study is needed before the required dose and clinical potential of flaxseed is understood (see Table 13.2), but it is discussed in detail since future studies may resolve the inconsistencies.

Introduction

Flaxseed, the seed of *Linum usitatissimum*, is widely used as food and as a bulking agent in treating constipation. It is also a rich source of dietary plant lignans. After ingestion, flaxseed lignans are metabolized by colonic bacteria to produce the two major mammalian lignans, enterodiol and enterolactone. In one human study, oral administration of 10 grams per day of flaxseed increased urinary excretion of enterodiol and enterolactone in women by about 18-fold and 9-fold, respectively.[82] These mammalian lignans are structurally similar to estrogens, and like isoflavones, they produce weak estrogenic or antiestrogenic activities, depending on estrogen availability. Their production may serve to protect women against breast cancer, presumably by competing with estrogen for estrogen-binding sites.[83] High urinary excretion of enterolactone has been associated with reduced risk of breast cancer in Australian women.[84] One study also observed that enterolactone competed for type II estrogen-binding sites (discussed in Chapter 19) in rat uterine tissues.[85]

Enterolactone may also produce an antiestrogenic effect by stimulating the production of sex hormone binding globulin (SHBG) in the liver.[85] In a study on 30 postmenopausal women taking flaxseed, higher levels of plasma SHBG were observed in women with high urinary excretion of diphenols, of the kind produced from flax lignans.[85] SHBG is a plasma protein that binds and transports sex hormones (estrogens and androgens); through its binding actions, it regulates the concentration of free sex hormones in the plasma. Sex hormone responsive cells exhibit receptors for SHBG. At least in estrogen-dependent human breast cancer cells, binding between estrogen, SHBG, and the SHBG receptor has caused an antiproliferative, antiestrogenic effect.[86] The flax lignan SECO also binds directly to SHBG and competes with sex hormones for binding sites. This action too may inhibit cell proliferation in some tissues.

In addition to these antiestrogenic mechanisms, flaxseed contains a high amount of fiber, which can increase estrogen excretion and SHBG levels.[87] Lastly, similar to flavonoids, enterolactone and enterodiol inhibit the enzyme aromatase, which is involved in estrogen synthesis.[88, 89]

The content of mammalian lignan precursors in flaxseed varies with plant variety and growing conditions.

The range of total mammalian lignan precursors in different flaxseed samples (measured after in-vitro fermentation of whole flaxseeds to produce enterodiol and enterolactone) varied from 0.03 to 0.1 percent, the average of these values being 0.052 percent. This average was roughly 29-fold greater than the lignan precursor content of lentils, which is the next richest source known.[90] The primary mammalian lignan precursor in flax is SECO, which is present in its diglycoside form (SD). The SECO content in flaxseed is about 0.1 percent, and the SD content is about 0.2 percent.[93]

TABLE 20.7 ESTIMATED THERAPEUTIC AND LOAEL DOSES FOR FLAXSEED*	
DESCRIPTION	**FLAXSEED DOSE (g/day)**
Required dose as scaled from animal antitumor studies	60
Required cytotoxic dose as determined from pharmacokinetic calculations	3,500
Target dose based on range from animal antitumor studies and pharmacokinetic calculations	60 to 3,500
Minimum required antitumor dose assuming 15-fold synergistic benefits	4 to 230
Commonly prescribed human dose in noncancerous conditions	10 to 30
Estimated LOAEL dose	greater than 60
Tentative dose recommendation for further research	**30 to 60**
Minimum degree of synergism required	**uncertain**

See Appendix J for details.

In-vitro and In-vivo Anticancer Studies

A small number of in-vitro studies have investigated the cytotoxic effects of enterodiol and enterodiol on cancer cells. In one study, enterolactone inhibited proliferation of human breast cancer cells by about 75 percent at 33 μM.[77] In another, enterolactone decreased proliferation of four human colon cancer cells lines at 50 to 100 μM, and it was more than twice as effective as enterodiol.[72] One other study reported that enterodiol was not effective against two human leukemia cell lines.[66] From these two studies, it would appear that enterolactone might be more potent than enterodiol in some situations. At least one in-vitro study reported that normal cells were not adversely affected by mammalian lignans; only high concentrations (about 330 μM) of enterolactone were cytotoxic to normal human lymphocytes.[91]

At lower concentrations, enterolactone stimulated proliferation of estrogen-dependent cancers, as seen in three studies on human breast cancer cells at concentrations below about 10 μM; above 10 to 20 μM, enterolactone inhibited cell proliferation.[73, 74, 76] It is uncertain if this stimulatory effect would appear in vivo, since one study reported that enterolactone, in the presence of estrogen, did not stimulate the proliferation of estrogen-dependent human breast cancer cells.[75] This is not unlike the effects of flavonoids discussed in Chapter 19, and it seems likely that the estrogenic effect of enterolactone and enterodiol is weaker than that of genistein. More research is needed, but it does not appear that flaxseed would be contraindicated in patients with estrogen-dependent cancers, especially if combined with other anticancer compounds.

Animal studies have reported that flaxseed can reduce cancer risk as well as the volume of established tumors. In one study, a 5 percent flaxseed diet given to rats decreased the number of breast tumors induced by a high fat diet and a carcinogen; urinary enterodiol and enterolactone excretion increased.[83] In another study, oral administration of SD at about 8 mg/kg (equivalent to a 5 percent flaxseed diet) inhibited growth of established breast cancer in rats during the late stages of carcinogenesis (greater than 50 percent reduction in tumor volume). This inhibitory effect correlated with the degree of urinary lignan excretion, indicating that flax lignans may have been partly responsible.[92, 93] A 5 percent flaxseed diet also reduced the lung metastasis of melanoma cells injected into mice, as well as tumor volumes.[94] In another study with melanoma cells, oral administration of SD also reduced the number of lung metastases in mice. Again, tumor volumes were decreased.[79] The 5 percent flaxseed diet used in these studies (3.8 g/kg in rats and 6 g/kg in mice) is roughly equivalent to a human flaxseed dose of 60 grams per day, which provides about 60 milligrams of SECO.

Estimated Therapeutic and LOAEL Doses of Flaxseed Lignans

The estimated required dose of flaxseed scaled from animal antitumor studies does not agree with the estimated dose calculated from pharmacokinetic and in-vitro data; therefore, the target human dose can be estimated only within a large range. The anticancer dose based on pharmacokinetic calculations is much higher than the one from animal studies. Using a target in-vivo concentration of 15 μM of mammalian lignans (30 μM after adjustment for conjugates), the required flaxseed dose is about 3,500 grams per day, which is far higher than 60 grams. Possible reasons for such a large difference are discussed in Appendix J. Lacking additional data, we estimate a target human dose between 60 and 3,500 grams per day.

The commonly prescribed flaxseed dose in noncancerous conditions is 10 to 30 grams per day, while the LOAEL dose is likely to be greater than 60 grams. In Table 20.7, the tentative dose recommendation is 30 to 60 grams, with the former value based on the high end of the commonly prescribed dose range and the latter on the estimated minimum LOAEL dose.

Because the target dose is uncertain, it is not clear whether synergistic interactions will be required to produce an anticancer effect in humans or if an anticancer effect could be produced even with synergism. In a worst-case scenario, where the target dose is 3,500 grams and the LOAEL dose is 60, the full 15-fold allowable increase in potency due to synergism would lower the target dose only to 230 grams, which is still above the LOAEL dose. Thus a dose of 60 grams may not produce an anticancer effect if the effective target dose is high.

Although the use of flaxseed is not recommended at this time due to uncertainties in the required dose and the possibility that even with synergism it may not be effective, dose details are still provided in the table. Because of the uncertainties, a beneficial effect cannot be ruled out. Moreover, the tentatively recommended dose would not be expected to cause harm.

A 60-gram flaxseed dose would contain about 12 grams per day of alpha-linolenic acid, which could be of some concern (see Chapter 17). Although alpha-linolenic acid is an omega-3 fatty acid, it is not reliably converted to EPA in vivo and may not be as effective as EPA. If the two fatty acids were administered together, alpha-linolenic acid might compete for cellular uptake and reduce the effectiveness of EPA. Therefore, if high doses of flaxseed are used, it may be prudent to use a defatted form. Alternatively, a semi-purified SECO or SD extract could be used.

Lastly, note that plant lignans other than those found in flaxseed may increase plasma enterolactone concentrations and inhibit tumor growth. For example, in a rat study, hydroxymatairesinol, a lignan from Norway spruce trees, was converted to enterodiol. At a dose of 240 milligrams (as scaled to humans) this lignan inhibited the growth of chemically induced breast cancer.[95] This lignan dose is higher than the 60-milligram dose of SECO in 60 grams of flaxseed. Not all lignans, however, can be expected to increase enterodiol plasma con-

centrations. For example, arctigenin belongs to a different family of lignans than SECO (dibenzyl butyrolactones versus dibenzyl butanes) and is not as likely to increase enterolactone concentrations.

STILBENES—RESVERATROL

Summary of Research and Conclusions

At least 18 in-vitro studies have reported that resveratrol produces cytotoxic effects against a variety of cancer cell lines.[96–100] In these studies, resveratrol was generally active at concentrations of 10 to 100 μM, with most studies showing activity at 10 to 30 μM. One review has also been published, as well as a number of studies on its cancer prevention effects.[101] In the one animal antitumor study conducted, resveratrol decreased the growth of ascites liver cancer cells transplanted into rats.[102]

Although the few in-vitro and in-vivo studies look promising, the pharmacokinetics and metabolism of resveratrol are uncertain. Based on the limited information available, there are inconsistencies between the dose found effective in the animal study and that calculated from in-vitro and pharmacokinetic data. Again, the required target dose can be estimated only within a large range. Even if the effective target dose were at the high end, however, resveratrol should still be effective at the maximum safe human dose with synergism.

Discussion

Stilbenes are related to flavonoids in their biosynthesis and are often referred to as stilbenoids for this reason. Unlike many of the other phenolics discussed in Chapters 19 and 20, they occur naturally in both their free and glycoside forms. The stilbene resveratrol is produced by plants in response to stress conditions. Its role in plant physiology is apparently to fight fungal infections; thus it is considered a phytoalexin, which is a class of antibiotics of plant origin. Other stilbenes besides resveratrol are also recognized phytoalexins.

Research on resveratrol was stimulated in 1992 when it was detected in wine and grapes. About 54 percent of the resveratrol in wine is in the aglycone form, and 46 percent occurs as piceid, its glycoside. The total resveratrol content in wine varies, but the average (including glycosides and isomers) is about 6.2 mg/L.[103, 104] Red wines tend to have much higher concentrations than white wines. Resveratrol is thought to be one of the compounds responsible for the decreased risk of cardiovascular disease seen in wine drinkers (the so-called French Paradox). It may do this by acting as an antioxidant and inhibiting platelet aggregation, both of which may also make it useful in cancer treatment. Resveratrol has also reduced inflammation and inhibited chemically induced carcinogenesis in rodents.[105, 109]

Resveratrol acts as a phytoestrogen in vitro at concentrations of 3 to 25 μM.[106, 107] As with other phytoestrogens discussed, at low concentrations it stimulated proliferation of estrogen-dependent breast cancer cells but inhibited them at higher ones. When estrogen was present, however, as it would be in vivo, stimulation did not occur. Moreover, some studies have indicated that its estrogenic effect is weaker than that of genistein. For example, one reported that resveratrol did not stimulate proliferation of estrogen-dependent pituitary cancer cells, whereas genistein did.[108] For these reasons, it does not seem that resveratrol is contraindicated in patients with estrogen-dependent cancers, especially if combined with other anticancer compounds, but more work is needed to fully understand its estrogenic potential.

The possible anticancer actions of resveratrol are listed in Table 20.8, and Table 20.9 summarizes some representative in-vitro studies that have been conducted. As shown in Table 20.9, most studies indicate that resveratrol is active in vitro at concentrations between about 10 and 30 μM.

In the one animal antitumor study completed, intraperitoneal administration of 1 mg/kg significantly reduced tumor growth in rats injected with ascites liver cancer cells. Resveratrol treatment did enhance tumor-induced cachexia even while decreasing tumor growth, but it is unclear whether the cachetic effect is limited to the rapid-growing, cachexia-inducing rat tumor used in the study. Healthy control mice showed no side effects of treatment.[109] The equivalent human oral dose is about 68 milligrams.

TABLE 20.8 POTENTIAL ANTICANCER ACTIONS OF RESVERATROL

ACTIVITY	KNOWN EFFECTS	AS AN ANTI-OXIDANT, MAY:	AS A PKC INHIBITOR, MAY:	AS A NF-κB INHIBITOR, MAY:	AS AN EICOSANOID INHIBITOR, MAY:	AS A HYALURONIDASE INHIBITOR, MAY:
Chapter 2: Mutations, Gene Expression, and Proliferation						
Act as an antioxidant	x	—				
Chapter 3: Results of Therapy at the Cellular Level						
Induce differentiation	x					
Induce apoptosis	x				x	
Increase TGF-beta	x					
Chapter 4: Growth Factors and Signal Transduction						
Inhibit PKC	variable					
Chapter 5: Transcription Factors and Redox Signaling						
Support p53 function		x				
Inhibit NF-κB activity	x	x	x	—	x	
Chapter 6: Cell-to-Cell Communication						
Affect CAMs	x		x	x	x	
Improve gap junction communication	x					
Chapters 7 and 8: Angiogenesis						
Inhibit angiogenesis		x	x	x	x	x
Inhibit bFGF effects						x
Inhibit histamine effects			x	x		
Inhibit eicosanoid effects	x			x	—	
Inhibit TNF effects		x	x	x		
Inhibit VEGF effects		x	x		x	
Inhibit insulin resistance		x				
Chapters 9 and 10: Invasion and Metastasis						
Inhibit invasion			x			x
Inhibit hyaluronidase, beta-glucuronidase, or elastase	x				x	—
Inhibit collagenase effects		x	x		x	
Inhibit cell migration			x			x
Inhibit metastasis			x			x
Inhibit platelet aggregation	x					

Estimated Therapeutic and LOAEL Doses of Resveratrol

The estimated required dose of resveratrol scaled from animal antitumor studies is not close to the estimated dose calculated from pharmacokinetic and in-vitro data, again suggesting that the target human dose can be estimated only within a large range. The required dose scaled from an animal antitumor experiment is about 68

TABLE 20.9   IN-VITRO CYTOTOXIC EFFECTS OF RESVERATROL

CELL LINE	COMMENT
Human breast cancer	Inhibited proliferation of estrogen-dependent and -independent cell lines at 22 to 175 µM.[110]
	Inhibited proliferation by 60% to 80% at 25 µM. Highly invasive breast cancer cells were inhibited more than less-invasive cells.[111]
Human leukemia	IC_{50} = 15 to 30 µM. Normal lymphocytes were not affected.[112]
	Complete inhibition of proliferation at 30 µM.[113]
	IC_{50} = about 20 µM.[96]
Human lung cancer	IC_{50} = about 10 µM.[114]
Human oral cancer	Cell proliferation was inhibited at 10 to 100 µM.[115]
Human prostate cancer	Proliferation of three different cell lines was inhibited at 25 µM.[98]
	Proliferation was inhibited and prostate-specific antigen (PSA) levels decreased at 25 µM.[116]

TABLE 20.10   ESTIMATED THERAPEUTIC AND LOAEL DOSES FOR RESVERATROL[*]

DESCRIPTION	DOSE (mg/day)
Required dose as scaled from an animal antitumor study	68
Required cytotoxic dose as determined from pharmacokinetic calculations	770
Target dose based on range from animal antitumor study and pharmacokinetic calculations	68 to 770
Minimum required antitumor dose assuming 15-fold synergistic benefits	4.5 to 51
Commonly prescribed human dose in noncancerous conditions	20
Estimated LOAEL dose	410
Tentative dose recommendation for further research	**68 to 410**
Minimum degree of synergism required	**uncertain**

[*] *See Appendix J for details.*

milligrams per day, and the one based on in-vitro and pharmacokinetic data is higher. Using a target in-vivo concentration of 15 µM (30 µM after adjustment for conjugates), the required resveratrol dose is about 770 milligrams per day. Without additional data, we estimate the target human dose at between 68 and 770 milligrams daily. Whether synergistic interactions would be needed to produce an anticancer effect in humans is not clear; at the low end of this range, synergism would not be needed, but it would be at the high end.

The commonly prescribed resveratrol dose in noncancerous conditions is about 20 milligrams per day. Based on LD_{50} predictions, the LOAEL dose is estimated to be about 410 milligrams per day, but this is a rough approximation; the high end of the tentative recommended range is based on this value (see Table 21.10). The low end, 68 milligrams, comes from the dose effective in the animal study.

Although the target dose is uncertain, even in a worst-case scenario an anticancer effect may still be possible within the recommended dose range, with the benefits of synergism. Given a target dose of 770 milligrams and a LOAEL dose of 410 milligrams, the full 15-fold allowable increase in potency due to synergism would lower the target dose to 51 milligrams, which is below the LOAEL dose. Thus, a 410-milligram dose could produce an anticancer effect. A 1.9-fold increase in potency would be necessary, which is similar to that required for other direct-acting compounds (see Table 13.1).

QUINONES

Quinones are a group of over 1,200 naturally occurring compounds. Many quinones have been reported to possess antibacterial and fungicidal properties. Quinone-rich plants have also been used as dyes (for example, henna), and as laxatives (rhubarb root, aloe resin, senna leaf, and *Cascara sagrada* bark). In this section, we discuss two anticancer quinones, emodin and hypericin.

Quinones are phenols that are comprised of a quinone nucleus conjugated to various oxidized aromatic structures. In the case of emodin, the aromatic structure is an anthracene group. Hence, emodin is known as an anthraquinone. Anthraquinones exist mainly as glycosides in nature and can join to form dimers (dianthrones). The aromatic structure of hypericin is a naphthodianthrone. Hypericin and emodin are closely related in that hypericin is biosynthetically derived from emodin. Structures for emodin, hypericin, the quinone nucleus, and other related compounds are illustrated in Figures A.53 to A.58 of Appendix A.

Emodin

Summary of Research and Conclusions

In 14 in-vitro studies, emodin inhibited proliferation of a variety of cancer cell lines, usually at concentrations of 2 to 76 μM, often below 40 μM.[117–121] Only three animal antitumor studies have been conducted; in these, emodin inhibited tumor growth and/or increased the survival of mice with transplanted leukemia, melanoma, and breast cancer cells.[122, 123, 124] In one, emodin acted synergistically with the chemotherapy drug Taxol, besides inhibiting tumor growth on its own. In-vitro studies have also reported synergistic effects with chemotherapy drugs (see Chapter 23).

Discussion

As mentioned, emodin is an anthraquinone. Other anthraquinone compounds have been approved by the FDA as anticancer drugs, including mitoxantrone and doxorubicin. Studies indicate that emodin has vasorelaxive, immunosuppressive, immunostimulatory, antibacterial, antitumor, anti-inflammatory, anti-ulcer, and hypolipidemic properties.[133–137]

Table 20.11 gives a few details on the in-vitro cytotoxicity of emodin. In some cases, the inhibitory effects of emodin may be selective to cancer cells, especially *ras*-transformed cells and *HER-2/neu*-overexpressing cells (common in breast cancer). As shown in the table, emodin is active in vitro at concentrations between 2 and 76 μM. Its potential anticancer actions are listed in Table 20.12.

Three animal antitumor studies have been published. Intraperitoneal administration of 40 mg/kg per day increased the survival time of leukemia-bearing mice by 47 percent.[122] The equivalent human oral dose is about 2.6 grams per day. Intraperitoneal administration of 40 mg/kg twice a week significantly reduced tumor growth and increased survival of mice with transplanted *HER-2/neu*-overexpressing human breast cancer cells.[123] The equivalent human oral dose is about 750 milligrams per day. Intraperitoneal administration of 5 mg/kg decreased melanoma growth in mice by 73 percent, and 75 mg/kg inhibited breast cancer in them by 45 percent.[124] Equivalent human oral doses are about 330 milligrams

TABLE 20.11 CYTOTOXICITY OF EMODIN	
CELL LINE	**IC$_{50}$ CONCENTRATION**
Ehrlich ascites cells	74 μM.[125]
Human cervical cancer cells	2 μM.[126]
Human breast cancer cells	5 to 40 μM.[118, 127]
Mouse breast cancer cells	4 to 37 μM.[120]
Human leukemia cells	19 μM.[128]
	49 μM.[129]
Human lung cancer cells	37 μM.[130]
Six different human cell lines	6 to 33 μM.[121]
54 nonhuman cell lines	4 to 68 μM; average is 23 μM.[132]
ras-transformed human bronchial epithelial cells	15 μM; normal human bronchial epithelial cells were inhibited only at high concentrations (370 μM).[131, 132]
Five *HER-2/neu* overexpressing human breast cancer cell lines	19 to 76 μM; normal cells were not affected.[132]

and 4.9 grams daily, respectively. The average of all these doses is 2.2 grams per day.

Herbs containing emodin have been used in cancer therapy in China. In one study, 67 patients with leukopenia who received radiotherapy also received crude extracts of *Polygonum cuspidatum* or its anthraquinones. Both agents significantly increased leukocyte counts.[138]

Estimated Therapeutic and LOAEL Doses of Emodin

The estimated required dose scaled from animal studies agrees with the required dose calculated from pharmacokinetic and in-vitro data, with the former at 330 milligrams to 4.9 grams per day (average of 2.2 grams per day) and the latter within this range. Using a target in-vivo concentration of 15 μM (30 μM after adjustment for conjugates), the required emodin dose is about 2.5 grams per day. We use the average of 2.2 and 2.5, or 2.4 grams per day, as a target human dose.

The commonly prescribed dose of emodin (as found in *Polygonum cuspidatum* extracts) in noncancerous conditions is about 20 milligrams. The LOAEL dose is estimated to be much larger, about 810 milligrams per day. Dose estimates are summarized in Table 20.13, with the tentative recommended range from 160 to 810 milligrams daily. The 160-milligram value assumes a full 15-fold increase in potency due to synergistic interactions, while the 810-milligram value is based on the estimated LOAEL dose.

It appears that synergistic interactions will be required for emodin to produce an anticancer effect in humans. In comparing the 2.4-gram target dose to the 810-milligram maximum dose, synergistic interactions will be needed to create about a 3-fold increase in potency.

TABLE 20.12   POTENTIAL ANTICANCER ACTIONS OF EMODIN

ACTIVITY	KNOWN EFFECTS	AS A PTK INHIBITOR, MAY:	AS A PKC INHIBITOR, MAY:	AS A COLLAGENASE INHIBITOR, MAY:
Chapter 3: Results of Therapy at the Cellular Level				
Induce differentiation	x			
Induce apoptosis		x		
Chapter 4: Growth Factors and Signal Transduction				
Inhibit PTK	x	—		
Inhibit PKC	x		—	
Chapter 5: Transcription Factors and Redox Signaling				
Inhibit NF-κB activity	weak	x	x	
Inhibit AP-1 activity		x		
Chapter 6: Cell-to-Cell Communication				
Affect CAMs		x	x	
Chapters 7 and 8: Angiogenesis				
Inhibit angiogenesis		x	x	x
Inhibit bFGF effects				x
Inhibit histamine effects		x	x	
Inhibit eicosanoid effects		x		
Inhibit TNF effects		x	x	
Inhibit VEGF effects		x	x	
Inhibit insulin resistance			x	
Chapters 9 and 10: Invasion and Metastasis				
Inhibit invasion			x	x
Inhibit collagenase effects	x		x	—
Inhibit GAG synthesis		x		
Inhibit cell migration		x	x	
Inhibit metastasis			x	x
Inhibit platelet aggregation	x	x		
Chapters 11 and 12: Immune System				
Inhibit tumor-induced immunosuppression		x		

This should be possible, since a 3-fold increase is well below the allowable 15-fold increase (see Chapter 13).

In some studies, emodin and other related anthraquinones were mutagenic in vitro.[120, 139, 140] The National Toxicology Program recently challenged the scientific community to predict the carcinogenicity potential of 30 chemicals currently under study in rodents, one of which was emodin. Most responses have predicted emodin will be carcinogenic.[139, 141, 142] On the other hand, several suggested that the evidence of carcinogenicity is weak and/or that its effects on DNA are secondary, rather than intrinsic to the chemical.[143, 144] Despite positive predictions and in-vitro tests then, some

investigators proposed it is unlikely to be of high risk in humans.[145] The mutagenic effect is diminished by the presence of plasma in vitro and is not seen at high oral doses (and at high plasma concentrations) in mice.[146, 147] The carcinogenicity of emodin-rich plant extracts must be further investigated, but at this point it seems improbable they will be carcinogenic, especially if used with other natural (antioxidant) compounds.

Note that other anthraquinones closely related to emodin have also shown antitumor activity. For example, aloe-emodin, found in *Aloe vera*, blocked proliferation of various cancer cell lines in-vitro at an IC_{50} of 1 to 13 µM. The effects were selective to cancer cells, since the IC_{50} for normal cells was much higher. An intraperitoneal dose of 50 mg/kg per day inhibited transplanted neuroectodermal cells in mice but not transplanted human colon cancer cells.[148] The equivalent human oral dose is about 3.3 grams per day, which is similar to the human dose scaled from animal antitumor studies for emodin (see Table 20.13).

Hypericin

Summary of Research and Conclusions

Approximately nine in-vitro studies have been conducted on the cytotoxic effects of hypericin against cancer cells.[149–153] In studies where it was effective, the concentration was generally under 25 µM.

Hypericin is a photoactive compound, and additional in-vitro studies have been done on the cytotoxic effects of photoactivated hypericin.[154, 155, 156] At least one review has been published, and at least three studies reported that photoactivated hypericin caused antitumor effects in animals.[157–160] Photoactivated hypericin has also been effective in human patients with skin cancer when injected intralesionally.[161] As a whole, these studies suggest that photoactivated hypericin is more potent and can affect a greater variety of cancer cell lines than nonphotoactivated hypericin.

There are inconsistencies between the doses that were effective in animal studies (for photoactivated hypericin) and the dose estimated from in-vitro and pharmacokinetic studies (for nonphotoactivated hypericin). Thus we can estimate the required target dose only within a large range. Moreover, for a target dose in the high end of this range, it is possible hypericin would not be effective at the maximum safe human dose, even with synergism. For these reasons, a relatively large amount of study is needed before the required dose and clinical potential of hypericin can be understood (see Table 13.2). We discuss it here because future studies may resolve the inconsistencies. It is also of interest since photoactivated hypericin, especially when used for superficial cancers, does hold some promise. In addition, an anticancer effect from orally administered nonphotoactivated hypericin cannot yet be ruled out.

Discussion

Hypericin seems most useful in its photoactivated form. In fact, most animal antitumor studies on hypericin used it in combination with laser light focused on the tumor. It effectively inhibits PTK and PKC activity and cancer cell proliferation in vitro, and exhibits other properties that could produce anticancer effects in vivo. Photoactivated hypericin appears to act via a prooxidant mechanism, causing oxidative damage to lipid membranes and proteins. In one in-vitro study, treatment with photoactivated hypericin killed mouse breast cancer cells and induced an antioxidant enzyme response.[162] Oxygen was necessary for the cytotoxic effect to occur. Nonphotoactivated hypericin may not be as useful; depending on the cell line, in-vitro cancer cell proliferation can be decreased or unaffected by hypericin under dark conditions.[163, 164]

Hypericin and its related compound pseudohypericin are derived from the plant St. John's wort (*Hypericum perforatum*); its extract has been used in humans to treat depression. It has also produced antiviral effects and improved wound healing, and it has been tested as anti-HIV agent because of its ability to block NF-κB activity.[157] Again, photoactivated hypericin is a more effective antiviral agent than the nonphotoactivated compound.

Hypericin inhibits proliferation of a number of cancer cell lines, with photoactivated hypericin being more potent. Cytotoxic studies on nonphotoactivated hypericin are listed in Table D.2 of Appendix D. Normal laboratory lighting could have been used in some of these studies, however, which may have affected results.

The potential anticancer actions of hypericin are listed in Table 20.14. Several animal studies have reported an antitumor effect from photoactivated hypericin. For example, in two mouse studies, the growth of transplanted human epidermoid carcinoma cells decreased after intraperitoneal doses of 2.5 to 20 mg/kg.[158, 165] The equivalent human oral dose is about 120 to 920 milligrams per day (average of 520 milligrams); we can assume the required dose of nonphotoactivated hypericin would be greater than this.

Estimated Therapeutic and LOAEL Doses of Hypericin

The estimated required dose of hypericin scaled from animal antitumor studies is not in close agreement with that calculated from pharmacokinetic and in-vitro data. This discrepancy implies the target human dose can be estimated only within a large range. The required dose scaled from animal antitumor experiments (on photoactivated hypericin) is about 520 milligrams per day (range of 120 to 920 milligrams), whereas the anticancer dose based on pharmacokinetic calculations is much lower. Using a target in-vivo concentration of 15 μM (30 μM after adjustment for conjugates), the required

TABLE 20.13   ESTIMATED THERAPEUTIC AND LOAEL DOSES FOR EMODIN*

DESCRIPTION	DOSE (g/day)
Required dose as scaled from animal antitumor studies	0.33 to 4.9 (average 2.2)
Required cytotoxic dose as determined from pharmacokinetic calculations	2.5
Target dose based on an average from animal antitumor studies and pharmacokinetic calculations	2.4
Minimum required antitumor dose assuming 15-fold synergistic benefits	0.16
Commonly prescribed human dose in noncancerous conditions	0.02
Estimated LOAEL dose	0.81
Tentative dose recommendation for further research	**0.16 to 0.81**
Minimum degree of synergism required	**3-fold potency increase**

See Appendix J for details.

TABLE 20.14 POTENTIAL ANTICANCER ACTIONS OF HYPERICIN					
ACTIVITY	KNOWN EFFECTS	AS A PTK INHIBITOR, MAY:	AS A PKC INHIBITOR, MAY:	AS A NF-κB INHIBITOR, MAY:	AS A COLLAGENASE INHIBITOR, MAY:
Chapter 3: Results of Therapy at the Cellular Level					
Induce apoptosis	x	x			
Chapter 4: Growth Factors and Signal Transduction					
Inhibit PTK	x	—			
Inhibit PKC	x		—		
Chapter 5: Transcription Factors and Redox Signaling					
Inhibit NF-κB activity	x	x	x	—	
Inhibit AP-1 activity		x			
Chapter 6: Cell-to-Cell Communication					
Affect CAMs		x	x	x	
Chapters 7 and 8: Angiogenesis					
Inhibit angiogenesis		x	x	x	x
Inhibit bFGF effects					x
Inhibit histamine effects		x	x	x	
Inhibit eicosanoid effects		x		x	
Inhibit TNF effects		x	x	x	
Inhibit VEGF effects		x	x		
Inhibit insulin resistance			x		
Chapters 9 and 10: Invasion and Metastasis					
Inhibit invasion			x		x
Inhibit collagenase effects	x		x		—
Inhibit GAG synthesis		x			
Inhibit cell migration	x	x	x		
Inhibit metastasis			x		x
Inhibit platelet aggregation		x			
Chapters 11 and 12: Immune System					
Inhibit tumor-induced immunosuppression		x			

dose (of nonphotoactivated hypericin) is about 130 milligrams daily. This relatively low dose is in conflict with the 520-milligram dose scaled from animal studies; we would expect the dose for photoactivated hypericin to be lower, not higher, than that of nonphotoactivated hypericin. Lacking additional data, we estimate a target human dose between 130 and 520 milligrams per day.

The commonly prescribed dose in noncancerous conditions is about 2.7 milligrams per day as contained in standardized *Hypericum* extracts. Commercial extracts are commonly standardized for 0.3 percent hypericin. The LOAEL dose is estimated to be 5.6 to 11 milligrams daily, with the primary adverse effect being photosensitivity (see Appendix J).

Dose calculations for hypericin are summarized in Table 20.15. The tentative recommended dose range is listed as 5.6 to 11 milligrams daily, based on the estimated LOAEL dose.

Whether synergistic interactions will be needed to produce an anticancer effect in humans, or if such effect could be produced even with synergism is uncertain. If the target dose is 520 milligrams and the LOAEL dose is 11 milligrams, the full 15-fold allowable increase in potency from synergism would lower the target dose to 35 milligrams, which is still above the LOAEL dose. Thus a dose of 11 milligrams may not produce an anticancer effect if the target dose is high.

Although the use of hypericin is not recommended at this time due to uncertainties in the required dose and the possibility that even with synergism hypericin may not be effective, dose details are still provided in the table. The tentatively recommended dose would not be expected to cause harm and because of the uncertainties, a beneficial effect cannot be ruled out.

CONCLUSION

Nonflavonoid phenolic compounds represent a diverse group of potential anticancer compounds that could inhibit cancer progression through several means. For many of these compounds, the metabolism and pharmacokinetics are uncertain in vivo, and doses scaled from animal studies and those calculated from pharmacokinetic and in-vitro data do not match. In most of these cases, the latter is higher, suggesting that other active metabolites might occur in the plasma that are not accounted for in the pharmacokinetic dose calculations. That discrepancies exist does not mean the compounds will not be useful; the dose calculations indicate that most could be effective with synergism. A few compounds, particularly flaxseed and hypericin, do not seem as promising as the

TABLE 20.15 ESTIMATED THERAPEUTIC AND LOAEL DOSES FOR HYPERICIN[*]	
DESCRIPTION	**DOSE (mg/day)**
Required dose as scaled from animal antitumor studies (photoactivated)	120 to 920 (average 520)
Required cytotoxic dose as determined from pharmacokinetic calculations (nonphotoactivated)	130
Target dose based on range from animal antitumor studies and pharmacokinetic calculations	130 to 520
Minimum required antitumor dose assuming 15-fold synergistic benefits	9 to 35
Commonly prescribed human dose in noncancerous conditions	2.7
Estimated LOAEL dose	5.6 to 11
Tentative dose recommendation for further research	**5.6 to 11**
Minimum degree of synergism required	**uncertain**

[*] *See Appendix J for details.*

others; based on preliminary data, they may not be effective when target doses are high, even with the benefits of synergism.

REFERENCES

[1] Grunberger D, Banerjee R, Eisinger K, et al. Preferential cytotoxicity on tumor cells by caffeic acid phenethyl ester isolated from propolis. Experientia 1988; 44:230–232.

[2] Hladon B, Bylka W, Ellnain-Wojtaszek M, et al. In-vitro studies on the cytostatic activiety of propolis extracts. Arzneimittel forschung 1980; 30(11):1847–8.

[3] Su ZZ, Lin J, Grunberger D, Fisher PB. Growth suppression and toxicity induced by caffeic acid phenethyl ester (CAPE) in type 5 adenovirus-transformed rat embryo cells correlate directly with transformation progression. Cancer Res 1994 Apr 1; 54(7):1865–70.

[4] Guarini L, Su ZZ, Zucker S, et al. Growth inhibition and modulation of antigenic phenotype in human melanoma and glioblastoma multiforme cells by caffeic acid phenethyl ester (CAPE). Cellular and Molecular Biology 1992; 38(5):513–527.

[5] Huang MT, Ma W, Yen P, et al. Inhibitory effects of caffeic acid phenethyl ester (CAPE) on 12-O-tetradecanoylphorbol-13-acetate-induced tumor promotion in mouse skin and the synthesis of DNA, RNA and protein in HeLa cells. Carcinogenesis 1996 Apr; 17(4):761–5.

[6] Scheller S, Krol W, Swiacik J, et al. Antitumoral property of ethanolic extract of propolis in mice-bearing Ehrlich carcinoma, as compared to bleomycin. Z Naturforsch [C] 1989 Nov–Dec; 44(11–12):1063–5.

[7] Greenaway W, Scaysbrook T, Whatley FR. The analysis of bud exudate of Populus euramericana, and of propolis, by gas chromatography-mass spectromety. Proc R. Soc Lond B 1987; 232:249–272.

[8] Serra Bonvehi J, Ventura Coll F. Phenolic composition of propolis from China and South America. Zeitschrift fuer naturforschung Section C Biosci 1994; 49(11–12):712–718.

[9] Markham KR, Mitchell KA, Wilkins AL, et al. HPLC and GC-MS identification of the major organic constituents in New Zealand propolis. Phytochemistry 1996; 42(1):205–211.

[10] Marcucci MC. Propolis: Chemical composition, biological properties and therapeutic activity. Apidologie 1995; 26:83–99.

[11] Dobrowolski JW, Vohora SB, Sharma K, et al. Antibacterial, antifungal, antiamoebic, antiinflammatory and antipyretic studies on propolis bee products. J Ethnopharmacol 1991 Oct; 35(1):77–82.

[12] Peluso G, De Feo V, De Simone F, et al. Studies on the inhibitory effects of caffeoylquinic acids on monocyte migration and superoxide ion production. J Nat Prod 1995 May; 58(5):639–46.

[13] Basnet P, Matsushige K, Hase K, et al. Potent antihepatotoxic activity of dicaffeoyl quinic acids from propolis. Biol Pharm Bull 1996 Apr; 19(4):655–7.

[14] Basnet P, Matsushige K, Hase K, et al. Four di-O-caffeoyl quinic acid derivatives from propolis. Potent hepatoprotective activity in experimental liver injury models. Biol Pharm Bull 1996 Nov; 19(11):1479–84.

[15] Amoros M, Simoes CM, Girre L, et al. Synergistic effect of flavones and flavonols against herpes simplex virus type 1 in cell culture. Comparison with the antiviral activity of propolis. J Nat Prod 1992 Dec; 55(12):1732–40.

[16] Burdock GA. Review of the biological properties and toxicity of bee propolis (propolis). Food and Chemical Toxicology 1998; 36(4):347–63.

[17] Grunberger, D. Personal communication. Sept 1997.

[18] Bailey D, Boik J. Unpublished observations. 1999.

[19] Park EH, Kim SH, Park SS. Anti-inflammatory activity of propolis. Arch Pharm Res 1996; 19(5):337–341.

[20] El-Ghazaly MA, Khayyal MT. The use of aqueous propolis extract against radiation-induced damage. Drugs Exp Clin Res 1995; 21(6):229–36.

[21] Grunberger D, Banerjee R, Eisinger K, et al. Preferential cytotoxicity on tumor cells by caffeic acid phenethyl ester isolated from propolis. Experientia 1988; 44:230–232.

[22] Chen JH, Shao Y, Huang MT, et al. Inhibitory effect of caffeic acid phenethyl ester on human leukemia HL-60 cells. Cancer Lett 1996 Nov 29; 108(2):211–4.

[23] Chiao C, Carothers AM, Grunberger D, et al. Apoptosis and altered redox state induced by caffeic acid phenethyl ester (CAPE) in transformed rat fibroblast cells. Cancer Res 1995 Aug 15; 55(16):3576–83.

[24] Su ZZ, Lin J, Prewett M, et al. Apoptosis mediates the selective toxicity of caffeic acid phenethyl ester (CAPE) toward oncogene-transformed rat embryo fibroblast cells. Anticancer Res 1995 Sep–Oct; 15(5B):1841–8.

[25] Mahmoud NN, Carothers AM, Grunberger D, et al. Plant phenolics decrease intestinal tumors in an animal model of familial adenomatous polyposis. Carcinogenesis 2000 May; 21(5):921–7.

[26] Lee SK, Song L, Mata-Greenwood E, et al. Modulation of in vitro biomarkers of the carcinogenic process by chemopreventive agents. Anticancer Res 1999 Jan–Feb; 19(1A):35–44.

[27] Ahn CH, Choi WC, Kong JY. Chemosensitizing activity of caffeic acid in multidrug-resistant MCF-7/Dox human breast carcinoma cells. Anticancer Res 1997 May–Jun; 17(3C):1913–7.

[28] Inayama S, Harimaya K, Hori H, et al. Studies on non-sesquiterpenoid constituents of Gaillardia pulchella. II. Less lipophilic substances, methyl caffeate as an antitumor catecholic. Chem Pharm Bull (Tokyo) 1984 Mar; 32(3):1135–41.

[29] Rao CV, Desai D, Simi B, et al. Inhibitory effect of caffeic acid esters on azoxymethane-induced biochemical changes and aberrant crypt foci formation in rat colon. Cancer Res 1993 Sep 15; 53(18):4182–8.

[30] Rao CV, Desai D, Kaul B, et al. Effect of caffeic acid esters on carcinogen-induced mutagenicity and human colon adenocarcinoma cell growth. Chem Biol Interact 1992 Nov 16; 84(3):277–90.

[31] Mehta K, Pantazis P, McQueen T, Aggarwal BB. Curcumin (diferuloylmethane) is a potent antiproliferative agent against human breast tumor cell lines. Anticancer Drugs 1997; 8:470–481.

[32] Ramachandran C, You W. Differential sensitivity of human mammary epithelial and breast carcinoma cell lines to curcumin. Breast Cancer Res Treat 1999 Apr; 54(3):269–78.

[33] Nagabhushan M, Bhide SV. Curcumin as an inhibitor of cancer. J Am College of Nutr 1992; 11:192–198.

[34] Gautam SC, Xu YX, Pindolia KR, et al. Nonselective inhibition of proliferation of transformed and nontransformed cells by the anticancer agent curcumin (diferuloylmethane). Biochem Pharmacol 1998 Apr 15; 55(8):1333–7.

[35] Syu WJ, Shen CC, Don MJ, et al. Cytotoxicity of curcuminoids and some novel compounds from Curcuma zedoaria. J Nat Prod 1998 Dec; 61(12):1531–4.

[36] Simon A, Allais DP, Duroux JL, et al. Inhibitory effect of curcuminoids on MCF-7 cell proliferation and structure-activity relationships. Cancer Lett 1998 Jul 3; 129(1):111–6.

[37] Lin LI, Ke YF, Ko YC, Lin JK. Curcumin inhibits SK-Hep-1 hepatocellular carcinoma cell invasion in vitro and suppresses matrix metalloproteinase-9 secretion. Oncology 1998 Jul–Aug; 55(4):349–53.

[38] Khafif A, Schantz SP, Chou TC, et al. Quantitation of chemopreventive synergism between (-)-epigallocatechin-3-gallate and curcumin in normal, premalignant and malignant human oral epithelial cells. Carcinogenesis 1998 Mar; 19(3):419–24.

[39] Hanif R, Qiao L, Shiff SJ, Rigas B. Curcumin, a natural plant phenolic food additive, inhibits cell proliferation and induces cell cycle changes in colon adenocarcinoma cell lines by a prostaglandin-independent pathway. J Lab Clin Med 1997 Dec; 130(6):576–84.

[40] Menon LG, Kuttan R, Kuttan G. Inhibition of lung metastasis in mice induced by B16F10 melanoma cells by polyphenolic compounds. Cancer Lett 1995 Aug 16; 95(1–2):221–5.

[41] Menon LG, Kuttan R, Kuttan G. Anti-metastatic activity of curcumin and catechin. Cancer Lett 1999 Jul 1; 141(1–2):159–65.

[42] Ruby AJ, Kuttan G, Babu KD, et al. Anti-tumour and antioxidant activity of natural curcuminoids. Cancer Lett 1995 Jul 20; 94(1):79–83.

[43] Kuttan R, Sudheeran PC, Josph CD. Turmeric and curcumin as topical agents in cancer therapy. Tumori 1987 Feb 28; 73(1):29–31.

44 Mahmoud NN, Carothers AM, Grunberger D, et al. Plant phenolics decrease intestinal tumors in an animal model of familial adenomatous polyposis. Carcinogenesis 2000 May; 21(5):921–7.

45 Bradlow HL, Telang NT, Sepkovic DW, Osborne MP. Phytochemicals as modulators of cancer risk. Adv Exp Med Biol 1999; 472:207–21.

46 Churchill M, Chadburn A, Bilinski RT, Bertagnolli MM. Inhibition of intestinal tumors by curcumin is associated with changes in the intestinal immune cell profile. J Surg Res 2000 Apr; 89(2):169–75.

47 Reddy S, Aggarwal BB. Curcumin is a non-competitive and selective inhibitor of phosphorylase kinase. FEBS 1994; 341:19–22.

48 Kuttan R, Bhanumathy P, Nirmala K, George MC. Potential anticancer activity of tumeric (Curcuma longa). Cancer Letters 1985; 29:197–202.

49 NCI, DCPC. Clinical development plan: Curcumin. J Cell Biochem 1996; 26S:72–85.

50 Sharma OP. Antioxidant activity of curcumin and related compounds. Biochemical Pharm 1976; 25:1811–1812.

51 Toda S, Miyase T, Arichi H, et al. Natural antioxidants. III. Antioxidative components isolated from rhizome of Curcuma longa L. Chem Pharm Bull 1985; 33(4):1725–1728.

52 Dixit VP, Jain P, Joshi SC. Hypolipidaemic effects of Curcuma longa L and Nardostachys fatamansi, DC in triton-induced hyperlipidamic rats. Indian J Physiol Pharm 1988; 32(4):299–304.

53 Bruneton J. Pharmacognosy, phytochemistry, and medicinal plants. Secaucus, NY: Lavoisier Publishing, 1995, p. 257.

54 Srimal RC, Dhawan BN. Pharmacology of diferuloyl methane (curcumin), a non-steroidal anti-inflammatory agent. J Pharm Pharmac 1973; 25:447–452.

55 Ammon HPT, Wahl MA. Pharmacology of Curcuma longa. Planta Medica 1991; 57:1–7.

56 Satoskar RR, Shah SJ, Shenoy SG. Evaluation of anti-inflammatory property of curcumin (diferuloyl methane) in patients with postoperative inflammation. Int J Clin Pharmacol Therapy Toxicol 1986; 24(12):651–654.

57 Thresiamma KC, George J, Kuttan R. Protective effect of curcumin, ellagic acid and bixin on radiation induced toxicity. Indian J Exp Biol 1996 Sep; 34(9):845–7.

58 Venkatesan N, Chandrakasan G. Modulation of cyclophosphamide-induced early lung injury by curcumin, an anti-inflammatory antioxidant. Mol Cell Biochem 1995 Jan 12; 142(1):79–87.

59 Venkatesan N, Punithavathi V, Chandrakasan G. Curcumin protects bleomycin-induced lung injury in rats. Life Sci 1997; 61(6):51–58.

60 Nirmala C, Puvanakrishnan R. Protective role of curcumin against isoproterenol induced myocardial infarction in rats. Mol Cell Biochem 1996 Jun 21; 159(2):85–93.

61 Rao CV, Simi B, Reddy BS. Inhibition by dietary curcumin of azoxymethane-induced ornithine decarboxylase, tyrosine protein kinase, arachidonic acid metabolism and aberrant crypt foci formation in the rat colon. Carcinogenesis 1993; 14(11):2219–2225.

62 Anto RJ, George J, Dinesh Babu KV, et al. Antimutagenic and anticarcinogenic activity of natural and synthetic curcuminoids. Mutation Res 1996; 370:127–131.

63 Sriganth INP, Premalatha B. Dietary curcumin with cisplatin administration modulates tumor marker indices in experimental fibrosarcoma. Pharm Res 1999; 39(3):175–9.

64 Bruneton J. Pharmacognosy, phytochemistry, and medicinal plants. Secaucus, NY: Lavoisier Publishing, 1995, p. 244.

65 Ryu SY, Ahn JW, Kang YH, et al. Antiproliferative effect of arctigenin and arctiin. Arch Pharm Res 1995; 18(6):462–3.

66 Hirano T, Gotoh M, Oka K. Natural flavanoids and lignans are potent cytostatic agents against human leukemic HL60 cells. Life Sciences 1994; 55(13):1061–9.

67 Moritani S, Nomura M, Takeda Y, Miyamoto KI. Cytotoxic components of Bardanae fructus (goboshi). Biol Pharm Bull 1996 Nov; 19(11):1515–7.

68 Umehara K, Sugawa A, Kuroyanagi M, et al. Studies on differentiation-inducers from Arctium fructus. Chem Pharm Bull 1993; 41(10):1774–9.

69 Umehara K, Nakamura M, Miyase T, et al. Studies on differentiation inducers. VI. Lignan derivatives from Arctium fructus. (2). Chem Pharm Bull (Tokyo) 1996 Dec; 44(12):2300–4.

70 Boik J, Newman R, Bailey D. Unpublished observations. 1999.

71 Cho JY, Kim AR, Yoo ES, et al. Immunomodulatory effect of arctigenin, a lignan compound, on tumour necrosis factor-alpha and nitric oxide production, and lymphocyte proliferation. J Pharm Pharmacol 1999 Nov; 51(11):1267–73.

72 Sung MK, Lautens M, Thompson LU. Mammalian lignans inhibit the growth of estrogen-independent human colon tumor cells. Anticancer Res 1998 May–Jun; 18(3A):1405–8.

73 Wang C, Kurzer MS. Effects of phytoestrogens on DNA synthesis in MCF-7 cells in the presence of estradiol or growth factors. Nutr Cancer 1998; 31(2):90–100.

74 Wang C, Kurzer MS. Phytoestrogen concentration determines effects on DNA synthesis in human breast cancer cells. Nutr Cancer 1997; 28(3):236–47.

75 Mousavi Y, Adlercreutz H. Enterolactone and estradiol inhibit each other's proliferative effect on MCF-7 breast cancer cells in culture. J Steroid Biochem Mol Biol 1992 Mar; 41(3–8):615–9.

76 Welshons WV, Murphy CS, Koch R, et al. Stimulation of breast cancer cells in vitro by the environmental estrogen enterolactone and the phytoestrogen equol. Breast Cancer Res Treat 1987 Nov; 10(2):169–75.

77 Hirano T, Fukuoka K, Oka K, et al. Antiproliferative activity of mammalian lignan derivatives against the human breast carcinoma cell line, ZR-75-1. Cancer Invest 1990; 8(6):595–602.

78 Yan L, Yee JA, Li D, et al. Dietary flaxseed supplementation and experimental metastasis of melanoma cells in mice. Cancer Lett 1998 Feb 27; 124(2):181–6.

79 Li D, Yee JA, Thompson LU, Yan L. Dietary supplementation with secoisolariciresinol diglycoside (SDG) reduces experimental metastasis of melanoma cells in mice. Cancer Lett 1999 Jul 19; 142(1):91–6.

[80] Thompson LU, Rickard SE, Orcheson LJ, Seidl MM. Flaxseed and its lignan and oil components reduce mammary tumor growth at a late stage of carcinogenesis. Carcinogenesis 1996 Jun; 17(6):1373–6.

[81] Thompson LU. Experimental studies on lignans and cancer. Baillieres Clin Endocrinol Metab 1998 Dec; 12(4):691–705.

[82] Lampe JW, Martini MC, Kurzer MS, et al. Urinary lignan and isoflavonoid excretion in premenopausal women consuming flaxseed powder. AM J Clin Nutr 1994; 60:122–8.

[83] Serraino M, Thompson L. The effect of flaxseed supplementation on the initiation and promotional stages of mammary tumorigenesis. Nutr Cancer 1992; 17:153–59.

[84] Ingram D, Sanders K, Kolybaba M, Lopez D. Case-control study of phyto-oestrogens and breast cancer. Lancet 1997; 350:990–94.

[85] Adlercreutz H, Mousavi Y, Clark J, et al. Dietary phytoestrogens and cancer: In vitro and in vivo studies. J Steroid Biochem Mol Biol 1992; 41(3–8):331–7.

[86] Fortunati N, Becchis M, Catalano MG, et al. Sex hormone-binding globulin, its membrane receptor, and breast cancer: A new approach to the modulation of estradiol action in neoplastic cells. J Steroid Biochem Mol Biol 1999 Apr–Jun; 69(1–6):473–9.

[87] Adlercreutz H. Western diet and Western diseases: Some hormonal and biochemical mechanisms and associations. Scand J Clin Lab Invest Suppl 1990; 201:3–23.

[88] Wang C, Makela T, Hase T, et al. Lignans and flavonoids inhibit aromatase enzyme in human preadipocytes. J Steroid Biochem Mol Biol 1994 Aug; 50(3–4):205–12.

[89] Adlercreutz H, Bannwart C, Wahala K, et al. Inhibition of human aromatase by mammalian lignans and isoflavonoid phytoestrogens. J Steroid Biochem Mol Biol 1993 Feb; 44(2):147–53.

[90] Thompson LU, Rickard SE, Cheung F, et al. Variability in anticancer lignan levels in flaxseed. Nutr Cancer 1997; 27(1):26–30.

[91] Setchell KD, Lawson AM, Borriello SP, et al. Lignan formation in man—microbial involvement and possible roles in relation to cancer. Lancet 1981 Jul 4; 2(8236):4–7.

[92] Thompson LU, Seidl MM, Rickard SE, et al. Antitumorigenic effect of a mammalian lignan precursor from flaxseed. Nutr Cancer 1996; 26(2):159–65.

[93] Thompson LU, Rickard SE, Orcheson LJ, Seidl MM. Flaxseed and its lignan and oil components reduce mammary tumor growth at a late stage of carcinogenesis. Carcinogenesis 1996 Jun; 17(6):1373–6.

[94] Yan L, Yrr JA, Li D, et al. Dietary flaxseed supplementation and experimental metastasis of melanoma cells in mice. Cancer Letters 1998; 124(2):181–186.

[95] Saarinen NM, Warri A, Makela SI, et al. Hydroxymatairesinol, a novel enterolactone precursor with antitumor properties from coniferous tree. Nutr Cancer 2000; 36(2):207–16.

[96] Surh YJ, Hurh YJ, Kang JY, et al. Resveratrol, an antioxidant present in red wine, induces apoptosis in human promyelocytic leukemia (HL-60) cells. Cancer Lett 1999 Jun 1; 140(1–2):1–10.

[97] Hsieh TC, Burfeind P, Laud K, et al. Cell cycle effects and control of gene expression by resveratrol in human breast carcinoma cell lines with different metastatic potentials. Int J Oncol 1999 Aug; 15(2):245–52.

[98] Hsieh TC, Wu JM. Differential effects on growth, cell cycle arrest, and induction of apoptosis by resveratrol in human prostate cancer cell lines. Exp Cell Res 1999 May 25; 249(1):109–15.

[99] Lu R, Serrero G. Resveratrol, a natural product derived from grape, exhibits antiestrogenic activity and inhibits the growth of human breast cancer cells. J Cell Physiol 1999 Jun; 179(3):297–304.

[100] Huang C, Ma WY, Goranson A, Dong Z. Resveratrol suppresses cell transformation and induces apoptosis through a p53-dependent pathway. Carcinogenesis 1999 Feb; 20(2):237–42.

[101] Fremont L. Biological effects of resveratrol. Life Sci 2000 Jan 14; 66(8):663–73.

[102] Carbo N, Costelli P, Baccino FM, et al. Resveratrol, a natural product present in wine, decreases tumour growth in a rat tumour model. Biochem Biophys Res Commun 1999 Jan 27; 254(3):739–43.

[103] Bertelli AAE. Modulatory effect of resveratrol, a natural phytoalexin, on endothelial adhesion molecules and intracellular signal transduction. Pharm Biol 1998; 36(Suppl):44–52.

[104] Lamuela-Raventos RM, Romero-Perez AI, Waterhouse AL, et al. Direct HPLC analysis of cis- and trans-resveratrol and piceid isomers in Spanish red Vitis vinifera wines. J. Agric Food Chem 1995; 43:281–283.

[105] Jang M, Cai L, Udeani GO, et al. Cancer chemopreventive activity of resveratrol, a natural product derived from grapes. Science 1997 Jan 10; 275(5297):218–20.

[106] Gehm BD, McAndrews JM, Chien PY, Jameson JL. Resveratrol, a polyphenolic compound found in grapes and wine, is an agonist for the estrogen receptor. Proc Natl Acad Sci USA 1997 Dec 9; 94(25):14138–43.

[107] Basly JP, Marre-Fournier F, Le Bail JC, et al. Estrogenic/antiestrogenic and scavenging properties of (E)- and (Z)-resveratrol. Life Sci 2000 Jan 21; 66(9):769–77.

[108] Stahl S, Chun TY, Gray WG. Phytoestrogens act as estrogen agonists in an estrogen-responsive pituitary cell line. Toxicol Appl Pharmacol 1998 Sep; 152(1):41–8.

[109] Carbo N, Costelli P, Baccino FM, et al. Resveratrol, a natural product present in wine, decreases tumour growth in a rat tumour model. Biochem Biophys Res Commun 1999 Jan 27; 254(3):739–43.

[110] Mgbonyebi OP, Russo J, Russo IH. Antiproliferative effect of synthetic resveratrol on human breast epithelial cells. Int J Oncol 1998 Apr; 12(4):865–9.

[111] Hsieh T, Burfeind P, Laud K, et al. Cell cycle effects and control of gene expression by resveratrol in human breast carcinoma cell lines with different metastatic potentials. Int J Oncol 1999; 15(2):245–52.

[112] Clement MV, Hirpara JL, Chawdhury SH, Pervaiz S. Chemopreventive agent resveratrol, a natural product derived from grapes, triggers CD95 signaling-dependent apoptosis in human tumor cells. Blood 1998 Aug 1; 92(3):996–1002.

[113] Ragione FD, Cucciolla V, Borriello A, et al. Resveratrol arrests the cell division cycle at S/G2 phase transition. Biochem Biophys Res Commun 1998 Sep 8; 250(1):53–8.

[114] Steele VE, Wargovich MJ, McKnee K, et al. Cancer chemoprevention drug development strategies for resveratrol. Pharmaceutical Biology 1998; 36(suppl):62–68.

[115] ElAttar TM, Virji AS. Modulating effect of resveratrol and quercetin on oral cancer cell growth and proliferation. Anticancer Drugs 1999 Feb; 10(2):187–93.

[116] Hsieh TC, Wu JM. Grape-derived chemopreventive agent resveratrol decreases prostate-specific antigen (PSA) expression in LNCaP cells by an androgen receptor (AR)-independent mechanism. Anticancer Res 2000 Jan–Feb; 20(1A):225–8.

[117] Zhang L, Lau YK, Xi L, et al. Tyrosine kinase inhibitors, emodin and its derivative repress HER-2/neu-induced cellular transformation and metastasis-associated properties. Oncogene 1998 Jun 4; 16(22):2855–63.

[118] Zhang L, Chang CJ, Bacus SS, Hung MC. Suppressed transformation and induced differentiation of HER-2/neu-overexpressing breast cancer cells by emodin. Cancer Res 1995 Sep 1; 55(17):3890–6.

[119] Chan TC, Chang CJ, Koonchanok NM, Geahlen RL. Selective inhibition of the growth of ras-transformed human bronchial epithelial cells by emodin, a protein-tyrosine kinase inhibitor. Biochem Biophys Res Commun 1993 Jun 30; 193(3):1152–8.

[120] Morita H, Umeda M, Masuda T, et al. Cytotoxic and mutagenic effects of emodin on cultured mouse carcinoma FM3A cells. Mutat Res 1988; 204(2):329–32.

[121] Kuo YC, Sun CM. Ou JC, Tsai WJ. A tumor cell growth inhibitor from Polygonum hypoleucum Ohwi. Life Sci 1997; 61(23):2335–2344.

[122] Lu M, Chen Q. Biochemical study of Chinese rhubarb; Inhibitory effects of anthraquinone derivatives on P388 leukemia in mice. Zhongguo Yaoke Daxue Xuebao 1989; 20(3):155–7.

[123] Zhang L, Lau YK, Xia W, et al. Tyrosine kinase inhibitor emodin suppresses growth of HER-2/neu-overexpressing breast cancer cells in athymic mice and sensitizes these cells to the inhibitory effect of paclitaxel. Clin Cancer Res 1999 Feb; 5(2):343–53.

[124] Chang HM, But PPH. Pharmacology and applications of Chinese materia medica. Vol. 1. Teaneck, NJ: World Scientific Publishing Company, 1986, p. 77.

[125] Chen Q, Liu C, Qui C. Studies of Chinese rhubarb: XII. Effect of anthraquinone derivatives on the respiration and glycolysis of Ehrlich ascites carcinoma cell. Yao Hsueh Hsueh Pao 1980; 15(2):65–70.

[126] Yim H, Lee YH, Lee CH, Lee SK. Emodin, an anthraquinone derivative isolated from the rhizomes of Rheum palmatum, selectively inhibits the activity of casein kinase II as a competitive inhibitor. Planta Med 1999 Feb; 65(1):9–13.

[127] Zhang L, Lau YK, Xi L, et al. Tyrosine kinase inhibitors, emodin and its derivatives repress HER-2/neu-induced cellular transformation and metastasis-associated properties. Oncogene 1998; 16:2855–2863.

[128] Yeh SF, Chou TC, Liu TS. Effects of anthraquinones of Polygonum cuspidatum on HL-60 Cells. Planta Med 1988; 413–14.

[129] Koyama M, Takahashi K, Chou TC, et al. Intercalating agents with covalent bond forming capability. A novel type of potential anticancer agents. 2. Derivatives of chrysophanol and emodin. J Med Chem 1989 Jul; 32(7):1594–9.

[130] Chen J, Wu Z, Yang H, et al. Cytokinetic effects of emodin on human lung cancer A-549 cell. Zhongcaoyao 1991; 22(12):543–6.

[131] Chan TCK, Chang CJ, Koonchanok NM, Geahlen RL. Selective inhibition of the growth of ras-transformed human bronchial epithelial cells by emodin, a protein-tyrosine kinase inhibitor. Biochemical and Biophysical Research Communications 1993; 193(3):1152–1158.

[132] Chang CJ, Ashendel CL, Geahlen RL, et al. Oncogene signal transduction inhibitors from medicinal plants. In Vivo 1996; 10:185–90.

[133] Huang HC, Chu SH, Lee Chao PD. Vasorelaxants from Chinese herbs, emodin and scoparone, possess immunosuppressive properties. European Journal of Pharmacology 1991; 198:211–13.

[134] Huang HC, Chang JH, Tung SF, et al. Immunosuppressive effect of emodin, a free radical generator. Eur J Pharmacol 1992a; 211(3):359–64.

[135] Goel RK, Das Gupta G, Ram SN, et al. Antiulcerogenic and anti-inflammatory effects of emodin, isolated from Rhamnus triquerta wall. J Exp Biol 1991; 29(3):230–2.

[136] Anton R, Haag-Berrurier M. Therapeutic use of natural anthraquinone for other than laxative actions. Pharmacology 1980; 20(suppl 1):104–12.

[137] Friedmann CA. Structure-activity relationships of anthraquinones in some pathological conditions. Pharmacology 1980; 20(suppl 1):113–22.

[138] Chang HM, But PPH. Pharmacology and applications of Chinese materia medica. Vol. 2. Teaneck, NJ: World Scientific Publishing Company, 1987, p. 783.

[139] Zhang YP, Sussman N, Macina OT, et al. Prediction of the carcinogenicity of a second group of organic chemicals undergoing carcinogenicity testing. Environ Health Perspect 1996 Oct; 104S(5):1045–50.

[140] Westendorf J, Marquardt H, Poginsky B, et al. Genotoxicity of naturally occurring hydroxyanthraquinones. Mutat Res 1990 Jan; 240(1):1–12.

[141] Marchant CA, DEREK collaborative group. Prediction of rodent carcinogenicity using the DEREK system for 30 chemicals currently being tested by the national toxicology program. Environmental Health Perspectives 1996; 104 (Suppl 5):1065–73.

[142] Lee Y, Buchanan BG, Rosenkranz HS. Carcinogenicity predictions for a group of 30 chemicals undergoing rodent cancer bioassays based on rules derived from subchronic organ toxicities. Environmental Health Perspectives 1996; 104 (Suppl 5):1059–63.

[143] Ashby J. Prediction of rodent carcinogenicity for 30 chemicals. Environmental Health Perspectives 1996; 104 (Suppl 5):1101–4.

[144] Lewis DFV, Ioannides C, Parke DV. COMPACT and molecular structure in toxicity assessment: A prospective evaluation of 30 chemicals currently being tested for rodent carcinogenicity by the NCI/NTP. Environ Health Perspect 1996 Oct; 104S(5):1011–6.

[145] Bosch R, Friederich U, Lutz WK, et al. Investigations on DNA binding in rat liver and in Salmonella and on mutagenicity in the Ames test by emodin, a natural anthraquinone. Mutat Res 1987 Jul; 188(3):161–8.

[146] Mengs U, Krumbiegel G, Volkner W. Lack of emodin genotoxicity in the mouse micronucleus assay. Mutat Res 1997; 393(3):289–293.

[147] Mueller SO, Lutz WK, Stopper H. Factors affecting the genotoxic potency ranking of natural anthraquinones in mammalian cell culture systems. Mutation Res 1998; 414:125–129.

[148] Pecere T, Gazzola MV, Mucignat C, et al. Aloe-emodin is a new type of anticancer agent with selective activity against neuroectodermal tumors. Cancer Res 2000 Jun 1; 60(11):2800–4.

[149] Kim JI, Park JH, Park HJ, et al. Induction of differentiation of the human histocytic lymphoma cell line U-937 by hypericin. Arch Pharm Res 1998 Feb; 21(1):41–5.

[150] Zhang W, Law RE, Hinton DR, Couldwell WT. Inhibition of human malignant glioma cell motility and invasion in vitro by hypericin, a potent protein kinase C inhibitor. Cancer Lett 1997 Nov 25; 120(1):31–8.

[151] Hamilton HB, Hinton DR, Law RE, et al. Inhibition of cellular growth and induction of apoptosis in pituitary adenoma cell lines by the protein kinase C inhibitor hypericin: Potential therapeutic application. J Neurosurg 1996 Aug; 85(2):329–34.

[152] Zhang W, Lawa RE, Hintona DR, et al. Growth inhibition and apoptosis in human neuroblastoma SK-N-SH cells induced by hypericin, a potent inhibitor of protein kinase C. Cancer Lett 1995 Sep 4; 96(1):31–5.

[153] Couldwell WT, Gopalakrishna R, Hinton DR, et al. Hypericin: A potential antiglioma therapy. Neurosurgery 1994 Oct; 35(4):705–9; discussion 709–10.

[154] Miccoli L, Beurdeley-Thomas A, De Pinieux G, et al. Light-induced photoactivation of hypericin affects the energy metabolism of human glioma cells by inhibiting hexokinase bound to mitochondria. Cancer Res 1998 Dec 15; 58(24):5777–86.

[155] Fox FE, Niu Z, Tobia A, Rook AH. Photoactivated hypericin is an anti-proliferative agent that induces a high rate of apoptotic death of normal, transformed, and malignant T lymphocytes: Implications for the treatment of cutaneous lymphoproliferative and inflammatory disorders. J Invest Dermatol 1998 Aug; 111(2):327–32.

[156] Johnson SA, Dalton AE, Pardini RS. Time-course of hypericin phototoxicity and effect on mitochondrial energies in EMT6 mouse mammary carcinoma cells. Free Radic Biol Med 1998 Jul 15; 25(2):144–52.

[157] Lavie G, Mazur Y, Lavie D, Meruelo D. The chemical and biological properties of hypericin—a compound with a broad spectrum of biological activities. Med Res Rev 1995 Mar; 15(2):111–9.

[158] Chen B, de Witte PA. Photodynamic therapy efficacy and tissue distribution of hypericin in a mouse P388 lymphoma tumor model. Cancer Lett 2000 Mar 13; 150(1):111–7.

[159] Martens A, de Moor A, Waelkens E, et al. In vitro and in vivo evaluation of hypericin for photodynamic therapy of equine sarcoids. Vet J 2000 Jan; 159(1):77–84.

[160] Vandenbogaerde AL, Geboes KR, Cuveele JF, et al. Antitumour activity of photosensitized hypericin on A431 cell xenografts. Anticancer Res 1996 Jul–Aug; 16(4A):1619–25.

[161] Alecu M, Ursaciuc C, Halalau F, et al. Photodynamic treatment of basal cell carcinoma and squamous cell carcinoma with hypericin. Anticancer Res 1998 Nov–Dec; 18(6B):4651–4.

[162] Johnson SA, Pardini RS. Antioxidant enzyme response to hypericin in EMT6 mouse mammary carcinoma cells. Free Radic Biol Med 1998; 24(5):817–826.

[163] Thomas C, Pardini RS. Oxygen dependence of hypericin-induced phototoxicity to EMT6 mouse mammary carcinoma cells. Photochem Photobiol 1992 Jun; 55(6):831–7.

[164] Colasanti A, Kisslinger A, Liuzzi R, et al. Hypericin photosensitization of tumor and metastatic cell lines of human prostate. J Photochem Photobiol B 2000 Feb; 54(2–3):103–7.

[165] Vandenbogaerde AL, Geboes KR, Cuveele JF, et al. Antitumour activity of photosensitized hypericin on A431 cell xenografts. Anticancer Res 1996 Jul–Aug; 16(4A):1619–25.

This chapter and the next discuss terpenes and related compounds. We focus here on three groups of terpenes: monoterpenes, triterpenes, and sesquiterpenes, each of which is composed of multiple isoprene units. The monoterpenes discussed are limonene, perillyl alcohol, and geraniol; the triterpenes discussed are asiatic acid and boswellic acid; and the sesquiterpene discussed is parthenolide.

The isoprene unit and the production of different terpenoids from it are illustrated in Figure 4.5. As shown there, the isoprenoid pathway is also the source for steroids. On the basis of that link, a number of steroidlike compounds are also discussed in this chapter. These are saponins, special glycosides of triterpene or steroidlike compounds. The saponins discussed are those from horse chestnut, butcher's broom, and ginseng. Structures for all compounds covered in this chapter are illustrated in Figures A.59 to A.74 of Appendix A.

MONOTERPENES

Summary of Research and Conclusions

Fifteen in-vitro studies have reported that monoterpenes inhibit a variety of cancer cell lines.[1-5] The minimum effective concentration varied greatly between different monoterpenes and between different studies, with the total range being roughly 50 to 5,000 µM and the average range being 160 to 1,300 µM. These concentrations are high relative to the effective concentrations for most other natural compounds. Nevertheless, due to favorable pharmacokinetics and relatively low toxicity, these high concentrations and the doses required to achieve them are not prohibitive.

At least seven antitumor studies on monoterpenes have been conducted in animals.[5-11] Two reviews discussing animal studies have also been published.[12, 13] As a whole, these studies suggest that orally administered monoterpenes are capable of causing the regression of several types of established tumors. In many cases, these regressions were complete (100 percent).

Two human phase I studies were done; these were designed to determine pharmacokinetic parameters and the highest safe dose in cancer patients, not efficacy.[14, 15]

In addition to the above, a number of other animal studies have reported that monoterpenes have cancer preventive effects.[16, 17, 18]

Introduction

Orally administered monoterpenes have produced some dramatic anticancer effects in tumor-bearing rodents. A variety of monoterpenes have this capacity, differing only by their potency. Three promising monoterpenes are limonene, perillyl alcohol, and geraniol.

Monoterpenes are the simplest compounds of the terpene series. These and other low-molecular-weight terpenes tend to be highly volatile and often constitute the primary components of essential oils, the fragrant principles of plants. Essential oils are used in perfumes and as flavoring agents for foods; an example of the latter is orange oil, which contains a high amount of the monoterpene limonene. Essential oils are generally antiseptic, and some, like limonene, are local irritants. Most monoterpenes occur naturally as aglycones, but glycosides have also been reported.

The monoterpenes limonene, perillyl alcohol, and geraniol decrease the proliferation of a variety of tumor cell lines both in vitro and in vivo; although the exact method for this is still not certain, many possibilities have been postulated. The potential anticancer actions of monoterpenes are listed in Table 21.1.

The first activity listed in the table is inhibition of isoprene synthesis. As a reminder, the lipid tail needed to make the ras protein functional is a product of the isoprene synthesis pathway. Plant monoterpenes can block this pathway by inhibiting HMGR, the rate-limiting enzyme in isoprene synthesis (see Figure 4.5).

The relative ability of monoterpenes to inhibit cell proliferation in six different cell lines in vitro is shown in Figure 21.1 (not all compounds were tested in all lines).[3, 19, 20] Included in the figure is perillic acid, the primary active metabolite of limonene and perillyl alcohol, and possibly geraniol. Of the three monoterpenes, perillyl alcohol is most efficiently converted to perillic acid. The geometric averages shown are 160 µM for perillyl alcohol, 200 µM for geraniol, 520 µM for perillic acid, and 1,300 µM for limonene. Perillyl alcohol would appear to be the most effective, but again, it is metabolized primarily to perillic acid in vivo. The ability of these compounds to inhibit HMGR is directly correlated with their ability to inhibit cancer cell proliferation.[19]

TABLE 21.1 POTENTIAL ANTICANCER ACTIONS OF MONOTERPENES

ACTIVITY	KNOWN EFFECTS
Chapter 3: Results of Therapy at the Cellular Level	
Inhibit isoprene synthesis	x
Chapter 4: Growth Factors and Signal Transduction	
Induce differentiation	x
Induce apoptosis	x
Improve TGF-beta signaling	x
Chapters 11 and 12: Immune System	
Inhibit tumor-induced immunosuppression	x

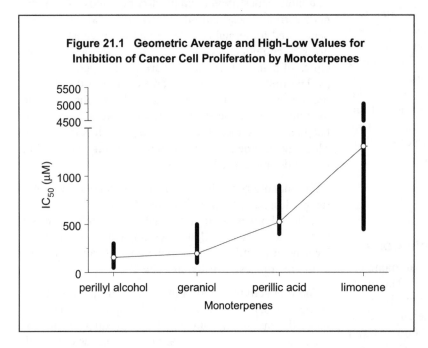

Figure 21.1 Geometric Average and High-Low Values for Inhibition of Cancer Cell Proliferation by Monoterpenes

Limonene

As mentioned, limonene is the primary constituent of orange oil. Midseason sweet orange oil may contain 80 to 96 percent limonene, with the remainder being other terpenes. The concentration can vary, however, and analysis of some commercial orange oil has revealed zero limonene content.[21] The anticarcinogenic and antitumor effects of limonene and other monoterpenes have been extensively studied at the University of Wisconsin, where limonene has been reported to hinder stomach, lung, skin, and liver cancers in rodent models. Oral administration of limonene at 10 percent of diet (about 7.5 g/kg per day) for three weeks caused regression of tumors in 89 percent of rats with chemically induced breast cancer. A minimum dose of 7.5 percent of diet (about 5.6 g/kg per day) was required for complete regression. This effect was observed in rats with both small and advanced tumors, and the majority of tumor regressions were complete. Regression was maintained

as long as limonene was continued, and little or no toxicity was observed.[22] The human equivalent of a 5.6 g/kg per day dose in rats is about 91 grams daily. Although little or no toxicity was seen in rats at this dose, it may still produce adverse effects in humans.

At lower doses (less than 1 percent of diet), limonene inhibited breast cancer development induced by a variety of carcinogens in rats. The anticarcinogenic effects of limonene and other monoterpenes are probably due to their ability to stimulate drug metabolism in the liver, thereby effectively detoxifying carcinogens. Drug detoxification is discussed in more detail in Chapter 23. Monoterpenes induce a wider spectrum of detoxification enzymes than does the classic enzyme inducer, phenobarbital.[23]

Perillyl Alcohol

Because a high dose of limonene is required for tumor regression, other related monoterpenes have been investigated. Perillyl alcohol, a common chemical used in the perfume industry, is a limonene analog that is more potent than limonene itself in inducing tumor regression—5 to 10 times more so in inhibiting breast cancer in rats.[8]

Both limonene and perillyl alcohol are rapidly metabolized in vivo to active terpene derivatives. One derivative in particular, perillic acid, appears to be responsible for most of the antitumor effects from oral administration of either limonene or perillyl alcohol. Within one hour after limonene administration to rats, more than 80 percent is metabolized to derivatives, the most common being perillic acid and dihydroperillic acid.[24, 25] In humans, approximately 40 percent of limonene is metabolized to perillic acid.[26] Perillyl alcohol is also metabolized to perillic acid, but the conversion is more complete than that for limonene.[8]

At high doses (2 to 2.5 percent of diet), perillyl alcohol induced regression of 81 percent of small breast tumors and 75 percent of advanced, chemically induced breast tumors in rats. The majority of these regressions were complete, and secondary tumors were prevented. Although no toxic effects occurred at a 2 percent diet, a 2.5 percent diet caused weight loss in rats, which may have been due to food aversion. (The human equivalent of a 2 percent diet, 1.5 g/kg, is 24 grams per day.) A 3 percent diet resulted in several deaths. A minimum of 1 percent (about 750 mg/kg per day) was required to produce a significant number of complete tumor regressions (55 percent).[8] The equivalent human dose is about 12 grams per day.

Other studies have confirmed the effect of these doses in rodents. At 2 percent of diet (about 1.5 g/kg), perillyl alcohol reduced tumor mass by a factor of 10 in rats with chemically induced liver tumors. Cell proliferation was not affected, but the rate of apoptosis was markedly increased.[27] This effect on apoptosis may be specific to cancer cells. For example, one study reported that perillyl alcohol was much more effective at inducing apoptosis in pancreatic cancer cells than in normal pancreas cells.[28] At 1.5 g/kg per day, perillyl alcohol reduced growth of pancreatic tumors in hamsters by more than 50 percent, and in 16 percent, complete regressions were seen. No regressions happened in controls.[29] The equivalent human dose is about 21 grams per day.

Much lower doses of perillyl alcohol (75 to 150 mg/kg) were effective at inhibiting the incidence of chemically induced colon cancer in rats.[30] As with limonene, the cancer preventive dose is lower than the antitumor one.

Geraniol

The monoterpene geraniol may be slightly more effective than perillyl alcohol in treating established tumors. In one study, a maximum response to geraniol was seen at approximately 740 mg/kg in rats, whereas a minimum response to perillyl alcohol took place at 750 mg/kg.[31] Even at doses as low as 360 mg/kg, geraniol was effective in decreasing transplanted liver cancer cells in rats. The equivalent human dose is about 5.8 grams per day. An oral dose of roughly 250 mg/kg reduced growth of transplanted melanoma and leukemia cells in mice.[32, 33] The equivalent human dose is about 2.4 grams per day. A larger geraniol dose of approximately 2.4 g/kg per day (2 percent of diet) completely inhibited the growth of transplanted pancreatic cancer cells in hamsters, without adverse effects.[34] The equivalent human dose is about 34 grams per day.

Estimated Therapeutic and Tolerated Doses of Monoterpenes

The estimated required limonene and perillyl alcohol doses scaled from animal antitumor studies roughly agree with those calculated from pharmacokinetic and in-vitro data. The former is about 91 grams for limonene and 12 to 24 (average 19 grams) grams for perillyl alcohol; doses based on pharmacokinetic data are 120

grams for limonene and 19 grams for perillyl alcohol. As discussed in Appendix J, however, the doses calculated from pharmacokinetic and in-vitro data do not provide a true corroboration of the animal data. Nonetheless, we still estimate target human doses by using an average of the values from both types of studies, or 110 grams for limonene and 19 grams for perillyl alcohol. Although pharmacokinetic data are not available for geraniol, the animal antitumor data indicate a dose of 2.4 to 34 grams would be required (average of 4.1 grams based on the two studies with the lowest dose).

The estimated maximum tolerated dose of limonene is about 14 grams per day, while the estimated LOAEL doses for perillyl alcohol and geraniol are 9 and 5.7 grams per day, respectively (see Appendix J). The dose-limiting adverse effects of monoterpenes are gastrointestinal problems like nausea, vomiting, and diarrhea. The three monoterpenes are not commonly used as therapeutic agents in noncancerous conditions, so a commonly prescribed dose cannot be determined.

The therapeutic dose estimates are summarized in Table 21.2. For all three monoterpenes, the low end of the tentative recommended dose range is equal to the dose calculated by assuming a full 15-fold increase in potency due to synergistic interactions. The high end of the range is the LOAEL dose or, in the case of limonene, the maximum tolerated dose. These are above the 1.8-gram general linear bioavailability limit, but this is not a problem for these compounds, since they were tested in pharmacokinetic studies at high doses.

Synergistic interactions are probably necessary for limonene and perillyl alcohol to produce an anticancer effect in humans. In comparing the target doses in Table 21.2 to the maximum tentative recommended doses, synergistic interactions will be needed to yield a minimum 7.9-fold and 2.1-fold increase in potency for these two compounds. This should be possible, since such increases are well below the allowable 15-fold increase. The 7.9-fold value for limonene is the highest of all direct-acting compounds (see Table 13.1). From this perspective, limonene is among the weakest direct-acting compounds discussed, and it may be prudent to place a low priority on its use relative to other compounds.

As with other drugs and natural compounds, tumor cells may develop resistance to monoterpenes. For example, resistance has been reported with other HMGR inhibitors in vitro.[35] Therefore, it may be helpful to combine monoterpenes with agents that reduce multidrug resistance (see Chapter 23). Lastly, because tumor regression due to monoterpenes is reversible, continual treatment may be necessary. It is not known,

TABLE 21.2 ESTIMATED THERAPEUTIC AND TOLERATED DOSES FOR MONOTERPENES[*]			
DESCRIPTION	LIMONENE DOSE (g/day)	PERILLYL ALCOHOL DOSE (g/day)	GERANIOL DOSE (g/day)
Required dose as scaled from animal antitumor studies	91	12 to 24 (average 19)	2.4 to 34 (average 4.1)[†]
Required cytotoxic dose as determined from pharmacokinetic calculations	120[‡]	19[‡]	uncertain
Target dose based on an average from animal antitumor studies and pharmacokinetic calculations	110	19	4.1
Minimum required antitumor dose assuming 15-fold synergistic benefits	7.3	1.3	0.27
Estimated LOAEL dose	14[§]	9	5.7
Tentative dose recommendation for further research	**7.3 to 14**	**1.3 to 9**	**0.27 to 5.7**
Minimum degree of synergism required	**7.9-fold potency increase**	**2.1-fold potency increase**	**none**

[*] *See Appendix J for details.*

[†] *The highest of the three available doses was omitted to calculate the average.*

[‡] *Assumes that other monoterpenes in the plasma besides perillic acid allow a threefold dose reduction.*

[§] *Maximum tolerated dose.*

however, if treatment will still be reversible if synergistic combinations are used.

As a practical point, monoterpenes are highly volatile and are local irritants. Therefore, adverse effects might be minimized if they are diluted with oil and placed in capsules. Monoterpenes are best stored in a closed, dark container to prevent evaporation and degradation. Like other compounds we discuss, monoterpenes will be most effective when taken in at least three divided doses per day. Additive toxicities can be avoided if different monoterpenes are not taken together.

TRITERPENOIDS

Although many triterpenoids inhibit cancer cell proliferation in vitro, they are not generally thought of as anticancer compounds. Rather, triterpenoid-rich plants have been used in herbal medicine traditions more for their anti-inflammatory effects and their protective effects on the vascular system. We included them here partly for these characteristics, which may inhibit angiogenesis (see Chapters 7 and 8) as well as invasion and metastasis (see Chapters 9 and 10). In addition, some triterpenoids, including those from the *Centella* and *Boswellia* species, produce cytotoxic effects against cancer cells. Like all triterpenoids, they contain six isoprene units, and their structure is quite similar to the steroids.

Centella asiatica

Summary of Research and Conclusions

The single study conducted on *Centella* reported that its extracts inhibited cancer cell growth in vitro and in animals.[36] Other in-vitro and animal studies on related compounds corroborate these results. The compounds include ursolic, oleanolic, and boswellic acids, all triterpenes related to asiatic acid, a primary triterpene in *Centella*. Moreover, additional mechanistic studies suggest that *Centella* triterpenoids have the capacity to fight cancer (for example, they counteract collagenase activity); thus *Centella* does have potential as an anticancer agent even though more studies are necessary to better define its effects and usefulness.

Discussion

Centella asiatica (gotu kola, Indian pennywort) is a tropical herb used in traditional medicines for a wide variety of conditions, including burns, venous disorders, and skin ulcers.[37] Studies have confirmed that oral or topical administration promotes wound healing, including surgical and nonhealing wounds, ulcerations, and leprosy sores.[38–42] *Centella* is used internally for venous insufficiency conditions such as varicose veins and edema. The most common formulation for oral administration is the standardized total triterpenic fraction of *Centella asiatica* (TTFCA), which contains about 30 percent asiatic acid, 30 percent madecassic acid, and 40 percent asiaticoside, a glycoside of asiatic acid.[a] Oral doses of TTFCA are commonly 60 to 180 milligrams per day, and the dose is generally well tolerated.

The content of total triterpenoids in the whole plant varies from 1.1 to 8 percent. Most samples yield a concentration between 2.2 and 3.4 percent.[43] A dose of about 2.1 grams of plant material is therefore needed to provide 60 mg of TTFCA.

Centella triterpenoids may be cytotoxic in vitro, but only one study has reported this so far. Although it indicated that fractions of *Centella* were cytotoxic in vitro to Dalton's lymphoma and Ehrlich ascites cancer cells, the content of terpenoids in the fractions was not specified.[36] The cytotoxic effects of the related ursane-type triterpenoids, ursolic and oleanolic acid, have received more attention, as has the triterpene boswellic acid.[b] It is likely that asiatic acid acts similarly to these compounds. In-vitro studies on ursolic and oleanolic acid indicate they are able to inhibit proliferation of a variety of cancer cell lines at an IC_{50} of 1 to 20 μM.[44–47] In addition, both oleanolic acid and ursolic acid decreased endothelial cell proliferation at an IC_{50} of 5 to 20 μM.[48] Therefore, these triterpenoids may be useful in preventing angiogenesis, which requires endothelial cell proliferation for building new blood vessels.

Oleanolic and ursolic acids have also produced antitumor effects in vivo. Intraperitoneal administration of 50 to 100 mg/kg of oleanolic or ursolic acid inhibited growth of established sarcoma tumors in mice by 30 percent. Lower doses were not effective. The compounds also protected the immune system of mice from radiation damage.[49] The equivalent human oral dose of a 100-mg/kg intraperitoneal dose in mice is about 1.3 grams per day. Because of its antitumor effects, a pharmaceutical preparation containing oleanolic acid is patented in Japan for treating nonlymphatic leukemia, although no data have been published on its clinical efficacy. Again, asiatic acid probably acts in a similar way to ursolic and oleanolic acids and could produce antitumor effects at similar doses and concentrations. We focus on *Centella* triterpenoids here rather than ursolic and oleanolic acids, in part because of the commercial availability of *Centella* and its history of safe use in hu-

mans. Nevertheless, ursolic and oleanolic acids remain potential treatment agents.

The possible anticancer actions of *Centella* are summarized in Table 21.3. Direct cytotoxic actions are not included because so little research on them exists, but such effects are certainly possible.

In the single animal antitumor study, oral administration of a terpenoid-rich extract (probably not as concentrated as TTFCA) at 1 g/kg on five alternate days inhibited tumor growth and increased survival in mice injected with lymphoma cells. Inhibition was most significant when mice were treated with the extract before tumor injection, and it was not significant when treatment was started 10 days after injection.[36] The equivalent human dose is about 4.8 grams per day. In this study, the inhibitory effect apparently was not due to cytotoxicity but to indirect antitumor effects (e.g., reduced vascular permeability).

Estimated Therapeutic and LOAEL Doses of *Centella* Triterpenoids

The estimated required dose scaled from animal studies is in rough agreement with that calculated from pharmacokinetic and in-vitro data. The dose for asiatic acid from animal studies is about 1.3 grams per day (based on studies for oleanolic and ursolic acids), and the one from pharmacokinetic calculations is somewhat higher; using a target in-vivo concentration of 15 μM, the required asiatic acid dose is about 2.1 grams per day. We use the average of 1.3 and 2.1, or 1.7 grams per day as our target human dose, which is equal to a TTFCA dose of about 3.1 grams daily. The commonly prescribed dose of asiatic acid in noncancerous conditions is 33 to 99 milligrams of asiatic acid (60 to 180 milligrams of TTFCA). The LOAEL dose for asiatic acid is roughly 2.7 grams per day (see Appendix J).

Dose calculations for asiatic acid are summarized in Table 21.4. The tentative recommended dose is 1.7 grams per day, a value equal to the target human dose calculated above. Because the target dose is achievable, synergistic interactions may not be required for asiatic acid to have an anticancer effect in humans. Nonetheless, asiatic acid may greatly benefit from synergistic interactions, and it makes sense to test it in combination with other compounds.

Side effects are possible at high doses. The juice of fresh *Centella* plants produced antifertility effects in mice at oral doses equivalent to about 10 grams of whole plant.[50] This amount of plant contains about 280 milligrams of triterpenoids. Antifertility effects were also caused by oleanolic acid in male rats (sperm production was inhibited).[51] Oleanolic acid and other

---

[a] *Because only about 62 percent of the glycoside is asiatic acid by weight (the rest being the sugar group), and because almost all of the glycoside can be cleaved in humans to produce asiatic acid and its sugar, TTFCA actually contains the equivalent of about 55 percent asiatic acid.*

[b] *Ursolic and oleanolic acid are isomers of one another, meaning they have the same chemical formula but a slightly different chemical structure.*

TABLE 21.3 POTENTIAL ANTICANCER ACTIONS OF *CENTELLA*

ACTIVITY	KNOWN EFFECTS	AS A COLLAGENASE INHIBITOR, MAY:	AS A HYALURONIDASE INHIBITOR, MAY:
Chapters 7 and 8: Angiogenesis			
Inhibit angiogenesis		x	x
Inhibit bFGF effects		x	x
Impede increased vascular permeability	x		
Chapters 9 and 10: Invasion and Metastasis			
Inhibit invasion		x	x
Inhibit hyaluronidase, beta-glucuronidase, or elastase	x		—
Inhibit collagenase effects	x	—	
Inhibit cell migration			x
Inhibit metastasis		x	x

TABLE 21.4 ESTIMATED THERAPEUTIC AND LOAEL DOSES FOR ASIATIC ACID*

DESCRIPTION	DOSE (g/day)
Required dose as scaled from animal antitumor studies (for oleanolic and ursolic acids)	1.3
Required cytotoxic dose as determined from pharmacokinetic calculations	2.1
Target dose based on an average from animal antitumor studies and pharmacokinetic calculations	1.7
Minimum required antitumor dose assuming 15-fold synergistic benefits	0.11
Commonly prescribed human dose in noncancerous conditions	0.03 to 0.09
Estimated LOAEL dose	2.7
Tentative dose recommendation for further research	**1.7**
Minimum degree of synergism required	**none**

* *See Appendix J for details.*

triterpenoids also hinder the enzyme testosterone 5 alpha-reductase, an action that can produce antifertility effects but may also make these compounds useful in prostate cancer treatment.[52] In addition to such antifertility effects, TTFCA applied topically to sensitive individuals can cause contact dermatitis.[53]

Since other ursane-type triterpenes reverse the inhibitory effects of boswellic acid on 5-lipoxygenase synthesis, it may be wise to avoid using TTFCA in combination with boswellic acid. Additional in-vitro and in-vivo studies are needed, however, to verify this inhibitory interaction.

Boswellic Acid

Summary of Research and Conclusions

Seven in-vitro studies have reported that boswellic acid inhibited proliferation and/or induced differentiation in leukemia or central nervous system cancer cell lines.[54–60] In addition, cytotoxic effects against two cancer cell lines have been observed by our research group.[61] At least three animal antitumor studies have been published, which found that boswellic acids inhibited the growth of transplanted brain cancer cells and leukemia cells in rodents.[62, 63, 64] Two human studies have also been conducted.[65, 66] These indicated that *Boswellia* extracts or boswellic acid could reduce brain edema or otherwise have a palliative effect in brain cancer patients.

Discussion

Frankincense is the gum resin secreted by the tree *Boswellia serrata* (or *B. carteri*). Frankincense and its close relative myrrh (*Commiphora* species.) have a history of use dating to ancient Egyptian civilizations 5,000 years ago.[67, 68] Both plants are used in Chinese herbal medicine for treating pain from trauma and other swellings. Frankincense is also applied topically to promote healing of sores. A primary active compound in frankincense is boswellic acid, which occurs naturally in both an alpha and beta form (see Figures A.65 and A.66 in Appendix A).

Numerous studies documented that boswellic acid and/or *Boswellia* extracts produce anti-inflammatory effects. For example, the alcohol extract of *Boswellia* produced anti-inflammatory effects in rats at oral doses of 50 mg/kg.[69] Mitigation of chronic arthritis (including a reduction in collagen degradation) was observed at an oral dose of 100 mg/kg in rats; in this study, alcohol extracts were just slightly more effective than boswellic acid alone.[70] Oral doses of 50 to 200 mg/kg of the alcohol extract reduced leukocyte migration at inflammatory sites in rats.[71] Oral administration of boswellic acid at 25 to 100 mg/kg improved chronic arthritis in rabbits.[72] The human equivalents to these animal doses range from about 0.73 to 3.2 grams per day.

Anti-inflammatory effects have also been observed in human studies. In arthritic patients, daily oral doses of about 600 milligrams of boswellic acid for eight weeks reduced symptoms and improved clinical parameters.[72] Oral doses of about 1.1 grams per day of *Boswellia* resin for six weeks reduced signs and symptoms in patients with ulcerative colitis (82 percent went into remission), while daily oral doses of about 900 milligrams for six weeks reduced symptoms in patients with bronchial asthma (70 percent showed improvement).[73, 74]

Boswellic acid has induced differentiation and/or decreased proliferation of leukemia or central nervous system cancer cells in vitro. The effective concentrations ranged from 2 to 40 μM:

TABLE 21.5 POTENTIAL ANTICANCER ACTIONS OF BOSWELLIC ACID			
ACTIVITY	**KNOWN EFFECTS**	**AS AN EICOSANOID INHIBITOR, MAY:**	**AS A HYALURONIDASE INHIBITOR, MAY:**
Chapter 2: Mutations, Gene Expression, and Proliferation			
Inhibit topoisomerases	x		
Chapter 3: Results of Therapy at the Cellular Level			
Induce differentiation	x		
Induce apoptosis	x	x	
Chapter 5: Transcription Factors and Redox Signaling			
Inhibit NF-κB activity		x	
Chapter 6: Cell-to-Cell Communication			
Affect CAMs		x	
Chapters 7 and 8: Angiogenesis			
Inhibit angiogenesis		x	x
Inhibit bFGF effects			x
Inhibit eicosanoid effects	x	—	
Inhibit VEGF effects		x	
Chapters 9 and 10: Invasion and Metastasis			
Inhibit invasion			x
Inhibit hyaluronidase, beta-glucuronidase, or elastase	x	x	—
Inhibit collagenase effects		x	
Inhibit GAG synthesis	x		
Inhibit cell migration	x		x
Inhibit metastasis			x

- Boswellic acid inhibited proliferation of four human brain cancer cell lines at an IC_{50} of 30 to 40 μM.[55]

- Boswellic acid inhibited proliferation of 11 lines of meningiomas obtained from patients at an IC_{50} of 2 to 8 μM.[60]

- Boswellic acid induced differentiation in human leukemia cells at 11 to 22 μM.[63, 75]

- Boswellic acid induced apoptosis in human leukemia cells at an IC_{50} of 30 μM.[58]

- Boswellic acid inhibited proliferation of human leukemia cells by 72 percent at 4 μM.[54]

- Boswellic acid acetate at concentrations of less than 24 μM induced differentiation in three of five leukemia cell lines; the proliferation of all five cell lines was inhibited at concentrations of about 40 μM or less.[57]

In addition to the above, at least one in-vitro study has reported that boswellic acid interacts synergistically with other natural compounds. In that study, boswellic acid was a weak inducer of differentiation in human leukemia cells, but its action greatly increased in the presence of daidzein.[56] The potential anticancer actions of boswellic acid are listed in Table 21.5.

Three animal studies reported that boswellic acid produced antitumor effects. In the first, oral doses of 75, 150, and 300 mg/kg per day reduced the growth of transplanted brain cancer cells in rats.[62] The human equivalent of 150 mg/kg per day in rats is 2.4 grams per day. In the second study, intraperitoneal administration of 25 to 50 mg/kg inhibited growth and induced the differentiation of transplanted leukemia cells in mice.[63, 75] The equivalent human oral dose is about 340 to 680 milligrams per day. In the third, oral administration of 720 mg/kg of *Boswellia* extract increased the survival of rats injected with brain cancer cells.[64] This extract contained 20 percent boswellic acid.[76] The dose of boswellic acid was then about 144 mg/kg, or about 2.3 grams as scaled to humans.

TABLE 21.6   ESTIMATED THERAPEUTIC AND LOAEL DOSES FOR BOSWELLIC ACID*

DESCRIPTION	DOSE (g/day)
Required dose as scaled from animal antitumor studies	0.34 to 2.4
Required dose as scaled from animal anti-inflammatory studies	0.73 to 3.2
Doses used in human anticancer studies	3.6 to 5.4 as *Boswellia* extract†
Required cytotoxic dose as determined from pharmacokinetic calculations	2.3
Target dose based on an average from animal antitumor studies and pharmacokinetic calculations	1.8
Minimum required antitumor dose assuming 15-fold synergistic benefits	0.12
Commonly studied human dose in noncancerous conditions	0.6 (boswellic acid) 0.9 to 1.1 (*Boswellia* extract)
Estimated LOAEL dose	2.7
Tentative dose recommendation for further research	**1.8**
Minimum degree of synergism required	**none**

* See Appendix J for details.
† The concentration of boswellic acid in the Boswellia *extracts used is uncertain.*

At least two human studies have also been conducted. In the first, oral administration of about 3.6 grams daily of *Boswellia* extract tablets reduced brain edema in brain tumor patients.[65] This effect could be attributed largely to its anti-inflammatory action. In another study, on 19 children with brain cancer, a boswellic acid product given orally at a daily average dose of 77 mg/kg for nine months produced palliative benefits, including relief of general symptoms and transient or sometimes longer-lasting regression of neurological symptoms.[66] The equivalent adult dosage would be about 5.4 grams. Because the concentration of boswellic acid in the products used in the human studies is uncertain, the doses of boswellic acid used are also uncertain.

Estimated Therapeutic and LOAEL Doses of Boswellic Acid

The required dose scaled from animal studies is similar to the one calculated from pharmacokinetic and in-vitro data. The former is 340 milligrams to 2.4 grams per day, and doses scaled from anti-inflammatory experiments are similar. Using a target in-vivo concentration of 15 µM, the required boswellic acid dose from pharmacokinetic calculations is about 2.3 grams per day. We use an average of 0.34, 2.4, 2.3, and 2.3 grams, or 1.8 grams per day as our target human dose, which is nearly the same target dose estimated for asiatic acid. This dose also seems reasonable in comparison to the

3.6-gram per day dose of *Boswellia* extract used in the human study on brain tumor patients; the actual boswellic acid content in the extract was not given.

The commonly prescribed dose of *Boswellia* resin for noncancerous conditions in Chinese herbal medicine is 3 to 9 grams per day, although the actual content of boswellic acid in the resin has not been reported. Human anti-inflammatory studies have used doses of 600 milligrams per day of boswellic acid and 0.9 to 1.1 grams of resin per day. The LOAEL dose for boswellic acid is estimated at 2.7 grams daily (see Appendix J).

Dose calculations for boswellic acid are summarized in Table 21.6, with the tentative recommended dose listed as 1.8 grams per day. This value is equal to the target human dose. *Boswellia* extract is the most common source of boswellic acid, and dose estimates for it will differ, depending on its boswellic acid content.

Because the target dose is achievable, synergistic interactions may not be required for boswellic acid to produce an anticancer effect in humans. Still, it may greatly benefit from synergistic interactions and is best tested in combinations.

The dose of 1.8 grams recommended in Table 21.6 might produce analgesic or sedative effects, which could be useful in some situations. Such effects occurred at an intraperitoneal dose of 55 mg/kg in rats but were slight at 20 mg/kg.[77] The equivalent human oral dose of a 55-mg/kg dose in rats is about 1.2 grams.

SAPONINS

Saponins are a special category of isoprenoid glycosides that form colloidal solutions with water and foam when shaken. Removing the glycoside fraction yields aglycones known as sapogenins, which have either a terpenoid or steroid structure.

In this section, we discuss two groups of saponin-rich plants: those generally used to treat vascular or inflammatory problems and those generally used as immune stimulants. Compounds from the first group are not commonly regarded as anticancer agents, but they seem to have promise as part of a multicompound approach.

Their vasoactive characteristics give them the potential for inhibiting angiogenesis, metastasis, and invasion. The two saponins reviewed from this first group come from horse chestnut and butcher's broom. The second group of saponin-rich plants, the immune stimulants, have been more widely studied as cancer treatment agents (see Chapter 12); saponins discussed from this group are from *Panax ginseng*.

Horse Chestnut

Summary of Research and Conclusions

Although horse chestnut has not generally been considered an anticancer agent, one in-vitro study found that horse chestnut saponins are cytotoxic to cancer cells.[78] In this book, we include horse chestnut not as a cytotoxic compound but as one that can protect the vasculature and reduce edema. Through these actions, it should be able to inhibit angiogenesis, metastasis, and invasion. Even though anticancer studies on animals and humans have not yet been done, it seems likely that horse chestnut has a role in cancer treatment.

Discussion

Horse chestnut (*Aesculus hippocastanum*) is used in Western herbal medicine to treat diseases of the venous system. In Germany, preparations of horse chestnut are approved to treat diseases such as thrombophlebitis, varicose veins, and many types of edema. *Aesculus* extracts are the second most prescribed herbal monopreparation in Germany, with annual retail sales of $103 million (U.S. dollars).[79] In Chinese herbal medicine, the seed of a related plant, *A. chinensis*, is used to treat malnutrition and other digestive difficulties at a dose of 3 to 9 grams in decoction. Japanese herbal medicine prescribes the seed of *A. turbinata*, another related plant, to treat digestive difficulties and promote absorption.[80]

Horse chestnut extract is effective against many forms of edema, including brain edema (see Tables 8.1 and F.1). For example, oral administration of 50 to 200 mg/kg in rats and 100 to 200 mg/kg in mice inhibited chemically induced increases in vascular permeability.[81] The human equivalents are about 810 milligrams to 3.2 grams. In a recent meta-analysis of placebo-controlled human trials, horse chestnut extract was superior to placebo in alleviating signs and symptoms of chronic ve-

TABLE 21.7 POTENTIAL ANTICANCER ACTIONS OF ESCIN AND HORSE CHESTNUT EXTRACT

ACTIVITY	KNOWN EFFECTS	AS A HYALURONIDASE INHIBITOR, MAY:
Chapters 7 and 8: Angiogenesis		
Inhibit angiogenesis		x
Inhibit bFGF effects		x
Impede increased vascular permeability	x	
Chapters 9 and 10: Invasion and Metastasis		
Inhibit invasion		x
Inhibit hyaluronidase, beta-glucuronidase, or elastase	x	—
Inhibit cell migration		x
Inhibit metastasis		x

nous insufficiency.[82] The primary active compound in horse chestnut extract is the saponin escin, although other compounds such as flavonoids and the coumarin derivative esculin may add to its effects. The common dose of escin itself is 100 to 150 milligrams per day. For example, an oral dose of 100 milligrams per day decreased leg edema in humans.[83] In animal experiments, escin was 600 times more potent than the flavonoid rutin in reducing edema.[84]

Escin is actually a group of related complex saponins. These saponins contain additional acids and a greater number of sugar molecules than other saponins or glycosides we discuss. The yield of escin from dried horse chestnut seeds is roughly 1.9 to 3.8 percent.[85, 86] Commercial standardized horse chestnut extracts usually contain 16 to 21 percent escin.[87]

The potential anticancer actions of escin are listed in Table 21.7. At least one in-vitro study reported that escin directly inhibited cancer cell proliferation. In that study, the IC_{50} for Ehrlich ascites cells was about 10 µM; normal cells were affected only at much higher concentrations.[78] Although escin is known to cause direct cytotoxicity, the actions in the table are those that may inhibit cancer by indirect, noncytotoxic means. Such actions will likely be the most prominent in vivo.

Estimated Therapeutic and LOAEL Doses of Escin

Because of the poor pharmacokinetic characteristics of escin, cytotoxic concentrations can probably not be achieved in the plasma. Indeed, based on pharmacokinetic and in-vitro data, the cytotoxic dose appears to be about 100 grams, which is 1,000-fold higher than the dose commonly prescribed in noncancerous conditions. Therefore, escin is best used for its potential to inhibit

TABLE 21.8 ESTIMATED THERAPEUTIC AND LOAEL DOSES FOR ESCIN*

DESCRIPTION	DOSE (mg/day)
Required dose as scaled from animal anti-edema studies	150 to 600
Required dose as determined from human anti-inflammatory or anti-edema studies	100 to 150
Required cytotoxic dose as determined from pharmacokinetic calculations	100 grams
Commonly prescribed human dose in noncancerous conditions	100 to 150
Estimated LOAEL dose	150
Tentative dose recommendation for further research	**150**

* *See Appendix J for details.*

TABLE 21.9 ESTIMATED THERAPEUTIC AND LOAEL DOSES FOR RUSCOGENINS*

DESCRIPTION	DOSE (mg/day)
Required cytotoxic dose as determined from pharmacokinetic calculations	1,500[†]
Commonly prescribed human dose in noncancerous conditions	100
Estimated LOAEL dose	130
Tentative dose recommendation for further research	**100 to 130**

* *See Appendix J for details.*

† *Based on an average clearance value obtained from other simple triterpenoids and saponins.*

cancer progression by indirect means. The commonly prescribed escin dose in noncancerous conditions is 100 to 150 milligrams per day. This dose might be sufficient to cause anticancer effects through indirect actions, if horse chestnut is used with other anticancer compounds. Although the LOAEL dose is uncertain, adverse effects may occur at doses significantly above 150 milligrams (see Appendix J).

Dose estimates for escin are summarized in Table 21.8. The tentative dose recommendation of 150 milligrams is based on the upper range of the commonly prescribed dose.

Butcher's Broom

Summary of Research and Conclusions

Like horse chestnut, butcher's broom has not generally been thought of as an anticancer agent. However, at least one in-vitro study suggested that saponins from butcher's broom are cytotoxic to cancer cells.[88] Here we are interested in its ability to protect the vasculature and reduce edema, and thus its potential to inhibit angiogenesis, metastasis, and invasion. As with horse chestnut, the efficacy of butcher's broom in cancer treatment remains to be proven in animals or humans.

Discussion

Butcher's broom (*Ruscus aculeatus*) is an evergreen bush native to the Mediterranean region. It has been used extensively in herbal medicine to treat varicose veins, hemorrhoids, and edema, although it has not received as much research in this area as horse chestnut. The active ingredients include a group of saponins known as ruscogenins, which have vasoconstrictive and anti-inflammatory effects in vivo (see Tables 8.1 and F.1).

The potential anticancer actions of butcher's broom are the same as those for horse chestnut (see Table 21.7). In addition, cytotoxic effects are possible. Some ruscogenins inhibited proliferation of human leukemia cells in vitro, with an IC_{50} of about 4 μM.[88]

Estimated Therapeutic and LOAEL Doses of Butcher's Broom

As stated, butcher's broom is regarded here as an indirect-acting, rather than a cytotoxic compound. Nonetheless, there is a possibility ruscogenins could induce direct cytotoxic effects, with the benefits of synergism. Using a target in-vivo concentration of 15 μM, the required ruscogenin dose needed to cause cytotoxic effects would be about 1.5 grams per day. This dose is greater than the approximate 100-milligram dose commonly prescribed in noncancerous conditions. It is also above the estimated LOAEL dose of 130 milligrams (see Appendix J). Accordingly, at least a 12-fold increase in potency due to synergism would be required to produce direct inhibitory effects. Although this size of increase is theoretically possible, the 1.5-gram target dose is based on very limited pharmacokinetic and in-vitro data. Therefore, while direct effects may be possible in synergistic combinations, it is best at this stage to think of ruscogenins as indirect-acting compounds.

Dose estimates for ruscogenins are summarized in Table 21.9. The tentative dose recommendation is listed as 100 to 130 milligrams, where the lower value is equal to the commonly prescribed dose and the higher is the estimated LOAEL dose.

TABLE 21.10 POTENTIAL ANTICANCER ACTIONS OF GINSENG	
ACTIVITY	**KNOWN EFFECTS**
Chapters 9 and 10: Invasion and Metastasis	
Inhibit cell migration	x
Inhibit platelet aggregation	x
Chapters 11 and 12: Immune System	
Stimulate the immune system	x

Ginseng

Summary of Research and Conclusions

Some 33 in-vitro studies have been conducted on the effects of ginseng extracts or isolated saponins on cancer cells.[89–93] As a whole, these suggest that ginseng or its isolated saponins can inhibit cancer cell proliferation and invasion, usually at 10 to 180 µM (for the saponins).

Fifteen animal studies have been conducted on the antitumor effects of ginseng extracts or its isolated saponins.[94–98] These studies suggest that the extracts and saponins can decrease tumor growth and metastasis and improve survival. The active constituent in the plasma apparently is a metabolite of ginseng saponins, rather than the saponins themselves.

Four anticancer studies have been done with humans using ginseng extracts.[99–102] All were published in the Chinese literature and were not available for review, and all used ginseng in combination with other herbs. Based on the abstracts, these herbal combinations helped cancer patients who were also treated with chemotherapy.

In addition to the above, a number of other animal and human studies have indicated that ginseng can reduce cancer risk.[103, 104, 105] Animal studies reported that it improved the effects of chemotherapy drugs. These will be discussed in Chapter 23.

Ginseng is characterized in this book as an immune stimulant, but it also has the capacity to operate as a direct-acting compound. It could be effective at safe doses when used alone as an immune stimulant or when used in synergistic combinations as a direct-acting compound. The pharmacokinetics and metabolism of ginseng are not well defined, and there are inconsistencies between the doses found effective in animal studies and those calculated from in-vitro and pharmacokinetic data. Due to the inconsistencies, we can estimate the target dose (for direct actions) only within a large range. Nonetheless, even if the effective target dose is at the high end of this range, ginseng could still have direct inhibitory effects at the maximum safe human dose, with the benefits of synergism.

Discussion

Panax ginseng is a commonly used medicinal herb. It is categorized as a *qi* (vital energy) tonic in Chinese herbal medicine, and its use dates back more than 3,000 years. The main active constituents of ginseng are ginsenoside saponins. Although at least 28 ginsenosides have been identified, these can be classified into one of three groups, Ro, Rb, and Rg.[a] The quantity of these saponins in four-year-old roots is about 0.4, 2.3, and 1.1 percent respectively, for a total saponin content of about 3.8 percent.[106] However, in another study on different ginseng samples obtained from herb shops in Taiwan, the average total saponin content was about half this amount, or 1.6 percent.[107]

In addition to the saponins, ginseng also contains a high-molecular-weight polysaccharide (ginsan), which has an immunostimulant effect, and an alcohol (panaxytriol), which causes a reversible cytotoxic effect against various cancer cell lines at about 45 µM.[108, 109] The latter also reduced melanoma growth in mice when administered at 40 mg/kg intramuscularly.[110, 111]

Pharmacological studies have reported that ginseng produces a variety of effects in animals and humans. These include antishock, immune stimulation, sedation, and antifatigue effects, as well as enhancement of memory, inhibition of platelet aggregation, and modulation of the endocrine system.[112–118, 126]

The potential anticancer actions of ginseng are listed in Table 21.10. In addition to these indirect actions, ginseng saponins, and especially a metabolite of ginseng saponins called M1, may cause direct cytotoxic effects against cancer cells.

Several in-vitro studies have reported that ginsenosides inhibited proliferation and invasion of a variety of cell lines at concentrations of roughly 10 to 180 µM, although some cell lines were not affected.[119–123] The metabolite M1 was effective at somewhat lower concen-

---

[a] *Ginsenosides are triterpenoid glycosides of the dammaran series. Ro ginsenosides are oleanolic-based glycosides, Rb ginsenosides are panaxadiol-based glycosides, and Rg ginsenosides are panaxatriol-based glycosides.*

TABLE 21.11 ESTIMATED THERAPEUTIC AND LOAEL DOSES FOR GINSENG[*]

DESCRIPTION	GINSENOSIDE DOSE (mg/day)	GINSENG ROOT DOSE (g/day)
Required dose as scaled from animal antitumor studies	120 to 610	3.2 to 16
Required cytotoxic dose as determined from pharmacokinetic calculations	1,800	47
Target dose based on range from animal antitumor studies and pharmacokinetic calculations	120 to 1,800	3.2 to 47
Minimum required antitumor dose assuming 15-fold synergistic benefits	8 to 120	0.21 to 3.1
Commonly prescribed human dose in noncancerous conditions	110 to 340	3 to 9
Estimated LOAEL dose	340	9
Tentative dose recommendation for further research	**110 to 340**	**3 to 9**
Minimum degree of synergism required for direct inhibition of cancer	uncertain	

[*] *See Appendix J for details.*

trations (one- to fivefold lower) and appeared to be effective on more cell lines. Based on data from three studies, M1 or a related metabolite decreased proliferation or invasion of six different cell lines at an average concentration of roughly 25 µM.[90, 124, 125] Normal cells were affected only at concentrations greater than 130 µM.

Ginseng extracts also inhibited tumor growth in animals. Oral administration of crude ginseng extracts (at 50 to 500 mg/kg) for 10 days significantly reduced tumor growth in melanoma- and sarcoma-bearing mice.[126] The actual content of saponins in these extracts was not specified. If we assume that these were crude extracts yielding 30 percent material (as discussed in Chapter 13), the equivalent human dose of 500 mg/kg in mice is about 16 grams of whole root per day.

Isolated ginseng saponins have also decreased tumor growth and/or metastasis in animals. In sarcoma-bearing mice, intraperitoneal administration of 20 mg/kg of ginsenosides for 8 days reduced tumor weights by as much as 75 percent and increased natural killer cell activity. Inhibition decreased when tumor loads were large.[127, a] The equivalent human oral dose is about 350 milligrams of ginsenosides, or 9.1 grams of root (assuming that the whole root contains about 3.8 percent ginsenosides and that all ginsenosides are equally active).

---

[a] *This article stated only that the ginsenosides were injected; we assume this refers to intraperitoneal injection.*

Daily oral administration of 12 mg/kg of Rb_2 reduced tumor size, metastasis, and angiogenesis in melanoma-bearing mice.[119] The equivalent human dose is about 120 milligrams of Rb_2 per day, or about 3.2 grams of root. Daily oral administration of Rb_1 (at 20 mg/kg) blocked metastasis but not tumor growth in mice injected with lung cancer cells.[128] The equivalent human dose is about 190 milligrams of Rb_2 per day, or 5.1 grams of root.

The in-vivo antitumor effects of ginseng saponins appear due to M1, the primary metabolite of ginsenosides. In one study, orally administered ginseng saponins (Rb_1, Rb_2, Rc) at 20 mg/kg were slightly more effective than 20 mg/kg of M1 in reducing lung metastasis of melanoma cells injected into mice.[124]

Ginseng may also reduce cancer risk. In one study, ginseng extracts inhibited cancer formation in hamster lung cells exposed to carcinogenic chemicals, apparently by inducing DNA repair.[129] Similar effects may occur in vivo. In a study of 4,600 people, those who consumed ginseng regularly had a decreased risk of most cancers.[115, 130] Those who took it more frequently had a lower risk than those taking it less frequently.

Estimated Therapeutic and LOAEL Doses of Ginseng

As discussed, in addition to immune effects ginseng may cause direct cytotoxic effects against cancer cells. Therefore, it is interesting to compare doses scaled from animal experiments to those calculated from pharmacokinetic and in-vitro data. The doses estimated by these two methods are not in close agreement. The required ginseng root dose from the former is 3.2 to 16 grams per day, while that from pharmacokinetic calculations is higher. Using a target in-vivo concentration of 25 µM of ginsenosides, the required ginseng root dose is about 47 grams per day. Considering the differences, we can estimate a target human dose between 3.2 and 47 grams per day. Since the target dose is uncertain, we are also unsure if synergism is necessary to create a direct anticancer effect in humans. At the low end of this range, it would not be, but it would be needed at the high end.

The commonly prescribed dose in noncancerous conditions is about 3 to 9 grams per day of ginseng root. The LOAEL dose is uncertain but, based on the LD_{50}, is estimated to be about 9 grams per day (see Appendix J).

The therapeutic dose estimates are summarized in Table 21.11. The tentative dose recommendation is 3 to 9 grams per day of ginseng root, which is based on the commonly prescribed dose and the estimated LOAEL dose.

Although the target dose is uncertain, a direct anticancer effect may still be possible within the recommended dose range, with the benefits of synergism. Consider a scenario where the target dose is 47 grams of ginseng root and the LOAEL dose is 9 grams. The full 15-fold allowable increase in potency due to synergism would lower the target dose to 3.1 grams, which is below the LOAEL dose. Thus a 9-gram dose could produce a direct anticancer effect, even in a worst-case scenario. A 5.2-fold increase in potency would be required, which is similar to that needed for other direct acting compounds (see Table 13.1).

SESQUITERPENES

Sesquiterpenes are compounds composed of three isoprene units. Like monoterpenes, some sesquiterpenes are found in the essential oils of plants, and like stilbenes, some are phytoalexins (antibiotics of plant origin).

A number of sesquiterpene lactones are cytotoxic in vitro, and some have shown antitumor effects in vivo. In this section, however, we focus exclusively on the sesquiterpene lactone parthenolide, because feverfew, the plant source of parthenolide, has a safe history of use in herbal medicine and commercial feverfew extracts are available that are standardized for parthenolide. In the future, other sesquiterpene lactones may be found promising for cancer treatment.

Many sesquiterpenes, including parthenolide from feverfew, contain a lactone element. One of medicinal interest is artemisinin, from *Artemisia annua* (sweet wormwood), which has been used successfully in treating malaria. There are approximately 3,000 known sesquiterpene lactones, many of which are antibacterial or antifungal.

Feverfew

Summary of Research and Conclusions

At least three in-vitro studies have reported that parthenolide inhibited the proliferation of multiple cancer cell lines.[131, 132, 133] In these studies, parthenolide was active at concentrations between 3 and 9 μM. In addition, cytotoxic effects against two cancer cell lines have been observed by our research group.[61] At least one animal antitumor study has been conducted; in it,

TABLE 21.12 POTENTIAL ANTICANCER ACTIONS OF PARTHENOLIDE				
ACTIVITY	**KNOWN EFFECTS**	**AS A PTK INHIBITOR, MAY:**	**AS A NF-κB INHIBITOR, MAY:**	**AS AN EICOSANOID INHIBITOR, MAY:**
Chapter 3: Results of Therapy at the Cellular Level				
Induce apoptosis		x		x
Chapter 4: Growth Factors and Signal Transduction				
Inhibit PTK	x	—		
Inhibit NF-κB activity	x	x	—	x
Chapter 5: Transcription Factors and Redox Signaling				
Inhibit AP-1 activity		x		
Chapter 6: Cell-to-Cell Communication				
Affect CAMs		x	x	x
Chapters 7 and 8: Angiogenesis				
Inhibit angiogenesis		x	x	x
Inhibit histamine effects		x	x	
Inhibit eicosanoid effects	x	x	x	—
Inhibit TNF effects		x	x	
Inhibit VEGF effects		x		x
Chapters 9 and 10: Invasion and Metastasis				
Inhibit hyaluronidase, beta-glucuronidase, or elastase				x
Inhibit collagenase effects				x
Inhibit GAG synthesis		x		
Inhibit cell migration		x		
Inhibit platelet aggregation	x	x		
Chapters 11 and 12: Immune System				
Inhibit tumor-induced immunosuppression		x		

TABLE 21.13 ESTIMATED THERAPEUTIC AND LOAEL DOSES FOR PARTHENOLIDE*	
DESCRIPTION	**DOSE (mg/day)**
Required dose as scaled from animal antitumor studies	96
Required cytotoxic dose as determined from pharmacokinetic calculations	57
Target dose based on an average from animal antitumor studies and pharmacokinetic calculations	77
Minimum required antitumor dose assuming 15-fold synergistic benefits	5.1
Commonly prescribed human dose in noncancerous conditions	0.54 to 5.8
Estimated LOAEL dose	17
Tentative dose recommendation for further research	**17**
Minimum degree of synergism required	**4.5-fold potency increase**

See Appendix J for details.

sesquiterpene lactones from *Parthenium hysterophorus* inhibited leukemia in mice.[134] Although their composition was not identified, we can assume the sesquiterpene lactones tested included parthenolide.

Discussion

Feverfew (*Tanacetum parthenium*) has been used for centuries as a treatment for migraines and arthritis. The primary active constituents are sesquiterpene lactones, the most important of which appears to be parthenolide. A small number of human clinical studies support the contention that the herb is useful for preventing migraines.[135, 136] In addition to parthenolide, feverfew also contains apigenin and luteolin glycosides.[137]

The parthenolide concentration in feverfew varies with geography and growing conditions. In addition, parthenolide itself is an unstable compound. Therefore, it is not surprising that the parthenolide content of commercial preparations varies greatly; in fact, one analysis of more than 26 feverfew preparations reported that about half contained very low or no parthenolide.[138] Clinical trials with this plant should use standardized extracts, and even then it might be wise to verify the concentration independently.

Although the mechanisms for its cytotoxic action are not well understood, parthenolide does inhibit proliferation of cancer cells in vitro. At concentrations above 5 μM, it irreversibly decreased proliferation of mouse fibrosarcoma and human lymphoma cell lines.[132] Parthenolide also reduced proliferation of human cervical cancer cells at an IC_{50} of 3 μM and nasopharyngeal cancer cells at an IC_{50} of 9.3 μM.[131, 133]

In the one animal antitumor study conducted, oral doses of sesquiterpene lactones (at 10 mg/kg) extracted from the related plant *Parthenium hysterophorus* markedly increased the life span and reduced tumor size in leukemia-bearing mice.[134] Given what we know about the makeup of *P. hysterophorus*, it is likely that parthenolide was a primary constituent in the extract. The equivalent human dose is about 96 milligrams per day of lactones.

The potential anticancer actions of parthenolide are listed in Table 21.12.

Estimated Therapeutic and LOAEL Doses of Parthenolide

The estimated required dose of parthenolide as scaled from animal antitumor studies is in rough agreement with that calculated from pharmacokinetic and in-vitro data, with the dose from animal experiments about 96 milligrams per day and that from pharmacokinetic calculations somewhat lower. Using a target in-vivo concentration of 5 μM, the required daily parthenolide dose is about 57 milligrams. We use an average of these two values, or 77 milligrams per day, as our target human dose.

The commonly prescribed dose in noncancerous conditions is about 5.8 milligrams, based on the labels of some feverfew products that are standardized for parthenolide. Lower doses of 0.54 milligrams were used in some successful studies on migraine patients.[138] At commonly prescribed doses, only mild adverse reactions to parthenolide have been reported, the most common being mouth ulcers, which seems to be a systemic effect. Allergic reactions also occur in some people.[139] The LOAEL dose is uncertain, but based on the LD_{50} of related compounds it is estimated to be about 17 milligrams daily (see Appendix J).

Therapeutic dose estimates for parthenolide are summarized in Table 21.13. The tentative recommended dose range is listed as 17 milligrams per day, which is based on the estimated LOAEL dose.

It appears that synergistic interactions will be required for parthenolide to have an anticancer effect in humans. In comparing the 77-milligram target dose to the 17-milligram one, synergistic interactions are needed to produce about a 4.5-fold increase in potency. This should be possible, since a 4.5-fold increase is well below the allowable 15-fold increase (see Chapter 13).

CONCLUSION

This chapter has focused on a number of terpene compounds. Some of these, such as monoterpenes, tend to inhibit isoprenoid synthesis via feedback inhibition of HMGR, and others, such as boswellic acid, tend to produce anti-inflammatory effects. Others may cause anti-cancer effects through other direct or indirect actions. As a whole, the terpenes do not suffer some of the drawbacks of the phenolic compounds discussed in the previous two chapters. Because they are lipid-soluble, they are more easily absorbed, and therefore lower doses can be used to reach the plasma target concentration. We see then that of the terpenes, only monoterpenes have a recommended dose as high as the 1.8-gram general bioavailability limit, whereas doses this high were common among the phenolics. The reason the monoterpene doses are higher than 1.8 grams is not that they are poorly absorbed, but rather that high plasma concentrations are necessary for cytotoxicity. Moreover, since terpenes are not metabolized to conjugates to the same degree that phenolic compounds are, there are fewer ambiguities regarding their pharmacokinetic characteristics, and therefore dose estimates may be more reliable. Terpenes are not favored over phenolic compounds, however; the use of both together will provide certain advantages. Phenolics and terpenes, because of their different structures and characteristics, will affect different targets in different cellular compartments, thereby helping to assure cancer cells are inhibited through diverse means.

REFERENCES

1 Sahin MB, Perman SM, Jenkins G, Clark SS. Perillyl alcohol selectively induces G0/G1 arrest and apoptosis in Bcr/Abl-transformed myeloid cell lines. Leukemia 1999 Oct; 13(10):1581–91.

2 Ariazi EA, Satomi Y, Ellis MJ, et al. Activation of the transforming growth factor beta signaling pathway and induction of cytostasis and apoptosis in mammary carcinomas treated with the anticancer agent perillyl alcohol. Cancer Res 1999 Apr 15; 59(8):1917–28.

3 Bardon S, Picard K, Martel P. Monoterpenes inhibit cell growth, cell cycle progression, and cyclin D1 gene expression in human breast cancer cell lines. Nutr Cancer 1998; 32(1):1–7.

4 Masuda Y, Nakaya M, Nakajo S, Nakaya K. Geranylgeraniol potently induces caspase-3-like activity during apoptosis in human leukemia U937 cells. Biochem Biophys Res Commun 1997 May 29; 234(3):641–5.

5 He L, Mo H, Hadisusilo S, et al. Isoprenoids suppress the growth of murine B16 melanomas in vitro and in vivo. J Nutr 1997 May; 127(5):668–74.

6 Broitman SA, Wilkinson J 4th, Cerda S, Branch SK. Effects of monoterpenes and mevinolin on murine colon tumor CT-26 in vitro and its hepatic "metastases" in vivo. Adv Exp Med Biol 1996; 401:111–30.

7 Yu SG, Hildebrandt LA, Elson CE. Geraniol, an inhibitor of mevalonate biosynthesis, suppresses the growth of hepatomas and melanomas transplanted to rats and mice. J Nutr 1995 Nov; 125(11):2763–7.

8 Haag JD, Gould MN. Mammary carcinoma regression induced by perillyl alcohol, a hydroxylated analog of limonene. Cancer Chemother Pharmacol 1994; 34(6):477–83.

9 Haag JD, Lindstrom MJ, Gould MN. Limonene-induced regression of mammary carcinomas. Cancer Res 1992 Jul 15; 52(14):4021–6.

10 Shoff SM, Grummer M, Yatvin MB, Elson CE. Concentration-dependent increase of murine P388 and B16 population doubling time by the acyclic monoterpene geraniol. Cancer Res 1991 Jan 1; 51(1):37–42.

11 Elegbede JA, Elson CE, Tanner MA, et al. Regression of rat primary mammary tumors following dietary d-limonene. J Natl Cancer Inst 1986 Feb; 76(2):323–5.

12 Crowell PL. Prevention and therapy of cancer by dietary monoterpenes. J Nutr 1999 Mar; 129(3):775S-778S.

13 Gould MN. Cancer chemoprevention and therapy by monoterpenes. Environ Health Perspect 1997 Jun; 105 Suppl 4:977–9.

14 Vigushin DM, Poon GK, Boddy A, et al. Phase I and pharmacokinetic study of d-limonene in patients with advanced cancer. Cancer Chemother Pharmacol 1998; 42(2):111–7.

15 Ripple GH, Gould MN, Stewart JA, et al. Phase I clinical trial of perillyl alcohol administered daily. Clin Cancer Res 1998 May; 4(5):1159–64.

16 Giri RK, Parija T, Das BR. d-limonene chemoprevention of hepatocarcinogenesis in AKR mice: Inhibition of c-jun and c-myc. Oncol Rep 1999 Sep–Oct; 6(5):1123–7.

17 Crowell PL. Monoterpenes in breast cancer chemoprevention. Breast Cancer Res Treat 1997 Nov–Dec; 46(2–3):191–7.

18 Reddy BS, Wang CX, Samaha H, et al. Chemoprevention of colon carcinogenesis by dietary perillyl alcohol. Cancer Res 1997 Feb 1; 57(3):420–5.

19 Elson CE. Suppression of mevalonate pathway activities by dietary isoprenoids: Protective roles in cancer and cardiovascular disease. J Nutr 1995; 125:1666S-1672S.

20 He L, Mo H, Hadisusilo S, et al. Isoprenoids suppress the growth of murine B16 melanomas in vitro and in vivo. J Nutr 1997; 127:668–674.

21 Gould MN. Personal communication, 1994.

22 Haag JD, Lindstrom MJ, Gould MN. Limonene-induced regression of mammary carcinomas. Cancer Research 1992 Jul 15; 52:4021–6.

23 Gould MN. Chemoprevention of mammary cancer by monoterpenes. Proceedings of the Am Assoc for Can Res 1993; 34:572.

24 Crowell PL, Lin S, Vedejs E, et al. Identification of metabolites of the antitumor agent d-limonene capable of

inhibiting protein isoprenylation and cell growth. Cancer Chemother Pharmacol 1992; 31(3):205–212.

25 Poon GK, Vigushin D, Griggs LJ, et al. Identification and characterization of limonene metabolites in patients with advanced cancer by liquid chromatography/mass spectrometry. Drug Metab Dispos 1996 May; 24(5):565–71.

26 Crowell PL, Elson CE, Bailey HH, et al. Human metabolism of the experimental cancer therapeutic agent d-limonene. Cancer Chemother Pharmacol 1994; 35:31–37.

27 Mills JJ, Chari RS, Boyer IJ, et al. Induction of apoptosis in liver tumors by the monoterpene perillyl alcohol. Cancer Res 1995 Mar 1; 55(5):979–83.

28 Stayrook KR, McKinzie JH, Burke YD, et al. Induction of the apoptosis-promoting protein Bak by perillyl alcohol in the pancreatic ductal adenocarcinoma relative to untransformed ductal epithelial cells. Carcinogeneis 1997; 18(8):1655–58.

29 Stark MJ, Burke YD, McKinzie JH, et al. Chemotherapy of pancreatic cancer with the monoterpene perillyl alcohol. Cancer Lett 1995 Sep 4; 96(1):15–21.

30 Reddy BS, Wang CX, Samaha H, et al. Chemoprevention of colon carcinogenesis by dietary perillyl alcohol. Cancer Res 1997 Feb 1; 57(3):420–5.

31 Anderson P, Yu SG, Kwon R, et al. A comparison of the anticarcinogenic activities of two monoterpenes d-limonene and geraniol. FASEB (Meeting Abstract) 1993; 7(3):A70.

32 Yu SG, Hildebrandt LA, Elson CE. Geraniol, an inhibitor of mevalonate biosynthesis, suppresses the growth of hepatomas and melanomas transplanted to rats and mice. J Nutr 1995 Nov; 125(11):2763–7.

33 Shoff SM, Grummer M, Yatvin MB, Elson CE. Concentration-dependent increase of murine P388 and B16 population doubling time by the acyclic monoterpene geraniol. Cancer Res 1991 Jan 1; 51(1):37–42.

34 Burke YD, Stark MJ, Roach SL, et al. Inhibition of pancreatic cancer growth by the dietary isoprenoids farnesol and geraniol. Lipids 1997; 32:151–156.

35 Gebhardt A, Niendorf A. Effects of pravastatin, a hydroxymethylglutaryl-CoA reductase inhibitor, on two human tumour cell lines. J Cancer Res Clin Oncol 1995; 121(6):343–9.

36 Babu TD, Kuttan G, Padikkala J. Cytotoxic and anti-tumour properties of certain taxa of Umbelliferae with special reference to Centella asiatica (L.) Urban. J Ethnopharmacol 1995 Aug 11; 48(1):53–7.

37 Murray MT. The healing power of herbs. Rocklin, CA: Prima Publishing, 1992, pp. 204–213.

38 Hausen BM. Centella asiatica (Indian pennywort), an effective therapeutic but a weak sensitizer. Contact Dermatitis 1993 Oct; 9(4):175–9.

39 Suguna L, Sivakumar P, Chandrakassan G. Effects of Centella aisiatica extract on dermal wound healing in rats. Indian J Exp Biology 1996; 34(12); 1208–1211.

40 Rao GV, Shivakumar HG, Parthasarathi G. Influence of the aqueous extract of Centella asiatica (brahmi) on experimental wounds in albino rats. Indian J Pharmacol 1996; 28(4):249–253.

41 Kartnig T. Clinical applications of Centella asiatica (L.) Urb. Herbs, Spices, and Medicinal Plants 1988; 3:146–73.

42 Shukla A, Rasik AM, Jain GK, Shankar R, et al. In vitro and in vivo wound healing activity of asiaticoside isolated from Centella asiatica. J Ethnopharmacol 1999 Apr; 65(1):1–11.

43 Rao PS, Seshadri TR. Variation in the chemical composition of Indian samples of Centella asiatica. Current Science 1969; 38:77–79.

44 Es-Saady D, Simon A, Jayat-Vignoles C, et al. MCF-7 cell cycle arrested at G1 through ursolic acid, and increased reduction of tetrazolium salts. Anticancer Res 1996 Jan–Feb; 16(1):481–6.

45 Es-saady D, Simon A, Ollier M, et al. Inhibitory effect of ursolic acid on B16 proliferation through cell cycle arrest. Cancer Lett 1996 Sep 10; 106(2):193–7.

46 Es-Saady D, Najid A, Simon A, et al. Effects of ursolic acid and its analogs on soybean 15-lipoxygenase activity and the proliferation of a human gastric tumor cell line. Mediators of Inflammation 1994; 3:181–184.

47 Njoku CJ, Zeng Lu, Asuzu IU, et al. Oleanolic acid, a bioactive component of the leaves of Ocimum gratissimum (Lamiaceae). Int J Pharmacognosy 1977; 35(2):134–137.

48 Paper DH. Natural products as angiogenesis inhibitors. Planta Medica 1998; 64:686–695.

49 Hsu HY, Yang JJ, Lin CC. Effects of oleanolic acid and ursolic acid on inhibiting tumor growth and enhancing the recovery of hematopoietic system postirradiation in mice. Cancer Lett 1997 Jan 1; 111(1–2):7–13.

50 Dutta T, Basu UP. Crude extract of Centella asiatica and products derived from its glycosides as oral antifertility agents. Indian J Exp Biol 1968 Jul; 6(3):181–2.

51 Rajasekaran M, Bapna JS, Lakshmanan S, et al. Antifertility effect in male rats of oleanolic acid, a triterpene from Eugenia jambolana flowers. J Ethnopharmacol 1988 Sep; 24(1):115–21.

52 Liu J. Pharmacology of oleanolic acid and ursolic acid. J Ethnopharmacol 1995 Dec 1; 49(2):57–68.

53 Eun HC, Lee AY. Contact dermatitis due to madecassol. Contact Dermatitis 1985 Nov; 13(5):310–3.

54 Shao Y, Ho CT, Chin CK, et al. Inhibitory activity of boswellic acids from Boswellia serrata against human leukemia HL-60 cells in culture. Planta Medica 1998; 64:328–331.

55 Glaser T, Winter S, Groscurth P, et al. Boswellic acids and malignant glioma: Induction of apoptosis but no modulation of drug sensitivity. Br J Cancer 1999 May; 80(5–6):756–65.

56 Jing YK, Han R. [Combination induction of cell differentiation of HL-60 cells by daidzein (S86019) and BC-4 or Ara-C.] Yao Hsueh Hsueh Pao 1993; 28(1):11–6.

57 Jing Y, Nakajo S, Xia L, et al. Boswellic acid acetate induces differentiation and apoptosis in leukemia cell lines. Leuk Res 1999 Jan; 23(1):43–50.

58 Hoernlein RF, Orlikowsky T, Zehrer C, et al. Acetyl-11-keto-beta-boswellic acid induces apoptosis in HL-60 and CCRF-CEM cells and inhibits topoisomerase I. J Pharmacol Exp Ther 1999 Feb; 288(2):613–9.

59 Jing Y, Xia L, Han R. Growth inhibition and differentiation of promyelocytic cells (HL-60) induced by BC-4, an active principle from Boswellia carterii Birdw. Chin Med Sci J 1992 Mar; 7(1):12–5.

[60] Park YS, Lee JH, Harwalkar JA, et al. Acetyl-11-keto-beta-boswellic acid (AKBA) is cytotoxic for meningioma cells and inhibits phosphorylation of the extracellular-signal regulated kinase 1 and 2. In press: Eicosanoids and other bioactive lipids in cancer, inflammation and related diseases. Proceedings of the 6th international conference on eicosanoids and other bioactive lipids in cancer inflammation and related diseases held in Boston, MA, Sept. 12–15, 1999.

[61] Boik J, Newman R, Bailey D. Unpublished observations. 1999.

[62] Winking M, Sarikaya S, Jodicke A, et al. Boswellic acids inhibit glioma growth. J Cancer Res Clin Oncol 1998; 124:R141.

[63] Jing Y, Xia L, Han R. Growth inhibition and differentiation of promyelocytic cells (HL-60) induced by BC-4, an active principle from Boswellia carterii Birdw. Chin Med Sci J 1992 Mar; 7(1):12–5.

[64] Winking M, Sarikaya S, Rahmanian A, et al. Boswellic acids inhibit glioma growth: A new treatment option? J Neurooncol 2000; 46(2):97–103.

[65] Safayhi H, Sailer ER. Anti-inflammatory actions of pentacyclic triterpenes. Planta Medica 1997; 63:487–493.

[66] Janssen G, Bode U, Breu H, et al. Boswellic acids in the palliative therapy of children with progressive or relapsed brain tumors. Klin Padiatr 2000 Jul–Aug; 212(4):189–95.

[67] Miller JM, Goodell HB. Frankincense and myrrh. Surg Gynecol Obstet 1968 Aug; 127(2):360–5.

[68] Greene DA. Gold, frankincense, myrrh, and medicine. N C Med J 1993 Dec; 54(12):620–2.

[69] Singh GB, Atal CK. Pharmacology of an extract of salai guggal ex-Boswellia serrata, a new non-steroidal anti-inflammatory agent. Agents Actions 1986 Jun; 18(3–4):407–12.

[70] Kesava Reddy G, Dhar SC, Singh GB. Urinary excretion of connective tissue metabolites under the influence of a new non-steroidal anti-inflammatory agent in adjuvant induced arthritis. Agents Actions 1987 Oct; 22(1–2):99–105.

[71] Sharma ML, Khajuria A, Kaul A, et al. Effect of salai guggal ex-Boswellia serrata on cellular and humoral immune responses and leucocyte migration. Agents Actions 1988 Jun; 24(1–2):161–4.

[72] Sharma ML, Bani S, Singh GB. Anti-arthritic activity of boswellic acids in bovine serum albumin (BSA)-induced arthritis. Int J Immunopharmacol 1989; 11(6):647–52.

[73] Gupta I, Parihar A, Malhotra P, Singh GB, et al. Effects of Boswellia serrata gum resin in patients with ulcerative colitis. Eur J Med Res 1997 Jan; 2(1):37–43.

[74] Gupta I, Gupta V, Parihar A, et al. Effects of Boswellia serrata gum resin in patients with bronchial asthma: Results of a double-blind, placebo-controlled, 6-week clinical study. Eur J Med Res 1998 Nov 17; 3(11):511–4.

[75] Han R. Recent progress in the study of anticancer drugs originating from plants and traditional medicines in China. Chin Med Sci J 1994 Mar; 9(1):61–9.

[76] Daum G. Personal communication with Pharmasan GmbH, Freiburg, Germany, December, 2000.

[77] Menon MK, Kar A. Analgesic and psychopharmacological effects of the gum resin of Boswellia serrata. Planta Med 1971 Apr; 19(4):333–41.

[78] Szydlowska H, Zaporowska E, Kuszlik-Jochym K, et al. Membranolytic activity of detergents as studied with cell viability tests. Folia Histochem Cytochem (Krakow) 1978; 16(2):69–78.

[79] Grunwald J. The European phytomedicines market figures, trends, analyses. Herbalgram Summer 1995; 34:60–5.

[80] Hsu HY, Chen YP, Shen SJ, et al. Oriental materia medica: A concise guide. Long beach, CA: Oriental Healing Arts Institute, 1986, pp. 400–1.

[81] Matsuda H, Li Y, Murakami T, et al. Effects of escins Ia, Ib, IIa, and IIb from horse chestnut, the seeds of Aesculus hippocastanum L., on acute inflammation in animals. Biol Pharm Bull 1997 Oct; 20(10):1092–5.

[82] Pittler MH, Ernst E. Horse-chestnut seed extract for chronic venous insufficiency. A criteria-based systematic review. Arch Dermatol 1998; 134(11):1356–60.

[83] Diehm C, Trampisch HJ, Lange S, Schmidt C. Comparison of leg compression stocking and oral horse-chestnut seed extract therapy in patients with chronic venous insufficiency. Lancet 1996; 347:292–94.

[84] Weiss RF. Herbal medicine. Beaconsfield, England: Beaconsfield Publishers, 1991, p. 188.

[85] Khan L, Ahmad N, Ahmad KD, et al. Commercial extraction of aescin. Int J Pharmacognosy 1995; 33(4):344–5.

[86] Ogawa S. Preparation of pure aescin from horse chestnut seeds. Patent application, Maruzen Chemical Company, Japan.

[87] Tyler V. Herbs of choice: The therapeutic use of phytomedicines. Binghamton, NY: Pharmaceutical Products Press, 1994, p. 113.

[88] Mimaki Y, Kuroda M, Kameyama A, et al. Steroidal saponins from the underground parts of Ruscus aculeatus and their cytostatic activity of HL-60 cells. Phytochemistry 1998; 48(3):485–93.

[89] Duda RB, Zhong Y, Navas V, et al. American ginseng and breast cancer therapeutic agents synergistically inhibit MCF-7 breast cancer cell growth. J Surg Oncol 1999 Dec; 72(4):230–9.

[90] Lee SJ, Sung JH, Lee SJ, et al. Antitumor activity of a novel ginseng saponin metabolite in human pulmonary adenocarcinoma cells resistant to cisplatin. Cancer Lett 1999 Sep 20; 144(1):39–43.

[91] Kim SE, Lee YH, Park JH, Lee SK. Ginsenoside-Rs4, a new type of ginseng saponin concurrently induces apoptosis and selectively elevates protein levels of p53 and p21WAF1 in human hepatoma SK-HEP-1 cells. Eur J Cancer 1999 Mar; 35(3):507–11.

[92] Kim HE, Oh JH, Lee SK, Oh YJ. Ginsenoside RH-2 induces apoptotic cell death in rat C6 glioma via a reactive oxygen- and caspase-dependent but Bcl-X(L)-independent pathway. Life Sci 1999; 65(3):PL33–40.

[93] Oh M, Choi YH, Choi S, et al. Anti-proliferating effects of ginsenoside Rh2 on MCF-7 human breast cancer cells. Int J Oncol 1999 May; 14(5):869–75.

[94] Hasegawa H, Uchiyama M. Antimetastatic efficacy of orally administered ginsenoside Rb1 in dependence on intestinal bacterial hydrolyzing potential and significance of treatment

with an active bacterial metabolite. Planta Med 1998 Dec; 64(8):696–700.

95 Nakata H, Kikuchi Y, Tode T, et al. Inhibitory effects of ginsenoside Rh2 on tumor growth in nude mice bearing human ovarian cancer cells. Jpn J Cancer Res 1998 Jul; 89(7):733–40.

96 Wakabayashi C, Hasegawa H, Murata J, Saiki I. In vivo antimetastatic action of ginseng protopanaxadiol saponins is based on their intestinal bacterial metabolites after oral administration. Oncol Res 1997; 9(8):411–7.

97 Mochizuki M, Yoo YC, Matsuzawa K, et al. Inhibitory effect of tumor metastasis in mice by saponins, ginsenoside-Rb2, 20(R)- and 20(S)-ginsenoside-Rg3, of red ginseng. Biol Pharm Bull 1995 Sep; 18(9):1197–202.

98 Sato K, Mochizuki M, Saiki I, et al. Inhibition of tumor angiogenesis and metastasis by a saponin of Panax ginseng, ginsenoside-Rb2. Biol Pharm Bull 1994 May; 17(5):635–9.

99 Lin SY, Liu LM, Wu LC. [Effects of Shenmai injection on immune function in stomach cancer patients after chemotherapy.] Chung Kuo Chung Hsi I Chieh Ho Tsa Chih 1995 Aug; 15(8):451–3.

100 Cha RJ, Zeng DW, Chang QS. [Non-surgical treatment of small cell lung cancer with chemo-radio-immunotherapy and traditional Chinese medicine.] Chung Hua Nei Ko Tsa Chih 1994 Jul; 33(7):462–6.

101 Li NQ. [Clinical and experimental study on shen-qi injection with chemotherapy in the treatment of malignant tumor of digestive tract.] Chung Kuo Chung Hsi I Chieh Ho Tsa Chih 1992 Oct; 12(10):588–92, 579.

102 Guo XP, Zhang XY, Zhang SD. [Clinical trial on the effects of shikonin mixture on later stage lung cancer.] Chung Hsi I Chieh Ho Tsa Chih 1991 Oct; 11(10):598–9, 580.

103 Kakizoe T. Asian studies of cancer chemoprevention. latest clinical results. Eur J Cancer 2000 Jun 1; 36(10):1303–1309.

104 Shin HR, Kim JY, Yun TK, et al. The cancer-preventive potential of Panax ginseng: A review of human and experimental evidence. Cancer Causes Control 2000 Jul; 11(6):565–76.

105 Keum YS, Park KK, Lee JM, et al. Antioxidant and anti-tumor promoting activities of the methanol extract of heat-processed ginseng. Cancer Lett 2000 Mar 13; 150(1):41–8.

106 Liu CX, Xiao PG. Recent advances on ginseng research in China. J Ethnopharmacol 1992 Feb; 36(1):27–38.

107 Chuang WC, Wu HK, Sheu SJ, et al. A comparative study on commercial samples of ginseng radix. Planta Medica 1995; 61:459–465.

108 Kim KH, Lee YS, Jung IS. Acidic polysaccharide from Panax ginseng, ginsan, induces Th1 cell and macrophage cytokines and generates LAK cells in synergy with rIL-2. Planta Medica 1998; 64:110–115.

109 Lee YS, Chung IS, Lee IR, et al. Activation of multiple effector pathways of immune system by the antineoplastic immunostimulator acidic polysaccharide ginsan isolated from Panax ginseng. Anticancer Res 1997 Jan–Feb; 17(1A):323–31.

110 Matsunaga H, Saita T, Nagumo F, et al. A possible mechanism for the cytotoxicity of a polyacetylenic alcohol,

panaxytriol: Inhibition of mitochondrial respiration. Cancer Chemother Pharmacol 1995; 35(4):291–6.

111 Katano M, Yamamoto H, Matsunaga H, et al. [Cell growth inhibitory substance isolated from Panax ginseng root: Panaxytriol.] Gan To Kagaku Ryoho 1990 May; 17(5):1045–9.

112 Rhee YH, Ahn JH, Choe J, et al. Inhibition of mutagenesis and transformation by root extracts of Panax ginseng in vitro. Planta Med 1991 Apr; 57(2):125–8.

113 Yun TK. Experimental and epidemiological evidence of the cancer-preventive effects of Panax ginseng C.A. Meyer. Nutr Rev 1996 Nov; 54(11 Pt 2):S71–81.

114 Wang LCH, Lee TF. Effect of ginseng saponins on exercise performance in non-trained rats. Planta Medica 1998; 64:130–133.

115 Yun TK, Choi SY. Preventive effect of ginseng intake against various human cancers: A case-control study on 1987 pairs. Cancer Epidemiol Biomarkers Prev 1995 Jun; 4(4):401–8.

116 Yun TK, Choi SY. A case-control study of ginseng intake and cancer. Int J Epidemiol 1990 Dec; 19(4):871–6.

117 Scaglione F, Ferrara F, Dugnani S, et al. Immunomodulatory effects of two extracts of Panax ginseng C.A. Meyer. Drugs Exp Clin Res 1990; 16(10):537–42.

118 Takagi K, Saito H, Tsuchiya M. Pharmacological studies of Panax Ginseng root: Pharmacological properties of a crude saponin fraction. Jpn J Pharmacol 1972 Jun; 22(3):339–46.

119 Mochizuki M, Yoo YC, Matsuzawa K, et al. Inhibitory effect of tumor metastasis in mice by saponins, ginsenoside-Rb2, 20(R)- and 20(S)-ginsenoside-Rg3, of red ginseng. Biol Pharm Bull 1995 Sep; 18(9):1197–202.

120 Hasegawa H, Sung JH, Matsumiya S, et al. Reversal of daunomycin and vinblastine resistance in multidrug-resistant P388 leukemia in vitro through enhanced cytotoxicity by triterpenoids. Planta Med 1995 Oct; 61(5):409–13.

121 Nakata H, Kikuchi Y, Tode T, et al. Inhibitory effects of ginsenoside Rh2 on tumor growth in nude mice bearing human ovarian cancer cells. Jpn J Cancer Res 1998; 89(7):733–40.

122 Park JA, Lee KY, Oh YJ, et al. Activation of caspase-3 protease via a Bcl-2-insensitive pathway during the process of ginsenoside Rh2-induced apoptosis. Cancer Lett 1997 Dec 16; 121(1):73–81.

123 Atoplina LN, Malinovskaya GV, Elyakov GB, et al. Cytotoxicity of natural ginseng glycosides and semisynthetic analogues. Planta Medica 1999; 65:30–40.

124 Wakabayashi C, Hasegawa H, Murata J, Saiki I. In vivo antimetastatic action of ginseng protopanaxadiol saponins is based on their intestinal bacterial metabolites after oral administration. Oncol Res 1997; 9(8):411–7.

125 Wakabayashi C, Murakami K, Hasegawa H, et al. An intestinal bacterial metabolite of ginseng protopanaxadiol saponins has the ability to induce apoptosis in tumor cells. Biochem Biophys Res Commun 1998; 246(3):725–30.

126 Chen X, Liu H, Lei X, et al. Cancer chemopreventive and therapeutic activities of red ginseng. J Ethnopharmacology 1998; 60:71–78.

127 Yang G, Yu Y. Effects of ginsenoside on the natural killer cell-interferon-interleukin-2 regulatory network and its tumor inhibiting effect. J of Trad Chin Med 1988; 8(2):135–140.

128 Hasegawa H, Uchiyama M. Antimetastatic efficacy of orally administered ginsenoside Rb1 in dependence on intestinal bacterial hydrolyzing potential and significance of treatment with an active bacterial metabolite. Planta Medica 1998; 64:696–700.

129 Rhee YH, Ahn JH, Choe J, et al. Inhibition of mutagenesis and transformation by root extracts of Panax ginseng in vitro. Planta Medica 1991; 57:125–28.

130 Yun TK, Choi SY. Non-organ specific cancer prevention of ginseng: A prospective study in Korea. Int J Epidemiol 1998; 27(3):359–64.

131 Hoffmann JJ, Torrance SJ, Widehopf RM, Cole JR. Cytotoxic agents from Michelia champaca and Talauma ovata: Parthenolide and costunolide. J Pharm Sci 1977 Jun; 66(6):883–4.

132 Ross JJ, Arnason JT, Birnboim HC. Low concentrations of the feverfew component parthenolide inhibit in vitro growth of tumor lines in a cytostatic fashion. Planta Med 1999 Mar; 65(2):126–9.

133 Woynarowski JM, Konopa J. Inhibition of DNA biosynthesis in HeLa cells by cytotoxic and antitumor sesquiterpene lactones. Mol Pharm 1981; 19:97–102.

134 Mukherjee B, Chatterjee M. Antitumor activity of Parthenium hysterophorus and its effect in the modulation of biotransforming enzymes in transplanted murine leukemia. Planta Med 1993 Dec; 59(6):513–6.

135 Murphy JJ, Heptinstall S, Mitchell JRA. Randomised double-blind placebo-controlled trial of feverfew in migraine prevention. Lancet 1988 Jul 23; 2(8604):189–92.

136 Johnson ES, Kadam MP, Hylands DM, et al. Efficacy of feverfew as prophylactic treatment of migraine. Br Med J (Clin Res Ed) 1985 Aug 31; 291(6495):569–73.

137 Williams CA, Hoult JR, Harborne JB, et al. A biologically active lipophilic flavonol from Tanacetum parthenium. Phytochemistry 1995 Jan; 38(1):267–70.

138 Heptinstall S, Awang DV, Dawson BA, et al. Parthenolide content and bioactivity of feverfew (Tanacetum parthenium (L.) Schultz-Bip.). Estimation of commercial and authenticated feverfew products. J Pharm Pharmacol 1992 May; 44(5):391–5.

139 Groenewegen WA, Knight DW, Heptinstall S. Progress in the medicinal chemistry of the herb feverfew. Prog Med Chem 1992; 29:217–38.

Three lipid-soluble vitamins, A, D₃, and E, are discussed here. Each is related to the terpene (isoprenoid) compounds covered in the previous chapter; vitamins A and E contain isoprene side chains, and vitamin D₃ is a hormone with a steroidlike structure. This chapter also reviews melatonin, another natural hormone. The structures of all four compounds are illustrated in Figures A.75 to A.81 of Appendix A.

VITAMIN A

Summary of Research and Conclusions

The active metabolite of vitamin A, all-*trans* retinoic acid, or ATRA, has received a fair amount of research as an anticancer compound. In fact, ATRA is now a prescription drug approved by the Food and Drug Administration for the treatment of some types of cancers. Because this book concentrates on compounds not yet approved as drugs (see Chapter 1), our discussions focus on vitamin A (retinol), covering ATRA only in its role as a metabolite. More specifically, we focus on the form of retinol commonly found in foods and supplements, the retinyl ester form (i.e., retinyl palmitate). ATRA remains a viable treatment compound, however, and it may be preferable in some situations. For information on the use of ATRA, the reader is referred to drug reference books and manufacturer's literature.

Each of the three forms of vitamin A—retinyl esters, retinol, and ATRA—can inhibit cancer cells in vitro and in vivo, and each is produced in the plasma after oral administration of retinyl esters; of the three, the retinyl ester form occurs at the highest concentration after retinyl ester administration, and seems to have the greatest inhibitory effect on cancer. Once taken up by the cancer cell, retinyl esters are metabolized to ATRA, and in that form they subsequently decrease proliferation.

Some 23 in-vitro studies have investigated the cytotoxicity of retinol or its retinyl ester forms against cancer cells.[1-5] These studies reported that concentrations between 1 and 30 μM of either compound inhibited proliferation of a variety of cell lines. At least 12 animal studies have also been conducted, and as a whole, they reported that oral or intraperitoneal administration of retinol or retinyl esters reduced tumor growth.[6-10]

Seven human studies have been conducted.[11-17] One of these was a phase I trial, and was therefore designed to determine the maximum safe dose. One reported that retinol was ineffective in late-stage cancer, but the remaining 5 found that oral retinol or retinyl esters inhibited acute non-lymphocytic leukemia or improved disease-free survival in patients previously treated for lung cancer.

A much larger number of in-vitro, animal, and human studies have investigated the anticancer effects of ATRA; overall, these reported that ATRA inhibited the growth of a variety of cancers. Several hundred such studies have been conducted in total.[18-22]

Roughly 10 animal and human studies examined the effects of retinol or retinyl esters in combination with immunotherapy and/or chemotherapy. These are discussed in Chapter 23.

A large number of in-vitro and animal studies have investigated the cancer-preventive effects of retinol or retinyl esters. In addition, several human cancer prevention trials have been conducted, and many more are in progress or being planned.[23-26] These have indicated that retinol or retinyl esters can reduce cancer risk, but many unknowns remain.

Because of inconsistent results between studies and a large variation in the maximum tolerated dose between individuals, the target and safe doses of retinyl esters can be estimated only within large ranges. Nevertheless, they could still be effective if used synergistically.

Introduction

To be precise, the term *vitamin A* refers to a group of compounds that possess the biologic activity of all-*trans* retinol, the fundamental dietary form of vitamin A. Actually, all-*trans* retinol (referred to hereafter simply as retinol) exists naturally in food as retinyl esters (retinol combined with a fatty acid), such as retinyl palmitate. The supplement forms of vitamin A are also composed of retinyl esters, usually retinyl acetate or retinyl palmitate. The metabolites of retinol are much more biologically active than retinol itself. The two primary groups of retinol metabolites are retinal, which is involved with vision and reproduction, and retinoic acid compounds, which are important in many other functions, including cell proliferation, differentiation, and immune function.[27, 28, a] The two primary retinoic acids are all-*trans*

---

[a] *The name* retinol *is derived from* retina, *signifying its effects on the eye.*

TABLE 22.1 CYTOTOXIC EFFECTS OF RETINOL	
CELL LINE	**COMMENTS**
Human breast cancer cells	Retinol inhibited proliferation at an IC_{50} of about 1 µM. Resistant clones of these cells were only marginally inhibited.[29]
	Retinol inhibited proliferation at an IC_{50} of about 3 µM. ATRA was less effective.[6]
Human leukemia cells	Retinol inhibited proliferation by 35 percent at 10 µM. ATRA inhibited proliferation by 50 percent at the same concentration.[30]
Human myeloid leukemia cells	At physiologic concentrations of retinol (1 to 3 µM), bound to its carrier protein, cell proliferation was inhibited after three to four days. At higher concentrations (10 µM), differentiation was induced in 40% of the cells.[41]
Human melanoma cells	Retinol was as effective as ATRA at inhibiting proliferation (about 40% inhibition at 1 µM), but clones of the melanoma cells exhibited variable sensitivity to both retinol and ATRA.[31]
Human retinoblastoma cells	Retinol inhibited proliferation at an IC_{50} of about 25 µM, whereas ATRA was only marginally effective.[32]
Mouse liver cancer cells	Retinol at 1 and 10 µM inhibited proliferation by about 38 and 50 percent, respectively. Retinol was less effective on human adenocarcinoma cells.[33]
Osteosarcoma cells	Retinol at 10 µM inhibited proliferation and invasion. Lower concentrations (10 nM) appeared to enhance invasion.[5]

retinoic acid (ATRA) and 9-*cis*-retinoic acid. Because of their effects on proliferation and differentiation, the retinoic acids, especially ATRA, have been studied as anticancer agents.

In this book, we focus on the potential of retinyl esters as anticancer compounds. Oral administration of retinyl esters results in elevated plasma concentrations of retinyl esters, retinol, and ATRA, as already mentioned. The metabolism, plasma transport, and tissue uptake of these vitamin A compounds is complex and occurs by mechanisms quite different from those of almost all other compounds we discuss (although there are some similarities with vitamin E). The details of these mechanisms are discussed in Appendix J. Briefly, orally administered retinyl esters are incorporated along with other fatty substances, such as triglycerides and cholesterol, into a group of fatty substances called chylomicrons. Chylomicrons, in turn, are transported into the general blood circulation via the lymphatic system. Once in the circulation, chylomicron remnants can be absorbed by the liver and other tissues. In many tissues, the uptake of chylomicron remnants is mediated by the low-density lipoprotein (LDL) receptor. After entering the tissues, and especially the liver, retinyl esters can be further metabolized to retinol and then to ATRA or other retinoic acids. Retinol and ATRA in turn leave the liver

and reenter the circulation bound to specific carrier proteins.

In recent years, cancer research on vitamin A has concentrated on the use of ATRA or other forms of retinoic acid. One reason is that direct administration of ATRA bypasses the need for its metabolism from retinol. Nonetheless, administration of retinyl esters can also be effective; these have shown cytotoxic effects in vitro at physiological concentrations as well as antitumor effects in animals and humans. Retinyl esters are attractive anticancer compounds for the following reasons:[34]

- They are present at much higher concentrations than ATRA in vivo. Furthermore, plasma concentrations of retinyl esters are consistently increased by oral administration. In contrast, when ATRA is administered, its bioavailability (as measured by the area under the concentration-time curve) tends to decrease with repeated administration, since detoxification enzymes are induced.

- Cancer cells, such as some leukemic cells, express specific uptake mechanisms for retinyl esters in chylomicrons.[35]

- In some cancer cell lines, retinyl esters in chylomicrons are at least as potent as ATRA in inhibiting proliferation and inducing differentiation.

- Retinyl esters are less likely to cause adverse effects than ATRA.

In-vitro Effects of Retinol and Retinyl Esters

Most in-vitro studies on vitamin A do not closely mimic in-vivo conditions.[34] In vivo, healthy tissues and cancer cells uptake retinyl esters in chylomicrons, but uptake retinol and ATRA as bound to carrier proteins. In most in-vitro studies, however, retinol, retinyl esters, and ATRA are generally dissolved in a solvent before being added to the culture. Thus most in-vitro systems do not account for the specific transport and uptake that occurs in vivo. In addition, the concentration of serum or albumin in the culture medium can greatly affect the results of the study.[36] For these reasons, results from most in-vitro studies should be interpreted carefully.

Well over a dozen studies have investigated the in-vitro cytotoxicity of retinol, some of which are summarized in Table 22.1. Note that the sensitivity of tumor clones to retinol varies, which is in keeping with the discussions in Appendix J. In general, the studies suggested that retinol concentrations of 1 to 25 μM (average of about 7 μM) inhibited proliferation of a variety of cancer cell lines. Although this average concentration is only slightly larger than normal retinol plasma concentrations of 1 to 3 μM, such cytotoxic concentrations are not easily achieved with oral administration. For example, one study reported that daily oral administration of 300,000 I.U. of retinol increased plasma concentrations only by about 20 percent.[41-44] For this and other reasons, the elevated plasma retinyl ester concentrations produced after oral administration of retinyl esters may be more effective than the retinol concentrations produced.

A smaller number of studies have noted the cytotoxic effects of retinyl esters (see Table 22.2). As shown, retinyl ester concentrations of 1 to 30 μM (average of about 10 μM) are effective in inhibiting cell proliferation. This is similar to the concentrations reported effective for retinol. After administration of retinyl esters, however, retinyl esters are present in much higher plasma concentrations than retinol. For example, one study reported that after a test meal containing about 90,000 I.U. of retinyl esters, peak concentrations were about 25 μM, whereas retinol concentrations remained at about 1 to 3 μM.[45]

The fourth study listed is of particular interest, since it suggests that retinyl esters bound to chylomicron remnants may be more effective than retinol bound to its carrier protein for some cell lines. In this study, the authors obtained chylomicron remnants from a patient who had been taking 50,000 I.U. of retinol daily for four years. At the concentration present in plasma, the chylomicrons induced differentiation and almost completely inhibited the proliferation of human leukemia cells in vitro.

TABLE 22.2	CYTOTOXIC EFFECTS OF RETINYL ESTERS
CELL LINE	**COMMENTS**
Human leukemia cells	At 10 μM, retinyl palmitate in chylomicron remnants induced differentiation and inhibited proliferation.[37]
Human leukemic cells	At 10 μM, retinyl esters in chylomicron remnants almost completely inhibited proliferation.[38]
Human myeloid and lymphoid leukemic cells	At 5 to 10 μM, retinyl esters in chylomicron remnants inhibited proliferation of three myeloid cell lines. Differentiation was induced in two of these lines. The same concentration inhibited proliferation of one of four lymphoid lines, and it also inhibited proliferation of three of six cell lines obtained from patients with leukemia. Acute lymphocytic leukemia cells were not inhibited, but myeloid leukemia cells were.[39]
Leukemic blast cells taken from a patient with acute promyelocytic leukemia	At 1 μM, retinyl palmitate bound to chylomicron remnants was far more effective in inhibiting cell proliferation than retinol bound to its carrier protein (at 3 μM) or retinyl esters bound to LDL (at 0.3 μM).[45]
Human lung cancer cells	Retinyl acetate inhibited invasion at a nontoxic IC_{50} of 0.27 μM and inhibited proliferation at an IC_{50} of about 30 μM. On a molar basis, retinyl palmitate was equally or more effective.[40]

Vitamin A, in whatever form, may inhibit cancer progression through a number of mechanisms; its potential anticancer actions are listed in Table 22.3.

In-vivo Effects

A number of animal studies have reported that administration of retinol or retinyl esters can inhibit tumor growth. For example, oral administration of 38,000 I.U. and above of retinol (as scaled to humans) decreased growth of transplanted human breast cancer cells in mice by more than 50 percent.[6, a] In another experiment, oral administration of 32,000 I.U. of retinol (as scaled to humans) produced a complete remission in 20 percent of rats with transplanted squamous cell carcinoma and a partial response in the other 80 percent.[7] (Oral retinol will also increase plasma retinyl ester concentrations.) Retinol was also effective when administered intraperitoneally.[9]

Oral or intraperitoneal administration of retinyl esters have been tested in at least three animal studies.[46, 47, 48] In all cases, however, only low doses were used (the human oral equivalent of about 190, 440, and 1,700 I.U.). Two of the studies reported reduced tumor

---

[a] One I.U. is equal to 0.3 μg of retinol, 0.344 μg of retinyl acetate, and 0.550 μg of retinyl palmitate. Retinyl esters in the plasma, as well as in supplements, tend to be primarily retinyl palmitate. We use a value of 0.49 μg per I.U. here for mixed retinyl esters.

TABLE 22.3 POTENTIAL ANTICANCER ACTIONS OF VITAMIN A		
ACTIVITY	KNOWN EFFECTS	AS A COLLAGENASE INHIBITOR, MAY:
Chapter 2: Mutations, Gene Expression, and Proliferation		
Inhibit topoisomerases	x	
Chapter 3: Results of Therapy at the Cellular Level		
Induce differentiation	x	
Induce apoptosis	x	
Improve TGF-beta signaling	x	
Chapter 4: Growth Factors and Signal Transduction		
Induce *p21* or *p27* activity	x	
Chapter 6: Cell-to-Cell Communication		
Affect CAMs	x	
Improve gap junction communication	x	
Chapters 7 and 8: Angiogenesis		
Inhibit angiogenesis	x	x
Inhibit bFGF effects		x
Chapters 9 and 10: Invasion and Metastasis		
Inhibit invasion		x
Inhibit collagenase effects	x	—
Inhibit metastasis		x

growth, an effect probably due to enhanced immune response.

Human studies have also suggested that retinol or retinyl esters may have anticancer effects; most of these were conducted on patients with acute nonlymphocytic leukemia. Four studies are summarized below:

- Administration of retinyl palmitate (at 16,000 I.U. per day) induced differentiation of bone marrow cells in five patients with acute nonlymphocytic leukemia. In three of the four patients who underwent conventional chemotherapy, the sequential treatment with retinyl palmitate resulted in complete remission.[49]

- In a case report, administration of retinyl palmitate (about 270,000 I.U. per day, or 150,000 I.U. per square meter) to one woman with acute myelogenous leukemia induced differentiation of her bone marrow cells.[17]

- In a case report, a woman with advanced promyelocytic leukemia showed a dramatic decrease in clinical symptoms (for example, a reduced leukocyte count) during daily administration of 210,000 I.U. of retinyl palmitate.[12] Her condition remained improved for six weeks of treatment until it was discontinued due to side effects, after which the proliferation of leukemic cells greatly increased.

- In a series of studies on children with acute myelogenous leukemia, a revised treatment protocol was compared against a protocol used by the authors

in previous years.[13] The original chemotherapy protocol produced an event-free rate of about 20 percent at six years. The revised protocol, which contained a change in chemotherapy and daily administration of 50,000 I.U. of retinyl palmitate during remission, resulted in an event-free rate of about 60 percent at six years. The authors speculated that adding retinyl esters to the treatment protocol contributed to the improved results. No side effects were seen at this dose.

Other human studies indicated that retinol or retinyl esters may be effective in preventing recurrence. In a 14-month trial in 181 patients with postsurgical non-small-cell lung cancer, recurrence rates were lower in the group receiving retinyl esters (at 300,000 I.U. per day) as compared to controls (18 percent versus 28 percent). Mild signs of toxicity were seen in some patients at this dose. After 46 months, the rates for tumor recurrence or the development of new primary tumors were 37 percent in the treated group and 48 percent in controls.[50, 51, 52]

Lastly, one phase II trial suggested that oral retinol may have no effect on cancer progression. Oral administration of about 360,000 I.U. (200,000 I.U. per square meter of surface area) did not appreciably affect tumor progression in 65 patients with a variety of advanced cancers (mostly lung cancer, melanoma, and colon cancer).[16] Side effects occurred in 38 percent, and although most of these were mild, 20 percent did develop acute central nervous system symptoms. In all cases, the side effects were reversible with discontinued treatment. The 360,000 I.U. dose was determined to be the maximum tolerated dose in a previous phase I trial.[15] The fact that retinol was not effective in this study is not of great concern. Both retinol and retinyl esters are likely to require synergistic interactions if they are to be consistently useful in humans. What is significant is that anticancer effects were observed in some human trials, even without synergism.

A larger number of human studies have been conducted on ATRA. It has undergone more than a dozen phase I and phase II trials for different cancers, both as a single agent and as a component of a multidrug regime.[53-58] ATRA is in fact approved for treating acute promyelocytic leukemia (PML) and is being evaluated as a treatment for a variety of other human cancers. In PML, orally administered ATRA produced complete remissions in as many as 80 percent of patients.[59]

Estimated Therapeutic and Tolerated Doses of Retinyl Esters

Of the three forms of vitamin A discussed here, we focus on retinyl esters. Retinyl esters are the form least toxic to the liver, and they occur naturally in foods, have unique means for plasma transport and tissue uptake, possess antitumor activity, and can be metabolized in vivo to retinol and ATRA.

At low doses, retinyl esters can support immune function or produce anticancer effects in other indirect ways. Antitumor effects were observed in two of three animal studies that used low doses (about 190 to 1,700 I.U. per day, as scaled to humans). Our calculations, however, are concerned with the dose needed to directly inhibit cancer, so we will not discuss the animal data further.

The estimated required dose of retinyl esters based on human anticancer studies does not closely agree with that calculated from pharmacokinetic and in-vitro data. Furthermore, the doses used in human studies cover a very wide range (16,000 to 270,000 I.U. per day, average of 140,000 I.U.). Again, the doses at the low end of this range would tend to have indirect, rather than direct effects on cancer. The required dose based on pharmacokinetic calculations is higher. Using a target in-vivo concentration of 10 μM for retinyl esters, the required retinyl ester dose is about 740,000 I.U. per day. Because the target human dose is uncertain, it can be estimated only within a large range—140,000 I.U. to 740,000 I.U. per day. It is also uncertain whether synergistic interactions will be needed for an anticancer effect in humans. At the low end of this range, synergism would not be needed but would be at the high end.

The commonly prescribed retinyl ester dose in noncancerous conditions (for general health maintenance) is 2,500 to 5,000 I.U. The maximum tolerated dose is estimated from 50,000 to 600,000 I.U. per day, which again is a large range. Therapeutic dose estimates are given in Table 22.4. The tentative dose recommendation is 50,000 to 600,000 I.U. daily of retinyl esters, which is based on the estimated maximum tolerated dose.

TABLE 22.4 ESTIMATED THERAPEUTIC AND LOAEL DOSES FOR RETINYL ESTERS*

DESCRIPTION	DOSE (I.U./day)
Required dose based on human anticancer studies	16,000 to 270,000 (average of 140,000)
Required cytotoxic dose as determined from pharmacokinetic calculations	740,000
Target dose based on range from human and animal studies and pharmacokinetic calculations	140,000 to 740,000
Minimum required antitumor dose assuming 15-fold synergistic benefits	9,300 to 49,000
Commonly prescribed human dose in noncancerous conditions	2,500 to 5,000
Estimated maximum tolerated dose	50,000 to 600,000
Tentative dose recommendation for further research	**50,000 to 600,000**
Minimum degree of synergism required	**uncertain**

* *See Appendix J for details.*

An anticancer effect may be possible within the recommended dose range, if synergism is employed. If the target dose is 740,000 I.U. and the maximum tolerated dose is only 50,000 I.U., the full 15-fold allowable increase in potency due to synergism would lower the target dose to 49,000 I.U., which is below the maximum tolerated dose. Thus a 50,000-I.U. dose could produce an anticancer effect, with the benefits of synergism. Still, a 15-fold increase in potency would be required, which is higher than that required for other direct-acting compounds, as listed in Table 13.1.

Signs of toxicity after retinyl ester supplementation include chapped lips and dry skin, followed later by headache, fatigue, joint pain, and emotional lability. Liver damage can occur with high doses, and children are more susceptible to toxicity than adults. Chronic doses greater than 5,000 I.U. per day are best monitored by a physician to assure safety. Although some references caution that women at risk of becoming pregnant should not take retinol supplements because of its potential to cause birth defects, others suggest that up to 30,000 I.U. could be safe for pregnant women.[60]

Beta-Carotene and Cancer

Even though beta-carotene is not fully covered in this book, it is of interest for several reasons: it can be converted to vitamin A in vivo, it may have an effect on cancer risk, and it is widely used as a supplement. However, the results of human trials using beta-carotene are conflicting. Although high plasma levels of beta-carotene from dietary intake tend to be associated with reduced cancer risk, studies also indicated that beta-carotene supplements may actually increase cancer risk, at least in smokers. The reasons are not clear but could be due to beta-carotene's effects on carcinogen metabolism, free radical production from oxidized beta-carotene, or both. Until more information is available, it seems reasonable for cancer patients, especially those who smoke, to avoid beta-carotene supplementation (especially as a sole supplement) but to continue eating beta-carotene-rich foods as usual. Selected studies on beta-carotene and cancer are summarized below:

- In a review of prediagnostic plasma levels of beta-carotene, selenium, vitamin A, and vitamin E from 10 study populations for 10 cancer sites, plasma levels were slightly lower for all four micronutrients among those diagnosed with cancer. The strongest association was between low levels of beta-carotene and the subsequent development of lung cancer. Results indicated it is unlikely that any single one of these micronutrients is associated with protection against all cancer types.[61]

- In a study of 5,200 Italians, breast cancer risk was lower for those eating diets rich in beta-carotene, vitamin E, and calcium.[62]

- In a study of 15,000 women, the risk of cervical cancer was nearly triple in those women with a low concentration of total plasma carotenoids (e.g., beta-carotene, lycopene) as compared to women with high levels.[63]

- A review of epidemiologic studies associated high plasma levels of beta-carotene with a reduced risk for a number of human cancers, especially epithelial cancers.[64]

- Analysis of blood samples of 26,000 adults in Maryland found that high levels of beta-carotene and vitamin E were associated with decreased cancer risk of oral and pharyngeal cancer. Persons with the highest levels of total carotenoids exhibited an approximate 66 percent reduction in risk compared to the group with the lowest levels.[65]

- Based on data obtained from 25,000 volunteers, high plasma beta-carotene levels were associated with decreased risk of lung cancer.[66]

- Other epidemiological studies of the cancer-preventive effects of beta-carotene and other antioxidants have been inconclusive, partially because the beneficial effects have been small and easily influenced by confounding factors.[67]

- In a study of 530 men with oral leukoplakia and/or chronic esophagitis (risk factors for cancers of the mouth and esophagus), administration of retinol, beta-carotene, and vitamin E reduced the prevalence of leukoplakia after 6 months and the risk of progression of chronic esophagitis after 20 months.[68]

- In the Alpha-Tocopherol, Beta-Carotene prevention study (ATBC), administration of beta-carotene (at 20 milligrams per day) for 5 to 8 years to 29,000 Finnish male smokers 50 to 69 years of age increased the rate of lung cancer by 18 percent.[69, 70, 71]

- In the Beta-Carotene and Retinol Efficiency Trial (CARET), about 4,000 men exposed to asbestos and 14,000 male and female smokers were administered a combination of 30 milligrams of beta-carotene and 25,000 I.U. of retinol per day. The trial was stopped 21 months early because of evidence of no benefit but substantial harm; there were 28 percent more lung cancers and 17 percent more deaths in the treatment group. Presumably, this adverse effect was caused by beta-carotene rather than vitamin A, as beta-carotene produced similar results in the ATBC study.[72-77]

VITAMIN D$_3$

Summary of Research and Conclusions

At least 133 in-vitro studies have been published on the cytotoxic effects of the active metabolite of vitamin D$_3$, 1,25-D$_3$.[78-82] Sixteen of these were conducted on a combination of 1,25-D$_3$ and retinoids, with most suggesting that the two compounds interact additively or synergistically.[83-87] In the studies on 1,25-D$_3$ alone, cell differentiation and inhibition of invasion and cell proliferation generally occurred in the concentration range of 0.01 to 1 μM.[88-93] 1,25-D$_3$ was effective against a wide range of cancer cell lines.

In addition, 27 animal studies suggested as a whole that 1,25-D$_3$ inhibited tumor growth, angiogenesis, and metastasis in vivo.[94-98] Unfortunately, the doses found useful in the animal studies were generally greater than those considered safe in humans. At least four human studies have been conducted, but the results have been mixed.[99-102] Other human studies have indicated that below-normal plasma concentrations of 1,25-D$_3$ may increase cancer risk and disease progression.

Lastly, a number of other in-vitro, animal, and human studies have investigated the effects of 1,25-D$_3$ in combination with chemotherapy. These studies are discussed in Chapter 23.

In some respects, the situation with vitamin D$_3$ is similar to that with vitamin A. For one thing, the active form (1,25-D$_3$ and ATRA) for both vitamins is a metabolite. For another, these metabolites are available only by prescription and therefore do not meet our selection criteria. Nonetheless, because of their potential usefulness, both are discussed.

Administration of vitamin D_3 by itself can also produce antitumor effects, as suggested by at least two animal studies, but its ability to do so may vary because its conversion to $1,25$-D_3 is unpredictable. For this reason, the use of $1,25$-D_3 would seem preferable in most cases. Still, vitamin D_3 potentially could add to an antitumor effect and be useful in cancer prevention, since only slightly elevated plasma concentrations of $1,25$-D_3 may reduce cancer risk.

With regard to the use of $1,25$-D_3, there are inconsistencies between the doses scaled from animal studies and those used in human studies. (Doses based on pharmacokinetic and in-vitro data were not calculated, for reasons given below.) The required target dose of $1,25$-D_3 can thus be estimated only within a large range, but even with a target dose in the high end of this range, it could still be effective at the maximum safe human dose with synergism. The situation with vitamin D_3 is more uncertain; because the conversion rate to $1,25$-D_3 is variable, it is not clear if it would be effective at the maximum safe human dose, even with synergism.

Introduction

Vitamin D_3 (cholecalciferol) is a hormone produced in the skin through the action of sunlight. After its production, it is converted first to an intermediate, 25-D_3, and then, with the help of an enzyme in the kidneys, to the active metabolite $1,25$-dihydroxyvitamin D_3 ($1,25$-D_3). The concentration of vitamin D_3 in the plasma is large relative to that of 25-D_3, which itself is large relative to the concentration of $1,25$-D_3. Vitamin D_3 is fully metabolized to $1,25$-D_3 only when the body senses that additional $1,25$-D_3 is needed. For this reason, administration of vitamin D_3 does not necessarily increase $1,25$-D_3 concentrations. However, $1,25$-D_3 concentrations would be increased if vitamin D_3 levels (and therefore $1,25$-D_3 levels) were initially low.

$1,25$-D_3 is best known for its ability to stimulate calcium absorption, but it also has antitumor properties. Like ATRA, it is believed to act by binding to receptors in the nucleus of cells. The antitumor effects of $1,25$-D_3 have been relatively well studied in vitro and in vivo, and although it shows great promise, its usefulness has been hampered by its toxicity. At elevated concentrations, it causes hypercalcemia (excess calcium in the blood), which can be life-threatening if severe. Many research groups are now searching for vitamin D_3 analogs that inhibit cancer progression but do not increase calcium absorption, and therefore have fewer side effects. Nevertheless, $1,25$-D_3 may still be useful, even at

TABLE 22.5 POTENTIAL ANTICANCER ACTIONS OF 1,25-D₃	
ACTIVITY	KNOWN EFFECTS
Chapter 3: Results of Therapy at the Cellular Level	
Induce differentiation	x
Increase TGF-beta	x
Induce apoptosis	x
Chapter 4: Growth Factors and Signal Transduction	
Induce p21 or p27 activity	x
Chapter 5: Transcription Factors and Redox Signaling	
Inhibit NF-κB activity	weak
Chapter 6: Cell-to-Cell Communication	
Affect CAMs	x
Improve gap junction communication	x
Chapters 7 and 8: Angiogenesis	
Inhibit angiogenesis	x
Chapters 9 and 10: Invasion and Metastasis	
Inhibit cell migration	x

lower, safe doses, if it is used in synergistic combinations.

$1,25$-D_3, may inhibit cancer through the actions listed in Table 22.5. In addition to these, it may also reduce the expression of estrogen receptors on breast cancer cells, thereby reducing the proliferative effects of estrogen.[103] This effect occurs, however, at about 10 nM, which is greater than achievable plasma concentrations. Administration of $1,25$-D_3 may have the additional benefit of increasing the half-life of ATRA in the body.[104]

In-vitro Studies

Effective concentrations of $1,25$-D_3 to decrease cancer cell proliferation or induce differentiation in vitro are 10 to 1,000 nM (see Table D.1 in Appendix D), but plasma $1,25$-D_3 concentrations cannot be increased above about 0.2 nM without causing serious adverse effects (hypercalcemia) in some individuals. Average plasma levels of $1,25$-D_3 range between 0.05 and 0.15 nM, but it may block cancer by indirect means at lower doses and concentrations.[105-108] For example, in one study, concentrations as low as 0.1 nM inhibited invasion of lung cancer cells in vitro.[109] In another, concentrations of 0.1 nM potentiated the cytotoxic effects of TNF against human breast cancer cells in vitro.[110]

Animal Studies

A number of animal studies have reported that high doses of vitamin D_3 and $1,25$-D_3 can inhibit tumor progression and that the latter can act synergistically with other compounds, as discussed in Chapters 3 and 13. Some of these and other studies are summarized below. The average dose based on the following 10 animal studies is about 10 micrograms per day of 1,25-D_3 (range of 0.24 to 39 micrograms), as scaled to humans. In two that tested vitamin D_3, the average dose was 31 micrograms per day (range of 19 to 39 micrograms), as scaled to humans:

- The combination of 1,25-D_3 (at 0.5 μg/kg intraperitoneal) and ATRA or other vitamin A analogs (at 2.5 mg/kg) synergistically inhibited tumor-induced angiogenesis in vitro and in mice. Treatment with 1,25-D_3 alone also decreased angiogenesis in vitro and in mice. The equivalent human oral doses are about 7.2 micrograms of 1,25-D_3 and 36 milligrams of ATRA.[111, 112]

- Intraperitoneal administration every other day of ATRA (at 300 mg/kg) and 1,25-D_3 (at 2 μg/kg) inhibited growth of human breast cancer cells injected into mice.[113] This was better than the effect caused by either agent separately. These doses were the highest that could be used without causing acute side effects. The equivalent human oral doses are about 2.2 grams of ATRA and 14 micrograms of 1,25-D_3 daily.

- Intraperitoneal administration of 0.52 μg/kg of 1,25-D_3 three times weekly decreased growth of chemically induced breast cancer cells in rats. The equivalent human oral dose is about 5.5 micrograms of 1,25-D_3 per day.[94]

- Administration of 0.02 to 0.5 μg/kg of 1,25-D_3 daily (intraperitoneal and oral, alternating every day) inhibited growth of liver cancer cells transplanted in mice. The equivalent human oral dose is about 0.24 to 6.0 micrograms of 1,25-D_3 per day.[95]

- Intraperitoneal administration of 0.5 to 1.0 μg/kg of 1,25-D_3 three times per week reduced growth of transplanted prostate cancer cells in rats. The equivalent human oral dose is about 5.2 to 10 micrograms of 1,25-D_3 per day.[96]

- Oral administration of 0.5 μg/kg of 1,25-D_3 three times a week inhibited the growth of chemically induced breast cancers in rats. The equivalent human dose is about 3.5 micrograms of 1,25-D_3 per day.[114]

- Subcutaneous administration of 0.21 μg/kg 1,25-D_3 blocked angiogenesis by transplanted breast cancer cells in mice.[115] The equivalent human oral dose is about 3.9 micrograms of 1,25-D_3.

- Intraperitoneal administration of 5.0 μg/kg vitamin D_3 every other day reduced tumor-induced immunosuppression and caused a marked reduction in metastasis in mice with lung tumors.[116] The equivalent

human oral dose is about 36 micrograms (1,400 I.U.) per day.[a]

- Subcutaneous administration of 1 and 2.1 μg/kg of 1,25-D_3 or vitamin D_3 inhibited angiogenesis in transplanted kidney cancer cells in mice.[117] The equivalent human oral dose is about 19 and 39 micrograms per day (for vitamin D_3, about 760 and 1,600 I.U.).

Lastly, combined treatment with the glucocorticoid dexamethasone may reduce the adverse effects (hypercalcemia) of 1,25-D_3 and increase the antitumor effect. In mice, an intraperitoneal dose of 2 μg/kg of 1,25-D_3 in combination with dexamethasone produced a greater antitumor effect in mice with transplanted squamous cell carcinoma than either compound alone; hypercalcemia was also reduced by the combination.[118] The equivalent human oral dose is about 12 micrograms of 1,25-D_3 per day.

Human Studies

Four human studies have been conducted on the anticancer effects of 1,25-D_3. Because of hypercalcemia, the doses were generally limited to 1 to 2.5 micrograms, which is lower than those used in most animal studies. The results of the human studies are mixed, with 1,25-D_3, even combined with ATRA, being ineffective in some cases; this would be expected based on our material. The most consistent and greatest anticancer effects of both 1,25-D_3 and ATRA are likely when they are used within *large* combinations that provide synergistic interactions. The studies are as follows:

- In 7 patients with prostate cancer, oral administration of 1.5 to 2.5 micrograms of 1,25-D_3 reduced the rise in prostate-specific antigen (PSA, a plasma tumor marker) in all patients, significantly in six of them. The dose was limited by hypercalcemia.[99]

- In a case report, oral administration of 0.5 micrograms of 1,25-D_3 appeared to contribute to a long-term, postsurgical remission in a woman with parathyroid cancer.[100]

- In 22 patients with ovarian cancer, a combination of ATRA (about 70 milligrams orally per day) and 1,25-D_3 (1 to 4 micrograms orally per day) did not effect tumor progression as measured by CA 125, a plasma tumor marker.[101]

- In 18 patients with preleukemia (myelodysplastic syndromes), oral administration of 1,25-D_3 (up to 2 micrograms orally per day) did not produce signifi-

---

[a] *One I.U. of vitamin D_3 is equal to about 25 nanograms of vitamin D_3.*

cant beneficial effects.[102] In addition, half of the patients developed hypercalcemia.

Estimated Therapeutic and Tolerated Doses of Vitamin D$_3$

We do not calculate a dose estimate for 1,25-D$_3$ using a combination of pharmacokinetic and in-vitro data because the range of active concentrations in vitro is so large (0.01 to 1 μM). Any specific target concentration that might be chosen would be somewhat arbitrary. Consequently, we calculate dose estimates based only on animal and human studies.

The estimated required dose of 1,25-D$_3$ scaled from animal antitumor studies is not in close agreement with doses used in human studies, suggesting that the target human dose is still uncertain and can be estimated only in a large range. The required dose scaled from animal antitumor experiments is 0.24 to 39 micrograms daily (average of 10 micrograms). Doses in human studies were lower, commonly 1 to 2.5 micrograms, and could not be increased above this range without adverse effects. Based on the animal and human studies, we estimate a target human dose between 1 and 10 micrograms per day. Since a range is used, it is uncertain whether synergistic interactions will be required to produce an anticancer effect in humans. At the low end of this range, synergism would not be needed, but it would be at the high end.

The maximum tolerated dose of 1,25-D$_3$ is about 1 to 2.5 micrograms per day. In most human anticancer studies, doses were started low (about 0.5 micrograms per day), then raised by 0.5 micrograms each week until hypercalcemia was reached; treatment was stopped and restarted a week later at a slightly lower dose. With this schedule, daily doses as high as 4 micrograms could be achieved in some patients.[101] In most studies, 1,25-D$_3$ was also given at least four hours after the last meal to reduce calcium uptake and the risk of hypercalcemia. Standard drug reference books and manufacturer's literature are available to guide the practitioner in using 1,25-D$_3$.

Table 22.6 summarizes therapeutic dose estimates and gives a tentative dose recommendation of 1 to 2.5 micrograms of 1,25-D$_3$ per day, based on the maximum tolerated dose.

If we consider a scenario where the target dose is 10 micrograms and the maximum tolerated dose is 1 microgram, the full 15-fold allowable increase in potency

TABLE 22.6 ESTIMATED THERAPEUTIC AND TOLERABLE DOSES FOR 1,25-D$_3$	
DESCRIPTION	**1,25-D$_3$ DOSE (μg/day)**
Doses used in human anticancer studies	commonly 1 to 2.5
Required dose as scaled from animal antitumor studies	0.24 to 39 (10 average)
Target dose based on range from human anticancer studies and average dose from animal studies	1 to 10
Minimum required antitumor dose assuming 15-fold synergistic benefits	0.066 to 0.93
Commonly prescribed human dose in noncancerous conditions	0.25 to 0.75
Maximum tolerated dose	1 to 2.5
Tentative dose recommendation for further research	0.75 to 2.5
Minimum degree of synergism required	**uncertain**

due to synergism would lower the target dose to 0.67 micrograms, which is below the maximum tolerated dose. Thus, a 1-microgram dose could produce an anticancer effect, even in a worst-case scenario, with synergism. Still, a 10-fold increase in potency would be required, which is greater than that for most other direct-acting compounds (see Table 13.1).

Aside from administering 1,25-D$_3$, there may also be some benefit to using vitamin D$_3$ to moderately increase 1,25-D$_3$ concentrations, or at least to avoid below-normal ones. The latter have been associated with increased cancer risk and increased disease progression. For example, one study associated low plasma concentrations of 1,25-D$_3$ with increased disease progression in breast cancer patients.[119] In another, the risk of palpable prostate cancer in men age 57 or above was greater in those with low 1,25-D$_3$ plasma concentrations.[120] In a study of 620 healthy volunteers, the risk of developing colon cancer decreased threefold in subjects with moderate 25-D$_3$ plasma concentrations as opposed to those with low concentrations.[121] Furthermore, low vitamin D$_3$ concentrations have been implicated as a risk factor in cancers of the breast, colon, and prostate.[122, 123, a] Taken together, these studies indicate that high normal plasma levels of 1,25-D$_3$ may reduce cancer risk and inhibit cancer progression. Thus it would seem prudent to maintain at least normal to high-normal plasma concentrations of 1,25-D$_3$, which could be accomplished through adequate sun exposure or taking vitamin D$_3$ or both.

---

[a] *Vitamin D$_3$ is produced naturally from sun exposure, and sunlight deprivation has been suggested as a risk factor for breast cancer.*

TABLE 22.7 ESTIMATED THERAPEUTIC AND NOAEL DOSES FOR VITAMIN D$_3$		
DESCRIPTION	**D$_3$ DOSE (µg/day)**	**D$_3$ DOSE (I.U./day)**
Required dose as scaled from animal antitumor studies	19 to 39 µg (31 µg average)	760 to 1,600 I.U. (1,200 I.U. average)
Commonly prescribed human dose as a general supplement	10 to 25 µg	400 to 1,000 I.U.
Commonly prescribed human dose in the treatment of rickets	25 to 125 µg	1,000 to 5,000 I.U.
Estimated NOAEL dose	50 to 250 µg	2,000 to 10,000 I.U.
Tentative dose recommendation for further research	**10 to 250 µg**[*]	**400 to 10,000 I.U.**[*]
Minimum degree of synergism required	**uncertain**	**uncertain**

[*] *Doses above 25 micrograms (1,000 I.U.) are best administered under medical supervision.*

As a general supplement, vitamin D$_3$ is usually given at doses of about 10 micrograms (400 I.U.) per day. The NOAEL (no-adverse-effects-level) dose is still being debated, but the currently accepted one is 50 micrograms (2,000 I.U.) per day. Recent papers have proposed that it may be at least fivefold higher, or 250 micrograms (10,000 I.U.) per day.[124] Although the NOAEL dose is well above the common supplement dose, excess vitamin D$_3$ can cause adverse effects, and more than 25 micrograms (1,000 I.U.) daily is best taken under the care of a practitioner.

The therapeutic dose estimates for vitamin D$_3$ are summarized in Table 22.7, with a tentative dose recommendation of 10 to 250 micrograms (400 to 10,000 I.U.) per day. Note that in two animal studies, relatively moderate doses of vitamin D$_3$ (about 31 micrograms or 1,200 I.U. per day) reduced tumor growth. As mentioned, however, the conversion of vitamin D$_3$ to 1,25-D$_3$ is variable. If additional animal studies were conducted, it would seem unlikely that moderate doses would consistently produce antitumor effects.

VITAMIN E

Summary of Research and Conclusions

At least five in-vitro studies have investigated the cytotoxic effects of vitamin E (alpha-tocopherol).[125–130] Two reviews have also been published.[131, 132] In general, these studies reported that concentrations between 50 and 250 µM are required to inhibit cancer cell proliferation. The effects appear to be cell-specific, since many cancer cell lines do not respond to this range of concentrations. Plasma concentrations as high as 120 µM of vitamin E can be safely achieved in humans.

In addition to the limited sensitivity of some cell lines to vitamin E, like some other antioxidants it can actually stimulate cell proliferation under some conditions, especially at relatively low concentrations. In one in-vitro study, vitamin E stimulated cancer cell proliferation at concentrations below 10 µM but inhibited it at 100 µM.[125] As with all antioxidants, it makes sense to avoid using vitamin E alone—combinations with other anticancer compounds are preferable.

Although alpha-tocopherol can inhibit proliferation of some cancer cell lines, other forms of vitamin E, such as vitamin E succinate (VES), are more effective. Some 39 in-vitro studies have been conducted on the cytotoxic effects of VES.[133–137] Two reviews have also been published.[138, 139] VES tends to reduce cancer cell proliferation at lower concentrations than alpha-tocopherol, commonly between about 2 and 38 µM. As with alpha-tocopherol, a small number of in-vitro studies have shown that VES can stimulate cell proliferation at some concentrations.[140, 141]

In addition to the above, three papers have been published on the efficacy of combinations of two to four antioxidants in vitro.[139, 142, 143] These studies reported that combinations of antioxidant vitamins containing VES inhibited cancer cell proliferation more effectively than single antioxidants.

While it is clear that alpha-tocopherol and VES can limit cancer cell proliferation in-vitro, their in-vivo antitumor effects are more uncertain. Five animal studies have reported that alpha-tocopherol or VES reduced tumor growth (some of these studies used combinations of antioxidant vitamins).[144–148] These studies used widely different experimental protocols, however, and many questions remain. A primary one is whether oral administration of VES increases plasma VES concentrations to the point where cytotoxicity can occur, since most of the ingested VES is converted to alpha-tocopherol in the intestines.

A number of studies have investigated the ability of vitamin E or VES to prevent cancer.[149–153] In two prevention studies, oral administration of a combination of antioxidant vitamins containing VES inhibited development of chemically induced cancers in rodents.[154, 155] In human trials, vitamin E reduced the risk of prostate and colorectal but not lung cancer, in smokers or recent quitters.[156–159] Vitamin E and other antioxidants may also be useful in preventing recurrence. One human study reported that a mixture of vitamins in conjunction with a bacterial immunostimulant reduced recurrence in patients with bladder cancer (see Chapter 15).[160]

Other animal studies have reported that vitamin E inhibited tumor growth promoted by a high-fat diet and inhibited cancer cachexia (see Chapter 17).[161, 162] In addition to the above, a number of in-vitro and animal studies have investigated the effects of vitamin E on chemotherapy treatment; these are discussed in Chapter 23.

As a whole, the research clearly indicates that alpha-tocopherol and VES can inhibit cancer proliferation in vitro and that both compounds can produce general beneficial effects in vivo, such as free radical scavenging and improvements in immune function. Through such indirect actions, alpha-tocopherol or VES could contribute to an anticancer effect, but it is not clear if either would also directly reduce tumor growth in vivo. Of the two, VES is more likely to have a direct inhibitory effect, but it appears unlikely that orally administered VES would sufficiently increase plasma VES concentrations. At present, it seems that direct anticancer effects after oral administration of vitamin E or VES would be limited to a few sensitive cell lines, while indirect effects are likely to be more prominent.

Introduction

Vitamin E is the generic name for eight different compounds—four tocopherols and four tocotrienols. The form of vitamin E most commonly used as a supplement is alpha-tocopherol, and we use the terms *vitamin E* and *alpha-tocopherol* interchangeably here. Alpha-tocopherol is available in both natural forms (*RRR*-alpha-tocopherol) and synthetic (all-*rac*-alpha-tocopherol), the two forms being mirror images of one another.[a] The natural form is preferred clinically, since it is absorbed better in the intestines and in some other tissues.[163, 164, 165]

Vitamin E is one of the most important fat-soluble antioxidants in the body, and one of its main functions is to prevent oxidation of fatty acids in cell membranes. Consequently, the most obvious sign of vitamin E deficiency in humans is red blood cell fragility. Through its antioxidant and other effects, vitamin E can reduce the risk of some cancers.

In-vitro Studies

Vitamin E can directly inhibit cancer cell proliferation in vitro, but unlike vitamin C, it does not require a prooxidant action to do so. Rather, this appears to occur through modulation of PKC activity or some other mechanism.

Although at high concentrations a prooxidant action is possible both in vitro and in vivo, vitamin E most likely acts as an antioxidant in vivo at common supplement doses.[166, 167] One study did suggest that prolonged administration of high doses (about 1,500 I.U. per day) in healthy, nonsmoking individuals may reduce plasma ascorbate levels and increase susceptibility of red blood cells to lipid peroxidation, indicating a prooxidant effect.[167] It may be possible to prevent this effect by lowering the dose and administering other antioxidants along with vitamin E.

Vitamin E decreased proliferation of a limited number of cell lines in vitro at concentrations of roughly 50 to 250 μM; this action appeared to be cell- and stimulant-specific, since many tumor cell lines did not respond.[132, 168] In one study, hormone-sensitive cancers, such as human breast and prostate cancers, were inhibited by more than 50 percent at concentrations of 100 μM. Other cell lines like erythroleukemia were inhibited at concentrations greater than 250 μM, and neuroblastoma at concentrations of approximately 150 μM.[169, 170] In part, its anticancer effects may be due to decreased PKC activity; depending on the experimental conditions, vitamin E inhibits PKC activity in normal and cancer cell lines at concentrations of about 50 to 450 μM in vitro (see Table E.2 in Appendix E).

Vitamin E succinate has inhibited proliferation of a greater variety of cancer cell lines in vitro, and does so at lower concentrations.[171–175] Inhibition was observed at relatively low concentrations, commonly between 2 and 38 μM. Although VES is metabolized to alpha-tocopherol in the intestines and in most cells, it appears that its effects have little to do with metabolism to vitamin E or with any antioxidant action. Other related forms of vitamin E that are not metabolized to alpha-tocopherol (specifically, TSE, or alpha-tocopheryloxy-butyric acid) are as effective as VES. The cytotoxic effects of VES are due to the unique properties of the intact compound and are aided by its high water-solubility and ease of cellular uptake.[139, 176] (VES is a water-soluble form of vitamin E.) One paper proposed that it acts by altering the fluidity of the plasma membrane.[177]

Lastly, in-vitro studies have reported that a combination of antioxidant vitamins is more effective in

---

[a] RRR-*alpha-tocopherol was formerly referred to as* d-*alpha-tocopherol, and* all-rac-*alpha-tocopherol was formerly referred to as* dl-*alpha tocopherol.*

TABLE 22.8   POTENTIAL ANTICANCER ACTIONS OF VITAMIN E

ACTIVITY	KNOWN EFFECTS	AS AN ANTIOXIDANT, MAY:	AS A PKC INHIBITOR, MAY:	AS AN EICOSANOID INHIBITOR, MAY:
Chapter 2: Mutations, Gene Expression, and Proliferation				
Act as an antioxidant	x	—		
Chapter 3: Results of Therapy at the Cellular Level				
Induce apoptosis	x			x
Chapter 4: Growth Factors and Signal Transduction				
Inhibit PKC	x	—		
Induce *p21* or *p27* activity	x			
Chapter 5: Transcription Factors and Redox Signaling				
Support p53 function	x	x		
Inhibit NF-κB activity	weak	x	x	x
Inhibit AP-1 activity	x			
Chapter 6: Cell-to-Cell Communication				
Affect CAMs	x		x	x
Chapters 7 and 8: Angiogenesis				
Inhibit angiogenesis		x	x	x
Inhibit histamine effects			x	
Inhibit eicosanoid effects	x			—
Inhibit TNF effects		x	x	
Inhibit VEGF effects		x	x	x
Inhibit insulin resistance			x	
Chapters 9 and 10: Invasion and Metastasis				
Inhibit invasion			x	
Inhibit hyaluronidase, beta-glucuronidase, or elastase				x
Inhibit collagenase effects		x	x	x
Inhibit cell migration			x	
Inhibit metastasis			x	
Inhibit platelet aggregation	x			
Chapters 11 and 12: Immune System				
Stimulate the immune system	x			
Inhibit tumor-induced immunosuppression	x			
Chapter 17: Lipids				
Inhibit cachexia	x			

reducing cancer cell proliferation than single antioxidants.[139, 142, 143, 178]   In these studies, various combinations of VES, carotenoids, vitamin C, and ATRA synergistically inhibited proliferation, and combinations with all four compounds were most effective.

The potential anticancer actions of vitamin E are listed in Table 22.8.

In-vivo Studies

Vitamin E and VES, especially combined with other antioxidant vitamins, have caused antitumor effects in animal studies. Widely different protocols were used, however, and much more work is needed to verify the means and degree of any antitumor effect produced. One study reported that a very low oral dose of VES and beta-carotene (1.6 mg/kg) dramatically inhibited growth of established carcinogen-induced oral cancers in hamsters.[147] The equivalent human dose is only about 23 milligrams of each compound, or 28 I.U. of VES.[a] No effect was seen for each compound alone at double the dose. In another study on VES, intraperitoneal administration of 150 mg/kg dramatically inhibited the growth of breast cancer in mice.[148] The equivalent human oral dose is about 2.2 grams (2,600 I.U.) of VES. Subcutaneous administration was not effective in this study, probably because the VES would have been metabolized to alpha-tocopherol in the skin.

As discussed in Chapter 15, one study on rats reported that a combination of vitamin E, vitamin C, selenium, and a thiol antioxidant was effective in inhibiting established chemically induced tumors only at very high doses.[146] In this study, high and very high doses of antioxidants were given in the drinking water. The high doses were 150 mg/kg of vitamin C and 50 mg/kg of vitamin E daily (the human of about 2.4 grams of vitamin C and 1,200 I.U. of vitamin E). The very high doses were 10-fold greater. Both groups received selenium (at 2 μg/kg) and a thiol antioxidant compound (2-MPG, at 15 mg/kg). The high-dose therapy did not increase life span, and in fact, secondary metastases were greater. Life span increased 1.4-fold in the very high dose group, but again secondary metastases developed, equal to the high-dose group. The doses used in the very high group (12,000 I.U. of vitamin E) would be prohibitive in humans.

---

[a] *One gram of Vitamin E is roughly equivalent to 1,500 I.U. Due to their differences in molecular weight, one gram of VES is roughly equal to 1,200 I.U.*

Two other animal studies have been conducted.[144, 145] In these, oral administration of vitamin E (about 870 and 2,100 I.U. per day as scaled to humans) inhibited growth of transplanted sarcoma and lymphoma cells in mice. In both cases, vitamin E was administered beginning at the same time tumors were implanted, and the authors postulated that the effects were mediated by the immune system. Vitamin E appeared to be most effective in the early stage of tumor growth after transplantation. Markedly higher doses were not helpful; no protective effect was seen against transplanted sarcoma cells at a 10-fold higher dose (8,700 I.U., as scaled to humans).

Also, vitamin E (at 11.4 mg/kg per day) inhibited growth of transplanted human prostate cancer cells in mice fed a high-fat diet (see Chapter 17).[162] The effect was likely from reduced lipid peroxidation. The equivalent human dose is about 110 milligrams, or 170 I.U., per day. As also discussed in Chapter 17, vitamin E (at approximately 640 mg/kg) hindered the development of TNF-induced cachexia in mice. The equivalent human dose is about 6.1 grams, or 9,200 I.U., per day.[179]

Although no human anticancer studies have been conducted on alpha-tocopherol or VES, cancer prevention studies have been done. In the Alpha-Tocopherol Beta-Carotene (ATBC) study mentioned previously, vitamin E at 50 milligrams (75 I.U.) per day reduced prostate cancer incidence in smokers by 34 percent. High serum levels of vitamin E were also associated with a 19 percent reduction in lung cancer incidence.[158, 180] Another large study reported similar protective effects for prostate cancer in smokers or recent quitters, although no such effect was seen in nonsmokers.[159] As mentioned in the discussion of beta-carotene above, some studies have reported that high plasma levels or high dietary intake of vitamin E (along with other nutrients) were associated with reduced risk of some cancers.

Estimated Therapeutic and LOAEL Doses of Vitamin E

The concentrations of vitamin E effective in vitro (50 to 250 µM) are above the normal plasma concentrations of 12 to 40 µM; however, plasma concentrations can be increased to 30 to 120 µM in patients taking supplements.[181, 182, 183] For example, in one study average peak plasma levels were roughly 70 µM in healthy subjects receiving a single dose of either 440, 880, or 1,320 I.U. of vitamin E.[184] In another, oral administration of 900 I.U. for 13 weeks produced a plasma concentration of about 51 µM, up from the baseline of 19 µM.[185] These data suggest two things. First, moderate doses (about 440 I.U.) may increase plasma concentrations into the range that is cytotoxic for a few cancer cell

lines. Second, doses above about 440 I.U. may not further increase plasma concentrations. Still, one study reported that a daily dose of 2,400 I.U. did generate a somewhat higher plasma concentration than did 600 I.U. (about twofold greater, or 97 versus 42 µM).[186] But again, this study pointed to limited gains from high doses.

VES is more effective than alpha-tocopherol in vitro, and if it is not fully metabolized to alpha-tocopherol, it may also be more effective in vivo. Although study results conflict, it appears, unfortunately, that it is heavily metabolized. The majority of orally administered VES is converted to alpha-tocopherol in the gastrointestinal tract before absorption.[187] Indeed, VES apparently is equipotent to alpha-tocopherol in increasing alpha-tocopherol plasma concentrations.[188] Nonetheless, one paper proposed that oral administration still adequately increases VES plasma concentrations. This paper, which referred to unpublished human data, stated that oral administration of 800 I.U. of VES per day produced a VES plasma concentration of about 11 µM and an alpha-tocopherol concentration of about 140 µM.[139] This concentration of VES would be sufficient to inhibit many cancer cell lines. In contrast, a rat study reported that VES was not detected in the plasma after oral administration of 100 mg/kg VES (the detection limit was 5 µM). The equivalent human dose is about 1.6 grams (1,900 I.U.). Although this rat study does not prove that VES is unable to increase VES plasma concentrations, it does make it seem likely. Further work is needed to better characterize the pharmacokinetics of VES. Other related forms of vitamin E like TSE, which are not metabolized to alpha-tocopherol, may prove to be most useful, but TSE is not commercially available at this time.

Both alpha-tocopherol and VES may be most useful for their indirect effects, although a few cancer cell lines may be directly inhibited. For direct effects, the estimated required dose scaled from animal studies is in reasonable agreement with that calculated from pharmacokinetic and in-vitro data. The required dose of alpha-tocopherol or VES from the five animal antitumor studies mentioned above ranges from 28 I.U. to 12,000 I.U. We can extract a reasonable dose estimate from this range by omitting the lowest and highest doses and averaging the remaining three, giving an estimate of 1,700 I.U., which could be expected to increase plasma alpha-tocopherol concentrations to about 30 to 120 µM in humans; this is within the cytotoxic range for a few cancer cell lines. And if VES administration significantly increases plasma VES concentrations, this same dose would generate concentrations within the cytotoxic range for a large number of cell lines. Since human

| TABLE 22.9   ESTIMATED THERAPEUTIC AND LOAEL DOSES FOR ALPHA-TOCOPHEROL OR VES ||
DESCRIPTION	DOSE (I.U./day)
Required dose as scaled from animal antitumor studies	28 to 12,000 (average of 1,700)
Required cytotoxic dose as determined from pharmacokinetic calculations	440 to 1,700
Target dose based on an average from animal antitumor studies and pharmacokinetic calculations	440 to 1,700
Commonly prescribed human dose in noncancerous conditions	400 to 800
Estimated LOAEL dose	4,800
Tentative dose recommendation for further research	**440 to 1,700**
Minimum degree of synergism required	**variable**

studies have indicated that vitamin E doses much greater than 440 I.U. do not greatly increase plasma concentrations, we use a range of 440 to 1,700 I.U. per day as a target dose.

Vitamin E is commonly used at doses of 270 to 530 milligrams daily (about 400 to 800 I.U. per day). A dose of 1 gram per day (about 1,500 I.U.) is considered safe.[189] Although vitamin E can lead to some adverse effects, primarily increased risk for bleeding, its use even at high doses appears safe in most healthy humans. For example, in one study oral doses as high as 3.2 grams per day (about 4,800 I.U.) resulted in few side effects.[189] We can estimate then that the LOAEL dose is about 4,800 I.U. per day.

Therapeutic dose estimates for alpha-tocopherol and VES are summarized in Table 22.9. The tentative recommended dose is 440 to 1,700 I.U. per day, which is equal to the target dose. In the table, the minimum degree of synergism needed for direct inhibitory effects is listed as variable because oral administration of both may increase alpha-tocopherol plasma concentrations, but only a limited number of cell lines may be inhibited at those concentrations.

For dose calculation, it is not clear if synergistic interactions would allow a lower dose of either compound to be effective. Moderate concentrations of alpha-tocopherol are already present in the plasma (oral administration increases concentrations from the range of 12 to 40 μM only to 30 to 120 μM), and so a low dose will probably not greatly affect plasma concentrations or contribute to synergistic effects. A low dose might, however, contribute to indirect anticancer effects.

MELATONIN

Summary of Research and Conclusions

At least 41 in-vitro studies have been conducted on the cytotoxic effects of melatonin against cancer cells.[190–194] These studies suggest that a number of cell lines, particularly breast cancer, are inhibited at peak physiological concentrations of melatonin (about 0.1 to 1 nM). Thirteen animal studies reported anticancer effects against a number of different cancers.[195–199]

Twenty-eight human studies have been conducted on melatonin alone or in conjunction with interleukin-2.[200–204] Seven were randomized controlled studies, and all reported that melatonin or melatonin plus IL-2 increased the survival of patients as compared to those given supportive care or IL-2 alone.

In addition to the above, a number of reviews on the anticancer effects of melatonin have been published.[205–209] Lastly, still other in-vitro, animal, and human studies have demonstrated that melatonin increased the effectiveness or decreased the adverse effects of chemotherapy or radiotherapy. These are discussed in Chapter 23.

Introduction

Melatonin has been studied in a number of clinical trials for its ability to inhibit cancer progression, and the results are encouraging. Its anticancer action may be due to its antioxidant capabilities, or its effects on estrogen receptors or the immune system, among others. Because melatonin augments the effects of IL-2, in many of the trials it was administered with IL-2 (see Chapter 12). Some immune cells, including CD4 helper T cells, also have specific melatonin-binding sites.[210]

Melatonin is a hormone produced by the pineal gland. In healthy humans, it is secreted in a day-night rhythm, with the highest plasma concentrations occurring during the evening. During the day, concentrations are about 0.07 nM, and at night they increase to about 0.4 nM, sometimes approaching 1 nM.[211, 212, 213] Melatonin influences a number of biological functions, the most studied being its ability to induce sleep. It is becoming increasingly popular as a nontoxic, nonaddictive remedy for jet lag and insomnia.

Melatonin is a powerful antioxidant—more potent than glutathione in scavenging the hydroxyl radical and more potent than vitamin E in scavenging the peroxyl radical.[214, 215] Furthermore, melatonin stimulates glutathione peroxidase (see Figure 5.2) and so plays a role in the glutathione antioxidant system.[214] Since it is both fat- and water-soluble, it is readily diffused into all tissues and cells of the body. In the cells, it protects DNA against free radical damage.[216]

In-vitro Studies

Melatonin has inhibited proliferation of breast cancer, melanoma, prostate cancer, and some other cancer cell lines in vitro, although the majority of studies have been conducted on breast cancer. In these studies, inhibition generally occurred at concentrations of 0.1 to 1 nM, which is within the range of normal nighttime concentrations.[217–221] Concentrations markedly above (i.e., 100 nM) or below physiologic concentrations were generally not effective. At least one study has reported that a concentration pattern mimicking the normal day-night cycle produced maximal inhibition of human breast cancer cells.[222]

TABLE 22.10 POTENTIAL ANTICANCER ACTIONS OF MELATONIN		
ACTIVITY	**KNOWN EFFECTS**	**AS AN ANTI-OXIDANT, MAY:**
Chapter 2: Mutations, Gene Expression, and Proliferation		
Act as an antioxidant	x	—
Chapter 3: Results of Therapy at the Cellular Level		
Increase TGF-beta	x	
Chapter 5: Transcription Factors and Redox Signaling		
Support p53 function		x
Inhibit NF-κB activity	weak	x
Chapter 6: Cell-to-Cell Communication		
Affect CAMs	x	
Improve gap junction communication	x	x
Chapters 7 and 8: Angiogenesis		
Inhibit angiogenesis		x
Inhibit eicosanoid effects	x	
Inhibit TNF effects	x	x
Inhibit VEGF effects		x
Chapters 9 and 10: Invasion and Metastasis		
Inhibit invasion	x	
Inhibit collagenase effects		x
Inhibit cell migration	x	
Chapters 11 and 12: Immune System		
Stimulate the immune system	x	
Chapter 17: Lipids		
Inhibit cachexia	x	

Although the exact mechanisms are still uncertain, recent research indicates that in breast cancer cells, the in-vitro actions of melatonin are mediated through two primary events: modulation of estrogen-receptor expression or activation, and stimulation of specific melatonin receptors (mt1 and MT2) on the cell's surface. Some human prostate cancer cells have also been reported to possess melatonin receptors.[223] Other postulated mechanisms active in vivo are modulation of immune activity, inhibition of eicosanoid production, and antioxidant activity.[209, 224, 225] The potential anticancer actions of melatonin are listed in Table 22.10.

Animal Studies

In animal studies, subnormal melatonin concentrations have facilitated the growth of various cancers.[226, 227] For example, removing the pineal gland in hamsters increased the progression rate of melanoma.[228] In others, oral intraperitoneal, intramuscular, or subcutaneous administration of moderate doses reduced the growth of a variety of cancers.[195, 229, 230] Selected studies are summarized below:

- Oral administration of 480 milligrams per day (as scaled to humans) reduced growth of Ehrlich ascites cancer cells injected into mice.[196]

- Oral administration of 12 milligrams per day (as scaled to humans) inhibited growth and reduced metastasis of lung cancer cells injected into mice.[198, 199]

- Oral administration of 48 milligrams per day (as scaled to humans) decreased growth of melanoma cells injected into mice.[197]

Although a few studies used very high levels, as a whole, the animal studies suggested a human oral equivalent of 10 to 50 milligrams was effective at reducing tumor growth.

Human Studies

A number of investigators have tried to determine if melatonin production is altered in cancer patients (reviewed in references 205 and 209). Although the results are somewhat inconsistent, it does appear that reduced melatonin production is associated with advanced cancers. This has been seen for both endocrine-dependent (breast cancer, for example) and endocrine-independent cancers (lung cancer, for example). The trend was most pronounced for patients with advanced localized primary tumors, such as breast and prostate cancer, where melatonin production was negatively associated with tumor size. Interestingly, melatonin levels tended to normalize with cancer regression but not with surgical removal, which indicates that the factors governing melatonin production are complex. In contrast to these findings, patients with ovarian cancer often show increased melatonin production, probably due to a different set of hormonal changes with this cancer.

A number of human studies have been published on the anticancer effects of melatonin. Eleven used melatonin as a single agent, although only three of these were randomized trials (where the control group received supportive care alone) and none were placebo controlled. The three studies are summarized below (melatonin was given once a day in the evening in all cases):

- In a study on 30 melanoma patients surgically treated for regional node recurrence, those who received 20 milligrams of melatonin showed increased disease-free survival at 31 months as compared to controls who received no treatment (71 versus 31 percent). No adverse effects were reported with the treatment.[231]

- In 50 patients with untreatable brain metastases, those receiving supportive care and 20 milligrams of melatonin exhibited greater survival at 12 months compared to controls who received only supportive care (37 versus 12 percent). In addition, the group that received melatonin experienced reduced side effects from steroid therapy.[200]

- In 63 patients with metastatic non-small-cell lung cancer who progressed after first-line chemotherapy, those who received 10 milligrams of melatonin showed increased one-year survival compared to controls who had supportive care only (26 versus 6 percent). No toxicity was observed.[201]

Like these results, the nonrandomized trials also reported beneficial effects on patients with a variety of cancers, including immune enhancing effects.[202, 203, 204] Similar doses were used in the nonrandomized studies.

At least 16 studies used melatonin in combination with low-dose IL-2. Only three of these were randomized trials (versus IL-2 alone or supportive care alone), and none were placebo controlled; these are summarized below (melatonin was given once per day in the evening in all cases):

- In a study of 100 patients with untreatable metastatic cancer, those who received supportive care, IL-2, and 40 milligrams of melatonin showed increased survival at 12 months compared to controls receiving supportive care only (40 versus 10 percent).[232]

- In 50 patients with metastatic colorectal cancer who were unresponsive to chemotherapy, those getting supportive care, IL-2, and 40 milligrams of melatonin demonstrated higher survival at 12 months compared to controls who had supportive care only (36 versus 12 percent).[233]

- In 80 patients with advanced cancers (other than kidney cancer or melanoma), those who took IL-2 and 40 milligrams of melatonin showed greater survival at 12 months compared to controls who took only IL-2 (46 versus 15 percent).[234]

In addition to these three randomized studies, a fourth one compared IL-2 plus melatonin with chemotherapy for patients with non-small-cell lung cancer. Again, one-year survival was greater in those receiving IL-2 plus melatonin, and toxicity was substantially lower.[235]

Similar to the above, the nonrandomized trials also noted beneficial effects of a combination of melatonin and IL-2 on patients with a variety of cancers.[236, 237, 238] We can speculate that a combination of melatonin and immunostimulant herbs, which also increase IL-2 concentrations, might be as effective as melatonin and IL-2 itself.

In the human studies, oral doses were usually 10 to 50 milligrams. As discussed in Appendix J, a 10-milligram dose would be expected to produce an average nighttime plasma concentration of about 14 nM (and a 54-nM peak concentration). It would seem reasonable that this average value is close enough to 1 nM, the optimal concentration seen in vitro, to produce cytotoxic effects against cancer cells. If true, it may be that a 50-milligram dose is less effective than a 10-milligram dose (since high concentrations in vitro were less effective). An even lower dose, such as 3 milligrams, could be even more effective than a dose of 10 milligrams.

Although cytotoxic effects may occur at a low dose, it is likely that other noncytotoxic mechanisms are also active. For one thing, melatonin appears to be useful for cancers that are not endocrine-dependent, even though endocrine-dependent ones were most easily inhibited in vitro. Potential mechanisms include inhibiting eicosanoid synthesis, facilitating the immune response, and other actions listed in Table 22.10.

Estimated Therapeutic and LOAEL Doses of Melatonin

Melatonin is characterized in this book as an immune stimulant (see Table 1.2), but in addition to immune effects it may also have direct cytotoxic effects against cancer cells. Therefore, it is interesting to compare doses scaled from animal and human experiments to those calculated from pharmacokinetic and in-vitro data. These doses are in agreement. The required melatonin dose from the animal experiments is 10 to 50 milligrams per day, the same as the range used in human studies; most of these used 10 to 20 milligrams. The anticancer dose based on pharmacokinetic calculations is similar. As discussed, a 10-milligram dose will produce an average nighttime melatonin concentration of about 14 nM, which is reasonably close to the 1-nM optimal concentration. Under normal circumstances, this 1-nM concentration can be reached in vivo with no external administration of melatonin. Thus pharmacokinetic calculations suggest that doses of 0 to 10 milligrams may be adequate and may produce both direct and immune-stimulating effects. We use a range of 0 to 20 milligrams per day as our target human dose.

TABLE 22.11 ESTIMATED THERAPEUTIC AND LOAEL DOSES FOR MELATONIN[*]	
DESCRIPTION	DOSE (mg/day)
Required dose as scaled from animal antitumor studies	commonly 10 to 50
Doses used in human anticancer studies	10 to 50 (commonly 10 to 20)
Required cytotoxic dose as determined from pharmacokinetic calculations	0 to 10
Target dose based on human studies and pharmacokinetic calculations	0 to 20
Minimum required antitumor dose assuming 15-fold synergistic benefits	0.67 to 1.3
Commonly prescribed human dose in noncancerous conditions	3
Estimated LOAEL dose	10 to 50
Tentative dose recommendation for further research	**3 to 20**
Minimum degree of synergism required	**none**

[*] *See Appendix J for details.*

The commonly prescribed dose in noncancerous conditions (insomnia and jet lag) is 3 milligrams. The LOAEL dose is uncertain but likely to be between 10 and 50 milligrams per day (see Appendix J). Severe drowsiness can occur at doses of 3 milligrams or less, however.

Therapeutic dose estimates for melatonin are summarized in Table 22.11, with a tentative recommended dose range of 3 to 20 milligrams daily. The 3-milligram value is based on the commonly prescribed dose, and the 20-milligram value on the highest common dose in human studies.

Because the target dose is achievable, synergistic interactions may not be required for melatonin to produce an anticancer effect in humans. Nevertheless, melatonin may greatly benefit from synergism, and it makes sense to continue testing it in combination with other compounds.

It is important to note that melatonin is best taken at night. Morning administration was reported to stimulate growth of two different cancer cell lines in rodents, whereas taken in the afternoon it inhibited growth.[239, 240, 241] Furthermore, melatonin induces drowsiness, which may be unwanted during the day.

As discussed above, normal levels of melatonin may impede tumor progression. Therefore, even without external melatonin, it may be worthwhile to maximize natural production. This can be done in at least two ways. First, the body's levels of melatonin can be maximized by reducing exposure to artificial light during the dark hours. Even short periods of light at night can dramatically reduce melatonin production for the remainder of the night.[242] Second, at least two studies indicate that meditation practices can increase melatonin concentrations.[243, 244] In addition to an effect on melatonin, meditation may have other beneficial effects, not the least being increased peace of mind. Several preliminary studies have in fact reported that deep meditation may prolong the lives of some cancer patients.[245–248]

CONCLUSION

Lipid-soluble vitamins represent a unique class of potential anticancer compounds. Two vitamins, A and D_3, in the form of their active metabolites, have the ability to enter the nucleus and directly affect gene transcription. Since few other natural compounds discussed here can do this, when used in combinations they offer valuable diversity. The effects of vitamin E are limited primarily to the plasma membrane. Since the membrane's characteristics govern antigen presentation, the uptake and transport of drugs and nutrients, as well as the functioning of growth factor receptors and other important structures, vitamin E, especially in its alternate forms such as VES, has the potential to directly inhibit cancer cell proliferation. At the same time, questions on VES pharmacokinetics must be answered before we can predict that its potential will be realized in treatment. Through its antioxidant characteristics, vitamin E can also inhibit cancer through indirect actions, such as by supporting immune function. Melatonin, which is not a vitamin but a hormone, is both water- and lipid-soluble, and for this reason it can enter several cellular compartments to affect change. It can inhibit cancer cells directly and, like vitamin E, also through indirect means.

REFERENCES

[1] Maziere S, Cassand P, Narbonne JF, Meflah K. Vitamin A and apoptosis in colonic tumor cells. Int J Vitam Nutr Res 1997; 67(4):237–41.

[2] Rosewicz S, Stier U, Brembeck F, et al. Retinoids: Effects on growth, differentiation, and nuclear receptor expression in human pancreatic carcinoma cell lines. Gastroenterology 1995 Nov; 109(5):1646–60.

[3] Ramanathan R, Tan CH, Das NP. Cytotoxic effect of plant polyphenols and fat-soluble vitamins on malignant human cultured cells. Cancer Lett 1992 Mar 15; 62(3):217–24.

[4] Halter SA, Fraker LD, Parl F, et al. Selective isolation of human breast carcinoma cells resistant to the growth-inhibitory effects of retinol. Nutr Cancer 1990; 14(1):43–56.

[5] Ferreri-Santi L, Agostacchio C, Rosellini C, et al. Effect of vitamin A on chemotactic and chemoinvasive behaviour of an osteosarcoma cell line. Boll Soc Ital Biol Sper 1990 Apr; 66(4):373–80.

[6] Fraker LD, Halter SA, Forbes JT. Growth inhibition by retinol of a human breast carcinoma cell line in vitro and in athymic mice. Cancer Res 1984 Dec; 44(12 Pt 1):5757–63.

[7] Huang CC. Effect of retinoids on the growth of squamous cell carcinoma of the palate in rats. Am J Otolaryngol 1986 Jan–Feb; 7(1):55–7.

[8] Wang CJ, Chou MY, Lin JK. Inhibition of growth and development of the transplantable C-6 glioma cells inoculated in rats by retinoids and carotenoids. Cancer Lett 1989 Nov 30; 48(2):135–42.

[9] Wetherall NT, Mitchell WM, Halter SA. Antiproliferative effect of vitamin A on xenotransplanted CaMa-15 cells. Cancer Res 1984 Jun; 44(6):2393–7.

[10] Malkovsky M, Hunt R, Palmer L, et al. Retinyl acetate-mediated augmentation of resistance to a transplantable 3-methylcholanthrene-induced fibrosarcoma. The dose response and time course. Transplantation 1984 Aug; 38(2):158–61.

[11] Tsutani H, Ueda T, Uchida M, Nakamura T. Pharmacological studies of retinol palmitate and its clinical effect in patients with acute non-lymphocytic leukemia. Leuk Res 1991; 15(6):463–71.

[12] Tsutani H, Iwasaki H, Kawai Y, et al. Reduction of leukemia cell growth in a patient with acute promyelocytic leukemia treated by retinol palmitate. Leuk Res 1990; 14(7):595–600.

[13] Lie SO, Wathne KO, Petersen LB, et al. High-dose retinol in children with acute myelogenous leukemia in remission. Eur J Haematol 1988 May; 40(5):460–5.

[14] Pastorino U, Infante M, Maioli M, et al. Adjuvant treatment of stage I lung cancer with high-dose vitamin A. J Clin Oncol 1993 Jul; 11(7):1216–22.

[15] Goodman GE, Alberts DS, Earnst DL, Meyskens FL. Phase I trial of retinol in cancer patients. J Clin Oncol 1983 Jun; 1(6):394–9.

[16] Goodman GE. Phase II trial of retinol in patients with advanced cancer. Cancer Treat Rep 1986 Aug; 70(8):1023–4.

[17] Nomura J, Endo K, Furuyama K, et al. [Differentiating effect of oral administration of retinol palmitate (Chocola-A) for an aged AML (M3) with severe complications.] Rinsho Ketsueki 1992 Nov; 33(11):1673–8.

[18] Hofmanova J, Soucek K, Dusek L, et al. Inhibition of the cytochrome P-450 modulates all-*trans* retinoic acid-induced differentiation and apoptosis of HL-60 cells. Cancer Detect Prev 2000; 24(4):325–42.

[19] Toma S, Raffo P, Nicolo G, et al. Biological activity of all-*trans* retinoic acid with and without tamoxifen and alpha-interferon 2a in breast cancer patients. Int J Oncol 2000 Nov; 17(5):991–1000.

[20] Zhang JW, Wang JY, Chen SJ, Chen Z. Mechanisms of all-*trans* retinoic acid-induced differentiation of acute promyelocytic leukemia cells. J Biosci 2000 Sep; 25(3):275–84.

[21] Liu J, Guo L, Luo Y, et al. All trans-retinoic acid suppresses in vitro growth and down-regulates LIF gene expression as well as telomerase activity of human medulloblastoma cells. Anticancer Res 2000 Jul–Aug; 20(4):2659–64.

[22] Faiderbe S, Chagnaud JL, De Seze R, Geffard M. Curative effects of all-*trans* retinoic acid on rat sarcomas. Anticancer Drugs 1992 Oct; 3(5):541–7.

[23] Khuri FR, Lippman SM. Lung cancer chemoprevention. Semin Surg Oncol 2000 Mar; 18(2):100–5.

[24] Biasco G, Paganelli GM. European trials on dietary supplementation for cancer prevention. Ann N Y Acad Sci 1999; 889:152–6.

[25] Goodman GE. Prevention of lung cancer. Crit Rev Oncol Hematol 2000 Mar; 33(3):187–97.

[26] Hong WK, Sporn MB. Recent advances in chemoprevention of cancer. Science 1997 Nov 7; 278(5340):1073–7.

[27] Bates CJ. Vitamin A [see comments]. Lancet 1995 Jan 7; 345(8941):31–5.

[28] Linder MC, ed. Nutritional biochemistry and metabolism 2nd ed. New York: Elsevier Science, 1991, pp. 153–6.

[29] Halter SA, Fraker LD, Parl F, Bradley R, Briggs R. Selective isolation of human breast carcinoma cells resistant to the growth-inhibitory effects of retinol. Nutr Cancer 1990; 14(1):43–56.

[30] Satyamoorthy K, Chitnis MP. Effect of vitamin A compounds on DNA biosynthesis in murine tumor models in vitro. Oncology 1987; 44(6):356–9.

[31] Meyskens FL Jr, Fuller BB. Characterization of the effects of different retinoids on the growth and differentiation of a human melanoma cell line and selected subclones. Cancer Res 1980 Jul; 40(7):2194–6.

[32] Kyritsis A, Joseph G, Chader GJ. Effects of butyrate, retinol, and retinoic acid on human Y-79 retinoblastoma cells growing in monolayer cultures. J Natl Cancer Inst 1984 Sep; 73(3):649–54.

33 Audette M, Page M. Growth modification of normal and tumor cell lines with retinol. Cancer Detect Prev 1983; 6(6):497–505.

34 Blomhoff R, Skrede B, Norum KR. Uptake of chylomicron remnant retinyl ester via the low density lipoprotein receptor: Implications for the role of vitamin A as a possible preventive for some forms of cancer. J Intern Med 1990 Sep; 228(3):207–10.

35 Wathne KO, Carlander B, Norum KR, Blomhoff R. Uptake of retinyl ester in HL-60 cells via the low-density-lipoprotein-receptor pathway. Biochem J 1989 Jan 1; 257(1):239–44.

36 Klaassen I, Brakenhoff RH, Smeets SJ, et al. Considerations for in vitro retinoid experiments: Importance of protein interaction. Biochim Biophys Acta 1999 Apr 19; 1427(2):265–75.

37 [No authors listed]. Effect of retinoids on growth and differentiation of myeloid leukemia cells. Nutr Rev 1989 May; 47(5):153–4.

38 Botilsrud M, Holmberg I, Wathne KO, et al. Effect of retinoids and 1,25(OH)2 vitamin D3 bound to their plasma transport proteins on growth and differentiation of HL-60 cells. Scand J Clin Lab Invest 1990 May; 50(3):309–17.

39 Skrede B, Blomhoff HK, Smeland EB, et al. Retinyl esters in chylomicron remnants inhibit growth of myeloid and lymphoid leukaemic cells. Eur J Clin Invest 1991 Dec; 21(6):574–9.

40 Fazely F, Ledinko N, Smith DJ. Inhibition by retinoids of in vitro invasive ability of human lung carcinoma cells. Anticancer Res 1988 Nov–Dec; 8(6):1387–91.

41 [No authors listed]. Effect of retinoids on growth and differentiation of myeloid leukemia cells. Nutr Rev 1989 May; 47(5):153–4.

42 Buss NE, Tembe EA, Prendergast BD, et al. The teratogenic metabolites of vitamin A in women following supplements and liver. Hum Exp Toxicol 1994 Jan; 13(1):33–43.

43 Copper MP, Klaassen I, Teerlink T, et al. Plasma retinoid levels in head and neck cancer patients: A comparison with healthy controls and the effect of retinyl palmitate treatment. Oral Oncol 1999 Jan; 35(1):40–4.

44 Infante M, Pastorino U, Chiesa G, et al. Laboratory evaluation during high-dose vitamin A administration: A randomized study on lung cancer patients after surgical resection. J Cancer Res Clin Oncol 1991; 117(2):156–62.

45 Wathne KO, Norum KR, Smeland E, Blomhoff R. Retinol bound to physiological carrier molecules regulates growth and differentiation of myeloid leukemic cells. J Biol Chem 1988 Jun 25; 263(18):8691–5.

46 Forni G, Cerruti Sola S, et al. Effect of prolonged administration of low doses of dietary retinoids on cell-mediated immunity and the growth of transplantable tumors in mice. J Natl Cancer Inst 1986 Mar; 76(3):527–33.

47 Wang CJ, Chou MY, Lin JK. Inhibition of growth and development of the transplantable C-6 glioma cells inoculated in rats by retinoids and carotenoids. Cancer Lett 1989 Nov 30; 48(2):135–42.

48 Pavelic ZP, Dave S, Bialkowski S, et al. Antitumor activity of Corynebacterium parvum and retinyl palmitate used in combination on the Lewis lung carcinoma. Cancer Res 1980 Dec; 40(12):4617–21.

49 Tsutani H, Ueda T, Uchida M, et al. Pharmacological studies of the retinol palmitate and its clinical effect in patients with acute non-lymphocytic leukemia. Leuk Res 1991; 15(6):463–71.

50 Pastorino U, Soresi M, Clerci G, et al. Lung cancer chemoprevention with retinol palimate: Preliminary data from a randomized trial on stage Ia non small-cell lung cancer. Acta Oncology 1988; 27:773–80.

51 Pastorino U, Infante M, Maioli M, et al. Adjuvant treatment of stage I lung cancer with high-dose vitamin A. J Clin Oncol 1993; 11(7):1216–22.

52 Infante M, Pastorino U, Chiesa G, et al. Laboratory evaluation during high-dose vitamin A administration: A randomized study on lung cancer patients after surgical resection. J Cancer Res Oncol 1991; 117:156–62.

53 Lee JS, Newman RA, Lippman SM, et al. Phase I evaluation of all-trans retinoic acid in adults with solid tumors. J Clin Oncol 1993 May; 11(5):959–66.

54 Budd GT, Adamson PC, Gupta M, et al. Phase I/II trial of all-trans retinoic acid and tamoxifen in patients with advanced breast cancer. Clin Cancer Res 1998 Mar; 4(3):635–42.

55 Estey EH, Thall PF, Pierce S, et al. Randomized phase II study of fludarabine + cytosine arabinoside + idarubicin +/- all-trans retinoic acid +/- granulocyte colony-stimulating factor in poor prognosis newly diagnosed acute myeloid leukemia and myelodysplastic syndrome. Blood 1999 Apr 15; 93(8):2478–84.

56 Culine S, Kramear A, Droz JP, Theodore C. Phase II study of all-trans retinoic acid administered intermittently for hormone refractory prostate cancer. J Urol 1999 Jan; 161(1):173–5.

57 Conley BA, Egorin MJ, Sridhara R, et al. Phase I clinical trial of all-trans retinoic acid with correlation of its pharmacokinetics and pharmacodynamics. Cancer Chemother Pharmacol 1997; 39(4):291–9.

58 Trump DL, Smith DC, Stiff D, et al. A phase II trial of all-trans retinoic acid in hormone-refractory prostate cancer: A clinical trial with detailed pharmacokinetic analysis. Cancer Chemother Pharmacol 1997; 39(4):349–56.

59 Cornic M, Agadir A, Degos L, Chomienne C. Retinoids and differentiation treatment: A strategy for treatment in cancer. Anticancer Res 1994 Nov–Dec; 14(6A):2339–46.

60 Wiegand UW, Hartmann S, Hummler H. Safety of vitamin A: Recent results. Int J Vitam Nutr Res 1998; 68(6):411–6.

61 Comstock GW, Bush TL, Helzlsouer K. Serum retinol, beta-carotene, vitamin E, and selenium as related to subsequent cancer of specific sites. American Journal of Epidemiology 1992; 135(2):115–21.

62 Franceschi S. Micronutrients and breast cancer. Eur J Cancer Prev 1997 Dec; 6(6):535–9.

63 Batieha AM, Armenian HK, Norkus EP, et al. Serum micronutrients and the subsequent risk of cervical cancer in a population-based nested case-control study. Cancer Epidemiol Biomarkers Prev 1993 Jul–Aug; 2(4):335–9.

64 Mayne ST, Graham S, Zheng TZ. Dietary retinol: Prevention or promotion of carcinogenesis in humans? Cancer Causes Control 1991; 2(6):443–50.

[65] Zheng W, Blot WJ, Diamond EL, et al. Serum micronutrients and the subsequent risk of oral and pharyngeal cancer. Cancer Res 1993 Feb 15; 53(4):795–8.

[66] Comstock G, et al. Prediagonostic serum levels of carotenoids and vitamin E as related to subsequent cancer in Washington County, Maryland. Am J Clin Nutr 1991; 53:260s-264s.

[67] Hennekens CH, Buring JE. Antioxidant vitamins—benefits not yet proved. New Engl J Med 1994; 330(15):1080–1.

[68] Zaridze D, Evstifeeva T, Boyle P. Chemoprevention of oral leukoplakia and chronic esophagitis in an area of high incidence of oral and esophageal cancer. Ann Epidemiol 1993 May; 3(3):225–34.

[69] Rautalahti M, Albanes D, Virtamo J, et al. Beta-carotene did not work: Aftermath of the ATBC study. Cancer Lett 1997 Mar 19; 114(1–2):235–6.

[70] The Alpha-Tocopherol, Beta Carotene Cancer Prevention Study Group. The effect of vitamin E and beta carotene on the incidence of lung cancer and other cancers in male smokers [see comments]. N Engl J Med 1994 Apr 14; 330(15):1029–35.

[71] Albanes D, Heinonen OP, Huttunen JK, et al. Effects of alpha-tocopherol and beta-carotene supplements on cancer incidence in the alpha-tocopherol beta-carotene cancer prevention study. Am J Clin Nutr 1995 Dec; 62(6 Suppl):1427S-1430S.

[72] Omenn GS, Goodman GE, Thornquist MD, et al. Risk factors for lung cancer and for intervention effects in CARET, the beta-carotene and retinol efficacy trial [see comments]. J Natl Cancer Inst 1996 Nov 6; 88(21):1550–9.

[73] Albanes D, Heinonen OP, Taylor PR, et al. Alpha-tocopherol and beta-carotene supplements and lung cancer incidence in the alpha-tocopherol, beta-carotene cancer prevention study: Effects of base-line characteristics and study compliance [see comments]. J Natl Cancer Inst 1996 Nov 6; 88(21):1560–70.

[74] Omenn GS, Goodman G, Thornquist M, et al. The beta-carotene and retinol efficacy trial (CARET) for chemoprevention of lung cancer in high risk populations: Smokers and asbestos-exposed workers. Cancer Res 1994 Apr 1; 54(7 Suppl):2038s-2043s.

[75] Omenn GS, Goodman GE, Thornquist M, Brunzell JD. Long-term vitamin A does not produce clinically significant hypertriglyceridemia: Results from CARET, the beta-carotene and retinol efficacy trial. Cancer Epidemiol Biomarkers Prev 1994 Dec; 3(8):711–3.

[76] Goodman GE, Omenn GS, Thornquist MD, et al. The carotene and retinol efficacy trial (CARET) to prevent lung cancer in high-risk populations: Pilot study with cigarette smokers. Cancer Epidemiol Biomarkers Prev 1993 Jul–Aug; 2(4):389–96.

[77] Omenn GS, Goodman GE, Thornquist MD, et al. The carotene and retinol efficacy trial (CARET) to prevent lung cancer in high-risk populations: Pilot study with asbestos-exposed workers. Cancer Epidemiol Biomarkers Prev 1993 Jul–Aug; 2(4):381–7.

[78] Suzuki S, Takenoshita S, Furukawa H, Tsuchiya A. Antineoplastic activity of 1,25(OH)2D3 and its analogue 22-oxacalcitriol against human anaplastic thyroid carcinoma cell lines in vitro. Int J Mol Med 1999 Dec; 4(6):611–4.

[79] Tong WM, Hofer H, Ellinger A, et al. Mechanism of antimitogenic action of vitamin D in human colon carcinoma cells: Relevance for suppression of epidermal growth factor-stimulated cell growth. Oncol Res 1999; 11(2):77–84.

[80] Gache C, Berthois Y, Cvitkovic E, et al. Differential regulation of normal and tumoral breast epithelial cell growth by fibroblasts and 1,25-dihydroxyvitamin D3. Breast Cancer Res Treat 1999 May; 55(1):29–39.

[81] Hershberger PA, Modzelewski RA, Shurin ZR, et al. 1,25-dihydroxycholecalciferol (1,25-D3) inhibits the growth of squamous cell carcinoma and down-modulates p21(Waf1/Cip1) in vitro and in vivo. Cancer Res 1999 Jun 1; 59(11):2644–9.

[82] Celli A, Treves C, Nassi P, Stio M. Role of 1,25-dihydroxyvitamin D3 and extracellular calcium in the regulation of proliferation in cultured SH-SY5Y human neuroblastoma cells. Neurochem Res 1999 May; 24(5):691–8.

[83] Li J, Finch RA, Sartorelli AC. Role of vitamin D3 receptor in the synergistic differentiation of WEHI-3B leukemia cells by vitamin D3 and retinoic acid. Exp Cell Res 1999 Jun 15; 249(2):279–90.

[84] Taimi M, Chateau MT, Cabane S, Marti J. Synergistic effect of retinoic acid and 1,25-dihydroxyvitamin D3 on the differentiation of the human monocytic cell line U937. Leuk Res 1991; 15(12):1145–52.

[85] Koga M, Sutherland RL. Retinoic acid acts synergistically with 1,25-dihydroxyvitamin D3 or antioestrogen to inhibit T-47D human breast cancer cell proliferation. J Steroid Biochem Mol Biol 1991 Oct; 39(4A):455–60.

[86] Camagna A, Testa U, Masciulli R, et al. The synergistic effect of simultaneous addition of retinoic acid and vitamin D3 on the in-vitro differentiation of human promyelocytic leukemia cell lines could be efficiently transposed in vivo. Med Hypotheses 1998 Mar; 50(3):253–7.

[87] James SY, Williams MA, Newland AC, Colston KW. Leukemia cell differentiation: Cellular and molecular interactions of retinoids and vitamin D. Gen Pharmacol 1999 Jan; 32(1):143–54.

[88] Yabushita H, Hirata M, Noguchi M, Nakanishi M. Vitamin D receptor in endometrial carcinoma and the differentiation-inducing effect of 1,25-dihydroxyvitamin D3 on endometrial carcinoma cell lines. J Obstet Gynaecol Res 1996 Dec; 22(6):529–39.

[89] Moore TB, Koeffler HP, Yamashiro JM, Wada RK. Vitamin D3 analogs inhibit growth and induce differentiation in LA-N-5 human neuroblastoma cells. Clin Exp Metastasis 1996 May; 14(3):239–45.

[90] Radhika S, Choudhary SK, Garg LC, Dixit A. Induction of differentiation in murine erythroleukemia cells by 1 alpha,25-dihydroxy vitamin D3. Cancer Lett 1995 Apr 14; 90(2):225–30.

[91] Defacque H, Dornand J, Commes T, et al. Different combinations of retinoids and vitamin D3 analogs efficiently promote growth inhibition and differentiation of myelomonocytic leukemia cell lines. J Pharmacol Exp Ther 1994 Oct; 271(1):193–9.

[92] Welsh J. Induction of apoptosis in breast cancer cells in response to vitamin D and antiestrogens. Biochem Cell Biol 1994 Nov–Dec; 72(11–12):537–45.

[93] Danielsson C, Fehsel K, Polly P, Carlberg C. Differential apoptotic response of human melanoma cells to 1 alpha,25-

dihydroxyvitamin D3 and its analogues. Cell Death Differ 1998 Nov; 5(11):946–52.

94 Saez S, Falette N, Guillot C, et al. 1,25(OH)2D3 modulation of mammary tumor cell growth in vitro and in vivo. Breast Cancer Res Treat 1993; 27(1–2):69–81.

95 Pourgholami MH, Akhter J, Lu Y, Morris DL. In vitro and in vivo inhibition of liver cancer cells by 1,25-dihydroxyvitamin D3. Cancer Lett 2000 Apr 3; 151(1):97–102.

96 Lokeshwar BL, Schwartz GG, Selzer MG, et al. Inhibition of prostate cancer metastasis in vivo: A comparison of 1,23-dihydroxyvitamin D (calcitriol) and EB1089. Cancer Epidemiol Biomarkers Prev 1999 Mar; 8(3):241–8.

97 Young MR, Ihm J, Lozano Y, et al. Treating tumor-bearing mice with vitamin D3 diminishes tumor-induced myelopoiesis and associated immunosuppression, and reduces tumor metastasis and recurrence. Cancer Immunol Immunother 1995 Jul; 41(1):37–45.

98 Shokravi MT, Marcus DM, Alroy J, et al. Vitamin D inhibits angiogenesis in transgenic murine retinoblastoma. Invest Ophthalmol Vis Sci 1995 Jan; 36(1):83–7.

99 Gross C, Stamey T, Hancock S, Feldman D. Treatment of early recurrent prostate cancer with 1,25-dihydroxyvitamin D3. J Urol 1998 Jun; 159(6):2035–9; discussion 2039–40.

100 Palmieri-Sevier A, Palmieri GM, Baumgartner CJ, Britt LG. Case report: Long-term remission of parathyroid cancer: Possible relation to vitamin D and calcitriol therapy. Am J Med Sci 1993 Nov; 306(5):309–12.

101 Rustin GJ, Quinnell TG, Johnson J, et al. Trial of isotretinoin and calcitriol monitored by CA 125 in patients with ovarian cancer. Br J Cancer 1996 Nov; 74(9):1479–81.

102 Koeffler HP, Hirji K, Itri L. 1,25-Dihydroxyvitamin D3: In vivo and in vitro effects on human preleukemic and leukemic cells. Cancer Treat Rep 1985 Dec; 69(12):1399–407.

103 Stoica A, Saceda M, Fakhro A, et al. Regulation of estrogen receptor-alpha gene expression by 1,25-dihydroxyvitamin D in MCF-7 cells. J Cell Biochem 1999 Dec 15; 75(4):640–651.

104 Reinhardt TA, Koszewski NJ, Omdahl J, et al. 1,25-dihydroxyvitamin D(3) and 9-cis-retinoids are synergistic regulators of 24-hydroxylase activity in the rat and 1, 25-dihydroxyvitamin D(3) alters retinoic acid metabolism in vivo. Arch Biochem Biophys 1999 Aug 15; 368(2):244–8.

105 Dubbelman R, Jonxis JHP, Muskiet FAJ, Saleh AEC. Age-dependent vitamin D status and vertebral conditions of white women living in Curacao (The Netherlands Antilles) as compared with their counterparts in The Netherlands. Am J Clin Nutr 1993; 58:106–9.

106 Gann PH, Ma J, Hennekens CH, et al. Circulating vitamin D metabolites in relation to subsequent development of prostate cancer. Cancer Epidem Biomark Preven 1996; 5:121–126.

107 Smith DC, Johnson CS, Freeman CC, et al. A phase I trial of calcitriol (1,25-dihydroxycholecalciferol) in patients with advanced malignancy. Clin Cancer Res 1999 Jun; 5(6):1339–45.

108 Koeffler HP, Hirji K, Itri L, et al. 1,25-dihydroxyvitamin D3: In vivo and in vitro effects on human preleukemic and leukemic cells. Cancer Treatment Reports 1985; 69(12):1399–1407.

109 Young MR, Lozano Y. Inhibition of tumor invasiveness by 1alpha,25-dihydroxyvitamin D3 coupled to a decline in protein kinase A activity and an increase in cytoskeletal organization. Clin Exp Metastasis 1997 Mar; 15(2):102–10.

110 Rocker D, Ravid A, Liberman UA, et al. 1,25-dihydroxyvitamin D3 potentiates the cytotoxic effect of TNF on human breast cancer cells. Mol Cell Endocrinol 1994 Dec; 106(1–2):157–62.

111 Majewski S, Marczak M, Szmurlo A, et al. Retinoids, interferon alpha, 1,25-dihydroxyvitamin D3 and their combination inhibit angiogenesis induced by non-HPV-harboring tumor cell lines. RAR alpha mediates the antiangiogenic effect of retinoids. Cancer Lett 1995 Feb 10; 89(1):117–24.

112 Majewski S, Skopinska M, Marczak M, et al. Vitamin D3 is a potent inhibitor of tumor cell-induced angiogenesis. J Investig Dermatol Symp Proc 1996; 1(1):97–101.

113 Koshizuka K, Kubota T, Said J, et al. Combination therapy of a vitamin D3 analog and all-trans retinoic acid: Effect on human breast cancer in nude mice. Anticancer Res 1999 Jan–Feb; 19(1A):519–24.

114 Iino Y, Yoshida M, Sugamata N, et al. 1 alpha-hydroxyvitamin D3, hypercalcemia, and growth suppression of 7,12-dimethylbenz[a]anthracene-induced rat mammary tumors. Breast Cancer Res Treat 1992; 22(2):133–40.

115 Mantell DJ, Owens PE, Bundred NJ, et al. 1 alpha,25-dihydroxyvitamin D(3) inhibits angiogenesis in vitro and in vivo. Circ Res 2000 Aug 4; 87(3):214–20.

116 Young MR, Ihm J, Lozano Y, et al. Treating tumor-bearing mice with vitamin D3 diminishes tumor-induced myelopoiesis and associated immunosuppression, and reduces tumor metastasis and recurrence. Cancer Immunol Immunotherapy 1995; 41:37–45.

117 Fujioka T, Hasegawa M, Ishikura K, et al. Inhibition of tumor growth and angiogenesis by vitamin D3 agents in murine renal cell carcinoma. J Urol 1998; 160:247–251.

118 Yu WD, McElwain MC, Modzelewski RA, et al. Enhancement of 1,25-dihydroxyvitamin D3-mediated antitumor activity with dexamethasone. J Natl Cancer Inst 1998 Jan 21; 90(2):134–41.

119 Mawer EB, Walls J, Howell A, et al. Serum 1,25-dihydroxyvitamin D may be related inversely to disease activity in breast cancer patients with bone metastases. J Clin Endocrinol Metab 1997 Jan; 82(1):118–22.

120 Corder EH, Guess HA, Hulka BS, et al. Vitamin D and prostate cancer: A prediagnostic study with stored sera [see comments]. Cancer Epidemiol Biomarkers Prev 1993; 2(5):467–72.

121 Garland CF, Comstock GW, Garland FC, et al. Serum 25-hydroxyvitamin D and colon cancer: Eight-year prospective study. Lancet 1989; 2(8673):1176–8.

122 Studzinski GP, Moore DC. Sunlight—can it prevent as well as cause cancer? Cancer Research 1995 Sep 15; 55:4014–4022.

123 Newmark HL. Vitamin D adequacy: A possible relationship to breast cancer. Adv Exp Med Biol 1994; 364:109–14.

124 Vieth R. Vitamin D supplementation, 25-hydroxyvitamin D concentrations, and safety. Am J Clin Nutr 1999 May; 69(5):842–56.

125 Odukoya O, Schwartz J, Shklar G. Vitamin E stimulates proliferation of experimental oral carcinoma cells in vitro. Nutr Cancer 1986; 8(2):101–6.

126 Pastori M, Pfander H, Boscoboinik D, Azzi A. Lycopene in association with alpha-tocopherol inhibits at physiological concentrations proliferation of prostate carcinoma cells. Biochem Biophys Res Commun 1998 Sep 29; 250(3):582–5.

127 Sigounas G, Anagnostou A, Steiner M. dl-alpha-tocopherol induces apoptosis in erythroleukemia, prostate, and breast cancer cells. Nutr Cancer 1997; 28(1):30–5.

128 Cornwell DG, Jones KH, Jiang Z, et al. Cytotoxicity of tocopherols and their quinones in drug-sensitive and multidrug-resistant leukemia cells. Lipids 1998 Mar; 33(3):295–301.

129 Slack R, Proulx P. Studies on the effects of vitamin E on neuroblastoma N1E 115. Nutr Cancer 1989; 12(1):75–82.

130 Boscoboinik D, Szewczyk A, Hensey C, Azzi A. Inhibition of cell proliferation by alpha-tocopherol. Role of protein kinase C. J Biol Chem 1991 Apr 5; 266(10):6188–94.

131 Azzi A, Boscoboinik D, Chatelain E, et al. d-alpha-tocopherol control of cell proliferation. Mol Aspects Med 1993; 14(3):265–71.

132 Traber MG, Packer L. Vitamin E: Beyond antioxidant function. Am J Clin Nutr 1995 Dec; 62(6 Suppl):1501S–1509S.

133 Israel K, Yu W, Sanders BG, Kline K. Vitamin E succinate induces apoptosis in human prostate cancer cells: Role for Fas in vitamin E succinate-triggered apoptosis. Nutr Cancer 2000; 36(1):90–100.

134 Yu W, Simmons-Menchaca M, Gapor A, et al. Induction of apoptosis in human breast cancer cells by tocopherols and tocotrienols. Nutr Cancer 1999; 33(1):26–32.

135 Yu W, Israel K, Liao QY, et al. Vitamin E succinate (VES) induces Fas sensitivity in human breast cancer cells: Role for Mr 43,000 Fas in VES-triggered apoptosis. Cancer Res 1999 Feb 15; 59(4):953–61.

136 Turley JM, Ruscetti FW, Kim SJ, et al. Vitamin E succinate inhibits proliferation of BT-20 human breast cancer cells: Increased binding of cyclin A negatively regulates E2F transactivation activity. Cancer Res 1997 Jul 1; 57(13):2668–75.

137 Turley JM, Fu T, Ruscetti FW, et al. Vitamin E succinate induces Fas-mediated apoptosis in estrogen receptor-negative human breast cancer cells. Cancer Res 1997 Mar 1; 57(5):881–90.

138 Prasad KN, Edwards-Prasad J. Vitamin E and cancer prevention: Recent advances and future potentials. J Am Coll Nutr 1992 Oct; 11(5):487–500.

139 Prasad KN, Kumar A, Kochupillai V, Cole WC. High doses of multiple antioxidant vitamins: Essential ingredients in improving the efficacy of standard cancer therapy. J Am Coll Nutr 1999 Feb; 18(1):13–25.

140 Elattar TM, Virji AS. Biphasic action of vitamin E on the growth of human oral squamous carcinoma cells. Anticancer Res 1999 Jan–Feb; 19(1A):365–8.

141 Yu W, Sanders BG, Kline K. Modulation of murine EL-4 thymic lymphoma cell proliferation and cytokine production by vitamin E succinate. Nutr Cancer 1996; 25(2):137–49.

142 Prasad KN, Kumar R. Effect of individual and multiple antioxidant vitamins on growth and morphology of human nontumorigenic and tumorigenic parotid acinar cells in culture. Nutr Cancer 1996; 26(1):11–9.

143 Prasad KN, Cole WC, Prasad JE. Multiple antioxidant vitamins as an adjunct to standard and experimental cancer therapies. J Oncol 1999; 31(4):101–8.

144 Dasgupta J, Sanyal U, Das S. Vitamin E—its status and role in leukemia and lymphoma. Neoplasma 1993; 40(4):235–40.

145 Kurek MP, Corwin LM. Vitamin E protection against tumor formation by transplanted murine sarcoma cells. Nutr Cancer 1982; 4(2):128–39.

146 Evangelou A, Kalpouzos G, Karkabounas S, et al. Dose-related preventive and therapeutic effects of antioxidants-anticarcinogens on experimentally induced malignant tumors in Wistar rats. Cancer Lett 1997 May 1; 115(1):105–11.

147 Shklar G, Schwartz J, Trickler D, Reid S. Regression of experimental cancer by oral administration of combined alpha-tocopherol and beta-carotene. Nutr Cancer 1989; 12(4):321–5.

148 Malafa MP, Neitzel LT. Vitamin E succinate promotes breast cancer tumor dormancy. J Surg Res 2000 Sep; 93(1):163–70.

149 Horvath PM, Ip C. Synergistic effect of vitamin E and selenium in the chemoprevention of mammary carcinogenesis in rats. Cancer Res 1983 Nov; 43(11):5335–41.

150 Woutersen RA, Appel MJ, Van Garderen-Hoetmer A. Modulation of pancreatic carcinogenesis by antioxidants. Food Chem Toxicol 1999 Sep–Oct; 37(9–10):981–4.

151 Shklar G, Schwartz JL, Trickler DP, Reid S. Prevention of experimental cancer and immunostimulation by vitamin E (immunosurveillance). J Oral Pathol Med 1990 Feb; 19(2):60–4.

152 Shklar G, Schwartz JL. Vitamin E inhibits experimental carcinogenesis and tumour angiogenesis. Eur J Cancer B Oral Oncol 1996 Mar; 32B(2):114–9.

153 Kelloff GJ, Crowell JA, Boone CW, et al. Clinical development plan: Vitamin E. J Cell Biochem Suppl 1994; 20:282–99.

154 Kallistratos GI, Fasske EE, Karkabounas S, Charalambopoulos K. Prolongation of the survival time of tumor bearing Wistar rats through a simultaneous oral administration of vitamins C + E and selenium with glutathione. Prog Clin Biol Res 1988; 259:377–89.

155 Shklar G, Schwartz J, Trickler D, Cheverie SR. The effectiveness of a mixture of beta-carotene, alpha-tocopherol, glutathione, and ascorbic acid for cancer prevention. Nutr Cancer 1993; 20(2):145–51.

156 [No authors listed]. The effect of vitamin E and beta carotene on the incidence of lung cancer and other cancers in male smokers. N Engl J Med 1994 Apr 14; 330(15):1029–35.

157 Albanes D, Malila N, Taylor PR, et al. Effects of supplemental alpha-tocopherol and beta-carotene on colorectal cancer: Results from a controlled trial. Cancer Causes Control 2000 Mar; 11(3):197–205.

158 Heinonen OP, Albanes D, Virtamo J, et al. Prostate cancer and supplementation with alpha-tocopherol and beta-carotene: Incidence and mortality in a controlled trial. J Natl Cancer Inst 1998 Mar 18; 90(6):440–6.

159 Chan JM, Stampfer MJ, Ma J, et al. Supplemental vitamin E intake and prostate cancer risk in a large cohort of men in the United States. Cancer Epidemiol Biomarkers Prev 1999 Oct; 8(10):893–9.

160 Lamm DL, Riggs DR, Shriver JS, et al. Megadose vitamins in bladder cancer: A double-blind clinical trial. J Urol 1994 Jan; 151(1):21–6.

161 Buck M, Chojkier M. Muscle wasting and dedifferentiation induced by oxidative stress in a murine model of cachexia is prevented by inhibitors of nitric oxide synthesis and antioxidants. EMBO J 1996 Apr 15; 15(8):1753–65.

162 Fleshner N, Fair WR, Huryk R, Heston WD. Vitamin E inhibits the high-fat diet promoted growth of established human prostate LNCaP tumors in nude mice. J Urol 1999 May; 161(5):1651–4.

163 Burton GW, Traber MG, Acuff RV, et al. Human plasma and tissue alpha-tocopherol concentrations in response to supplementation with deuterated natural and synthetic vitamin E. Am J Clin Nutr 1998 Apr; 67(4):669–84.

164 Traber MG. Utilization of vitamin E. Biofactors 1999; 10(2–3):115–20.

165 Behrens WA, Madere R. Tissue discrimination between dietary RRR-alpha- and all-rac-alpha-tocopherols in rats. J Nutr 1991 Apr; 121(4):454–9.

166 Kontush A, Finckh B, Karten B, et al. Antioxidant and prooxidant activity of alpha-tocopherol in human plasma and low density lipoprotein. J Lipid Res 1996 Jul; 37(7):1436–48.

167 Brown KM, Morrice PC, Duthie GG. Erythrocyte vitamin E and plasma ascorbate concentrations in relation to erythrocyte peroxidation in smokers and nonsmokers: Dose response to vitamin E supplementation [see comments]. Am J Clin Nutr 1997 Feb; 65(2):496–502.

168 Azzi A, Boscoboinik D, Chatelain E, et al. d-alpha-tocopherol control of cell proliferation. Mol Aspects Med 1993; 14(3):265–71.

169 Sigounas G, Anagnostou A, Steiner M. dl-alpha-tocopherol induces apoptosis in erythroleukemia, prostate, and breast cancer cells. Nutr Cancer 1997; 28(1):30–5.

170 Boscoboinik D, Szewczyk A, Hensey C, Azzi A. Inhibition of cell proliferation by alpha-tocopherol. Role of protein kinase C. J Biol Chem 1991 Apr 5; 266(10):6188–94.

171 Zhao B, Yu W, Qian M, et al. Involvement of activator protein-1 (AP-1) in induction of apoptosis by vitamin E succinate in human breast cancer cells. Mol Carcinog 1997 Jul; 19(3):180–90.

172 Prasad KN, Cohrs RJ, Sharma OK. Decreased expressions of c-myc and H-ras oncogenes in vitamin E succinate induced morphologically differentiated murine B-16 melanoma cells in culture. Biochem Cell Biol 1990 Nov; 68(11):1250–5.

173 Yu W, Heim K, Qian M, et al. Evidence for role of transforming growth factor-beta in RRR-alpha-tocopheryl succinate-induced apoptosis of human MDA-MB-435 breast cancer cells. Nutr Cancer 1997; 27(3):267–78.

174 Charpentier A, Groves S, Simmons-Menchaca M, et al. RRR-alpha-tocopheryl succinate inhibits proliferation and enhances secretion of transforming growth factor-beta (TGF-beta) by human breast cancer cells. Nutr Cancer 1993; 19(3):225–39.

175 Turley JM, Sanders BG, Kline K. RRR-alpha-tocopheryl succinate modulation of human promyelocytic leukemia (HL-60) cell proliferation and differentiation. Nutr Cancer 1992; 18(3):201–13.

176 Fariss MW, Fortuna MB, Everett CK, et al. The selective antiproliferative effects of alpha-tocopheryl hemisuccinate and cholesteryl hemisuccinate on murine leukemia cells result from the action of the intact compounds. Cancer Res 1994 Jul 1; 54(13):3346–51.

177 Djuric Z, Heilbrun LK, Lababidi S, et al. Growth inhibition of MCF-7 and MCF-10A human breast cells by alpha-tocopheryl hemisuccinate, cholesteryl hemisuccinate and their ether analogs. Cancer Lett 1997 Jan 1; 111(1–2):133–9.

178 Shklar G, Schwartz JL. Ascorbic acid and cancer. Subcell Biochem 1996; 25:233–47.

179 Buck M, Chojkier M. Muscle wasting and dedifferentiation induced by oxidative stress in a murine model of cachexia is prevented by inhibitors of nitric oxide synthesis and antioxidants. EMBO J 1996 Apr 15; 15(8):1753–65.

180 Woodson K, Tangrea JA Barrett MK, et al. Serum alpha-tocopherol and subsequent risk of lung cancer among male smokers. J Natl Cancer Inst 1999; 91(20):1738–43.

181 Mahoney CW, Azzi A. Vitamin E inhibits protein kinase C activity. Biochem Biophys Res Commun 1988 Jul 29; 154(2):694–7.

182 Freedman JE, Farhat JH, Loscalzo J, Keaney JF Jr. Alpha-tocopherol inhibits aggregation of human platelets by a protein kinase C-dependent mechanism. Circulation 1996 Nov 15; 94(10):2434–40.

183 Chon W. Bioavailability of vitamin E. Eur J Clin Nutr 1997; 51(Suppl 1): S80–5.

184 Dimitrov NV, Meyer C, Gilliland D, et al. Plasma tocopherol concentrations in response to supplemental vitamin E. Am J Clin Nutr 1991 Mar; 53(3):723–9.

185 Kitagawa M, Mino M. Effects of elevated d-alpha(RRR)-tocopherol dosage in man. J Nutr Sci Vitaminol (Tokyo) 1989 Apr; 35(2):133–42.

186 Machlin LJ, Gabriel E. Kinetics of tissue alpha-tocopherol uptake and depletion following administration of high levels of vitamin E. Ann NY Acad Sci 1982; 393:48–60.

187 Nakamura T, Aoyama Y, Fujita T, Katsui G. Studies on tocopherol derivatives: V. Intestinal absorption of several d,l-3,4-3 H_2-α-tocopheryl esters in the rat. Lipids 1975; 10:627–33.

188 Cheeseman KH, Holley AE, Kelly FJ, et al. Biokinetics in humans of RRR-alpha-tocopherol: The free phenol, acetate ester, and succinate ester forms of vitamin E. Free Radic Biol Med 1995 Nov; 19(5):591–8.

189 Diplock AT. Safety of antioxidant vitamins and β-carotene. Am J Clin Nutr 1995; 62(suppl):1510S-6S.

190 Shiu SY, Li L, Xu JN, et al. Melatonin-induced inhibition of proliferation and G1/S cell cycle transition delay of human choriocarcinoma JAr cells: Possible involvement of MT2 (MEL1B) receptor. J Pineal Res 1999 Oct; 27(3):183–92.

191 Mediavilla MD, Cos S, Sanchez-Barcelo EJ. Melatonin increases p53 and p21WAF1 expression in MCF-7 human breast cancer cells in vitro. Life Sci 1999; 65(4):415–20.

[192] Petranka J, Baldwin W, Biermann J, et al. The oncostatic action of melatonin in an ovarian carcinoma cell line. J Pineal Res 1999 Apr; 26(3):129–36.

[193] Karasek M, Pawlikowski M. Antiproliferative effects of melatonin and CGP 52608. Biol Signals Recept 1999 Jan–Apr; 8(1–2):75–8.

[194] Papazisis KT, Kouretas D, Geromichalos GD, et al. Effects of melatonin on proliferation of cancer cell lines. J Pineal Res 1998 Dec; 25(4):211–8.

[195] Pawlikowski M, Kunert-Radek J, Winczyk K, et al. The antiproliferative effects of melatonin on experimental pituitary and colonic tumors. Possible involvement of the putative nuclear binding site? Adv Exp Med Biol 1999; 460:369–72.

[196] El-Missiry MA, Abd El-Aziz AF. Influence of melatonin on proliferation and antioxidant system in Ehrlich ascites carcinoma cells. Cancer Lett 2000 Apr 14; 151(2):119–25.

[197] Narita T, Kudo H. Effect of melatonin on B16 melanoma growth in athymic mice. Cancer Res 1985 Sep; 45(9):4175–7.

[198] Mocchegiani E, Perissin L, Santarelli L, et al. Melatonin administration in tumor-bearing mice (intact and pinealectomized) in relation to stress, zinc, thymulin and IL-2. Int J Immunopharmacol 1999 Jan; 21(1):27–46.

[199] Rapozzi V, Perissin L, Zorzet S, Giraldi T. Effects of melatonin administration on tumor spread in mice bearing Lewis lung carcinoma. Pharmacol Res 1992 Feb–Mar; 25 Suppl 1:71–2.

[200] Lissoni P, Barni S, Ardizzoia A, et al. A randomized study with the pineal hormone melatonin versus supportive care alone in patients with brain metastases due to solid neoplasms. Cancer 1994 Feb 1; 73(3):699–701.

[201] Lissoni P, Barni S, Ardizzoia A, et al. Randomized study with the pineal hormone melatonin versus supportive care alone in advanced nonsmall cell lung cancer resistant to a first-line chemotherapy containing cisplatin. Oncology 1992; 49(5):336–9.

[202] Neri B, de Leonardis V, Gemelli MT, et al. Melatonin as biological response modifier in cancer patients. Anticancer Res 1998 Mar–Apr; 18(2B):1329–32.

[203] Lissoni P, Barni S, Crispino S, et al. Endocrine and immune effects of melatonin therapy in metastatic cancer patients. Eur J Cancer Clin Oncol 1989 May; 25(5):789–95.

[204] Lissoni P, Barni S, Cattaneo G, et al. Clinical results with the pineal hormone melatonin in advanced cancer resistant to standard antitumor therapies. Oncology 1991; 48(6):448–50.

[205] Bartsch C, Bartsch H. Melatonin in cancer patients and in tumor-bearing animals. Adv Exp Med Biol 1999; 467:247–64.

[206] Maestroni GJ. Therapeutic potential of melatonin in immunodeficiency states, viral diseases, and cancer. Adv Exp Med Biol 1999; 467:217–26.

[207] Conti A, Maestroni GJ. The clinical neuroimmunotherapeutic role of melatonin in oncology. J Pineal Res 1995 Oct; 19(3):103–10.

[208] Panzer A, Viljoen M. The validity of melatonin as an oncostatic agent. J Pineal Res 1997 May; 22(4):184–202.

[209] Cos S, Sanchez-Barcelo EJ. Melatonin and mammary pathological growth. Front Neuroendocrinol 2000 Apr; 21(2):133–70.

[210] Gonzalez-Haba MG, Garcia-Maurino S, Calvo JR, et al. High-affinity binding sites of melatonin by human circulating T lymphocytes (CD4+). FASEB J 1995; 9:1331–1335.

[211] Voultsios A, Kennaway DJ, Dawson D. Salivary melatonin as a circadian phase marker: Validation and comparison to plasma melatonin. J Biol Rhythms 1997 Oct; 12(5):457–66.

[212] Shirakawa S, Tsuchiya S, Tsutsumi Y, et al. Time course of saliva and serum melatonin levels after ingestion of melatonin. Psychiatry Clin Neurosci 1998 Apr; 52(2):266–7.

[213] Kane MA, Johnson A, Nash AE, et al. Serum melatonin levels in melanoma patients after repeated oral administration. Melanoma Res 1994; 4:59–65.

[214] Reiter RJ, Melchiorri D, Sewerynek E, Poeggeler B, et al. A review of the evidence supporting melatonin's role as an antioxidant. J Pineal Res 1995; 18(1):1–11.

[215] Pieri C, Marra M, Moroni F, Recchioni R, Marcheselli F. Melatonin: A peroxyl radical scavenger more effective than vitamin E. Life Sci 1994; 55(15):PL271–6.

[216] Reiter RJ. Interactions of the pineal hormone melatonin with oxygen-centered free radicals: A brief review. Braz J Med Biol Res 1993; 26(11):1141–55.

[217] Cos S, Fernandez F, Sanchez-Barcelo EJ. Melatonin inhibits DNA synthesis in MCF-7 human breast cancer cells in vitro. Life Sci 1996 May 24; 58(26):2447–53.

[218] Crespo D, Fernandez-Viadero C, Verduga R, et al. Interaction between melatonin and estradiol on morphological and morphometric features of MCF-7 human breast cancer cells. J Pineal Res 1994 May; 16(4):215–222.

[219] Hill SM, Spriggs LL, Simon MA. The growth inhibitory action of melatonin on human breast cancer cells is linked to the estrogen response system. Cancer Lett 1992 Jul 10; 64(3):249–56.

[220] Cos S, Sanchez-Barcelo EJ. Differences between pulsatile or continuous exposure to melatonin on MCF-7 human breast cancer cell proliferation. Cancer Lett 1994 Sep 30; 85(1):105–109.

[221] Furuya Y, Yamamoto K, Kohno N, et al. 5-fluorouracil attenuates an oncostatatic effect of melatonin on estrogen-sensitive human breast cancer cells (MCF7). Cancer Lett 1994 June 15; 81(1):95–8.

[222] Cos S, Sanchez-Barcelo EJ. Differences between pulsatile or continuous exposure to melatonin on MCF-7 human breast cancer cell proliferation. Cancer Lett 1994 Sep 30; 85(1):105–9.

[223] Gilad E, Laufer M, Matzkin H, Zisapel N. Melatonin receptors in PC3 human prostate tumor cells. J Pineal Res 1999 May; 26(4):211–20.

[224] Steinhilber D, Brungs M, Werz O, et al. The nuclear receptor for melatonin represses 5-lipoxygenase gene expression in human B lymphocytes. J Biol Chem 1995 Mar 31; 270(13):7037–40.

[225] Blask DE, Sauer LA, Dauchy R, et al. New actions of melatonin on tumor metabolism and growth. Biol Signals Recept 1999 Jan–Apr; 8(1–2):49–55.

[226] Dauchy RT, Blask DE, Sauer LA, et al. Dim light during darkness stimulates tumor progression by enhancing tumor fatty acid uptake and metabolism. Cancer Lett 1999 Oct 1; 144(2):131–6.

227 Dauchy RT, Sauer LA, Blask DE, Vaughan GM. Light contamination during the dark phase in "photoperiodically controlled" animal rooms: Effect on tumor growth and metabolism in rats. Lab Anim Sci 1997 Oct; 47(5):511–8.

228 Stanberry LR, Das Gupta TK, Beattie CW. Photoperiodic control of melanoma growth in hamsters: Influence of pinealectomy and melatonin. Endocrinology 1983 Aug; 113(2):469–75.

229 Cini G, Coronnello M, Mini E, Neri B. Melatonin's growth inhibitory effect on hepatoma AH 130 in the rat. Cancer Letters 1998; 125:51–59.

230 Philo R, Berkowitz AS. Inhibition of Dunning tumor growth by melatonin. J Urol 1988 May; 139(5):1099–102.

231 Lissoni P, Brivio O, Brivio F, et al. Adjuvant therapy with the pineal hormone melatonin in patients with lymph node relapse due to malignant melanoma. J Pineal Res 1996 Nov; 21(4):239–42.

232 Lissoni P, Barni S, Fossati V, et al. A randomized study of neuroimmunotherapy with low-dose subcutaneous interleukin-2 plus melatonin compared to supportive care alone in patients with untreatable metastatic solid tumour. Support Care Cancer 1995 May; 3(3):194–7.

233 Barni S, Lissoni P, Cazzaniga M, et al. A randomized study of low-dose subcutaneous interleukin-2 plus melatonin versus supportive care alone in metastatic colorectal cancer patients progressing under 5-fluorouracil and folates. Oncology 1995 May–Jun; 52(3):243–5.

234 Lissoni P, Barni S, Tancini G, et al. A randomised study with subcutaneous low-dose interleukin 2 alone vs interleukin 2 plus the pineal neurohormone melatonin in advanced solid neoplasms other than renal cancer and melanoma. Br J Cancer 1994 Jan; 69(1):196–9.

235 Lissoni P, Meregalli S, Fossati V, et al. A randomized study of immunotherapy with low-dose subcutaneous interleukin-2 plus melatonin vs chemotherapy with cisplatin and etoposide as first-line therapy for advanced non-small cell lung cancer. Tumori 1994 Dec 31; 80(6):464–7.

236 Lissoni P, Barni S, Tancini G, et al. Immunotherapy with subcutaneous low-dose interleukin-2 and the pineal indole melatonin as a new effective therapy in advanced cancers of the digestive tract. Br J Cancer 1993 Jun; 67(6):1404–7.

237 Lissoni P, Barni S, Rovelli F, et al. Neuroimmunotherapy of advanced solid neoplasms with single evening subcutaneous injection of low-dose interleukin-2 and melatonin: Preliminary results. Eur J Cancer 1993; 29A(2):185–9.

238 Aldeghi R, Lissoni P, Barni S, et al. Low-dose interleukin-2 subcutaneous immunotherapy in association with the pineal hormone melatonin as a first-line therapy in locally advanced or metastatic hepatocellular carcinoma. Eur J Cancer 1994; 30A(2):167–70.

239 Bartsch H, Bartsch C. Effect of melatonin on experimental tumors under different photoperiods and times of administration. J Neural Transmission 1981; 52:269–279.

240 Bartsch C, Bartsch H, Lippert TH. Rationales to consider the use of melatonin as a chrono-oncotherapeutic drug. in vivo 1995; 9:305–310.

241 Blask DE. Neuroendocrine aspects of circadian pharmacodynamics. In Circadian cancer therapy. Hrushesky WJ, ed. Ann Arbor: CRC Press, 1994, pp. 43–59.

242 Morin LP. History of biological clock research. Light treatment and biological rhythms. Bulletin of the Society for Light Treatment and Biological Rhythms 1996; 8(2):20–29.

243 Massion AO, Teas J, Hebert JR, et al. Meditation, melatonin and breast/prostate cancer: Hypothesis and preliminary data. Med Hypotheses 1995 Jan; 44(1):39–46.

244 Tooley GA, Armstrong SM, Norman TR, Sali A. Acute increases in night-time plasma melatonin levels following a period of meditation. Biol Psychol 2000 May; 53(1):69–78.

245 Meares A. A form of intensive meditation associated with the regression of cancer. Am J Clin Hypn 1982 Oct-1983 Jan; 25(2–3):114–21.

246 Meares A. Stress, meditation and the regression of cancer. Practitioner 1982 Sep; 226(1371):1607–9.

247 Meares A. Regression of recurrence of carcinoma of the breast at mastectomy site associated with intensive meditation. Aust Fam Physician 1981 Mar; 10(3):218–9.

248 Meares A. Meditation: A psychological approach to cancer treatment. Practitioner 1979 Jan; 222(1327):119–22.

NATURAL COMPOUNDS, CHEMOTHERAPY, AND RADIOTHERAPY

Although the main focus of this book is the use of natural compounds in combination with one another or, more generally, of the mechanism-based approach, it also seems important to investigate using natural compounds to improve the efficacy and safety of current chemotherapy drugs and radiotherapy. As discussed in the preface, within the next decade cancer chemotherapy will undergo radical changes, as mechanism-based drugs that effectively inhibit cancer without harming normal cells begin to be utilized. Natural compounds, similar in many ways to this new generation of drugs, would likely complement their actions; for example, those that inhibit PTK activity could be expected to complement drugs that do the same. The advent of such drugs is still some years off, however, and the more practical question now is whether natural compounds can maximize the efficacy or minimize the adverse effects of currently used drugs. While the majority of animal studies conducted thus far do suggest that natural compounds could perform one or both functions, the data are still limited, and much more work is needed to determine how and when they might best be used and when they should not be. In particular, additional animal studies are needed in which natural compounds are administered in ways that humans would use them (i.e., orally, at moderate doses, in combination with one another, and for prolonged time periods). Many animal studies used other routes of administration, doses, and/or schedules.

Using natural compounds with chemotherapy or radiotherapy is a controversial issue, and of all natural compounds, antioxidants in such combinations are the most controversial. On one hand, there is concern antioxidants might protect cancer cells from conventional therapies. On the other, there is evidence antioxidants can support the immune system and protect normal cells from the adverse effects of conventional treatments. Studies are currently under way or are being planned that will help shed more light on when and where antioxidants may be beneficial or detrimental. The preliminary evidence available, however, suggests that antioxidants will be beneficial (or at least not harmful) in most situations.

Antioxidants receive much attention from researchers and the public, but they are by no means the only compounds of importance. In fact, exploring the effects of antioxidants is best viewed as the first and most superficial layer of an examination into the effects of natural compounds as a whole. As discussed below, a great many natural compounds may be useful that either are not antioxidants (EPA, for example) or are secondary antioxidants, those that show antioxidant activity but also inhibit cancer through other non-redox-mediated means. To give an example, quercetin is an antioxidant compound, but it stops cancer cell proliferation primarily through inhibition of kinase activity. Even a compound like vitamin E succinate is a secondary antioxidant because its primary effect on cancer cells is not mediated through an antioxidant action. As indicated in previous chapters, these nonantioxidant and secondary antioxidant compounds are likely to produce the greatest anticancer effects. Similarly, they may have the greatest impact on the efficacy of chemotherapy and radiotherapy.

In this chapter we first review the effects of natural compounds on chemotherapy, then on radiotherapy. Finally we examine their effects on drug metabolism. Although little is currently known regarding this last topic, it is important because natural compounds that alter drug metabolism can alter the concentration of chemotherapy drugs in the plasma. Note that dose recommendations are not given in this chapter; those provided in previous chapters can be used as a guide for new studies on the effects of natural compounds on conventional treatment. As emphasized previously, the benefits of natural compounds are likely to be maximized when they are used in large combinations. There is also reason to believe that combinations of natural compounds will be more beneficial than single compounds when used with chemotherapy and radiotherapy.

INTRODUCTION

Natural compounds could conceivably increase the efficacy of chemotherapy and radiotherapy through several means. For example, a compound that interferes with signal transduction could be expected to act additively or synergistically with a chemotherapy drug that interferes with DNA synthesis. Animal studies have reported, in fact, that beneficial interactions can be produced between natural compounds and chemotherapy/radiotherapy. Such studies have also reported that beneficial interactions occur between chemotherapy/radiotherapy and other agents that share properties with natural compounds. For example, additive or synergistic antitumor effects have been reported for combinations of HMGR inhibitors and cisplatin; MMP (matrix metalloproteinase) inhibitors and cisplatin; epidermal growth factor receptor inhibitors (i.e., PTK inhibitors) and doxorubicin; agents that induce cytokine production and radiotherapy; and cytokines in combination with mitomycin, cyclophosphamide, or carboplatin.[1-7] Thus there is reason to think that natural compounds that inhibit cancer cell proliferation or affect the immune system by some of these same mechanisms could increase the efficacy of chemotherapy and radiotherapy.

To understand how natural compounds might best be employed, it is worthwhile to consider the possible goals for combining natural compounds with chemotherapy and radiotherapy. At least six different goals can be envisioned (adapted from reference 8):

1. Natural compounds could diminish the side effects of chemotherapy/radiotherapy so that higher, more effective doses could be given with more safety.

2. Natural compounds might overcome cell resistance to chemotherapy/radiotherapy or otherwise increase drug accumulation in cancer cells.

3. They could produce additive or synergistic cytotoxic effects with chemotherapy/radiotherapy.

4. They could modify the tumor environment to enhance local delivery of chemotherapy drugs.

5. Immune stimulant drugs could be used to enhance the antitumor effects of natural compounds.

6. Chemotherapy/radiotherapy could be utilized to maximally reduce tumor volume, then followed by natural compounds to restore the immune system and enhance immunologic elimination of any remaining microscopic tumors.

This chapter is concerned with the first three types of interactions. There are few data on the fourth and fifth types of interactions, and these are not discussed further, other than to mention that fibrinolytic agents may help increase delivery of chemotherapy drugs to cancer cells within a solid tumor. The last type of interaction involves the immune system; see Chapters 11 and 12 for more information.

The first three interactions are not mutually exclusive and can occur simultaneously. For instance, compounds like EPA may both increase drug accumulation within a cancer cell and reduce the cell's proliferation by inhibiting PKC activity. Moreover, multiple submechanisms can exist for each of these interactions; for example, drug resistance could be reduced through at least four submechanisms, as discussed below. Therefore, the ways that natural compounds interact with chemother-

apy drugs or radiotherapy are complex. This is particularly true if large combinations of natural compounds are used. The benefits of combinations probably will be proven long before the exact means of action are understood.

Before discussing the effects of individual compounds on chemotherapy and radiotherapy, we first examine the first three primary interactions to provide some idea of how natural compounds might be useful and to help envision optimal combinations.

Use of Natural Compounds to Reduce Adverse Effects of Chemotherapy

Many chemotherapy drugs induce necrosis or apoptosis in cancer cells by generating free radicals, but at the same time, these prooxidant mechanisms are responsible for adverse effects on normal cells. For example, doxorubicin, one of the most widely used chemotherapy drugs, induces DNA damage in cancer cells through a prooxidant mechanism. One of its primary side effects is heart damage that is also caused by its prooxidant action.[9, 10, 11] Because doxorubicin treatment can reduce total antioxidant stores in the body, antioxidant treatment might maintain these stores and protect normal tissues from adverse effects.[12, 13] This has in fact been reported in a large number of animal studies that tested doxorubicin in combination with antioxidants such as melatonin, vitamin E, vitamin C, combinations of vitamins C and E, beta-carotene, curcumin, catechin, the antioxidant drugs dexrazoxane and probucol, and others.[14-23]

If antioxidants can help prevent adverse effects of prooxidant chemotherapy drugs, can they also reduce the ability of such drugs to destroy cancer cells? Although some in-vitro studies have suggested antioxidants can prevent chemotherapy-induced apoptosis, a growing number of them report that antioxidants increase the cytotoxic effects of chemotherapy drugs against cancer cells. A recent in-vitro study on lymphoma cells in fact identified several ways antioxidants could improve the effects of chemotherapy; it reported that oxidative stress reduced the total amount of cell kill from apoptosis and necrosis that was induced by etoposide, doxorubicin, cisplatin, and cytarabine. Moreover, it reported that oxidative stress shifted the mechanism of cell kill away from apoptosis and toward necrosis.[24] As discussed in Chapter 15, apoptosis is the preferred method of cell kill during cancer treatment because, unlike necrotic cells, apoptotic cells do not rupture in the extracellular space. Before apoptotic cells can spill their contents, they are ingested by macrophages; such ingestion reduces the spillage of iron stores as well as that of other cellular compounds that lead to inflammation and the generation of free radicals. Both iron and inflammation, as we have seen, can facilitate cancer progression. This same study reported that antioxidant treatment increased the efficacy of the four chemotherapy drugs by favoring the induction of apoptosis over necrosis and by improving the ingestion of apoptotic cells by macrophages.

In addition to this in-vitro study, most animal studies have also indicated that antioxidants could produce a beneficial effect when used with chemotherapy. For example, antioxidants such as melatonin, vitamin C, vitamin E, and the antioxidant drugs probucol and amifostine have protected animals from doxorubicin- or cisplatin-induced toxicity without interfering with the drug's antitumor effects, and in some cases improving them.[14, 20, 21, 23, 25–27]

Antioxidants have potential to improve the efficacy of chemotherapy or reduce its adverse effects through the following mechanisms:

- They can protect normal tissues from free radical damage induced by chemotherapy.

- Because immune cells need a high concentration of antioxidants to function, antioxidants can produce healthier immune cells, which are more likely to inhibit cancer than unhealthy ones.

- They could reduce the mutation rate, resulting, over time, in cancers that are less aggressive and less adaptable to changing conditions.

- They could reduce the proliferation rate of cancer cells by normalizing the activity of growth factor receptors and transcription factors.

- In conditions of high oxidative stress (such as caused by chemotherapy), antioxidants could reduce lipid peroxidation, thereby increasing the proliferation rate. (Lipid peroxidation acts as a negative growth regulator for most cells, including most cancer cells.[28–31]) Increased proliferation could actually improve the efficacy of chemotherapy drugs, since cancer cells must be in the cell cycle for most chemotherapy drugs to work.[32]

- By reducing oxidative stress, they could assist cancer cells to die of apoptosis rather than necrosis, which has at least two primary advantages: First, it helps minimize iron release and inflammation, and second, apoptotic cells are ingested more efficiently by macrophages than necrotic cells are. Since antioxidants favor apoptosis and support macrophage activity, they can help macrophages to present the cancer's antigens to T cells efficiently. This allows

T cells to target the remaining cancer cells more effectively.

Use of Natural Compounds to Increase Drug Accumulation or Reduce Drug Resistance

Cancer cells are better able to adapt to stress than normal cells. In cancer treatment, this adaptation results in tumor cells that develop resistance to chemotherapy drugs, which is a primary obstacle to treatment success. Cancer cells often develop resistance not only to the drug to which they have been exposed but also to other drugs and noxious agents they have not encountered. Development of this nonspecific or multidrug resistance might be likened to a battleship crew placed on "battle stations" after a surprise attack; in this state of alertness, they are prepared for any new onslaught, whatever its form. Once a cancer cell becomes stressed and develops multidrug resistance, it is not easily harmed.

To devise strategies for reversing multidrug resistance with natural compounds, we must first understand how resistance develops. At least four mechanisms have been described that mediate multidrug resistance:[33]

1. *Decreased drug sensitivity.* A cancer cell's sensitivity to a drug can be reduced if the cell produces mutated targets of the drug, such as a mutated enzyme, that are no longer sensitive to the drug's actions. Sensitivity can also be reduced if the cell overproduces the intended target (again, such as an enzyme). Lastly, it can be lowered if the cancer cell overproduces certain proteins that protect the cell from damage. Examples include altered production/activity of the antiapoptotic protein Bcl-2 (see Table 2.1), topoisomerase II (see Chapter 2), and heat-shock proteins. The latter are produced in response to stress and prepare the cell for additional stress.

2. *Increased repair of intended drug targets.* Drug resistance can develop if the cancer cell increases the repair of drug targets. For example, many drugs target DNA, and some cancer cells can increase DNA repair. In some cases, this may take the form of greater *p53* expression, since *p53* facilitates repair of damaged genes.

3. *Increased drug expulsion.* Drug resistance can develop if export of the drug from the cell is increased. The required pumping action is commonly mediated through two proteins called P-glycoprotein and the multidrug resistance protein (MRP).[a] When one or both these proteins are overactive, drug concentra-

---

[a] *A series of MRP proteins exist named MRP1, MRP2, and so on.*

tions within the cell are minimized. Note that the functions of these proteins are still not fully understood, and reports on their activities vary.[34]

4. *Altered metabolism and drug detoxification.* Cancer cells can gain resistance by increasing their ability to detoxify drugs. A common example is increased resistance due to enhanced activity of the glutathione *S*-transferase drug detoxification system; recall that this enzyme catalyzes the formation of drug-glutathione conjugates (see Figure 18.1). Once formed, these water-soluble conjugates can be expelled from the cell.[a] Increased glutathione concentrations and/or glutathione *S*-transferase activity have been associated with resistance to many drugs. Multiple means are available by which the conjugates can be expelled from the cell; the primary mechanism in most appears to be via the glutathione-xenobiotic (GSH-X) pump. Increasing evidence indicates this pump is closely related to, if not identical with, the multidrug resistance protein (MRP) mentioned above. If they are indeed identical, this implies that MRP is able to expel both conjugated and unconjugated compounds.

Inhibition of drug resistance has a strong parallel with inhibition of cancer in general. Multiple mechanisms are at work both in cancer cell survival and multidrug resistance, and neither has yet been adequately inhibited by targeting a single mechanism. For example, two drugs, verapamil and cyclosporin, have received the most study as modifiers of multidrug resistance. Both inhibit drug resistance primarily through a single mechanism, inhibition of P-glycoprotein.[35, 36] The results of clinical studies using these drugs in patients with solid tumors have been disappointing, although some promising results were seen with hematological cancers.[37] A recent review postulates that the poor results were likely due to the multitude of mechanisms occurring in multidrug resistance and the fact that it is affected by other factors such as cell proliferation, angiogenesis, and apoptosis, as well.[37]

The complexity of multiple mechanisms in drug resistance has been investigated by other authors. In a study on leukemia patients, no relationship was found between the resistance to chemotherapy and the expression of any single protein involved in drug resistance (MRP, p53, heat-shock protein, P-glycoprotein, and so on). A correlation to resistance was found, however, when groups of two or more of these proteins were analyzed together, indicating that a number of events occur simultaneously to confer multidrug resistance.[38] Consequently, combinations of compounds that can inhibit drug resistance through multiple pathways may provide the greatest effect.

Although each of the four mechanisms listed could conceivably be affected by natural compounds, most research has focused on three areas: inhibition of P-glycoprotein, inhibition of the glutathione *S*-transferase drug detoxification system, and inhibition of heat-shock proteins. Each of these is discussed separately below.

Inhibition of P-glycoprotein

As mentioned, P-glycoprotein acts as a pump to export drugs and other noxious compounds from a cell. It has at least three characteristics that make it susceptible to inhibition by natural compounds. First, its actions are regulated largely through PKC activity, and as we know, many natural compounds inhibit PKC. Tumor cell variants that overexpress *mdr* (the gene that encodes for P-glycoprotein) tend to have several-fold higher levels of PKC activity compared to their drug-responsive counterparts. Consequently, PKC inhibitors reduce multidrug resistance in a variety of cell lines.[39, 40] For example, one study reported that PKC inhibitors reduced resistance of brain cancer cells to vincristine in vitro.[41]

A similar PKC-dependent effect is seen in cells surviving radiation exposure. Like chemotherapy, radiation is a noxious agent that stimulates multidrug resistance. Ionizing radiation rapidly and transiently activates PKC in a dose-dependent fashion.[40] Since PKC activity is important for cell survival following radiation, PKC inhibitors can sensitize cells to radiation-induced killing.[42] For example, hypericin, which decreases PKC activity, increased the sensitivity of brain cancer cells to radiation in vitro.[43]

The second means by which natural compounds can inhibit P-glycoprotein is by blocking ATP binding. ATP is the energy source within cells. As discussed in Chapter 4, the pluripotent activity of several natural compounds against various ATP-dependent enzymes such as PTK and PKC may be due to their ability to decrease the binding of ATP, thereby reducing the enzyme's energy source. Other ATP-dependent enzymes like MRP/GSH-X might also be inhibited with these natural compounds.

The third means of inhibiting P-glycoprotein is through inhibition of NF-κB. In some cancer cell lines, the expression of the *mdr* gene is associated with prior increases in NF-κB activity and can be diminished by NF-κB antagonists.[44, 45] NF-κB activity can be reduced

---

[a] *In some cases, glutathione conjugates can form spontaneously, without the activity of glutathione-S-transferase, but the reactions occur more readily when it is present.*

by a number of natural compounds, including antioxidants (see Chapter 5).

Inhibition of the Glutathione S-Transferase Drug Detoxification System

As already stated, the glutathione S-transferase drug detoxification system involves the formation of drug-glutathione conjugates and expulsion of these conjugates from the cell. Adequate glutathione must therefore be present for this system to function, and it is possible to reduce this form of drug resistance by lowering intracellular concentrations of glutathione. Compounds such as glutamine and whey may be well suited for this task (see Chapter 18). It is true that by lowering glutathione concentrations, cancer cells might come under considerable oxidative stress, and for several reasons we do not advocate the production of oxidative stress as a treatment strategy. If chemotherapy is being used, however, a commitment has likely already been made for a prooxidant therapy.

Drug resistance may also be lowered by reducing the activity of the MRP/GSH-X pump. Since this protein is dependent on ATP, a number of natural compounds may be able to affect its activity, as discussed previously.

Inhibition of Heat-shock Proteins

Heat-shock proteins are those that protect the cell from death due to adverse conditions. Heat-shock proteins are induced by stress, including that caused by chemotherapy drugs. Once produced, these proteins assist the cell to withstand future insults. The production of heat-shock proteins is stimulated by the binding of a transcription factor (called heat-shock factor) to DNA.

Natural compounds can inhibit heat-shock proteins through at least two mechanisms. First, some natural compounds, including quercetin, prevent heat-shock factor from activating gene transcription, thereby averting the production of heat-shock proteins.[46, 47] Second, increased heat-shock factor activity and gene expression are positively associated with increased NF-κB activity.[48, 49, 50] It follows then that inhibitors of NF-κB activity could inhibit production of heat-shock proteins.

Producing Synergistic Cytotoxic Effects

We now turn to the final primary interaction between natural compounds and chemotherapy drugs: the production of synergistic cytotoxic effects. We know that natural compounds can produce cytotoxic effects in cancer cells through a variety of mechanisms. Not sur-

prisingly, when they are combined with chemotherapy drugs, the cytotoxic effects are often additive or synergistic. The exact means by which synergistic interactions occur is usually not obvious; in some cases, natural compounds and chemotherapy drugs may simply damage the cancer cell through different but complementary mechanisms. In others, they may cooperate to inhibit the same mechanism, and in still others, natural compounds may reduce resistance to the drug. Many interactions are possible.

Whether they act by reducing adverse reactions, increasing drug accumulation or reducing drug resistance, producing synergistic cytotoxic effects, or some other means, a number of natural compounds have been reported to increase the safety and efficacy of chemotherapy and radiotherapy. These studies are discussed below.

EFFECTS OF NATURAL COMPOUNDS ON CHEMOTHERAPY

Selenium

In animal and human studies, selenium reduced both the adverse effects of cisplatin and multidrug resistance induced by cisplatin.

Intraperitoneal administration of 2 mg/kg of selenium given one hour before injection of cisplatin protected mice against kidney toxicity but did not reduce cisplatin's antitumor effects.[51] The equivalent human dose is about 19 milligrams of selenium by intraperitoneal administration, which is prohibitively large. Other studies also reported protective effects in mice at similar high doses.[52, 53, 54] The protective effect appeared due to the formation of a selenium-cisplatin complex in the kidneys.[55]

A similar selenium dose (1.5 mg/kg intraperitoneal) prevented drug resistance in tumor-bearing mice if it was given at the time of cisplatin treatment. The effect was attributed to prevention of cisplatin-induced increases in glutathione synthesis in the cancer cells.[56]

Although the selenium doses used in these studies were prohibitively high for human use, selenium may also be helpful at somewhat lower doses. In a study on 41 patients with various cancers, those who received 4,000 micrograms of selenium orally for eight days, beginning four days before treatment with cisplatin, exhibited higher leukocyte counts and reduced kidney toxicity as compared to controls (same patients at a different time) treated only with cisplatin.[57] Although this dose is far above the 1,100-microgram maximum dose recommended in Table 14.2, it did not cause adverse effects, probably because it was given for only a short period of time and in a relatively nontoxic organic form (kappa-selenocarrageenan).

Vitamin C

Vitamin C increased the cytotoxicity of some chemotherapy drugs in vitro. Some of these studies used high concentrations (roughly 200 µM and above), and we can suppose the vitamin produced prooxidant effects that acted in conjunction with the drugs to improve cell kill. However, at least one in-vitro study reported that much lower concentrations of vitamin C also enhanced the effects of chemotherapy. In this study, nontoxic concentrations (1 µM) improved the cytotoxicity of doxorubicin, cisplatin, and paclitaxel against human breast cancer cells.[58] It seems unlikely a prooxidant effect was produced at this low concentration, and other mechanisms apparently were involved.

Vitamin C has also reduced the adverse effects and/or increased the efficacy of chemotherapy drugs in animals. Based on the two oral studies summarized below, doses of up to 2 grams per day appeared to be effective in reducing adverse effects. This is a small number of studies, however, and many more are needed.

- Vitamin C prolonged survival of mice and guinea pigs inoculated with leukemia and treated with doxorubicin; in addition, it did not inhibit the antitumor effect of doxorubicin.[23] A related experiment reported similar beneficial results.[59] The applicability of these studies in humans is uncertain, however, since vitamin C was initially injected intraperitoneally with the doxorubicin and then injected alone afterward, a system that would not be used in humans. The intraperitoneal doses of vitamin C were about 19 grams per day in mice and 2.9 grams per day in guinea pigs (as scaled to humans).

- Subcutaneous injections of vitamin C (at 580 milligrams per day as scaled to humans) reduced the adverse effects of N-methylformamide and increased survival of leukemia- and sarcoma-bearing mice as compared with treatment by the chemotherapy agent alone.[60]

- Orally administered vitamin C at a single dose of 1.6 grams (as scaled to humans) reduced lipid peroxidation and kidney toxicity in rats given a single intraperitoneal dose of cisplatin.[61] Doses half this amount were not effective, and twice as much was no more effective.

- Vitamin C inhibited genotoxicity in mice induced by cyclophosphamide, mitomycin, and cisplatin. The

effective oral doses ranged from 15 milligrams to 3.7 grams, as scaled to humans.[62, 63] Intraperitoneal administration (at doses ranging from about 16 to 67 grams, as scaled to humans) also protected mice from genotoxicity due to cyclophosphamide and mitomycin.[64, 65]

Polysaccharides

A large number of studies have reported that the mushroom polysaccharides PSK or PSP increased survival of tumor-bearing rodents treated with chemotherapy or protected them from its adverse effects or both.[66–71] Most of the studies used oral administration. We do not discuss these here, however, since many human studies using PSK/PSP in combination with chemotherapy were already described in Chapter 16. In most animal and human studies, PSK/PSP was reported beneficial when used in conjunction with chemotherapy drugs.

Herbal formulas containing *Astragalus* and other immunostimulant herbs in combination with various chemotherapy drugs have also been tested in animals. For example, oral administration of the herbal formula *Ba Zhen Tang*, which contains ginseng, *Astragalus*, and other herbs, reduced cisplatin-induced adverse effects and lethality in mice injected with sarcoma and bladder cancer cells. Moreover, the formula did not reduce the antitumor effect of cisplatin and may have improved it. Effects were seen at doses of 0.6 to 1.7 g/kg.[72, 73] The formula had a similar protective effect after mitomycin administration.[74, 75] Also, a polysaccharide fraction isolated from the formula and given orally protected mice from kidney toxicity and death induced by cisplatin.[76] Other herbal formulas have also been reported beneficial; oral administration of *Bu Zhong Yi Qi Tang*, containing ginseng, *Astragalus*, and other herbs, reduced cyclophosphamide-induced toxicity and increased the antitumor effect in sarcoma-bearing mice.[77]

Lastly, a number of human studies summarized in Chapter 12 indicated that herbal formulas containing immunostimulant herbs may improve survival of cancer patients receiving chemotherapy while reducing its adverse effects.

EPA/DHA

Many in-vitro studies have examined the effects of EPA/DHA or fish oil on the cytotoxicity of chemotherapy drugs. Most of these reported that EPA/DHA enhanced the cytotoxicity of chemotherapy drugs, including mitomycin, cisplatin, and vincristine.[78–81] Enhanced cytotoxicity could have occurred through at least four mechanisms. First, if vitamin E or other antioxidants were not given with the fatty acids, the fatty acids could have directly induced cytotoxicity through a prooxidant mechanism.[82] Second, the fatty acids could have inhibited cell proliferation through other means such as inhibition of signal transduction (see Chapters 4 and 17). Third, the fatty acids could have increased the uptake of chemotherapy drugs by altering the fluidity of the plasma membrane, and fourth they could have reversed multidrug resistance through inhibiting PKC activity.[83, 84, 85]

Several animal studies have also documented that EPA/DHA or fish oil, at very high doses, increased the efficacy or decreased the adverse effects of chemotherapy drugs or both. These are summarized below:

- A diet of 3 or 6 percent fish oil (about 3.6 and 7.2 g/kg) enhanced the antitumor effect and reduced the adverse effects of irinotecan in mice with transplanted human breast cancer cells.[86] Treatment with the drug alone caused inhibition of tumor growth only, whereas co-administration with fish oil led to tumor regression. The equivalent human dose is about 34 and 69 grams per day.

- In a randomized, double-blind, placebo-controlled study, a diet of about 6 percent fish oil and 3 percent arginine enhanced the antitumor effect of doxorubicin in dogs with spontaneous lymphoma. Disease-free intervals and survival time were increased by the treatment as compared to dogs receiving only doxorubicin. Mean survival times were 318 versus 227 days, respectively. The effect was dependent on stage, as dogs at stage III received benefit but dogs at stage IV did not. In stage III dogs, survival time was directly related to plasma concentrations of EPA, DHA, and arginine. Treatment also reduced plasma concentrations of lactic acid, and low lactic acid concentrations were associated with greater survival. Plasma concentrations of insulin were also decreased by the experimental diet.[87] The equivalent human dose of a 6 percent fish oil diet is about 69 grams per day.

- A diet of 20 percent fish oil (about 24 g/kg) enhanced the antitumor effect of mitomycin in mice with transplanted human breast cancer cells. The effect was due to increased lipid peroxidation.[88] The equivalent human dose is about 230 grams per day.

- A diet of 20 percent fish oil (about 24 g/kg) enhanced the antitumor effect of cyclophosphamide and reduced its acute adverse effects in mice with transplanted human breast cancer cells.[89] The equivalent human dose is about 230 grams per day.

- A diet of 19 percent fish oil (about 23 g/kg) enhanced the antitumor effect of doxorubicin (with ferric citrate) in mice with transplanted human lung cancer cells.[86] The equivalent human dose is about 220 grams per day.

The above studies appear irrelevant to human use, given the prohibitively large doses of fish oil involved. As discussed in Chapter 17, the recommended maximum dose of fish oil is about 21 grams per day. Still, one animal and one human study have suggested that relatively low doses could be beneficial. In the animal study, oral administration of DHA (at 5 to 50 mg/kg) protected mice from methotrexate-induced small intestine damage, with the 50-mg/kg dose more effective than the 5-mg/kg one.[90] The human equivalent of 50 mg/kg in mice is about 480 milligrams per day. The human study found that normal dietary levels of fish oil or other sources of EPA/DHA increased the efficacy of chemotherapy drugs; breast cancer patients with higher fat tissue levels of omega-3 fatty acids, especially DHA, were more likely to respond to combinations of chemotherapy drugs than were patients with low tissue levels of DHA.[91] This effect was apparently due partly to increased drug uptake by tumor cells.

Glutamine

Glutamine has reduced the gastrointestinal-related adverse effects of a variety of chemotherapy drugs in animals. Human studies also suggested a protective effect, which seemed to occur in part due to glutamine's ability to act as a fuel for intestinal cells. In addition, glutamine improved the efficacy of some chemotherapy drugs by decreasing intracellular glutathione concentrations in cancer cells, while increasing glutathione concentrations in normal ones. These results were discussed in Chapter 18.

Garlic

Few animal studies have investigated the ability of garlic or its primary constituent, DADS, to alter the efficacy or safety of chemotherapy drugs. In one study, intraperitoneal administration of garlic extract (equivalent to 2 g/kg of garlic) reduced the toxicity of cyclophosphamide in mice but not its antitumor effects. The effect might have been from an antioxidant mechanism, since lipid peroxidation in the liver was reduced.[92] The equivalent human dose is about 19 grams of garlic by intraperitoneal administration, which is high compared to dose estimates given in Table 18.4.

Enzyme mixtures

Orally administered proteolytic enzymes increased absorption and tissue diffusion of drugs, including some antibiotics and chemotherapy drugs.[93] In part, this may be due to the moderate fibrinolytic effects of the enzymes, which assist the free flow of therapeutic drugs to inflamed sites. It may also come from the ability of proteolytic enzymes, especially mixed enzymes, to open tight junctions in the intestinal lining and allow the passage of large drug molecules.[94] Combinations of enzyme therapy and chemotherapy have been used in Germany in preliminary experiments with some success, including more rapid remissions, reduced side effects, and reductions in therapy costs.[95–99] Reduced side effects appear to be due partly to inhibition of chemotherapy-induced production of inflammatory substances. One human study reported that orally administered enzymes (WOBE-MUGOS) also reduced the acute side effects of radiation therapy in patients with head and neck cancers.[100]

Quercetin, Apigenin, and Genistein

Quercetin, apigenin, and genistein have all been reported to affect production or activity of multidrug resistance protein (MRP) and P-glycoprotein in vitro. In some studies, MRP and/or P-glycoprotein were inhibited and in others, they were stimulated or there was a biphasic effect, where one or both proteins were inhibited at high concentrations and stimulated at low concentrations. Thus, based on the in-vitro studies, the effects of these flavonoids on multidrug resistance is somewhat unpredictable and more study is necessary.

At 20 μM, genistein inhibited multidrug resistance in human leukemia cells active for P-glycoprotein.[101] At 100 to 200 μM, it reduced multidrug resistance in human MRP and/or P-glycoprotein breast and lung cancer cells and colon cells (lower concentrations were not tested).[102–105] Apigenin, daidzein, quercetin, and other flavonoids were also effective. Genistein concentrations of 11 μM also increased drug accumulation and markedly reduced resistance to a variety of chemotherapy agents in human leukemia cells that were not active for P-glycoprotein.[106] Quercetin (at 100 μM) inhibited production of P-glycoprotein and reduced multidrug resistance in human liver cancer cells and other neoplastic cell lines in response to toxic compounds such as arsenite, vincristine, and vinblastine (lower concentrations were not tested).[107, 108] At 1 to 10 μM, quercetin lowered multidrug resistance in human breast cancer cells and potentiated the effects of doxorubicin.[109] A number of studies reported that quercetin reduced the activity of heat-shock proteins, which help facilitate drug resistance.[108, 110–112] A similar inhibitory effect on heat-shock proteins may be produced by genistein and luteolin.[113]

In contrast to the above, flavonoids (at least genistein) can also increase drug resistance in some cases. Gen-

istein at 50 μM decreased methotrexate uptake and its cytotoxicity in drug-resistant leukemia cells.[114] Other drugs may also be affected since in one study, treatment with genistein at 25 μM caused 25 out of 26 samples of acute lymphoblastic leukemia cells ex vivo to be about twofold more resistant to inhibition by daunorubicin.[115]

Apart from studies specifically on drug resistance, quercetin and genistein have been reported to act synergistically with many chemotherapy drugs. For example, quercetin at 0.01 to 2.5 μM acted synergistically with cisplatin against human ovarian cancer cells in vitro.[116] Quercetin (at about 25 μM) acted synergistically with busulphan against human leukemia cells in vitro.[117] Quercetin (at 0.01 nM to 10 μM) acted synergistically with cytarabine against human leukemia cells in vitro, however, another study reported that quercetin did not affect the cytotoxicity of cytarabine in leukemia cells.[118, 119] Genistein (at about 4 μM) and doxorubicin produced synergistic effects in human estrogen-dependent and -independent breast cancer cells in vitro.[120] Genistein (at 10 to 20 μM) acted synergistically with tiazofurin against human leukemia and ovarian cancer cells.[121, 122]

Quercetin has also been reported to be active in animals. Intraperitoneal administration of 20 mg/kg of quercetin every three days enhanced the antitumor effect of cisplatin in mice injected with human lung cancer cells, but it did not appear to protect against adverse toxicity induced by cisplatin.[123] The equivalent human oral dose is about 410 milligrams daily. Genistein has also shown beneficial effects in vivo. Intraperitoneal administration of cyclophosphamide or 100 mg/kg of genistein inhibited growth of transplanted melanoma cells and lung cancer cells in mice; the greatest effect was seen when both agents were used in combination.[124] The equivalent human oral dose of genistein is about 4.5 grams per day.

Green tea or EGCG

At least one in-vitro study has reported that EGCG increased the efficacy of chemotherapy. EGCG (at 22 to 44 μM) sensitized doxorubicin-resistant mouse sarcoma cells and human colon cancer cells to doxorubicin treatment. The effect was attributed to PKC inhibition and subsequent inhibition of P-glycoprotein and other proteins related to drug resistance.[125]

Effects have also been seen in vivo. Oral administration of green tea extract (at 1 g/kg per day for 10 days) increased efficacy of doxorubicin by 2.5-fold in mice bearing Ehrlich ascites cancer. The doxorubicin content in cancer cells but not normal cells was increased by the green tea.[126] The equivalent human dose is 9.6 grams of green tea extract per day, or about 1.2 grams of EGCG. In addition, oral administration of EGCG (at 1.9 grams per day as scaled to humans) reduced the number of tumors induced by cisplatin treatment as well as the weight loss caused by cisplatin. Cisplatin treatment induces secondary tumors in about 1 to 10 percent of treated lung cancer patients.[127]

Curcumin

Curcumin has shown protective effects in animals in combination with chemotherapy. Oral administration of curcumin (at 200 mg/kg) reduced inflammation and lipid peroxidation and increased antioxidant defense mechanisms in the lung tissue of rats treated with cyclophosphamide.[128] Similar effects were observed in the lung tissue of bleomycin-treated rats given the same oral dose.[129] This same dose reduced doxorubicin-induced heart and kidney toxicity in rats.[130, 131] The human equivalent of 200 mg/kg in rats is about 3.2 grams daily. Curcumin has also increased the effectiveness of chemotherapy; 28 mg/kg given orally in combination with cisplatin reduced the progression of fibrosarcoma in rats (based on analysis of tumor marker enzymes) more effectively than cisplatin alone.[132] The equivalent human dose is about 450 milligrams per day.

Emodin

Emodin has shown synergistic effects both in vitro and in animals. Emodin (at 30 µM) acted synergistically with cisplatin, doxorubicin, and etoposide in inhibiting HER-2/neu-overexpressing human lung cancer cells in vitro.[133] Intraperitoneal injection of emodin (40 mg/kg twice a week for eight weeks) with Taxol significantly inhibited the growth of HER-2/neu-overexpressing human breast cancer cells injected into mice, compared with Taxol treatment alone. The same effect was seen in vitro.[134] The equivalent human oral dose is about 750 milligrams per day.

Ginseng

Ginseng has interacted beneficially with chemotherapy drugs both in vitro and in animals. For example, selected ginseng triterpenoids at 25 to 100 µM reversed multidrug resistance to daunomycin and vinblastine in mouse leukemia cells in vitro.[135]

Oral administration of a crude extract of ginseng (at 500 mg/kg) increased the cytotoxicity of mitomycin in mice with transplanted Ehrlich ascites cancer cells and increased survival time of the mice as compared to those receiving only mitomycin. In-vitro experiments also reported that the extract increased the uptake of mitomycin and enhanced its cytotoxicity.[136] The equivalent human dose is about 4.8 grams per day.

In rats with transplanted liver cancer cells, a combination of mitomycin and a crude ginseng extract (given orally at 200 to 500 mg/kg) produced a greater antitumor effect than mitomycin alone.[137, 138] The equivalent human dose is about 3.2 to 8.1 grams per day.

Vitamin A

Vitamin A in the form of retinol or retinyl esters has enhanced the effect of chemotherapy drugs in vitro. For example, retinol (at 2.5 to 15 µM) increased the cytotoxicity of doxorubicin against human leukemia cells; this occurred despite the fact that retinol produced an antioxidant effect in the cells, as shown by reduced lipid peroxidation.[139] In another study, retinyl acetate (at 30 to 60 µM) increased the cytotoxicity of vincristine against drug-resistant leukemia cells, partly due to increased drug uptake by the cells.[140] ATRA has also been reported to enhance the effects of chemotherapy drugs in vitro. For example, it acted synergistically (at about 0.5 to 50 µM) with cisplatin against human ovarian cell lines.[141] In another study, ATRA (at 1 µM) increased the sensitivity of three human leukemia cell lines to cytarabine.[119]

Retinol or retinyl esters have also produced beneficial effects in animals, but unfortunately, only intraperitoneal doses have been tested, and the results may be different for oral administration. In addition, several studies used doses that would be excessive in humans (the LOAEL dose is about 50,000 to 600,000 I.U.). Five studies are summarized below:

- A combination of fluorouracil and retinyl palmitate (at 5,000 I.U./kg per day intraperitoneal) increased the survival of mice with transplanted sarcoma cells, compared with 5-fluorouracil alone.[142] The equivalent human oral dose is about 72,000 I.U. per day.

- A combination of immunotherapy (IL-2 plus low-dose cyclophosphamide) and retinyl palmitate (at 100,000 I.U./kg every four days, intraperitoneal) increased the survival of mice with transplanted neuroblastoma cells, compared with any of the three therapies alone.[143] The equivalent human oral dose is about 360,000 I.U. per day.

- In a series of tests on combinations of retinyl palmitate and various chemotherapy drugs, retinyl palmitate enhanced the drug's antitumor effects, depending on the type of cancer and the dose. An intraperitoneal dose of 3.3 mg/kg per day improved the antitumor effects of fluorouracil, methotrexate, and nimustine hydrochloride but not doxorubicin in mice with transplanted sarcoma cells. An intraperitoneal dose of 167 or 330 mg/kg improved the antitumor effects of methotrexate, doxorubicin, nimustine, and cisplatin but not fluorouracil, in mice with transplanted leukemia cells.[144] The equivalent human oral doses of 3.3, 167, and 330 mg/kg intraperitoneal in mice are about 85,000, 2.9 million, and 8.7 million I.U. per day.

- A combination of vincristine and retinyl acetate (at 42 or 84 mg/kg, intraperitoneal) increased the survival of mice with transplanted vincristine-sensitive and -resistant leukemia cells, compared with vincristine alone. The equivalent human oral dose is about 1.8 to 3.6 million I.U. per day.[140]

- A combination of 6-mercaptopurine and retinyl palmitate (at 270 mg/kg, intraperitoneal) increased the survival of mice with transplanted leukemia cells more than 6-mercaptopurine alone.[145] The equivalent human oral dose is about 7 million I.U. per day.

Human phase II studies have also been conducted. Because these do not use a control group, the exact contribution of retinyl esters to the results seen is difficult to determine. Still, the studies did suggest that the combinations were beneficial overall. Doses ranged from 30,000 to 300,000 I.U. per day (oral doses were used in all cases):

- Twenty-three patients with pancreatic cancer were given combination chemotherapy, interferon, and retinyl palmitate (at 100,000 I.U. per day). Nine percent achieved a complete response and 26 percent a partial response.[146]

- Forty patients with advanced non-small-cell lung cancer were given combination chemotherapy, interferon, and retinyl palmitate (at 100,000 I.U. per day). Eight percent achieved a complete response and 35 percent a partial one.[147]

- Thirty-three patients with advanced breast cancer received a combination of tamoxifen and retinyl acetate (at 300,000 I.U. per day). Nine percent had a complete response and 27 percent a partial one.[148]

- Forty-nine patients with advanced breast cancer received a combination of interferon, tamoxifen and retinyl palmitate (at 100,000 I.U. per day). Twenty-four percent achieved a complete response and 31 percent achieved a partial one.[149] In a similar study, the numbers were 31 percent complete and 33 percent partial.[150]

- Twenty-three patients with oral cancer took a combination of cisplatin, fluorouracil, radiotherapy, and retinyl palmitate (at 30,000 I.U. per day). Thirty-two percent had a complete response and 32 percent had a partial response.[151]

Vitamin D$_3$

In a number of in-vitro studies, 1,25-D$_3$ increased the cytotoxicity of chemotherapy drugs. Unfortunately, nearly all the studies summarized below used concentrations of 10 nM or larger. Plasma concentrations of 1,25-D$_3$ cannot exceed about 0.2 nM without causing adverse effects.

- 1,25-D$_3$ at 10 nM enhanced the susceptibility of human breast cancer cells to doxorubicin in vitro. The effects apparently were due to increased ROS generation with the combined treatment.[152]

- Exposure of human leukemia cells to cytarabine or hydroxyurea followed by exposure to 1,25-D$_3$ (at 0.1 µM) increased cytotoxicity compared with treatment by the drugs alone. If treatment with 1,25-D$_3$ occurred first, however, there was a slight decrease in the cytotoxicity of the chemotherapy drugs.[153]

- A combination of 1,25-D$_3$ (at about 1 nM) and cisplatin or carboplatin acted synergistically to inhibit proliferation of prostate cancer cells.[154]

- 1,25-D$_3$ (at 100 nM) and tamoxifen together inhibited proliferation of human breast cancer cells more than either compound used alone.[155]

- 1,25-D$_3$ (at 10 to 50 nM) and carboplatin inhibited proliferation of endometrial cancer cells more than either compound used alone.[156]

- 1,25-D$_3$ (at 10 and 100 nM) and carboplatin inhibited proliferation of human breast cancer cells more than either compound used alone.[157]

- A combination of 1,25-D$_3$ (at 10 nM) and methotrexate, mitomycin, cisplatin, or doxorubicin inhibited proliferation of osteosarcoma cells more then any of the compounds used alone.[158]

In a phase II study, a combination of low-dose cytarabine, hydroxyurea, and 1,25-D$_3$ (at 0.5 micrograms per day orally) was given to 29 elderly patients with myeloid leukemia. Forty-five percent had a complete response and 34 percent a partial one.[159] In a case series study on two patients with multiple myeloma receiving combination chemotherapy, treatment with 1,25-D$_3$ combined with bisphosphonates appeared to help curtail disease progression and stimulate bone healing.[160] Although intravenous treatment was used initially, most of the 1,25-D$_3$ doses were oral at 0.5 micrograms.

Vitamin E

Numerous in-vitro studies have observed that vitamin E (alpha-tocopherol) or VES (vitamin E succinate) increased the effectiveness of chemotherapy against cancer cells or protected normal cells or both:

- VES (at concentrations greater than about 9.2 μM) produced a synergistic effect with doxorubicin against human prostate cancer cells. At lower concentrations, it had an additive effect.[161]

- VES (at 50 μM), with or without beta-carotene (at 50 μM), increased the cytotoxicity of melphalan toward human squamous cell carcinoma, but VES did not alter the effects of cisplatin against this cell line.[162]

- Vitamin E and VES (at 0.1 to 10 μM) protected normal leukocytes from patients with head and neck cancers against genotoxicity induced by bleomycin.[163]

- Vitamin E (at 140 μM) inhibited doxorubicin-induced lipid peroxidation in Ehrlich ascites cancer cells in vitro but did not decrease the cytotoxic effect of doxorubicin.[164]

Detrimental results have also been seen in vitro. In one study, vitamin E (at 58 μM) antagonized the beneficial effects of five different sensitizing agents to the cytotoxicity of doxorubicin and vinblastine against drug-resistant human lung cancer cells. The effect was not caused by its antioxidant actions, as other lipid- and water-soluble antioxidants did not share the effect.[165]

Several animal studies have reported that vitamin E enhanced the effectiveness of chemotherapy or protected normal cells; however, most of these used very high doses (1,600 to 52,000 I.U.). As listed in Table 22.9, the tentative recommended dose is 440 to 1,700 I.U. per day, although larger doses are likely to be safe. In many of the following, the administration scheme may not reflect human treatment conditions, since the doses were high, were given intraperitoneally, and were often given only once or for only a few days:

- Intraperitoneal administration of vitamin E (a single dose of 1,600 I.U. as scaled to humans) reduced doxorubicin toxicity and enhanced the antitumor and antimetastatic effect of cyclophosphamide, doxorubicin, and methotrexate in rats injected with prostate cancer cells.[166]

- Intraperitoneal administration of vitamin E (at 240 I.U. per day, as scaled to humans) for three days before doxorubicin treatment increased the life span of mice with transplanted leukemia cells and reduced doxorubicin organ toxicity. The same dose given orally did not affect survival.[167]

- Intraperitoneal administration of vitamin E (at 288 I.U. as scaled to humans) increased the cytotoxic effects of cisplatin against one line of neuroblastoma cells in mice. Taken orally at about double the dose it did not statistically alter the drug's effectiveness. Vitamin E did not increase the antitumor effects against a second cisplatin-resistant cell line.[168]

- Intraperitoneal administration of vitamin E (at 2,500 I.U. per day, as scaled to humans) prevented bleomycin-induced lung fibrosis in mice.[169]

- An extremely large, single dose of vitamin E (33,000 I.U. intraperitoneal, as scaled to humans) given prior to doxorubicin treatment reduced lipid peroxidation but not the efficacy of doxorubicin against leukemia in mice.[170]

- Vitamin E increased the antitumor effect of doxorubicin in rats with transplanted prostate cancer cells; however, this was seen only when a single, high intraperitoneal dose (1,600 I.U., as scaled to humans) was given on day one after transplantation. At lower doses given every day for three days, mortality increased over treatment with doxorubicin alone.[171]

- An extremely large, single dose of vitamin E (52,000 I.U. subcutaneous, as scaled to humans) given before doxorubicin, reduced heart toxicity caused by the drug. This dose did not reduce the efficacy of a combination of doxorubicin and cytarabine against acute myeloid leukemia in rats.[172]

- Intraperitoneal administration of vitamin E (at about 290 I.U., as scaled to humans) protected mice from the acute lethal effects of high-dose doxorubicin but not the delayed lethal effects.[173]

- Intraperitoneal administration of vitamin E (at about 27,000 I.U., as scaled to humans) protected rats from cisplatin-induced kidney damage.[174]

- Vitamin E given orally (at 3,600 I.U. per day, as scaled to humans) improved the antitumor activity of doxorubicin in mice with transplanted Ehrlich ascites cancer cells. Vitamin E treatment also improved the antioxidant status of the heart.[14]

- Vitamin E (at 9,700 I.U. per day orally, as scaled to humans) reduced doxorubicin-induced organ toxicity in rats.[175]

Detrimental effects have occurred in vivo. As mentioned above, low doses of vitamin E increased the mortality of mice treated with doxorubicin. In addition, extremely large doses of vitamin E (33,000 I.U., intraperitoneal, as scaled to humans) increased the toxicity of doxorubicin to bone marrow cells in mice.[176] Similarly, an extremely large dose of vitamin E (7,200 I.U. per day, subcutaneous, as scaled to humans) increased the mortality of and tissue drug concentrations in mice treated with doxorubicin.[177, 178, 179] It would appear that at some doses, vitamin E can increase drug uptake, possibly through modifying the plasma membrane.

Lastly, some in-vivo studies reported no protective effects for vitamin E:

- In one single-arm study, prolonged oral administration of vitamin E acetate (at 1,600 I.U. per day) did not protect patients from doxorubicin-induced hair loss.[180]

- In a single-arm trial, prolonged oral administration of vitamin E (at about 5,400 I.U. per day) did not reduce heart or other forms of toxicity in patients treated with doxorubicin.[181]

- Intraperitoneal administration of vitamin E (at about 15,000 I.U., as scaled to humans) failed to protect rabbits from death due to doxorubicin injections.[182]

- Intraperitoneal administration of vitamin E (at about 1,200 I.U., as scaled to humans) failed to alter the severity and incidence of skin lesions in dogs chronically injected with doxorubicin.[183]

The studies showing no effect on hair loss or skin toxicity may actually be considered a good sign. Like cancer cells, skin and hair cells are fast growing. If vitamin E had protected those against death, it may have also protected cancer cells. With regard to heart toxicity, it seems likely that a combination of antioxidants may be more useful than vitamin E alone.

To sum up the animal studies, beneficial, detrimental, and no effects have been observed with combinations of chemotherapy and vitamin E. Many of these studies, however, did not give the vitamin the way humans would generally use it (e.g., oral doses of about 400 to 800 I.U. per day, prolonged administration, and in combination with other antioxidants). Furthermore, it is not clear whether other vitamin E compounds such as VES would have different effects than those for alpha-tocopherol. Therefore, additional study is warranted using protocols that more closely reflect how vitamin E is used in humans. Some studies on the combined use of antioxidants have in fact already been conducted, and these are discussed below.

Combined Antioxidant Vitamins

A small number of in-vitro studies have reported that combinations of antioxidant vitamins (for example, vitamin C, VES, ATRA, and beta-carotene) used in conjunction with chemotherapy drugs produced a greater cytotoxic effect against cancer cells than the chemotherapy drugs alone. For example, these four vitamins in-

creased the cytotoxic effect of cisplatin and tamoxifen in human melanoma cells in vitro.[184, 185, 186]

In animal studies that have been conducted:

- Liver toxicity to daunorubicin in rats was inhibited by a combination of vitamin C (at 570 milligrams per day, intramuscular, as scaled to humans) and vitamin E (at 970 I.U., orally, as scaled to humans).[187]

- Oral administration of both vitamin C (at about 9.6 grams, as scaled to humans) and vitamin E (at about 1,100 I.U., as scaled to humans) reduced the genotoxic effects of bleomycin in mice.[188]

- Both intramuscular administration of vitamin E (at about 440 I.U., as scaled to humans) and intravenous administration of vitamin C (at about 150 milligrams, as scaled to humans) reduced hydroxyurea-induced organ toxicity in rabbits.[189]

- Oral administration of vitamins A and E (about 3,600 I.U. and 870 I.U., respectively, as scaled to humans) reduced doxorubicin-induced heart toxicity in rabbits.[190]

Lastly, at least two human studies have been conducted. In a nonrandomized uncontrolled study, oral administration of vitamin A (at 15,000 to 40,000 I.U., as retinyl palmitate), vitamin C (at 2 to 5 grams), vitamin E (at 300 to 800 I.U.), along with other vitamins and minerals, appeared to increase the mean survival time of patients with small-cell lung cancer treated with combination chemotherapy and radiotherapy. The two-year survival was 33 percent, compared with about 15 percent from historical data.[191] The second study was a prospective, randomized, double-blind, and placebo-controlled study on 26 patients receiving radiotherapy or chemotherapy that investigated the effects of antioxidants on heart damage. Twelve of these patients were receiving radiotherapy and 13 had individually tailored chemotherapy regimes. The experimental group received 900 I.U. per day of vitamin E orally, starting on the first day of chemotherapy/radiotherapy, and 1 gram of vitamin C and 200 milligrams of *N*-acetylcysteine only on days that chemotherapy/radiotherapy was applied. The small number of patients in the study precluded a definite statement, but preliminary results suggested the antioxidants provided heart protection.[192]

Melatonin

Animal studies have reported that at doses applicable to humans, or larger ones, melatonin caused an antioxidant effect and protected normal cells from the adverse effects of chemotherapy drugs. At the same time, melatonin treatment did not reduce the antitumor activity of chemotherapy drugs, even at high doses that would have produced a profound antioxidant effect.

- Oral administration of melatonin (at about 48 milligrams per day, as scaled to humans) improved the antitumor activity of doxorubicin in mice with transplanted Ehrlich ascites cancer cells. Melatonin also improved the antioxidant status of the heart.[14]

- Oral administration of melatonin (at about 20 milligrams per day, as scaled to humans) reduced damage to auditory neurons caused by cisplatin in rats.[193]

- Intraperitoneal administration of 4 mg/kg melatonin reduced oxidative damage in the heart induced by doxorubicin treatment in mice and decreased mortality after doxorubicin treatment.[17] The equivalent human oral dose is about 300 milligrams.

- Subcutaneous administration of 2 mg/kg melatonin reduced oxidative damage in the liver induced by doxorubicin treatment in mice.[194] The equivalent human oral dose is about 120 milligrams.

- Subcutaneous administration of 10 mg/kg melatonin reduced mortality caused by doxorubicin and prevented oxidative damage from it in mice with transplanted lymphoma cells. The antitumor activity of doxorubicin was not reduced by melatonin treatment.[195] The equivalent human oral dose is about 580 milligrams.

- Subcutaneous administration of 5 mg/kg melatonin reduced genetic damage of normal cells induced by N-nitrosomethylurea, cyclophosphamide, and dimethylhydrazine in mice. The antitumor effects of these drugs in mice with transplanted Ehrlich carcinoma cells were not diminished by melatonin treatment.[196] The equivalent human oral dose is about 290 milligrams.

As with the animal studies, most human studies also indicated that melatonin acted as an antioxidant and reduced the adverse effects of chemotherapy without lessening its antitumor actions:

- In a randomized, nonblinded study on 250 patients with different advanced metastatic cancers receiving combination chemotherapy, those who also took melatonin (at 20 milligrams per day, orally) showed fewer adverse effects, particularly less myelosuppression, neuropathy, and heart toxicity. One-year survival was increased in the group receiving melatonin (51 percent versus 23 percent).[197]

- In a randomized, nonblinded study on 80 patients with different metastatic cancers receiving combination chemotherapy, those who received melatonin (at 20 milligrams per day, orally) showed fewer adverse effects, particularly less myelosuppression and neu-

ropathy. The incidence of hair loss and vomiting was not affected.[198]

- In a randomized, nonblinded study on 70 patients with advanced non-small-cell lung cancer treated with cisplatin and etoposide, the addition of melatonin (at 20 milligrams per day, orally) increased the one-year survival as compared to those getting chemotherapy only (44 percent versus 19 percent, respectively). The adverse effects of drug treatment, particularly myelosuppression, neuropathy, and cachexia, were reduced in the melatonin group.[199]

- In a phase II study, the addition of melatonin (at 20 milligrams per day, orally) to treatment with epirubicin appeared to reduce drug-induced thrombocytopenia.[200]

In contrast to the above, a randomized, double-blind study on 20 patients with advanced lung cancer receiving carboplatin and etoposide reported that those who received melatonin (at 40 milligrams per day, orally) did not experience reduced myelotoxic effects.[201]

Alpha-lipoic acid

Alpha-lipoic acid is a potent water- and fat-soluble thiol antioxidant mentioned briefly in previous chapters. It is discussed here in more detail as an example of an antioxidant that can reduce the side effects of chemotherapy without reducing its antitumor effects.

Alpha-lipoic acid effectively increases glutathione concentrations in vitro and in vivo. For example, intraperitoneal administration (at 4 to 16 mg/kg) increased the glutathione content in liver and kidney cells in mice, while this same dose protected mice from adverse effects of radiotherapy.[202] The equivalent human oral dose of 4 to 16 mg/kg intraperitoneal in mice is about 110 to 430 milligrams. This is about equal to the commonly prescribed dose of alpha-lipoic acid in noncancerous conditions, which is about 200 milligrams; higher doses are used to treat diseases such as diabetes.

In addition to (or because of) its antioxidant effects, alpha-lipoic acid also inhibits NF-κB in vitro and in vivo. Although in-vitro studies suggest that very high concentrations (about 4 mM) are required, daily oral doses of 600 milligrams in diabetic patients did reduce NF-κB activity in ex-vivo lymphocytes.[203, 204]

Similar doses have been tested in animals in conjunction with chemotherapy. These studies generally reported that alpha-lipoic acid did not inhibit the drug's antitumor effect and may have improved it in some cases:

- Oral administration (at 10 to 40 mg/kg) did not inhibit effectiveness of cyclophosphamide or vincristine sulfate in treating transplanted sarcoma and Walker carcinoma in rats. The treatment did, however, reduce adverse effects of vincristine sulfate (but not cyclophosphamide) to such a degree that the combined treatment increased median survival as compared to animals treated only with vincristine sulfate.[205] The equivalent human dose is 160 to 650 milligrams.

- Single intraperitoneal administrations of alpha-lipoic acid (at 25 to 100 mg/kg) reduced auditory and kidney damage in rats treated with cisplatin. The protective effects were associated with improved antioxidant status.[206, 207, 208] The equivalent human dose is 410 milligrams to 1.6 grams, intraperitoneal.

- A single intraperitoneal administration of 16 mg/kg of alpha-lipoic acid did not statistically affect the survival of mice with transplanted leukemia cells that were treated with doxorubicin, although there was a slight gain in survival in the group treated with both compounds.[209] The human equivalent is 150 milligrams, intraperitoneal.

We digress for a moment to examine the dose of alpha-lipoic acid that might be required to directly inhibit cancer cells. In vitro, concentrations of 10 μM and above inhibited proliferation of melanoma and neuroblastoma cells when exposure lasted for six days.[202] Inhibition occurred in spite of increased intracellular glutathione concentrations. In a human pharmacokinetic study, an oral dose of 200 milligrams produced an oral clearance of about 280 L/hr and a very short half-life of less than 30 minutes.[210] Based on these values, the oral dose needed to produce a 10-μM average plasma concentration is about 14 grams per day.

The LOAEL dose of alpha-lipoic acid is uncertain but may be about 2 grams per day. Daily oral doses of 1.2 to 1.8 grams have been used in human studies (treatment of diabetic polyneuropathy) with little ill effect, although intravenous administration of doses as high as 1.2 grams did cause nausea and vomiting.[211, 212, 213] The oral LD_{50} of alpha-lipoic acid is about 500 mg/kg in mice and 1.1 g/kg in rats, or the human equivalent of 4.8 and 18 grams.[213] Based on this, an oral dose of 14 grams would be prohibitive, and we can conclude that oral administration could not safely increase plasma concentration to cytotoxic levels. Synergism would be needed to produce direct effects.

At lower doses alpha-lipoic acid acts as an antioxidant in vivo, as mentioned above, and as seen in humans after an oral dose of 600 milligrams per day.[214] This antioxidant effect may be useful in inhibiting cancer through indirect means. Moderate doses of alpha-lipoic acid alone have in fact increased the life span of tumor-bearing animals in some but not all studies. In one study, a single oral administration of 10 to 40 mg/kg prolonged survival of rats with transplanted sarcoma cells but not Walker carcinoma cells.[215] The equivalent human dose is about 160 to 650 milligrams. Intravenous, subcutaneous, or intraperitoneal doses of 100 mg/kg (about 960 milligrams, as scaled to humans) for five days did not affect the survival of mice with transplanted Ehrlich ascites cancer cells, except for decreased survival due to alpha-lipoic acid toxicity with some routes of administration.[216] A single intraperitoneal administration of 16 mg/kg (about 150 milligrams, as scaled to humans) did not improve survival of mice with transplanted leukemia cells.[209] Higher doses have been effective in some studies; for example, intraperitoneal administration of 250 mg/kg for 10 days extended the life span of rats with transplanted Walker carcinoma by 25 percent.[217] The equivalent human oral dose is about 11 grams per day, which is prohibitive.

EFFECTS OF NATURAL COMPOUNDS ON RADIOTHERAPY

Radiotherapy causes DNA damage to cancer cells by inducing free radical production. Unfortunately, it also damages normal cells by the same mechanism. Antioxidants can protect normal cells against the damaging effects of radiotherapy, but there is some concern they might also protect cancer cells. Of the limited in-vivo studies available, most suggested that antioxidants do not interfere with the efficacy of radiotherapy; only two studies (on coenzyme Q10 and vitamin E) indicated that antioxidants do interfere. The unfavorable results in the one study on vitamin E may in fact have been an anomaly due to the experimental conditions, since several other studies found that vitamin E actually improved the efficacy of radiotherapy. In addition to not interfering with the cytotoxicity of radiotherapy in cancer cells, most animal studies also reported that antioxidants help limit adverse effects in normal tissues. While the majority of animal studies saw beneficial effects, few studies have been conducted and a small number reported detrimental effects. More studies are therefore needed to predict decisively the results of antioxidants in patients undergoing radiotherapy.

Several in-vivo studies, summarized below, suggest that antioxidants improve or do not interfere with the efficacy of radiotherapy. Note that only one human study is reported and many of the animal studies did not use a protocol that resembles how antioxidants would be used by humans (i.e., orally, in combinations, at moderate doses, and for prolonged periods); therefore, many uncertainties remain. The studies are as follows:

- High intraperitoneal doses of vitamin C (43 grams as scaled to humans) protected normal cells and reduced the lethality of radiation treatment but did not reduce its antitumor effect against transplanted fibrosarcoma cells in mice. Lower doses of vitamin C were not effective at providing radiation protection in any tissue.[218, 219, 220]

- Oral administration of 1.9 grams per day of vitamin C (as scaled to humans) in drinking water increased the efficacy of radiotherapy in mice inoculated with Ehrlich ascites cancer cells, as compared with mice receiving only distilled water.[221] However, these authors reported that this same dose in drinking water increased the mortality of mice receiving whole-body radiation.[222] The mechanisms causing these results are uncertain but it appears that vitamin C may have produced a prooxidant effect. As discussed in Chapter 15, vitamin C dissolved in water can lead to a prooxidant effect in some cases.

- In a study on mice, oral (1.2 g/kg) and intraperitoneal (0.4 to 4 g/kg) administration of either (+)-catechin or the flavonoid rutin did not reduce or improve the effectiveness of radiation treatment for three different types of implanted tumors.[223] Both natural compounds possess antioxidant properties.

- In a study on rats with transplanted sarcoma and Crocker carcinoma cells, administration of unspecified citrus flavonoids at 100 mg/kg did not interfere with the efficacy of radiotherapy but did reduce its adverse effects (the route of administration was not specified). The greatest reduction in mortality from lethal radiation occurred when the flavonoids were given both before and after treatment.[224]

- A combination of low-dose antioxidant vitamins (retinyl esters 1,300 I.U., intraperitoneal; vitamin E, 41 I.U., intraperitoneal; and vitamin C, 38 milligrams, intramuscular) given daily reduced the toxicity of radio-antibody therapy and bone marrow transplantation in mice. Antioxidant treatment did not reduce the antitumor effects of combined radio-antibody therapy and bone marrow transplantation in mice injected with human colon cancer cells.[225]

- A series of papers have been published on vitamin E's effects on the antitumor activity of radiotherapy. All reported a beneficial effect when the vitamin was given at moderate doses 24 hours or more before irradiation (reviewed in reference 226). For example, intraperitoneal administration of 50 to 500 mg/kg as a single dose seven days before irradiation increased antitumor effects of radiotherapy in mice with trans-

planted sarcoma cells. The equivalent human oral dose is about 720 and 7,200 I.U. An oral dose of 37 mg/kg (about 530 I.U. as scaled to humans) produced similar beneficial effects, as did a single intraperitoneal dose of 50 mg/kg given seven days before irradiation.[227, 228] These results are surprising considering the low dose and the length of time before irradiation, and other studies are needed to verify them. In contrast, a higher intraperitoneal dose of 1 g/kg did not enhance the antitumor effects.[229]

- In a randomized study on 30 patients with brain cancer receiving radiotherapy, those who also took melatonin (at 20 milligrams per day, orally) showed a higher one-year survival than those receiving only radiotherapy (43 percent versus 6 percent). In addition, adverse effects were lower in the melatonin group.[230]

In contrast, at least two studies have suggested that antioxidants may impair the efficacy of radiotherapy. In mice, oral administration of coenzyme Q10 at doses greater than 20 mg/kg per day reduced the effectiveness of radiation against lung cancer.[231] The equivalent human dose is about 190 milligrams per day. Intraperitoneal administration of 1 g/kg vitamin E in a single dose 30 minutes before radiation reduced antitumor activity in mice with transplanted squamous cell carcinoma.[232] The equivalent human dose is about 14,000 I.U. of vitamin E, intraperitoneal, which is prohibitive. As mentioned, other animal studies reported that such a large dose of vitamin E did not improve the efficacy of radiotherapy and that it was more effective when given seven days before irradiation than one day before. Thus it is possible these negative results may have come from the excessive dose and the fact it was administered so close to the time of irradiation.

Apart from any positive or negative effects antioxidants may have during radiotherapy, they may be beneficial after it. In particular, they may protect patients from the later impacts of radiation exposure, including ulceration and fibrosis. Preliminary data suggest that late effects are due to inflammatory processes and that antioxidants and other anti-inflammatory compounds can inhibit these.[218] Tumor cell destruction continues for a prolonged period after radiotherapy, possibly many months, and the optimum time to begin postradiation antioxidant treatment has not been established.

Radiation-induced chronic fibrosis is the most devastating long-term complication of radiotherapy. Fibrotic lesions do not regress spontaneously, and there is no accepted treatment known to cause regression. In a series of studies, a combination of vitamin E and pentoxifylline (a drug that improves blood flow by de-

TABLE 23.1 EFFECTS OF NATURAL COMPOUNDS ON PHASE I AND PHASE II ENZYMES

COMPOUND	EFFECTS ON P450 ENZYMES	EFFECTS ON PHASE II ENZYMES	REFERENCES
Apigenin	inhibits		237
Caffeic acid		induces	238
Curcumin	inhibits/induces	inhibits/induces	239–242
EPA/DHA	induces	induces	243, 244
Garlic and DADS	inhibits/induces	induces	238, 245–248
Genistein and daidzein		induces	249
Ginseng saponins	inhibits/induces		250, 270
Green tea and EGCG	inhibits/induces	induces	251, 252, 253
Limonene and perillyl alcohol	inhibits/induces	induces	254–257
Luteolin	inhibits	inhibits	258, 259
Melatonin	inhibits	induces	260, 261
PSP (polysaccharide)		induces	262
Quercetin	inhibits	induces	237, 249
Resveratrol	inhibits		263, 264, 265
Retinol and ATRA	inhibits		266, 267, 271
Selenium	induces	induces	268, 269
Silymarin, from milk thistle	inhibits		270
Vitamin D_3	inhibits		271

creasing its viscosity) caused marked regressions of fibrotic lesions in patients treated with radiotherapy.[233, 234] For example, in a study on 43 patients, oral administration of vitamin E (at 1,000 I.U. per day) and pentoxifylline for one year caused lesions to regress in 83 percent of patients. The lesions slowly diminished over time, and after a year their surface areas had shrunk an average of 66 percent.[235]

In one other postradiotherapy study, a retrospective one on 405 advanced patients with brain metastases who received radiotherapy, 143 patients who took 2.5 grams of omega-3 fatty acids from fish oil and 200 milligrams of silymarin daily showed longer average survival (54 days versus 89 days respectively) and fewer adverse delayed effects (14 percent versus 4 percent showing radionecrosis, respectively). The fish oil and silymarin treatment was started two weeks after completion of radiotherapy and lasted up to 20 weeks.[236]

DRUG METABOLISM

Before ending this discussion on the interactions of natural compounds and conventional treatment, we must consider the possibility that natural compounds will influence the metabolism of chemotherapy drugs. These interactions are important when determining chemotherapy doses. Until 1991, little attention was paid to the prospect of altered metabolism, but this changed with the first publication that grapefruit juice could alter the pharmacokinetics of felodipine and nifedipine, two drugs used to treat hypertension.[272] Many papers on the topic have since been published but the effects of natural compounds on drug uptake and disposition, and the clinical ramifications of these effects, are still largely unknown. Quite likely, many natural compounds besides grapefruit juice can affect drug pharmacokinetics in humans; potential mechanisms include effects on oxidative metabolism, detoxification enzymes, and drug transport proteins such as P-glycoprotein.[273] The largest impact on drug pharmacokinetics by natural compounds is probably from altering prehepatic drug metabolism in the intestines.

Drugs and other foreign compounds are removed from the body through detoxification. This process, which occurs mostly in the liver and to a lesser extent the intestines and other tissues, is divided into two phases; depending on the chemical structure, drugs may go through one or both. In phase I detoxification, compounds are oxidized or reduced to a less reactive form. In phase II detoxification, a polar group, like glutathione or glucuronic acid, is conjugated to the drug, which greatly increases its water-solubility. (Conjugation is discussed in some detail in Chapter 13 and Appendix J.) Enzymes important in phase II detoxification include glutathione *S*-transferase and UDP-glucuronosyl-transferase (UGT); the latter is the primary enzyme catalyzing the formation of glucuronide conjugates.

Cytochrome P450 is an important enzyme in phase I detoxification, and it can be induced by a variety of drugs and other compounds. Once induced, it is available to act not only on the inducing agent but also on any other compound metabolized by cytochrome P450. For example, when people drink alcohol regularly, they stimulate cytochrome P450 activity, which allows them to drink more alcohol without feeling its effects. At the same time, the increase in P450 enzymes also causes them to metabolize a variety of prescription drugs more readily.

The ability of natural compounds to induce cytochrome P450 or other phase I or phase II enzymes is important, since this can influence the concentration of chemotherapy drugs in the plasma. If detoxification enzymes are induced and if the chemotherapy drug is metabolized by them to an inactive form, the drug dose may need to be increased to reach the effective concentration. On the other hand, if the chemotherapy drug is metabolized to an active form by the induced enzymes, an overdose could occur.

Reports are beginning to surface on modulating drug detoxification with natural compounds. For example, altered plasma concentrations were observed in two recent studies on *Hypericum* (St. John's wort). In the first, oral administration of 900 milligrams per day of *Hypericum* extract (standardized for 3 percent hypericin) reduced the plasma concentration of indinavir in healthy volunteers by an average of 57 percent; indinavir is a HIV-1 protease inhibitor used in HIV treatment.[274] In the second study, the authors described two cases where *Hypericum* initiated the rejection of heart transplants in patients being treated with cyclosporin, an immune suppressant.[275] We can see from these studies that such drug/natural compound interactions can be life threatening in some situations.

Natural compounds that affect either phase I or phase II enzymes are listed in Table 23.1. Quite likely, future research will find that a high percentage of natural compounds can affect phase I or phase II enzymes, at least to some degree. For this reason, it is wise to use caution when combining natural compounds and chemotherapy or other drugs, and in many cases additional monitoring of plasma drug concentrations may be warranted.

CONCLUSION

Based on the studies cited in this chapter, it appears that natural compounds have the potential to improve the efficacy of chemotherapy and radiotherapy and/or reduce their adverse effects. Indeed, very few of the studies found that natural compounds are detrimental. While these results are very encouraging, caution is still necessary. Relatively few in-vivo studies have been completed, and most were on animals. Moreover, many of these did not use protocols that accurately reflect the general human use of natural compounds (i.e., orally, at moderate doses, in combinations, and for prolonged periods). In addition, the effects natural compounds might have on the metabolism of chemotherapy drugs have barely been investigated, and these effects could play an important role in determining proper drug doses. Thus, while the benefits of combining natural compounds with chemotherapy appear to be great, additional study is needed to determine their best and safest use.

REFERENCES

[1] Feleszko W, Zagozdzon R, Golab J, Jakobisiak M. Potentiated antitumour effects of cisplatin and lovastatin against MmB16 melanoma in mice. Eur J Cancer 1998 Feb; 34(3):406–11.

[2] Giavazzi R, Garofalo A, Ferri C, et al. Batimastat, a synthetic inhibitor of matrix metalloproteinases, potentiates the antitumor activity of cisplatin in ovarian carcinoma xenografts. Clin Cancer Res 1998 Apr; 4(4):985–92.

[3] Nishisaka N, Maini A, Kinoshita Y, et al. Immunotherapy for lung metastases of murine renal cell carcinoma: Synergy between radiation and cytokine-producing tumor vaccines. J Immunother 1999 Jul; 22(4):308–14.

[4] Ishihara M, Kubota T, Watanabe M, et al. Interferon gamma increases the antitumor activity of mitomycin C against human colon cancer cells in vitro and in vivo. Oncol Rep 1999 May–Jun; 6(3):621–5.

[5] Yu WD, Chang MJ, Trump DL, Johnson CS. Interleukin-1alpha synergistic in vivo enhancement of cyclophosphamide- and carboplatin-mediated antitumor activity. Cancer Immunol Immunother 1997 Aug; 44(6):316–22.

[6] Roh H, Hirose CB, Boswell CB, et al. Synergistic antitumor effects of HER2/neu antisense oligodeoxynucleotides and conventional chemotherapeutic agents. Surgery 1999 Aug; 126(2):413–21.

[7] Baselga J, Norton L, Masui H, et al. Antitumor effects of doxorubicin in combination with anti-epidermal growth factor receptor monoclonal antibodies. J Natl Cancer Inst 1993 Aug 18; 85(16):1327–33.

[8] Dillman RO. Rationales for combining chemotherapy and biotherapy in the treatment of cancer. Mol Biother 1990; 2(4):201–7.

[9] Taatjes DJ, Fenick DJ, Gaudiano G, Koch TH. A redox pathway leading to the alkylation of nucleic acids by doxorubicin and related anthracyclines: Application to the design of antitumor drugs for resistant cancer. Curr Pharm Des 1998 Jun; 4(3):203–18.

[10] Gustafson DL, Swanson JD, Pritsos CA. Modulation of glutathione and glutathione dependent antioxidant enzymes in mouse heart following doxorubicin therapy. Free Radic Res Commun 1993; 19(2):111–20.

[11] Singal PK, Li T, Kumar D, et al. Adriamycin-induced heart failure: Mechanism and modulation. Mol Cell Biochem 2000 Apr; 207(1–2):77–86.

[12] Faure H, Coudray C, Mousseau M. 5-Hydroxymethyluracil excretion, plasma TBARS and plasma antioxidant vitamins in adriamycin-treated patients. Free Radic Biol Med 1996; 20(7):979–83.

[13] Erhola M, Kellokumpu-Lehtinen P, Metsa-Ketela T. Effects of anthracyclin-based chemotherapy on total plasma antioxidant capacity in small cell lung cancer patients. Free Radic Biol Med 1996; 21(3):383–90.

[14] Wahab MH, Akoul ES, Abdel-Aziz AA. Modulatory effects of melatonin and vitamin E on doxorubicin-induced

cardiotoxicity in Ehrlich ascites carcinoma-bearing mice. Tumori 2000 Mar–Apr; 86(2):157–62.

[15] Lu HZ, Geng BQ, Zhu YL, Yong DG. Effects of beta-carotene on doxorubicin-induced cardiotoxicity in rats. Chung Kuo Yao Li Hsueh Pao 1996 Jul; 17(4):317–20.

[16] Herman EH, Ferrans VJ. Preclinical animal models of cardiac protection from anthracycline-induced cardiotoxicity. Semin Oncol 1998 Aug; 25(4 Suppl 10):15–21.

[17] Morishima I, Matsui H, Mukawa H, et al. Melatonin, a pineal hormone with antioxidant property, protects against adriamycin cardiomyopathy in rats. Life Sci 1998; 63(7):511–21.

[18] Venkatesan N. Curcumin attenuation of acute adriamycin myocardial toxicity in rats. Br J Pharmacol 1998 Jun; 124(3):425–7.

[19] Kozluca O, Olcay E, Surucu S, et al. Prevention of doxorubicin induced cardiotoxicity by catechin. Cancer Lett 1996 Jan 19; 99(1):1–6.

[20] Siveski-Iliskovic N, Hill M, Chow DA, Singal PK. Probucol protects against adriamycin cardiomyopathy without interfering with its antitumor effect. Circulation 1995 Jan 1; 91(1):10–5.

[21] Shimpo K, Nagatsu T, Yamada K, et al. Ascorbic acid and adriamycin toxicity. Am J Clin Nutr 1991 Dec; 54(6 Suppl):1298S-1301S.

[22] Geetha A, Catherine J, Shyamala Devi CS. Effect of alpha-tocopherol on the microsomal lipid peroxidation induced by doxorubicin: Influence of ascorbic acid. Indian J Physiol Pharmacol 1989 Jan–Mar; 33(1):53–8.

[23] Fujita K, Shinpo K, Yamada K, et al. Reduction of adriamycin toxicity by ascorbate in mice and guinea pigs. Cancer Res 1982 Jan; 42(1):309–16.

[24] Shacter E, Williams JA, Hinson RM, et al. Oxidative stress interferes with cancer chemotherapy: Inhibition of lymphoma cell apoptosis and phagocytosis. Blood 2000 Jul 1; 96(1):307–313.

[25] Nagata Y, Takata J, Karube Y, Matsushima Y. Effects of a water-soluble prodrug of vitamin E on doxorubicin-induced toxicity in mice. Biol Pharm Bull 1999 Jul; 22(7):698–702.

[26] Foster-Nora JA, Siden R. Amifostine for protection from antineoplastic drug toxicity. Am J Health Syst Pharm 1997 Apr 1; 54(7):787–800.

[27] Santini V, Giles FJ. The potential of amifostine: From cytoprotectant to therapeutic agent. Haematologica 1999 Nov; 84(11):1035–42.

[28] Bartoli GM, Galeotti T. Growth-related lipid peroxidation in tumour microsomal membranes and mitochondria. Biochim Biophys Acta 1979 Sep 28; 574(3):537–41.

[29] Chajes V, Sattler W, Stranzl A, Kostner GM. Influence of n-3 fatty acids on the growth of human breast cancer cells in vitro: Relationship to peroxides and vitamin-E. Breast Cancer Res Treat 1995 Jun; 34(3):199–212.

[30] Morisaki N, Lindsey JA, Stitts JM, et al. Fatty acid metabolism and cell proliferation. V. Evaluation of pathways for the generation of lipid peroxides. Lipids 1984 Jun; 19(6):381–94.

[31] Muzio G, Salvo RA, Trombetta A, et al. Dose-dependent inhibition of cell proliferation induced by lipid peroxidation products in rat hepatoma cells after enrichment with arachidonic acid. Lipids 1999 Jul; 34(7):705–11.

[32] Conklin KA. Dietary antioxidants during cancer chemotherapy: Impact on chemotherapeutic effectiveness and development of side effects. Nutr Cancer 2000; 37(1):1–18.

[33] O'Brien ML, Tew KD. Glutathione and related enzymes in multidrug resistance. Eur J Cancer 1996 Jun; 32A(6):967–78.

[34] Grech KV, Davey RA, Davey MW. The relationship between modulation of MDR and glutathione in MRP-overexpressing human leukemia cells. Biochem Pharmacol 1998 Apr 15; 55(8):1283–9.

[35] Yu DS, Ma CP, Chang SY. Verapamil modulation of multidrug resistance in renal cell carcinoma. J Formos Med Assoc 2000 Apr; 99(4):311–6.

[36] Grey M, Borg AG, Wood P, et al. Effect on cell kill of addition of multidrug resistance modifiers cyclosporin A and PSC 833 to cytotoxic agents in acute myeloid leukaemia. Leuk Res 1997 Sep; 21(9):867–74.

[37] Volm M. Multidrug resistance and its reversal. Anticancer Res 1998 Jul–Aug; 18(4C):2905–17.

[38] Kasimir-Bauer S, Ottinger H, Meusers P, et al. In acute myeloid leukemia, coexpression of at least two proteins, including P-glycoprotein, the multidrug resistance-related protein, bcl-2, mutant p53, and heat-shock protein 27, is predictive of the response to induction chemotherapy. Exp Hematol 1998 Nov; 26(12):1111–7.

[39] Blobe GC, Obeid LM, Hannun YA. Regulation of protein kinase C and role in cancer biology. Cancer Metastasis Rev 1994 Dec; 13(3–4):411–31.

[40] Philip PA, Harris AL. Potential for protein kinase C inhibitors in cancer therapy. Cancer Treat Res 1995; 78:3–27.

[41] Baltuch GH, Dooley NP, Villemure JG, Yong VW. Protein kinase C and growth regulation of malignant gliomas. Can J Neurol Sci 1995 Nov; 22(4):264–71.

[42] Tsuchida E, Urano M. The effect of UCN-01 (7-hydroxystaurosporine), a potent inhibitor of protein kinase C, on fractionated radiotherapy or daily chemotherapy of a murine fibrosarcoma. Int J Radiat Oncol Biol Phys 1997 Dec 1; 39(5):1153–61.

[43] Zhang W, Anker L, Law RE, et al. Enhancement of radiosensitivity in human malignant glioma cells by hypericin in vitro. Clin Cancer Res 1996 May; 2(5):843–6.

[44] Thevenod F, Friedmann JM, Katsen AD, Hauser IA. Up-regulation of multidrug resistance P-glycoprotein via nuclear factor-kappaB activation protects kidney proximal tubule cells from cadmium- and reactive oxygen species-induced apoptosis. J Biol Chem 2000 Jan 21; 275(3):1887–96.

[45] Zhou G, Kuo MT. NF-kappaB-mediated induction of mdr1b expression by insulin in rat hepatoma cells. J Biol Chem 1997 Jun 13; 272(24):15174–83.

[46] Hansen RK, Oesterreich S, Lemieux P, et al. Quercetin inhibits heat shock protein induction but not heat shock factor DNA-binding in human breast carcinoma cells. Biochem Biophys Res Commun 1997 Oct 29; 239(3):851–6.

[47] Lee YJ, Erdos G, Hou ZZ, et al. Mechanism of quercetin-induced suppression and delay of heat shock gene expression and thermotolerance development in HT-29 cells. Mol Cell Biochem 1994 Aug 31; 137(2):141–54.

[48] Winyard PG, Blake DR. Antioxidants, redox-regulated transcription factors, and inflammation. Advances in Pharmacology 1997; 38:403–421.

[49] Zhou G, Kuo MT. NF-kappaB-mediated induction of mdr1b expression by insulin in rat hepatoma cells. J Biol Chem 1997 Jun 13; 272(24):15174–83.

[50] Guzhova IV, Darieva ZA, Melo AR, Margulis BA. Major stress protein Hsp70 interacts with NF-κB regulatory complex in human T-lymphoma cells. Cell Stress Chaperones 1997 Jun; 2(2):132–9.

[51] Baldew GS, van den Hamer CJ, Los G, et al. Selenium-induced protection against cis-diamminedichloroplatinum(II) nephrotoxicity in mice and rats. Cancer Res 1989 Jun 1; 49(11):3020–3.

[52] Ohkawa K, Tsukada Y, Dohzono H, et al. The effects of co-administration of selenium and cis-platin (CDDP) on CDDP-induced toxicity and antitumour activity. Br J Cancer 1988 Jul; 58(1):38–41.

[53] Naganuma A, Satoh M, Yokoyama M, Imura N. Selenium efficiently depressed toxic side effect of cis-diamminedichloroplatinum. Res Commun Chem Pathol Pharmacol 1983 Oct; 42(1):127–34.

[54] Berry JP, Pauwells C, Tlouzeau S, Lespinats G. Effect of selenium in combination with cis-diamminedichloroplatinum(II) in the treatment of murine fibrosarcoma. Cancer Res 1984 Jul; 44(7):2864–8.

[55] Baldew GS, Mol JG, de Kanter FJ, et al. The mechanism of interaction between cisplatin and selenite. Biochem Pharmacol 1991 May 15; 41(10):1429–37.

[56] Caffrey PB, Frenkel GD. Selenium compounds prevent the induction of drug resistance by cisplatin in human ovarian tumor xenografts in vivo. Cancer Chemother Pharmacol 2000; 46(1):74–8.

[57] Hu YJ, Chen Y, Zhang YQ, et al. The protective role of selenium on the toxicity of cisplatin-contained chemotherapy regimen in cancer patients. Biol Trace Elem Res 1997 Mar; 56(3):331–41.

[58] Kurbacher CM, Wagner U, Kolster B, et al. Ascorbic acid (vitamin C) improves the antineoplastic activity of doxorubicin, cisplatin, and paclitaxel in human breast carcinoma cells in vitro. Cancer Lett 1996 Jun 5; 103(2):183–9.

[59] Shimpo K, Nagatsu T, Yamada K, et al. Ascorbic acid and adriamycin toxicity. Am J Clin Nutr 1991 Dec; 54(6 Suppl):1298S-1301S.

[60] Osswald H, Herrmann R, Youssef M. The influence of sodium ascorbate, menadione sodium bisulfite or pyridoxal hydrochloride on the toxic and antineoplastic action of N-methylformamide in P 388 leukemia or M 5076 sarcoma in mice. Toxicology 1987 Feb; 43(2):183–91.

[61] Greggi Antunes LM, Darin JD, Bianchi MD. Protective effects of vitamin c against cisplatin-induced nephrotoxicity and lipid peroxidation in adult rats: A dose-dependent study. Pharmacol Res 2000 Apr; 41(4):405–11.

[62] Ghaskadbi S, Rajmachikar S, Agate C, et al. Modulation of cyclophosphamide mutagenicity by vitamin C in the in vivo rodent micronucleus assay. Teratog Carcinog Mutagen 1992; 12(1):11–7.

[63] Giri A, Khynriam D, Prasad SB. Vitamin C mediated protection on cisplatin induced mutagenicity in mice. Mutat Res 1998 Nov 3; 421(2):139–48.

[64] Krishna G, Nath J, Ong T. Inhibition of cyclophosphamide and mitomycin C-induced sister chromatid exchanges in mice by vitamin C. Cancer Res 1986 Jun; 46(6):2670–4.

[65] Rivas-Olmedo G, Barriga-Arceo SD, Madrigal-Bujaidar E. Inhibition of mitomycin C-induced sister chromatid exchanges by vitamin C in vivo. J Toxicol Environ Health 1992 Feb; 35(2):107–13.

[66] Mickey DD, Carvalho L, Foulkes K. Combined therapeutic effects of conventional agents and an immunomodulator, PSK, on rat prostatic adenocarcinoma. J Urol 1989 Dec; 142(6):1594–8.

[67] Takenoshita S, Hashizume T, Asao T, et al. Inhibitory effects of combined administration of 5-FU and Krestin on liver cancer KDH-8 in WKA/H rats. J Invest Surg 1995 Jan–Feb; 8(1):1–5.

[68] Qian ZM, Xu MF, Tang PL. Polysaccharide peptide (PSP) restores immunosuppression induced by cyclophosphamide in rats. Am J Chin Med 1997; 25(1):27–35.

[69] Mickey DD. Combined therapeutic effects of an immunomodulator, PSK, and chemotherapy with carboquone on rat bladder carcinoma. Cancer Chemother Pharmacol 1985; 15(1):54–8.

[70] Fujii T, Sugita N, Kobayashi Y, et al. Treatment with Krestin combined with mitomycin C, and effect on immune response. Oncology 1989; 46(1):49–53.

[71] Iino Y, Takai Y, Sugamata N, Morishita Y. PSK (krestin) potentiates chemotherapeutic effects of tamoxifen on rat mammary carcinomas. Anticancer Res 1992 Nov–Dec; 12(6B):2101–3.

[72] Sugiyama K, Ueda H, Ichio Y, Yokota M. Improvement of cisplatin toxicity and lethality by juzen-taiho-to in mice. Biol Pharm Bull 1995 Jan; 18(1):53–8.

[73] Ebisuno S, Hirano A, Kyoku I, et al. [Basal studies on combination of Chinese medicine in cancer chemotherapy: Protective effects on the toxic side effects of CDDP and antitumor effects with CDDP on murine bladder tumor (MBT-2).] Nippon Gan Chiryo Gakkai Shi 1989 Jun 20; 24(6):1305–12.

[74] Iijima OT, Fujii Y, Funo S, et al. [Protective effects of the Chinese medicine Juzentaiho-to from the adverse effects of mitomycin C and cisplatin.] Gan To Kagaku Ryoho 1989 Apr; 16(4 Pt 2–2):1525–32.

[75] Komiyama K, Hirokawa Y, Zhibo Y, et al. [Potentiation of chemotherapeutic activity by a Chinese herb medicine juzen-taiho-toh.] Gan To Kagaku Ryoho 1988 May; 15(5):1715–9.

[76] Kiyohara H, Matsumoto T, Komatsu Y, Yamada H. Protective effect of oral administration of a pectic polysaccharide fraction from a Kampo (Japanese herbal) medicine "Juzen-Taiho-To" on adverse effects of cis-diaminedichloroplatinum. Planta Med 1995 Dec; 61(6):531–34.

[77] Ji YB, Jiang WX, Zhang XJ. [Effects of buzhong yiqi decoction on the anticancer activity and toxicity induced by cyclophosphamide.] Chung Kuo Chung Yao Tsa Chih 1989 Mar; 14(3):48–51, 64.

78 Tsai WS, Nagawa H, Muto T. Differential effects of polyunsaturated fatty acids on chemosensitivity of NIH3T3 cells and its transformants. Int J Cancer 1997 Jan 27; 70(3):357–61.

79 Timmer-Bosscha H, de Vries EG, Meijer C, et al. Differential effects of all-*trans* retinoic acid, docosahexaenoic acid, and hexadecylphosphocholine on cisplatin-induced cytotoxicity and apoptosis in a cisplantin-sensitive and resistant human embryonal carcinoma cell line. Cancer Chemother Pharmacol 1998; 41(6):469–76.

80 Guffy MM, North JA, Burns CP. Effect of cellular fatty acid alteration on adriamycin sensitivity in cultured L1210 murine leukemia cells. Cancer Res 1984 May; 44(5):1863–6.

81 Kinsella JE, Black JM. Effects of polyunsaturated fatty acids on the efficacy of antineoplastic agents toward L5178Y lymphoma cells. Biochem Pharmacol 1993 May 5; 45(9):1881–7.

82 Germain E, Chajes V, Cognault S, et al. Enhancement of doxorubicin cytotoxicity by polyunsaturated fatty acids in the human breast tumor cell line MDA-MB-231: Relationship to lipid peroxidation. Int J Cancer 1998 Feb 9; 75(4):578–83.

83 Ikushima S, Fujiwara F, Todo S, Imashuku S. Effects of polyunsaturated fatty acids on vincristine-resistance in human neuroblastoma cells. Anticancer Res 1991 May–Jun; 11(3):1215–20.

84 Zijlstra JG, de Vries EG, Muskiet FA, et al. Influence of docosahexaenoic acid in vitro on intracellular adriamycin concentration in lymphocytes and human adriamycin-sensitive and -resistant small-cell lung cancer cell lines, and on cytotoxicity in the tumor cell lines. Int J Cancer 1987 Dec 15; 40(6):850–6.

85 Das UN, Madhavi N, Sravan Kumar G, et al. Can tumour cell drug resistance be reversed by essential fatty acids and their metabolites? Prostaglandins Leukot Essent Fatty Acids 1998 Jan; 58(1):39–54.

86 Hardman WE, Moyer MP, Cameron IL. Dietary fish oil sensitizes A549 lung xenografts to doxorubicin chemotherapy. Cancer Lett 2000 Apr 14; 151(2):145–51.

87 Ogilvie GK, Fettman MJ, Mallinckrodt CH, et al. Effect of fish oil, arginine, and doxorubicin chemotherapy on remission and survival time for dogs with lymphoma: A double-blind, randomized placebo-controlled study. Cancer 2000 Apr 15; 88(8):1916–28.

88 Shao Y, Pardini L, Pardini RS. Dietary menhaden oil enhances mitomycin C antitumor activity toward human mammary carcinoma MX-1. Lipids 1995 Nov; 30(11):1035–45.

89 Shao Y, Pardini L, Pardini RS. Intervention of transplantable human mammary carcinoma MX-1 chemotherapy with dietary menhaden oil in athymic mice: Increased therapeutic effects and decreased toxicity of cyclophosphamide. Nutr Cancer 1997; 28(1):63–73.

90 Horie T, Nakamaru M, Masubuchi Y. Docosahexaenoic acid exhibits a potent protection of small intestine from methotrexate-induced damage in mice. Life Sci 1998; 62(15):1333–8.

91 Bougnoux P, Germain E, Chajes V, et al. Cytotoxic drugs efficacy correlates with adipose tissue docosahexaenoic acid level in locally advanced breast carcinoma. Br J Cancer 1999 Apr; 79(11–12):1765–9.

92 Unnikrishnan MC, Soudamini KK, Kuttan R. Chemoprotection of garlic extract toward cyclophosphamide toxicity in mice. Nutr Cancer 1990; 13(3):201–7.

93 Stankler L. Tetracycline and proteolytic enzymes combined compared with tetracycline alone in acne vulgaris. Br J Clin Pract 1976 Mar; 30(3):65–6.

94 Bock U, Kolac C, Borchard G, et al. Transport of proteolytic enzymes across Caco-2 cell monolayers. Pharm Res 1998 Sep; 15(9):

95 Wrba H, Pecher O. Enzymes: A drug of the future. Strengthening the immunological system with enzyme therapy. MUCOS Pharma GmbH, 1996. http://www.mucos.de

96 Lahousen M. [Modification of liver parameters by adjuvant administration of proteolytic enzymes following chemotherapy in patients with ovarian carcinoma.] Wien Med Wochenschr 1995; 145(24):663–8.

97 Schedler M, Lind A, Schatzle W, Stauder G. Adjuvant therapy with hydrolytic enzymes in oncology—a hopeful effort to avoid bleomycin induced pneumotoxicity? J Cancer Res Clin Oncol 1990; 116 (Suppl 1):697.

98 Klaschka, F. Oral enzymes in oncology: Clinical studies on Wobe-MuGos. MUCOS Pharma GmbH, 1997. http://www.mucos.de

99 Lotz-Winter H. On the pharmacology of bromelain: An update with special regard to animal studies on dose-dependent effects. Planta Med 1990; 56:249–53.

100 Kaul R, Mishra BK, Sutradar P, et al. The role of WOBE-MUGOS in reducing acute sequele of radiation in head and neck cancers—a clinical phase-III randomized trial. Indian J Cancer 1999 Jun–Dec; 36(2–4):141–8.

101 Sedlak J, Hunakova L, Sulikova M, Chorvath B. Protein kinase inhibitor-induced alterations of drug uptake, cell cycle and surface antigen expression in human multidrug-resistant (Pgp and MRP) promyelocytic leukemia HL-60 cells. Leuk Res 1997 May; 21(5):449–58.

102 Castro AF, Altenberg GA. Inhibition of drug transport by genistein in multidrug-resistant cells expressing P-glycoprotein. Biochem Pharmacol 1997 Jan 10; 53(1):89–93.

103 Versantvoort CH, Schuurhuis GJ, Pinedo HM, et al. Genistein modulates the decreased drug accumulation in non-P-glycoprotein mediated multidrug resistant tumour cells. Br J Cancer 1993 Nov; 68(5):939–46.

104 Versantvoort CH, Rhodes T, Twentyman PR. Acceleration of MRP-associated efflux of rhodamine 123 by genistein and related compounds. Br J Cancer 1996 Dec; 74(12):1949–54.

105 Critchfield JW, Welsh CJ, Phang JM, Yeh GC. Modulation of adriamycin accumulation and efflux by flavonoids in HCT-15 colon cells. Activation of P-glycoprotein as a putative mechanism. Biochem Pharmacol 1994 Oct 7; 48(7):1437–45.

106 Takeda Y, Nishio K, Niitani H, Saijo N. Reversal of multidrug resistance by tyrosine-kinase inhibitors in a non-P-glycoprotein-mediated multidrug-resistant cell line. Int J Cancer 1994 Apr 15; 57(2):229–39.

107 Kioka N, Hosokawa N, Komano T, et al. Quercetin, a bioflavonoid, inhibits the increase of human multi-drug resistance gene (MDR1) expression caused arsenite. Federation of European Biochemical Societies 1992; 301(3):307–9.

108 Kim SH, Yeo GS, Lim YS, et al. Suppression of multidrug resistance via inhibition of heat shock factor by quercetin in MDR cells. Exp Mol Med 1998 Jun 30; 30(2):87–92.

109 Scambia G, Ranelletti FO, Panici PB, et al. Quercetin potentiates the effect of adriamycin in a multidrug-resistant MCF-7 human breast-cancer cell line: P-glycoprotein as a possible target [see comments]. Cancer Chemother Pharmacol 1994; 34(6):459–64.

110 Hosokawa N, Hirayoshi K, Kudo H, et al. Inhibition of the activation of heat shock factor in vivo and in vitro by flavonoids. Mol Cell Biol 1992 Aug; 12(8):3490–8.

111 Elia G, Santoro MG. Regulation of heat shock protein synthesis by quercetin in human erythroleukaemia cells. Biochem J 1994 May 15; 300 (Pt 1):201–9.

112 Wei YQ, Zhao X, Kariya Y, et al. Induction of apoptosis by quercetin: Involvement of heat shock protein. Cancer Res 1994 Sep 15; 54(18):4952–7.

113 Hosokawa N, Hirayoshi K, Nakai A, et al. Flavonoids inhibit the expression of heat shock proteins. Cell Structure Function 1990; 15:393–401.

114 Xuan Y, Hacker MP, Tritton TR, Bhushan A. Modulation of methotrexate resistance by genistein in murine leukemia L1210 cells. Oncol Rep 1998; 5(2):419–421.

115 den Boer ML, Pieters R, Kazemier KM, et al. The modulating effect of PSC 833, cyclosporin A, verapamil and genistein on in vitro cytotoxicity and intracellular content of daunorubicin in childhood acute lymphoblastic leukemia. Leukemia 1998 Jun; 12(6):912–20.

116 Scambia G, Ranelletti FO, Benedetti Panici P, et al. Synergistic antiproliferative activity of quercetin and cisplatin on ovarian cancer cell growth. Anticancer Drugs 1990 Oct; 1(1):45–8.

117 Hoffman R, Graham L, Newlands ES. Enhanced anti-proliferative action of busulphan by quercetin on the human leukaemia cell line K562. Br J Cancer 1989 Mar; 59(3):347–8.

118 Teofili L, Pierelli L, Iovino MS, et al. The combination of quercetin and cytosine arabinoside synergistically inhibits leukemic cell growth. Leuk Res 1992; 16(5):497–503.

119 Freund A, Boos J, Harkin S, et al. Augmentation of 1-beta-D-arabinofuranosylcytosine (Ara-C) cytotoxicity in leukaemia cells by co-administration with antisignalling drugs. Eur J Cancer 1998 May; 34(6):895–901.

120 Monti E, Sinha BK. Antiproliferative effect of genistein and adriamycin against estrogen-dependent and -independent human breast carcinoma cell lines. Anticancer Res 1994 May–Jun; 14(3A):1221–6.

121 Li W, Weber G. Synergistic action of tiazofurin and genistein on growth inhibition and differentiation of K-562 human leukemic cells. Life Sci 1998; 63(22):1975–81.

122 Li W, Weber G. Synergistic action of tiazofurin and genistein in human ovarian carcinoma cells. Oncol Res 1998; 10(3):117–22.

123 Hofmann J, Fiebig HH, Winterhalter BR, et al. Enhancement of the antiproliferative activity of cis-diamminedichloroplatinum(II) by quercetin. Int J Cancer 1990 Mar 15; 45(3):536–9.

124 Wietrzyk J, Opolski A, Madej J, Radzikowski C. Antitumour and antimetastatic effect of genistein alone or combined with cyclophosphamide in mice transplanted with various tumours depends on the route of tumour transplantation. In Vivo 2000 Mar–Apr; 14(2):357–62.

125 Stammler G, Volm M. Green tea catechins (EGCG and EGC) have modulating effects on the activity of doxorubicin in drug-resistant cell lines. Anticancer Drugs 1997 Mar; 8(3):265–8.

126 Sadzuka Y, Sugiyama T, Hirota S. Modulation of cancer chemotherapy by green tea. Clin Cancer Res 1998 Jan; 4(1):153–6.

127 Mimoto J, Kiura K, Matsuo K, et al. (-)-Epigallocatechin gallate can prevent cisplatin-induced lung tumorigenesis in A/J mice. Carcinogenesis 2000 May; 21(5):915–9.

128 Venkatesan N, Chandrakasan G. Modulation of cyclophosphamide-induced early lung injury by curcumin, an anti-inflammatory antioxidant. Mol Cell Biochem 1995 Jan 12; 142(1):79–87.

129 Venkatesan N, Punithavathi V, Chandrakasan G. Curcumin protects bleomycin-induced lung injury in rats. Life Sci 1997; 61(6):51–58.

130 Venkatesan N. Curcumin attenuation of acute adriamycin myocardial toxicity in rats. Br J Pharmacol 1998 Jun; 124(3):425–7.

131 Venkatesan N, Punithavathi D, Arumugam V. Curcumin prevents adriamycin nephrotoxicity in rats. Br J Pharmacol 2000 Jan; 129(2):231–4.

132 Sriganth INP, Premalatha B. Dietary curcumin with cisplatin administration modulates tumor marker indices in experimental fibrosarcoma. Pharm Res 1999; 39(3):175–9.

133 Zhang L, Hung MC. Sensitization of HER-2/neu-overexpressing non-small cell lung cancer cells to chemotherapeutic drugs by tyrosine kinase inhibitor emodin. Oncogene 1996 Feb 1; 12(3):571–6.

134 Zhang L, Lau YK, Xia W, et al. Tyrosine kinase inhibitor emodin suppresses growth of HER-2/neu-overexpressing breast cancer cells in athymic mice and sensitizes these cells to the inhibitory effect of paclitaxel. Clin Cancer Res 1999 Feb; 5(2):343–53.

135 Hasegawa H, Sung JH, Matsumiya S, et al. Reversal of daunomycin and vinblastine resistance in multidrug-resistant P388 leukemia in vitro through enhanced cytotoxicity by triterpenoids. Planta Med 1995 Oct; 61(5):409–13.

136 Kubo M, Tong CN, Matsuda H. Influence of the 70% methanolic extract from red ginseng on the lysosome of tumor cells and on the cytocidal effect of mitomycin C. Planta Med 1992 Oct; 58(5):424–8.

137 Matsuda H, Tong CN, Kubo M. [Pharmacological study on Panax ginseng C. A. Meyer. XIV. Effect of 70% methanolic extract from red ginseng on the cytocidal effect of mitomycin C against rat ascites hepatoma AH 130.] Yakugaku Zasshi 1992 Nov; 112(11):846–55.

138 Hau DM, You ZS. Therapeutic effects of ginseng and mitomycin C on experimental liver tumors. Int J of Oriental Med 1990; 15(1):10–14.

139 Ciaccio M, Tesoriere L, Pintaudi AM, et al. Vitamin A preserves the cytotoxic activity of adriamycin while counteracting its peroxidative effects in human leukemic cells in vitro. Biochem Mol Biol Int 1994 Sep; 34(2):329–35.

[140] Nogae I, Kikuchi J, Yamaguchi T, et al. Potentiation of vincristine by vitamin A against drug-resistant mouse leukaemia cells. Br J Cancer 1987 Sep; 56(3):267–72.

[141] Caliaro MJ, Vitaux P, Lafon C. Multifactorial mechanism for the potentiation of cisplatin (CDDP) cytotoxicity by all-*trans* retinoic acid (ATRA) in human ovarian carcinoma cell lines. Br J Cancer 1997; 75(3):333–40.

[142] Tomita Y, Himeno K, Nomoto K, et al. Combined treatments with vitamin A and 5-fluorouracil and the growth of allotransplantable and syngeneic tumors in mice. J Natl Cancer Inst 1982 May; 68(5):823–7.

[143] Fowler CL, Brooks SP, Squire R, et al. Enhanced resection and improved survival in murine neuroblastoma (C1300-NB) after preoperative immunotherapy. J Pediatr Surg 1991 Apr; 26(4):381–7; discussion 387–8.

[144] Nakagawa M, Yamaguchi T, Ueda H, et al. Potentiation by vitamin A of the action of anticancer agents against murine tumors. Jpn J Cancer Res 1985 Sep; 76(9):887–94.

[145] Akiyama S, Masuda A, Tabuki T, et al. Enhancement of the antitumor effect of 6-mercaptopurine by vitamin A. Gann 1981 Oct; 72(5):742–6.

[146] Recchia F, Sica G, Casucci D, et al. Advanced carcinoma of the pancreas: Phase II study of combined chemotherapy, beta-interferon, and retinoids. Am J Clin Oncol 1998 Jun; 21(3):275–8.

[147] Recchia F, Sica G, De Filippis S, et al. Combined chemotherapy and differentiation therapy in the treatment of advanced non-small-cell lung cancer. Anticancer Res 1997 Sep–Oct; 17(5B):3761–5.

[148] Boccardo F, Canobbio L, Resasco M, et al. Phase II study of tamoxifen and high-dose retinyl acetate in patients with advanced breast cancer. J Cancer Res Clin Oncol 1990; 116(5):503–6.

[149] Recchia F, Sica G, de Filippis S, et al. Interferon-beta, retinoids, and tamoxifen in the treatment of metastatic breast cancer: A phase II study. J Interferon Cytokine Res 1995 Jul; 15(7):605–10.

[150] Recchia F, Frati L, Rea S, et al. Minimal residual disease in metastatic breast cancer: Treatment with IFN-beta, retinoids, and tamoxifen. J Interferon Cytokine Res 1998 Jan; 18(1):41–7.

[151] Recchia F, Lelli S, Di Matteo G, et al. [5-fluorouracil, cisplatin and retinol palmitate in the management of advanced cancer of the oral cavity. Phase II study.] Clin Ter 1993 May; 142(5):403–9.

[152] Ravid A, Rocker D, Machlenkin A, et al. 1,25-dihydroxyvitamin D3 enhances the susceptibility of breast cancer cells to doxorubicin-induced oxidative damage. Cancer Res 1999 Feb 15; 59(4):862–7.

[153] Studzinski GP, Bhandal AK, Brelvi ZS. Potentiation by 1-alpha,25-dihydroxyvitamin D3 of cytotoxicity to HL-60 cells produced by cytarabine and hydroxyurea. J Natl Cancer Inst 1986 Apr; 76(4):641–8.

[154] Moffatt KA, Johannes WU, Miller GJ. 1Alpha,25dihydroxyvitamin D3 and platinum drugs act synergistically to inhibit the growth of prostate cancer cell lines. Clin Cancer Res 1999 Mar; 5(3):695–703.

[155] Vink-van Wijngaarden T, Pols HA, Buurman CJ, et al. Combined effects of 1,25-dihydroxyvitamin D3 and tamoxifen on the growth of MCF-7 and ZR-75-1 human breast cancer cells. Breast Cancer Res Treat 1994 Feb; 29(2):161–8.

[156] Saunders DE, Christensen C, Wappler NL, et al. Additive inhibition of RL95-2 endometrial carcinoma cell growth by carboplatin and 1,25 dihydroxyvitamin D3. Gynecol Oncol 1993 Nov; 51(2):155–9.

[157] Cho YL, Christensen C, Saunders DE, et al. Combined effects of 1,25-dihydroxyvitamin D3 and platinum drugs on the growth of MCF-7 cells. Cancer Res 1991 Jun 1; 51(11):2848–53.

[158] Tanaka H, Yamamuro T, Kotoura Y, et al. 1 alpha,25(OH)2D3 exerts cytostatic effects on murine osteosarcoma cells and enhances the cytocidal effects of anticancer drugs. Clin Orthop 1989 Oct; (247):290–6.

[159] Slapak CA, Desforges JF, Fogaren T, Miller KB. Treatment of acute myeloid leukemia in the elderly with low-dose cytarabine, hydroxyurea, and calcitriol. Am J Hematol 1992 Nov; 41(3):178–83.

[160] Imseis RE, Palmieri GM, Holbert JM, et al. Effect of calcitriol and pamidronate in multiple myeloma. Am J Med Sci 1999 Jul; 318(1):61–6.

[161] Ripoll EA, Rama BN, Webber MM. Vitamin E enhances the chemotherapeutic effects of adriamycin on human prostatic carcinoma cells in vitro. J Urol 1986 Aug; 136(2):529–31.

[162] Schwartz JL, Tanaka J, Khandekar V, et al. Beta-carotene and/or vitamin E as modulators of alkylating agents in SCC-25 human squamous carcinoma cells. Cancer Chemother Pharmacol 1992; 29(3):207–13.

[163] Trizna Z, Hsu TC, Schantz SP. Protective effects of vitamin E against bleomycin-induced genotoxicity in head and neck cancer patients in vitro. Anticancer Res 1992 Mar–Apr; 12(2):325–7.

[164] Okamoto K, Ogura R. Effects of vitamins on lipid peroxidation and suppression of DNA synthesis induced by adriamycin in Ehrlich cells. J Nutr Sci Vitaminol (Tokyo) 1985 Apr; 31(2):129–37.

[165] Van Rensburg CE, Joone G, Anderson R. Alpha-tocopherol antagonizes the multidrug-resistance-reversal activity of cyclosporin A, verapamil, GF120918, clofazimine and B669. Cancer Lett 1998 May 15; 127(1–2):107–12.

[166] Drago JR, Nesbitt JA, Badalament RA, Smith J. Chemotherapy and vitamin E in treatment of Nb rat prostate tumors. In Vivo 1988 Nov–Dec; 2(6):399–401.

[167] Tanigawa N, Katoh H, Kan N, et al. Effect of vitamin E on toxicity and antitumor activity of adriamycin in mice. Jpn J Cancer Res 1986 Dec; 77(12):1249–55.

[168] Sue K, Nakagawara A, Okuzono S, et al. Combined effects of vitamin E (alpha-tocopherol) and cisplatin on the growth of murine neuroblastoma in vivo. Eur J Cancer Clin Oncol 1988 Nov; 24(11):1751–8.

[169] Kilinc C, Ozcan O, Karaoz E, et al. Vitamin E reduces bleomycin-induced lung fibrosis in mice: Biochemical and morphological studies. J Basic Clin Physiol Pharmacol 1993 Jul–Sep; 4(3):249–69.

170 Myers CE, McGuire WP, Liss RH, et al. Adriamycin: The role of lipid peroxidation in cardiac toxicity and tumor response. Science 1977 Jul 8; 197(4299):165–7.

171 Nesbitt JA, Smith J, McDowell G, Drago JR. Adriamycin-vitamin E combination therapy for treatment of prostate adenocarcinoma in the Nb rat model. J Surg Oncol 1988 Aug; 38(4):283–4.

172 Sonneveld P. Effect of alpha-tocopherol on the cardiotoxicity of adriamycin in the rat. Cancer Treat Rep 1978 Jul; 62(7):1033–6.

173 Hermansen K, Wassermann K. The effect of vitamin E and selenium on doxorubicin (Adriamycin) induced delayed toxicity in mice. Acta Pharmacol Toxicol (Copenh) 1986 Jan; 58(1):31–7.

174 Sugihara K, Gemba M. Modification of cisplatin toxicity by antioxidants. Jpn J Pharmacol 1986 Feb; 40(2):353–5.

175 Geetha A, Sankar R, Marar T, Devi CS. Alpha-tocopherol reduces doxorubicin-induced toxicity in rats—histological and biochemical evidences. Indian J Physiol Pharmacol 1990 Apr; 34(2):94–100.

176 Alberts DS, Peng YM, Moon TE. Alpha-tocopherol pretreatment increases adriamycin bone marrow toxicity. Biomedicine 1978 Oct; 29(6):189–91.

177 Shinozawa S, Gomita Y, Araki Y. Effect of high dose alpha-tocopherol acetate on the toxicity and tissue distribution of adriamycin (doxorubicin). Acta Med Okayama 1988 Oct; 42(5):253–8.

178 Shinozawa S, Gomita Y, Araki Y. Effect of high dose alpha-tocopherol and alpha-tocopherol acetate pretreatment on adriamycin (doxorubicin) induced toxicity and tissue distribution. Physiol Chem Phys Med NMR 1988; 20(4):329–35.

179 Shinozawa S, Gomita Y, Araki Y. Tissue concentration of doxorubicin (adriamycin) in mouse pretreated with alpha-tocopherol or coenzyme Q10. Acta Med Okayama 1991 Jun; 45(3):195–9.

180 Perez JE, Macchiavelli M, Leone BA, et al. High-dose alpha-tocopherol as a preventive of doxorubicin-induced alopecia. Cancer Treat Rep 1986 Oct; 70(10):1213–4.

181 Legha SS, Wang YM, Mackay B, et al. Clinical and pharmacologic investigation of the effects of alpha-tocopherol on adriamycin cardiotoxicity. Ann N Y Acad Sci 1982; 393:411–8.

182 Breed JG, Zimmerman AN, Dormans JA, Pinedo HM. Failure of the antioxidant vitamin E to protect against adriamycin-induced cardiotoxicity in the rabbit. Cancer Res 1980 Jun; 40(6):2033–8.

183 Van Vleet JF, Ferrans VJ. Clinical observations, cutaneous lesions, and hematologic alterations in chronic adriamycin intoxication in dogs with and without vitamin E and selenium supplementation. Am J Vet Res 1980 May; 41(5):691–9.

184 Prasad KN, Hernandez C, Edwards-Prasad J, et al. Modification of the effect of tamoxifen, cis-platin, DTIC, and interferon-alpha 2b on human melanoma cells in culture by a mixture of vitamins. Nutr Cancer 1994; 22(3):233–45.

185 Prasad KN, Kumar A, Kochupillai V, Cole WC. High doses of multiple antioxidant vitamins: Essential ingredients in improving the efficacy of standard cancer therapy. J Am Coll Nutr 1999 Feb; 18(1):13–25.

186 Prasad KN, Cole WC, Prasad JE. Multiple antioxidant vitamins as an adjunct to standard and experimental cancer therapies. J Oncol 1999; 31(4):101–8.

187 Chibowska I, Chibowski D, Celinski K, Pokora J. Ultrastructural studies of daunorubicin hepatotoxicity in rats including protective effects of tocopherol and ascorbic acid. Pol J Pathol 1996; 47(3):119–26.

188 Anderson D, Basaran N, Blowers SD, Edwards AJ. The effect of antioxidants on bleomycin treatment in in vitro and in vivo genotoxicity assays. Mutat Res 1995 Jun; 329(1):37–47.

189 Malec J, Szczepanska I, Grabarczyk M, et al. Hydroxyurea-induced toxic side-effects in animals and an attempt at reducing them with vitamins E and C. Neoplasma 1989; 36(4):427–35.

190 Milei J, Boveris A, Llesuy S, et al. Amelioration of adriamycin-induced cardiotoxicity in rabbits by prenylamine and vitamins A and E. Am Heart J 1986 Jan; 111(1):95–102.

191 Jaakkola K, Lahteenmaki P, Laakso J, et al. Treatment with antioxidant and other nutrients in combination with chemotherapy and irradiation in patients with small-cell lung cancer. Anticancer Res 1992 May–Jun; 12(3):599–606.

192 Wagdi P, Fluri M, Aeschbacher B, et al. Cardioprotection in patients undergoing chemo- and/or radiotherapy for neoplastic disease. A pilot study. Jpn Heart J 1996 May; 37(3):353–9.

193 Lopez-Gonzalez MA, Guerrero JM, Rojas F, Delgado F. Ototoxicity caused by cisplatin is ameliorated by melatonin and other antioxidants. J Pineal Res 2000 Mar; 28(2):73–80.

194 Rapozzi V, Comelli M, Mavelli I, et al. Melatonin and oxidative damage in mice liver induced by the prooxidant antitumor drug, adriamycin. In Vivo 1999 Jan–Feb; 13(1):45–50.

195 Rapozzi V, Zorzet S, Comelli M, et al. Melatonin decreases bone marrow and lymphatic toxicity of adriamycin in mice bearing TLX5 lymphoma. Life Sci 1998; 63(19):1701–13.

196 Musatov SA, Rosenfeld SV, Togo EF, et al. [The influence of melatonin on mutagenicity and antitumor action of cytostatic drugs in mice.] Vopr Onkol 1997; 43(6):623–7.

197 Lissoni P, Barni S, Mandala M, et al. Decreased toxicity and increased efficacy of cancer chemotherapy using the pineal hormone melatonin in metastatic solid tumour patients with poor clinical status. Eur J Cancer 1999 Nov; 35(12):1688–92.

198 Lissoni P, Tancini G, Barni S, et al. Treatment of cancer chemotherapy-induced toxicity with the pineal hormone melatonin. Support Care Cancer 1997 Mar; 5(2):126–9.

199 Lissoni P, Paolorossi F, Ardizzoia A, et al. A randomized study of chemotherapy with cisplatin plus etoposide versus chemoendocrine therapy with cisplatin, etoposide and the pineal hormone melatonin as a first-line treatment of advanced non-small cell lung cancer patients in a poor clinical state. J Pineal Res 1997 Aug; 23(1):15–9.

200 Lissoni P, Tancini G, Paolorossi F, et al. Chemoneuroendocrine therapy of metastatic breast cancer with persistent thrombocytopenia with weekly low-dose epirubicin plus melatonin: A phase II study. J Pineal Res 1999 Apr; 26(3):169–73.

201 Ghielmini M, Pagani O, de Jong J, et al. Double-blind randomized study on the myeloprotective effect of melatonin in combination with carboplatin and etoposide in advanced lung cancer. Br J Cancer 1999 Jun; 80(7):1058–61.

202 Busse E, Zimmer G, Schopohl B, Kornhuber B. Influence of alpha-lipoic acid on intracellular glutathione in vitro and in vivo. Arzneimittelforschung 1992 Jun; 42(6):829–31.

203 Suzuki YJ, Aggarwal BB, Packer L. Alpha-lipoic acid is a potent inhibitor of NF-kappa B activation in human T cells. Biochem Biophys Res Commun 1992 Dec 30; 189(3):1709–15.

204 Hofmann MA, Schiekofer S, Isermann B, et al. Peripheral blood mononuclear cells isolated from patients with diabetic nephropathy show increased activation of the oxidative-stress sensitive transcription factor NF-kappaB. Diabetologia 1999 Feb; 42(2):222–32.

205 Berger M, Habs M, Schmahl D. [Effect of thioctic acid (alpha-limpoic acid) on the chemotherapeutic efficacy of cyclophosphamide and vincristine sulfate.] Arzneimittelforschung 1983; 33(9):1286–8.

206 Somani SM, Husain K, Whitworth C, et al. Dose-dependent protection by lipoic acid against cisplatin-induced nephrotoxicity in rats: Antioxidant defense system. Pharmacol Toxicol 2000 May; 86(5):234–41.

207 Rybak LP, Husain K, Whitworth C, Somani SM. Dose dependent protection by lipoic acid against cisplatin-induced ototoxicity in rats: Antioxidant defense system. Toxicol Sci 1999 Feb; 47(2):195–202.

208 Rybak LP, Whitworth C, Somani S. Application of antioxidants and other agents to prevent cisplatin ototoxicity. Laryngoscope 1999 Nov; 109(11):1740–4.

209 Dovinova I, Novotny L, Rauko P, Kvasnicka P. Combined effect of lipoic acid and doxorubicin in murine leukemia. Neoplasma 1999; 46(4):237–41.

210 Teichert J, Kern J, Tritschler HJ, et al. Investigations on the pharmacokinetics of alpha-lipoic acid in healthy volunteers. Int J Clin Pharmacol Ther 1998 Dec; 36(12):625–8.

211 Ruhnau KJ, Meissner HP, Finn JR, et al. Effects of 3-week oral treatment with the antioxidant thioctic acid (alpha-lipoic acid) in symptomatic diabetic polyneuropathy. Diabet Med 1999 Dec; 16(12):1040–3.

212 Ziegler D, Reljanovic M, Mehnert H, Gries FA. Alpha-lipoic acid in the treatment of diabetic polyneuropathy in Germany: Current evidence from clinical trials. Exp Clin Endocrinol Diabetes 1999; 107(7):421–30.

213 Biewenga GP, Haenen GR, Bast A. The pharmacology of the antioxidant lipoic acid. Gen Pharmacol 1997 Sep; 29(3):315–31.

214 Marangon K, Devaraj S, Tirosh O, et al. Comparison of the effect of alpha-lipoic acid and alpha-tocopherol supplementation on measures of oxidative stress. Free Radic Biol Med 1999 Nov; 27(9–10):1114–21.

215 Berger M, Habs M, Schmahl D. [Effect of thioctic acid (alpha-limpoic acid) on the chemotherapeutic efficacy of cyclophosphamide and vincristine sulfate.] Arzneimittelforschung 1983; 33(9):1286–8.

216 Kunstler K. [The influence of thioctic acid on the growth of Ehrlich ascites carcinoma.] Arzneimittelforschung 1980; 30(10):1717–8.

217 Karpov LM, Dvuzhil'naia ED, Savvov VI, Phan Van Thuy. [S35 lipoic acid distribution and its effect on pyruvate dehydrogenase activity in rats with Walker carcinoma.] Vopr Onkol 1977; 23(10):87–90.

218 Okunieff P. Interactions between ascorbic acid and the radiation of bone marrow, skin, and tumor. Am J Clin Nutr 1991; 54:1281S-3S.

219 Okunieff P, Suit HD. Toxicity, radiation sensitivity modification, and combined drug effects of ascorbic acid with misonidazole in vivo on FSaII murine fibrosarcomas. J Natl Cancer Inst 1987 Aug; 79(2):377–81.

220 Okunieff P. Personal communication, 1995.

221 Tewfik FA, Tewfik HH, Riley EF. The influence of ascorbic acid on the growth of solid tumors in mice and on tumor control by X-irradiation. Int J Vitam Nutr Res Suppl 1982; 23:257–63.

222 Tewfik HH, Tewfik FA, Riley EF. The influence of ascorbic acid on survival of mice following whole body X-irradiation. Int J Vitam Nutr Res Suppl 1982; 23:265–76.

223 Fritz-Niggli H, Rao KR. Rutosides and radiation induced regression of experimental tumours. Arzneimittelforschung 1977; 27(5):1057–64.

224 Arons I, Freeman J, Sokoloff B, Eddy W. Bio-flavonoids in radiation injury II. Contact radiation in experimental cancer. Br. J Radiol 1954; 27:642–44.

225 Blumenthal RD, Lew W, Reising A, et al. Anti-oxidant vitamins reduce normal tissue toxicity induced by radio-immunotherapy. Int J Cancer 2000 Apr 15; 86(2):276–80.

226 Kagerud A, Peterson HI. Tocopherol in tumor irradiation (review). Anticancer Res 1981; 1:35–38.

227 Kagerud A, Lund N, Peterson HI. Tocopherol in irradiation of temporary hypoxic tumours. Acta Radiol Oncol 1981; 20(1):1–4.

228 Kagerud A, Holm G, Larsson H, Peterson HI. Tocopherol and local X-ray irradiation of two transplantable rat tumours. Cancer Lett 1978 Sep; 5(3):123–9.

229 Kagerud A, Peterson HI. Tocopherol in irradiation of experimental neoplasms. Influence of dose and administration. Acta Radiol Oncol 1981; 20(2):97–100.

230 Lissoni P, Meregalli S, Nosetto L, et al. Increased survival time in brain glioblastomas by a radioneuroendocrine strategy with radiotherapy plus melatonin compared to radiotherapy alone. Oncology 1996 Jan–Feb; 53(1):43–6.

231 Lund EL, Quistorff B, Spang-Thompsen M, Kristjansen PE. Effect of radiation therapy on small-cell lung cancer is reduced by ubiquinone intake. Folia Microbiol (Praha) 1998; 43(5):505–6.

232 Sakamoto K, Sakka M. Reduced effect of irradiation on normal and malignant cells irradiated in vivo in mice pretreated with vitamin E. Br J Radiol 1973 Jul; 46(547):538–40.

233 Delanian S. Striking regression of radiation-induced fibrosis by a combination of pentoxifylline and tocopherol. Br J Radiol 1998 Aug; 71(848):892–4.

234 Baillet F. Alpha-tocopherol treatment of radio-fibrosis post-brachytherapy for breast cancer. Radiother Oncol 1997; 43:S3.

235 Delanian S, Balla-Mekias S, Lefaix JL. Striking regression of chronic radiotherapy damage in a clinical trial of combined pentoxifylline and tocopherol. J Clin Oncol 1999 Oct; 17(10):3283–90.

236 Gramaglia A, Loi GF, Mongioj V, Baronzio GF. Increased survival in brain metastatic patients treated with stereotactic radiotherapy, omega three fatty acids and bioflavonoids. Anticancer Res 1999 Nov–Dec; 19(6C):5583–6.

237 Moon JY, Lee DW, Park KH. Inhibition of 7-ethoxycoumarin O-deethylase activity in rat liver microsomes by naturally occurring flavonoids: Structure-activity relationships. Xenobiotica 1998 Feb; 28(2):117–26.

238 Manson MM, Ball HW, Barrett MC, et al. Mechanism of action of dietary chemoprotective agents in rat liver: Induction of phase I and II drug metabolizing enzymes and aflatoxin B1 metabolism. Carcinogenesis 1997 Sep; 18(9):1729–38.

239 Dinkova-Kostova AT, Talalay P. Relation of structure of curcumin analogs to their potencies as inducers of phase 2 detoxification enzymes. Carcinogenesis 1999 May; 20(5):911–4.

240 Ciolino HP, Daschner PJ, Wang TT, et al. Effect of curcumin on the aryl hydrocarbon receptor and cytochrome P450 1A1 in MCF-7 human breast carcinoma cells. Biochem Pharmacol 1998 Jul 15; 56(2):197–206.

241 Firozi PF, Aboobaker VS, Bhattacharya RK. Action of curcumin on the cytochrome P450-system catalyzing the activation of aflatoxin B1. Chem Biol Interact 1996 Mar 8; 100(1):41–51.

242 Oetari S, Sudibyo M, Commandeur JN, et al. Effects of curcumin on cytochrome P450 and glutathione S-transferase activities in rat liver. Biochem Pharmacol 1996 Jan 12; 51(1):39–45.

243 Valdes E, Vega P, Avalos N, et al. Dietary fish oil and cytochrome P-450 monooxygenase activity in rat liver and kidney. Lipids 1995 Oct; 30(10):955–8.

244 Kravchenko LV, Kuz mina EE, Avren eva LI, et al. [Xenobiotic-metabolizing enzymes in rat liver and small intestinal mucosa with varying combinations of polyunsaturated omega-6 and omega-3 fatty acids in the diet.] Vopr Med Khim 1992 Nov–Dec; 38(6):53–6.

245 Siess MH, Le Bon AM, Canivenc-Lavier MC, et al. Modification of hepatic drug-metabolizing enzymes in rats treated with alkyl sulfides. Cancer Lett 1997 Dec 9; 120(2):195–201.

246 Jeong HG, Lee YW. Protective effects of diallyl sulfide on N-nitrosodimethylamine-induced immunosuppression in mice. Cancer Lett 1998 Dec 11; 134(1):73–9.

247 Guyonnet D, Siess MH, Le Bon AM, et al. Modulation of phase II enzymes by organosulfur compounds from allium vegetables in rat tissues. Toxicol Appl Pharmacol 1999 Jan 1; 154(1):50–8.

248 Maurya AK, Singh SV. Differential induction of glutathione transferase isoenzymes of mice stomach by diallyl sulfide, a naturally occurring anticarcinogen. Cancer Lett 1991 May 1; 57(2):121–9.

249 Yannai S, Day AJ, Williamson G, et al. Characterization of flavonoids as monofunctional or bifunctional inducers of quinone reductase in murine hepatoma cell lines. Food Chem Toxicol 1998 Aug; 36(8):623–30.

250 Kuong DD, Dovgii AI, Adrianov NV, et al. [Induction of cytochrome P-450 by triterpensaponins in Vietnamese ginseng.] Biokhimiia 1991 Apr; 56(4):707–13.

251 Dashwood RH, Xu M, Hernaez JF, et al. Cancer chemopreventive mechanisms of tea against heterocyclic amine mutagens from cooked meat. Proc Soc Exp Biol Med 1999 Apr; 220(4):239–4.

252 Bu-Abbas A, Clifford MN, Walker R, et al. Contribution of caffeine and flavanols in the induction of hepatic phase II activities by green tea. Food Chem Toxicol 1998 Aug; 36(8):617–21.

253 Obermeier MT, White RE, Yang CS. Effects of bioflavonoids on hepatic P450 activities. Xenobiotica 1995 Jun; 25(6):575–84.

254 Morse MA, Toburen AL. Inhibition of metabolic activation of 4-(methylnitrosamino)-1-(3-pyridyl)-1-butanone by limonene. Cancer Lett 1996 Jul 12; 104(2):211–7.

255 Reicks MM, Crankshaw D. Effects of d-limonene on hepatic microsomal monooxygenase activity and paracetamol-induced glutathione depletion in mouse. Xenobiotica 1993 Jul; 23(7):809–19.

256 Elegbede JA, Maltzman TH, Elson CE, et al. Effects of anticarcinogenic monoterpenes on phase II hepatic metabolizing enzymes. Carcinogenesis 1993 Jun; 14(6):1221–3.

257 Maltzman TH, Christou M, Gould MN, et al. Effects of monoterpenoids on in vivo DMBA-DNA adduct formation and on phase I hepatic metabolizing enzymes. Carcinogenesis 1991 Nov; 12(11):2081–7.

258 Yokoi T, Narita M, Nagai E, et al. Inhibition of UDP-glucuronosyltransferase by aglycons of natural glucuronides in kampo medicines using SN-38 as a substrate. Jpn J Cancer Res 1995 Oct; 86(10):985–9.

259 Siess MH, Le Bon AM, Suschetet M, et al. Inhibition of ethoxyresorufin deethylase activity by natural flavonoids in human and rat liver microsomes. Food Addit Contam 1990; 7 Suppl 1:S178–81.

260 Tan D, Reiter RJ, Chen LD, et al. Both physiological and pharmacological levels of melatonin reduce DNA adduct formation induced by the carcinogen safrole. Carcinogenesis 1994 Feb; 15(2):215–8.

261 Kothari L, Subramanian A. A possible modulatory influence of melatonin on representative phase I and II drug metabolizing enzymes in 9,10-dimethyl-1,2-benzanthracene induced rat mammary tumorigenesis. Anticancer Drugs 1992 Dec; 3(6):623–8.

262 Yeung JH, Chiu LC, Ooi VE. Effect of polysaccharide peptide (PSP) on in vivo sulphation and glucuronidation of paracetamol in the rat. Eur J Drug Metab Pharmacokinet 1995 Oct–Dec; 20(4):287–92.

263 Casper RF, Quesne M, Rogers IM, et al. Resveratrol has antagonist activity on the aryl hydrocarbon receptor: Implications for prevention of dioxin toxicity. Mol Pharmacol 1999 Oct; 56(4):784–90.

264 Ciolino HP, Yeh GC. Inhibition of aryl hydrocarbon-induced cytochrome P-450 1A1 enzyme activity and CYP1A1 expression by resveratrol. Mol Pharmacol 1999 Oct; 56(4):760–7.

265 Chun YJ, Kim MY, Guengerich FP. Resveratrol is a selective human cytochrome P450 1A1 inhibitor. Biochem Biophys Res Commun 1999 Aug 19; 262(1):20–4.

266 Inouye K, Mae T, Kondo S, et al. Inhibitory effects of vitamin A and vitamin K on rat cytochrome P4501A1-dependent monooxygenase activity. Biochem Biophys Res Commun 1999 Aug 27; 262(2):565–9.

267 Huang DY, Ohnishi T, Jiang H, et al. Inhibition by retinoids of benzo(A)pyrene metabolism catalyzed by 3-methylcholanthrene-induced rat cytochrome P-450 1A1. Metabolism 1999 Jun; 48(6):689–92.

268 Mukherjee B, Sarkar A, Chatterjee M. Biochemical basis of selenomethionine-mediated inhibition during 2-acetylaminofluorene-induced hepatocarcinogenesis in the rat. Eur J Cancer Prev 1996 Dec; 5(6):455–63.

269 Liu JZ, Zhang BZ, Milner JA. Dietary selenite modifies glutathione metabolism and 7,12-dimethylbenz(a)anthracene conjugation in rats. J Nutr 1994 Feb; 124(2):172–80.

270 Beckmann-Knopp S, Rietbrock S, Weyhenmeyer R, et al. Inhibitory effects of silibinin on cytochrome P-450 enzymes in human liver microsomes. Pharmacol Toxicol 2000 Jun; 86(6):250–6.

271 Yamazaki H, Shimada T. Effects of arachidonic acid, prostaglandins, retinol, retinoic acid and cholecalciferol on xenobiotic oxidations catalysed by human cytochrome P450 enzymes. Xenobiotica 1999 Mar; 29(3):231–41.

272 Bailey DG, Spence JD, Munoz C, et al. Interaction of citrus juices with felodipine and nifedipine. Lancet 1991 Feb 2; 337(8736):268–9.

273 Evans AM. Influence of dietary components on the gastrointestinal metabolism and transport of drugs. Ther Drug Monit 2000 Feb; 22(1):131–6.

274 Piscitelli SC, Burstein AH, Chaitt D, et al. Indinavir concentrations and St John's wort. Lancet 2000 Feb 12; 355(9203):547–8.

275 Ruschitzka F, Meier PJ, Turina M, et al. Acute heart transplant rejection due to Saint John's wort. Lancet 2000 Feb 12; 355(9203):548–9.

CHEMICAL DATA ON NATURAL COMPOUNDS

This appendix provides information on the chemistry of natural compounds, beginning with a set of figures depicting the structural diagrams for most natural compounds discussed in this book and some related compounds of interest. The diagrams for large and complex molecules, such as high-molecular-weight polysaccharides, bromelain, and the saponin ruscogenin, are not included because of the difficulty of depicting their structures. The figures are listed roughly in the order the compounds are discussed in Part III. Diagrams for DNA bases and nucleotides (see Chapter 2) are also shown, and these occur first.

In addition, Table A.1 lists the molecular weights of most natural compounds discussed, along with weights for related compounds. Such values are needed, for example, for conversion of concentration units (e.g., for converting from µg/ml to µM) and for dose or clearance calculations in which the raw data or desired concentration contains units of moles.

STRUCTURAL DIAGRAMS FOR SELECTED NATURAL COMPOUNDS

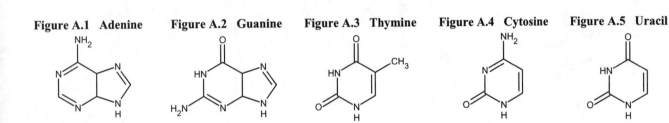

Figure A.1 Adenine

Figure A.2 Guanine

Figure A.3 Thymine

Figure A.4 Cytosine

Figure A.5 Uracil

Figure A.6 Adenosine Diphosphate

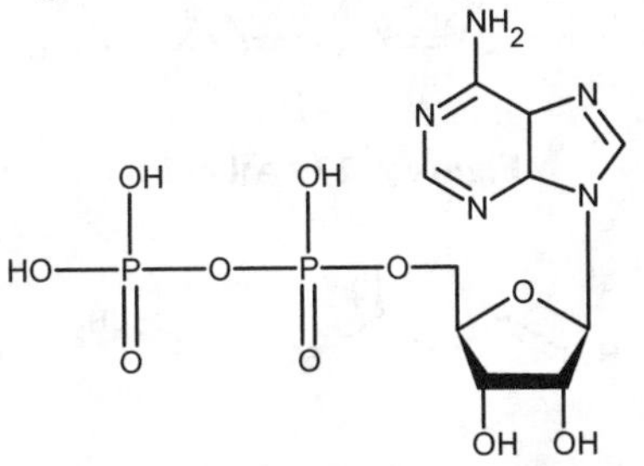

Figure A.7 Deoxyadenosine Diphosphate

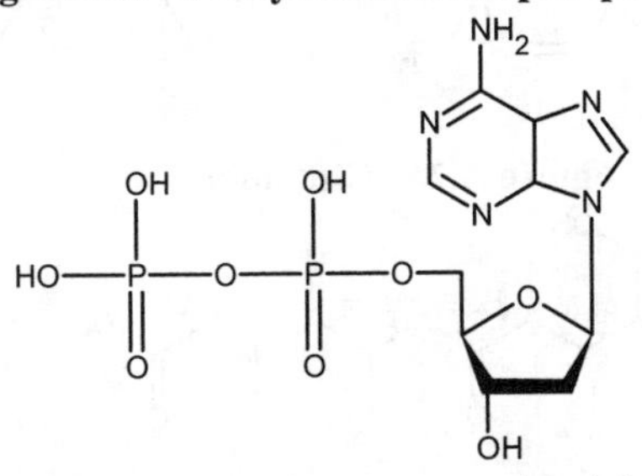

Figure A.8 Methylated Cytosine

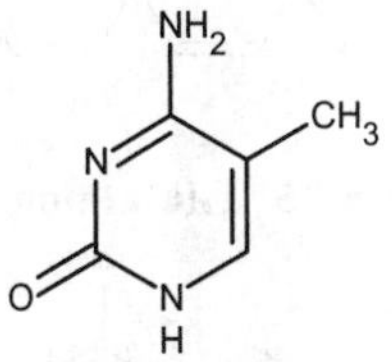

(occurs during epigenetic changes)

(Adenosine is used here as a sample nucleotide and is shown in its oxygenated and deoxy form. The diphosphate is shown, but nucleotides also exist in mono- and triphosphate forms.)

Figure A.9
S-adenosylmethionine (SAM)

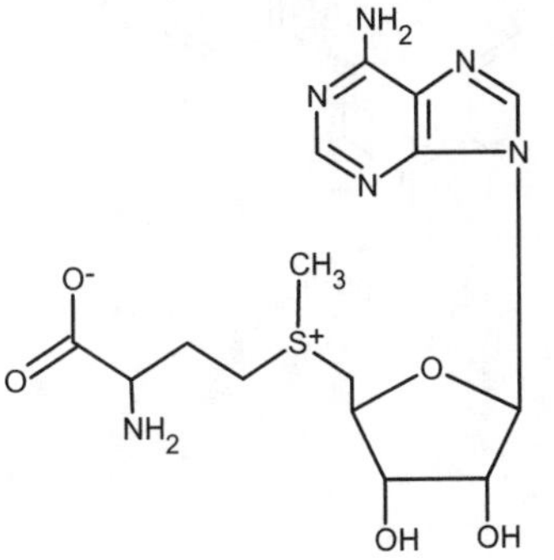

Figure A.10 Spermidine

Figure A.11
Sodium Selenite

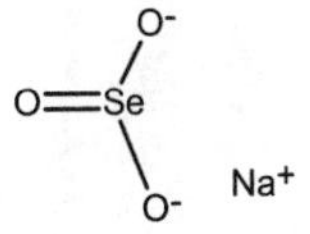

Figure A.12 Cysteine

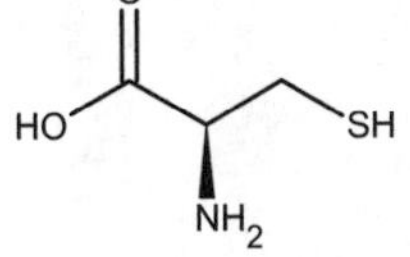

**Figure A.13
Selenocysteine**

Figure A.14   Methionine

**Figure A.15
Selenomethionine**

**Figure A.16
Methylselenocysteine**

Figure A.17   D-Glucose

Figure A.18   Ascorbic Acid

**Figure A.19   Ascorbate
(Ionized Form)**

**Figure A.20   Ascorbate Free
Radical**

Figure A.21   Dehydroascorbate

Figure A.22   Arachidonic Acid

Figure A.23   EPA

Figure A.24   DHA

Figure A.25   Glutathione

Figure A.26   Glutamine

Figure A.27   Allicin

Figure A.28   DADS

**Figure A.29   Basic Flavonoid
Structure**

Figure A.30   Chalcone (Isoliquirtigenin)

Figure A.31   Flavanone (Naringenin)

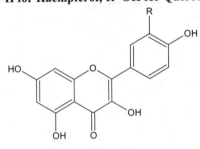

Figure A.32   Flavones
R=H for Apigenin; R=OH for Luteolin

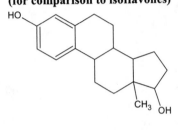

Figure A.33   Isoflavones
R=H for Daidzein; R=OH for Genistein

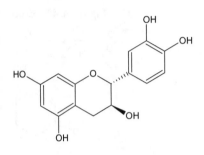

Figure A.34   Flavonols
R=H for Kaempferol; R=OH for Quercetin

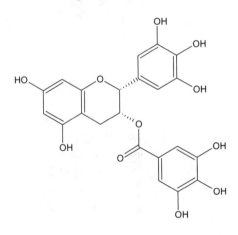

Figure A.35   Estradiol
(for comparison to isoflavones)

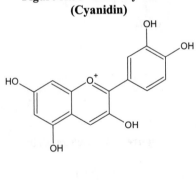

Figure A.36   Catechin

Figure A.37   EGCG

Figure A.38   Anthocyanidins
(Cyanidin)

Figure A.39   Cyanidin-3-*O*-glucoside

Figure A.40   Proanthocyanidins
(Proanthocyanidin B1)

Figure A.41
Caffeic Acid

Figure A.42   CAPE

Figure A.43 Curcumin

Figure A.44 Podophyllotoxin

Figure A.45 Etoposide

Figure A.46 Silybin

Figure A.47 Arctigenin

Figure A.48 Schizandrin

Figure A.49 SECO
(Secoisolariciresinol)

Figure A.50   Enterodiol

Figure A.51   Enterolactone

Figure A.52   Resveratrol

Figure A.53   Anthraquinone =
p-**Quinone   +   Anthracene**

Figure A.54   Emodin

Figure A.55   Emodin Dianthrone

Figure A.56   Rhein

Figure A.57   Aloe-Emodin

Figure A.58   Hypericin

Figure A.59   (-)-Limonene

Figure A.60   Perillyl Alcohol

Figure A.61   Geraniol

Figure A.62 Perillic Acid

Figure A.63 Asiatic Acid

Figure A.64 Ursolic Acid

Figure A.65 Alpha-Boswellic Acid

Figure A.66 Beta-Boswellic Acid

Figure A.67 Ruscogenin

Figure A.68 Steroid Structure

Figure A.69 Ginsenoside Rb₂

Figure A.70 Ginseng Metabolite M1

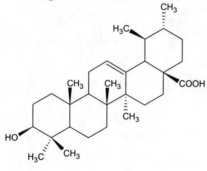

Figure A.71   Glycyrrhetic Acid

**Figure A.72
Parthenolide**

Figure A.73   Artemisinin

**Figure A.74
Helenalin**

Figure A.75   ATRA

Figure A.76   Vitamin D$_3$

Figure A.77   1,25-D$_3$

Figure A.78   Alpha-Tocopherol

Figure A.79   Vitamin E Succinate

Figure A.80   Gamma-Tocotrienol

Figure A.81   Melatonin

TABLE A.1 MOLECULAR WEIGHTS OF SELECTED COMPOUNDS			
COMPOUND	**MOLECULAR WEIGHT (grams/mole)**	**COMPOUND**	**MOLECULAR WEIGHT (grams/mole)**
Allicin	162	Glycyrrhetic acid	470
Allinin	177	Glycyrrhizin = glycyrrhizic acid	823
Aloe-emodin	270	Hypericin	504
Alpha-lipoic acid	206	Kaempferol	286
Anthocyanidin	467	Limonene	136
Apigenin	270	Luteolin	286
Arctigenin	372	Melatonin	232
Arctiin	534	Parthenolide	248
Artemisinin	282	Perillic acid	166
Asiatic acid	488	Perillyl alcohol	152
Boswellic acid	457	*P*-hydroxybenzoic acid	138
Bromelain	33,000 (approx.)	Plenolin	264
Caffeic acid	180	Proanthocyanidin dimers	576 (approx.)
CAPE	284	Protocatechuic acid	154
Catechin	290	Pseudohypericin	520
Chondroitin sulfate	16,000	PSK (range 50,000 to 200,000)	94,000
Curcumin	368	Quercetin	302
Cyanidin	287	Resveratrol	228
Cyanidin-3-glucoside	449	Rhein	284
DADS	146	Ruscogenin	430
Daidzein	254	S-allylcysteine	161
EGCG	458	S-allylmercaptocysteine	193
Emodin	270	Schizandrin (average of A,B,C)	432
Enterodiol	302	Secoisolariciresinol (SECO)	362
Enterolactone	298	Secoisolariciresinol glucoside (SD)	722 (approx.)
EPA	302	Selenium (elemental)	79
Epicatechin	290	Silybin	482
Escin	1,100	Tangeretin	370
Escin prosapogenin	630	TTFCA (assumed)	681
Estradiol	272	Ursolic acid and oleanolic acid	456
Etoposide	588	Vitamin A (ATRA)	300
Gamma-tocotrienol	411	Vitamin A (retinol)	286
Genistein	270	Vitamin B_{12}	1,355
Geraniol	154	Vitamin C	176
Ginsenoside derivative M1	622	Vitamin D_3 (1,25-D3)	416
Ginsenoside Rb_2	1,078	Vitamin E (alpha-tocopherol)	430
Ginsenoside Rh_2	622	Vitamin K_3	172
Glucose	180		
Glutathione	307		
		Geometric mean of all compounds:	**385**
		Average of all compounds that are less than 10,000 grams/mole:	**372**
		(all nonprotein, nonpolysaccharide compounds)	

PHARMACOKINETICS, PHARMACODYNAMICS, AND DOSE SCALING

It has been said that pharmacokinetics is what the body does to a drug, and pharmacodynamics is what the drug does to the body.[1] Pharmacokinetics is the study of tissue concentrations of an administered drug over time. Pharmacodynamics is the study of the effects of a drug produced by different tissue concentrations. In this book, we use pharmacokinetic and pharmacodynamic data to predict the dose of natural compounds needed to produce an anticancer effect.

Although some of the human doses reported in Part III were calculated using pharmacokinetic and pharmacodynamic models, a detailed understanding of these models is not necessary to use this book. The only message in this appendix important to all readers is that since the available pharmacokinetic and pharmacodynamic data are limited for most natural compounds, and since most were obtained from rodent rather than human studies, the dose estimates we make are in most cases only preliminary. Clearly, any dose calculation based on limited data must be viewed with healthy skepticism.

This appendix first discusses the pharmacokinetic and pharmacodynamic models used in this book, then the scaling of doses and clearance values from animals to humans. This material forms the background for Appendices I and J, which contain information on the models used to estimate clearance and other values and information on dose calculations, respectively.

PHARMACOKINETIC MODELS

Pharmacokinetics is a branch of pharmacology concerned with the movement of drugs within the body. The tissue concentration of a drug at any particular time is dependent on at least five factors:

- The route of administration (for example, oral, intravenous, or intraperitoneal).
- The degree and rate of absorption of the drug.
- The degree and rate of distribution within body tissues.

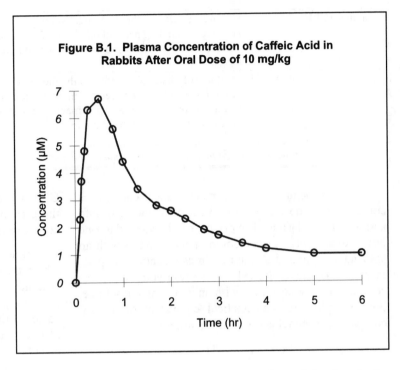

Figure B.1. Plasma Concentration of Caffeic Acid in Rabbits After Oral Dose of 10 mg/kg

- The degree and rate of metabolism of the drug in the liver and other tissues.
- The rate of excretion of the drug and its metabolites.

Commonly, a pharmacokinetic study of a drug will measure its plasma concentration over time. For example, a pharmacokinetic study of caffeic acid in rabbits produced the data illustrated in Figure B.1 (based on reference 2). The oral dose given was 10 mg/kg, and each rabbit weighed about 2.5 kilograms. Therefore, the total dose was 25 milligrams (139 micromoles) of caffeic acid per rabbit. The data points in this figure are connected by straight lines; later we connect them with a smooth curve based on an equation.

The first step in pharmacokinetic analysis is to choose a general model that adequately describes the data; there are two types in common use: compartmental and noncompartmental. Various specialized computer programs are available for compartmental and noncompartmental analysis of data. In this book, the software program WinNonlin® was used (see Appendix L).[a] Noncompartmental models were used for the analysis in this book, but we will discuss compartmental models first.

---

[a] *WinNonlin® is a registered trademark of Pharsight Corporation.*

TABLE B.1 SELECTED PARAMETERS CALCULATED IN PHARMACOKINETIC ANALYSIS		
PARAMETER	**DESCRIPTION**	**EQUATION**[*]
Area under the curve (AUC)	A measure of the area under the concentration-time curve	$$AUC = \int_0^\infty C(t)dt$$
Clearance (CL)	Clearance refers to the theoretical volume of fluid that is cleared of the drug per unit time. In oral pharmacokinetic studies, CL/F (oral clearance) is calculated rather than CL alone.	$$CL = \frac{F \times Dose}{AUC}$$ where F is the fraction absorbed.
Volume of distribution (Vd)	Volume of distribution refers to the theoretical volume of fluid that would be required to uniformly contain the administered dose. In oral pharmacokinetic studies, Vd/F is calculated rather than Vd alone.	$$Vd = \frac{F \times Dose}{AUC \times \beta}$$ where β is the elimination rate constant of the terminal phase.
[*] *A variety of equations can be used to derive these parameters; the ones shown are chosen for convenience.*		

In compartmental models, a mathematical equation is constructed to describe the movement of the drug into and out of the plasma. The plasma can be viewed as one large compartment (a one-compartment model) with an associated input and output rate or as a central compartment with an attached side reservoir (a two-compartment model), each with an input and output rate. For example, the mathematical equivalent of a two-compartment model is given in Equation B.1.

$$C(t) = A \times e^{-\alpha t} + B \times e^{-\beta t} - (A + B) \times e^{-k t}$$

Equation B.1

In Equation B.1, $C(t)$ is the plasma concentration over time (t), A and B are constants, and α, β, and k are rate constants. The first term of the equation governs the initial distribution period, where the drug fills the compartments, and the second term governs the terminal decay period, where the drug is eliminated from them. The last term governs the absorption rate, where the drug enters the compartments. Models with more than two compartments also can be used. The choice of how many compartments to use depends on what model best fits the data and the distributions that the model is intended to predict. A number of pharmacokinetic parameters can be calculated from compartmental models. Some of these are listed in Table B.1.

Although clearance and volume of distribution are theoretical values, they provide clues to the physical behavior of the drug. The clearance (CL) from an organ cannot exceed the rate of blood flow into the organ. For example, the rate of blood flow into the human liver is about 90 L/hr and that into the kidneys is about 72 L/hr. The extreme upper limit of clearance is the cardiac output, which is about 300 L/hr. Of course, CL/F can be higher, since the fraction absorbed can be low. For example, if the clearance is 300 L/hr and F is 5 percent,

CL/F would be 6,000 L/hr. The higher the clearance, the greater the dose needed to produce a given plasma concentration.

Volume of distribution (Vd) provides an estimate of where the drug is distributed in the body. The physical volume of different tissues in the human body is 3 to 4 liters for plasma, 10 to 13 liters for interstitial fluid, and 25 to 28 liters for intracellular fluids. The total volume of body fluids is 40 to 46 liters. If, for example, Vd is calculated to be 2 liters, it is likely that the drug is contained solely within the plasma. As another example, if Vd is calculated to be 10 liters, the drug is likely distributed to both the plasma and interstitial fluids. In some cases, a drug may bind to tissues such as those of the vascular system, and this can increase its Vd by a factor of 10 or more. Also, as with clearance, Vd/F can be larger than Vd alone.

Using a two-compartment model and the caffeic acid data mentioned above, Equation B.1 can be used to generate a curve to fit the data points, as illustrated in Figure B.2. In this example, the AUC is 18.8 µM-hr, CL/F is 7.4 L/hr, and Vd is 28.5 liters. As seen, the derived equation reasonably fits all the data points.

As mentioned, noncompartmental models were used for calculations in this book. Unlike compartmental models, these models do not directly calculate an equation for $C(t)$ as in Equation B.1; rather, they estimate the AUC and elimination rate constants by graphical methods. Noncompartmental models can therefore be used with data that do not easily fit compartmental models. As with the latter, noncompartmental models can also calculate values for CL/F and Vd/F.

LINKING PHARMACODYNAMIC AND PHARMACOKINETIC MODELS

The data obtained from pharmacokinetic models can be used in conjunction with pharmacodynamic models to predict the effect of a drug over time. One of the simplest pharmacokinetic-pharmacodynamic link models in common use is called the E_{max} (maximum effect) model. We can use this model to illustrate how pharmacokinetics and pharmacodynamics can be related for natural compounds that reversibly inhibit cancer proliferation.[1, 3] Although this model was not explicitly used in our dose calculations, the general theory behind it is implied in the calculations. The E_{max} model is based on the following equation derived from receptor theory for a drug and its receptor at equilibrium:

$$E = \frac{E_{max} \times C}{E_{50} + C}$$

Equation B.2

In Equation B.2, E is the effect, E_{50} is the IC_{50}, and C is the concentration. To illustrate the use of the link model, we will imagine a hypothetical compound (compound Z, molecular weight 360 grams/mole) with a plasma concentration curve as shown in Figure B.3 after oral administration of 1 gram in humans. Based on noncompartmental analysis, the oral clearance (CL/F) of compound Z is 30 L/hr, which is not unlike that of some natural compounds discussed here.

Compound Z will be administered once every eight hours, as is recommended for most natural compounds. On multiple dosing, the average plasma concentration is a function of the dose, dose interval (τ), and oral clearance. The average concentration at steady state (C_{ss}) can be calculated as follows:

$$C_{ss} = \frac{AUC}{\tau} = \frac{Dose}{\frac{CL}{F} \times \tau}$$

Equation B.3

We can use this equation to predict the required dose if we know the target plasma concentration (C_{ss}). We have generally based the target plasma concentration on the

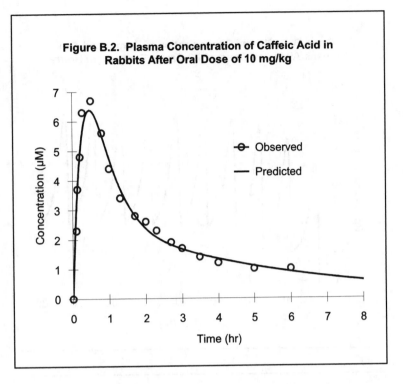

Figure B.2. Plasma Concentration of Caffeic Acid in Rabbits After Oral Dose of 10 mg/kg

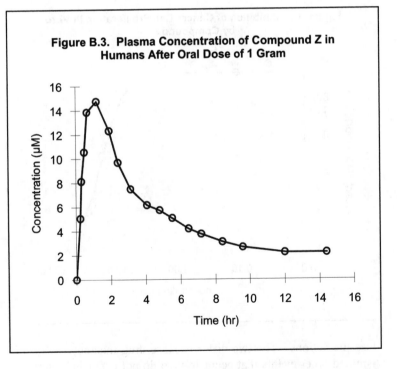

Figure B.3. Plasma Concentration of Compound Z in Humans After Oral Dose of 1 Gram

IC_{50} of the natural compound for inhibiting cell proliferation in vitro. Actually, since the IC_{50} varies for different studies on different cell lines, we use an estimate of the IC_{50}, which for convenience is taken to be 15 μM for most compounds discussed.

Although it does not necessarily follow that a concentration effective in vitro will also be effective in vivo, it is reasonable to assume so in order to make preliminary

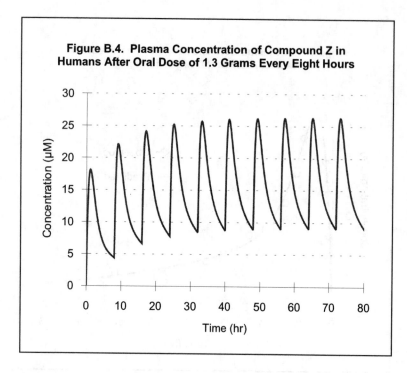

Figure B.4. Plasma Concentration of Compound Z in Humans After Oral Dose of 1.3 Grams Every Eight Hours

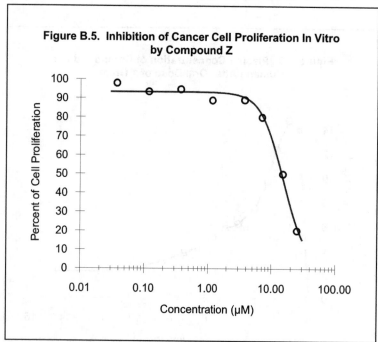

Figure B.5. Inhibition of Cancer Cell Proliferation In Vitro by Compound Z

was added to the culture dish. Adding plasma helps account for changes in the IC_{50} due to protein binding.

Using a target concentration of 15 μM, a dose interval of eight hours, and an oral clearance of 30 L/hr, the required dose predicted by Equation B.3 for compound Z is 1.3 grams every eight hours. Figure B.4 illustrates the effect of this dose on the plasma concentration curve. As seen, the average concentration at steady state is just over 15 μM. In this case, it is not exactly equal to 15 μM, since the AUC from noncompartmental analysis was slightly higher than the AUC from compartmental analysis, on which the curve in Figure B.4 is based.

We can now examine the effects this plasma concentration curve will have on cell inhibition. Let us assume that compound Z inhibits cancer cells in vitro according to the curve shown in Figure B.5. The general shape of this curve is typical of that for most natural agents with an IC_{50} of about 15 μM.

The E_{max} pharmacokinetic-pharmacodynamic link model now allows us to view reversible cell inhibition as a function of plasma concentration. The growth inhibition curves resulting from single and multiple doses of 1.3 grams of compound Z are shown in Figures B.6 and B.7. As seen in Figure B.7, the average cell inhibition at steady state is just over 50 percent, which is as expected since we used a target in-vivo concentration equal to the IC_{50}.

Note that the larger the dosing interval, the larger the fluctuation between the maximum and minimum concentration (and maximum and minimum effect). Therefore, to maintain plasma concentrations as close to the average as possible, the shortest practical dosing interval is needed. For compounds with a very low clearance value, a short dosing interval is particularly important. Dosing intervals similar to the elimination half-life are preferred but are sometimes too short to be practical; for example, the half-life of some phenolic compounds in humans may be four to nine hours. The shortest, most practical dosing interval is about once every eight hours, which is a reasonable interval for the compounds discussed here. The dose required per day will not vary with the dosing interval chosen, only the dose per administration will vary. A longer dosing interval requires a proportionally larger

dose predictions. The two differ because drug metabolism and other events that occur in vivo do not occur in vitro. For example, unlike in-vivo conditions, drugs in vitro are not metabolized to conjugate forms and may not be bound to serum proteins. We compensate for in-vivo metabolism to some degree by modifying the dose for the presence of conjugates (as discussed in Appendix J, this modification pertains only to phenolic compounds). In addition, many of the IC_{50} values cited here were based on studies where plasma (and its proteins) dose at each administration to maintain the average concentration.

SCALING BETWEEN SPECIES

We have discussed above how a required dose can be calculated based on a combination of in-vitro and pharmacokinetic data. To make this calculation, a value is needed for the oral clearance. For many compounds, however, the pharmacokinetic studies were conducted in rodents or other small mammals, not humans. Therefore, it is necessary to scale the animal clearance values to their human equivalents. Similar scaling is also needed to determine an equivalent human antitumor dose based on animal data. Scaling of both clearance and dose is necessary because animals metabolize drugs at a different rate than humans.

The Allometric Equation

It does not necessarily follow that a 10-mg/kg dose in rabbits is equivalent to a 10-mg/kg dose in humans. Due to their higher metabolism, small animal species often metabolize and excrete compounds faster than humans. In most cases, the speed at which metabolism and excretion occur is exponentially related to the body weight of the animal. An "allometric" equation can be used to describe this relationship:

$$Y = aW^b$$

Equation B.4

In Equation B.4, Y is the dose, W is the body weight, and a and b are constants. It is a fascinating pattern of nature that many physical functions and parameters are scaled equally across species according to this equation. These include water intake, urine output, drug clearance, heartbeat duration, kidney weight, blood volume, and others.[4] For example, kidney weight in various species can be estimated using the equation Y (kidney weight) = 0.0212 $W^{0.85}$ (where kidney weight and body weight is in grams).

Allometric equations accurately scale pharmacokinetic data between species only under specific conditions. In order for the allometric equations to be valid, a number of biologic conditions must be met:

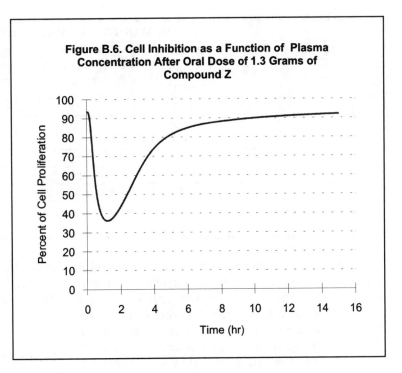

Figure B.6. Cell Inhibition as a Function of Plasma Concentration After Oral Dose of 1.3 Grams of Compound Z

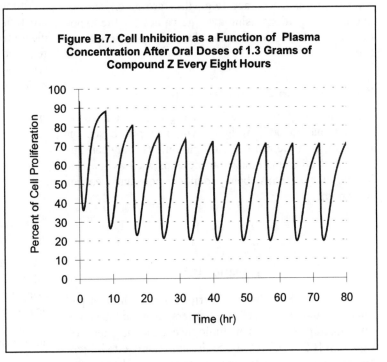

Figure B.7. Cell Inhibition as a Function of Plasma Concentration After Oral Doses of 1.3 Grams of Compound Z Every Eight Hours

- The pharmacokinetics must be first order in each species.

- Drug elimination must be through physical processes (i.e., via the bile or kidneys rather than through metabolism).

- The percentage of drug-protein binding must be similar between species and linear over the concentration range.

TABLE B.2 HUMAN TO MAMMAL BIOLOGIC TIME RATIOS			
MAMMAL	**WEIGHT (kg)**	**FOOD INTAKE (grams/day)**	**WATER INTAKE (ml/day)**	**HUMAN TO MAMMAL TIME RATIO**
Mouse	0.025*	3	5	7.3 to 1
Hamster	0.125	15	10	4.9 to 1
Rat	0.2	15	25	4.3 to 1
Guinea pig	0.5	30	85	3.4 to 1
Rabbit	2	60	330	2.4 to 1
Dog	10	250	500	1.6 to 1
Human	70	900 (calculated)	—	—

* *A value of 0.02 kilograms was used in some calculations in this book.*
Source: Reference 5.

In addition, to obtain accurate estimates of *a* and *b*, sufficient data must be available in multiple species to allow drug-specific linear regression analysis. Lastly, the equations do not work for all dosing regimes. Allometric equations are most accurate for intravenous dosing. Although most compounds discussed here exhibit characteristics that do not meet the requirements for validity and accuracy (e.g., they are given orally), allometric equations using average values for the exponent can still provide useful, albeit rough, approximations.

Time and the Allometric Equation

The time required for a biologic process tends to be proportional to body weight. For example, based on Equation B.4, the ratio of biologic time (*t*) between humans and other mammals can be expressed as the following (the *a* terms, being identical constants, cancel one another):

$$\frac{t_h}{t_m} = \frac{(w_h)^b}{(w_m)^b}$$

Equation B.5

In Equation B.5, the *h* subscript refers to human parameters and the *m* subscript refers to parameters for other mammals. For many biologic events, the *b* term of Equation B.5 is equal to 0.25, the commonly cited interspecies time-scaling factor.[6] If common body weights are used, then the ratio of biologic time between species can be readily calculated. For example, the ratio of biologic time between humans and rats is about 4.3/1. Once the time factor is equalized, other parameters that depend on time will be relatively equal for different species.[4, 7–11] For example, the heartbeat rate of rats is about 4.3-fold faster than that of humans.

Using a *b* term of 0.25 and average body weights, Table B.2 provides ratios of equivalent biologic time be-

tween humans and other mammals. For additional reference, data on water and food intake are also provided. This information is useful when an animal dose is specified as a function of food or water intake.

Scaling Clearance Between Species

Although we have determined a *b* term for time, we are more interested in the *b* term for clearance, since clearance can be used in Equation B.3 to determine the required dose. (It is assumed that the fraction absorbed will be similar in all species.) The commonly cited empirical value for the *b* term for clearance is between 0.6 and 0.8.[12, 13] In this book, we use a *b* term of 0.7, as shown in Equation B.6.[a]

$$\frac{CL_h}{CL_m} = \frac{(w_h)^{0.7}}{(w_m)^{0.7}}$$

Equation B.6

Using a *b* term of 0.7, Table B.3 provides clearance ratios between humans and other mammals.

To sum up, oral clearance values that were obtained from animal studies can be scaled to human equivalents using the ratios listed in Table B.3. For example, if a rat pharmacokinetic study reported that the oral clearance of a compound was 2 L/hr, then we can estimate that the human oral clearance is about 2 x 60, or 120 L/hr.

Scaling of Doses Between Species

In many instances in Part III, a human dose was estimated based on that given to a small animal. For example, an anticancer effect might be produced in rats after a daily dose of 10 mg/kg of some compound, and we would like to know what the equivalent human dose

---

[a] *Volume of distribution ratios can be estimated by using a* b *term of 0.8 to 1.0, and AUC can be estimated using a* b *term of 0.25.*

would be. The scaling of doses between species has been studied by many scientists, particularly in regards to scaling acute toxicity data. A number of studies have been conducted in multiple animal species to measure the acute toxic dose of various compounds. These studies found that, like clearance, toxicity can be scaled between species using the allometric equation. Based on a variety of studies, two b terms, 0.25 and 0.33, have come into common use.[14, 15]

The b term of 0.25 scales biologic time between species, as discussed above. If the definition of equal pharmacologic doses is taken to be those that produce equal areas under the concentration-time curve, a b term of 0.25 naturally makes sense (since AUC is related to time). Some studies have found that toxicity can best be scaled based on relative body surface areas, and a b term of 0.33 scales body surface area between species. When scaling a dose from rats to humans and using a b term of 0.25, for example, we have the following equation:

$$human\ dose\left(\frac{mg}{kg}\right) = \frac{rat\ dose\left(\frac{mg}{kg}\right)}{\dfrac{(70)^{0.25}}{(0.2)^{0.25}}}$$

Equation B.7

Not surprisingly, using b terms of 0.25 and 0.33 produces somewhat different results, as illustrated in Figure B.8; the contrast shown between the two methods illustrates the point that the generic methods commonly used to scale doses between species provide only rough estimates. In this book, we use a b term of 0.25 to scale doses (the solid lines in the figure). A simple equation for scaling doses based on a b term of 0.25 is presented in Chapter 1 (Equation 1.1).

TABLE B.3 HUMAN TO MAMMAL CLEARANCE RATIOS		
MAMMAL	**WEIGHT (KG)**	**HUMAN TO MAMMAL CLEARANCE RATIO**
Mouse	0.025	260 to 1
Hamster	0.13	82 to 1
Rat	0.20	60 to 1
Guinea pig	0.50	32 to 1
Rabbit	2.0	12 to 1
Dog	10	3.9 to 1
Human	70	—

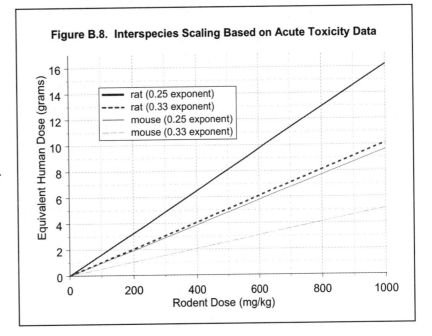

Figure B.8. Interspecies Scaling Based on Acute Toxicity Data

- rat (0.25 exponent)
- rat (0.33 exponent)
- mouse (0.25 exponent)
- mouse (0.33 exponent)

(y-axis: Equivalent Human Dose (grams); x-axis: Rodent Dose (mg/kg))

REFERENCES

[1] Meibohm B, Derendorf H. Basic concepts of pharmacokinetic/pharmacodynamic (PK/PD) modelling. Int J Clin Pharmacol Ther 1997 Oct; 35(10):401–13.

[2] Uang YS, Kang FL, Hsu KY. Determination of caffeic acid in rabbit plasma by high-performance liquid chromatography. J Chromatogr B Biomed Appl 1995 Nov 3; 673(1):43–9.

[3] Cawello W. Connection of pharmacokinetics and pharmacodynamics—how does it work? Int J Clin Pharmacol Ther 1997 Oct; 35(10):414–7.

[4] Mordinti J. Man versus beast: Pharmacokinetic scaling in mammals. J Pharm Sci 1986; 75(11):1028–1040.

[5] Lewis RJ. Sax's dangerous properties of industrial materials. 9th ed. New York: Van Nostrand Reinhold, 1996, p. xix.

[6] West GB, Brown JH, Enquist BJ. The fourth dimension of life: Fractal geometry and allometric scaling of organisms. Science 1999; 284(5420):1677–9.

[7] Boxenbaum H. Interspecies scaling, allometry, physiological time, and the ground plan of pharmacokinetics. J Pharmacokinet Biopharm 1982 Apr; 10(2):201–27.

[8] Boxenbaum H. Evolutionary biology, animal behavior, fourth-dimensional space, and the raison d'etre of drug metabolism and pharmacokinetics. Drug Metab Rev 1983; 14(5):1057–97.

[9] Boxenbaum H. Time concepts in physics, biology, and pharmacokinetics. J Pharm Sci 1986 Nov; 75(11):1053–62.

[10] Boxenbaum H. Interspecies pharmacokinetic scaling and the evolutionary-comparative paradigm. Drug Metab Rev 1984; 15(5–6):1071–121.

[11] Boxenbaum H, Ronfeld R. Interspecies pharmacokinetic scaling and the Dedrick plots. Am J Physiol 1983 Dec; 245(6):R768–75.

[12] Mordenti J, Chen SA, Moore JA, et al. Interspecies scaling of clearance and volume of distribution data for five therapeutic proteins. Pharm Res 1991 Nov; 8(11):1351–9.

[13] Ings RM. Interspecies scaling and comparisons in drug development and toxicokinetics. Xenobiotica 1990 Nov; 20(11):1201–31.

[14] Travis CC, Morris JM. On the use of 0.75 as an interspecies scaling factor. Risk Anal 1992 Jun; 12(2):311–3.

[15] Watanabe K, Bois FY, Zeise L. Interspecies extrapolation: A reexamination of acute toxicity data. Risk Anal 1992 Jun; 12(2):301–10.

SUPPLEMENTAL MATERIAL FOR CHAPTER 2

Supplemental material for Chapter 2, "Mutations, Gene Expression, and Proliferation," includes Table C.1, which summarizes studies on the inhibition of topoisomerase activity by natural compounds. The role of polyamines in cancer cell proliferation is also discussed, as is natural compounds that block polyamine synthesis.

TABLE C.1 NATURAL COMPOUNDS THAT INHIBIT TOPOISOMERASE ACTIVITY		
COMPOUND	**TOPOISOMERASE I INHIBITION**	**TOPOISOMERASE II INHIBITION**
Apigenin	• Ineffective at 18 and 180 μM.[1] • Ineffective at 370 μM.[2] • About 1.7-fold inhibition at 1,000 μM.[3]	• Ineffective at 370 μM.[2] • Substantial (10–50%) DNA cleavage at 0–185 μM.[4] • 28% inhibition at 18 μM and 45% at 180 μM. Marked cell death occurred at 180 μM even though PTK activity was not affected. The effect was thought to be due to inhibition of topoisomerase II.[1]
ATRA (vitamin A)		• ATRA at 3 μM repressed the synthesis of topoisomerase II in human liver cancer cells. At this concentration it did not inhibit cell proliferation (IC_{50} = about 17 μM) and did not affect topoisomerase protein levels even after 72 hours.[5]
Boswellic acids	• Alpha-boswellic acid acetate (BC-4-1) was more potent than camptothecin at inhibiting topoisomerase I (>80% inhibition at 5 μM).[1, 6] Camptothecin is a natural compound that is a known topoisomerase inhibitor. • Acetyl-11-keto-beta boswellic acid reduced proliferation of human leukemia cells at an IC_{50} of 30 μM. This was thought to be due to topoisomerase I inhibition, which took place at concentrations greater than or equal to 10 μM.[7]	• BC-4-1 was more potent than etoposide (>25% inhibition at 5 μM) at blocking topoisomerase II activity. BC-4-1 reduced the proliferation of nasopharynx carcinoma cells at 12 μM and an etoposide-resistant cell line at 3 μM.[1, 6]
Genistein	• Ineffective at 18 and 180 μM.[1] • Ineffective at 370 μM.[2] • Ineffective at 1,000 μM.[3] • Less then 50% inhibition at 3,700 μM.[8]	• IC_{50} = 111 μM.[2, 8] • Inhibited topoisomerase II at concentrations greater than 7 μM and selectively reduced proliferation of transformed but not normal mouse fibroblast cells at 37 μM.[9] • 34% inhibition at 18 μM, 49% at 180 μM. Marked cell death occurred at 180 μM even though PTK activity was not affected. The effect was apparently due to inhibition of topoisomerase II.[1] • Gradual inhibition starting at 20 μM, complete at 80 to 370 μM.[10] • Inhibited topoisomerase II and doubled the amount of DNA cleavage at 5 μM.[11] • In some cell lines, cell death induced by genistein may be due more to inhibition of topoisomerase activity than to that of PTK.[10, 12]
Luteolin		• Substantial (10–50%) DNA cleavage at 0–175 μM.[4]
Quercetin	• IC_{50} = 42 μM.[2]	• IC_{50} = 23 μM.[2] • IC_{50} = 40 μM.[11]

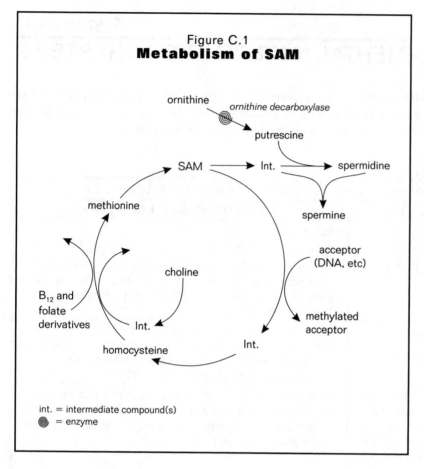

Figure C.1
Metabolism of SAM

int. = intermediate compound(s)

◎ = enzyme

methyl (CH_3) groups for DNA and other compounds (the circular branch shown), SAM is transformed into the amino acid homocysteine and then into the amino acid methionine. More than 99 percent of SAM follows this circular branch.[15]

In the second branch, SAM is metabolized into the polyamines: spermidine, spermine, and putrescine. These three are similar compounds, differing only in the length of their chains. The structure of spermidine is illustrated in Figure A.10 of Appendix A as an example. Spermidine and spermine derive their name from sperm, the cells in which they were first found.

As shown in Figure C.1, production of polyamines from SAM requires the amino acid ornithine and the actions of the enzyme ornithine decarboxylase (ODC). In fact, ODC is a rate-limiting enzyme in polyamine synthesis, and its overproduction is one of the early signs of transformation of a normal cell to a cancer cell.[16] Because of ODC's involvement in carcinogenesis, many studies have been performed to find natural sources of ODC inhibitors.

POLYAMINES

Polyamines are short carbon chains interspersed with nitrogen molecules; they help stabilize or otherwise assist DNA molecules. Although their exact role is uncertain, it is clear they are required for cell survival and that increased polyamine synthesis is one of the early events of cell proliferation. Furthermore, compounds that prevent polyamine synthesis also inhibit cancer cell proliferation. Recent research suggests that polyamines may play a pivotal role by functioning as a point of convergence of multiple signal transduction pathways leading to cell proliferation. This event occurs early after cell stimulation by proliferative signals, soon after the expression of *fos, myc,* and *jun* genes. Polyamines themselves may also act as signals in regulating later events of cell proliferation.[13]

Polyamines are related to cytosine methylation in that both polyamine synthesis and that of the primary methyl donor, *S*-adenosylmethionine (SAM) involve the same cycle. The SAM cycle is illustrated in Figure C.1 (adapted from references 14 and 15). Briefly, the cycle consists of two branches. In the branch that provides

A number of natural compounds have been reported to inhibit ODC activity and reduce polyamine concentrations in cancer cells. In some cases, however, inhibition of ODC activity may be secondary to a decrease in proliferation caused by other means. Nonetheless, in many cases the effects of natural compounds appear to be specific for ODC or for the signal transduction cascades that regulate ODC gene activity. By inhibiting ODC production or activity, these natural compounds have the potential to act as both cancer preventive and cancer therapy compounds. Table C.2 lists compounds reported to inhibit ODC and polyamine synthesis.

TABLE C.2 NATURAL COMPOUNDS THAT INHIBIT POLYAMINE SYNTHESIS

COMPOUND	EFFECTS
Apigenin	• Topical application of apigenin inhibited tumor formation and ODC activity in mice treated with a carcinogen and tumor promoter.[17]
ATRA	• Topical and oral application of ATRA inhibited injury-induced ODC activity in rat skin. The oral IC_{50} was 80 mg/kg.[18]
CAPE	• Topical application of CAPE inhibited promoter-induced ODC activity in mouse skin.[19] Oral administration of other propolis compounds related to CAPE (at about 40 mg/kg) inhibited ODC activity in the colon of rats fed a promoting agent.[20] Similar effects were seen in vitro.[21]
Curcumin	• Oral administration of 0.2 percent curcumin in the diet (about 150 mg/kg) reduced ODC activity in the liver and colon of rats treated with a promoting agent.[22] • Topical administration of curcumin inhibited promoter-induced ODC activity in mice.[23]
Genistein and other kinase inhibitors	• Genistein inhibited promoter-induced ODC activity at an IC_{50} of 20 µM. The effect appeared to be due to inhibition of kinases involved in the signal transduction cascade that regulates transcription and translation of ODC RNA.[24] In contrast, and unexpectedly, genistein has also increased ODC activity in some in-vitro conditions.[13] Still other studies on topical application of genistein reported it had modest inhibitory effects against promoter-induced ODC activity in mice.[25]
Green tea and EGCG	• Topical administration of green tea extract, and especially its primary constituent EGCG, inhibited promoter-induced ODC activity in mice.[26, 27] • Oral administration of green tea in drinking water to mice (at 400 mg/kg) and rats (at 250 mg/kg) inhibited testosterone-induced ODC activity in prostate cells. A similar effect was seen in vitro with prostate cancer cells.[28] • Green tea extracts and EGCG inhibited promoter-induced ODC activity over a wide range of concentrations in cancer cells in vitro. This effect appeared due in part to kinase inhibition.[29, 30]
Limonene	• Oral administration of 1 percent limonene in the diet (about 750 mg/kg) reduced tumor formation and ODC activity in rats fed a carcinogen and promoting agent.[31] A similar effect was seen in rats given 0.5 percent limonene and a different promoting agent.[32]
Lipoxygenase inhibitors	• Lipoxygenase inhibitors, including quercetin, inhibited promoter-induced increases in ODC activity in mouse skin cells in vitro. A number of natural compounds are lipoxygenase inhibitors (see Table 8.2). In this study, quercetin was effective at <10 µM.[33]
Proanthocyanidins and anthocyanidins	• Topical application of proanthocyanidins inhibited promoter-induced ODC activity in mouse skin.[34, 35] • Proanthocyanidins and anthocyanidins inhibited promoter-induced ODC activity in vitro.[36]
SAM	• Intramuscular administration of SAM (at 25 mg/kg) reduced both the number of preneoplastic lesions and polyamine synthesis in rats fed a carcinogen and tumor-promoting agent. Furthermore, SAM decreased ODC activity in vitro, probably via some metabolite.[37]
Selenium	• The effects of selenium on cancer are complex and may depend on the form used. In some studies, selenium reduced polyamine synthesis, possibly because of inhibition of ODC activity or that of other enzymes involved in converting SAM to polyamines.[38]
Silymarin	• Topical application of silymarin decreased ODC production caused by a variety of tumor-promoting agents in mice.[39]
Ursolic acid	• Topical application of ursolic acid inhibited promoter-induced ODC activity in mouse skin. Ursolic acid is similar in structure to boswellic acid and other triterpenes discussed in this book.[40]
Vitamin E and other prostaglandin inhibitors	• Oral administration of vitamin E (at 400 mg/kg) decreased promoter-induced ODC activity in mice, apparently by inhibiting signal transduction.[41] The equivalent human dose is about 5,700 I.U. per day, which is prohibitively large. • Oral administration of vitamin E (at 400 to 500 mg/kg) prevented lung tumor formation, ODC activity, and polyamine synthesis in mice treated with a carcinogen.[42, 43] The effects appeared related to prostaglandin inhibition. A number of natural compounds are prostaglandin inhibitors (see Table 8.2). • Oral administration of 400 I.U. vitamin E per day inhibited ODC activity in precancerous stomach cells and caused regression of precancerous intestinal lesions in humans.[44]

REFERENCES

[1] Azuma Y, Onishi Y, Sato Y, Kizaki H. Effects of protein tyrosine kinase inhibitors with different modes of action on topoisomerase activity and death of IL-2 dependent CTLL-2 cells. J Biochem (Tokyo) 1995 Aug; 118(2):312–8.

[2] Constantinou A, Mehta R, Runyan C, et al. Flavonoids as DNA topoisomerase antagonists and poisons: Structure-activity relationships. J Nat Prod 1995 Feb; 58(2):217–25.

[3] Boege F, Straub T, Kehr A, et al. Selected novel flavones inhibit the DNA binding or the DNA religation step of eukaryotic topoisomerase I. J Biol Chem 1996 Jan 26; 271(4):2262–70.

[4] Austin CA, Patel S, Ono K, et al. Site-specific DNA cleavage by mammalian DNA topoisomerase II induced by novel flavone and catechin derivatives. Biochem J 1992; 282(3):883–889.

[5] Tsao YP, Tsao LT, Hsu SH, Chen SL. Retinoic acid represses the gene expression of topoisomerase II in HEP3B cells. Cancer Letters 1994; 87:73–77.

[6] Liu SY, Lee YW, Han FS, et al. Identification of novel inhibitor of human DNA topoisomerase I and II from Chinese herb medicine. Proc Am Assoc Cancer Res 1990; 31:438.

[7] Hoernlein RF, Orlikowsky T, Zehrer C, et al. Acetyl-11-keto-beta-boswellic acid induces apoptosis in HL-60 and CCRF-CEM cells and inhibits topoisomerase I. J Pharmacol Exp Ther 1999; 288(2):613–19.

[8] Constantinou A, Kiguchi K, Huberman E. Induction of differentiation and DNA strand breakage in human HL-60 and K-562 leukemia cells by genistein. Cancer Res 1990; 50(9):2618–24.

[9] Okura A, Arakawa H, Oka H, et al. Effect of genistein on topoisomerase activity and on the growth of [VAL 12]Ha-ras-transformed NIH 3T3 cells. Biochem Biophys Res Communications 1988; 157(1):183–189.

[10] Markovits J, Linassier C, Fosse P, et al. Inhibitory effects of the tyrosine kinase inhibitor genistein on mammalian DNA topoisomerase II. Cancer Res 1989; 49:5111–7.

[11] Robinson MJ, Corbett AH, Osheroff N. Effects of topoisomerase II-targeted drugs on enzyme-mediated DNA cleavage and ATP hydrolysis: Evidence for distinct drug interaction domains on topoisomerase II. Biochemistry 1993; 32:3638–3643.

[12] Markovits J, Junqua S, Goldwasser F, et al. Genistein resistance in human leukaemic CCRF-CEM cells: Selection of a diploid cell line with reduced DNA topoisomerase II beta isoform. Biochem Pharmacol 1995 Jul 17; 50(2):177–86.

[13] Tacchini L, Dansi P, Matteucci E, Desiderio MA. Hepatocyte growth factor signal coupling to various transcription factors depends on triggering of met receptor and protein kinase transducers in human hepatoma cells HepG2. Exp Cell Res 2000 Apr 10; 256(1):272–281.

[14] Zingg JM, Jones PA. Genetic and epigenetic aspects of DNA methylation on genome expression, evolution, mutation and carcinogenesis. Carcinogenesis 1997 May; 18(5):869–82.

[15] Chiang PK, Gordon RK, Tal J, et al. S-Adenosylmethionine and methylation. FASEB J 1996 Mar; 10(4):471–80.

[16] Shantz LM, Pegg AE. Translational regulation of ornithine decarboxylase and other enzymes of the polyamine pathway. Int J Biochem Cell Biol 1999 Jan; 31(1):107–22.

[17] Wei H, Tye L, Bresnick E, Birt DF. Inhibitory effect of apigenin, a plant flavonoid, on epidermal ornithine decarboxylase and skin tumor promotion in mice. Cancer Res 1990 Feb 1; 50(3):499–502.

[18] Bouclier M, Shroot B, Eustache J, Hensby CN. A rapid and simple test system for the evaluation of the inhibitory activity of retinoids on induced ornithine decarboxylase activity in the hairless rat epidermis. J Pharmacol Methods 1986 Sep; 16(2):151–60.

[19] Frenkel K, Wei H, Bhimani R, et al. Inhibition of tumor promoter-mediated processes in mouse skin and bovine lens by caffeic acid phenethyl ester. Cancer Res 1993 Mar 15; 53(6):1255–61.

[20] Rao CV, Desai D, Simi B, et al. Inhibitory effect of caffeic acid esters on azoxymethane-induced biochemical changes and aberrant crypt foci formation in rat colon. Cancer Res 1993 Sep 15; 53(18):4182–8.

[21] Rao CV, Desai D, Kaul B, et al. Effect of caffeic acid esters on carcinogen-induced mutagenicity and human colon adenocarcinoma cell growth. Chem Biol Interact 1992 Nov 16; 84(3):277–90.

[22] Rao CV, Simi B, Reddy BS. Inhibition by dietary curcumin of azoxymethane-induced ornithine decarboxylase, tyrosine protein kinase, arachidonic acid metabolism and aberrant crypt foci formation in the rat colon. Carcinogenesis 1993 Nov; 14(11):2219–25.

[23] Huang MT, Newmark HL, Frenkel K. Inhibitory effects of curcumin on tumorigenesis in mice. J Cell Biochem Suppl 1997; 27:26–34.

[24] Tseng CP, Verma AK. Inhibition of 12-O-tetradecanoylphorbol-13-acetate-induced ornithine decarboxylase activity by genistein, a tyrosine kinase inhibitor. Mol Pharmacol 1996 Aug; 50(2):249–57.

[25] Wei H, Bowen R, Zhang X, Lebwohl M. Isoflavone genistein inhibits the initiation and promotion of two-stage skin carcinogenesis in mice. Carcinogenesis 1998 Aug; 19(8):1509–14.

[26] Agarwal R, Katiyar SK, Zaidi SI, Mukhtar H. Inhibition of skin tumor promoter-caused induction of epidermal ornithine decarboxylase in SENCAR mice by polyphenolic fraction isolated from green tea and its individual epicatechin derivatives. Cancer Res 1992 Jul 1; 52(13):3582–8.

[27] Hu G, Han C, Chen J. Inhibition of oncogene expression by green tea and (-)-epigallocatechin gallate in mice. Nutr Cancer 1995; 24(2):203–9.

[28] Gupta S, Ahmad N, Mohan RR, et al. Prostate cancer chemoprevention by green tea: In vitro and in vivo inhibition of testosterone-mediated induction of ornithine decarboxylase. Cancer Res 1999 May 1; 59(9):2115–20.

[29] Steele VE, Kelloff GJ, Balentine D, et al. Comparative chemopreventive mechanisms of green tea, black tea and selected polyphenol extracts measured by in vitro bioassays. Carcinogenesis 2000 Jan; 21(1):63–7.

[30] Kennedy DO, Nishimura S, Hasuma T, et al. Involvement of protein tyrosine phosphorylation in the effect of green tea

polyphenols on Ehrlich ascites tumor cells in vitro. Chem Biol Interact 1998 Apr 3; 110(3):159–72.

[31] Yano H, Tatsuta M, Iishi H, et al. Attenuation by d-limonene of sodium chloride-enhanced gastric carcinogenesis induced by N-methyl-N'-nitro-N-nitrosoguanidine in Wistar rats. Int J Cancer 1999 Aug 27; 82(5):665–8.

[32] Kawamori T, Tanaka T, Hirose Y, et al. Inhibitory effects of d-limonene on the development of colonic aberrant crypt foci induced by azoxymethane in F344 rats. Carcinogenesis 1996 Feb; 17(2):369–72.

[33] Yamamoto S, Sasakawa N, Kiyoto I, et al. The induction of ornithine decarboxylase caused by 12-O-tetradecanoylphorbol-13-acetate in isolated epidermal cells is inhibited by lipoxygenase inhibitors but not by cyclooxygenase inhibitors. Eur J Pharmacol 1987 Nov 24; 144(1):101–3.

[34] Gali HU, Perchellet EM, Gao XM, et al. Comparison of the inhibitory effects of monomeric, dimeric, and trimeric procyanidins on the biochemical markers of skin tumor promotion in mouse epidermis in vivo. Planta Med 1994 Jun; 60(3):235–9.

[35] Chen G, Perchellet EM, Gao XM, et al. Ability of m-chloroperoxybenzoic acid to induce the ornithine decarboxylase marker of skin tumor promotion and inhibition of this response by gallotannins, oligomeric proanthocyanidins, and their monomeric units in mouse epidermis in vivo. Anticancer Res 1995 Jul–Aug; 15(4):1183–9.

[36] Bomser J, Madhavi DL, Singletary K, Smith MA. In vitro anticancer activity of fruit extracts from Vaccinium species. Planta Med 1996 Jun; 62(3):212–6.

[37] Feo F, Garcea R, Daino L, et al. Early stimulation of polyamine biosynthesis during promotion by phenobarbital of diethylnitrosamine-induced rat liver carcinogenesis. The effects of variations of the S-adenosyl-L-methionine cellular pool. Carcinogenesis 1985 Dec; 6(12):1713–20.

[38] Redman C, Xu MJ, Peng YM, et al. Involvement of polyamines in selenomethionine induced apoptosis and mitotic alterations in human tumor cells. Carcinogenesis 1997 Jun; 18(6):1195–202.

[39] Agarwal R, Katiyar SK, Lundgren DW, Mukhtar H. Inhibitory effect of silymarin, an anti-hepatotoxic flavonoid, on 12-O-tetradecanoylphorbol-13-acetate-induced epidermal ornithine decarboxylase activity and mRNA in SENCAR mice. Carcinogenesis 1994 Jun; 15(6):1099–103.

[40] Huang MT, Ho CT, Wang ZY, et al. Inhibition of skin tumorigenesis by rosemary and its constituents carnosol and ursolic acid. Cancer Res 1994 Feb 1; 54(3):701–8.

[41] Yano T, Yano Y, Uchida M, et al. The modulation effect of vitamin E on prostaglandin E2 level and ornithine decarboxylase activity at the promotion phase of lung tumorigenesis in mice. Biochem Pharmacol 1997 Jun 1; 53(11):1757–9.

[42] Yano Y, Yano T, Uchida M, et al. The inhibitory effect of vitamin E on pulmonary polyamine biosynthesis, cell proliferation and carcinogenesis in mice. Biochim Biophys Acta 1997 Mar 27; 1356(1):35–42.

[43] Ichikawa T, Uchida M, Murakami A, et al. The inhibitory effect of vitamin E on arachidonic acid metabolism during the process of urethane-induced lung tumorigenesis in mice. J Nutr Sci Vitaminol (Tokyo) 1997 Aug; 43(4):471–7.

[44] Bukin YV, Draudin-Krylenko VA, Kuvshinov YP, et al. Decrease of ornithine decarboxylase activity in premalignant gastric mucosa and regression of small intestinal metaplasia in patients supplemented with high doses of vitamin E. Cancer Epidemiol Biomarkers Prev 1997 Jul; 6(7):543–6.

SUPPLEMENTAL MATERIAL FOR CHAPTER 3

Supplemental material for Chapter 3, "Results of Therapy at the Cellular Level," contains Table D.1, which summarizes studies on the induction of differentiation by natural compounds, and Table D.2, which summarizes studies on the induction of apoptosis.

TABLE D.1 NATURAL COMPOUNDS THAT INDUCE DIFFERENTIATION IN VITRO	
COMPOUND	**EFFECTS**
Apigenin	• Induced differentiation of mouse erythroleukemia cells at a minimal concentration of 30 μM. At higher concentrations, up to 80% of cells were induced to differentiate.[1] • Induced differentiation of human leukemia cells by more than 40% at 40 μM.[2] • Induced differentiation in human leukemia cells at 20 to 50 μM.[3]
Arctigenin	• Arctigenin inhibited cell proliferation and induced differentiation in mouse leukemia cells at concentrations as low as 0.5 μM. The proliferation rate was reduced by 74% at 5 μM and 88% at 20 μM.[4] • At 10 and 50 μM arctigenin induced differentiation and inhibited proliferation of mouse leukemia cells by 60% and 79%, respectively. Other *Arctium* lignans, although less active, also produced the same effect.[5]
ATRA and 1,25-D_3	• Both compounds induced differentiation in a range of cell lines in vitro, including human leukemia, melanoma, breast cancer, prostate cancer, neuroblastoma, and colon cancer.[6–15] Induction of differentiation occurred in a dose-dependent fashion at concentrations ranging from 0.01 to 1 μM for either compound tested separately.[16–23] • These two compounds interacted synergistically in inducing differentiation and were therefore more effective when used in combination.[24–28] Furthermore, combinations of ATRA and 1,25-D_3 produced persistent differentiation after drug withdrawal, whereas each compound used separately produced reversible differentiation.[29] A number of studies have reported that synergism occurred when each compound was used at about 100 nM. In other studies, optimal synergism occurred at concentrations as low as 10 nM, and still others reported that 1,25-D_3 at concentrations as low as 0.15 nM acted synergistically with ATRA.[30, 31] • Few studies have been done on retinol itself; in one, it induced differentiation in some but not all embryonal carcinoma cells at concentrations between 0.35 and 0.87 μM.[32]
Boswellic acid	• Although acetyl-boswellic acid was a weak inducer of differentiation in human leukemia cells, its ability to do this was greatly increased in the presence of daidzein.[33] • Boswellic acid acetate (BC-4) at concentrations less than 24 μM induced differentiation in three of five leukemia cell lines. The proliferation of all five cell lines was inhibited at concentrations of about 40 μM or less.[34] • Boswellic acid induced differentiation in human leukemia cells at 11 to 22 μM. Intraperitoneal administration of 25 to 50 mg/kg inhibited proliferation and induced differentiation of leukemia cells in mice. Proliferation was inhibited by 69% and 82%, respectively.[35, 36] The equivalent human oral dose is about 340 to 680 milligrams per day.
Bromelain and other proteolytic enzymes	• Bromelain induced differentiation and inhibited proliferation of three different leukemia cell lines. IC_{50}s were approximately 3, 8, and >30 μM, respectively. In the last cell line, a different batch of bromelain with higher purity inhibited cell proliferation at an IC_{50} of approximately 4 μM; however, in this same cell line lower concentrations of bromelain both induced differentiation and stimulated cell proliferation. A maximum of 40% growth stimulation was observed at 3 to 6 μM.[37] • A variety of proteases (at 25 to 50 μM) acted synergistically with retinoic acid and other compounds to induce differentiation in a variety of leukemia cell lines.[38] *(row continues next page)*

TABLE D.1 NATURAL COMPOUNDS THAT INDUCE DIFFERENTIATION IN VITRO *(continued)*	
COMPOUND	**EFFECTS**
	• The proliferation of ascites tumor cells was stimulated by about 50% at bromelain concentrations of 0.2 μM. Concentrations as high as 1.5 μM stimulated cell proliferation. Other proteases besides bromelain are known to stimulate proliferation and/or differentiation in some cell lines. In theory, this occurs due to the induction of new membrane transport components, which facilitate uptake of nutrients into the cell.[39] • Papain induced differentiation of mouse or human leukemia cells in vitro.[40]
CAPE	• CAPE at 9 μM inhibited proliferation and induced differentiation of human melanoma cells.[41]
Daidzein	• Induced differentiation and inhibited proliferation of mouse melanoma cells at 40 to 80 μM.[42] • Induced differentiation and inhibited proliferation of human leukemia cells. Differentiation was induced in >50% of cells and proliferation was inhibited by >50% at 80 μM. Concentrations of 40 μM daidzein increased both ATRA-induced (at 0.1 μM) and 1,25-D_3-induced (at 0.15 μM) differentiation by about 55%. Intraperitoneal administration of 25 to 50 mg/kg daidzein reduced tumor volume (>50% reduction) and induced differentiation of leukemia cells held in chambers in mice.[43] The human oral equivalent of 25 to 50 mg/kg is about 1.1 to 2.3 grams per day. • Induced differentiation and inhibited proliferation of mouse leukemia cells in a dose-dependent fashion. Differentiation was induced in approximately 50% of cells at about 67 μM. The IC_{50} for growth inhibition was about 78 μM. PTK inhibition did not appear to play a role in inducing differentiation. Little cytotoxic effect was observed.[44] • Induced differentiation of mouse erythroleukemia cells at a minimal concentration of <4 μM. A maximum of 55% of cells were induced to differentiate.[1] • Induced differentiation and inhibited proliferation of human leukemia cells. The IC_{50} was approximately 55 μM.[45]
Emodin	• Induced differentiation and inhibited cell proliferation in three different human breast cancer cell lines that overexpress *HER-2/neu*. The IC_{50} ranged from 20 to 30 μM, and cells were not affected at 10 μM. Cell lines that do not overexpress this gene were minimally affected at these concentrations. The effect was apparently due to PTK inhibition, as this occurs in a similar concentration range.[46]
EPA and DHA	• Low concentrations of DHA (10 μM) markedly accelerated ATRA-induced differentiation in human leukemic cells. The concentration of ATRA used was 1 μM. The effect appeared to be due to DHA's ability to alter the fluidity of the cell membrane.[47] • EPA at 120 μM induced differentiation and inhibited proliferation of human leukemia cells. Its effect was not reduced by antioxidant treatment and was not mediated by eicosanoids (see Chapter 7 for a discussion on eicosanoids). This effect may be specific to this cell line, as similar results were not seen in two different monocytic leukemia cell lines or in one colon cancer cell line exposed to 60 μM.[48]
Genistein	• Inhibited proliferation of high-grade mouse monocytic leukemia cells at an IC_{50} of 14 μM. Treatment with more than 19 μM produced cytotoxic effects. In a lower-grade cell line, genistein was less cytotoxic but was highly cytostatic, almost completely inhibiting cell proliferation by inducing differentiation at 9 μM. The growth-inhibitory effects were closely associated with inhibition of PTK activity.[49] • Induced differentiation and inhibited proliferation of two human leukemia cell lines. The IC_{50}s were approximately 56 and 63 μM, respectively. The effects of genistein on differentiation were dose dependent from zero to 37 μM.[50] • Induced differentiation of human breast cancer cells. The optimum effect was seen at 30 μM after 9 days.[51] • Induced differentiation and inhibited proliferation of human myelogenous leukemia cells. The IC_{50} was 25 μM. The effect was thought due to PTK inhibition.[52] • Induced differentiation and inhibited proliferation of mouse leukemia cells in a dose-dependent fashion. Differentiation was induced in approximately 50% of cells at about 59 μM. The IC_{50} for growth inhibition was about 22 μM. PTK inhibition did not appear to play a role in inducing differentiation. Minor cytotoxic effects were observed (30% at 59 μM).[44] *(row continues next page)*

TABLE D.1 NATURAL COMPOUNDS THAT INDUCE DIFFERENTIATION IN VITRO *(continued)*	
COMPOUND	**EFFECTS**
	• Induced differentiation and inhibited proliferation of a mouse megakaryoblastic cell line transformed by a leukemia virus. The IC_{50} was 5 µM. The effect was thought due to PTK inhibition.[53]
	• Potentiated 1,25-D_3-induced differentiation in human leukemia cells. At 0.05 µM of 1,25-D_3, the optimum concentration of genistein to potentiate differentiation was 37 µM. At these concentrations, differentiation was increased threefold as compared to D_3 alone. The authors believed the effect was due to PTK inhibition.[54]
	• Induced differentiation in five different human melanoma cell lines at 45 µM. The authors believed the effect was due to inhibition of topoisomerase II.[55]
	• Induced differentiation in mouse embryonal carcinoma cells at an optimal concentration of 35 to 55 µM. Mutant cells resistant to ATRA-induced differentiation were susceptible to genistein, and efforts to obtain mutant lines resistant to both were unsuccessful.[56]
	• At 60 µM genistein potentiated chemically induced differentiation in colon cancer cells. The authors believed the effect was due more to inhibition of topoisomerase activity than inhibition of PTK.[57]
	• In addition to its role in blood coagulation, the protease thrombin inhibits differentiation of brain and nervous system cells. Genistein blocked thrombin-induced inhibition of differentiation at an IC_{50} of about 20 µM.[58]
	• At 370 µM genistein induced differentiation in pheochromocytoma cells that were primed by nerve growth factor. Other PTK inhibitors had a similar effect, and daidzein, which is not a PTK inhibitor, had no effect.[59]
	• Inhibited cell proliferation by 20% to 50% and induced differentiation in one human melanoma and two human leukemia cell lines at concentrations of 37 to 56 µM. The authors believed the effect was due to inhibition of topoisomerase II activity rather than PTK inhibition.[60]
	• Induced differentiation in human leukemia cells at 18 µM. The authors believed the effect was due more to inhibition of inositol phospholipid breakdown than to PTK inhibition.[61]
	• Induced differentiation and inhibited proliferation of a mouse erythroleukemia cell line. Approximately 50% of the cells were induced to differentiate at about 30 µM. The effect was thought due to PTK inhibition.[62]
Luteolin	• Induced differentiation of human leukemia cells by more than 40% at 40 µM.[2]
	• Induced differentiation in human leukemia cells at 20 to 50 µM.[3]
Monoterpenes	• Perillyl alcohol induced differentiation and inhibited proliferation of neuroblastoma cells in the concentration range of 500 to 1,000 µM.[63]
	• Oral administration of about 8 g/kg of limonene to rats with transplanted breast cancer cells resulted in inhibition of tumor growth and increased differentiation and apoptosis of tumors.[64]
Quercetin	• Of 27 flavonoids, quercetin was one of 10 that were active in inducing differentiation in human leukemia cells.[65]
	• Induced differentiation in leukemia blast cells at 5.5 µM, with prolonged exposure.[66]
Resveratrol	• Induced differentiation in human leukemia cells at an IC_{50} of 18 µM.[67]
	• Induced differentiation of human leukemia cells at 30 µM.[68]

TABLE D.2 NATURAL COMPOUNDS THAT INDUCE APOPTOSIS IN CANCER CELLS IN VITRO	
COMPOUND	**EFFECTS**
Apigenin	• Induced apoptosis in human leukemia cells at 60 µM.[69]
	• Induced apoptosis in human thyroid cancer cells at 12 to 50 µM.[70]
ATRA (vitamin A)	• ATRA downregulated IL-6 receptors on myeloma cells; IL-6 is a growth factor for these cells. Growth inhibition and apoptosis were induced in two human myeloma cell lines at an IC_{50} of about 0.01 µM at seven days (about 1 µM at four days). Administration of 40 mg/kg (by injection) three times per week induced regression of tumors in 40% of treated mice.[71]
	• ATRA inhibited proliferation of hormone-dependent but not hormone-independent human breast cancer cells. In two hormone-independent cell line variants, ATRA induced apoptosis and inhibited proliferation by 40% at about 0.1 µM.[72]
	• At 0.1 µM, ATRA inhibited proliferation of two estrogen-dependent human breast cancer cell lines by 58% to 62%. Apoptosis was induced in about 55% of cells. In an estrogen-independent cell line, proliferation was inhibited by only about 30%.[73]
	• At 1 µM, ATRA inhibited proliferation of three human cervical cancer cell lines by 80%. Two other cell lines were inhibited by 30% to 48%, and two others responded poorly. Although ATRA does induce apoptosis in a variety of cell lines, inhibition of proliferation in these lines did not involve induction of apoptosis.[74]
	• ATRA induced apoptosis in human liver cancer cells at 100 µM. No apoptotic effect was seen at lower concentrations.[75]
Boswellic acid	• Induced apoptosis in four human brain cancer cell lines at an IC_{50} of 30 to 40 µM.[76]
	• Induced apoptosis in human leukemia cells at an IC_{50} of 30 µM.[77]
CAPE	• Caffeic acid phenethyl ester (CAPE), found in propolis, induced apoptosis in several kinds of transformed rat fibroblast cells but not normal cells. This effect was seen at 4 to 35 µM.[78]
	• CAPE induced apoptosis in a transformed rat fibroblast cell line but not in normal cells. This effect was seen at 4 µM. As with gallic acid, the effect appeared due to generation of free radicals.[79] (Whereas CAPE appears to act as an antioxidant in vivo, it can produce prooxidant effects in vitro.)
	• CAPE induced apoptosis in transformed rat fibroblast cells. This effect was selective to cancer cells (normal cells were spared) and appeared due to increased free radical damage.[80]
Curcumin	• Oral administration of approximately 150 mg/kg curcumin to rats with chemically induced colon cancer approximately doubled the number of tumor cells entering apoptosis.[81]
	• Curcumin induced apoptosis in transformed mouse fibroblast cells at 30 to 90 µM. Cytotoxicity was induced at an IC_{50} of 25 µM. At 50 µM curcumin also induced apoptosis in human liver, kidney, and colon cancer cells, and mouse sarcoma cells in vitro. Cell death was observed at concentrations as low as 9 µM (but not 3 µM). Curcumin did not induce apoptosis in normal mouse or human fibroblast cells at this concentration, indicating a selective effect on cancer cells.[82]
	• Curcumin inhibited proliferation and induced apoptosis in human myeloid leukemia cells starting at 10 µM. The IC_{50} was about 13 µM. This effect did not appear to be due to PTK or PKC inhibition and was prevented by antioxidants, suggesting that curcumin induced oxidative stress. One possibility is that curcumin inhibited intracellular antioxidant enzymes such as catalase in a manner analogous to kinase inhibition. The proliferation of other human cell lines (breast, cervical, colon, and liver) was inhibited to a lesser extent (about 12% to 33% inhibition at 13 µM).[83]
	• Curcumin induced apoptosis in a wide variety of human and mouse cancer cells at 30 to 90 µM.[84]
EGCG	• EGCG induced apoptosis in human lung cancer cells at 50 µM. This effect was enhanced fourfold when EGCG was combined with other green tea catechins.[85]
	• EGCG induced apoptosis in human leukemia cells. Proliferation was inhibited by 18% at 50 µM and 93% at 100 µM.[86]
	• EGCG inhibited proliferation and induced apoptosis in two human lung cancer cell lines at an IC_{50} of 22 µM. It was two- to threefold less effective against another human lung cancer line and human colon cancer cells.[87]
	• EGCG induced apoptosis in human epidermoid, keratinocyte, and prostate cancer lines at 87 to 170 µM.[88]
	• EGCG induced apoptosis in three human prostate cancer cell lines at an IC_{50} of 1 to 25 µM.[89]

TABLE D.2 NATURAL COMPOUNDS THAT INDUCE APOPTOSIS IN CANCER CELLS IN VITRO *(continued)*	
COMPOUND	**EFFECTS**
EPA	• EPA induced apoptosis (19% of cells) and necrosis (32% of cells) in a human myelocytic leukemia cell line at an IC_{50} of 60 μM. Its effect was not reduced by antioxidant treatment and was not mediated by eicosanoids. This effect may be specific to this cell line, as similar results were not seen in two different monocytic leukemia cell lines or in one colon cancer cell line.[48] • EPA induced apoptosis and inhibited proliferation of human prostate cancer cells. At 30 and 50 μM for 72 hours, EPA inhibited viability of the cells by 20% and 25%, respectively. At 50 μM for 72 hours, apoptosis occurred in 10% of cells and necrosis occurred in 26%.[90]
Garlic compounds	• Diallyl trisulfide (DATS) induced apoptosis in human lung cancer cells at 1 μM.[91] • S-allylmercaptocysteine (SAMC) induced apoptosis in leukemia cells at 46 to 93 μM.[92] • Ajoene induced apoptosis in human leukemia cells at an IC_{50} of roughly 40 μM.[93] • Allicin induced apoptosis in human leukemia cells at concentrations at or above 31 μM.[94]
Genistein	• In T-lymphocyte leukemia cells, genistein induced apoptosis at 18 to 110 μM.[95] • In two human myelogenous leukemia cell lines stimulated with growth factors (IL-3 and GM-CSF), genistein induced apoptosis at 110 μM. The action was primarily due to inhibition of PTK activity, but genistein may also inhibit topoisomerase II.[96] • In rat ovarian granulosa cells, genistein completely blocked the ability of EGF, TGF-alpha, and bFGF to suppress apoptosis.[97] • In 10 human gastrointestinal cell lines, genistein and the isoflavone biochanin A strongly inhibited some cell lines and moderately inhibited others. The compounds were cytostatic at low concentrations (approximately <37 μM and <74 μM, respectively) and induced apoptosis at high concentrations (>74 and >150 μM, respectively).[98] • In human myelogenous leukemia and human lymphocytic leukemia cells, genistein induced apoptosis in 50% of cells at 31 to 48 μM. Genistein did not induce apoptosis in normal human lymphocytes.[99] • In two human colon cancer cell lines, genistein induced apoptosis and inhibited proliferation. The IC_{50} was approximately 40 and 90 μM. Normal rat intestinal cells were also inhibited at an IC_{50} of 30 μM.[100] • Genistein induced DNA fragmentation and apoptosis in healthy human thymocytes at concentrations as low as 11 μM, probably due to its ability to inhibit topoisomerase II. Other topoisomerase inhibitors also induced apoptosis in these cells.[101] • In human estrogen-dependent and estrogen-independent breast cancer cell lines, genistein induced apoptosis and inhibited proliferation by about 50% at 74 μM.[102] • In human non-small-cell lung cancer cells, genistein induced apoptosis at 30 μM.[103]
Hypericin	• Induced apoptosis in three different human brain cancer cell lines. Proliferation was inhibited by approximately 74% at 10 μM, but 1 μM was not effective. The effects were only slightly sensitive to moderate light, which inhibited proliferation 13% more than dark conditions.[104] • Hypericin at 0.1 to 100 μM did not induce apoptosis in human leukemia cells, although other PKC inhibitors did. However, at 25 μM hypericin did inhibit further proliferation of these cells.[105] • Induced apoptosis in two human neuroblastoma cell lines, probably by PKC inhibition. Cell proliferation was inhibited by 82% at 5 μM but only by 4% at 1 μM.[106] • Inhibited proliferation and induced apoptosis in two rat pituitary adenoma cell lines. Greater than 80% inhibition was observed at concentrations of >5 μM. The authors believed the effect was due to PKC inhibition.[107]
Leukotriene inhibitors	• Apoptosis was induced in rat Walker carcinoma cells by treatment with various 12-lipoxygenase inhibitors but not cyclooxygenase inhibitors.[108]
Luteolin	• Induced apoptosis in human thyroid cancer cells at 12 to 50 μM.[70] • Induced apoptosis in skin cancer cells at 20 μM.[109]
Monoterpenes	• Oral administration of about 2 g/kg perillyl alcohol produced a 10-fold reduction in tumor weight in rats with chemically induced liver tumors. The effect was due to a 10-fold increase in apoptosis in the tumor cells of treated rats. Receptors for TGF-beta were also increased in the tumors of treated rats.[110]

TABLE D.2 NATURAL COMPOUNDS THAT INDUCE APOPTOSIS IN CANCER CELLS IN VITRO *(continued)*

COMPOUND	EFFECTS
Quercetin	• Induced apoptosis in human leukemia cells at 60 µM.[69] • Induced apoptosis in skin cancer cells at 20 µM.[109]
Resveratrol	• Induced apoptosis in human leukemia cells at an IC_{50} of 15 to 30 µM.[111] • Prevented transformation and induced apoptosis through activation of *p53* in mouse epidermal cells at concentrations at or above 5 µM.[112] • Induced apoptosis in human prostate cancer cells at 25 µM.[113] • Induced apoptosis in human leukemia cells at an IC_{50} of about 20 µM.[114]
Selenium	• Methylselenocysteine induced apoptosis in mouse breast cancer cells at 50 µM.[115] • Selenite induced apoptosis in human liver cancer cells at 10 µM.[116] • Selenite induced apoptosis in human colon cancer cells at concentrations greater than 10 µM.[117] • Selenium compounds differ in their ability to induce free radical damage and apoptosis. Inorganic selenium compounds were the most reactive and most effective at inducing apoptosis in vitro.[118]
Vitamin C	• Vitamin C, especially at high concentrations (1 to 10 mM), induced apoptosis in cancer cells by a free-radical-mediated mechanism. Normal cells were less susceptible.[119–123]
Vitamin D₃ (1,25-D₃)	• Induced apoptosis in human breast cancer cells at 100 nM.[124, 125] • Induced apoptosis in human breast cancer cells at 10 to 100 nM.[126] • Induced apoptosis in mouse breast cancer cells at 10 to 100 nM.[127] • Induced apoptosis in human breast cancer cells at 10 to 50 nM.[128]
Vitamin E	• Induced apoptosis in leukemia, prostate, and breast cancer cells at 100 to 250 µM.[129]

REFERENCES

[1] Kinoshita T, Sankawa U, Takuma T, et al. Induction of differentiation in murine erythroleukemia cells by flavonoids. Chem Pharm Bull 1985; 33(9):4109–4112.

[2] Kawaii S, Tomono Y, Katase E, et al. Effect of citrus flavonoids on HL-60 cell differentiation. Anticancer Res 1999 Mar–Apr; 19(2A):1261–9.

[3] Takahashi T, Kobori M, Shinmoto H, et al. Structure-activity relationships of flavonoids and the induction of granulocytic- or monocytic-differentiation in HL60 human myeloid leukemia cells. Biosci Biotechnol Biochem 1998 Nov; 62(11):2199–204.

[4] Umehara K, Sugawa A, Kuroyanagi M, et al. Studies on differentiation-inducers from Arctium fructus. Chem Pharm Bull 1993; 41(10):1774–9.

[5] Umehara K, Nakamura M, Miyase T, et al. Studies on differentiation inducers. VI. Lignan derivatives from Arctium fructus. (2). Chem Pharm Bull (Tokyo) 1996 Dec; 44(12):2300–4.

[6] Ferrari AC, Waxman S. Differentiation agents in cancer therapy. Cancer Chemother Biol Response Modif 1994; 15:337–66.

[7] Schwartz GG, Hill CC, Oeler TA, et al. 1,25-dihydroxy-16-ene-23-yne-vitamin D₃ and prostate cancer cell proliferation in vivo. Urology 1995; 46(3):365–369.

[8] Reichel H, Koeffler P, Norman AW. The role of the vitamin D endocrine system in health and disease. The New England Journal of Medicine 1989 April 13; 320(15):980–991.

9 Kane KF, Langman MJS, Williams GR. Antiproliferative responses of two human colon cancer cell lines to Vitamin D_3 are differentially modified by 9-cis-retinoic acid. Cancer Research 1996 Feb 1; 56:623–632.

10 Love JM, Gudas LJ. Vitamin A, differentiation and cancer. Current Opinion in Cell Biology 1994; 6:825–831.

11 Feldman D, Skowronski R, Peehl DM. Vitamin D and prostate cancer. Adv Exp Med Biol 1995; 375:53–63.

12 DeLuca HF. Vitamin D3 as a possible chemopreventive and therapeutic agent of cancers. Jpn J Cancer Res 1996 Apr; 87(4):inside front cover.

13 Christakos S. Vitamin D and breast cancer. Adv Exp Med Biol 1994; 364:115–8.

14 Lupulescu A. The role of hormones, growth factors and vitamins in carcinogenesis. Crit Rev Oncol Hematol 1996 Jun; 23(2):95–130.

15 Vanderwalle B, Wattez N, Lefebvre J. Effects of vitamin D3 derivatives on growth, differentiation and apoptosis in tumoral colonic HT 29 cells: Possible implication of intracellular calcium. Cancer Letters 1995; 97:99–106.

16 Yen A, Reece SL, Albright KL. Membrane origin for a signal eliciting a program of cell differentiation. Exp. Cell Res 1984; 152:493–499.

17 Breitman TR, He RY. Combinations of retinoic acid with either sodium butyrate, dimethyl sulfoxide, or hexamethylene bisacetamide synergistically induce differentiation of the human myeloid leukemia cell line HL60. Cancer Res 1990 Oct 1; 50(19):6268–73.

18 Yabushita H, Hirata M, Noguchi M, Nakanishi M. Vitamin D receptor in endometrial carcinoma and the differentiation-inducing effect of 1,25-dihydroxyvitamin D3 on endometrial carcinoma cell lines. J Obstet Gynaecol Res 1996 Dec; 22(6):529–39.

19 Moore TB, Koeffler HP, Yamashiro JM, Wada RK. Vitamin D3 analogs inhibit growth and induce differentiation in LA-N-5 human neuroblastoma cells. Clin Exp Metastasis 1996 May; 14(3):239–45.

20 Radhika S, Choudhary SK, Garg LC, Dixit A. Induction of differentiation in murine erythroleukemia cells by 1 alpha,25-dihydroxy vitamin D3. Cancer Lett 1995 Apr 14; 90(2):225–30.

21 Defacque H, Dornand J, Commes T, et al. Different combinations of retinoids and vitamin D3 analogs efficiently promote growth inhibition and differentiation of myelomonocytic leukemia cell lines. J Pharmacol Exp Ther 1994 Oct; 271(1):193–9.

22 Esquenet M, Swinnen JV, Heyns W, Verhoeven G. Control of LNCaP proliferation and differentiation: Actions and interactions of androgens, 1alpha,25-dihydroxycholecalciferol, all-trans retinoic acid, 9-cis retinoic acid, and phenylacetate. Prostate 1996 Mar; 28(3):182–94.

23 Danielsson C, Fehsel K, Polly P, Carlberg C. Differential apoptotic response of human melanoma cells to 1 alpha,25-dihydroxyvitamin D3 and its analogues. Cell Death Differ 1998 Nov; 5(11):946–52.

24 Defacque H, Commes T, Sevilla C, et al. Synergistic differentiation of U937 cells by all-trans retinoic acid and 1 alpha, 25-dihydroxyvitamin D3 is associated with the expression of retinoid X receptor alpha. Biochem Biophys Res Commun 1994 Aug 30; 203(1):272–80.

25 Bollag W, Majewski S, Jablonska S. Cancer combination chemotherapy with retinoids: Experimental rationale. Leukemia 1994 Sep; 8(9):1453–7.

26 Bollag W. Experimental basis of cancer combination chemotherapy with retinoids, cytokines, 1,25-dihydroxyvitamin D3, and analogs. J Cell Biochem 1994 Dec; 56(4):427–35.

27 Marti J, Commes T, Defacque H, Sevilla C. Vitamin D and 9-cis retinoic acid: An efficient partnership for the induction of myelomonocytic cell growth inhibition and differentiation. Leuk Res 1997 Feb; 21(2):173–6.

28 Blutt SE, Allegretto EA, Pike JW, Weigel NL. 1,25-dihydroxyvitamin D3 and 9-cis-retinoic acid act synergistically to inhibit the growth of LNCaP prostate cells and cause accumulation of cells in G1. Endocrinology 1997 Apr; 138(4):1491–7.

29 Verstuyf A, Mathieu C, Verlinden L, et al. Differentiation induction of human leukemia cells (HL60) by a combination of 1,25-dihydroxyvitamin D3 and retinoic acid (all trans or 9-cis). J Steroid Biochem Mol Biol 1995 Jun; 53(1–6):431–41.

30 Taimi M, Chateau MT, Cabane S, Marti J. Synergistic effect of retinoic acid and 1,25-dihydroxyvitamin D3 on the differentiation of the human monocytic cell line U937. Leuk Res 1991; 15(12):1145–52.

31 Ferrero D, Carlesso N, Bresso P, et al. Suppression of in vitro maintenance of non-promyelocytic myeloid leukemia clonogenic cells by all-trans retinoic acid: Modulating effects of dihydroxylated vitamin D3, alpha interferon and "stem cell factor." Leuk Res 1997 Jan; 21(1):51–8.

32 Eglitis MA, Sherman MI. Murine embryonal carcinoma cells differentiate in vitro in response to retinol. Exp Cell Res 1983 Jul; 146(2):289–96.

33 Jing YK, Han R. [Combination induction of cell differentiation of HL-60 cells by daidzein (S86019) and BC-4 or Ara-C.] Yao Hsueh Hsueh Pao 1993; 28(1):11–6.

34 Jing Y, Nakajo S, Xia L, et al. Boswellic acid acetate induces differentiation and apoptosis in leukemia cell lines. Leuk Res 1999 Jan; 23(1):43–50.

35 Jing Y, Xia L, Han R. Growth inhibition and differentiation of promyelocytic cells (HL-60) induced by BC-4, an active principle from Boswellia carterii Birdw. Chin Med Sci J 1992 Mar; 7(1):12–5.

36 Han R. Recent progress in the study of anticancer drugs originating from plants and traditional medicines in China. Chin Med Sci J 1994 Mar; 9(1):61–9.

37 Maurer HR, Hozumi M, Honma Y, et al. Bromelain induces the differentiation of leukemic cells in vitro: An explanation for its cytostatic effects? Planta Med 1988; 377–81.

38 Fibach E, Treves A, Kidron M, Mayer M. Induction of differentiation in human myeloid leukemia cells by proteolytic enzymes. J Cellular Physiol 1985; 123:228–234.

39 Adamietz IA, Kurfurst F, Muller U, et al. Growth acceleration of Ehrlich ascites tumor cells treated by proteinase in vitro. Eur J Cancer Clin Oncol 1989; 25(12):1837–41.

40 Slosberg EA, Scher BM, Scher W, et al. Induction of differentiation in mouse erythroleukaemia cells by the action

of papain at the cell surface. Cell Tissue Kinet 1987 Nov; 20(6):571–81.

[41] Guarini L, Su ZZ, Zucker S, et al. Growth inhibition and modulation of antigenic phenotype in human melanoma and glioblastoma multiforme cells by caffeic acid phenethyl ester (CAPE). [Published erratum appears in Cell Mol Biol 1992 Sep; 38(6):615]. Cell Mol Biol 1992 Aug; 38(5):513–27.

[42] Jing YK, Han R. Differentiation of B16 melanoma cells induced by daidzein. Chinese Journal of Pharmacology and Toxicology 1992; 6(4):278–80.

[43] Jing Y, Nakaya K, Han R. Differentiation of promyeloctic leukemia cells HL-60 induced by daidzen in vitro and in vivo. Anticancer Res 1993; 13(4):1049–54.

[44] Jing Y, Waxman S. Structural requirements for differentiation-induction and growth-inhibition of mouse erythroleukemia cells by isoflavones. Anticancer Res 1995 Jul–Aug; 15(4):1147–52.

[45] Han R, Jiao L, Liu H. Effects of S86019, an active component from Puralia lobata, on cell differentiation and cell cycle traverse of HL-60 cells. Chinese J Cancer Res 1990; 2(3):51–553.

[46] Zhang L, Chang CJ, Bacus SS, Hung MC. Suppressed transformation and induced differentiation of HER-2/neu-overexpressing breast cancer cells by emodin. Cancer Res 1995; 55:3890–3896.

[47] Burns CP, Petersen ES, North JA, et al. Effect of docosahexaenoic acid on rate of differentiation of HL-60 human leukemia. Cancer Research 1989; 49:3252–58.

[48] Finstad HS, Kolset SO, Holme JA, et al. Effect of n-3 and n-6 fatty acids on proliferation and differentiation of promyelocytic leukemic HL-60 cells. Blood 1994 Dec 1; 84(11):3799–3809.

[49] Kanatani Y, Kasukabe T, Hozumi M, Motoyoshi K, et al. Genistein exhibits preferential cytotoxity to a leukemogenic variant but induces differentiation of a non-leukemogenic variant of the mouse monocytic leukemia Mm cell line. Leuk Res 1993; 17(10):847–53.

[50] Constantinou A, Kiguchi K, Huberman E. Induction of differentiation and DNA strand breakage in human HL-60 and K-562 leukemia cells by genistein. Cancer Res 1990; 50(9):2618–24.

[51] Constantinou AI, Krygier AE, Mehta RR. Genistein induces maturation of cultured human breast cancer cells and prevents tumor growth in nude mice. Am J Clin Nutr 1998 Dec; 68(6 Suppl):1426S-1430S.

[52] Honma Y, Okabe-Kado J, Kasukabe T, et al. Inhibition of abl oncogene tyrosine kinase induces erythroid differentiation of human myelogenous leukemia K562 cells. Jpn J Cancer Res 1990; 81:1132–1136.

[53] Honma Y, Okabe-Kado J, Kasukabe T, et al. Induction of some protein kinase inhibitors of differentiation of a mouse megakaryoblastic cell line established by coinfection with Abelson murine leukemia virus and recombinant SV40 retrovirus. Cancer Res 1991; 51:4649–4655.

[54] Katagiri K, Katagiri T, Kajiyama K, et al. Modulation of monocytic differentiation of HL-60 cells by inhibitors of protein tyrosine kinases. Cell Immunol 1992 Apr; 140(2):282–94.

[55] Kiguchi K, Constantinou AI, Huberman E. Genistein-induced cell differentiation and protein-linked DNA strand breakage in human melanoma cells. Cancer Commin 1990; 2(8):271–7.

[56] Kondo K, Tsuneizumi K, Watanabe T, Oishi M. Induction of in vitro differentiation of mouse embryonal carcinoma F9 cells. Cancer Res 1991; 51(19):5398–404.

[57] Kuo ML, Huang TS, Lin JK. Preferential requirement for protein tyrosine phosphatase activity in the 12-O-tetradecanoylphorbol-13-acetate-induced differentiation of human colon cancer cells. Biochemical Pharmacology 1995; 50(8):1217–1222.

[58] Jalink K, Moolenaar WH. Thrombin receptor activation causes rapid neural cell rounding and neurite retraction independent of classic second messengers. J Cell Biol 1992; 118(2):411–9.

[59] Miller DR, Lee GM, Manes PF. Increased neurite outgrowth induced by inhibition of protein tyrosine kinase activity in PC12 pheochromocytoma cells. J Neurochem 1993; 60:2134–2144.

[60] Constantinou A, Huberman E. Genistein as an inducer of tumor cell differentiation: Possible mechanisms of action. Proc Soc Exp Biol Med 1995 Jan; 208(1):109–15.

[61] Makishima M, Honma Y, Hozumi M, et al. Effects of inhibitors of protein tyrosine kinase activity and/or phosphatidylinositol turnover on differentiation of some leukemia myelomonocytic leukemia cells. Leukemia Res 1991; 15(8):701–708.

[62] Watanabe T, Kondo K, Oishi M. Induction of in vitro differentiation of mouse erythroleukemia cells by genistein, an inhibitor of tyrosine protein kinases. Cancer Res 1991; 51:764–768.

[63] Shi W, Gould MN. Induction of differentiation in neuro-2A cells by the monoterpene perillyl alcohol. Cancer Letters 1995; 95:1–6.

[64] Ariazi EA, Gould MN. Identifying differential gene expression in monoterpene-treated mammary carcinomas using subtractive display. J Biol Chem 1996; 271(46):29286–94.

[65] Kawaii S, Tomono Y, Katase E, et al. Effect of citrus flavonoids on HL-60 cell differentiation. Anticancer Res 1999 Mar–Apr; 19(2A):1261–9.

[66] Csokay B, Prajda N, Weber G, Olah E. Molecular mechanisms in the antiproliferative action of quercetin. Life Sci 1997; 60(24):2157–63.

[67] Jang M, Cai L, Udeani GO, et al. Cancer chemopreventive activity of resveratrol, a natural product derived from grapes. Science 1997 Jan 10; 275(5297):218–20.

[68] Ragione FD, Cucciolla V, Borriello A, et al. Resveratrol arrests the cell division cycle at S/G2 phase transition. Biochem Biophys Res Commun 1998; 250(1):53–8.

[69] Wang IK, Lin-Shiau SY, Lin JK. Induction of apoptosis by apigenin and related flavonoids through cytochrome c release and activation of caspase-9 and caspase-3 in leukaemia HL-60 cells. Eur J Cancer 1999 Oct; 35(10):1517–25.

[70] Yin F, Giuliano AE, Van Herle AJ. Signal pathways involved in apigenin inhibition of growth and induction of apoptosis of human anaplastic thyroid cancer cells (ARO). Anticancer Res 1999 Sep–Oct; 19(5B):4297–303.

[71] Levy Y, Labaume S, Colombel M, Brouet JC. Retinoic acid modulates the in vivo and in vitro growth of IL-6 autocrine

human myeloma cell lines via induction of apoptosis. Clin Exp Immunol 1996 Apr; 104(1):167–72.

[72] Liu Y, Lee MO, Wang HG, et al. Retinoic acid receptor beta mediates the growth-inhibitory effect of retinoic acid by promoting apoptosis in human breast cancer cells. Mol Cell Biol 1996 Mar; 16(3):1138–49.

[73] Toma S, Isnardi L, Raffo P, et al. Effects of all-*trans* retinoic acid and 13-cis-retinoic acid on breast-cancer cell lines: Growth inhibition and apoptosis induction. Int J Cancer 1997 Mar 4; 70(5):619–27.

[74] Oridate N, Lotan D, Mitchell MF, et al. Inhibition of proliferation and induction of apoptosis in cervical carcinoma cells by retinoids: Implications for chemoprevention. J Cell Biochem Suppl 1995; 23:80–6.

[75] Kim DG, Jo BH, You KR, Ahn DS. Apoptosis induced by retinoic acid in Hep 3B cells in vitro. Cancer Lett 1996 Oct 1; 107(1):149–59.

[76] Glaser T, Winter S, Groscurth P, et al. Boswellic acids and malignant glioma: Induction of apoptosis but no modulation of drug sensitivity. Br J Cancer 1999 May; 80(5–6):756–65.

[77] Hoernlein RF, Orlikowsky T, Zehrer C, et al. Acetyl-11-keto-beta-boswellic acid induces apoptosis in HL-60 and CCRF-CEM cells and inhibits topoisomerase I. J Pharmacol Exp Ther 1999 Feb; 288(2):613–9.

[78] Su ZZ, Lin J, Prewett M, et al. Apoptosis mediates the selective toxicity of caffeic acid phenethyl ester (CAPE) toward oncogene-transformed rat embryo fibroblast cells. Anticancer Research 1995; 15(58):1841–1848.

[79] Chiao C, Carothers AM, Grunberger D, et al. Apoptosis and altered redox state induced by caffeic acid phenethyl ester (CAPE) in transformed rat fibroblast cells. Cancer Res 1995 Aug 15; 55(16):3576–83.

[80] Mirzoeva OK, Sud'ina GF, Pushkareva MA, et al. [Lipophilic derivatives of caffeic acid as lipoxygenase inhibitors with antioxidant properties.] Bioorg Khim 1995 Feb; 21(2):143–51.

[81] Samaha HS, Kelloff GJ, Steele V, et al. Modulation of apoptosis by sulindac, curcumin, phenylethyl-3-methylcaffeate, and 6-phenylhexyl isothiocyanate: Apoptotic index as a biomarker in colon cancer chemoprevention and promotion. Cancer Res 1997 Apr 1; 57(7):1301–5.

[82] Jiang MC, Yang-Yen HF, Yen JJ, Lin JK. Curcumin induces apoptosis in immortalized NIH 3T3 and malignant cancer cell lines. Nutr Cancer 1996; 26(1):111–20.

[83] Kuo ML, Huang TS, Lin JK. Curcumin, an antioxidant and anti-tumor promoter, induces apoptosis in human leukemia cells. Biochim Biophys Acta 1996; 1317:95–100.

[84] Lin JK, Chen YC, Huang YT, Lin-Shiau SY. Suppression of protein kinase C and nuclear oncogene expression as possible molecular mechanisms of cancer chemoprevention by apigenin and curcumin. J Cell Biochem Suppl 1997; 28/29:39–48.

[85] Suganuma M, Okabe S, Kai Y, et al. Synergistic effects of (--)-epigallocatechin gallate with (--)-epicatechin, sulindac, or tamoxifen on cancer-preventive activity in the human lung cancer cell line PC-9. Cancer Res 1999 Jan 1; 59 (1):44–7.

[86] Hibasami H, Achiwa Y, Fujikawa T, Komiya T. Induction of programmed cell death (apoptosis) in human lymphoid leukemia cells by catechin compounds. Anticancer Res 1996 Jul–Aug; 16(4A):1943–6.

[87] Yang GY, Liao J, Kim K, et al. Inhibition of growth and induction of apoptosis in human cancer cell lines by tea polyphenols. Carcinogenesis 1998 Apr; 19(4):611–6.

[88] Ahmad N, Feyes DK, Nieminen AL, et al. Green tea constituent epigallocatechin-3-gallate and induction of apoptosis and cell cycle arrest in human carcinoma cells. J Natl Cancer Inst 1997 Dec 17; 89(24):1881–6.

[89] Paschka AG, Butler R, Young CYF. Induction of apoptosis in prostate cancer cell lines by the green tea component, (-)-epigallocatechin-3-gallate. Cancer Lett 1998 Aug 14; 130(1–2):1–7.

[90] Lai PB, Ross JA, Fearon KC, et al. Cell cycle arrest and induction of apoptosis in pancreatic cancer cells exposed to eicosapentaenoic acid in vitro. Br J Cancer 1996 Nov; 74(9):1375–83.

[91] Sakamoto K, Lawson LD, Milner JA. Allyl sulfides from garlic suppress the in vitro proliferation of human A549 lung tumor cells. Nutr Cancer 1997; 29(2):152–6.

[92] Sigounas G, Hooker JL, Li W, et al. S-allylmercaptocysteine, a stable thioallyl compound, induces apoptosis in erythroleukemia cell lines. Nutr Cancer 1997; 28(2):153–9.

[93] Dirsch VM, Gerbes AL, Vollmar AM. Ajoene, a compound of garlic, induces apoptosis in human promyeloleukemic cells, accompanied by generation of reactive oxygen species and activation of nuclear factor kappaB. Mol Pharmacol 1998 Mar; 53(3):402–7.

[94] Zheng S, Yang H, Zhang S, et al. Initial study on naturally occurring products from traditional Chinese herbs and vegetables for chemoprevention. J Cell Biochem Suppl 1997; 27:106–12.

[95] Spinozzi F, Pagliacci MC, Migliorati G, et al. The natural tyrosine kinase inhibitor genistein produces cell cycle arrest and apoptosis in Jurkat T-leukemia cells. Leuk Res 1994; 18(6):431–9.

[96] Bergamaschi G, Rosti V, Danova M, Ponchio L, et al. Inhibitors of tyrosine phosphorylation induce apoptosis in human leukemic cell lines. Leukemia 1993 Dec; 7(12):20–8.

[97] Tilly JL, Billig H, Kowalski KI, Hsueh AJ. Epidermal growth factor and basic fibroblast growth factor supress the spontaneous onset of apoptosis in cultured rat ovarian granulosa cells and follicles by a tyrosine kinase-dependent mechanism. Mol Endocrinol 1992; 6(11):1942–50.

[98] Yanagihara K, Ito A, Toge T, Numoto M. Antiproliferative effects isoflavones on human cancer cell lines established from the gastrointestinal tract. Cancer Res 1993 Dec 1; 53(23):5815–21.

[99] Traganos F, Ardelt B, Halko N, Bruno S, Darzynkiewicz Z. Effects of genistein on the growth and cell cycle progression of normal human lymphocytes and human leukemic MOLT-4 and HL-60 cells. Cancer Res 1992; 52(22):6200–8.

[100] Kuo SM. Antiproliferative potency of structurally distinct dietary flavonoids on human colon cancer cells. Cancer Letters 1996; 110:41–48.

[101] McCabe MJ, Orrenius S. Genistein induces apoptosis in immature human thymocytes by inhibiting topoisomerase II. Biochem Biophysical Res Commun 1993; 194(2):944–950.

[102] Shao ZM, Alpaugh ML, Fontana JA, et al. Genistein inhibits proliferation similarly in estrogen receptor-positive and

negative human breast carcinoma cell lines characterized by p21[WAF1/CIP1] induction, G_2M arrest, and apoptosis. J Cell Biochem 1998; 69:44–54.

[103] Lian F, Bhuiyan M, Li YW, et al. Genistein-induced G2-M arrest, p21WAF1 upregulation, and apoptosis in a non-small-cell lung cancer cell line. Nutr Cancer 1998; 31(3):184–91.

[104] Couldwell WT, Gopalakrishna R, Hinton DR, et al. Hypericin: A potential antiglioma therapy. Neurosurgery 1994 Oct; 35(4):705–9; discussion 709–10.

[105] Jarvis WD, Turner AJ, Povirk LF, et al. Induction of apoptotic DNA fragmentation and cell death in HL- 60 human promyelocytic leukemia cells by pharmacological inhibitors of protein kinase C. Cancer Res 1994 Apr 1; 54(7):1707–14.

[106] Zhang W, Lawa RE, Hintona DR, et al. Growth inhibition and apoptosis in human neuroblastoma SK-N-SH cells induced by hypericin, a potent inhibitor of protein kinase C. Cancer Letters 1995; 96:31–35.

[107] Hamilton HB, Hinton DR, Law RE, et al. Inhibition of cellular growth and induction of apoptosis in pituitary adenoma cell lines by the protein kinase C inhibitor hypericin: Potential therapeutic application. J Neurosurgery 1996; 85:329–334.

[108] Tang DG, Chen YQ, Honn KV. Arachidonate lipoxygenases as essential regulators of cell survival and apoptosis. Proc Natl Acad Sci USA 1996 May 28; 93(11):5241–6.

[109] Huang YT, Hwang JJ, Lee PP, et al. Effects of luteolin and quercetin, inhibitors of tyrosine kinase, on cell growth and metastasis-associated properties in A431 cells overexpressing epidermal growth factor receptor. Br J Pharmacol 1999 Nov; 128(5):999–1010.

[110] Mills JJ, Chari RS, Boyer IJ, et al. Induction of apoptosis in liver tumors by the monoterpene perillyl alcohol. Cancer Res 1995 Mar 1; 55(5):979–83.

[111] Clement MV, Hirpara JL, Chawdhury SH, Pervaiz S. Chemopreventive agent resveratrol, a natural product derived from grapes, triggers CD95 signaling-dependent apoptosis in human tumor cells. Blood 1998 Aug 1; 92(3):996–1002.

[112] Huang C, Ma WY, Goranson A, Dong Z. Resveratrol suppresses cell transformation and induces apoptosis through a p53-dependent pathway. Carcinogenesis 1999 Feb; 20(2):237–42.

[113] Hsieh TC, Wu JM. Differential effects on growth, cell cycle arrest, and induction of apoptosis by resveratrol in human prostate cancer cell lines. Exp Cell Res 1999 May 25; 249(1):109–15.

[114] Surh YJ, Hurh YJ, Kang JY, et al. Resveratrol, an antioxidant present in red wine, induces apoptosis in human promyelocytic leukemia (HL-60) cells. Cancer Lett 1999 Jun 1; 140(1–2):1–10.

[115] Sinha R, Kiley SC, Lu JX, et al. Effects of methylselenocysteine on PKC activity, cdk2 phosphorylation and gadd gene expression in synchronized mouse mammary epithelial tumor cells. Cancer Lett 1999 Nov 15; 146(2):135–45.

[116] Shen HM, Yang CF, Ong CN. Sodium selenite-induced oxidative stress and apoptosis in human hepatoma HepG2 cells. Int J Cancer 1999 May 31; 81(5):820–8.

[117] Stewart MS, Davis RL, Walsh LP, Pence BC. Induction of differentiation and apoptosis by sodium selenite in human colonic carcinoma cells (HT29). Cancer Lett 1997 Jul 15; 117(1):35–40.

[118] Stewart MS, Spallholz JE, Neldner KH, Pence BC. Selenium compounds have disparate abilities to impose oxidative stress and induce apoptosis. Free Radic Biol Med 1999 Jan; 26(1–2):42–8.

[119] Maramag C, Menon M, Balaji KC, et al. Effect of vitamin C on prostate cancer cells in vitro: Effect on cell number, viability, and DNA synthesis. Prostate 1997 Aug 1; 32(3):188–95.

[120] Leung PY, Miyashita K, Young M, Tsao CS. Cytotoxic effect of ascorbate and its derivatives on cultured malignant and nonmalignant cell lines. Anticancer Res 1993 Mar–Apr; 13(2):475–80.

[121] Sakagami H, Satoh K, Ohata H, et al. Relationship between ascorbyl radical intensity and apoptosis-inducing activity. Anticancer Res 1996 Sep–Oct; 16(5A):2635–44.

[122] Bishun N, Basu TK, Metcalfe S, Williams DC. The effect of ascorbic acid (vitamin C) on two tumor cell lines in culture. Oncology 1978; 35(4):160–2.

[123] Park CH, Amare M, Savin MA, Hoogstraten B. Growth suppression of human leukemic cells in vitro by L-ascorbic acid. Cancer Res 1980 Apr; 40(4):1062–5.

[124] Welsh J. Induction of apoptosis in breast cancer cells in response to vitamin D and antiestrogens. Biochem Cell Biol 1994 Nov–Dec; 72(11–12):537–45.

[125] Simboli-Campbell M, Narvaez CJ, Tenniswood M, Welsh J. 1,25-Dihydroxyvitamin D3 induces morphological and biochemical markers of apoptosis in MCF-7 breast cancer cells. J Steroid Biochem Mol Biol 1996 Jul; 58(4):367–76.

[126] Simboli-Campbell M, Narvaez CJ, van Weelden K, et al. Comparative effects of 1,25(OH)2D3 and EB1089 on cell cycle kinetics and apoptosis in MCF-7 breast cancer cells. Breast Cancer Res Treat 1997 Jan; 42(1):31–41.

[127] Furuya Y, Ohta S, Shimazaki J. Induction of apoptosis in androgen-independent mouse mammary cell line by 1, 25-dihydroxyvitamin D3. Int J Cancer 1996 Sep 27; 68(1):143–8.

[128] James SY, Mackay AG, Colston KW. Effects of 1,25 dihydroxyvitamin D3 and its analogues on induction of apoptosis in breast cancer cells. J Steroid Biochem Mol Biol 1996 Jul; 58(4):395–401.

[129] Sigounas G, Anagnostou A, Steiner M. dl-alpha-tocopherol induces apoptosis in erythroleukemia, prostate, and breast cancer cells. Nutr Cancer 1997; 28(1):30–5.

SUPPLEMENTAL MATERIAL FOR CHAPTER 4

Supplemental material for Chapter 4, "Growth Factors and Signal Transduction," consists of two tables that summarize studies on the inhibition of protein tyrosine kinase (Table E.1) and protein kinase C (Table E.2), as well as one that summarizes studies on the induction of *p21* or *p27* activity (Table E.3).

TABLE E.1 NATURAL COMPOUNDS THAT INHIBIT PROTEIN TYROSINE KINASE ACTIVITY	
COMPOUND	**EFFECTS**
Apigenin and luteolin	• Apigenin inhibited PTK intrinsic to insulin receptor: $IC_{50} = 10$ μM.[1] • Apigenin inhibited PTK intrinsic to FGF receptor: $IC_{50} = 20$ μM.[28] • Apigenin inhibited PTK isolated from bovine thymocytes: $IC_{50} = 24$ μM.[2] • Apigenin inhibited PTK intrinsic to IGF-I receptor: $IC_{50} = 48$ μM.[1] • Apigenin inhibited PTK intrinsic to PDGF receptor: $IC_{50} = 87$ μM.[28] • Apigenin inhibited PTK intrinsic to EGF receptor: $IC_{50} =$ about 91 μM.[3, 28] • Apigenin and luteolin inhibited PTK isolated from bovine thymocytes: $IC_{50} = 15$ and 14 μM, respectively.[4] • Apigenin inhibited PTK intrinsic to EGF receptor of human epidermoid carcinoma cells: $IC_{50} = 3$ μM. For PTK intrinsic to EGF receptor of sarcoma virus-transformed rat cells, the IC_{50} was 30 μM. A metabolite of apigenin, *p*-hydroxybenzoic acid, inhibited PTK intrinsic to the EGF receptor at an IC_{50} of 72 μM.[5] • Apigenin inhibited PTK intrinsic to EGF, FGF, and PDGF receptors at IC_{50}s of 90, 20, and 87 μM respectively.[6] • Luteolin (at 20 μM) inhibited PTK intrinsic to EGF receptor in epidermal cells. Quercetin was equally effective.[7]
CAPE and other caffeic acid esters	• Oral administration of CAPE (at about 45 mg/kg) inhibited PTK activity in the colon and liver of rats treated with a tumor-promoting agent.[8] • Phenylethyl dimethylcaffeate (PEDMC) and CAPE (at 50 μM) inhibited PTK activity in human colon cancer cells by 43% and 48%, respectively. Inhibition became significant at 20 and 30 μM, respectively.[9] • Inhibited PTK activity in human skin cells at concentrations of 1.8 to 18 μM.[30]
Curcumin	• Oral administration of approximately 170 mg/kg inhibited PTK intrinsic to rat liver and colon cells by an average of 31% in control rats and 42% in rats treated with a tumor-promoting agent.[10] • Inhibited PTK isolated from EGF receptor of human epidermoid carcinoma cells by 85% at 10 μM after four hours.[11] • Inhibited PTK intrinsic to the EGF receptor in human prostate cancer cells at 5 to 50 μM.[12]
EGCG	• Inhibited PTK intrinsic to EGF and PDGF receptors at IC_{50}s of 1.1 and 2.2 μM, respectively.[13]
Emodin	• Inhibited PTK isolated from bovine thymocytes: $IC_{50} = 19$ μM.[14] • Inhibited PTK in *HER-2/neu*-overexpressing human lung cancer cells at 30 μM. At this concentration, emodin inhibited cell proliferation by 67%.[15] • Inhibited PTK isolated from bovine thymocytes: $IC_{50} = 19$ μM.[4] • Inhibited PTK isolated from bovine thymocytes: $IC_{50} = 37$ μM.[16]
Genistein	• Inhibited PTK intrinsic to EGF receptor: $IC_{50} = 3$ μM. 90% inhibition at 550 μM.[3, 17] • Inhibited PTK intrinsic to EGF receptor: $IC_{50} = 22$ μM.[18] • Inhibited PTK isolated from human spleen: $IC_{50} = 125$ μM.[19] • Not effective at inhibiting PTK isolated from bovine thymocytes.[2] • Inhibited PTK isolated from human colon cancer cells treated with a tumor-promoting agent: 32% decrease at 60 μM.[20]

TABLE E.1 NATURAL COMPOUNDS THAT INHIBIT PROTEIN TYROSINE KINASE ACTIVITY *(continued)*

COMPOUND	EFFECTS
Hypericin[*]	• **Hypericin:** • Inhibited PTK intrinsic to insulin receptor: IC_{50} = about 0.02 μM (under high light).[21, 43] • Inhibited PTK intrinsic to EGF receptor: IC_{50} = about 0.07 μM (under high light).[21, 22, 43] • Inhibited PTK intrinsic to EGF receptor: IC_{50} = 0.4 μM (under subdued light).[22] **Pseudohypericin:** • Inhibited PTK intrinsic to insulin receptor: IC_{50} = 0.01 μM (under high light).[43] • Inhibited PTK intrinsic to EGF receptor: IC_{50} = 0.03 μM (under high light).[43]
Parthenolide	• Inhibited PTK activity in stimulated macrophages at 20 μM.[23]
Quercetin	• Inhibited kinases such as PTK (EGF-stimulated) and PKC at an IC_{50} of about 10 μM.[24] • Inhibited membrane PTK of leukemia cells at an IC_{50} of 24 μM.[25] • In five studies, inhibited PTK intrinsic to EGF receptor at 0.4 to 50 μM (average 22 μM).[26]
Resveratrol	• Inhibited PTK in stimulated human leukocytes at 110 μM and above.[27] • Inhibited PTK from bovine thymocytes: IC_{50} = 263 μM.[16]

[*] *Unlike that caused by flavonoids such as quercetin, the inhibition of PTK by hypericin is irreversible. High light conditions resemble light on a sunny summer day, and subdued light conditions resemble light on a cloudy winter day.*

TABLE E.2 NATURAL COMPOUNDS THAT INHIBIT PROTEIN KINASE C ACTIVITY

COMPOUND	EFFECTS
Apigenin	• Inhibited PKC isolated from mouse skin cells: IC_{50} = 10 μM. The IC_{50} of PKC in intact cells was 40 μM. At 25 μM, inhibited proliferation of mouse cells stimulated with a tumor-promoting agent.[28] • Inhibited PKC isolated from rat brain: about 35% inhibition at 50 μM.[29] • Inhibited PKC isolated from fibroblast cells: IC_{50} = 10 μM. In intact cells, the IC_{50} was approximately 40 μM.[6]
CAPE	• Inhibited PKC activity in human skin cells at concentrations of 1.8 to 18 μM.[30]
Curcumin	• At 15 μM, curcumin inhibited PKC produced by mouse fibroblast cells in response to stimulation with a tumor-promoting agent. Membrane-bound PKC activity was inhibited by 69%. Cytosolic PKC activity was not affected. (Curcumin is lipophilic, and therefore has its greatest effects on membrane-bound PKC.[31]) • Did not inhibit PKC isolated from rat brain at concentrations as high as 200 μM.[32] • Curcumin's ability to inhibit PKC may be affected by the iron content of cells. Curcumin alone reversibly inhibited isolated PKC with an IC_{50} of 15 μM. In the presence of thiol agents, however, the IC_{50} was 105 μM. When curcumin was in the form of an iron complex, irreversible inhibition was observed at an IC_{50} of 3 μM. In cells with ample intracellular iron, the ability of curcumin to inhibit PKC may be increased dramatically.[33] • PKC in intact fibroblast cells: 69% inhibition in particulate fraction at 15 μM after 30 minutes.[6]
EGCG	• Inhibited PKC at an IC_{50} of 14 to 60 μM.[34] • Inhibited PKC at an IC_{50} of about 3 μM.[35] • Green tea polyphenol extract (80% EGCG) inhibited PKC at an IC_{50} of 5.5 μM.[36]
Emodin	• Inhibited PKC isolated from rat brain: IC_{50} = 25 μM. The IC_{50} of a related anthraquinone, chrysophanic acid, was 32 μM.[37] • Not effective at inhibiting PKC.[4] • Not effective at inhibiting PKC.[38]

TABLE E.2 NATURAL COMPOUNDS THAT INHIBIT PROTEIN KINASE C ACTIVITY *(continued)*	
COMPOUND	**EFFECTS**
Hypericin	**Hypericin:** • Inhibited PKC isolated from rat brain: $IC_{50} = 4$ µM (subdued light). Inhibited proliferation of *ras*-transformed mouse fibroblast cells at an IC_{50} of about 12 µM.[39, 40] • Inhibited PKC isolated from rat brain at 0.1 µM (under subdued light).[41] • Inhibited PKC isolated from rat pituitary adenoma cells: 60% inhibition after two hours at 10 µM (dark conditions).[42] • Inhibited PKC at an IC_{50} of about 0.02 µM (under strong light). Hypericin also inhibited two other related kinases: CK-2, at an IC_{50} of 0.006 µM, and MAPK, at an IC_{50} of 0.004 µM.[21, 43] • Inhibited PKC in bovine retinal cells: 72% inhibition at 2.5 µM (under light).[44] **Pseudohypericin:** • Inhibited PKC isolated from rat brain: $IC_{50} = 29$ µM (subdued light). Inhibited the proliferation of *ras*-transformed mouse cells at an IC_{50} of 54 µM.[39] • Inhibited PKC at an IC_{50} of 0.01 µM (under strong light).[43]
Luteolin	• Inhibited PKC isolated from rat brain: 70% inhibition at 50 µM.[29]
Omega-3 fatty acids (EPA and DHA)	• A number of studies have suggested that omega-3 fatty acids reduce PKC activity.[45] In contrast, diets high in omega-6 fatty acids increased PKC activity in mouse skin. Unsaturated fatty acids induced greater activation than saturated fatty acids.[46] • EPA inhibited PKC isolated from a variety of sources. The effect became apparent at about 100 µM and reached 50% inhibition at about 800 µM. • DHA facilitated PKC activity in vitro at an optimal concentration of 20 to 50 µM.[47, *] In mice fed either EPA- or DHA-enriched diets, however, DAG production in lymphocytes was suppressed relative to mice fed arachidonic or omega-6-fatty-acid-enriched diets.[48] • Rats treated with a cancer-promoting agent and a diet high in corn oil (which contains omega-6 fatty acids) showed increased level of colon cell PKC as compared to rats fed the tumor promoter and a diet high in fish oil.[49]
Quercetin	• Inhibited kinases such as PTK and PKC (from rat brain) at an IC_{50} of about 10 µM.[24] • Inhibited cytosolic PKC of leukemia cells at an IC_{50} of 31 µM.[25] • In four experiments, quercetin inhibited PKC at 8 to 83 µM (average 33 µM). A fifth experiment reported no effect.[26]
Selenium	• Inhibited PKC activity and neoplastic transformation at about 2 to 10 µM.[50, 51] • Methylselenocysteine inhibited PKC activity in mouse breast cancer cells at 50 µM.[52]
Vitamin E	• Physiologic concentrations of vitamin E inhibited PKC activity in a variety of cells. Intraperitoneal administration of 40 mg/kg also reduced PKC activity in vascular tissues of rats.[53] • Inhibited bovine brain PKC at an IC_{50} of 450 µM; however, inhibition may start as low as 10 µM in some cases.[54] • Inhibited PKC activity in stimulated smooth muscle cells by 30% to 70% at 50 µM.[55, 56] • Inhibited PKC in smooth muscle cells at 50 µM.[57] • Inhibited PKC activity in hamster ovary cells by 30% at 50 µM.[58] • Administration of 400 I.U. of vitamin E inhibited platelet aggregation in humans, due to a reduction in PKC activity.[59]

This increase in PKC activity was observed in the presence of low concentrations of phospholipids (phosphatidylserine, 8 µg/ml). Omega-3 fatty acids appear to inhibit PKC activity by competing with phospholipids, which are PKC stimulators. Therefore, at higher phospholipid concentrations, DHA may also inhibit PKC, as was demonstrated with EPA (using 100 µg/ml phospholipids). At low phospholipid concentrations, EPA also stimulated PKC activity but did so 30% less than arachidonic acid.

TABLE E.3 NATURAL COMPOUNDS THAT INDUCE *p21* OR *p27* ACTIVITY	
COMPOUND	**EFFECTS**
1,25-D$_3$	• Induced *p21* and *p27* in leukemia cells at 100 nM.[60] • Induced *p21* in osteosarcoma cells at 10 nM.[61] • Induced *p21* and *p27* in breast cancer cells at 500 nM.[62] • Induced *p21* and *p27* in leukemia cells at 0.1 to 100 nM.[63]
Apigenin	• Induced *p21* in human fibroblasts at 10 to 70 μM.[64]
ATRA	• Induced *p21* in leukemia cells at 100 nM.[65]
EGCG	• Induced *p21* in breast cancer cells at 30 μM.[66] • At 50 μM EGCG induced *p21* in breast epithelial cells stimulated by EGF.[67]
Genistein	• Induced *p21* in melanoma cells at 10 to 30 μM.[68] • Induced *p21* in lung cancer cells at 30 μM.[69]
Silymarin	• Induced *p21* in breast cancer cells at about 52 μM.[70]
Vitamin E*	• Induced *p21* in colorectal cancer cells at 500 to 10,000 μM.[71]
* *Vitamin E succinate (VES), a water-soluble form of vitamin E.*	

REFERENCES

[1] Fujita-Yamaguchi Y, Kathuria S. Characterization of receptor tyrosine-specific protein kinases by the use of inhibitors. Staurosporine is a 100-times more potent inhibitor of insulin receptor than IGF-I receptor. Biochem and Biophys Res Commun 1988 Dec 30; 157(3):955–62.

[2] Geahlen RL, Koonchanok NM, McLaughlin JL, Pratt DE. Inhibition of protein-tyrosine kinase activity by flavanoids and related compounds. J Nat Prod 1989 Sep–Oct; 52(5):982–6.

[3] Akiyama T, Ishida J, Nakagawa S, et al. Genistein, a specific inhibitor of tyrosine-specific protein kinases. J Biol Chem 1987; 262(12):5592–5595.

[4] Chang CJ, Ashendel CL, Geahlen RL, et al. Oncogene signal transduction inhibitors from medicinal plants. In Vivo 1996; 10:185–90.

[5] Ogawara H, Akiyama T, Ishida J, et al. A specific inhibitor for tyrosine protein kinase from Pseudomonas. J Antibiotics 1986; 39:606–608.

[6] Lin JK, Chen YC, Huang YT, Lin-Shiau SY. Suppression of protein kinase C and nuclear oncogene expression as possible molecular mechanisms of cancer chemoprevention by apigenin and curcumin. J Cell Biochem Suppl 1997; 28/29:39–48.

[7] Huang Y, Hwang JJ, Lee PP, et al. Effects of luteolin and quercetin, inhibitors of tyrosine kinase, on cell growth and metastasis-associated properties in A431 cells overexpressing epidermal growth factor receptor. Br J Pharmacol 1999 Nov; 128(5):999–1010.

[8] Rao CV, Desai D, Simi B, et al. Inhibitory effect of caffeic acid esters on azoxymethane-induced biochemical changes and aberrant crypt foci formation in rat colon. Cancer Res 1993 Sep 15; 53(18):4182–8.

[9] Rao CV, Desai D, Kaul B, et al. Effect of caffeic acid esters on carcinogen-induced mutagenicity and human colon adenocarcinoma cell growth. Chem Biol Interact 1992 Nov 16; 84(3):277–90.

[10] Rao CV, Simi B, Reddy BS. Inhibition by dietary curcumin of azoxymethane-induced ornithine decarboxylase, tyrosine protein kinase, arachidonic acid metabolism and aberrant crypt foci formation in the rat colon. Carcinogenesis 1993; 14(11):2219–2225.

[11] Korutla L, Kumar R. Inhibitory effect of curcumin on epidermal growth factor receptor kinase activity in A431 cells. Biochimica Biophysica Acta 1994; 1224:597–600.

[12] Dorai T, Gehani N, Katz A. Therapeutic potential of curcumin in human prostate cancer. II. Curcumin inhibits tyrosine kinase activity of epidermal growth factor receptor and depletes the protein. Mol Urol 2000; 4(1):1–6.

[13] Liang YC, Lin-shiau SY, Chen CF, et al. Suppression of extracellular signals and cell proliferation through EGF receptor binding by (-)-epigallocatechin gallate in human A431 epidermoid carcinoma cells. J Cell Biochem 1997 Oct 1; 67(1):55–65.

[14] Jayasuriya H, Koonchanok NM, Geahlen RL, et al. Emodin, a protein tyrosine kinase inhibitor from Polygonum cuspidatum. J Nat Prod 1992; 55(5):696–8.

[15] Zhang L, Hung MC. Sensitization of HER-2/neu-overexpressing non-small cell lung cancer cells to chemotherapeutic drugs by tyrosine kinase inhibitor emodin. Oncogene 1996 Feb 1; 12(3):571–6.

[16] Jayatilake GS, Jayasuriya H, Lee ES, et al. Kinase inhibitors from Polygonum cuspidatum. J Natural Prod 1993; 56(10):1805–1810.

[17] Constantinou A, Kiguchi K, Huberman E. Induction of differentiation and DNA strand breakage in human HL-60 and K-562 leukemia cells by genistein. Cancer Res 1990; 50(9):2618–24.

[18] Akiyama T, Ogawara H. Use and specificity of genistein as inhibitor of protein tyrosine kinases. Methods in Enzymology 1991; 201:362–370.

[19] Lazaro I, Palacios C, Gonzalez M, Gonzalez-Porque P. Inhibition of human spleen protein tyrosine kinases by phenolic compounds. Analytical Biochemistry 1995; 225:180–183.

[20] Kuo ML, Huang TS, Lin JK. Preferential requirement for protein tyrosine phosphatase activity in the 12-O-tetradecanoylphorbol-13-acetate-induced differentiation of human colon cancer cells. Biochemical Pharmacology 1995; 50(8):1217–1222.

[21] Agostinis P, Vandenbogaerde A, Donella-Deana A, et al. Photosensitized inhibition of growth factor-regulated protein kinases by hypericin. Biochemical Pharmacology 1995; 49(11):1615–1622.

[22] DeWitte P, Agostinis P, Van Lint J, et al. Inhibition of epidermal growth factor receptor tyrosine kinase activity by hypericin. Biochemical Pharmacology 1993; 46(11):1929–1936.

[23] Hwang D, Fischer NH, Jang BC, et al. Inhibition of the expression of inducible cyclooxygenase and proinflammatory cytokines by sesquiterpene lactones in macrophages correlates with the inhibition of MAP kinases. Biochem Biophys Res Commun 1996 Sep 24; 226(3):810–8.

[24] End DW, Look RA, Shaffer NL, et al. Non-selective inhibition of mammalian protein kinases by flavinoids in vitro. Res Commun Chem Pathol Pharmacol 1987 Apr; 56(1):75–86.

[25] Kang TB, Liang NC. Effect of quercetin on activities of protein kinase C and tyrosine protein kinase from HL-60 cells. Chung Kuo Yao Li Hsueh Pao 1997 Jul; 18(4):374–6.

[26] Barret JM, Ernould AP, Ferry G, et al. Integrated system for the screening of the specificity of protein kinase inhibitors. Biochem Pharmacol 1993 Aug 3; 46(3):439–48.

[27] Rotondo S, Rajtar G, Manarini S, et al. Effect of trans-resveratrol, a natural polyphenolic compound, on human polymorphonuclear leukocyte function. Br J Pharmacol 1998 Apr; 123(8):1691–9.

[28] Huang YT, Kuo ML, Liu JY, et al. Inhibitions of protein kinase C and proto-oncogene expressions in NIH 3T3 cells by apigenin. European Journal of Cancer 1996; 32A(1):146–151.

[29] Ferriola PC, Cody V, Middleton E Jr. Protein kinase C inhibition by plant flavonoids. Kinetic mechanisms and structure-activity relationships. Biochem Pharmacol 1989 May 15; 38(10):1617–24.

[30] Zheng ZS, Xue GZ, Grunberger D, et al. Caffeic acid phenethyl ester inhibits proliferation of human keratinocytes and interferes with the EGF regulation of ornithine decarboxylase. Oncol Res 1995; 7(9):445–52.

[31] Liu JY, Lin SJ, Lin JK. Inhibitory effects of curcumin on protein kinase C activity induced by 12-O-tetradecanoyl-phorbol-13-acetate in NIH 3T3 cells. Carcinogenesis 1993; 14(5):857–861.

[32] Huang MT, Lysz T, Ferraro T, et al. Inhibitory activities of curcumin on in vitro lipoxygenase and cyclooxygenase activities in mouse epidermis. Cancer Res 1991; 51:813–819.

[33] Gopalakrishna R, Gundimeda U, Chen ZH. Curcumin irreversibly inactivates protein kinase C activity and phorbol ester binding: Its possible role in cancer chemoprevention. Advances in Exp Med and Biol 1996; 401:275.

[34] Kitano K, Nam KY, Kimura S, et al. Sealing effects of (-)-epigallocatechin gallate on protein kinase C and protein phosphatase 2A. Biophys Chem 1997 Apr 22; 65(2–3):157–64.

[35] Yoshizawa S, Horiuchi T, Fujiki H, et al. Antitumor promoting activity of (-)-epigallocatechin gallate, the main constituent of "tannin" in green tea. Phytotherapy Res 1987; 1(1):44–47.

[36] Komori A, Yatsunami J, Okabe S, et al. Anticarcinogenic activity of green tea polyphenols. Jpn J Clin Oncol 1993; 23(3):186–90.

[37] Jinsart W, Ternai B, Polya GM. Inhibition of myosin light chain kinase, cAMP-dependent protein kinase, protein kinase C and of plant Ca2-dependent protein kinase by anthraquinones. Biol. Chem 1992; 373:903–910.

[38] Yim H, Lee YH, Lee CH, Lee SK. Emodin, an anthraquinone derivative isolated from the rhizomes of Rheum palmatum, selectively inhibits the activity of casein kinase II as a competitive inhibitor. Planta Med 1999 Feb; 65(1):9–13.

[39] Takahashi I, Nakanishi S, Kobayashi E, et al. Hypericin and pseudohypericin specifically inhibit protein kinase C: Possible relation to their antiretroviral activity. Biochem Biophys Res Commun 1989 Dec 29; 165(3):1207–12.

[40] Tamaoki T, Takahashi I, Kobayashi E, et al. Calphostin (UCN1028) and calphostin related compounds, a new class of specific and potent inhibitors of protein kinase C. Adv Second Messenger Phosphoprotein Res 1990; 24:497–501.

[41] Utsumi T, Okuma M, Utsumi T, et al. Light-dependent inhibition of protein kinase C and superoxide generation of neutrophils by hypericin, an antiretroviral agent. Arch Biochem Biophys 1995 Jan 10; 316(1):493–7.

[42] Hamilton HB, Hinton DR, Law RE, et al. Inhibition of cellular growth and induction of apoptosis in pituitary adenoma cell lines by the protein kinase C inhibitor hypericin: Potential therapeutic application. J Neurosurgery 1996; 85:329–334.

[43] Agostinis P, Donella-Deana A, Cuveele J. A comparative analysis of the photosensitized inhibition of growth-factor regulated protein kinases by hypericin-derivatives. Biochem Biophys Res Commun 1996 Mar 27; 220(3):613–7.

[44] Harris MS, Sakamoto T, Kimura H, et al. Hypericin inhibits cell growth and induces apoptosis in retinal pigment epithelial cells: Possible involvement of protein kinase C. Curr Eye Res 1996; 15(3):255–262.

[45] McCarty MF. Fish oil may impede tumour angiogenesis and invasiveness by down-regulating protein kinase C and modulating eicosanoid production. Med Hypotheses 1996 Feb; 46(2):107–15.

[46] Birt DF. Dietary modulation of epidermal protein kinase C: Mediation by diacylglycerol. J Nutr 1995 Jun; 125(6 Suppl):1673S-1676S.

[47] Shinomura T, Asaoka Y, Oka M, et al. Synergistic action of diacylglycerol and unsaturated fatty acids for protein kinase C activation: Its possible implications. Proc Natl Acad Sci USA 1991; 99:5149–5153.

[48] Jolly CA, Jiang YH, Chapkin RS, McMurray DN. Dietary (n-3) polyunsaturated fatty acids suppress murine lymphoproliferation, interleukin-2 secretion, and the formation of diacylglycerol and ceramide. J Nutr 1997 Jan; 127(1):37–43.

[49] Reddy BS, Simi B, Patel N, et al. Effect of amount and types of dietary fat on intestinal bacterial 7 alpha-dehydroxylase and phosphatidylinositol-specific phospholipase C and colonic mucosal diacylglycerol kinase and PKC activities during stages of colon tumor promotion. Cancer Res 1996 May 15; 56(10):2314–20.

[50] Su HD, Shoji M, Mazzei GJ, et al. Effects of selenium compounds on phospholipid/Ca2+-dependent protein kinase (protein kinase C) system from human leukemic cells. Cancer Res 1986 Jul; 46(7):3684–7.

[51] Gopalakrishna R, Chen ZH, Gundimeda U. Selenocompounds induce a redox modulation of protein kinase C in the cell, compartmentally independent from cytosolic glutathione: Its role in inhibition of tumor promotion. Arch Biochem Biophys 1997 Dec 1; 348(1):37–48.

[52] Sinha R, Kiley SC, Lu JX, et al. Effects of methylselenocysteine on PKC activity, cdk2 phosphorylation and gadd gene expression in synchronized mouse mammary epithelial tumor cells. Cancer Lett 1999 Nov 15; 146(2):135–45.

[53] Traber MG, Packer L. Vitamin E: Beyond antioxidant function. Am J Clin Nutr 1995 Dec; 62(6 Suppl):1501S-1509S.

[54] Mahoney CW, Azzi A. Vitamin E inhibits protein kinase C activity. Biochem Biophys Res Commun 1988 Jul 29; 154(2):694–7.

[55] Boscoboinik DO, Chatelain E, Bartoli GM. Inhibition of protein kinase C activity and vascular smooth muscle cell growth by d-alpha-tocopherol. Biochim Biophys Acta 1994 Dec 30; 1224(3):418–26.

[56] Clement S, Tasinato A, Boscoboinik D, Azzi A. The effect of alpha-tocopherol on the synthesis, phosphorylation and activity of protein kinase C in smooth muscle cells after phorbol 12-myristate 13-acetate down-regulation. Eur J Biochem 1997 Jun 15; 246(3):745–9.

[57] Ricciarelli R, Tasinato A, Clement S, et al. Alpha-tocopherol specifically inactivates cellular protein kinase C alpha by changing its phosphorylation state. Biochem J 1998 Aug 15; 334 (Pt 1):243–9.

[58] Fazzio A, Marilley D, Azzi A. The effect of alpha-tocopherol and beta-tocopherol on proliferation, protein kinase C activity and gene expression in different cell lines. Biochem Mol Biol Int 1997 Jan; 41(1):93–101.

[59] Freedman JE, Farhat JH, Loscalzo J, Keaney JF Jr. Alpha-tocopherol inhibits aggregation of human platelets by a protein kinase C-dependent mechanism. Circulation 1996 Nov 15; 94(10):2434–40.

[60] Liu M, Lee MH, Cohen M, et al. Transcriptional activation of the Cdk inhibitor p21 by vitamin D3 leads to the induced differentiation of the myelomonocytic cell line U937. Genes Dev 1996 Jan 15; 10(2):142–53.

[61] Matsumoto T, Sowa Y, Ohtani-Fujita N, et al. p53-independent induction of WAF1/Cip1 is correlated with osteoblastic differentiation by vitamin D3. Cancer Lett 1998 Jul 3; 129(1):61–8.

[62] Verlinden L, Verstuyf A, Convents R, et al. Action of 1,25(OH)2D3 on the cell cycle genes, cyclin D1, p21 and p27 in MCF-7 cells. Mol Cell Endocrinol 1998 Jul 25; 142(1–2):57–65.

[63] Muto A, Kizaki M, Yamato K, et al. 1,25-Dihydroxyvitamin D3 induces differentiation of a retinoic acid-resistant acute promyelocytic leukemia cell line (UF-1) associated with expression of p21(WAF1/CIP1) and p27(KIP1). Blood 1999 Apr 1; 93(7):2225–33.

[64] Lepley DM, Pelling JC. Induction of p21/WAF1 and G1 cell-cycle arrest by the chemopreventive agent apigenin. Mol Carcinog 1997 Jun; 19(2):74–82.

[65] Liu M, Iavarone A, Freedman LP. Transcriptional activation of the human p21(WAF1/CIP1) gene by retinoic acid receptor. Correlation with retinoid induction of U937 cell differentiation. J Biol Chem 1996 Dec 6; 271(49):31723–8.

[66] Liang YC, Lin-Shiau SY, Chen CF, Lin JK. Inhibition of cyclin-dependent kinases 2 and 4 activities as well as induction of Cdk inhibitors p21 and p27 during growth arrest of human breast carcinoma cells by (-)-epigallocatechin-3-gallate. J Cell Biochem 1999 Oct 1; 75(1):1–12.

[67] Liberto M, Cobrinik D. Growth factor-dependent induction of p21(CIP1) by the green tea polyphenol, epigallocatechin gallate. Cancer Lett 2000 Jun 30; 154(2):151–61.

[68] Kuzumaki T, Kobayashi T, Ishikawa K. Genistein induces p21(Cip1/WAF1) expression and blocks the G1 to S phase transition in mouse fibroblast and melanoma cells. Biochem Biophys Res Commun 1998 Oct 9; 251(1):291–5.

[69] Lian F, Li Y, Bhuiyan M, Sarkar FH. p53-independent apoptosis induced by genistein in lung cancer cells. Nutr Cancer 1999; 33(2):125–31.

[70] Zi X, Feyes DK, Agarwal R. Anticarcinogenic effect of a flavonoid antioxidant, silymarin, in human breast cancer cells MDA-MB 468: Induction of G1 arrest through an increase in Cip1/p21 concomitant with a decrease in kinase activity of cyclin-dependent kinases and associated cyclins. Clin Cancer Res 1998 Apr; 4(4):1055–64.

[71] Chinery R, Brockman JA, Peeler MO, et al. Antioxidants enhance the cytotoxicity of chemotherapeutic agents in colorectal cancer: A p53-independent induction of p21WAF1/CIP1 via C/EBPbeta. Nat Med 1997 Nov; 3(11):1233–41.

SUPPLEMENTAL MATERIAL FOR CHAPTER 8

This appendix contains three tables that provide supplemental material for Chapter 8, "Natural Inhibitors of Angiogenesis." Table F.1 summarizes studies on the prevention of increased vascular permeability. Table F.2 summarizes studies on the ability of natural compounds to beneficially affect prostanoid and leukotriene synthesis; such compounds increase production of 3-series prostanoids and 5-series leukotrienes, derived from omega-3 fatty acids, or inhibit production of 2-series prostanoids and 4-series leukotrienes, derived from omega-6 fatty acids. Table F.3 summarizes studies on the inhibition of mast cell granulation by natural compounds.

TABLE F.1 NATURAL COMPOUNDS THAT INHIBIT INCREASED VASCULAR PERMEABILITY	
COMPOUND	**EFFECTS**
Anthocyanidins	Anthocyanidins from bilberry inhibited increased vascular permeability and protected vascular tone in hamsters and rats. Oral doses of standardized bilberry extracts (25% anthocyanins) reduced skin vascular permeability elevated by chloroform in rabbits.[1–5] These effects may be due to the ability of anthocyanidins to protect collagen, which in blood vessel walls provides structural integrity and plays an important role in controlling vascular permeability.
Butcher's broom	Butcher's broom has a long history of use in treating hemorrhoids and varicose veins in humans. It is reported to be effective after oral administration.[6–12] Both in vitro and in vivo, it caused vasoconstriction and inhibited increased vascular permeability induced by a variety of agents.
Centella asiatica	The total triterpene fraction of *Centella asiatica* (TTFCA) has been used clinically for venous insufficiency. Double-blind studies have provided strong evidence of its effectiveness. It reduced edema and capillary permeability, and improved other microcirculatory parameters.[13–17]
Horse chestnut	Horse chestnut has been used orally in humans to treat hemorrhoids and edema. It improves venous tone, scavenges free radicals, and may inhibit the enzymatic breakdown of the basement membrane. In vitro, it also decreased capillary permeability that was increased by a variety of agents. Given orally or intravenously, it inhibited experimentally induced brain and paw edema, and lowered capillary permeability in rodents. It has effectively treated venous insufficiency in humans.[6, 18–27]
Proanthocyanidins	Proanthocyanidins have a high affinity for vascular tissue and have improved the integrity of the vascular wall.[28, 29] In vitro and in vivo, they have lowered both vascular permeability and the enzymatic breakdown of basement membrane induced by a variety of agents.[30] Oral administration of 30 mg/kg prevented chemically induced increases in blood-brain barrier permeability in rats; the human equivalent is about 490 milligrams. Oral administration of 200 mg/kg per day prevented chemically induced brain infarction in rats.[31, 32] The human equivalent is about 3.2 grams. Oral administration of 400 mg/kg per day protected rats from acute postoperative edema.[33] The human equivalent is about 6.4 grams. An oral dose of 300 mg/day inhibited postoperative edema in humans.[34] An oral dose of 100 mg/day was effective at reducing uncomplicated venous insufficiency in humans.[35] An oral dose of 150 mg/day increased capillary resistance in hypertensive and diabetic patients.[36]

TABLE F.2   NATURAL COMPOUNDS THAT BENEFICIALLY AFFECT PROSTANOID AND LEUKOTRIENE SYNTHESIS

COMPOUND	EFFECTS
Boswellic acid	• Boswellic acid inhibited the lipoxygenase pathway, specifically 5-lipoxygenase activity and 5-HETE production. It also produced anti-inflammatory effects in animals. The IC_{50} for 5-lipoxygenase was 1.5 to 33 µM. The effects of boswellic acid on lipoxygenase appeared to be independent of any antioxidant activity.[37–48]
CAPE and bee propolis	• Propolis has a history of use as an anti-inflammatory agent. Oral administration of propolis extract (at 240 mg/kg) significantly suppressed prostaglandin and leukotriene generation by mouse macrophages in vivo and suppressed the lipoxygenase pathway during inflammation. The equivalent human dose is about 2.3 grams per day. Of its constituents, caffeic acid phenethyl ester (CAPE) was the most potent inhibitor.[49–52] • CAPE inhibited 5-lipoxygenase at an IC_{50} of about 8 µM.[53] • Oral administration (about 45 mg/kg) of CAPE inhibited leukotriene synthesis in the colon and liver of rats treated with a tumor-promoting agent.[54] • At 9 µM, CAPE suppressed production of PGE_2 in stimulated human skin cells, and at concentrations above 35 µM it inhibited COX-2 activity. An intraperitoneal dose of 30 mg/kg inhibited PGE_2 production in rats, and an intraperitoneal dose of 100 mg/kg reduced COX-2 expression.[55] The equivalent human oral doses are about 1.1 and 3.6 grams, respectively.
Curcumin	• Curcumin inhibited 5-lipoxygenase, 12-lipoxygenase, and cyclooxygenase in vitro. Its effect on lipoxygenases may be due in part to its antioxidant activity.[41, 56, 57] • Oral administration of approximately 170 mg/kg of curcumin inhibited synthesis of various leukotrienes in rat liver and colon cells. In vitro, it inhibited leukotriene production in these cells by an average of 28% at 10 µM and 64% at 50 µM.[58] • In stimulated mouse skin cells, curcumin (at 3 µM) decreased the production of 5-HETE and 8-HETE by 40% and PGE_2 production by 42%.[59] • Curcumin inhibited 5-HETE production at an IC_{50} between 3 and 10 µM.[60] • Curcumin inhibited COX-2 expression in epithelial cells at 10 to 20 µM.[61]
EPA and DHA	• EPA inhibited leukotriene B_4 synthesis in rat lung macrophages at an IC_{50} of about 2 µM. Low concentrations of EPA may compete with arachidonic acid as a phospholipase A_2 (PLA_2) substrate.[62, 63] PLA_2 is the enzyme that releases fatty acids for the synthesis of eicosanoids. • EPA reduced the ability of rat macrophages to produce 5-HETE in vitro.[64] • EPA (at 1 µM) inhibited COX-2 activity in human mast cells in vitro.[65] • DHA (at 4% in diet) partially suppressed the growth of human breast cancer cells in mice and reduced angiogenesis. Inhibition of angiogenesis appeared due to reduced PGE_2 and 12- and 15-HETE synthesis.[66] The equivalent human dose is about 46 grams per day. • Oral administration of fish oil (at 18% of diet) inhibited COX-1 and COX-2 synthesis in chemically induced breast cancers in rats by 28% and 36%, respectively.[67] • Fish oil administration (at 20% of diet) reduced COX-2 expression in chemically induced colon tumors and in colon tissue in rats. COX-1 expression was not affected.[68]
Flavonoids	• As a group, flavonoids inhibit the cyclooxygenase and lipoxygenase pathways and also the activity of other enzymes involved with arachidonic acid metabolism, such as phospholipase A_2. Enzyme inhibition has been reported for quercetin, luteolin, and apigenin. Although the potency varies for different enzymes under different conditions, inhibition is generally in the low micromolar range. Through inhibition of these and other enzymes, topical and intraperitoneal administration of flavonoids decreased the inflammatory response in rodents. In in-vitro studies, genistein, apigenin, and quercetin all inhibited COX-2 activity at concentrations below 40 µM (often below 15 µM).[69–79] • EGCG inhibited leukotriene LTB_4 release from stimulated rat peritoneal cells at concentrations above 10 µM. EGCG was the most potent of the green tea catechins.[80]

TABLE F.2 NATURAL COMPOUNDS THAT BENEFICIALLY AFFECT PROSTANOID AND LEUKOTRIENE SYNTHESIS *(continued)*	
COMPOUND	**EFFECTS**
Garlic	• Inhibited the cyclooxygenase and lipoxygenase pathways of eicosanoid production.[56, 81]
Glutathione-enhancing agents	• Cellular redox may modulate arachidonic acid metabolism, and in some studies prostaglandin synthesis was inhibited by normal concentrations of intracellular glutathione.[82, 83] A number of antioxidants, including vitamin C, are able to increase intracellular glutathione levels.
Melatonin	• Melatonin (at 100 nM) markedly downregulated the expression of the 5-lipoxygenase gene in human B lymphocyte; it appears to affect the gene via its ability to bind to retinoid nuclear receptors.[84] • Melatonin inhibited linoleic acid (omega-6 fatty acid) uptake and eicosanoid metabolism by liver cancer cells at physiologic concentrations (1 nM) in vivo. Tumor growth was also inhibited.[85]
NF-κB Inhibitors (see Tables 5.1 and 5.2)	• NF-κB activity can affect the expression of cyclooxygenase genes. In many cases, PGE_2 production by macrophages may be dependent on NF-κB activation.[86] Thus, NF-κB inhibitors may reduce eicosanoid production. For example, melatonin inhibited 5-lipoxygenase production in vitro.[84, 87]
Parthenolide	• Inhibited 5-lipoxygenase activity at an IC_{50} of 20 to 200 μM in rat and human leukocytes.[88] • Inhibited 5-lipoxygenase activity at an IC_{50} of 33 μM in human platelets.[89] • Inhibited COX-2 activity at an IC_{50} of 0.8 μM.[90]
PTK inhibitors (see Table 4.2 and the entry for flavonoids above)	• PTK activity may mediate the activation of phospholipase A_2, which releases arachidonic acid from the plasma membrane for use in the production of prostanoids and leukotrienes. This has been demonstrated for genistein, which inhibited PGE_2 production (IC_{50} = 20 μM) and leukotriene LTC_4 production.[91, 92] • Genistein inhibited leukotriene LTB_4 production by stimulated leukocytes.[93] • Genistein (at 37 μM) completely inhibited leukotriene production in leukemia cells.[94] • Genistein inhibited the activities of LTB_4 once it was produced. This leukotriene appears to require PTK activity to exert its effect.[95, 96, 97]
Resveratrol	• Inhibited 5-HETE production in human and rat leukocytes at an IC_{50} of 3 to 9 μM.[98, 99] • Inhibited 5-lipoxygenase activity in human leukocytes at an IC_{50} of 48 μM.[100] • Inhibited COX-2 activity in human breast cells at concentrations above 2.5 μM.[101] • Inhibited COX-1 activity at an IC_{50} of 15 μM but did not affect COX-2 activity.[102]
Vitamin E	• Oral administration of vitamin E decreased production of 5-HETE by rat leukocytes.[103] • In vitamin E deficient rats, increased macrophage 5-HETE production was observed.[104] • Vitamin E inhibited phospholipase A_2 activity both in vitro and in vivo.[105]

TABLE F.3 NATURAL COMPOUNDS THAT INHIBIT MAST CELL GRANULATION IN VITRO	
COMPOUND	**EFFECTS**
Eleutherococcus senticosus	• Fractions of this herb strongly inhibited histamine release from rat mast cells in a concentration-dependent manner. The most active fraction was 6,800 times stronger than disodium cromoglycate, a successful flavonoid-like antiallergy drug.[106]
Flavonoids	• Genistein inhibited histamine release from mast cells at concentrations of 10 to 100 μM.[95] • Luteolin inhibited histamine release in human basophils exposed to tumor-promoting agents. The IC_{50} was about 15 μM.[108] • Apigenin inhibited histamine release in human basophils and rat mast cells exposed to tumor-promoting agents. The IC_{50} was about 35 μM.[107–110] • Quercetin, luteolin, and apigenin inhibited mast cell degranulation at IC_{50}s of less than 10 μM.[111] Some in-vitro studies suggested that quercetin was the most effective of these flavonoids.[112, 113] • Proanthocyanidins reduced histamine levels in blood vessel tissue in vitro.[28, 114] • EGCG inhibited histamine release from stimulated rat peritoneal cells in vitro at concentrations above 10 μM.[80] • EGCG inhibited histamine release from rat basophilic leukemia cells at 100 μM.[115]
Vitamin C	• Oral administration of vitamin C (at 2 grams per day) reduced blood histamine levels by 38% in healthy humans.[116, 117] A similar effect was seen in guinea pigs.[118]

REFERENCES

[1] Bertuglia S, Malandrino S, Colantuoni A. Effect of Vaccinium myrtillus anthocyanosides on ischaemia reperfusion injury in hamster cheek pouch microcirculation. Pharmacol Res 1995 Mar–Apr; 31(3–4):183–7.

[2] Detre Z, Jellinek H, Miskulin M, Robert AM. Studies on vascular permeability in hypertension: Action of anthocyanosides. Clin Physiol Biochem 1986; 4(2):143–9.

[3] Lietti A, Cristoni A, Picci M. Studies on Vaccinium myrtillus anthocyanosides. I. Vasoprotective and antiinflammatory activity. Arzneimittelforschung 1976; 26(5):829–32.

[4] Robert AM, Godeau G, Moati F, Miskulin M. Action of anthocyanosides of Vaccinium myrtillis on the permeability of the blood brain barrier. J Med 1977; 8(5):321–32.

[5] Kadar A, Robert L, Miskulin M, et al. Influence of anthocyanoside treatment on the cholesterol-induced atherosclerosis in the rabbit. Paroi Arterielle 1979 Dec; 5(4):187–205.

[6] Murray M, Pizzorno J. Encyclopedia of natural medicine. Rocklin, CA: Prima Publishing, 1991, p. 538.

[7] Bouskela E, Cyrino FZ, Marcelon G. Inhibitory effect of the Ruscus extract and of the flavonoid hesperidine methylchalcone on increased microvascular permeability induced by various agents in the hamster cheek pouch. J Cardiovasc Pharmacol 1993 Aug; 22(2):225–30.

[8] Rudofsky G. Improving venous tone and capillary sealing. Effect of a combination of Ruscus extract and hesperidine methyl chalcone in healthy probands in heat stress. Fortschr Med 1989 Jun 30; 107(19):52, 55–8.

[9] Cluzan RV, Alliot F, Ghabboun S, Pascot M. Treatment of secondary lymphedema of the upper limb with CYCLO 3 FORT. Lymphology 1996 Mar; 29(1):29–35.

[10] Bouskela E, Cyrino FZ, Marcelon G. Possible mechanisms for the inhibitory effect of Ruscus extract on increased microvascular permeability induced by histamine in hamster cheek pouch. J Cardiovasc Pharmacol 1994 Aug; 24(2):281–5.

[11] Bouskela E, Cyrino FZ, Marcelon G. Possible mechanisms for the venular constriction elicited by Ruscus extract on hamster cheek pouch. J Cardiovasc Pharmacol 1994 Jul; 24(1):165–70.

[12] Cappelli R, Nicora M, Di Perri T. Use of extract of Ruscus aculeatus in venous disease in the lower limbs. Drugs Exp Clin Res 1988; 14(4):277–83.

[13] Cesarone MR, Laurora G, De Sanctis MT, Belcaro G. [Activity of Centella asiatica in venous insufficiency.] Minerva Cardioangiol 1992 Apr; 40(4):137–43.

[14] Cesarone MR, Laurora G, De Sanctis MT, et al. [The microcirculatory activity of Centella asiatica in venous insufficiency. A double-blind study.] Minerva Cardioangiol 1994 Jun; 42(6):299–304.

[15] Pointel JP, Boccalon H, Cloarec M, et al. Titrated extract of Centella asiatica (TECA) in the treatment of venous insufficiency of the lower limbs. Angiology 1987 Jan; 38(1 Pt 1):46–50.

[16] Belcaro GV, Rulo A, Grimaldi R. Capillary filtration and ankle edema in patients with venous hypertension treated with TTFCA. Angiology 1990 Jan; 41(1):12–8.

[17] Belcaro GV, Grimaldi R, Guidi G. Improvement of capillary permeability in patients with venous hypertension after treatment with TTFCA. Angiology 1990 Jul; 41(7):533–40.

[18] Bisler H, Pfeifer R, Kluken, et al. Effects of horse-chestnut seed extract on transcapillary filtration in chronic venous insufficiency. Dtsch Med Wochenschr 1986 Aug 29; 111(35):1321–9.

[19] Guillaume M, Padioleau F. Veinotonic effect, vascular protection, antiinflammatory and free radical scavengering properties of horse chestnut extract. Arzneim-Forsch 1994; 44(1):25–35.

[20] Longiave D, Omini C, Nicosia S, et al. The mode of action aescin on isolated veins: Relationship with PGF2.alpha. Pharmacol Res Commun 1978; 10(2):145–52.

[21] Czernicki Z. Effects of agents which increase the resistance of the vascular wall and the proteinase inhibitor trasylol on experimental brain edema. Neurol Neurochir Pol 1977; 11(4):457–60.

[22] Arnold M, Przerwa M. Therapeutic effects on experimentally induced edemas. Arzneim-Forsch 1976; 26(3):402–9.

[23] Ogura M, Suzuki K, Terumi T, et al. Antiinflammatory action of the horse chestnut saponin (amorphous aescin). Oyo Yakuri 1975; 9(6):883–94.

[24] Vogel G, Marek ML, Oertner R. Mechanisms of therapeutic and toxic actions of the horse chestnut saponin escin. Arzneim-Forsch 1970; 20(5):699–703.

[25] Vogel G, Stroecker H. Effect of pharmacologically active principles, especially flavonoids and escine, on lymph flow and permeability of the intact plasma-lymph barrier for fluids and defined macromolecules in rats. Arzneim-Forsch 1966; 16(12):1630–4.

[26] Diehm C, Trampisch HJ, Lange S, Schmidt C. Comparison of leg compression stocking and oral horse-chestnut seed extract therapy in patients with chronic venous insufficiency. Lancet 1996; 347:292–94.

[27] Hitzenberger G. The therapuetic effectiveness of chestnut extract. Wein Med Wochenschr (Austria) 1989; 139:385–9.

[28] Schwitters B, Masquelier J. OPC in practice; bioflavinoids and their application. Rome, Italy: Alfa Omega Publishers, 1993, p. 52.

[29] Facino RM, Carini M, Aldini G, et al. Free radicals scavenging action and anti-enzyme activities of procyanidines from Vitis vinifera. A mechanism for their capillary protective action. Arzneimittelforschung 1994 May; 44(5):592–601.

[30] Robert L, Godeau G, Gavignet-Jeannin C, et al. [The effect of procyanidolic oligomers on vascular permeability. A study using quantitative morphology.] Pathol Biol (Paris) 1990 Jun; 38(6):608–16.

[31] Cahn J, Borzeix MG. [Administration of procyanidolic oligomers in rats. Observed effects on changes in the permeability of the blood-brain barrier.] Sem Hop 1983; 59:2031–4.

[32] Cahn J, Borzeix MG. [Administration of procyanidolic oligomers in rats. Observed effects on changes in the cerebral biochemistry, secondary to multiple infarction.] Sem Hop 1983 Jul 7; 59(27–28):2035–8.

[33] Doutremepuich JD, Barbier A, Lacheretz F. Effect of Endotelon (procyanidolic oligomers) on experimental acute lymphedema of the rat hindlimb. Lymphology 1991 Sep; 24(3):135–9.

[34] Baruch J. Effects of endotelon in postoperative edema. Results of a double-blind study with placebo on a group of thirty-two female patients. Ann Chir Plast Esthet 1984; 29(4):393–5.

[35] Costantini A, De Bernardi T, Gotti A. [Clinical and capillaroscopic evaluation of chronic uncomplicated venous insufficiency with procyanidins extracted from vitis vinifera.] Minerva Cardioangiol 1999 Jan–Feb; 47(1–2):39–46.

[36] Lagrua G, Olivier-Martin F, Grillot A. A study of the effects of procyanidololigomers on capillary resistance in hypertension and in certain nephropathies. Sem Hop 1981; 57:1399–1401

[37] Sailer ER, Subramanian LR, Rall B, et al. Acetyl-11-keto-beta-boswellic acid (AKBA): Structure requirements for binding and 5-lipoxygenase inhibitory activity. Br J Pharmacol 1996 Feb; 117(4):615–8.

[38] Safayhi H, Sailer ER, Ammon HP. Mechanism of 5-lipoxygenase inhibition by acetyl-11-keto-beta-boswellic acid. Mol Pharmacol 1995 Jun; 47(6):1212–6.

[39] Safayhi H, Mack T, Sabieraj J, et al. Boswellic acids: Novel, specific, nonredox inhibitors of 5-lipoxygenase. J Pharmacol Exp Ther 1992 Jun; 261(3):1143–6.

[40] Gupta OP, Sharma N, Chand D. A sensitive and relevant model for evaluating anti-inflammatory activity-papaya latex-induced rat paw inflammation. J Pharmacol Toxicol Methods 1992 Aug; 28(1):15–9.

[41] Gupta OP, Sharma N, Chand D. Application of papaya latex-induced rat paw inflammation: Model for evaluation of slowly acting antiarthritic drugs. J Pharmacol Toxicol Methods 1994 Apr; 31(2):95–8.

[42] Ammon HP, Mack T, Singh GB, Safayhi H. Inhibition of leukotriene B4 formation in rat peritoneal neutrophils by an

ethanolic extract of the gum resin exudate of Boswellia serrata. Planta Med 1991 Jun; 57(3):203–7.

[43] Ammon HP, Safayhi H, Mack T, Sabieraj J. Mechanism of antiinflammatory actions of curcumine and boswellic acids. J Ethnopharmacol 1993 Mar; 38(2–3):113–9.

[44] Kulkarni RR, Patki PS, Jog VP, et al. Treatment of osteoarthritis with a herbomineral formulation: A double-blind, placebo-controlled, cross-over study. J Ethnopharmacol 1991 May–Jun; 33(1–2):91–5.

[45] Sharma ML, Bani S, Singh GB. Anti-arthritic activity of boswellic acids in bovine serum albumin (BSA)-induced arthritis. Int J Immunopharmacol 1989; 11(6):647–52.

[46] Singh GB, Atal CK. Pharmacology of an extract of salai guggal ex-Boswellia serrata, a new non-steroidal anti-inflammatory agent. Agents Actions 1986 Jun; 18(3–4):407–12.

[47] Kar A, Menon MK. Analgesic effect of the gum resin of Boswellia serata Roxb. Life Sci 1969 Oct 1; 8(19):1023–8.

[48] Safayhi H, Boden SE, Schweizer S, Ammon HP. Concentration-dependent potentiating and inhibitory effects of Boswellia extracts on 5-lipoxygenase product formation in stimulated PMNL. Planta Med 2000 Mar; 66(2):110–3.

[49] Mirzoeva OK, Calder PC. The effect of propolis and its components on eicosanoid production during the inflammatory response. Prostaglandins Leukot Essent Fatty Acids 1996 Dec; 55(6):441–9.

[50] Mirzoeva OK, Sud'ina GF, Pushkareva MA, et al. [Lipophilic derivatives of caffeic acid as lipoxygenase inhibitors with antioxidant properties.] Bioorg Khim 1995 Feb; 21(2):143–51.

[51] Khayyal MT, el-Ghazaly MA, el-Khatib AS. Mechanisms involved in the antiinflammatory effect of propolis extract. Drugs Exp Clin Res 1993; 19(5):197–203.

[52] Kimura Y, Okuda H, Okuda T, et al. Studies on the activities of tannins and related compounds X. Effects of caffeetannins and related compounds on arachidonate metabolism in human polymorphonuclear leukocytes. J Nat Prod 1987 May–Jun; 50(3):392–9.

[53] Sud'ina GF, Mirzoeva OK, Pushkareva MA. Caffeic acid phenethyl ester as a lipoxygenase inhibitor with antioxidant properties. FEBS Lett 1993 Aug 23; 329(1–2):21–4.

[54] Rao CV, Desai D, Simi B, et al. Inhibitory effect of caffeic acid esters on azoxymethane-induced biochemical changes and aberrant crypt foci formation in rat colon. Cancer Res 1993 Sep 15; 53(18):4182–8.

[55] Michaluart P, Masferrer JL, Carothers AM, et al. Inhibitory effects of caffeic acid phenethyl ester on the activity and expression of cyclooxygenase-2 in human oral epithelial cells and in a rat model of inflammation. Cancer Res 1999 May 15; 59(10):2347–52.

[56] Srivastava KC, Mustafa T. Spices: Antiplatelet activity and prostanoid metabolism. Prostaglandins Leukot Essent Fatty Acids 1989 Dec; 38(4):255–66.

[57] Flynn DL, Rafferty MF, Boctor AM. Inhibition of 5-hydroxy-eicosatetraenoic acid (5-HETE) formation in intact human neutrophils by naturally-occurring diarylheptanoids: Inhibitory activities of curcuminoids and yakuchinones. Prostaglandins Leukot Med 1986 Jun; 22(3):357–60.

[58] Rao CV, Simi B, Reddy BS. Inhibition by dietary curcumin of azoxymethane-induced ornithine decarboxylase, tyrosine protein kinase, arachidonic acid metabolism and aberrant crypt foci formation in the rat colon. Carcinogenesis 1993; 14(11):2219–2225.

[59] Huang MT, Lysz T, Ferraro T, et al. Inhibitory activities of curcumin on in vitro lipoxygenase and cyclooxygenase activities in mouse epidermis. Cancer Res 1991; 51:813–819.

[60] Conney AH, Lou YR, Xie JG, et al. Some perspectives on dietary inhibition of carcinogenesis: Studies with curcumin and tea. Proc Soc Exp Biol Med 1997 Nov; 216(2):234–45.

[61] Zhang F, Altorki NK, Mestre JR, et al. Curcumin inhibits cyclooxygenase-2 transcription in bile acid- and phorbol ester-treated human gastrointestinal epithelial cells. Carcinogenesis 1999 Mar; 20(3):445–51.

[62] Rosenthal MD, Rzigalinski BA, Blackmore PF, Franson RC. Cellular regulation of arachidonate mobilization and metabolism. Prostaglandins Leukot Essent Fatty Acids 1995 Feb–Mar; 52(2–3):93–8.

[63] Kobayashi J, Yokoyama S, Kitamura S. Eicosapentaenoic acid modulates arachidonic acid metabolism in rat alveolar macrophages. Prostaglandins Leukot Essent Fatty Acids 1995 Apr; 52(4):259–62.

[64] Chang KJ, Saito H, Tatsuno I, et al. Role of 5-lipoxygenase products of arachidonic acid in cell-to-cell interaction between macrophages and natural killer cells in rat spleen. J Leukoc Biol 1991 Sep; 50(3):273–8.

[65] Obata T, Nagakura T, Masaki T, et al. Eicosapentaenoic acid inhibits prostaglandin D2 generation by inhibiting cyclo-oxygenase-2 in cultured human mast cells. Clin Exp Allergy 1999 Aug; 29(8):1129–35.

[66] Rose DP, Connolly JM. Antiangiogenicity of docosahexaenoic acid and its role in the suppression of breast cancer cell growth in nude mice. Int J Oncol 1999 Nov; 15(5):1011–1015.

[67] Hamid R, Singh J, Reddy BS, Cohen LA. Inhibition by dietary menhaden oil of cyclooxygenase-1 and -2 in N-nitrosomethylurea-induced rat mammary tumors. Int J Oncol 1999 Mar; 14(3):523–8.

[68] Singh J, Hamid R, Reddy BS. Dietary fat and colon cancer: Modulation of cyclooxygenase-2 by types and amount of dietary fat during the postinitiation stage of colon carcinogenesis. Cancer Res 1997 Aug 15; 57(16):3465–70.

[69] Buck AC. Phytotherapy for the prostate. Br J Urol 1996 Sep; 78(3):325–36.

[70] Della Loggia R, Ragazzi E, Tubaro A, et al. Anti-inflammatory activity of benzopyrones that are inhibitors of cyclo- and lipo-oxygenase. Pharmacol Res Commun 1988 Dec; 20 Suppl 5:91–4.

[71] Welton AF, Hurley J, Will P. Flavonoids and arachidonic acid metabolism. Prog Clin Biol Res 1988; 280:301–12.

[72] Welton AF, Tobias LD, Fiedler-Nagy C, et al. Effect of flavonoids on arachidonic acid metabolism. Prog Clin Biol Res 1986; 213:231–42.

[73] Tordera M, Ferrandiz ML, Alcaraz MJ. Influence of anti-inflammatory flavonoids on degranulation and arachidonic acid release in rat neutrophils. Z Naturforsch [C] 1994 Mar–Apr; 49(3–4):235–40.

[74] Laughton MJ, Evans PJ, Moroney MA, et al. Inhibition of mammalian 5-lipoxygenase and cyclo-oxygenase by flavonoids and phenolic dietary additives. Relationship to antioxidant activity and to iron ion-reducing ability. Biochem Pharmacol 1991 Oct 9; 42(9):1673–81.

[75] Della Loggia R, Tubaro A, Dri P, et al. The role of flavonoids in the antiinflammatory activity of Chamomilla recutita. Prog Clin Biol Res 1986; 213:481–4.

[76] Goel RK, Pandey VB, Dwivedi SPD, Rao YV. Antiinflammatory and antiulcer effects of kaempferol, a flavone, isolated from Rhamnus procumbens. Ind J Exp Biol 1988; 26:121–24.

[77] Pagonis C, Tauber AI, Pavlotsky N, Simons ER. Flavonoid impairment of neutrophil response. Biochem Pharmacol 1986 Jan 15; 35(2):237–45.

[78] Liang YC, Huang YT, Tsai SH, et al. Suppression of inducible cyclooxygenase and inducible nitric oxide synthase by apigenin and related flavonoids in mouse macrophages. Carcinogenesis 1999 Oct; 20(10):1945–52.

[79] Mutoh M, Takahashi M, Fukuda K, et al. Suppression of cyclooxygenase-2 promoter-dependent transcriptional activity in colon cancer cells by chemopreventive agents with a resorcin-type structure. Carcinogenesis 2000 May; 21(5):959–963.

[80] Matsuo N, Yamada K, Yamashita K, et al. Inhibitory effect of tea polyphenols on histamine and leukotriene B4 release from rat peritoneal exudate cells. In Vitro Cell Dev Biol Anim 1996 Jun; 32(6):340–4.

[81] Sendl A, Elbl G, Steinke B, et al. Comparative pharmacological investigations of Allium ursinum and Allium sativum. Planta Med 1992 Feb; 58(1):1–7.

[82] Buckley BJ, Kent RS, Whorton AR. Regulation of endothelial cell prostaglandin synthesis by glutathione. J Biol Chem 1991; 266(25):16659–16666.

[83] Klimberg VS, Kornbluth J, Cao Y, et al. Glutamine suppresses PGE2 synthesis and breast cancer growth. J Surg Res 1996 Jun; 63(1):293–7.

[84] Steinhilber D, Brungs M, Werz O, et al. The nuclear receptor for melatonin represses 5-lipoxygenase gene expression in human B lymphocytes. J Biol Chem 1995 Mar 31; 270(13):7037–40.

[85] Blask DE, Sauer LA, Dauchy RT, et al. Melatonin inhibition of cancer growth in vivo involves suppression of tumor fatty acid metabolism via melatonin receptor-mediated signal transduction events. Cancer Res 1999 Sep 15; 59(18):4693–701.

[86] Lo CJ, Cryer HG, Fu M, Lo FR. Regulation of macrophage eicosanoid generation is dependent on nuclear factor kappaB. J Trauma 1998 Jul; 45(1):19–23; discussion 23–4.

[87] Carlberg C, Wiesenberg I. The orphan receptor family RZR/ROR, melatonin and 5-lipoxygenase: An unexpected relationship. J Pineal Res 1995 May; 18(4):171–8.

[88] Sumner H, Salan U, Knight DW, Hoult JR. Inhibition of 5-lipoxygenase and cyclo-oxygenase in leukocytes by feverfew. Involvement of sesquiterpene lactones and other components. Biochem Pharmacol 1992 Jun 9; 43(11):2313–20.

[89] Groenewegen WA, Heptinstall S. A comparison of the effects of an extract of feverfew and parthenolide, a component of feverfew, on human platelet activity in-vitro. J Pharm Pharmacol 1990 Aug; 42(8):553–7.

[90] Hwang D, Fischer NH, Jang BC, et al. Inhibition of the expression of inducible cyclooxygenase and proinflammatory cytokines by sesquiterpene lactones in macrophages correlates with the inhibition of MAP kinases. Biochem Biophys Res Commun 1996 Sep 24; 226(3):810–8.

[91] Glaser KB, Sung A, Bauer J, Weichman BM. Regulation of eicosanoid biosynthesis in the macrophage. Involvement of protein tyrosine phosphorylation and modulation by selective protein tyrosine kinase inhibitors. Biochem Pharmacol 1993 Feb 9; 45(3):711–21.

[92] Currie S, Roberts EF, Spaethe SM, et al. Phosphorylation and activation of Ca(2+)-sensitive cytosolic phospholipase A2 in MCII mast cells mediated by high-affinity Fc receptor for IgE. Biochem J 1994 Dec 15; 304 (Pt 3):923–8.

[93] Atluru D, Gudapaty S. Genistein, a selective protein tyrosine kinase inhibitor, inhibits interleukin-2 and leukotriene B4 production from human mononuclear cells. Clin Immunol Immunopathol 1991 Jun; 59(3):379–87.

[94] Hagmann W. Cell proliferation status, cytokine action and protein tyrosine phosphorylation modulate leukotriene biosynthesis in a basophil leukaemia and a mastocytoma cell line. Biochem J 1994 Apr 15; 299 (Pt 2):467–72.

[95] Wong WS, Koh DS, Koh AH, et al. Effects of tyrosine kinase inhibitors on antigen challenge of guinea pig lung in vitro. J Pharmacol Exp Ther 1997 Oct; 283(1):131–7.

[96] Gronroos E, Schippert A, Engstrom M, Sjolander A. The regulation of leukotriene D4-induced calcium influx in human epithelial cells involves protein tyrosine phosphorylation. Cell Calcium 1995 Mar; 17(3):177–86.

[97] Massoumi R, Sjolander A. The inflammatory mediator leukotriene D4 triggers a rapid reorganisation of the actin cytoskeleton in human intestinal epithelial cells. Eur J Cell Biol 1998 Jul; 76(3):185–91.

[98] Kimura Y, Okuda H, Kubo M. Effects of stilbenes isolated from medicinal plants on arachidonate metabolism and degranulation in human polymorphonuclear leukocytes. J Ethnopharmacol 1995 Feb; 45(2):131–9.

[99] Kimura Y, Okuda H, Arichi S. Effects of stilbenes on arachidonate metabolism in leukocytes. Biochim Biophys Acta 1985 Apr 25; 834(2):275–8.

[100] Rotondo S, Rajtar G, Manarini S, et al. Effect of trans-resveratrol, a natural polyphenolic compound, on human polymorphonuclear leukocyte function. Br J Pharmacol 1998 Apr; 123(8):1691–9.

[101] Subbaramaiah K, Chung WJ, Michaluart P, et al. Resveratrol inhibits cyclooxygenase-2 transcription and activity in phorbol ester-treated human mammary epithelial cells. J Biol Chem 1998 Aug 21; 273(34):21875–82.

[102] Jang M, Cai L, Udeani GO, et al. Cancer chemopreventive activity of resveratrol, a natural product derived from grapes. Science 1997 Jan 10; 275(5297):218–20.

[103] Chan AC, Tran K, Pyke DD, Powell WS. Effects of dietary vitamin E on the biosynthesis of 5-lipoxygenase products by rat polymorphonuclear leukocytes (PMNL). Biochim Biophys Acta 1989 Oct 17; 1005(3):265–9.

[104] Eskew ML, Zarkower A, Scheuchenzuber WJ, et al. Effects of inadequate vitamin E and/or selenium nutrition on the release of arachidonic acid metabolites in rat alveolar macrophages. Prostaglandins 1989 Jul; 38(1):79–89.

[105] Traber MG, Packer L. Vitamin E: Beyond antioxidant function. Am J Clin Nutr 1995 Dec; 62(6 Suppl):1501S–1509S.

[106] Umeyama A, Shoji N, Takei M, et al. Ciwujianosides D1 and C1; powerful inhibitors of histamine release induced by anti-immunoglobulin E from rat peritoneal mast cells. J Pharm Sci 1992; 81(7):661–2.

[107] Middleton E Jr; Drzewiecki G. Flavonoid inhibition of human basophil histamine release stimulated by various agents. Biochem Pharmacol 1984 Nov 1; 33(21):3333–8.

[108] Pearce FL, Befus AD, Bienenstock J. Mucosal mast cells. III. Effect of quercetin and other flavonoids on antigen-induced histamine secretion from rat intestinal mast cells. J Allergy Clin Immunol 1984 Jun; 73(6):819–23.

[109] Ogasawara H, Fujitani T, Drzewiecki G, Middleton E Jr. The role of hydorgen peroxide in pasophil histamine release and the effect of selected flavonoids. J Allergy Clin Immunol 1986 Aug; 78(2):321–8.

[110] Middleton E Jr. Some biological properties of plant flavonoids. Ann Allergy 1988 Dec; 61(6 Pt 2):53–7.

[111] Cheong H, Ryu SY, Oak MH, et al. Studies of structure activity relationship of flavonoids for the anti-allergic actions. Arch Pharm Res 1998 Aug; 21(4):478–80.

[112] Middleton E Jr, Drzewiecki G. Effects of flavonoids and transitional metal cations on antigen-induced histamine release from human basophils. Biochem Pharmacol 1982 Apr 1; 31(7):1449–53.

[113] Pearce FL, Befus AD, Bienenstock J. Mucosal mast cells. III. Effect of quercetin and other flavonoids on antigen-induced histamine secretion from rat intestinal mast cells. J Allergy Clin Immunol 1984 Jun; 73(6):819–23.

[114] Masquelier J. Natural products as medicinal agents. Planta Med 1980; 242S–256S.

[115] Matsuo N, Yamada K, Shoji K, et al. Effect of tea polyphenols on histamine release from rat basophilic leukemia (RBL-2H3) cells: The structure-inhibitory activity relationship. Allergy 1997 Jan; 52(1):58–64.

[116] Johnston CS, Martin LJ, Cai X. Antihistamine effect of supplemental ascorbic acid and neutrophil chemotaxis. J Am Coll Nutr 1992 Apr; 11(2):172–6.

[117] Johnston CS. The antihistamine action of ascorbic acid. Subcell Biochem 1996; 25:189–207.

[118] Johnston CS, Huang SN. Effect of ascorbic acid nutriture on blood histamine and neutrophil chemotaxis in guinea pigs. J Nutr 1991 Jan; 121(1):126–30.

SUPPLEMENTAL MATERIAL FOR CHAPTER 9

Supplemental material for Chapter 9, "Invasion," contains three tables. Table G.1 lists natural compounds that inhibit hyaluronidase, its assistant enzymes, or elastase; Table G.2 lists those that affect collagen; and Table G.3 those that affect immune cell and cancer cell migration.

TABLE G.1 NATURAL COMPOUNDS THAT INHIBIT HYALURONIDASE, ITS ASSISTANT ENZYMES, OR ELASTASE	
COMPOUND	**EFFECTS**
Apigenin	• Inhibited hyaluronidase by 50% or more at 50 to 250 μM.[1, 2, 3] • When mixed with injected tumor cells, apigenin (at 4 μM) inhibited tumor angiogenesis in mice.[4] • Inhibited beta-glucuronidase at an IC_{50} of about 40 μM.[5]
Boswellic acids[*]	• Oral administration of boswellic acids (at 100 mg/kg) reduced the activity of plasma beta-glucuronidase and *N*-acetylglucosaminidase and GAG synthesis and degradation in arthritic rats.[6, 7, 8] • The IC_{50} for inhibition of leukocyte elastase was 15 μM.[9]
Centella asiatica[*]	• Oral administration of the total triterpenic fraction (TTFCA) at 60 mg/day for three months to patients with varicose veins reduced the concentration of plasma beta-glucuronidase by 33%.[10]
Escin, from horse chestnut	• The IC_{50} for hyaluronidase was 150 μM.[11]
Luteolin	• Inhibited hyaluronidase by 50% or more at 100 to 250 μM.[1, 3] • Inhibited beta-glucuronidase at an IC_{50} of about 40 μM.[5]
Proanthocyanidins	• Inhibited hyaluronidase by 50% or more at 50 to 80 μM.[3, 12] • IC_{50} for porcine pancreatic elastase was 4 μM.[12] • Inhibited beta-glucuronidase at an IC_{50} of 1 μM.[12]
Resveratrol	• Inhibited secretion of elastase and beta-glucuronidase from stimulated leukocytes at IC_{50}s of 37 and 25 μM, respectively.[13]
Ruscogenin, from butcher's broom	• The IC_{50} for porcine pancreatic elastase was 120 μM.[11]
Vitamin C	• Oral administration of 1.5 grams/day reduced urinary beta-glucuronidase activity in humans. Vitamin C also inhibited this enzyme in vitro.[14] • Vitamin C inhibited *N*-acetyl-beta-glucosaminidase in vitro.[15]
[*] *Two other related triterpenes, oleanolic acid and ursolic acid, were also active as hyaluronidase and elastase inhibitors at similar concentrations.[11, 16, 17]*	

| TABLE G.2 NATURAL COMPOUNDS THAT AFFECT COLLAGEN ||
COMPOUND	EFFECTS
Anthocyanidins and proanthocyanidins	• Anthocyanidins promote collagen synthesis and stability. Anthocyanidins from *Vaccinium myrtillus* (bilberry) protected cartilage (a collagen-rich substance) by stimulating collagen cross-linking, inhibiting free radical damage and inflammation, inhibiting enzymatic degradation, and stimulating collagen synthesis. Proanthocyanidins protected collagen and inhibited collagenase activity by similar mechanisms.[12, 18–21]
Centella asiatica	• *Centella* triterpenes (at 15 to 30 μM) stimulated production of collagen by human fibroblasts in vitro and in wound chambers in rats.[22, 23, 24] Production of both collagen and fibronectin was stimulated at roughly 37 μM. GAG production was not affected.[25] Other related ursane triterpenes are also active. Ursolic acid reduced invasion of highly metastatic human fibrosarcoma cells in vitro by 80% after treatment with 10 μM. This was associated with a marked reduction in MMP-9.[26]
Curcumin	• Curcumin (at 10 μM) inhibited the invasion of liver cancer cells in vitro. This effect was associated with inhibition of MMP-9.[27]
EGCG	• EGCG (at an IC_{50} of about 9 μM) inhibited collagenases (probably MMP-2 and MMP-9) produced by mouse lung cancer cells.[28] EGCG also stimulated collagen synthesis and cross-linking.[29]
Emodin	• Inhibited bacterial collagenase at an IC_{50} 40 μM.[30]
EPA	• EPA inhibited production of type IV collagenase by mouse melanoma and human fibrosarcoma cells in vitro. Invasion of these cells was inhibited by 50% at about 1 μM. The effect may have been related to inhibition of prostaglandin and/or leukotriene production and subsequent inhibition of collagenase production. Collagenase production and invasion were restored by the addition of certain leukotrienes.[31] EPA at 3 μM reduced collagenase production by human breast cancer cells by 30%. Oral administration of about 6 g/kg EPA reduced the metastasis of breast cancer cells injected into mice. In contrast, administration of linoleic acid (found in many vegetable oils) stimulated invasion and collagenase production.[32] In other studies, DHA, but not EPA, reduced MMP-9 production in mice injected with colon cancer cells.[33]
Genistein	• Genistein (at 50 to 100 μM) reduced secretion of MMP-9 and urokinase-type plasminogen activator (uPA) in mouse breast cancer cells.[34] (Like MMP-9, uPA is involved in tumor cell invasion.) • Genistein (at 50 μM) inhibited production of MMPs and uPA in multiple cancer cell lines and increased production of TIMPs and uPA inhibitors.[35] • Genistein (at 37 to 74 μM) inhibited in-vitro invasion of human breast cancer cells via downregulation of MMP-9 and up-regulation of TIMP-1.[36] • In addition to their inhibitory effects against MMPs, TIMPs also stimulate proliferation in a wide range of cells. Genistein (at 10 μM) and other PTK inhibitors reduced TIMP-induced proliferation in human osteosarcoma cells.[37]
Leukotriene inhibitors (see Table 8.2)	• Diets rich in omega-6 fatty acids stimulated the metastasis of human breast cancer cells in mice. Omega-6 fatty acids act as a substrate for production of various eicosanoids, including the leukotriene 12-HETE. Both omega-6 fatty acids and 12-HETE induced collagenase activity in human breast cancer cells and stimulated invasion in vitro. 12-lipoxygenase inhibitors suppressed this effect.[38]
Luteolin and quercetin	• Luteolin (at 20 μM) suppressed secretion of MMP-2 and MMP-9 by epithelial cells. Quercetin was equally effective, while genistein was less effective.[39]
PSK and other mushroom polysaccharides	• PSK inhibited the attachment of tumor cells to the basement membrane, degradation of the basement membrane, and tumor cell invasion in vitro and in vivo. Metastasis of melanoma cells in mice was decreased by intraperitoneal administration of 500 mg/kg PSK every other day. The human oral equivalent is about 12 grams per day. In-vitro invasion was inhibited by about 60% at about 6 μM. A related compound, PSP (also from *Coriolus versicolor*) has shown antitumor activity in animals and has prolonged the life span of cancer patients. Although much of PSP's activity may be due to immunostimulation, enzyme inhibition may also be occurring.[40–45]

TABLE G.2 NATURAL COMPOUNDS THAT AFFECT COLLAGEN *(continued)*	
COMPOUND	**EFFECTS**
Vitamin A	• Retinoids (at 1 µM) increased the amount of collagenase inhibitors produced by growing capillary cells in vitro. ATRA tended to increase molecules similar to TIMP-2, and retinol tended to increase molecules similar to TIMP-1.[46] ATRA (at 10 µM) preferentially inhibited migration and invasion of highly invasive human melanoma cell lines as compared to less invasive melanoma cell lines. ATRA increased production of TIMP-2 and reduced production of MMP-1.[47] The effects of ATRA on invasion are complex, however, and in one study on human breast cancer cells, ATRA actually increased invasion in vitro.[48]
Vitamin C	• Vitamin C is necessary for maintenance of the extracellular matrix; it stimulated collagen synthesis in human fibroblast cells in vitro and enhanced angiogenesis in CAM assays.[49–54] It is uncertain whether it would enhance tumor angiogenesis in vivo.

TABLE G.3 EFFECTS OF NATURAL COMPOUNDS ON CELL MIGRATION	
COMPOUND	**EFFECTS**
1,25-D$_3$	• Oral administration of 0.5 µg/kg reduced invasion and metastasis of melanoma cells in mice. The effects were apparently due to reduced cell adhesion to the ECM and reduced degradation of the ECM by tumor cells.[55] The equivalent human dose is about 48 micrograms per day. • Concentrations as low as 1 nM reduced invasion of lung cancer cells in vitro.[56] • Concentrations as low as 1 nM reduced migration of human lymphocytes in response to IL-2 in vitro.[57]
Apigenin, luteolin, and quercetin	• Apigenin, luteolin, and quercetin (at 2 to 24 mg/kg, intraperitoneal) inhibited immune cell migration in a rat model of acute inflammation.[58] The equivalent human oral dose is about 0.19 to 5.1 grams. These effects appeared to be unrelated to their ability to inhibit prostaglandin synthesis. (Some prostaglandins act as attractants for immune cells.)
Boswellic acid	• Alcohol extracts of *Boswellia* inhibited immune cell migration in rats and mice.[59] • Oral administration (at 25 to 100 mg/kg per day) reduced leukocyte migration to arthritic joints in rabbits and inhibited leukocyte migration in vitro.[60] The human equivalent is about 0.73 to 2.9 grams/day.
Bromelain and other proteolytic enzymes	• Bromelain and other proteolytic enzymes such as trypsin cleaved CD44 molecules from the surface of T lymphocytes and reduced their migration.[61, 62] • Intravenous administration of bromelain (at 10 mg/kg) reduced colony-stimulating factor-induced neutrophil migration in rats.[63]
EPA/DHA	• Intraperitoneal administration of EPA, and especially DHA, decreased migration of eosinophils in response to leukotrienes in guinea pigs.[64] • Oral administration of EPA/DHA (at 9.4 and 5 grams/day, respectively) reduced migration of neutrophils in humans. This effect was due to both decreased production of leukotrienes and inhibition of leukotriene-induced and platelet activating factor-induced migration.[65] • Oral administration of EPA and DHA (at 3.2 and 2.2 grams/day, respectively) reduced neutrophil migration in heart disease patients.[66] • Oral administration of EPA (at 4 grams/day) inhibited migration of granulocytes, but not macrophages, in asthmatic humans.[67]
Genistein	• Genistein (at 37 µM) inhibited the motility of *ras*-dependent human bladder cancer cells in vitro.[68] • Low concentrations of genistein (0.37 µM) reversed the stimulatory effects of EGF and TNF on thyroid cancer cell invasion and proliferation. At higher concentrations (3.7 µM), genistein inhibited invasion and proliferation of unstimulated cancer cells.[69] • Genistein (at 37 µM) reduced hyaluronic acid-induced and RHAMM-mediated migration of *ras*-transformed fibroblasts.[70]
Hyaluronidase inhibitors (see Table 9.1)	• Compounds that inhibit hyaluronidase may decrease tumor cell migration by interfering with the ability of CD44 and RHAMM proteins to grip and release hyaluronic acid. In addition, inhibition of hyaluronidase may reduce the spread of compounds that attract immune or cancer cells (chemotactic compounds) through the extracellular matrix.

TABLE G.3 EFFECTS OF NATURAL COMPOUNDS ON CELL MIGRATION *(continued)*	
COMPOUND	**EFFECTS**
Melatonin	• At concentrations slightly higher than physiological (about 1 nM), melatonin inhibited invasion of human breast cancer cells in vitro. Very high concentrations (10 µM) were not effective.[71]
Panax ginseng	• Metabolites of ginseng inhibited migration and metastasis of lung cancer cells in vitro and in tumor-bearing mice.[72] On the other hand, oral administration of a ginseng extract (at 100 mg/day) increased leukocyte migration and phagocytosis.[73]
PKC inhibitors (see Table 4.3)	• In six human melanoma cell lines and five human brain cancer cell lines, PKC activity was directly correlated with migration and invasive ability. PKC inhibitors suppressed both migration and invasion.[74, 75] • Human neuroblastoma cells produced excessive quantities of CD44 variants in response to stimulation by insulin-like growth factor (IGF), which resulted in increased binding to hyaluronic acid. This process was prevented by treatment with PKC inhibitors.[82] • Hypericin (at 1 µM under standard laboratory light) and other PKC inhibitors reduced the motility and invasiveness of human brain cancer cells in vitro. Cell proliferation was not affected.[76]
PSK	• PSK enhanced macrophage migration but decreased tumor cell migration in vitro.[77] • Oral administration of PSK enhanced leukocyte migration and phagocytic activity and prolonged post-surgical disease-free survival periods in patients with colorectal cancer.[78] • PSK prevented sarcoma-induced suppression of macrophage migration in mice.[79]
PTK inhibitors (see Table 4.2)	• Genistein (at 37 µM) and other PTK inhibitors reduced migration of human bladder cancer cells that overexpress the EGF receptor more than that of other bladder cancer cells that overexpress the *ras* gene and not the EGF receptor.[80] • Genistein (at 10 µM) and other PTK inhibitors reduced EGF-mediated invasion of brain cancer cells in vitro at much lower concentrations than required to suppress proliferation.[81] • Phosphatidylinositol 3-kinase inhibitors (see Chapter 4) reduced the stimulatory effects of platelet-derived growth factor and IGF on CD44 variant expression in cancer cells.[82] • Genistein (at 100 µM) inhibited migration of human neutrophils in response to insulin in vitro. The effect was due to kinase inhibition.[83] • Genistein (at greater than 74 µM) inhibited random migration of human T cells in vitro. The effect was due to PTK inhibition.[84] • Genistein (at 37 µM) and PKC inhibitors reduced migration of T lymphocytes through the vascular wall in vitro. The effects of genistein were due to PTK inhibition.[85]

REFERENCES

1 Kuppusamy UR, Das NP. Inhibitory effects of flavonoids on several venom hyaluronidases. Experientia 1991 Dec 1; 47(11–12):1196–200.

2 Tung JS, Mark GE, Hollis GF. A microplate assay for hyaluronidase and hyaluronidase inhibitors. Anal Biochem 1994 Nov 15; 223(1):149–52.

3 Kuppusamy UR, Khoo HE, Das NP. Structure-activity studies of flavonoids as inhibitors of hyaluronidase. Biochem Pharmacol 1990 Jul 15; 40(2):397–401.

4 Liu D, Pearlman E, Diaconu E, et al. Expression of hyaluronidase by tumor cells induces angiogenesis in vivo. Proc Natl Acad Sci USA 1996 Jul 23; 93(15):7832–7.

5 Tordera M, Ferrandiz ML, Alcaraz MJ. Influence of anti-inflammatory flavonoids on degranulation and arachidonic acid release in rat neutrophils. Z Naturforsch [C] 1994 Mar–Apr; 49(3–4):235–40.

6 Kesava Reddy G, Dhar SC, Singh GB. Urinary excretion of connective tissue metabolites under the influence of a new

non-steroidal anti-inflammatory agent in adjuvant induced arthritis. Agents Actions 1987 Oct; 22(1–2):99–105.

[7] Kesava Reddy G, Dhar SC. Effect of a new non-steroidal anti-inflammatory agent on lysosomal stability in adjuvant induced arthritis. Ital J Biochem 1987 Jul–Aug; 36(4):205–17.

[8] Reddy GK, Chandrakasan G, Dhar SC. Studies on the metabolism of glycosaminoglycans under the influence of new herbal anti-inflammatory agents. Biochem Pharmacol 1989 Oct 15; 38(20):3527–34.

[9] Safayhi H, Rall B, Sailer ER, Ammon HPT. Inhibition by boswellic acids of human leukocyte elastase. J Pharm Exp Ther 1997; 281(1):460–63.

[10] Arpaia MR, Ferrone R, Amitrano M, et al. Effects of Centella asiatica extract on mucopolysaccharide metabolism in subjects with varicose veins. Int J Clin Pharmacol Res 1990; 10(4):229-33.

[11] Facino RM, Carini M, Stefani R, et al. Anti-elastase and anti-hyaluronidase activities of saponins and sapogenins from Hedera helix, Aesculus hippocastanum, and Ruscus aculeatus: Factors contributing to their efficacy in the treatment of venous insufficiency. Arch Pharm (Weinheim) 1995 Oct; 328(10):720–4.

[12] Facino RM, Carini M, Aldini G, et al. Free radicals scavenging action and anti-enzyme activities of procyanidines from Vitis vinifera. A mechanism for their capillary protective action. Arzneimittelforschung 1994 May; 44(5):592–601.

[13] Rotondo S, Rajtar G, Manarini S, et al. Effect of trans-resveratrol, a natural polyphenolic compound, on human polymorphonuclear leukocyte function. Br J Pharmacol 1998 Apr; 123(8):1691–9.

[14] Young JC, Kenyon EM, Calabrese EJ. Inhibition of beta-glucuronidase in human urine by ascorbic acid. Hum Exp Toxicol 1990; 9(3):165–70.

[15] Cameron E, Pauling L, Leibovitz B. Ascorbic acid and cancer: A review. Cancer Research 1979 March; 39:663–681.

[16] Safayhi H, Rall B, Sailer ER, Ammon HP. Inhibition by boswellic acids of human leukocyte elastase. J Pharmacol Exp Ther 1997 Apr; 281(1):460–3.

[17] Ying QL, Rinehart AR, Simon SR, Cheronis JC. Inhibition of human leucocyte elastase by ursolic acid. Evidence for a binding site for pentacyclic triterpenes. Biochem J 1991 Jul 15; 277 (Pt 2):521–6.

[18] Murray MT. The healing power of herbs. Rocklin, CA: Prima Publishing, 1992, pp. 224–5.

[19] Monboisse JC, Braquet P, Randoux A, et al. Non-enzymatic degradation of acid-soluble calf skin collagen by superoxide ion: Protective effect of flavonoids. Biochem Pharmacol 1983; 32(1):53–8.

[20] Pizzorno J, Murray M. Vaccinium myrtillus. In A textbook of natural medicine. Seattle: John Bastyr College Publications, 1987.

[21] Schwitters B, Masquelier J. OPC in practice; bioflavinoids and their application. Rome, Italy: Alfa Omega Publishers, 1993, pp. 40–43.

[22] Maquart FX, Bellon G, Gillery P, et al. Stimulation of collagen synthesis in fibroblast cultures by a triterpene extracted from Centella asiatica. Connect Tissue Res 1990; 24(2):107–20.

[23] Maquart FX, Chastang F, Simeon A, et al. Triterpenes from Centella asiatica stimulate extracellular matrix accumulation in rat experimental wounds. Eur J Dermatol 1999 Jun; 9(4):289–96.

[24] Bonte F, Dumas M, Chaudagne C, Meybeck A. Influence of asiatic acid, madecassic acid, and asiaticoside on human collagen I synthesis. Planta Med 1994 Apr; 60(2):133–5.

[25] Tenni R, Zanaboni G, De Agostini MP, et al. Effect of the triterpenoid fraction of Centella asiatica on macromolecules of the connective matrix in human skin fibroblast cultures. Ital J Biochem 1988 Mar–Apr; 37(2):69–77.

[26] Cha HJ, Bae SK, Lee HY, et al. Anti-invasive activity of ursolic acid correlates with the reduced expression of matrix metalloproteinase-9 (MMP-9) in HT1080 human fibrosarcoma cells. Cancer Res 1996 May 15; 56(10):2281–4.

[27] Lin LI, Ke YF, Ko YC, Lin JK. Curcumin inhibits SK-Hep-1 hepatocellular carcinoma cell invasion in vitro and suppresses matrix metalloproteinase-9 secretion. Oncology 1998 Jul–Aug; 55(4):349–53.

[28] Sazuka M, Imazawa H, Shoji Y, et al. Inhibition of collagenases from mouse lung carcinoma cells by green tea catechins and black tea theaflavins. Biosci Biotechnol Biochem 1997 Sep; 61(9):1504–6.

[29] Beretz A, Cazenave JP. The effect of flavonoids on blood-vessel wall interactions. In Plant flavonoids in biology and medicine II. New York: Alan R. Liss, Inc., 1988, pp. 187–200.

[30] Tanaka T, Metori K, Mineo S, et al. [Studies on collagenase inhibitors. II. Inhibitory effects of anthraquinones on bacterial collagenase.] Yakugaku Zasshi 1990 Sep; 110(9):688–92.

[31] Reich R, Royce L, Martin GR. Eicosapentaenoic acid reduces the invasive and metastic activities of malignant tumor cells. Biochem Biophys Res Commun 1989; 160(2):559–64.

[32] Liu XH, Rose DP. Suppression of type IV collagenase in MDA-MB-435 human breast cancer cells by eicosapentaenoic acid in vitro and in vivo. Cancer Letters 1995; 92:21–26.

[33] Suzuki I, Iigo M, Ishikawa C, et al. Inhibitory effects of oleic and docosahexaenoic acids on lung metastasis by colon-carcinoma-26 cells are associated with reduced matrix metalloproteinase-2 and -9 activities. Int J Cancer 1997 Nov 14; 73(4):607–12.

[34] Aguirre Ghiso JA, Farias EF, Alonso DF, et al. Secretion of urokinase and metalloproteinase-9 induced by staurosporine is dependent on a tyrosine kinase pathway in mammary tumor cells. Int J Cancer 1998; 76(3):362–367.

[35] Fajardo I, Quesada AR, Nunez de Castro I, et al. A comparative study of the effects of genistein and 2-methoxyestradiol on the proteolytic balance and tumour cell proliferation. Br J Cancer 1999 Apr; 80(1–2):17–24.

[36] Shao ZM, Wu J, Shen ZZ, Barsky SH. Genistein inhibits both constitutive and EGF-stimulated invasion in ER-negative human breast carcinoma cell lines. Anticancer Res 1998 May–Jun; 18(3A):1435–9.

[37] Yamashita K, Suzuki M, Iwata H, et al. Tyrosine phosphorylation is crucial for growth signaling by tissue inhibitors of metalloproteinases (TIMP-1 and TIMP-2). FEBS Lett 1996 Oct 28; 396(1):103–7.

[38] Liu XH, Connolly JM, Rose DP. Eicosanoids as mediators of linoleic acid-stimulated invasion and type IV collagenase

production by a metastatic human breast cancer cell line. Clin Exp Metastasis 1996; 14:145–152.

39 Huang Y, Hwang JJ, Lee PP, et al. Effects of luteolin and quercetin, inhibitors of tyrosine kinase, on cell growth and metastasis-associated properties in A431 cells overexpressing epidermal growth factor receptor. Br J Pharmacol 1999 Nov; 128(5):999–1010.

40 Parish CR, Coombe DR, Jakobsen KB, et al. Evidence that sulphated polysaccharides inhibit tumour metastasis by blocking tumour-cell-derived heparanases. Int J Cancer 1987; 40:511–518.

41 Coombe DR, Parish CR, Ramshaw IA, Snowden JM. Analysis of the inhibition of tumour metastasis by sulphated polysaccharides. Int J Cancer 1987; 39:82–88.

42 Ebina T, Murata K. Antitumor effect of intratumoral administration of a Coriolus preparation, PSK: Inhibition of tumor invasion in vitro. Gan To Kagaku Ryoho 1994; 21:2241–3.

43 Yang QY, Kwok CY, eds. PSP international symposium 1993. Shanghai: Fudan University Press, 1993.

44 Matsunaga K, Ohhara M, Oguchi Y, et al. Antimetastatic effect of PSK, a protein-bound polysaccharide, against the B16-BL6 mouse melanoma. Invasion Metastasis 1996; 16(1):27–38.

45 Kobayashi H, Matsunaga K, Oguchi Y. Antimetastatic effects of PSK (Krestin), a protein-bound polysaccharide obtained from basidiomycetes: An overview. Cancer Epidemiol Biomarkers Prev 1995 Apr–May; 4(3):275–81.

46 Braunhut SJ, Moses MA. Retinoids modulate endothelial cell production of matrix-degrading proteases and tissue inhibitors of metalloproteinases (TIMP). J Biol Chem 1994; 269(18):13472–9.

47 Jacob K, Wach F, Holzapfel U, et al. In vitro modulation of human melanoma cell invasion and proliferation by all-trans retinoic acid. Melanoma Res 1998 Jun; 8(3):211–9.

48 Sapi E, Flick MB, Tartaro K, et al. Effect of all-trans retinoic acid on c-fms proto-oncogene [colony-stimulating factor 1 (CSF-1) receptor] expression and CSF-1-induced invasion and anchorage-independent growth of human breast carcinoma cells. Cancer Res 1999 Nov 1; 59(21):5578–85.

49 Chan D, Lamande SR, Cole WG, et al. Regulation of procollagen synthesis and processing during ascorbate-induced extracellular matrix accumulation in vitro. Biochem J 1990; 269(1):175–81.

50 Heino J, Kahari VM, Jaakkola S, et al. Collagen in the intracellular matrix of cultured scleroderma skin fibroblasts: Changes related to ascorbic acid-treatment. Matrix 1989; 9(1):34–9.

51 Grinnell F, Fukamizu H, Pawelek P, et al. Collagen processing, crosslinking, and fibril bundle assembly in matrix produced by fibroblasts in long-term cultures supplemented with ascorbic acid. Exp Cell Res 1989; 181(2):483–91.

52 McDevitt CA, Lipman JM, Ruemer RJ, et al. Stimulation of matrix formation in rabbit chondrocyte cultures by ascorbate. J Orthop Res 1988; 6(4):518–24.

53 Nicosia RF, Belser P, Bonanno E, Diven J. Regulation of angiogenesis in vitro by collagen metabolism. In Vitro Cell Dev Biol 1991 Dec; 27 A(12):961–6.

54 Ingber D, Folkman J. Inhibition of angiogenesis through modulation of collagen metabolism. Lab Invest 1988 Jul; 59(1):44–51.

55 Yudoh K, Matsuno H, Kimura T. 1alpha,25-dihydroxyvitamin D3 inhibits in vitro invasiveness through the extracellular matrix and in vivo pulmonary metastasis of B16 mouse melanoma. J Lab Clin Med 1999 Feb; 133(2):120–8.

56 Young MR, Lozano Y. Inhibition of tumor invasiveness by 1alpha,25-dihydroxyvitamin D3 coupled to a decline in protein kinase A activity and an increase in cytoskeletal organization. Clin Exp Metastasis 1997 Mar; 15(2):102–10.

57 Fraher LJ, Caveney AN, McFadden RG. Calcitriol and its synthetic analogue MC 903 inhibit the interleukin-2-induced migration of human lymphocytes. Am J Respir Cell Mol Biol 1995 Jun; 12(6):669–75.

58 Mascolo N, Pinto A, Capasso F. Flavonoids, leukocyte migration and eicosanoids. J Pharm Pharmacol 1988 Apr; 40(4):293–5.

59 Sharma ML, Khajuria A, Kaul A, et al. Effect of salai guggal ex-Boswellia serrata on cellular and humoral immune responses and leucocyte migration. Agents Actions 1988 Jun; 24(1–2):161–4.

60 Sharma ML, Bani S, Singh GB. Anti-arthritic activity of boswellic acids in bovine serum albumin (BSA)-induced arthritis. Int J Immunopharmacol 1989; 11(6):647–52.

61 Hale LP, Haynes BF. Bromelain treatment of human T cells removes CD44, CD45RA, E2/MIC2, CD6, CD7, CD8, and Leu 8AM1 surface molecules and markedly enhances CD2-mediated T cell activation. J Immunol 1992 Dec 15; 149(12):3809–16.

62 Munzig E, Eckert K, Harrach T, et al. Bromelain protease F9 reduces the CD44 mediated adhesion of human peripheral blood lymphocytes to human umbilical vein endothelial cells. FEBS Lett 1994 Sep 5; 351(2):215–8.

63 Ogino M, Majima M, Kawamura M, et al. Increased migration of neutrophils to granulocyte-colony stimulating factor in rat carrageenin-induced pleurisy: Roles of complement, bradykinin, and inducible cyclooxygenase-2. Inflamm Res 1996 Jul; 45(7):335–46.

64 Kikuchi S, Sakamoto T, Ishikawa C, et al. Modulation of eosinophil chemotactic activities to leukotriene B4 by n-3 polyunsaturated fatty acids. Prostaglandins Leukot Essent Fatty Acids 1998 Mar; 58(3):243–8.

65 Sperling RI, Benincaso AI, Knoell CT, et al. Dietary omega-3 polyunsaturated fatty acids inhibit phosphoinositide formation and chemotaxis in neutrophils. J Clin Invest 1993 Feb; 91(2):651–60.

66 Mehta JL, Lopez LM, Lawson D, et al. Dietary supplementation with omega-3 polyunsaturated fatty acids in patients with stable coronary heart disease. Effects on indices of platelet and neutrophil function and exercise performance. Am J Med 1988 Jan; 84(1):45–52.

67 Payan DG, Wong MY, Chernov-Rogan T, et al. Alterations in human leukocyte function induced by ingestion of eicosapentaenoic acid. J Clin Immunol 1986 Sep; 6(5):402–10.

68 Lu HQ, Niggemann B, Zanker KS. Suppression of the proliferation and migration of oncogenic ras-dependent cell lines, cultured in a three-dimensional collagen matrix, by

flavonoid-structured molecules. J Cancer Res Clin Oncol 1996; 122(6):335–42.

[69] Holting T, Siperstein AE, Clark OH, Duh QY. Epidermal growth factor (EGF)- and transforming growth factor alpha-stimulated invasion and growth of follicular thyroid cancer cells can be blocked by antagonism to the EGF receptor and tyrosine kinase in vitro. Eur J Endocrinol 1995 Feb; 132(2):229–35.

[70] Hall CL, Wang C, Lange LA, Turley EA. Hyaluronan and the hyaluronan receptor RHAMM promote focal adhesion turnover and transient tyrosine kinase activity. J Cell Biol 1994 Jul; 126(2):575–88.

[71] Cos S, Fernandez R, Guezmes A, et al. Influence of melatonin on invasive and metastatic properties of MCF-7 human breast cancer cells. Cancer Res 1998 Oct 1; 58(19):4383–90.

[72] Wakabayashi C, Hasegawa H, Murata J, Saiki I. In vivo antimetastatic action of ginseng protopanaxadiol saponins is based on their intestinal bacterial metabolites after oral administration. Oncol Res 1997; 9(8):411–7.

[73] Scaglione F, Ferrara F, Dugnani S, et al. Immunomodulatory effects of two extracts of Panax ginseng C.A. Meyer. Drugs Exp Clin Res 1990; 16(10):537–42.

[74] Mapelli E, Banfi P, Sala E, et al. Effect of protein kinase C inhibitors on invasiveness of human melanoma clones expressing different levels of protein kinase C isoenzymes. Int J Cancer 1994 Apr 15; 57(2):281–6.

[75] Uhm JH, Dooley NP, Villemure JG, Yong VW. Glioma invasion in vitro: Regulation by matrix metalloprotease-2 and protein kinase C. Clin Exp Metastasis 1996 Oct; 14(5):421–33.

[76] Zhang W, Law RE, Hinton DR, Couldwell WT. Inhibition of human malignant glioma cell motility and invasion in vitro by hypericin, a potent protein kinase C inhibitor. Cancer Letters 1997; 120(1):31–38.

[77] Katano M, Yamamoto H, Torisu M. [A suppressive effect of PSK, a protein-bound polysaccharide preparation, on tumor growth: A new effect of PSK on cell motility.] Gan To Kagaku Ryoho 1987 Jul; 14(7):2321–6.

[78] Torisu M, Hayashi Y, Ishimitsu T, et al. Significant prolongation of disease-free period gained by oral polysaccharide K (PSK) administration after curative surgical operation of colorectal cancer. Cancer Immunol Immunother 1990; 31(5):261–8.

[79] Ando T, Mastuda Y, Matsunaga K, et al. [Effect of PSK on the recovery of macrophage function in tumor-bearing mice.] Gan To Kagaku Ryoho 1984 Apr; 11(4):827–34.

[80] Theodorescu D, Laderoute KR, Calaoagan JM, Guilding KM. Inhibition of human bladder cancer cell motility by genistein is dependent on epidermal growth factor receptor but not p21ras gene expression. Int J Cancer 1998 Dec 9; 78(6):775–82.

[81] Penar PL, Khoshyomn S, Bhushan A, Tritton TR. Inhibition of epidermal growth factor receptor-associated tyrosine kinase blocks glioblastoma invasion of the brain. Neurosurgery 1997 Jan; 40(1):141–51.

[82] Fichter M, Hinrichs R, Eissner G, et al. Expression of CD44 isoforms in neuroblastoma cells is regulated by PI 3-kinase and protein kinase C. Oncogene 1997 Jun 12; 14(23):2817–24.

[83] Oldenborg PA, Sehlin J. Insulin-stimulated chemokinesis in normal human neutrophils is dependent on D-glucose concentration and sensitive to inhibitors of tyrosine kinase and phosphatidylinositol 3-kinase. J Leukoc Biol 1998 Feb; 63(2):203–8.

[84] Entschladen F, Niggemann B, Zanker KS, Friedl P. Differential requirement of protein tyrosine kinases and protein kinase C in the regulation of T cell locomotion in three-dimensional collagen matrices. J Immunol 1997 Oct 1; 159(7):3203–10.

[85] Hauzenberger D, Klominek J, Holgersson J, et al. Triggering of motile behavior in T lymphocytes via cross-linking of alpha 4 beta 1 and alpha L beta 2. J Immunol 1997 Jan 1; 158(1):76–84.

SUPPLEMENTAL MATERIAL FOR CHAPTER 12

Tables H.1 and H.2 provide supplemental material for Chapter 12, "Natural Compounds That Affect the Immune System." The first summarizes studies on how natural compounds stimulate or support the immune system, and the second lists the ingredients of herbal formulas discussed in Chapter 12.

TABLE H.1 NATURAL COMPOUNDS THAT AFFECT THE IMMUNE SYSTEM	
COMPOUND	**EFFECTS**
HERBAL COMPOUNDS	
Astragalus membranaceus	• Fractions of the herb caused a 10-fold potentiation of IL-2 activity in vitro, which increased LAK cell cytotoxicity. Because the success of IL-2 has been hampered by its severe toxicity, cotreatment with *Astragalus* may allow its use at lower, less toxic doses.[1, 2, 3] • Extracts of *Astragalus* injected into mice and rats immunosuppressed by chemotherapy, radiotherapy, or aging increased the antibody response to antigens and increased helper T-lymphocyte activity.[4] • Extracts induced interferon and IL-2 production in mouse lymphocytes in vitro, as well as in animals and humans.[5–9] • Polysaccharide fractions of the herb increased production of TNF by monocytes in vitro.[10] • A combination of *Astragalus* and *Ligustrum lucidum* extracts added to cultures of human immune cells restored T-cell function in cells from 9 out of 10 cancer patients; in a second experiment, T-cell function was restored in cells from 9 out of 13. The degree of the immune restoration appeared to be complete, as reactions of test cells equaled the levels found in cells from healthy donors.[11] • A combination of *Astragalus* and *Panax ginseng* extracts markedly enhanced the cytotoxic action of LAK cells in vitro.[12] • Fractions of the herb improved the function of T cells obtained from 13 cancer patients by 260%, as compared to untreated cells, and by 160% compared to cells from normal healthy donors.[13, 14] • Extracts of *Astragalus* and *Ligustrum lucidum* reversed macrophage suppression caused by kidney cancer in mice. Intraperitoneal administration of the extracts (at 20 mg/kg each, daily for 10 days) inhibited proliferation of kidney cancer cells transplanted into mice, reaching a 100% cure rate in mice with small tumor loads.[15, 16] • Extracts of *Astragalus* and *Ligustrum lucidum* reversed macrophage suppression caused by kidney and bladder cancer cells in vitro.[17]
Eleutherococcus senticosus	• Polysaccharide fractions stimulated macrophage, T-cell, and B-cell activity, and interleukin and interferon production in vitro. Extracts protected mice from the immunosuppressive effects of radiation. Administration of polysaccharide fractions to sarcoma-bearing mice inhibited tumor growth by up to 67% and prolonged their survival by up to 71%. Up to 33% of the mice obtained complete remission. Other tumors were also inhibited. The extract also enhanced the activity of mouse macrophages in vitro. In a four-week double-blind study in humans, *Eleutherococcus* extract drastically increased the number of immunocompetent cells, especially helper T cells and NK cells.[18–24]

TABLE H.1 NATURAL COMPOUNDS THAT AFFECT THE IMMUNE SYSTEM *(continued)*	
COMPOUND	**EFFECTS**
Ganoderma lucidum	• Polysaccharide fractions potentiated production of IL-1, IL-6, interferon, and TNF by human macrophages and T cells in vitro. Oral administration increased production of IL-2 in mice. Oral administration of a polysaccharide fraction increased the number of white blood cells in humans; this effect was thought to be due to stimulation of T cells and increased production of IL-2 and interferon. Polysaccharide fractions markedly inhibited sarcoma tumor cells transplanted into mice. Injection of the extract into mice bearing transplanted lung tumor cells increased life spans up to 200%; this effect was observed whether the extract was administered alone or in conjunction with chemotherapy drugs. The extract was nontoxic to cell cultures, and the antitumor action was believed to occur through T-cell activation. *Ganoderma* extract also enhanced immune recovery in mice treated with radiation.[25–31]
Panax ginseng	• The physiological effects of ginseng include sedation, antifatigue action, stimulation of protein biosynthesis in the liver and kidneys, stimulation of carbohydrate and fat metabolism, stimulation of macrophage phagocytosis, promotion of antibody and complement production, and restoration of sexual behavior in stressed animals. Researchers have referred to the overall effect as being "adaptogenic." (An adaptogen is an agent that helps increase the nonspecific resistance of an organism to adverse influences.) Ginseng saponins increased the NK cell activity of mouse spleen cells by 40% in vitro. IL-2 and interferon production each increased approximately 100%. Ginseng extracts induced IL-2 and interferon-gamma production in mouse lymphocytes. In healthy mice, NK activity increased as much as 600%. Extracts improved a wide range of immune indices in humans after oral ingestion; they enhanced the function of NK cells taken from healthy patients, as well as those suffering from HIV and chronic fatigue syndrome. Antibody-dependent cellular cytotoxicity (ADCC) was also improved.[6, 14, 32–37]
Shiitake (*Lentinus edodes*), PSK, and other mushroom polysaccharides	• Hundreds of studies have been conducted on the immunostimulating and antitumor effects of mushroom polysaccharides such as lentinan (from shiitake), and PSK (Krestin) and PSP (from *Coriolus versicolor*). Studies have suggested that about half of all cultivated mushrooms may have medicinal properties, the most common one being an immunomodulatory effect. As a group, these polysaccharides stimulate immune cells in vitro and in vivo, increase production of a variety of cytokines (including IL-1, IL-3, TNF, interferons, and CSF), and produce antitumor effects in rodents. These polysaccharides also inhibit the actions of immunosuppressive cytokines such as TGF-beta. In conjunction with radiotherapy or chemotherapy, PSK improved the survival of patients with a variety of cancers, in some cases by as much as 320%. Not all patients appear to be responsive to lentinan and PSK treatment, however, and immune system monitoring may be useful to determine those who are suitable for therapy. Orally administered PSK also normalized colonic lactobacillus populations decreased by the presence of sarcoma or treatment with chemotherapy.[38–42]
ANTIOXIDANTS AND NUTRITIONAL COMPOUNDS	
Glutamine	• Glutamine stimulates the immune response and inhibits tumor growth through a variety of mechanisms. It increases glutathione synthesis, which is required for optimal IL-2 activity. High doses of oral glutamine (8 g/kg) markedly increased serum IL-2 concentrations in mice. Glutamine is also a major fuel for immune cells; it increased cell-mediated cytotoxicity in vitro and NK cell cytotoxicity in vivo. In addition, in-vitro studies suggest that the cytotoxic effect of TNF in some tumor cell lines is dependent on adequate glutamine. Removal of glutamine reduced TNF cytotoxicity. Lastly, because of its effects on glutathione, glutamine may also reduce prostaglandin production by tumors. PGE_2 is one of the primary immunosuppressive substances found at tumor sites.[43–48]

TABLE H.1 NATURAL COMPOUNDS THAT AFFECT THE IMMUNE SYSTEM *(continued)*	
COMPOUND	**EFFECTS**
Glutathione-enhancing compounds	• Glutathione may be a rate-limiting component in IL-2 and LAK immunotherapy. Glutathione-deficient lymphocytes exhibit subnormal activation in response to stimuli. Furthermore, the addition of IL-2 cannot restore their activity, although glutathione can. Even a partial depletion in the intracellular glutathione pool dramatically reduced generation of cytotoxic T cells. The amino acid cysteine is a component of the tripeptide glutathione. Oral administration of *N*-acetylcysteine (NAC) in conjunction with IL-2 and LAK reduced the progression of refractory tumors in mice; complete regression was observed in 11% to 17%. Glutathione can also potentially inhibit cancer, as well as cancer-induced immunosuppression, via its ability to inhibit PGE_2 production.[49–55]
Selenium	• In human subjects, selenium (at 200 micrograms per day) enhanced lymphocyte and natural killer cell response and proliferation. Supplementation increased tumor cytotoxicity of lymphocytes and natural killer cells and reversed age-related immune deficiencies; these effects were partly due to enhanced expression of IL-2 receptors.[56, 57, 58] In addition, both vitamin E and selenium enhanced migration and activity of human and bovine leukocytes in vitro. Selenium deficiency inhibited macrophage-mediated tumor destruction and tumor necrosis factor production in animals. Dietary supplementation with selenium produced the opposite effects.[59–62]
Vitamins C and E	• Oral administration of vitamin C (at 1 gram/day) and vitamin E (at 200 mg/day) to aged women improved a variety of immune indices, including T-cell proliferation, phagocytic functions, and immune-cell migration. Both vitamins also improved macrophage phagocytosis, migration, and free radical production in vitro. Leukocytes contain a relatively high percentage of vitamin C, possibly to protect them from auto-oxidation during activation. The ability of neutrophils to kill bacteria is reduced when vitamin C is deficient. Although the most striking immunomodulating effects of antioxidant vitamins have been in the elderly, antioxidants also improved immune response in younger individuals. Even a marginal deficiency of vitamin E reduced immune response, and antioxidant supplementation enhanced innate and adaptive immunity.[63–67]

TABLE H.2 COMPOSITION OF HERBAL FORMULAS	
FORMULA	**COMPOSITION** *(Chinese names are in parentheses)*
Bu Zhong Yi Qi Tang	*Astragalus membranaceus* (huang qi), *Panax ginseng* (ren shen), *Atractylodes macrocephala* (bai zhu), *Glycyrrhiza uralensis* (zhi gan cao), *Angelica sinensis* (dang gui), *Cimicifuga foetida* (sheng ma), *Bupleurum chinense* (chai hu), *Citrus reticulata* (chen pi)
Fei Liu Ping	*Astragalus membranaceus* (huang qi), *Codonopsis pilosula* (dang shen), *Oldenlandia diffusa* (bai hua she ye cao), *Prunus armeniaca* (xing ren), *Paris polyphylla* (cao he che), *Houttuynia cordata* (yu xing cao), *Patrina villosa* (bai jian cao), *Glehnia littoralis* (bei sha shen)
Formula #1	*Paeonia lactiflora* (chi shao), *Ligusticum chuanxiong* (chuan xiong), *Angelica sinensis* (dang gui), *Prunus persica* (tao ren), *Carthamus tinctorius* (hong hua), *Millettia reticulata* (ji xue teng), *Pueraria lobata* (ge gen), *Citrus reticulata* (chen pi), *Salvia miltiorrhiza* (dan shen), *Astragalus membranaceus* (huang qi)
Formula #2	*Codonopsis pilosula* (dang shen), *Astragalus membranaceus* (huang qi), *Atractylodes macrocephala* (bai zhu), *Solanum lyrati* (shu yang quan), *Hedyosis diffusae* (bai hua she she cao), *Salvia chinensis* (shi jian chuan)
Li Wei Hua Jie Tang	*Codonopsis pilosula* (dang shen), *Atractylodes macrocephala* (bai zhu), *Poria cocos* (fu ling), *Glycyrrhiza uralensis* (gan cao), *Astragalus membranaceus* (sheng huang qi), *Rehmannia glutinosa* (shu di huang), *Polygonatum sibricum* (huang jing), *Solanum lyratum* (bai mao teng), *Oldenlandia diffusa* (bai hua she she cao), *Euryale ferox* (qian shi), *Nelumbo nucifera* (lian rou), *Panax notoginseng* (tian san qi), *Ziziphus jujuba* (da zao), *Adenophora tetraphylla* (sha shen), *Ovine calculi* (yang du zao), *Lycium barbarum* (gou qi zi)

TABLE H.2 COMPOSITION OF HERBAL FORMULAS *(continued)*	
FORMULA	**COMPOSITION** *(Chinese names are in parentheses)*
Pishen Fang (also known as *Jian Pi Yi Shen*)	*Codonopsis pilosula* (dang shen), *Atractylodes macrocephala* (bai zhu), *Cuscuta chinensis* (tu si zi), *Psoralen corylifolia* (bu gu zhi), *Ligusticum lucidum* (nu zhen zi), *Lycium chinense* (gou qi zi)
Shen Xue Tang	*Astragalus membranaceus* (huang qi), *Pseudostellaria heterophylla* (tai zi shen), *Atractylodes macrocephala* (bai zhu), *Poria cocos* (fu ling), *Ligustrum lucidum* (nu zhen zi), *Cuscuta chinensis* (tu si zi), *Lycium chinensis* (gou qi zi), *Millettia reticulata* (ji xue teng)
Shi Quan Da Bu Tang	*Astragalus membranaceus* (huang qi), *Cinnamomum cassia* (rou gui), *Panax ginseng* (ren shen), *Rehmannia glutinosa* (shu di huang), *Atractylodes macrocephala* (bai zhu), *Angelica sinensis* (dang gui), *Paeonia lactiflora* (bai shao yao), *Ligusticum chuanxiong* (chuan xiong), *Poria cocos* (fu ling), *Glycyrrhiza uralensis* (zhi gan cao), *Zingiber officinale* (sheng jiang), *Ziziphus jujuba* (da zao)
Si Jun Zi Tang	*Panax ginseng* (ren shen), *Atractylodes macrocephala* (bai zhu), *Poria cocos* (fu ling), *Glycyrrhiza uralensis* (zhi gan cao)
Xiao Chai Hu Tang	*Bupleurum chinense* (chai hu), *Scutellaria baicalensis* (huang qin), *Pinellia ternata* (ban xia), *Zingiber officinale* (sheng jiang), *Panax ginseng* (ren shen), *Glycyrrhiza uralensis* (gan cao), *Ziziphus jujuba* (da zao)
Ye Qi Sheng Xue Tang	*Astragalus membranaceus* (huang qi), *Angelica sinensis* (dang gui), *Equus asinus* (e jiao), *Spatholobi spp.*, *Pyrrosia lingua* (shi wei), *Ziziphus jujuba* (da zao), *Hordeum vulgare* (mai ya), *Citrus reticulata* (chen pi), *Glycyrrhiza uralensis* (gan cao)
Yi Qi Yang Yin Tang	*Pseudostellaria heterophylla* (tai zi shen), *Scrophularia ningpoensis* (xuan shen), *Ophiopogon japonicus* (mai men dong), *Rehmannia glutinosa* (shu di huang), *Ligusticum lucidum* (nu zhen zi), *Dendrobium officinale* (shi hu), *Trichosanthes kirilowii* (gua lou), *Hedyosis diffusa* (bai hua she she cao), *Scutellaria barbata* (ban zhi lian), *Glycyrrhiza uralensis* (gan cao)

REFERENCES

[1] Chu D, Sun Y, Lin J, et al. F3, a fractionated extract of Astragalus membranaceus, potentiates lymphokine-activated killer cell cytotoxicity generated by low-dose recombinant interleukin-2. Chung Hsi I Chieh Ho Tsa Chih 1990; 10(1):34–6.

[2] Wang Y, Qian XJ, Hadley HR, et al. Phytochemicals potentiate interleukin-2 generated lymphokine activated killer cell cytotoxicity against murine renal cell carcinoma. Mol Biother 1992; 4(3):143–6.

[3] Chu DT, Lepe-Zuniga J, Wong WL, et al. Fractionated extract of Astragalus membranaceus, a Chinese medicinal herb, potentiates LAK cell cytotoxicity generated by a low dose of recombinant interleukin-2. J Clin Lab Immunol 1988; 26(4):183–7.

[4] Zhao KS, Mancini C, Doria G. Enhancement of the immune response in mice by Astragalus membranaceus extracts. Immunopharmacology 1990; 20(3):225–33.

[5] Hou Y, Ma GL, Wu SH, et al. Effect of radix Astralagi seu hedysari on the interferon system. Chinese Medical Journal (Engl) 1981; 94(1):35–40.

[6] Jin R, Kurashige S. Effect of shi-ka-ron on cytokine production of lymphocytes in mice treated with cyclophosphamide. Am J Chin Med 1996; 24(1):37–44.

[7] Jin R, Wan LL, Mitisuishi T, et al. Effect of shi-ka-ron and Chinese herbs on cytokine production of macrophage in immunocompromised mice. American Journal of Chinese Medicine 1994; XXII(3–4):255–266.

8 Chen YC. [Experimental studies on the effects of danggui buxue decoction on IL-2 production of blood-deficient mice.] Chung Kuo Chung Yao Tsa Chih 1994 Dec; 19(12):739–41, 763.

9 Liang H, Zhang Y, Geng B. [The effect of Astragalus polysaccharides (APS) on cell mediated immunity (CMI) in burned mice.] Chung Hua Cheng Hsing Shao Shang Wai Ko Tsa Chih 1994 Mar; 10(2):138–41.

10 Zhao KW, Kong HY. Effect of astragalan on secretion of tumor necrosis factors in human peripheral blood mononuclear cells. Chung Kuo Chung Hsi I Chieh Ho Tsa Chih 1993; 13(5):263–5.

11 Sun Y, Hersh EM, Talpaz M, et al. Immune restoration and/or augmentation of local graft versus host reaction by traditional Chinese medicinal herbs. Cancer 1983; 52(1):70–3.

12 Zhao TH. Positive modulating action of shenmaisan with Astralagus membranaceus on anti-tumor activity of LAK cells. Chung Kuo Chung Hsi Chieh Ho Tsa Chih 1993; 13(8):471–2.

13 Chu DT, Wong WL, Mavlight GM. Immunotherapy with Chinese medicinal herbs: Immune restoration of local xenogeneic graft-versus-host reaction in cancer patients by fractionated Astragalus membranaceus in vitro. Journal of Clinical Laboratory Immunology 1988; 25(3):119–23.

14 Chu DT, Sun Y, Lin JR. Immune restoration of local xenogeneic graft-versus-host reaction in cancer patients in vitro and reversal of cyclophosphamide-induced immune suppression in the rat in vivo by fractionated Astragalus membranaceus. Chung Hsi I Chieh Ho Tsa Chih 1989; 9(6):351–4.

15 Lau BH, Ruckle HC, Botolazzo T, Lui PD. Chinese medicinal herbs inhibit growth of murine renal cell carcinoma. Cancer Biother 1994 Summer; 9(2):153–61.

16 Lau BH, Qian XJ, Wong BY, et al. Chinese medicinal herbs restore tumor-associated immunosuppression (Meeting abstract). FASEB J 1992; 6(5):A1930.

17 Rittenhouse JR, Lui PD, Lau BH. Chinese medicinal herbs reverse macrophage suppression induced by urological tumors. J Urol 1991; 146(2):486–90.

18 Wagner H. Immunostimulants from medicinal plants. In Advances in Chinese medicinal materials research. Chang HM, Yeung W, Tso W, Koo A, eds. Singapore: World Scientific, 1985.

19 Bohn B, Nebe CT, Birr C. Flow-cytometric studies with Eleutherococcus senticosus extract as an immunomodulatory agent. Arzneimittelforschung 1987 Oct; 37(10):1193–6.

20 Miyanomae T, Frindel E. Radioprotection of hemopoiesis conferred by Acanthopanax senticosus Harms (Shigoka) administered before or after irradiation. Exp Hematol 1988 Oct; 16(9):801–6.

21 Wang JZ, Tsumura H, Shimura K, et al. Antitumor activity of polysaccharide from a Chinese medicinal herb, Acanthopanax giraldii Harms. Cancer Lett 1992; 65(1):79–84.

22 Wang JZ, Tsumura H, Ma N, et al. Biochemical and morphological alterations of macrophages and spleen cells produced by antitumor polysaccharide from Acanthopanax obovatus roots. Planta Med 1993; 59(1):54–8.

23 Williams M. Eleutherococcus senticosus: The use of biological response modifiers in oncology. British J of Phytotherapy 1993; 3(1):32–37.

24 Xie SS. [Immunoregulatory effect of polysaccharide of Acanthopanax senticosus (PAS). I. Immunological mechanism of PAS against cancer.] Chung Hua Chung Liu Tsa Chih 1989 Sep; 11(5):338–40.

25 Zhang LX, Mong H, Zhou XB. Effect of Japanese Ganoderma lucidum (GL) planted in Japan on the production of interleukin-2 from murine splenocytes. Chung Kuo Chung Hsi I Chieh Ho Tsa Chih 1993; 13(10):613–5.

26 Haak-Frendscho M, Kino K, Sone T, et al. Ling Zhi-8: A novel T cell mitogen induces cytokine production and upregulation of ICAM-1 expression. Cell Immunol 1993; 150(1):101–13.

27 Chen WC, Hau DM, Lee SS. Effects of Ganoderma lucidum and krestin on cellular immunocompetence in gamma-ray-irradiated mice. Am J Chin Med 1995; 23(1):71–80.

28 Wang SY, Hsu ML, Hsu HC, et al. The anti-tumor effect of Ganoderma lucidum is mediated by cytokines released from activated macrophages and T lymphocytes. Int J Cancer 1997 Mar 17; 70(6):699–705.

29 Maruyama H, Yamazaki K, Murofushi S, et al. Antitumor activity of Sarcodon aspratus (Berk.) S. Ito and Ganoderma lucidum (Fr.) Karst. J Pharmacobiodyn 1989; 12(2):118–23.

30 Furusawa E, Chou SC, Furusawa S, et al. Antitumor activity of Ganoderma lucidium, an edible mushroom, on intraperitoneally implanted Lewis lung carcinoma in synergenic mice. Phytotherapy Research 1992; 6:300–304.

31 Zhang J, Wang G, Li H, et al. Antitumor active protein-containing glycans from the Chinese mushroom songshan lingzhi, Ganoderma tsugae mycelium. Biosci Biotechnol Biochem 1994 Jul; 58(7):1202–5.

32 Shibata S. Chemical studies on Chinese medicinal materials. In Advances in Chinese medicinal materials research. Chang HM, Yeung HW, Tso WW, Koo A, eds. Singapore: World Scientific, 1985.

33 Hiai, S. Chinese medicinal medicine material and the secretion of ACTH and corticosteroid. In Advances in Chinese medicinal materials research. Chang HM, Yeung HW, Tso WW, Koo A, eds. Singapore: World Scientific, 1985, pp. 49–60.

34 Wang B, Cui J, Lui A. The effect of ginseng on immune responses. In Advances in Chinese medicinal materials research. Singapore: World Scientific, 1985.

35 Yang G, Yu Y. Effects of ginsenoside on the natural killer cell-interferon-interleukin-2 regulatory network and its tumor inhibiting effect. J of Trad Chin Med 1988; 8(2):135–140.

36 Scaglione F, Ferrara F, Dugnani S, et al. Immunomodulatory effects of two extracts of Panax ginseng C.A. Meyer. Drugs Exp Clin Res 1990; 16(10):537–42.

37 See DM, Broumand N, Sahl L, Tilles JG. In vitro effects of echinacea and ginseng on natural killer and antibody-dependent cell cytotoxicity in healthy subjects and chronic fatigue syndrome or acquired immunodeficiency syndrome patients. Immunopharmacology 1997 Jan; 35(3):229–35.

38 Suzuki H, Iiyama K, Yoshida O, et al. Structural characterization of the immunoactive and antiviral water-solubilized lignin in an extract of the culture medium of

Lentinus edodes mycelia (LEM). Agric Biol Chem 1990 Feb; 54(2):479–87.

[39] Takehara M, Kuida K, Mori K. Antiviral activity of virus-like particles from Lentinus edodes (Shiitake). Brief report. Arch Virol 1979; 59(3):269–74.

[40] Liu M, Li J, Kong F, et al. Induction of immunomodulating cytokines by a new polysaccharide-peptide complex from culture mycelia of Lentinus edodes. Immunopharmacology 1998 Nov; 40(3):187–98.

[41] Chang R. Functional properties of edible mushrooms. Nutr Rev 1996 Nov; 54(11 Pt 2):S91–3.

[42] Aoki T, Usuda Y, Miyakoshi H, et al. Low natural killer syndrome: Clinical and immunologic features. Nat Immun Cell Growth Regul 1987; 6(3):116–28.

[43] Klimberg VS, McClellan JL. Glutamine, cancer and its therapy. Am J Surg 1996 Nov; 172(5):418–24.

[44] Fahr MJ, Kornbluth J, Blossom S, et al. Harry M. Vars Research Award. Glutamine enhances immunoregulation of tumor growth. JPEN J Parenter Enteral Nutr 1994 Nov–Dec; 18(6):471–6.

[45] Gismondo MR, Drago L, Fassina MC, et al. Immunostimulating effect of oral glutamine. Dig Dis Sci 1998 Aug; 43(8):1752–4.

[46] Shewchuk LD, Baracos VE, Field CJ. Dietary L-glutamine supplementation reduces the growth of the Morris Hepatoma 7777 in exercise-trained and sedentary rats. J Nutr 1997 Jan; 127(1):158–66.

[47] Goossens V, Grooten J, Fiers W. The oxidative metabolism of glutamine. A modulator of reactive oxygen intermediate-mediated cytotoxicity of tumor necrosis factor in L929 fibrosarcoma cells. J Biol Chem 1996 Jan 5; 271(1):192–6.

[48] Klimberg VS, Kornbluth J, Cao Y, et al. Glutamine suppresses PGE2 synthesis and breast cancer growth. J Surg Res 1996 Jun; 63(1):293–7.

[49] Hamilos DL, Mascali JJ, Wedner HJ. The role of glutathione in lymphocyte activation—II. Effects of buthionine sulfoximine and 2-cyclohexene -1-one on early and late activation events. Int J Immunopharmacol 1991; 13(1):75–90.

[50] Donnerstag B, Ohlenschlager G, Cinatl J, et al. Reduced glutathione and S-acetylglutathione as selective apoptosis-inducing agents in cancer therapy. Cancer Lett 1996 Dec 20; 110(1–2):63–70.

[51] Yim CY, Hibbs JB Jr, MeGregor JR, et al. Use of N-acetyl cysteine to increase intracellular glutathione during the induction of antitumor responses by IL-2. J Immunol 1994; 152:5796–5805.

[52] Liang CM, Lee N, Cattell D, Liang SM. Glutathione regulates interleukin-2 activity on cytotoxic T-cells. J Biol Chem 1989; 264(23):13519–523.

[53] Walsh AC, Lawrence DA. N-ras mRNA expression is unaffected in glutathione-depleted cells of hematopoietic origin. Cancer Lett 1995 Aug 16; 95(1–2):105–12.

[54] Palomares T, Alonso-Varona A, Alvarez A, et al. Interleukin-2 increases intracellular glutathione levels and reverses the growth inhibiting effects of cyclophosphamide on B16 melanoma cells. Clin Exp Metastasis 1997 May; 15(3):329–37.

[55] Margalit A, Hauser SD, Zweifel BS, et al. Regulation of prostaglandin biosynthesis in vivo by glutathione. Am J Physiol 1998 Feb; 274(2 Pt 2):R294–302.

[56] Kiremidjian-Schumacher L, Roy M, et al. Regulation of cellular immune responses by selenium. Biol Trace Elem Res 1992 Apr–Jun; 33:23–35.

[57] Kiremidjian-Schumacher L, Roy M, Wishe HI, et al. Supplementation with selenium and human immune cell functions. II. Effect on cytotoxic lymphocytes and natural killer cells. Biol Trace Elem Res 1994 Apr–May; 41(1–2):115–27.

[58] Roy M, Kiremidjian-Schumacher L, Wishe HI, et al. Supplementation with selenium and human immune cell functions. I. Effect on lymphocyte proliferation and interleukin 2 receptor expression. Biol Trace Elem Res 1994 Apr–May; 41(1–2):103–14.

[59] Funke AM. [No title available]. Med Klin 1999 Oct 15; 94 Suppl 3:42–4.

[60] Ndiweni N, Rinch JM. Effects of in vitro supplementation with alpha-tocopherol and selenium on bovine neutrophil functions: Implications for resistance to mastitis. Vet Immunol Immunopathol 1996 May; 51(1–2):67–78.

[61] Ventura MT, Serlenga E, Tortorella C, et al. In vitro vitamin E and selenium supplementation improves neutrophil-mediated functions and monocyte chemoattractant protein-1 production in the elderly. Cytobios 1994; 77(311):225–32.

[62] Kiremidjian-Schumacher L, Roy M. Selenium and immune function. Z Ernahrungswiss 1998; 37 Suppl 1:50–6.

[63] Henson DE, Block G, Levine M. Ascorbic acid: Biologic functions and relation to cancer. Journal of the National Cancer Institute 1991; 83(8):547–50.

[64] de la Fuente M, Ferrandez MD, Burgos MS, et al. Immune function in aged women is improved by ingestion of vitamins C and E. Can J Physiol Pharmacol 1998 Apr; 76(4):373–80.

[65] Del Rio M, Ruedas G, Medina S, et al. Improvement by several antioxidants of macrophage function in vitro. Life Sci 1998; 63(10):871–81.

[66] Hughes DA. Effects of dietary antioxidants on the immune function of middle-aged adults. Proc Nutr Soc 1999 Feb; 58(1):79–84.

[67] Beharka A, Redican S, Leka L, et al. Vitamin E status and immune function. Methods Enzymol 1997; 282:247–63.

This appendix provides information on four predictive models. The first is a linear regression model used to predict oral clearance of a free (unchanged) compound. For convenience, we call this the "free oral clearance" or FOC model. The second, which is a simple model specific for phenolic compounds, uses values for free oral clearance to predict ones for total (free plus conjugate) oral clearance; this is called this the "total oral clearance" or TOC model. Both the TOC and FOC models were created for this book. Third is the TOPKAT model, which predicts toxicology data; it was developed by the Oxford Molecular Group, who supplied TOPKAT predictions for the natural compounds discussed here. Finally, the fourth is the "oral-intraperitoneal" or ORIN model, used to predict an equivalent oral dose based on an intraperitoneal one; it was also created for this book. Although these models, especially the FOC, TOC, and ORIN ones, provide only rough estimates, they are still useful as a starting point for further research.

FREE ORAL CLEARANCE (FOC) MODEL

The FOC model estimates oral clearance based on chemical structure and related descriptors. It appears to be unique, since no other such linear regression model seems to have been published in pharmacology journals. It is not the first time, however, that linear regression or other mathematical techniques have been used to model other pharmacokinetic parameters related to oral clearance. For example, linear regression models have been used to predict intestinal absorption and total body clearance of drugs based on chemical descriptors.[1-8] The latter is the clearance after intravenous administration. Oral clearance depends on both intestinal absorption and total body clearance, since its definition is the total body clearance divided by the fraction of the drug absorbed.

The FOC model was designed to predict oral clearance of the free, unchanged compound, as opposed to oral clearance of the total (free plus conjugate) compound. Thus we use the FOC model to predict oral clearance for all compounds except phenolic ones, which appear in the plasma primarily in conjugate forms; for those we use a combination of the FOC model and the total oral clearance (TOC) model. The process of developing the FOC can be divided into five steps:

1. Collection of oral clearance data for numerous drugs.

2. Generation of descriptors based on the chemical structure.

3. Use of linear regression techniques to correlate oral clearance with structural descriptors.

4. Verification of the model.

5. Application of the model to natural compounds of interest.

Each step is described in more detail below.

Collection of Oral Clearance Data

Oral clearance values for more than 300 conventional or experimental drugs were obtained from the literature. In some cases, these values came directly from the published articles, and in others they were calculated based on the reported values for total clearance (CL) and bioavailability (F, fraction absorbed) or, using the formula below, on dose and area under the concentration-time curve (AUC):

$$oral\ clearance = \frac{CL}{F} = \frac{dose}{AUC}$$
Equation I.1

The drugs used were not preselected. Rather, any drug was included for which oral clearance values (and chemical structures) were easily obtained. For some drugs, more than one article served as a reference, and for others, reviews were used that summarized multiple studies. In any case, if a range of values was found, midrange values were used.

The frequency of oral clearance values in the final data set of 247 drugs is illustrated in Figure I.1. (Not all of the 300+ drugs reviewed had complete data sets or were amenable to analysis by the software used, and therefore some were omitted.) As seen, the majority of drugs used in the data set had a clearance value of 400 L/hr or less, as is the case with most natural compounds. The geometric average oral clearance for the 247 drugs was about 25 L/hr. The x-axis is split at 800 L/hr to show that a few compounds had an oral clearance higher than 4,400 L/hr.

Generation of Structural Descriptors

Over 200 chemical descriptors were generated for each compound. These descriptors included such items as

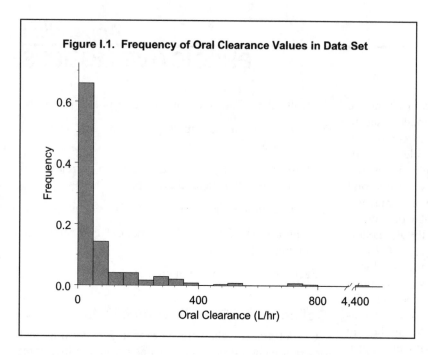

Figure I.1. Frequency of Oral Clearance Values in Data Set

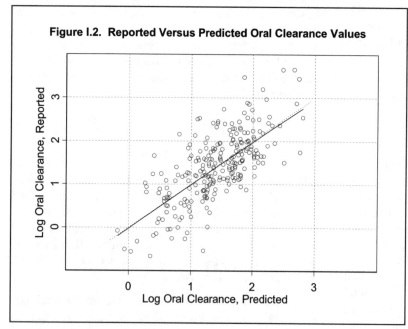

Figure I.2. Reported Versus Predicted Oral Clearance Values

number of carbon atoms, oxygen atoms, and double bonds, as well as log P values and solubility parameters. The descriptors were generated by the software programs Molecular Modeling Pro™ and Topix (see Appendix L for additional information on these programs). Prior to generation of the descriptors, the three-dimensional geometry of the structures was optimized by the MM2 routine in Molecular Modeling Pro.™

Because of limitations of the software, certain types of drugs were not analyzed, for example, those containing over 100 atoms or atoms with an atomic number greater than 19. For various reasons, over 50 drugs were omit-

ted from calculations, leaving 247 for which chemical descriptors and oral clearance values were obtained.

Linear Regression Technique

Linear regression was performed using the software program Axum (see Appendix L). A stepwise linear regression technique was used in an iterative fashion to choose meaningful descriptors out of the more than 300 possibilities; this pool included over 200 unmodified descriptors, as well as about 100 other ones derived through log transformation of the original data. (Log transformation was used to make the data for certain descriptors more linear.) Oral clearance values were also log-transformed.

The results from each round of stepwise regression were compared to a correlation matrix of all 300 descriptors. Descriptors that were chosen by the stepwise regression but were heavily correlated with other chosen descriptors (correlation index greater than 0.7) were removed from the pool of possibilities. The final result, after the last round of stepwise regression, was a linear regression model containing 24 unique descriptors, some of which were in their unmodified form and some were log-transformed. Figure I.2 illustrates the degree that predicted values for each drug were similar to values in the data set.

As shown, there is a moderate correlation between reported and predicted values. The R^2 value is 0.50, which means the model was able to account for 50 percent of the observed deviation from the average.

Model Verification

To verify the model, 10 percent of the data set was randomly chosen and set aside as a verification set. The linear regression model was then regenerated using the remaining data (the test set), and the verification set was run through the resulting model. This process was repeated three times. The R^2 values for the three test sets were 0.49, 0.50, and 0.49, and the R^2 values for the corresponding verification sets were 0.57, 0.50, and 0.57.

Therefore, prediction of the verification sets was at least as accurate as prediction of the test sets.

In addition to the linear regression technique, one test set was used as input to a neural network. Neural network optimization was performed using the software program NeuroGenetic Optimizer (see Appendix L). Modeling by an optimized neural network produced R^2 values for the test and verification sets similar to those produced by the linear regression model.

The average R^2 value for the three verification sets was 0.55. This is not a high R^2 value, and clearly, the model was not able to predict oral clearance with high accuracy. Based on data from the three verification sets, there is about an 80 percent probability that the predicted value will be within a factor of eight of the reported value (see Figure I.3). However, the FOC model is more accurate if we consider only drugs whose oral clearance is within the range of 2 to 1,600 L/hr. The model is more accurate in this range because the oral clearance values for most drugs in the data set fell into this range (see Figure I.1). (The oral clearance values for most natural compounds of interest also fall within this range.) Considering compounds that have a reported clearance within the range of 2 to 1,600 L/hr, there is an 80 percent probability that the predicted value will be within a factor of about five of the reported value (and a 50 percent probability the oral clearance will be predicted within a factor of two).

It is not surprising that the model would have only a moderate accuracy, since oral clearance values are themselves inherently variable (and thus there was variation within the data set). Many factors may be responsible for the variability of oral clearance values. Differences in absorption, metabolism, protein binding, and excretion may be involved, and these may depend on race, age, body weight, sex, state of health, and other factors.[9, 10] For example, in one study the oral clearance for the antimalaria drug quinine was 2.4-fold lower in patients with acute disease as opposed to patients in convalescence.[11] In another study, the oral clearance of the antimalaria drug atovaquone varied 2.8-fold due to differences in race.[12] In a study on patients with cystic fibrosis, the oral clearance of ibuprofen varied more than 5-fold among subjects, mostly due to differences in age and weight.[13] Oral clearance for some drugs can vary 15-fold between individuals.[14] Therefore, while predictions by the FOC model are only moderately accurate (in

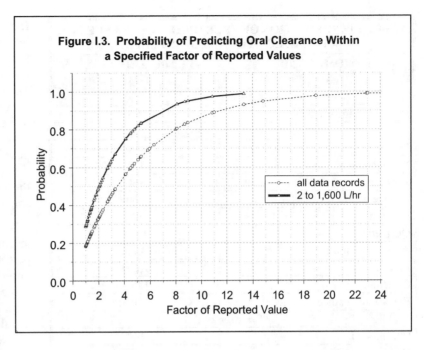

Figure I.3. Probability of Predicting Oral Clearance Within a Specified Factor of Reported Values

comparison to the data set), they are still reasonable given the inherent variability of oral clearance. With the understanding that we are making only ballpark estimates for oral clearance (and dose), the predictions made by this model are accurate enough to be useful.

Model Application

Once the model was developed and verified, data for the 24 descriptors were calculated using the software described above for natural compounds of interest. These descriptors were then used as input to the linear regression model. The predictions made by the model are listed in Table I.1 according to the chapter in which they are discussed in Part III of the text. Related natural compounds not discussed in Part III are also listed.

The use of these values and comparisons between them and the values obtained from animal and human pharmacokinetic studies are discussed below and in Appendix J.

TOTAL ORAL CLEARANCE (TOC) MODEL

Phenolic compounds exist in plasma primarily in their conjugate forms. Therefore, we base the dose calculations for phenolic compounds in Appendix J on clearance values obtained from total (free plus conjugate) plasma concentrations, rather than plasma concentrations for the free compound alone. Unfortunately, the oral clearance based on the total plasma concentration is unknown for many phenolic compounds of interest; the TOC model is designed to estimate these values. It is

TABLE I.1   PREDICTION OF FREE ORAL CLEARANCE FOR NATURAL COMPOUNDS OF INTEREST

COMPOUND	PREDICTED VALUE (L/HR)
Chapter 18	
Diallyl disulfide (DADS)	1.5
Chapter 19	
Daidzein	58
Naringenin	130
Apigenin	160
Genistein	180
Luteolin	490
Quercetin	2,000
Proanthocyanidin	63,000
Epicatechin	1,200
Catechin	1,200
Epicatechin gallate	24,000
Chapter 20	
Caffeic acid	140
CAPE	240
Curcumin	200
Silybin	260
Arctigenin	44
Schizandrin	110
Enterodiol	770
Enterolactone	57
Resveratrol	310
Rhein	55
Emodin	110
Chapter 21	
Limonene	0.10
Perillic acid	7.7
Geraniol	45
Perillyl alcohol	51
Asiatic acid	76
Ursolic acid	29
Beta boswellic acid	27
Glycyrrhetic acid	20
Parthenolide	1.9
Helenalin	5.1
Artemisinin	6.0
Chapter 22	
ATRA	2,100

$$total\ oral\ clearance = free\ oral\ clearance \times \frac{percent\ free\ in\ plasma}{100}$$

Equation I.2

reasonable to assume that the total oral clearance is directly related to both the free oral clearance and the percentage of the total that occurs in plasma in the free

form. This is because oral clearance is directly related to plasma concentration. As an extreme example, if the total plasma concentration is composed only of the free form (as we assume it is with nonphenolic compounds), then the total oral clearance would be expected to be equal to the free oral clearance. Likewise, if half the total concentration were composed of the free form, we would expect that the total oral clearance would be half that of the free oral clearance. This simple relationship is modeled by Equation I.2.

To use this equation, we must of course determine values for free oral clearance and the percentage that is free in the plasma. For our purposes, we can obtain free oral clearance values from the FOC model or, when available, from animal or human studies. Choosing a value for percent free in plasma is more problematic, since little information is available for many compounds. Moreover, for any given compound, values for percent free in plasma are likely to vary between studies at least as much as values for free oral clearance. Like free oral clearance, percent free in plasma can vary depending on the magnitude of the dose, the gut microflora of the individual, the species tested, and other factors. Not surprisingly, there is variation in the percent free in plasma values reported for different phenolic compounds, as shown in Table J.4 of Appendix J for flavonoids.

Thus the use of Equation I.2 requires as much art as science. As a guide, we can experiment with the values for free and total oral clearance for the nine phenolic compounds listed in Table I.2. Most of the free oral clearance values were obtained from the FOC model. The value for daidzein is an average of that from the FOC model (58 L/hr) and a human study (400 L/hr).[15] The 460-L/hr value for epicatechin is scaled from a rat study, and the 490-L/hr value for EGCG is taken from the human studies listed in Table J.10.[16]

To simplify the choice of a percentage, we limit our available values to the following somewhat arbitrary series: 0.5, 1.5, 3, 6, 12, 18, and 24 percent. Next, using the known values for free and total oral clearance, we can choose percentages that both seem reasonable based on the literature and provide the best result. Percentage values from the literature are discussed in Appendix J. The second column of numbers in Table I.2 lists the resulting percentages estimated by the above method.

As would be expected with a model using massaged input, the model quite accurately predicts the total clearance for these nine compounds ($R^2 = 0.99$). Figure I.4 is a graph of the observed versus predicted values for total oral clearance (the last two columns of Table I.2). As can be seen, the observed and predicted values are very similar. There is, on average, a 17 percent difference between observed and predicted values.

The values for percentage of free compound listed in Table I.2 are useful as an aid in predicting total clearance values for other compounds. This is because some of the other compounds are similar in structure to those in Table I.2, and we can assume the percentages are similar for both. For example, apigenin is similar to luteolin. Since we are estimating that free luteolin accounts for about 3 percent of the total plasma concentration, we can also estimate that the percent for free apigenin is similar. Using such inductive reasoning and using the values obtained from the literature as a guide (see Table J.4 and the text of Appendix J), we can estimate total oral clearance values for the phenolic compounds listed in Table I.3. Values in bold type are used in the dose calculations of Appendix J.

TOPKAT MODEL

Oxford Molecular Group (see Appendix L) has contributed predictions of rat oral toxicity for many compounds discussed in this book. These predictions were generated using their TOPKAT toxicity assessment software program, which predicts toxicity based on the two-dimensional chemical structure. This program calculates structural and electronic descriptors for each compound, compares this information against information calculated for compounds with experimentally derived toxicity values, and then predicts the query compound's toxicity based on the degree of similarity. The software is used to compute probable toxicity for compounds that have not been studied (or are impractical to study) in vivo. Although the software can predict many types of toxic effects, only rat oral lethal doses (LD_{50}) and rat oral lowest-observable-adverse-effects-level (LOAEL) doses have been predicted here.

TABLE I.2 DATA FOR CONSTRUCTION OF THE TOC MODEL AND PREDICTIONS OF TOTAL ORAL CLEARANCE				
COMPOUND	FREE ORAL CLEARANCE (L/Hr)	FREE COMPOUND IN PLASMA (% OF TOTAL)[†]	OBSERVED TOTAL ORAL CLEARANCE (L/Hr)[‡]	PREDICTED TOTAL ORAL CLEARANCE (L/Hr)
Genistein	180[*]	1.5	3.7	2.7
Daidzein	230	1.5	4.9	3.5
Enterolactone	57[*]	12	8.3	6.8
Quercetin	2,000[*]	0.5	24	10
Luteolin	490[*]	3	14	15
Epicatechin	460	4	22	18
Silybin	260[*]	12	32	31
EGCG	490	18	90	88
Proanthocyanidin	63,000[*]	0.5	410	320

[*] *Obtained from the FOC model. See text for explanations of other values in this column.*

[†] *See text for explanations of values.*

[‡] *Values obtained from literature; see Appendix J.*

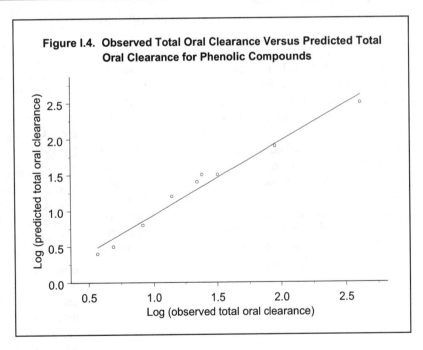

Figure I.4. Observed Total Oral Clearance Versus Predicted Total Oral Clearance for Phenolic Compounds

TABLE I.3 PREDICTED TOTAL ORAL CLEARANCE FOR VARIOUS PHENOLIC COMPOUNDS			
COMPOUND	**FREE CLEARANCE (L/Hr)**	**FREE COMPOUND IN PLASMA (% OF TOTAL)***	**PREDICTED TOTAL CLEARANCE (L/Hr)**
Naringenin	130	1.5	2.0
Resveratrol	310	1.5	**4.7**
Apigenin	160	3	**4.8**
Arctigenin	44	12	**5.3**
Rhein	55	12	6.6
Schizandrin	110	12	13
Emodin	110	12	**13**
Curcumin	6,500[†]	0.5	**33**
Caffeic acid	140	24	34
Catechin	1,200	3	36
CAPE	240	24	**58**
Enterodiol	770	12	92

* *Method for estimation of these values is discussed in the text.*

† *Estimated from literature, see Appendix J. All other values in this column were obtained from the FOC model.*

TOPKAT Predictions

The TOPKAT model provided LD_{50} and LOAEL dose predictions for the 26 natural compounds listed in Table I.4.[a] However, since some of these predictions may be of questionable validity due to lack of similar compounds in the database or for other reasons, the model assesses each prediction as being of acceptable, tentative, or unacceptable validity *within the accuracy of the model*. Predictions deemed of unacceptable or tentative validity are marked in the table as such. In a few cases, the test compounds were already included in the program's experimental database, and for these compounds the experimental animal data are given, as marked in the table. The table also provides equivalent doses as scaled to humans, using the method discussed in Chapter 1; this scaling method can be considered to provide only rough estimates.

Accuracy of TOPKAT's LOAEL Dose Predictions

For our purposes, we are more interested in LOAEL dose predictions than LD_{50} predictions, since we use the LOAEL dose to estimate the upper safe dose for humans. Therefore, we would like to know how accurate the LOAEL dose predictions are. The accuracy of the model has been determined by its creators during development. It consists of five separate submodels, each is used to make predictions for a different class of chemicals. The computations in the submodels are based on a total of 393 critically reviewed experimental LOAEL values. The model has been cross-validated using the leave-one-out method, in which each compound is removed once from the database, and its LOAEL dose is predicted by the model. The result is that for all five submodels, there is on average a 93 percent probability the model will predict the correct LOAEL dose within a factor of 3. Of course, the accuracy could be lower for compounds significantly different from the 393 compounds used as the basis for the model, and it will likely be lower for compounds with a tentative prediction.

Predicting the LOAEL Dose Based on the LD_{50}

For a few compounds, LOAEL dose estimates are not available, but LD_{50} data are, using animal studies or TOPKAT predictions. In these cases, it is useful to estimate the LOAEL dose based on the LD_{50}. Unfortunately, this estimate cannot be made with great accuracy, and the best we can do is provide a probable range. Using data from Table I.4, Table I.5 lists the predicted LD_{50} and LOAEL doses (as scaled to humans) and the ratios between these doses. (Compounds for which one or both of these doses could not be predicted are omitted.) As shown, ratios for quercetin and arctigenin are extremes; the ratio for quercetin is excessively low (values less than 1 imply that the LD_{50} is lower than the LOAEL dose), and the ratio for arctigenin is excessively high. These extremes are due to errors in the LD_{50} and LOAEL dose predictions. If these questionable ratios are omitted, then the geometric mean of all other ratios is 13. In other words, the LD_{50} is generally about 13 times higher than the LOAEL dose.

---

[a] *In animal studies, the LD_{50} test generally consists of a single administration to several groups of rats at different dosages. The LD_{50} is calculated as the dose that causes 50 percent of the animals to die. In contrast, the LOAEL test is based on chronic administration, and it measures the lowest dose that causes a statistically significant number of adverse effects. The database used by the TOPKAT model to predict LOAEL doses consists of rat experiments that lasted at least one year.*

Figure I.5 illustrates the probability of observing different LD_{50} to LOAEL dose ratios (again, excluding data for quercetin and arctigenin). As shown, there is a 75 percent chance the ratio will be less than about 75. This is not too different from probabilities reported in other studies. For example, in a study in rats, the LD_{50} to LOAEL dose ratio was about 120 for 75 percent of the 20 diverse compounds tested, while the average ratio for all compounds was only about 12.[17, a] Based on all the above, we assume here that when predicting the LOAEL dose from the LD_{50}, the LD_{50} to LOAEL dose ratio will be within the range of 13 to 75. Therefore, for example, if the LD_{50} is 10 grams, we assume the LOAEL dose is 1.3 to 7.7 grams.

As a point of interest, note the difference between the no-observable-adverse-effects-level (NOAEL) dose and the lowest-observable-adverse-effects-level (LOAEL) dose. As the names imply, the NOAEL dose is the largest dose for which no adverse effects are seen, and the LOAEL dose is the smallest dose at which adverse effects are seen. These doses are usually different. Rodent studies have suggested that the NOAEL dose is roughly 1- to 10-fold lower than the LOAEL dose for many compounds.[17, 18]

TABLE I.4 RESULTS OF TOPKAT PREDICTIONS WITH SCALING TO HUMAN EQUIVALENTS				
COMPOUND	PREDICTED RAT ORAL LD_{50} (mg/kg)	SCALED HUMAN LD_{50} (grams)	PREDICTED RAT ORAL LOAEL DOSE (mg/kg-day)	SCALED HUMAN LOAEL DOSE (grams/day)
Chapter 18				
Allicin	3,600	58	240(tent)	3.9
DADS	8,300	130	590 (tent)	10
Chapter 19				
Genistein	170	2.8	97	1.6
Daidzein	270	4.4	69	1.1
Quercetin	160 (exp)	2.6	400 (exp)	6.5
Apigenin	370	6.0	200	3.2
Luteolin	520	8.4	270	4.4
Epicatechin	(unacceptable)	—	34	0.55
EGCG	74 (tent)	1.2	(unacceptable)	—
Chapter 20				
CAPE	>10,000	>160	(unacceptable)	—
Curcumin	6,700	110	(unacceptable)	—
Silybin	(unacceptable)	—	16	0.26
Arctigenin	3,000	49	2.4	.039
Resveratrol	1,900	31	(unacceptable)	—
Emodin	2,100	34	180	2.9
Hypericin	2,700	44	260	4.2
Chapter 21				
Perillyl alcohol	2,100 (exp)	34	16	0.26
Limonene	4,400 (exp)	71	75 (exp)	1.2
Perillic acid	2,400	39	250	4.1
Geraniol	3,300	53	(unacceptable)	—
Boswellic acid	(unacceptable)	—	160 (tent)	2.6
Asiatic acid	(unacceptable)	—	460 (tent)	7.5
Ursolic acid	(unacceptable)	—	120 (tent)	1.9
Ruscogenin	(unacceptable)	—	7.8	0.13
Helenalin	130 (exp)	2.1	(unacceptable)	—
Parthenolide	5,000	81	12	0.19

Notes: exp= based on experimental animal studies; tent= tentative validity (associated doses scaled to humans are also tentative); unacceptable= unacceptable validity

ORAL-INTRAPERITONEAL (ORIN) MODEL

A number of studies mentioned in this book administered a natural compound by the intraperitoneal (i.p.) route. In these studies, the dose is injected into the intraperitoneal cavity surrounding the intestines. Compared with oral administration, intraperitoneal administration bypasses the degrading effects of stomach acids and intestinal bacteria; metabolism of the drug by intestinal bacteria and intestinal enzymes; and any possible limitations in intestinal absorption. Because we are interested in oral administration, however, we wish to convert an intraperitoneal dose to its oral equivalent. To accomplish this conversion, the oral-intraperitoneal (ORIN) model was developed for this book.

Unfortunately, the relationship between equivalent i.p. and oral doses is unknown for most compounds in this book. In general, an equivalent oral dose will be larger than the given intraperitoneal dose. For one thing, orally administered compounds are more readily excreted in the feces, although this can also happen to compounds

---

[a] *In this study, the LOAEL dose was called the two-year minimum effect dose.*

TABLE I.5 COMPARISON OF LD₅₀ AND LOAEL DOSES AS SCALED TO HUMANS

COMPOUND	HUMAN LD$_{50}$ (grams)[*]	HUMAN LOAEL DOSE (grams)[*]	LD$_{50}$/LOAEL RATIO
Quercetin	2.6	6.5[†]	0.4
Genistein	2.8	1.6	1.8
Apigenin	6.0	3.2	1.9
Luteolin	8.4	4.4	1.9
Daidzein	4.4	1.1	4.0
Perillic acid	39	4.1	9.5
Hypericin	44	4.2	10
Emodin	34	2.9	12
DADS	130[†]	10[†]	13
Allicin	58	3.9	15
Limonene	71	1.2	59
Perillyl alcohol	34	0.26	130
Parthenolide	81	0.19[†]	430
Arctigenin	49	0.039[†]	1,300[†]
Average:	**40**	**3.1**	
Standard deviation:	**37**	**2.8**	
		Geometric average:	**13[‡]**

[*] *Data from TOPKAT predictions listed in Table I.4.*

[†] *More than one standard deviation from average.*

[‡] *Excludes the two extremes of quercetin and arctigenin.*

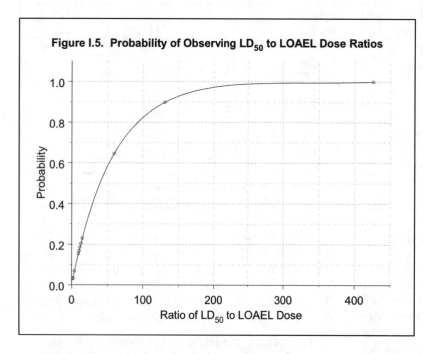

Figure I.5. Probability of Observing LD₅₀ to LOAEL Dose Ratios

in the plasma can differ after oral or i.p. administration; thus it is not easy to determine equivalent doses. Nonetheless, it is worth the attempt because so many antitumor studies have used i.p. administration.

Table I.6 lists the oral bioavailability and the ratio between oral and i.p. bioavailability for 30 different drugs. Calculations of oral bioavailability were generally made by comparing the area under the concentration-time curve after oral administration to that after intravenous administration. Calculations for intraperitoneal bioavailability were made in the same way (i.e., by comparing the AUC after i.p. and intravenous administration). Note that these bioavailabilities were calculated for the free form of the compound in the plasma, rather than the free plus conjugated forms.

The relationship between the bioavailabilities listed in Table I.6 is illustrated in Figure I.6. The curve and associated formula shown in the figure reasonably predict the values in the data set. The R^2 value is 0.81, which means the model was able to account for 81 percent of the observed deviation from the average. As shown, a high oral bioavailability is associated with a low i.p. to oral bioavailability ratio (the ratio approaches 1 at very high oral bioavailabilities). This is as would be expected, since a compound that is well absorbed after oral administration is likely to be equally well absorbed after i.p. administration. Also, a low oral bioavailability is associated with a high i.p. to oral bioavailability ratio; again this is as expected, since a compound that is poorly absorbed after oral administration would be easily excreted, whereas a compound administered by the i.p. route would not be.

administered by the i.p. route if they are excreted in the bile. In addition, compounds given orally must pass through the intestinal lining, which is a site of metabolism for many compounds. Therefore, not only the amount but also the form in which a compound appears

The required dose for a compound is inversely related to its bioavailability. As the latter increases, the re-

TABLE I.6 ORAL BIOAVAILABILITY AND INTRAPERITONEAL/ORAL RATIOS OF VARIOUS COMPOUNDS

COMPOUND	ORAL BIOAVAILABILITY (%)	I.P./ORAL BIOAVAILABILITY	REFERENCES
1,25-D_3	70	1.0	19, 20
14C-1	40	2.5	21
4,6-Benzylidene-d1-D-glucose	87	1.4	22
Acebutolol	61	1.4	23
AMD473	40	2.2	24
Bestatin	48	1.5	25
BMD188	8	8.8	26
Busulphan	5.6	6.6	27
Caffeine	16	2.8	28
CGP 64128A	2	14	29
Clocapramine	16	2.4	30
Cocaine	19	3.7	31
Glycyrrhizin	7.3	16	32
Halomon	4	11	33
Hexobarbitone	18	2.2	34
HI-240	1	24	35
ICI D 1694	15	6.7	36
Imexon	21	4.9	37
Melatonin	54	1.4	38
Midazolam	3.9	4.6	39
N-0923	0.3	24	40
Nicotine-1'-N-oxide	15	5.2	41
Norendimide	80	1.2	42
Pafenolol	33	3.0	43
Plenolin	87	1.7	44
PMPA	17	4.3	45
Propafenone	37	1.3	46
Propyl gallate	5	3.8	47
WHI-P131	30	3.2	48
WHI-P180	8.3	3.3	49

quired dose decreases. This relationship is shown in Equation I.3, where A is some constant:

$$oral\ dose = \frac{A}{oral\ bioavailability}$$

Equation I.3

A similar equation could be written for the relationship between i.p. dose and i.p. bioavailability, using the same value for the constant A. By considering the ratio between these two equations, we obtain Equation I.4 (the two constants, being equal, cancel one another):

$$\frac{oral\ dose}{i.p.\ dose} = \frac{i.p.\ bioavailability}{oral\ bioavailability}$$

Equation I.4

Equation I.4 can easily be solved for the oral dose, given the i.p. dose and the ratio for i.p. to oral bioavail-

ability. For example, if the given i.p. dose in a rodent study is 100 mg/kg, and the ratio of the i.p. to oral bioavailability is 4, this model predicts that the equivalent oral dose is 100 times 4, or 400 mg/kg. To be clear, this model only accounts for differences in bioavailability between i.p. and oral doses; it does not take into account any differences in metabolism that may occur, since doing so would be excessively complicated and the appropriate data are not available for constructing such a model. Even so, the simple model described here is reasonable for making rough estimates of an equivalent oral dose.

To use Equation I.4 for natural compounds, we must know the ratio of the i.p. to oral bioavailability. This ratio is not known for most of our compounds, however, and therefore must be estimated using the oral bioavailability and the relationships shown in Figure I.6.

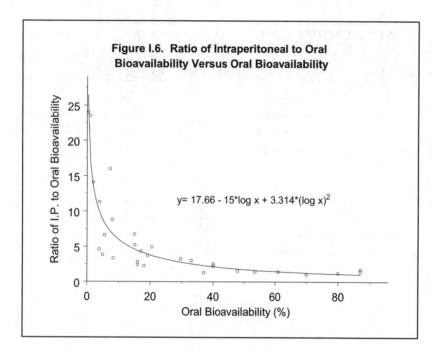

Figure I.6. Ratio of Intraperitoneal to Oral Bioavailability Versus Oral Bioavailability

$y = 17.66 - 15*\log x + 3.314*(\log x)^2$

Although the oral bioavailability is known for only a few of the natural compounds of interest, it can readily be estimated for others based on known bioavailabilities for similar compounds and discussions of oral clearance in Appendix J. Table I.7 lists estimates for bioavailability and oral to i.p. dose ratios for several natural compounds. For example, the oral bioavailability of DADS is estimated to be 65 percent, the same as that for the similar compound allicin. Using the data in Figure I.6 and Equation I.4, the ratio of the oral to i.p. dose is then 1.4. Note that the bioavailability of each phenolic compound is based on its total plasma concentration, consisting of free compound plus conjugates. For many phenolics, essentially no free compound exists in the plasma.

TABLE I.7 ORAL BIOAVAILABILITIES AND RATIOS OF ORAL TO INTRAPERITONEAL DOSES			
COMPOUND	**ORAL BIOAVAILABILITY (%)**	**RATIO OF ORAL TO I.P. DOSE**	**REFERENCES**
Chapter 16			
High-molecular-weight polysaccharides	13	5.1	
	Bioavailability is estimated based on 13% for chondroitin sulfate.		50
Chapter 18			
DADS	65	1.4	
	Bioavailability is estimated based on 65% for allicin.		51
Chapter 19			
Genistein and daidzein	15	4.7	
	Bioavailability is estimated based on average of 12% for genistein and 17% for daidzein.[*]		52
Quercetin	9[†]	6.4	53
Apigenin and luteolin	13	5.1	
	Bioavailability is estimated based on average of that for genistein, daidzein, and quercetin.		
Chapter 20			
Propolis (CAPE)	39	2.2	
	Bioavailability is estimated based on 39% for caffeic acid. (That for rosmarinic acid is similar, at 32%.)		54 55
Curcumin	8	6.8	
	Bioavailability is estimated based on 63% for curcumin in a radiolabeled study.[‡]		56
Resveratrol	17	4.2	
	Bioavailability is estimated based on average of that for all phenolic compounds listed here.		

TABLE I.7 ORAL BIOAVAILABILITIES AND RATIOS OF ORAL TO INTRAPERITONEAL DOSES *(continued)*			
COMPOUND	**ORAL BIOAVAILABILITY (%)**	**RATIO OF ORAL TO I.P. DOSE**	**REFERENCES**
Emodin	8[†]	6.8	57
	Bioavailability is similar to that of 14% for hypericin.		58
Chapter 21			
Oleanolic acid	61	1.4	
	Bioavailability is estimated based on average of that for ginseng, plenolin, ATRA, and 1,25-D_3 (see below), and 43% for limonene.		59
Boswellic acid	61	1.4	
	Bioavailability is estimated based on that for oleanolic acid.		
Ginseng (ginsenosides)	49[†]	1.8	60
Parthenolide	87[†]	1.4 average	
	Ratio of oral to i.p. dose is estimated based on an average of 1.7 (as obtained from a rodent study on plenolin that measured a bioavailability of 87%) and 1.0 (as determined by the ORIN model using an oral bioavailability of 87%).		44
Chapter 22			
ATRA	58[†]	1.5	61
1,25-D_3	NA	1.5[§]	62
	Ratio of oral to i.p. dose is estimated as 1.5 based on a human study. This is similar to the ratio of 1.0 measured in other human studies (in which the oral bioavailability was found to be 70%).		19, 20
Vitamin E	NA	1.5	
	Ratio of oral to i.p. dose is based on values for ATRA and 1,25-D_3		
Melatonin	15[‖]	4.6	63
Chapter 23			
Alpha-lipoic acid	29[†]	2.8	64

[*] *Based on urinary excretion.*

[†] *Based on experimental data.*

[‡] *Assumes 7.5-fold overestimate by radiolabeled study, as listed in Table J.2 of Appendix J.*

[§] *Based on repeated administration.*

[‖] *Measured in humans after a dose of 2 to 4 milligrams. At much larger doses in animals, the bioavailability was much higher (50 to 100%), suggesting that high doses may saturate metabolism pathways.[65]*

NA: Not available

TABLE I.8 SUBCUTANEOUS BIOAVAILABILITIES AND RATIOS OF SUBCUTANEOUS TO INTRAPERITONEAL BIOAVAILABILITIES			
COMPOUND	**S.C. BIOAVAILABILITY (%)**	**S.C./I.P. BIOAVAILABILITY**	**REFERENCES**
Cyclosporine	59	1.0	66
Bestatin	91	1.3	25
Halomon	47	1.0	33
CGP 64128A	31	1.1	29
Midazolam	3.9	2.1	39
Average:		**1.3**	

In some studies mentioned in this book, the subcutaneous (s.c.) route of administration was used. Based on the few studies listed in Table I.8, we can estimate that the ratio of the s.c. to i.p. bioavailability may be about 1.3/1. Again, an inverse relationship can be applied, so that the ratio of the i.p. to s.c. dose is then 1.3/1. Therefore, to obtain the oral equivalent for an s.c. dose, it is multiplied by 1.3 to obtain the equivalent i.p. dose, then the i.p. dose is converted to the oral dose as per the ORIN model above. The value of 1.3 used in this method is, of course, based only on the five data points in Table I.8, thus this method can be expected to produce only rough estimates. Nonetheless, these estimates can still be useful.

REFERENCES

[1] Winiwarter S, Bonham NM, Ax F, et al. Correlation of human jejunal permeability (in vivo) of drugs with experimentally and theoretically derived parameters. A multivariate data analysis approach. J Med Chem 1998 Dec 3; 41(25):4939–49.

[2] Ghuloum AM, Sage CR, Jain AN. Molecular hashkeys: A novel method for molecular characterization and its application for predicting important pharmaceutical properties of molecules. J Med Chem 1999 May 20; 42(10):1739–48.

[3] Palm K, Luthman K, Ungell AL, et al. Evaluation of dynamic polar molecular surface area as predictor of drug absorption: Comparison with other computational and experimental predictors. J Med Chem 1998 Dec 31; 41(27):5382–92.

[4] Palm K, Luthman K, Ungell AL, et al. Correlation of drug absorption with molecular surface properties. J Pharm Sci 1996 Jan; 85(1):32–9.

[5] Wessel MD, Jurs PC, Tolan JW, et al. Prediction of human intestinal absorption of drug compounds from molecular structure. J Chem Inf Comput Sci 1998 Jul–Aug; 38(4):726–35.

[6] Hirono S, Nakagome I, Hirano H, et al. Non-congeneric structure-pharmacokinetic property correlation studies using fuzzy adaptive least-squares: Oral bioavailability. Biol Pharm Bull 1994 Feb; 17(2):306–9.

[7] Gobburu JV, Shelver WH. Quantitative structure-pharmacokinetic relationships (QSPR) of beta blockers derived using neural networks. J Pharm Sci 1995 Jul; 84(7):862–5.

[8] Herman RA, Veng-Pedersen P. Quantitative structure-pharmacokinetic relationships for systemic drug distribution kinetics not confined to a congeneric series. J Pharm Sci 1994 Mar; 83(3):423–8.

[9] Johnson JA. Influence of race or ethnicity on pharmacokinetics of drugs. J Pharm Sci 1997 Dec; 86(12):1328–33.

[10] de Vries JD, Salphati L, Horie S, et al. Variability in the disposition of chlorzoxazone. Biopharm Drug Dispos 1994 Oct; 15(7):587–97.

[11] Babalola CP, Bolaji OO, Ogunbona FA, et al. Pharmacokinetics of quinine in African patients with acute falciparum malaria. Pharm World Sci 1998 Jun; 20(3):118–22.

[12] Hussein Z, Eaves J, Hutchinson DB, et al. Population pharmacokinetics of atovaquone in patients with acute malaria caused by Plasmodium falciparum. Clin Pharmacol Ther 1997 May; 61(5):518–30.

[13] Murry DJ, Oermann CM, Ou CN, et al. Pharmacokinetics of ibuprofen in patients with cystic fibrosis. Pharmacotherapy 1999 Mar; 19(3):340–5.

[14] Fontana RJ, deVries TM, Woolf TF, et al. Caffeine based measures of CYP1A2 activity correlate with oral clearance of tacrine in patients with Alzheimer's disease. Br J Clin Pharmacol 1998 Sep; 46(3):221–8.

[15] Lapcik O, Hampl R, al-Maharik N, et al. A novel radioimmunoassay for daidzein. Steroids 1997 Mar; 62(3):315–20.

[16] Piskula MK, Terao J. Accumulation of (-)-epicatechin metabolites in rat plasma after oral administration and distribution of conjugation enzymes in rat tissues. J Nutr 1998 Jul; 128(7):1172–8.

[17] Weil CS, Woodside MD, Bernard JR, Carpenter CP. Relationship between single-peroral, one-week, and ninety-day rat feeding studies. Toxicol Appl Pharmacol 1969; 14(3):426–31.

[18] Venman BC, Flaga C. Development of an acceptable factor to estimate chronic end points from acute toxicity data. Toxicol Ind Health 1985; 1(4):261–9.

[19] Jones CL, Vieth R, Spino M, et al. Comparisons between oral and intraperitoneal 1,25-dihydroxyvitamin D3 therapy in children treated with peritoneal dialysis. Clin Nephrol 1994 Jul; 42(1):44–9.

[20] Jongen M, van der Vijgh WJ, Netelenbos JC, et al. Pharmacokinetics of 24,25-dihydroxyvitamin D3 in humans. Horm Metab Res 1989 Oct; 21(10):577–80.

[21] Schieweck A, Offchert HH, Morgenroth U, et al. [The pharmacokinetics of Z-2-amino-5-chlorobenzophenoneamidinohydrazone in the rat.] Pharmazie 1993 May; 48(5):370–3.

[22] Dunsaed CB, Dornish JM, Pettersen EO. The bioavailability and dose dependency of the deuterated anti-tumour agent 4,6-benzylidene-d1-D-glucose in mice and rats. Cancer Chemother Pharmacol 1995; 35(6):464–70.

[23] Piquette-Miller M, Jamali F. Pharmacokinetics and multiple peaking of acebutolol enantiomers in rats. Biopharm Drug Dispos 1997 Aug; 18(6):543–56.

[24] Raynaud FI, Boxall FE, Goddard PM, et al. cis-Amminedichloro(2-methylpyridine) platinum(II) (AMD473), a novel sterically hindered platinum complex: In vivo activity, toxicology, and pharmacokinetics in mice. Clin Cancer Res 1997 Nov; 3(11):2063–74.

[25] Abe F, Alvord G, Koyama M, et al. Pharmacokinetics of bestatin and oral activity for treatment of experimental metastases. Cancer Immunol Immunother 1989; 28(1):29–33.

[26] Li L, Zhu Z, Joshi B, et al. A novel hydroxamic acid compound, BMD188, demonstrates anti-prostate cancer effects by inducing apoptosis. II: In vivo efficacy and pharmacokinetic studies. Anticancer Res 1999 Jan–Feb; 19(1A):61–9.

[27] Boland I, Vassal G, Morizet J, et al. Busulphan is active against neuroblastoma and medulloblastoma xenografts in

athymic mice at clinically achievable plasma drug concentrations. Br J Cancer 1999 Feb; 79(5–6):787–92.

28 Lau CE, Ma F, Falk JL. Oral and IP caffeine pharmacokinetics under a chronic food-limitation condition. Pharmacol Biochem Behav 1995 Feb; 50(2):245–52.

29 Nicklin PL, Bayley D, Giddings J, et al. Pulmonary bioavailability of a phosphorothioate oligonucleotide (CGP 64128A): Comparison with other delivery routes. Pharm Res 1998 Apr; 15(4):583–91.

30 Ishigooka J, Murasaki M, Wakatabe H, et al. Pharmacokinetic study of iminodibenzyl antipsychotic drugs, clocapramine and Y-516 in dog and man. Psychopharmacology (Berl) 1989; 97(3):303–8.

31 Pan WJ, Hedaya MA. An animal model for simultaneous pharmacokinetic/pharmacodynamic investigations: Application to cocaine. J Pharmacol Toxicol Methods 1998 Feb; 39(1):1–8.

32 Yamamura Y, Santa T, Kotaki H, et al. Administration-route dependency of absorption of glycyrrhizin in rats: Intraperitoneal administration dramatically enhanced bioavailability. Biol Pharm Bull 1995 Feb; 18(2):337–41.

33 Egorin MJ, Sentz DL, Rosen DM, et al. Plasma pharmacokinetics, bioavailability, and tissue distribution in CD2F1 mice of halomon, an antitumor halogenated monoterpene isolated from the red algae Portieria hornemannii. Cancer Chemother Pharmacol 1996; 39(1–2):51–60.

34 Van der Graaff M, Vermeulen NP, Breimer DD. Route- and dose-dependent pharmacokinetics of hexobarbitone in the rat: A re-evaluation of the use of sleeping times in metabolic studies. J Pharm Pharmacol 1985 Aug; 37(8):550–4.

35 Chen CL, Uckun FM. Evaluation of the pharmacokinetic features and tissue distribution of the potent nonnucleoside inhibitor of HIV-1 reverse transcriptase, N-[2-(2-fluorophenethyl)]-N'-[2-(5-bromopyridyl)]-thiourea (HI-240) with an analytical HPLC method. Pharm Res 1999 Aug; 16(8):1226–32.

36 Jodrell DI, Newell DR, Gibson W, et al. The pharmacokinetics of the quinazoline antifolate ICI D 1694 in mice and rats. Cancer Chemother Pharmacol 1991; 28(5):331–8.

37 Dorr RT, Liddil JD, Klein MK, et al. Preclinical pharmacokinetics and antitumor activity of imexon. Invest New Drugs 1995; 13(2):113–6.

38 Yeleswaram K, McLaughlin LG, Knipe JO, et al. Pharmacokinetics and oral bioavailability of exogenous melatonin in preclinical animal models and clinical implications. J Pineal Res 1997 Jan; 22(1):45–51.

39 Lau CE, Ma F, Wang Y, et al. Pharmacokinetics and bioavailability of midazolam after intravenous, subcutaneous, intraperitoneal and oral administration under a chronic food-limited regimen: Relating DRL performance to pharmacokinetics. Psychopharmacology (Berl) 1996 Aug; 126(3):241–8.

40 Swart PJ, de Zeeuw RA. Pharmacokinetics of the dopamine D2 agonist S(-)-2-(N-propyl-N-2-thienylethylamino)-5-hydroxytetralin in freely moving rats. J Pharm Sci 1993 Feb; 82(2):200–3.

41 Duan MJ, Yu L, Savanapridi C, et al. Disposition kinetics and metabolism of nicotine-1'-N-oxide in rabbits. Drug Metab Dispos 1991 May–Jun; 19(3):667–72.

42 Koch HP, Pischek G, Czejka M, et al. Pharmacokinetic evaluation of norendimide in rats. Methods Find Exp Clin Pharmacol 1982; 4(8):581–5.

43 Lennernas H, Renberg L, Jurgen K, et al. Presystemic elimination of the beta-blocker pafenolol in the rat after oral and intraperitoneal administration and identification of a main metabolite in both rats and humans. Drug Metab Dispos 1993 May–Jun; 21(3):435–40.

44 Grippo AA, Wyrick SD, Lee KH, et al. Disposition of an antineoplastic sesquiterpene lactone, [3H]-plenolin, in BDF1 mice. Planta Medica 1991; 57:309–14.

45 Cundy KC, Sueoka C, Lynch GR, et al. Pharmacokinetics and bioavailability of the anti-human immunodeficiency virus nucleotide analog 9-[(R)-2-phosphonomethoxy)propyl]adenine (PMPA) in dogs. Antimicrob Agents Chemother 1998 Mar; 42(3):687–90.

46 Mehvar R. Pharmacokinetics of propafenone enantiomers in rats. Drug Metab Dispos 1990 Nov–Dec; 18(6):987–91.

47 Vora J, Wu Z, Montague M, et al. Influence of dosing vehicles on the preclinical pharmacokinetics of phenolic antioxidants. Res Commun Mol Pathol Pharmacol 1999; 104(1):93–106.

48 Uckun FM, EK O, Liu XP, et al. In vivo toxicity and pharmacokinetic features of the janus kinase 3 inhibitor WHI-P131 [4-(4'hydroxyphenyl)-amino-6,7-dimethoxyquinazoline]. Clin Cancer Res 1999 Oct; 5(10):2954–62.

49 Chen CL, Malaviya R, Navara C, et al. Pharmacokinetics and biologic activity of the novel mast cell inhibitor, 4-(3-hydroxyphenyl)-amino-6,7-dimethoxyquinazoline in mice. Pharm Res 1999 Jan; 16(1):117–22.

50 Conte A, de Bernardi M, Palmieri L, et al. Metabolic fate of exogenous chondroitin sulfate in man. Arzneimittelforschung 1991; 41(7):768–72.

51 Lachmann G, Lorenz D, Radeck W, Steiper M. [The pharmacokinetics of the S35 labeled labeled garlic constituents alliin, allicin and vinyldithiine.] Arzneimittelforschung 1994 Jun; 44(6):734–43.

52 King RA. Daidzein conjugates are more bioavailable than genistein conjugates in rats. Am J Clin Nutr 1998 Dec; 68(6 Suppl):1496S-1499S.

53 Ader P, Wessmann A, Wolffram S. Bioavailability and metabolism of the flavonol quercetin in the pig. Free Radic Biol Med 2000 Apr 1; 28(7):1056–67.

54 Uang YS, Kang FL, Hsu KY. Determination of caffeic acid in rabbit plasma by high-performance liquid chromatography. J Chromatogr B Biomed Appl 1995 Nov 3; 673(1):43–9.

55 Nakazawa T, Ohsawa K. Metabolism of rosmarinic acid in rats. J Nat Prod 1998 Aug; 61(8):993–6.

56 Ravindranath V, Chandrasekhara N. Metabolism of curcumin—studies with [3H]curcumin. Toxicology. 1981–82; 22(4):337–44.

57 Lang W. Pharmacokinetic-metabolic studies with 14C-aloe emodin after oral administration to male and female rats. Pharmacology 1993; 47(suppl 1):110–119.

58 Kerb R, Brockmoller J, Staffeldt B, et al. Single-dose and steady-state pharmacokinetics of hypericin and pseudohypericin. Antimicrobial Agents and Chemotherapy 1996; 40(9):2087–2093.

[59] Chen H, Chan KK, Budd T. Pharmacokinetics of d-limonene in the rat by GC-MS assay. J Pharm Biomed Anal 1998 Aug; 17(4–5):631–40.

[60] Liu CX, Xiao PG. Recent advances on ginseng research in China. J Ethnopharmacol 1992 Feb; 36(1):27–38.

[61] el Mansouri S, Tod M, Leclerq M, et al. Time- and dose-dependent kinetics of all-*trans* retinoic acid in rats after oral or intravenous administration(s). Drug Metab Dispos 1995 Feb; 23(2):227–31.

[62] Vieth R, Kooh SW, Balfe JW, et al. Tracer kinetics and actions of oral and intraperitoneal 1,25-dihydroxyvitamin D3 administration in rats. Kidney Int 1990 Nov; 38(5):857–61.

[63] DeMuro RL, Nafziger AN, Blask DE, et al. The absolute bioavailability of oral melatonin. J Clin Pharmacol 2000 Jul; 40(7):781–4.

[64] Teichert J, Kern J, Tritschler HJ, et al. Investigations on the pharmacokinetics of alpha-lipoic acid in healthy volunteers. Int J Clin Pharmacol Ther 1998 Dec; 36(12):625–8.

[65] Yeleswaram K, McLaughlin LG, Knipe JO, Schabdach DJ. Pharmacokinetics and oral bioavailability of exogenous melatonin in preclinical animal models and clinical implications. Pineal Res 1997 Jan; 22(1):45–51.

[66] Wassef R, Cohen Z, Langer B. Pharmacokinetic profile of cyclosporine in rats. Transplantation 40(5):489–93.

This appendix provides technical information on the metabolism, pharmacokinetics, and toxicity of most natural compounds discussed in this book, with a focus on dose calculations based on pharmacokinetic and in-vitro data. This material builds on information on pharmacokinetic modeling in Appendix B and that on predictive modeling in Appendix I. Nearly all dose calculations in this book (including most LOAEL dose calculations) are based on preliminary evidence and are therefore uncertain. The dose calculations given here are not intended as definitive but rather as ones that provide rough, ballpark values. Although the usefulness of such estimates is limited, they are the best available to date. A few compounds, such as vitamins E and D_3, are not discussed here because dose calculations for these are less involved and were covered in Part III.

As discussed in Chapter 13, dose estimates can be based on three types of data: 1) human anticancer data; 2) animal antitumor data, as scaled to human equivalents; and 3) a combination of pharmacokinetic and in-vitro data. In comparing dose estimates from each, we begin to comprehend the general magnitude of the required dose for each compound, as well as the relative uncertainty of the estimates. If the dose estimates are in general agreement (considered as within a factor of two from each other), we assume the target dose is relatively well known. In these cases, our target dose is generally an average of the available estimates. If they are not in agreement, we use a range of target doses.

Of the three types of data, basing an effective dose on human anticancer and animal antitumor data is relatively straightforward. The only adjustment is that doses used in animal studies must be scaled to humans. The procedures to do this are discussed in Chapter 1 and Appendix B. Basing a dose on a combination of pharmacokinetic and in-vitro data is more complex and is discussed in detail below.

ESTIMATING DOSES BASED ON PHARMACOKINETIC AND IN-VITRO DATA

Oral Clearance Values in Dose Estimates

One of the most important pharmacokinetic parameters of a drug is its clearance (CL) because it can be used to estimate a required dose. Clearance values are not directly measured in pharmacokinetic studies; they are calculated based on other values that are measured. Clearance refers to the theoretical volume of body fluid that is cleared of a drug per unit time, and so it represents the rate at which a drug is removed from the body. Additional information on clearance is in Appendix B, along with a more detailed explantation of other pharmacokinetic and pharmacodynamic issues of importance. In brief, clearance can be calculated using the following equation:

$$clearance\,(CL) = \frac{F \times dose}{AUC}$$

Equation J.1

In this equation, F is the fraction absorbed and AUC is the area under the concentration-time curve after oral dosing. Many examples of concentration-time curves are found in Appendix B and in this appendix (see Figure J.1). To determine the value of F, both intravenous and oral pharmacokinetic studies are required; however, for most of the natural compounds we discuss, both types of studies have not been conducted. Therefore, we limit our clearance investigation to oral clearance (CL/F), which can be readily estimated from oral pharmacokinetic studies. Throughout this book, the term *clearance* refers to oral clearance unless stated otherwise. Rearrangement of Equation J.1 allows oral clearance to be calculated:

$$oral\ clearance \left(\frac{CL}{F} \right) = \frac{dose}{AUC}$$

Equation J.2

Note in Equation J.2 that, for a given dose, the oral clearance decreases as AUC increases. In other words, a compound that is well absorbed and slowly cleared (large AUC) will have a low oral clearance, and a compound that is poorly absorbed and quickly cleared (small AUC) will have a high oral clearance.

Oral clearance can be used to estimate a required dose if the target plasma concentration is known. The required dose can be calculated from the following equation:

$$dose = \frac{CL}{F} \times C_{SS} \times dose\ schedule$$

Equation J.3

In this equation, C_{ss} is the average plasma concentration at steady state (the average concentration after equilibrium has been established following multiple doses), and dose schedule is the number of hours between doses. For our dose estimates, we use a schedule of once every eight hours. Such reasonably short schedules are desirable because, compared to once a day, they allow a lower and therefore safer dose at each administration. This also minimizes the difference in concentration between the maximum plasma peak, which occurs shortly after the dose, and the minimum trough, which occurs just before the next dose.

The majority of compounds discussed here have a half-life of about four to nine hours. (The geometric average for 18 compounds is about 7.6 hours.) If dosed only once per day at the full daily dose, the patient would experience very high initial plasma concentrations followed later by concentrations approaching zero. Both high and low concentrations have obvious drawbacks. One more advantage of a short dose schedule is that the bioavailability of some compounds decreases with large doses, as discussed below. We use an eight-hour schedule for dose calculations, because a schedule of less than that is inconvenient and an eight hour-schedule is similar to the half-lives of most compounds.

Estimating Target Plasma Concentrations

The dose calculations based on Equation J.3 assume that the effective plasma concentration is known. Since we are mostly calculating doses that cause direct inhibition of cancer, we are referring to the effective cytotoxic concentration. Unfortunately, the concentration effective in vivo is not accurately known for most compounds. To obtain a target concentration, we assume that, for any given compound, the concentration that is effective in vivo is the one effective in vitro. Although this method of estimating a target concentration is not necessarily accurate, it does provide a reasonable first guess and allows us to make dose estimates using Equation J.3.

Determining the effective in-vitro concentration is not easy. Studies have used different techniques under various experimental conditions, and therefore the in-vitro results vary. For example, one study may report that apigenin inhibited cancer cell proliferation at 10 μM and another that it inhibited proliferation at 40 μM. Still, the effective concentrations for most natural compounds do fall within the relatively narrow range of 1 to 30 μM.[a]

Given the variable and often limited data, it is difficult to rank the potency of individual compounds, and so we choose an in-vivo target value of 15 μM for the majority of them. The 15-μM value is based on a rough estimate of the average IC_{50} for all direct-acting compounds. Exceptions to the 15-μM target are noted where applicable.

Estimating Oral Clearance Values

The dose calculations based on Equation J.3 also assume the oral clearance value is accurately known, but for our compounds, this is not usually the case. Human pharmacokinetic studies have been conducted for a few of the compounds of interest, and although this information is valuable, the oral clearance values reported do vary between studies. Oral clearance is dependent upon a number of parameters, including the dose absorbed (F), the actual clearance (CL), and the extent of metabolism; each can vary between individuals and so can oral clearance. Indeed, for some drugs, the latter can vary 15- to 20-fold among individuals.[1, 2] Even though most studies use multiple subjects and therefore provide average oral clearance values, average values can still vary between studies, although generally not so much as between individuals. As a very rough approximation, we estimate that studies usually agree with one another within a factor of about two or three. Depending on the drug, some can be in very close agreement.

Although human pharmacokinetic studies have been conducted only for a few natural compounds, there are a larger number of animal pharmacokinetic studies. The data from these are almost always less reliable than human data, however, since animals absorb and metabolize compounds differently than humans. To some degree, these differences can be quantified, and clearance values can be scaled from animals to humans (methods for scaling are described in Appendix B). The scaling process itself adds an additional degree of uncertainty to the resulting human clearance value. Thus, animal data scaled to humans is useful but generally not as accurate as data from humans.

For some natural compounds, neither human nor animal pharmacokinetic data are available. To overcome this obstacle, oral clearance values for these compounds

---

[a] *It is interesting that this effective range is so common among our natural compounds. One might suppose that other natural compounds commonly used in medicine might be effective within this same concentration range, and indeed, this seems to be the case. Most herbs are used at a dose of 5 to 10 grams per day. Assuming that an average active compound from an average herb has a molecular weight of 360 grams per mole and an oral clearance of 11 L/hr (the geometric average of all direct-acting com-*

pounds discussed in Appendix J), and assuming that the herb contains 1% of the active compound (roughly the average for most compounds discussed here), then the common dose of 10 grams per day would produce a plasma concentration for the active compound of about 1 μM, which is at the low end of the 1 to 30 μM range. When herbs are used in combination, as they are traditionally, additive and synergistic effects likely occur that would make the 1 μM concentration more effective.

can be estimated using the FOC (free oral clearance) and TOC (total oral clearance) models discussed in Appendix I. The terms *free clearance* and *total clearance* refer to values for the unchanged compound and the unchanged compound plus its conjugates, respectively. Total oral clearance values primarily come into play with phenolic compounds, since these compounds occur mostly as conjugates in the plasma.

The FOC and TOC models were able to predict oral clearance values for most of the compounds of interest. These models contain their own level of inaccuracy, however. For example, there is about an 80 percent chance that the value predicted by the FOC model will be within a factor of five of the reported value, and the error could be higher if the actual clearance value is outside the range where the model is most accurate (about 2 to 1,600 L/hr). Despite the uncertainties of their predictions, given the inherent variation of oral clearance and the lack of animal or human clearance data for some compounds, the models are still useful here.

In summary then, we can estimate oral clearance by three different means (human pharmacokinetic studies, animal pharmacokinetic studies, and the FOC and TOC models). None of these is perfect for determining oral clearance, but some are better than others. For the dose calculations in this appendix, data from all available sources were considered, and a single oral clearance value was chosen that seemed most reasonable for each compound. Because the data are limited or conflicting in many cases, the chosen clearance value should be viewed only as a rough estimate.

MODIFICATIONS TO THE ESTIMATED REQUIRED DOSE

We now have three methods to estimate a required dose (by using human data, animal data, and/or a combination of pharmacokinetic and in-vitro data), but this is not the end to our dose calculations. In most cases, the resulting doses must be modified to assure safety or for other reasons. In general, the procedures used to determine tentative dose recommendations are as follows:

1. Estimate an effective dose from human studies, when those are available.

2. Estimate an effective dose from animal studies, when available, and scale this dose to humans.

3. Estimate a target plasma concentration (usually 15 μM) and an oral clearance value (using human and animal pharmacokinetic data and/or the FOC model).

With this information, use Equation J.3 to estimate an effective dose.

4. Compare the dose estimates from steps 1, 2, and 3. If they are within a factor of two of one another, average them to obtain a target dose. If they are not, note the discrepancy and provide a range of possible target doses.

5. Estimate the minimum target dose based on the results of step 4 by assuming a full 15-fold allowable dose decrease for synergism, as discussed in Chapter 13.

6. Estimate the maximum safe dose. In most cases, this will be the lowest-observable-adverse-effects-level dose; the procedure for estimating the LOAEL dose is discussed later.

7. Base the tentative recommended dose for each compound on a comparison of the above doses and on the human dose commonly prescribed in noncancerous conditions, when it is known. (The results of this comparison for each compound are provided in Part III. To give an example, if the LOAEL dose is lower than the target dose obtained from step 4, the maximum tentative recommended dose is set equal to the LOAEL dose, thereby allowing safe use of the compound.)

8. If the maximum tentative recommended dose is larger than 1.8 grams per day, reduce it to 1.8 grams to account for nonlinearities in bioavailability at high doses. The reasoning for this is explained below. (Exceptions to the 1.8-gram daily limit are noted where applicable.)

9. For direct-acting compounds (see Table 1.2), calculate the minimum degree of synergism required. This is calculated as the ratio between the target dose estimated in step 4 and the maximum tentative recommended dose estimated in steps 7 and 8. For example, if the target dose is 6 grams per day and the maximum recommended dose is 2 grams per day, then synergism will be required to produce at least a threefold increase in potency.

Note that the above procedures will change slightly for phenolic compounds, since they exist in the plasma as conjugates. Procedures for phenolic compounds are discussed later.

LOAEL DOSE CALCULATION METHODS

It is likely that the best clinical results will be produced when the largest safe dose of a compound is used. In this book, we view the largest safe dose as that where adverse effects just begin. This is referred to as the lowest-observable-adverse-effects level (LOAEL) dose.

Unfortunately, the actual value of the oral LOAEL dose is unknown for the majority of natural compounds. LOAEL doses as determined from animal or human studies are available for only a few compounds discussed here. Some natural compounds do not have LOAEL data, but do have lethal dose (LD_{50}) data available. The latter is the dose causing death in 50 percent of the test animals after a single administration. As discussed in Appendix I, the LOAEL dose can be estimated from the LD_{50}.

In addition to animal and human studies, LOAEL doses can be estimated from the chemical structure, much as oral clearance values can be. Oxford Molecular Group, creators of the TOPKAT toxicity assessment software program, has contributed estimates for rat oral LD_{50} and LOAEL doses for many of the compounds discussed in this book. (Information on the TOPKAT model and a listing of its predictions are in Appendix I.) These estimates, along with data from animal and human toxicity studies, are used to estimate the human LOAEL dose. Of course, the human data are the most accurate; animal studies and TOPKAT predictions provide only rough estimates.

DOSE-DEPENDENT BIOAVAILABILITY

The bioavailability of a compound, and hence its oral clearance, is in some cases dependent on the dose given. The magnitude of the dose can affect both the fraction of the compound absorbed and the way it is metabolized. In many cases, the bioavailability decreases (and the oral clearance increases) as the dose increases. Thus normal dietary amounts of most natural compounds are reasonably well absorbed, but high therapeutic doses of some may be poorly absorbed or their metabolism may be altered. In other words, as doses increase, less and less gain in plasma concentration may be achieved per milligram of compound given. For example, reduced bioavailability has been reported for the semisynthetic lignan anticancer drug etoposide at doses above 200 milligrams; for EGCG (in green tea extract) at doses above 380 milligrams; for vitamin C at doses above 250 milligrams; for polyenzymes (bromelain and trypsin) at doses above 200 milligrams; and for hyperforin (a component of St John's wort) at doses above 600 milligrams.[3–10] In addition, the bioavailability of soy isoflavonoids has been reduced at high doses.[11] Moreover, one study reported that the bioavailability of quercetin was reduced at doses above about 2.6 grams (as scaled from a study on pigs). Since lower doses

were not tested, it is possible the bioavailability was affected at even lower doses.[12]

In addition, many compounds, especially phenolic ones, may show a nonlinear metabolism over different dose ranges. For example, at relatively low doses, a certain type of conjugate may be prominent in the plasma, and at higher concentrations, a different type may be present. These different conjugates may produce somewhat divergent biologic effects.

Unfortunately, the linearity of the bioavailability at different doses has been studied only for a few natural compounds of interest; still we can expect that a significant number of our natural compounds have a nonlinear pattern similar to those above. Lacking additional information, we make a broad and conservative assumption that bioavailability (and metabolism) is linear at doses up to about 600 milligrams for most natural compounds. This limit does not imply that zero bioavailability occurs at higher does, but rather that there may be markedly different (usually diminishing) gains in plasma concentrations at higher doses. Since an eight-hour dose schedule is recommended for most compounds (three administrations per day), the assumed general linear bioavailability limit is then 1.8 grams per day. A 1.8-gram per day linear bioavailability limit is of course a crude approximation, and conservative, but it is still useful until further information is available. Exceptions to this limit are discussed where applicable. Much additional study remains to be done to determine the actual dose-dependent linearity of bioavailability for individual compounds and for groups of compounds.

With the 600-milligram single-dose limit in mind, ideally we would like the doses used in the pharmacokinetic studies and the dose calculated for cancer treatment all to be either below the 600-milligram limit or above the limit (and roughly equal to one another). Unfortunately, this is not always the case. For example, let us say that two human pharmacokinetic studies tested a compound at 300 and 400 milligrams, respectively, but that dose calculations suggest the required dose for cancer treatment is 2 grams every eight hours. Such a situation may be problematic, since the oral clearance value used in the calculations may not be accurate at a dose of 2 grams. In these cases, we apply the 600-milligram (1.8 gram per day) limit. Note that this limit applies to doses of an isolated compound, such as the amount of CAPE contained in a dose of propolis, but it would not apply to the total propolis dose.

THERAPEUTIC AND LOAEL DOSE ESTIMATES FOR NATURAL COMPOUNDS

Natural compounds are discussed below in the order they appear in Part III: polysaccharides (from Chapter 16); garlic (from Chapter 18); flavones, isoflavones, EGCG, anthocyanidins, and proanthocyanidins (from Chapter 19); CAPE, arctigenin, flaxseed, resveratrol, emodin, and hypericin (from Chapter 20); monoterpenes, *Centella*, boswellic acid, horse chestnut, butcher's broom, ginseng, and parthenolide (from Chapter 21); and vitamin A and melatonin (from Chapter 22). Dose estimates for compounds not discussed in this appendix appear in Part III.

Chapter 16: Polysaccharides

High-Molecular-Weight Polysaccharides

Polysaccharides stimulate immune cell activity in vitro at concentrations of about 100 to 800 µg/ml, or roughly 0.5 to 4.0 µM, assuming an average molecular weight of 200,000.[13–17] We use a midrange target of 2.2 µM in our calculations here.

This target concentration will first be used in combination with oral pharmacokinetic data for the polysaccharide chondroitin sulfate (molecular weight 16,000) to estimate a polysaccharide dose. Figure J.1 illustrates the concentration-time curve for an oral dose of 3 grams in humans (figure based on reference 18). Also shown in the figure is the curve for its lower-molecular-weight (LMW, molecular weight less than 5,000) degradation products. From the limited data available, it appears that a sizable percentage of the polysaccharide dose is degraded in vivo to LMW products and that these constitute the bulk of the plasma concentration. In general, LMW polysaccharide fractions have less effect on the immune system and a weaker antitumor effect in animals than the unchanged higher-molecular-weight (HMW) fractions.[19] Other authors have shown degradation of HMW aloe polysaccharides into LMW fractions after oral and intravenous administration in mice.[20] The oral clearance of the HMW fraction shown in Figure J.1 is 16 L/hr. Using equation J.3, to achieve a serum concentration of 2.2 µM, a dose of roughly 6.9 grams of chondroitin sulfate would be needed every eight hours, or 14 grams per day, which is reasonably close to the 6.6-gram polysaccharide dose scaled from the animal antitumor experiments mentioned in Chapter 16.

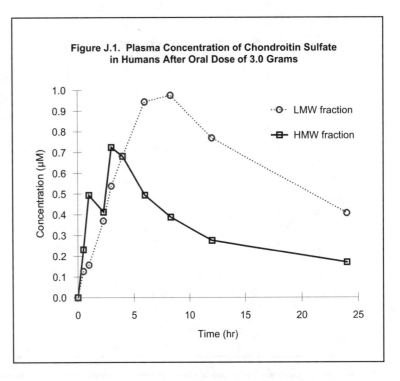

Figure J.1. Plasma Concentration of Chondroitin Sulfate in Humans After Oral Dose of 3.0 Grams

We can make a similar dose calculation based on pharmacokinetic data obtained from a radiolabeled study of PSK (molecular weight 94,000) in rabbits.[21, a] Unfortunately, this study did not clearly identify the ratio of high-molecular-weight to lower-molecular-weight degradation products in the plasma. It is reasonable to assume, however, that the ratio follows a similar pattern over time as that of chondroitin sulfate.[b] The resulting concentration-time curve is shown in Figure J.2. The human oral clearance based on the HMW curve is 1.9 L/hr. Using Equation J.3, the human dose required to produce a 2.2 µM plasma concentration is roughly 3.1 grams every eight hours, or 9.3 grams per day, which is quite similar to that calculated for chondroitin sulfate.

Table J.1 summarizes the therapeutic dose estimates for polysaccharides made in this appendix and Chapter 16.

---

[a] *This rabbit study measured PSK in blood. For polysaccharides and a number of other compounds discussed in this book, we estimate the plasma concentration to be twice that of the blood concentration. This difference occurs because the plasma volume in humans is a little more than half the total blood volume, and many of the compounds we discuss tend to be concentrated in the plasma rather than within red blood cells.*

[b] *In scaling the chondroitin sulfate data from humans to rabbits, we estimate that in rabbits the high-molecular-weight fraction varies from roughly 50% at one hour to 17% at 24 hours.*

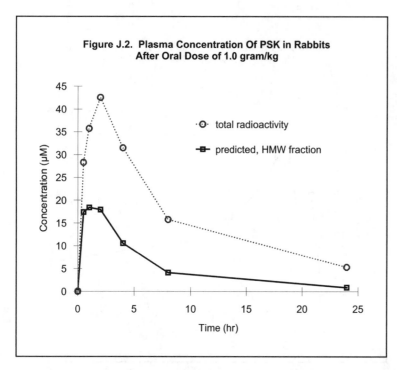

Figure J.2. Plasma Concentration Of PSK in Rabbits After Oral Dose of 1.0 gram/kg

labeled one. This is because radiolabeled studies track the concentration of isotopes initially associated with a test drug but make no distinction between isotopes that remain with the unchanged drug and those that travel with the drug when it is metabolized and degraded. Since the metabolites and degradation products generally remain in the animal longer than the unchanged drug, the half-life of the compound is artificially extended in a radiolabeled study. Consequently, the AUC for the radiolabeled study is higher and the oral clearance is lower.

Because several more radiolabeled studies are discussed here, we would like to estimate the "true" oral clearance based on the oral clearance obtained from radiolabeled studies. Unfortunately, few studies are available on which to base systematic estimates. Lacking additional data, we assume that the oral clearance from a given radiolabeled study is about 7.5-fold lower than the true value; this is based on the average of five observations shown in Table J.2. Values for the individual half-life and clearance values are taken or derived from data discussed elsewhere in this appendix. Half-lives are included in the table, since we can assume a rough correlation between half-life and oral clearance. (For a given compound, both radiolabeled and nonradiolabeled studies are likely to produce a similar initial peak concentration, but the half-life measured in the radiolabeled study is likely to be longer.) As the table shows, most studies suggest that the oral clearance is higher (or the half-life is shorter) in a nonradiolabeled study, the average difference being 7.5-fold. Of course, using the 7.5-fold value to estimate the true oral clearance provides only an extremely rough estimate, as each individual compound will be metabolized differently.

TABLE J.1 ESTIMATED THERAPEUTIC AND LOAEL DOSES FOR POLYSACCHARIDES	
DESCRIPTION	**DOSE (g/day)**
Required dose as scaled from animal antitumor studies	6.6 (midrange)
Common human dose in cancer treatment	2 to 6
Required dose as determined from pharmacokinetic calculations (for PSK)	9.3
Estimated LOAEL dose	much greater than 6
Tentative dose recommendation for further research	**2 to 9**

A 2- to 9-gram range for the tentative recommended polysaccharide dose is above the general linear bioavailability limit of 1.8 gram per day. In this case, however, a dose of 2 to 9 grams does not pose a significant bioavailability problem, since the PSK pharmacokinetic study used an even larger dose of 29 grams (as scaled to humans). Furthermore, the chondroitin sulfate pharmacokinetic study used a dose of 3 grams and produced a similar oral clearance value, after accounting for differences in molecular weight. Therefore, it does not appear there would be dose-dependent bioavailability differences at doses of 9 grams or less.

A Note on Radiolabeled Studies

We take a moment here to discuss the clearance values obtained from radiolabeled and nonradiolabeled studies, since the topic comes up again later. In general, the oral clearance of a compound determined in a radiolabeled study will be lower than that determined in a nonradio-

Chapter 18: Amino Acids and Related Compounds

Garlic Compounds—DADS

As discussed in Chapter 18, the principal garlic constituent of interest is DADS. Unfortunately, the pharmacokinetic parameters of DADS have not been well characterized. One study has been conducted on radiolabeled allicin in rats, however, and this information can be used to make rough estimates, since DADS and allicin probably display somewhat similar pharmacokinetics.

The blood concentration curve of radiolabeled allicin in rats is shown in Figure J.3 (adapted from reference 22).[a] The estimated human clearance based on this study is 0.75 L/hr. The curve shown is for blood concentrations, and plasma concentrations are likely to be about twice as high, as discussed with reference to PSK above. The clearance is then half as large, or 0.38 L/hr. In comparison, the oral clearance of DADS as estimated by the FOC model is 1.5 L/hr. The clearance from the radiolabeled study is lower than that predicted by the FOC model, as would be expected, and we use the value of 1.5 L/hr in dose calculations. Clearly, additional pharmacokinetics studies in humans are needed to determine whether this value is accurate. (Note that using a lower clearance value would reduce the estimated target doses.)

As mentioned in Chapter 18, DADS is active in vitro at about 100 μM. Using Equation J.3, a dose of 190 milligrams would be needed every eight hours, or 580 milligrams per day, to produce a plasma concentration of 100 μM. This is within the range of 210 to 780 milligrams as scaled from mouse antitumor experiments (see Chapter 18).

Unfortunately, it is difficult to determine the amount of whole garlic necessary to provide a 580-milligram dose of DADS per day. Garlic cloves contain approximately 3.7 mg/g allicin and another 1.7 mg/g related thiosulfinates, for a total of 5.4 mg/g thiosulfinates.[23] A majority of this can be converted to DADS in vivo, but it is uncertain exactly how much. Although not all thiosulfinates will be fully converted to DADS, those that are not could still add to the cytotoxic effect and so we will as-

TABLE J.2 RATIO OF ORAL CLEARANCE FROM NONRADIOLABELED TO RADIOLABELED STUDIES.			
OBSERVATION	**VALUE 1[*]**	**VALUE 2[*]**	**RATIO**
Ratio of half-life for PSK (radiolabeled) to chondroitin sulfate (nonradiolabeled)	13 hours	14 hours	0.93
Ratio of half-life of proanthocyanidin (radiolabeled) to anthocyanidin (nonradiolabeled)	27 hours	4.1 hours	6.7
Ratio of geometric average half-life for five natural compounds (radiolabeled) to 18 natural compounds (nonradiolabeled)	110 hours	7.6 hours	14
Ratio of allicin clearance predicted by FOC model to a radiolabeled study	1.5 L/hr	0.38 L/hr	3.9
Ratio of parthenolide clearance predicted by FOC model to a radiolabeled study	1.9 L/hr	0.16 L/hr	12
		Average:	**7.5**

[*] *Descriptions are given in the first column. Values are reported as human equivalents.*

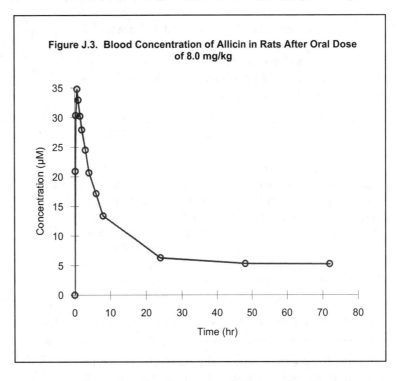

Figure J.3. Blood Concentration of Allicin in Rats After Oral Dose of 8.0 mg/kg

sume that essentially all of the 5.4 mg/g will be converted. The resulting required dose is then 110 grams, which is within the dose range of 19 to 150 grams as scaled from rodent antitumor experiments in Chapter 18. We can average 110 grams and the three highest doses scaled from animals (40, 62, and 150 grams) to obtain a target dose of 91 grams per day.

The LOAEL dose for garlic is uncertain. On the one hand, common experience suggests that garlic is quite benign. Indeed, oral doses of about 81 mg/kg per day of DADS did not produce noticeable adverse effects in mice. According to the assumptions above, this would

---

[a] *This study measured the plasma concentration in alliin equivalents (allicin is a metabolite of alliin, as illustrated in Figure 18.2). In constructing Figure J.3, the allicin yield is assumed to be 75 percent of the alliin content. This is typical of commercial garlic preparations.*

TABLE J.3 ESTIMATED THERAPEUTIC AND LOAEL DOSES FOR GARLIC	
DESCRIPTION	**DOSE (g/day)**
Required dose as scaled from animal antitumor studies	19 to 150
Required dose as determined from pharmacokinetic calculations	110
Target dose based on an average from animal antitumor studies (higher dose range) and pharmacokinetic calculations	91
Minimum required antitumor dose assuming 15-fold synergistic benefits	6.1
Commonly prescribed human dose in noncancerous conditions	4 to 15
Estimated LOAEL dose	15
Tentative dose recommendation for further research	**6 to 15**
Minimum degree of synergism required	**6.1-fold potency increase**

translate to a human garlic dose of about 150 grams.[a] In addition, many human studies on garlic's cardiovascular effects have used doses of about 15 to 70 grams per day.[24] The commonly prescribed garlic dose in Chinese herbal medicine is 6 to 15 grams daily.[25]

On the other hand, some studies suggest that high garlic doses would not be safe, especially for multiple administrations. Oral garlic doses as low as 500 mg/kg damaged lung and liver tissue in rats.[26] The human equivalent is only about 8.1 grams per day, or about 2 cloves of garlic. Similar results were seen in another rat study, where oral doses of 300 to 600 mg/kg per day of an aqueous garlic extract for 21 days produced toxic effects.[27] Lacking additional data, we estimate the garlic LOAEL dose is at least equal to the 15-gram per day dose commonly used in Chinese medicine. This would supply a DADS dose of about 57 milligrams.

Table J.3 summarizes the therapeutic dose estimates for garlic made in this appendix and Chapter 18.

Standardized commercial garlic products are preferable to whole garlic cloves. Such products typically contain 4 milligrams per capsule of allicin potential, which is about equal to a gram of whole garlic; for example, six capsules would be equivalent to a garlic dose of 6 grams. The best products may be enteric-coated ones because these dissolve in the intestines rather than the stomach. Stomach acids are likely to inactivate allinase, the enzyme that converts alliin to allicin.

The dose estimates presented here are not likely to be in error due to dose-dependent bioavailability issues. A 15-gram dose of garlic contains about 57 milligrams of DADS, which is well below the general linear bioavailability limit of 1.8 grams per day. Furthermore, the allicin pharmacokinetic study used a similar dose (77 milligrams, as scaled to humans).

Chapter 19: Phenolic Compounds—Flavonoids

Metabolism and Absorption of Phenolic Compounds

Before calculating doses for flavonoids, we first discuss their metabolism and absorption. The important point to remember is that flavonoids are extensively metabolized in vivo, and they occur in the plasma primarily in their glucuronide conjugate forms. These characteristics were first mentioned in Chapter 13 and are examined in more detail here. As discussed in that chapter, the production of conjugates is not limited to flavonoids but is shared by many other phenolic compounds. Therefore, this information applies to all the phenolic compounds covered in Chapters 19 and 20.

The absorption and metabolism of many phenolic compounds after oral administration follows the pathway shown in Figure J.4. In most cases, the natural compound will be taken in a glycoside form, since most phenolic compounds exist in plants as glycosides. Glycosides consist of the pure compound conjugated to a sugar molecule.[b] The pure compound is referred to as the aglycone of the glycoside. Administration of the aglycone is also possible. For example, quercetin is available commercially as an aglycone supplement. As a dietary example, the fermentation process used in making tempeh and miso from soybeans results in the cleavage of isoflavonoid (e.g., genistein) glycosides into their aglycones.

Some aglycones can be absorbed in the stomach, as was reported for daidzein and genistein in rats.[28] After leaving the stomach and entering the small intestine, the aglycones (and glycosides) are transported to the liver through the enterohepatic circulation. In the past, it was

---

[a] *The TOPKAT model tentatively predicts that the LOAEL dose of DADS in rats is 590 mg/kg, which translates to a human garlic dose of about 1,800 grams. The TOPKAT model clearly overestimated the DADS' LOAEL dose.*

[b] *Depending on the type of sugar molecule, glycosides may more specifically be called glucosides, rutinosides, galactosides, arabinosides, rhamnosides, or xylosides.*

believed that only the aglycone was absorbed from the small intestine; however, recent studies on quercetin and anthocyanins suggest that absorption of certain glycosides occurs in the small intestine. In the case of quercetin, absorption of glycosides may be about twice as great as absorption of the aglycone.[29, 30] At least in rats, however, the genistein aglycone was absorbed slightly better than its soy-based glycosides.[31]

The aglycones are heavily metabolized while passing through the lining of the small intestine on their way to the liver. Most of this metabolism is in the form of glucuronidation (the formation of glucuronide conjugates). Since conjugation is an important event, we discuss it in more detail here.

Conjugates are produced during what is known as phase II metabolism (detoxification). Conjugation is the body's attempt to make a foreign compound more water-soluble and thus more easily excreted in the urine. Conjugates are comprised of the parent molecule or its metabolites linked to a second, more water-soluble molecule like glutathione, sulfate, or glucuronic acid. The latter is related to glucose and the conjugates it forms are referred to as glucuronides. Conjugation can also result in glucuronide-sulfate biconjugates. Glutathione conjugation predominates in electrophilic (positively charged) compounds such as allicin (from garlic). Glucuronic acid or sulfate conjugation predominates in nucleophilic (negatively charged) compounds like most phenolic ones. Although there are exceptions, glucuronide conjugation is generally more prevalent than sulfate conjugation for phenolic compounds. Most sulfate conjugation occurs in the liver, whereas most glucuronide conjugation occurs in the intestinal wall.

Any glycosides or aglycones not absorbed in the small intestine travel down to the large intestine. Here, glycosides are cleaved by intestinal bacteria to produce aglycones, which can then be absorbed and undergo glucuronidation. The aglycones in the large intestine can also be degraded by bacteria to other inactive (or active) metabolites. The type and amount of intestinal bacteria influence the degradation that occurs.[32] Therefore, individuals may metabolize phenolic compounds somewhat differently. Note that some degradation products produced by gut bacteria might be bioactive. For example, *p*-hydroxybenzoic acid, produced after degradation of some flavonoids, is a PTK inhibitor (see Table E.1). This compound is produced after oral administration of kaempferol and quercetin in humans and apigenin in rats and is a common component of human urine.[33–36]

The aglycones absorbed from the large and small intestine enter the liver primarily as glucuronide conjugates. There they may be further metabolized by sulfation (the production of sulfate conjugates) and methylation (the addition of methyl groups, such as occurs during selenium detoxification). From the liver, the metabolites enter the blood, where they are recycled back to the liver. The liver sequesters some of these in the bile, which is then secreted into the large intestine. Metabolites in the blood also travel to the kidneys, where further methylation and excretion into the urine can occur.

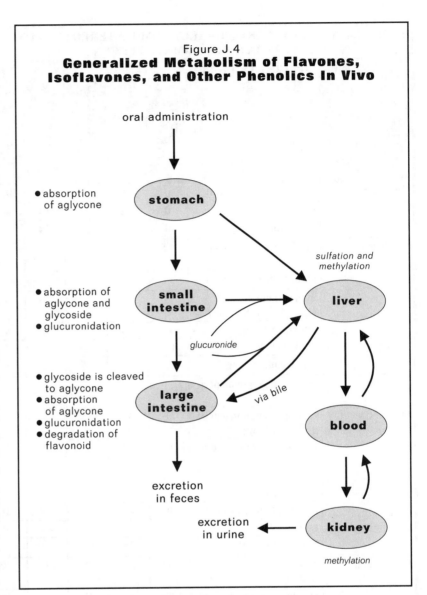

Figure J.4
Generalized Metabolism of Flavones, Isoflavones, and Other Phenolics In Vivo

TABLE J.4 METABOLITES OF ORALLY ADMINISTERED FLAVONOIDS IN PLASMA (APPROXIMATE PERCENT)		FREE COMPOUND	GLUCURONIDES	GLUCURONIDE-SULFATES	SULFATES	REFERENCES
COMPOUND	**SPECIES AND DOSE**					
Daidzein	human (dietary levels)	—	73[*]	—	12[†]	40, 55
	human (36 mg)	0	52	34	14	41
	Daidzein, average	**0**	**52**	**34**	**14**	
Genistein	rat (human equivalent of 65 mg)	4.8	36 to 78	—	0	42
	human (dietary levels)	—	83[*]	—	6[†]	40, 55
	mouse (human equivalent of 870 mg)	11	—	—	—	43
	human (5.6 mg)	0	85	15	0	41
	human (1.1 g)	1.3	—	—	—	44
	Genistein, average	**4**	**79**	**15**	**2**	
Luteolin	rat (human equivalent of 230 mg)	11	—	—	—	45
Quercetin	rat (human equivalent of 160 to 810 mg)	0	30	65	5	46
	rat (human equivalent of 2.4 g)	0	40	60	0	47
	rat (human equivalent of 93 to 371 mg)	1.5	—	—	—	48
	human (dietary levels)	0	—	—	—	49
	human (87 mg)	0	—	—	—	50
	Quercetin, average	**0**	**35**	**63**	**3**	
Epicatechin	rat (human equivalent of 810 mg)	10	86	0	3	37
	rat (human equivalent of 810 mg)[‡]	3	36	47	13	39
	human (dose of 32 mg)	0				51
	Epicatechin, average	**4**	**61**	**24**	**8**	
Overall average		**4**	**57**	**34**	**7**	

[*] *Glucuronide plus glucuronide-sulfates.*

[†] *Free plus sulfate, but consists mainly of sulfate.*

[‡] *Values are approximate. Includes methylated conjugates, which account for about half of the total conjugates.*

example, high doses of some compounds like epicatechin may overwhelm metabolizing enzymes, resulting in higher concentrations of aglycone in the blood.[37] High doses may also alter the pattern of glucuronide and sulfate conjugation and methylation.[38, 39]

Lastly, the metabolite profile can be much different after intraperitoneal or subcutaneous administration. A few intraperitoneal or subcutaneous studies are reported in Chapters 19 and 20, and equivalent oral dose estimates are provided. Because of differences in metabolite profiles and other differences discussed in Appendix I, these estimates should be viewed with healthy skepticism.

Reported percentages for different flavonoid conjugates in plasma are listed in Table J.4; note that the values in the table are only approximate. Based on the data presented for each compound, average values are also given. Methylated metabolites are not reported, since they were analyzed in very few studies.[52]

Dose Calculations for Phenolic Compounds

Almost all in-vitro studies on phenolic compounds tested the free (aglycone) form; however, this is not the form found in vivo. We can assume that on a weight-for-weight basis, the potency of conjugates will be different from that of the free compound. Indeed, examples exist of drug conjugates that are less potent than, equal to, and more potent than their aglycones.[41] For the phenolic compounds discussed here, the most bioactive form is likely to be the free form, followed by the sulfate conjugate form, and finally by the glucuronide conjugate one.[53, 54, 55] Since most phenolic compounds exist as conjugates in vivo, we must modify our dose calculations to account for their different potencies.

From the above, we see that most phenolic compounds in the blood are in the form of glucuronide conjugates, sulfate conjugates, glucuronide-sulfate biconjugates, or methylated derivatives including methylated conjugates. The primary circulating form of most phenolics is glucuronide conjugates. The production of different metabolites is dynamic and can be dose-dependent. For

Although most drugs and natural compounds undergo some degree of conjugation, we make dose modifications only for phenolic compounds. Other than for sex hormones, licorice, and vitamin A, relatively little is known regarding conjugation of most nonphenolic natural compounds. Because the available data suggests that glucuronide conjugates of these nonphenolic compounds represent a relatively small percentage of the total plasma concentration, we will not modify dose calculations for these.[56–62]

To modify calculations for phenolic compounds, we must know the relative potency of the free compound versus its conjugates. The first step in estimating this value is to look at the in-vitro studies that measured the activity of each form. The few studies available indicate that glucuronides tend to be about 1- to 4-fold less effective than their aglycones (on a μM basis). In one study, the IC_{50} for inhibiting EGF receptor expression in rat prostate tissue in vivo for total genistein (free form plus conjugates) was 4-fold higher than for the free form alone.[63] In a second study, the IC_{50} for inhibition of cancer cell proliferation by isorhamnetin glucuronide was about 2.5-fold higher than isorhamnetin aglycone (isorhamnetin is a flavonoid similar to quercetin).[64] In others, quercetin conjugates were about 2.6-fold less potent as antioxidants than free quercetin, with sulfates being slightly more potent than glucuronides, and glucuronides were about 4-fold less potent on geometric average than free quercetin in inhibiting lipoxygenase.[47, 65] Lastly, although ATRA is not a phenolic compound, glucuronide conjugates of ATRA were 1- to 2-fold less active at inhibiting cancer cell proliferation than the free form.[66, 67, 68]

We can also estimate conjugate potencies from the relative potencies of glycosides. Glucuronide conjugates and glycosides are similar, in that both consist of a free molecule with an attached sugarlike molecule.[a] We know from in-vitro studies on genistein, quercetin, anthocyanidins, and arctigenin that glycosides of phenolic compounds tend to be roughly two to four times less cytotoxic than their aglycones (on a μM basis).[69–76] Other activities besides cytotoxicity are also affected by conjugation. For example, one study reported that a quercetin glycoside (quercitrin) was 2.6-fold less active than quercetin in inducing topoisomerase II–mediated DNA cleavage in vitro.[77] Another study found apiin, a glycoside of apigenin, about 3.4-fold less potent than apigenin in inhibiting nitric oxide production by macrophages in vitro.[78]

Considering all the above data, we can estimate that glycosides and glucuronide conjugates are on average about 2- to 4-fold less potent than the free phenolic compound. For simplicity, we assume that all glucuronide conjugates are 3-fold less active.

It is not surprising that glycosides or glucuronide or sulfate conjugates would be less potent than the free compound, since on a weight-for-weight basis they contain less free compound. The average molecular weight of the phenolic compounds discussed in this book is about 312 grams per mole. Since the molecular weight of glucuronic acid is about 194 grams per mole, most glucuronide conjugates of phenolics are roughly 488 grams per mole.[b] Thus every 100 grams of glucuronide conjugate contains only about 64 grams of free compound. The same is true for glycosides because the average molecular weight of the primary sugar units (glucose, xylose, rutinose, rhamnose, and arabinose) is also 194 grams per mole.

Assuming that glucuronide conjugates are about 3-fold less potent than the free compound, since conjugates are only about 64 percent pure, they are actually only about 1.9-fold less potent, when normalized for the mass of free compound present. We thus assume that the total mix of glucuronide and sulfate conjugates are roughly 2-fold less potent than the free compound, when normalized for the mass of free compound present.

The need to view relative potencies on a mass-normalized basis comes from the fact that the pharmacokinetic studies reported here that measured the plasma concentration of total (free plus conjugate) phenolics did so by enzymatically digesting the plasma sample to convert the conjugates to the free compound. Therefore, in these studies, total plasma concentrations are given in terms of the free compound. For example, genistein exists in the plasma primarily as glucuronide conjugates. If a study reported that the plasma concentration of total genistein was 10 μM, this means the actual plasma concentration of genistein in the conjugate form was about 16 μM (about 1.6-fold higher due to the differences in molecular weights). By the same token, 10 μM of total genistein as measured in the plasma after enzymatic digestion would be equal to about 5 μM of free genistein (a 2-fold difference in potency). Seen another way, 16-μM of actual conjugates in the plasma would also be equal to about 5 μM of free genistein (about a 3-fold difference in potency). Any way it is viewed, the equivalent concentration of free genistein is about 5 μM.

---

[a] *The result of glucuronide conjugation in animals and glucose conjugation in plants is that a compound becomes more water-soluble, more easily transported, and less toxic.*

[b] *488 = 312 + 194 (for glucuronic acid) – 16 (for a shared oxygen atom) –2 (for two deleted hydrogen atoms).*

TABLE J.5 ORAL CLEARANCE OF FLAVONOIDS IN HUMANS BASED ON TOTAL PLASMA CONCENTRATIONS			
FLAVONOID	**DOSE**	**ORAL CL (L/Hr)**	**REFERENCES**
Daidzein	49 mg daidzein aglycone contained in soy flour	4.9	79
	6 mg daidzein aglycone contained in soy flour	4.6	80
	29 mg daidzein aglycone contained in baked soy flour	5.2	81
	Daidzein, average	**4.9**	
Genistein	71 mg genistein aglycone contained in soy flour	4.3	79
	8 mg genistein aglycone contained in soy flour	4.5	80
	28 mg genistein aglycone contained in baked soy flour	2.2	81
	Genistein, average	**3.7**	
Quercetin	150 grams of fried onions, containing 64 mg aglycone	22	82
	225 grams of fried onions, containing 50 mg aglycone	32	83
	150 mg quercetin glucosides	18	84
	Quercetin, average	**24**	

Again, since all pharmacokinetic studies on phenolic compounds that measured total concentrations used enzymatic digestion, we assume that the target plasma concentration (and hence the dose) of phenolic compounds must be increased 2-fold relative to what it would be for the free compound alone. Therefore, in estimating doses for phenolic compounds, we use the same nine-step procedure employed for nonphenolic compounds (see above) but with one exception. In step 3, the target plasma concentration is increased by a factor of 2 (generally, from 15 µM to 30 µM).

Methylated Conjugates of Phenolic Compounds

We have mentioned little about the potency and presence of methylated metabolites. Although these can occur in sizable concentrations, few pharmacokinetic studies have specifically measured them. Moreover, the available data sometimes conflict or are difficult to interpret. For example, depending on the magnitude of the dose and the adaptation to it over time, as well as the animal species tested and other factors, quercetin can appear in a plasma metabolite mix of anywhere from 0 to about 83 percent methylated quercetin (and methylated conjugates).[12, 46, 47, 85] In one human study, oral administration of about 87 milligrams of quercetin (in plant products) produced a metabolite mix that was about 30 percent methylated quercetin in three subjects and zero percent in seven.[50] To make matters more complicated, the percentage of methylated metabolites (or sulfate and glucuronide conjugates) can also be influenced by the amount of food in the stomach, or the gut microflora in an individual, or both.[86] Thus the production of methylated metabolites is dependent on many factors and is difficult to predict. In addition, the relative potencies of methylated metabolites are largely uncertain. Some methylated metabolites of quercetin possess about half the antioxidant activity of free quercetin, but conjugates of some methylated metabolites show little antioxidant activity.[50] One study found that methylated glucuronide conjugates of catechin and epicatechin possess almost no antioxidant ability, whereas glucuronide conjugates were only slightly less potent than the free compounds.[87] Moreover, it is known that the relative placement of glucuronic acid groups can affect the antioxidant activity of flavonoids.[88] (Methyl, glucuronic acid, and sulfate groups can attach to a number of different carbons in phenolic compounds.)

Considering the above, the magnitude of methylated metabolites in the plasma during treatment and the role they may play in the total biologic effect of phenolic compounds is still uncertain. Clearly, additional work is needed to fully identify the active metabolites of phenolic compounds and characterize their pharmacokinetics and biologic activity.

Apigenin, Luteolin, Quercetin, Genistein, and Daidzein

Oral Clearance Values

A limited number of studies have investigated the oral clearance of apigenin, luteolin, quercetin, genistein, and daidzein in humans, although more studies have been conducted in rodents. Because of their complex metabolism and the analytical difficulty of measuring the various metabolites, many questions remain. Some details on the available human studies are listed in Table J.5.

Some discrepancy exists in the literature regarding the relative bioavailabilities of genistein and daidzein. The data in Table J.5 suggest that genistein is slightly more bioavailable than daidzein (the average oral clearance of genistein is lower). This trend is supported by a number of human studies that measured peak plasma concentrations.[41, 89, 90] However, two human studies and one rat study that measured urinary output suggested daidzein is more bioavailable than genistein.[90, 91, 92] The human urinary studies indicated that daidzein is 1.4- to 2.3-fold more bioavailable than genistein. Interestingly, the FOC model produced a somewhat similar result; it predicted free daidzein was 3.1-fold more bioavailable than free genistein (see Table I.1). Nonetheless, since the studies using human plasma suggest that genistein is slightly more bioavailable than daidzein, we use the values in Table J.5 for further dose calculations.

TABLE J.6 ESTIMATED ORAL CLEARANCE VALUES OF FLAVONOIDS	
FLAVONOID	ESTIMATED TOTAL ORAL CLEARANCE OF FLAVONOID (L/Hr)
Apigenin	4.8
Genistein	3.7[*]
Daidzein	4.9[*]
Luteolin	14
Quercetin	24[*]

[*] *Data from Table J.5.*

TABLE J.7 REQUIRED DOSE FOR FLAVONOIDS BASED ON PHARMACOKINETIC DATA		
FLAVONOID	ORAL CLEARANCE[*] (L/Hr)	REQUIRED DOSE (grams/day)
Genistein	3.7	0.72
Daidzein	4.9	0.90
Apigenin	4.8	0.93
Luteolin	14	2.9
Quercetin	24	5.2

[*] *From Table J.6.*

Unfortunately, the pharmacokinetic parameters of apigenin and luteolin have not been studied in humans, and only one study on luteolin in rats is available. In that one, the oral clearance for total luteolin was approximately 0.23 L/hr. The human equivalent is about 14 L/hr.

We can estimate the total oral clearance values for apigenin and luteolin by using the TOC model from Appendix I. As listed in Tables I.2 and I.3, the total oral clearance values predicted for apigenin and luteolin are 4.8 and 15 L/hr, respectively.[a] The value of 15 L/hr for luteolin is nearly identical with the 14-L/hr value scaled above from a rat study, so we use the 14-L/hr value. For apigenin, we use the value predicted by the TOC model. Based on the above, the total oral clearance values for daidzein, genistein, and quercetin are shown in Table J.6.

Dose Calculations

The aglycones for all flavonoids listed in Table J.6 are active in vitro at a concentration of roughly 15 μM. Therefore, we use a target in-vivo concentration of 30 μM, after adjustment for conjugates. For genistein and daidzein, 30 μM is larger than the normal total (free plus conjugate) plasma concentrations of about 0.28 μM that occurs in subjects consuming a high-soy diet.[40] The same is true for quercetin, where average fasting total plasma concentrations are about 0.07 μM.[49, 93] We can confidently assume that 30 μM is also much larger than normal apigenin and luteolin plasma concentrations. We see then that therapeutic concentrations are well above normal concentrations, as would be expected. Table J.7 shows the resulting dose estimates based on a 30-μM target.

The dose estimates calculated above are similar to doses scaled from animal antitumor studies mentioned in Chapter 19. The 720-milligram dose of genistein is within the range of 250 milligrams to 9.9 grams scaled from animal antitumor experiments. The 930-milligram dose for apigenin is just below the range of 1.2 to 2.5 grams scaled from an animal antitumor experiment. The 2.9-gram dose for luteolin is within the range of 1.1 to 3.4 grams scaled from an animal antitumor experiment. The 5.2-gram dose for quercetin is just above the range of 1.2 to 4.9 grams scaled from animal antitumor experiments.

In addition, the calculated doses for apigenin, luteolin, and quercetin are similar to those scaled from animal anti-inflammatory experiments. Intraperitoneal administration of apigenin and luteolin (at 8 to 50 mg/kg) produced anti-inflammatory effects in rats; the equivalent

---

[a] *In using Equation I.2, the percent of free apigenin in the plasma chosen was 3 percent, the same for luteolin.*

DESCRIPTION	GENISTEIN DOSE (g/day)	APIGENIN DOSE (g/day)	LUTEOLIN DOSE (g/day)	QUERCETIN DOSE (g/day)
Required dose as scaled from animal antitumor studies	0.25 to 9.9 (average 2.3)	1.2 to 2.5	1.1 to 3.4	1.2 to 4.9
Required dose as scaled from animal anti-inflammatory studies	none	0.66 to 4.1	0.66 to 4.1	1 to 4
Required dose as estimated from pharmacokinetic calculations	0.72	0.93	2.9	5.2
Target dose based on an average from animal antitumor studies and pharmacokinetic calculations	1.5	1.5	2.5	3.8
Minimum required antitumor dose assuming 15-fold synergistic benefits	0.1	0.1	0.17	0.25
Commonly prescribed human dose in noncancerous conditions	0.05	0.01	uncertain	1
Estimated LOAEL dose	1.6	3.2	4.4	6.5
Tentative dose recommendation for further research	**0.1 to 1.1**[*]	**0.1 to 1.5**	**0.17 to 1.8**[†]	**0.25 to 1.8**[†]
Minimum degree of synergism required	**1.4-fold potency increase**	**none**	**1.4-fold potency increase**	**2.1-fold potency increase**

TABLE J.8   ESTIMATED THERAPEUTIC AND LOAEL DOSES FOR ISOFLAVONES, FLAVONES, AND FLAVONOLS

[*] *Upper value based on daidzein LOAEL.*
[†] *Upper value based on the general linear bioavailability limit of 1.8 grams per day.*

human oral dose is about 0.66 to 4.1 grams.[94, 95] Quercetin produced anti-inflammatory effects within the range of 1 to 4 grams, as scaled to humans, after oral administration in mice, rats, and guinea pigs. Anti-inflammatory effects were also produced at a dose of 2.6 grams, scaled to humans (oral equivalent), after intraperitoneal administration in rats.[96, 97]

To obtain target doses for these flavonoids, we can use an average of the doses calculated from pharmacokinetic and in-vitro data and those scaled from animal antitumor experiments. The results are in Table J.8.

Also in this table are the minimum required doses based on a full 15-fold increase in potency due to synergism. These minimum daily doses are 100 milligrams for genistein, 100 milligrams for apigenin, 170 milligrams for luteolin, and 250 milligrams for quercetin. Although these doses are above normal dietary intake, they are likely to be safe. One study reported that the dietary intake of genistein in Japanese subjects averaged about 20 milligrams per day (daidzein intake was 12 milligrams daily).[98] The average dietary intake of apigenin, luteolin, and quercetin in subjects from the Netherlands was smaller, at about 0.69, 0.92, and 16 milligrams per day, respectively.[99]

The minimum dose of 100 milligrams for genistein is larger than the commonly prescribed dose for noncan-

cerous conditions. The recommended genistein dose based on the label of some products is about 50 milligrams. The commonly prescribed doses of apigenin and luteolin are more difficult to determine. Chamomile products that are standardized for 1 percent apigenin are commercially available. When used according to the manufacturer's recommendations, the daily dose would provide about 10 milligrams of apigenin. No products standardized for luteolin are commercially available, although other herbs besides chamomile contain apigenin and/or luteolin. The commonly prescribed dose for quercetin supplements, as provided on the label of some products, is about 1 gram per day.

The exact LOAEL doses for these flavonoids are uncertain. Animal and human studies suggest that the human LOAEL dose for genistein is greater than 1.1 grams per day:

- In rat studies, the NOAEL dose for genistein was about 1.6 grams per day, as scaled to humans.[100] The LOAEL dose can be expected to be equal to or somewhat higher than the NOAEL dose.

- In a study on dogs, no adverse acute effects were seen after oral administration of 63 mg/kg of genistein.[101] The human equivalent is about 2.7 grams.

- Preliminary results of a phase I human clinical trial on genistein (as given in a soy isoflavone mixture) indicate that subjects can safely receive doses of at least 1.1 grams (16 mg/kg).[102]

The LOAEL dose for genistein predicted by the TOPKAT model is similar to the above doses. The TOPKAT model predicted LOAEL doses for genistein, apigenin, luteolin, and quercetin in rats of 97, 200, 270, and 400 mg/kg. These correspond to human doses of about 1.6, 3.2, 4.4, and 6.5 grams per day. Because this model appears to accurately predict the LOAEL dose for genistein, we base our LOAEL dose estimates for all these flavonoids on the TOPKAT results.

Since genistein occurs naturally with

TABLE J.9 AVERAGE AMOUNTS OF CATECHINS IN GREEN TEA EXTRACT						
SAMPLE	**UNITS**	**EGCG**	**EGC**	**EC**	**ECG**	**REFERENCES**
One gram tea extract (GTE) containing 35% (350 mg) catechins	mg	120	92	34	32	5, 51, 106–109
	% of total catechins*	34	26	9.7	9.1	
	% of total tea solids	12	9.2	3.4	3.2	
Dried tea leaf	% of total	2	1.5	0.57	0.53	

* *This assumes that 20% of total catechins are from catechin compounds not listed.*
EGC = epigallocatechin, EC = epicatechin, ECG = epicatechin gallate

TABLE J.10 SUMMARY OF HUMAN PHARMACOKINETIC STUDIES ON EGCG			
DOSE	**MEASURED SUBSTANCE**	**ORAL CLEARANCE (L/Hr)**	**REFERENCES**
220 mg of EGCG in 3 grams of GTE	total EGCG	110	5
88 mg of EGCG in 1.2 grams of GTE	total EGCG	69*	103
Average clearance for total EGCG		**90**	
370 mg of EGCG in 3 grams of GTE	free catechins	580†	104
110 mg in 5 grams of GTE	free EGCG	400	105
Average clearance for free EGCG		**490**	

* *Analysis required the estimation of one data point, which was done based on relative values from reference 5.*
† *Assumes that the average molecular weight of catechins is 370 grams/mole and that plasma concentrations are twice as great as blood concentrations.*

daidzein in soy (in about a 1 to 1 ratio), the toxicity of daidzein is also of interest. The TOPKAT model predicted a LOAEL dose of daidzein in rats of 69 mg/kg. The corresponding human dose is about 1.1 grams. This suggests that administration of a mixed soy isoflavone product should not exceed about 1.1 grams for daidzein, or subsequently, 1.1 grams for genistein.

The estimates presented in Table J.8 are not likely to be in error due to dose-dependent bioavailability issues. The human pharmacokinetic studies for genistein and quercetin used doses of 8 to 71 milligrams, which is below the linear bioavailability limit of 600 milligrams per administration (1.8 grams per day). The same is true for the rat pharmacokinetic study for luteolin, which used a dose of 230 milligrams, as scaled to humans.

Green Tea and EGCG

Phenolic compounds, of which catechins are the largest single group, account for about 35 percent of the weight of GTE (green tea extract). The measured concentration of catechins and the relative levels of different catechins in green tea can vary greatly, perhaps partly from differences in growing and processing con-

ditions and different handling and analytical procedures. Average values of catechins in GTE and dried tea leaf are shown in Table J.9. As a beverage, a cup of green tea is made from about 2 grams of dried leaves. Since it takes about 6 grams of leaves to make 1 gram of GTE, a cup of tea is equivalent to about 0.33 grams of GTE, which would contain about 40 milligrams of EGCG.[51]

The pharmacokinetics of EGCG and other green tea catechins have been investigated in humans, and the results of three such studies are summarized in Table J.10; these results are in rough agreement. Unlike estimates for other phenolics, about 20 percent of the total EGCG may exist as the free form in human plasma (as measured after a dose of 88 milligrams EGCG in GTE).[51] Therefore, the clearance for total EGCG would be expected to be about fivefold lower than that for the free form, which is nearly the case for the average values listed in the table. Although one study that measured the free form did so for free catechins rather than EGCG itself, we can assume a similar value for free EGCG. In another human study, the oral clearance of free EGCG was about 190 L/hr, less than would be expected, but the EGCG dose used in this study was not

TABLE J.11 ESTIMATED THERAPEUTIC AND LOAEL DOSES FOR EGCG	
DESCRIPTION	**DOSE (g/day)**
Required dose as scaled from animal antitumor studies	0.46 to 1.3
Required cytotoxic dose as determined from pharmacokinetic calculations	12
Target dose based on range from animal antitumor studies and pharmacokinetic calculations	0.46 to 12
Minimum required antitumor dose assuming 15-fold synergistic benefits	0.031 to 0.8
Commonly prescribed human dose in noncancerous conditions	0.2
Estimated LOAEL dose	0.21 to 0.55
Tentative dose recommendation for further research	**0.46 to 0.55**
Minimum degree of synergism required	**uncertain**

entirely certain.[110] Additional human studies are needed to clarify the pharmacokinetics of EGCG in humans. For dose calculations, we use the average value for total EGCG clearance listed in the table.

As discussed in Chapter 19, EGCG appears to be active via cytotoxic mechanisms in vitro at concentrations of roughly 50 to 80 µM. However, since it may be active through noncytotoxic mechanisms at lower concentrations (about 9 to 25 µM) and through cytotoxic ones at lower concentrations if exposure is prolonged, we still use a target concentration of 15 µM to estimate the required dose. If we assume the conjugates are 2-fold less potent than the free form, the modified in-vivo target concentration becomes 30 µM. Based on these values, the estimated required EGCG dose is 9.9 grams every eight hours, or 30 grams per day. We presume the other catechin compounds in GTE will increase the cytotoxicity of EGCG; as mentioned in Chapter 19, associated catechins may increase the cytotoxicity of EGCG 2.6-fold. The EGCG dose then becomes 12 grams per day, which is still prohibitively large.

A 12-gram dose is much higher than the range of 0.46 to 1.3 grams scaled from mouse antitumor experiments (see Chapter 19). The differences between these two doses are perplexing and point to large uncertainties regarding the pharmacokinetics of EGCG. Two rat studies indicate that the oral clearance of total EGCG (after oral administration of 240 milligrams and 2.2 grams of EGCG in GTE, as scaled to humans) is 35 and 27 L/hr, respectively.[103, 111] The data in the second study are less reliable because it used a relatively large dose and measured steady-state plasma levels after multiple dosing (rather than AUC values); the measurement of steady-state concentrations is less accurate in determining clearance. Therefore, we take the oral clearance of

total EGCG in rats to be 35 L/hr. When scaled to humans, this is an oral clearance of about 2,100 L/hr, which is 23-fold larger than the 90 L/hr estimated above. Based on this rat data, the required human EGCG dose would be 270 rather than 12 grams per day, a dose 270-fold larger than the approximate 1-gram daily dose scaled from mouse antitumor studies! Other studies have also suggested that the clearance of EGCG in rats may be much higher than in humans. One study reported that the bioavailability of free EGCG in rats was 27-fold lower than in humans (after oral administration of 5 grams of pure EGCG to rats, as scaled to humans, and oral administration of 97 milligrams of EGCG to humans).[112] The large differences in the doses may have accounted for some of the differences in bioavailability, however. Also note that the clearance of free and total EGCG in the rat studies above were similar (42 and 35 L/hr, respectively). We would have expected a value for free EGCG about five-fold higher than total EGCG, or about 180 L/hr. This unexpected finding is an additional concern about the rat data.

In summary, rat pharmacokinetic data suggest that extremely high doses of EGCG (and GTE) would be necessary to produce an anticancer effect in humans. This is in direct contrast with the low doses found effective in mouse antitumor studies. Additional study is required to determine the reasons for this inconsistency. The potential usefulness of green tea extract in cancer treatment, and the target dose, will remain uncertain until these issues are resolved.

We have calculated that the required human EGCG dose based on pharmacokinetic studies is about 12 grams per day, but mouse antitumor studies suggest an effective human dose of 460 milligrams to 1.3 grams per day. Lacking additional data, we estimate the human target dose falls within the range of 460 milligrams to 12 grams.

The LOAEL dose is also uncertain. The TOPKAT model was unable to predict a rat LOAEL dose for EGCG, but it did predict a value for epicatechin of 34 mg/kg; the human equivalent is about 550 milligrams per day. We can assume the LOAEL dose for EGCG is similar, and for further verification, we can estimate it from the lethal dose. The TOPKAT model tentatively predicted the oral LD$_{50}$ of EGCG would be 740 mg/kg in rats, or the human equivalent of about 12 grams. Similarly, one mouse study reported a LD_{50} for EGCG of about 20 grams, as scaled to humans.[151] We use an average of the two, or 16 grams, as the LD_{50}. If we assume the LOAEL dose is 13- to 75-fold lower than the LD_{50} (see Appendix I), the LOAEL dose of EGCG in humans is 210 milligrams to 1.2 grams per day. Lacking additional data, we will estimate the LOAEL dose to be between 210 and 550 milligrams per day. This dose is similar to the one commonly prescribed in noncancerous conditions. One standardized green tea product recommends an EGCG dose of 200 milligrams per day.

Table J.11 summarizes the therapeutic dose estimates for EGCG from this appendix and Chapter 19. The dose estimates presented are not likely to be inaccurate because of dose-dependent bioavailability issues. The human pharmacokinetic studies used doses of 88 to 220 milligrams, which are below the assumed linear bioavailability limit of 600 milligrams and similar to the tentative dose recommendation in the table.

Anthocyanidins and Proanthocyanidins

The pharmacokinetics of anthocyanidins and proanthocyanidins are discussed together here because their pharmacokinetic characteristics are similar. Although the data are limited, it appears the oral clearance values for both compounds are high enough that cytotoxic concentrations would be difficult to achieve in the plasma after oral dosing. This does not preclude their use in cancer treatment, however, since both compounds may be able to inhibit cancer through noncytotoxic means. In particular, both have a high affinity for vascular tissue and can reduce high vascular permeability, as discussed in Chapter 8. Further investigation of their pharmacokinetic properties is warranted to validate the high clearance values noted here.

The pharmacokinetic properties of anthocyanins have been investigated in rats and humans. It appears that anthocyanins (the glycoside form) are absorbed partially or mostly intact. In a rat study, after oral administration of about 140 mg/kg (the human equivalent of 2.3 grams), about 10 prominent anthocyanins were identified in the plasma.[113] These same compounds were also seen in the bilberry extract that was given. Based on this study, the oral clearance of bilberry anthocyanins in humans is about 760 L/hr. Apparently, the analytical techniques used in this study would have detected both the glycosides in plasma and any conjugates formed;

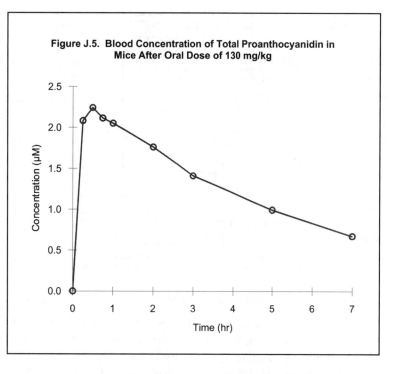

Figure J.5. Blood Concentration of Total Proanthocyanidin in Mice After Oral Dose of 130 mg/kg

therefore it appears total anthocyanin plasma concentrations were measured.

A clearance of 760 L/hr for anthocyanins is roughly similar to that determined from a mouse study on radiolabeled proanthocyanidins. The blood concentration curve for this study is shown in Figure J.5.[114] The proanthocyanidin dose was about 1.2 grams, scaled to humans. The estimated human oral clearance based on this study is 110 L/hr; however, since it measured blood rather than plasma clearance, we can estimate the plasma clearance by dividing by a factor of two (see the discussion on PSK). The adjusted clearance is then 55 L/hr. Furthermore, because this is a radiolabeled study and is likely to underestimate the clearance, we can multiply the clearance by 7.5 (see Table J.2). The adjusted human oral clearance then becomes 410 L/hr, which is about half the 760 L/hr value calculated for anthocyanins. Both values are similar in that they are much higher than those of other flavonoids discussed. We can roughly corroborate the 410-L/hr value for proanthocyanidin by using the TOC model (see Table I.2), which predicted the total oral clearance would be 320 L/hr. The high clearance values are likely due to extensive metabolism and extensive binding to vascular tissues.[115]

We could try to refine our 760- and 410-L/hr values for anthocyanins and proanthocyanidins by using different assumptions, but this is unnecessary. As we see in the calculations below, these large clearance values dictate that prohibitively large doses are needed to produce cytotoxic effects in vivo, a result not likely to change through any minor adjustments to the clearance values.

TABLE J.12 ESTIMATED THERAPEUTIC AND LOAEL DOSES FOR ANTHOCYANINS	
DESCRIPTION	**DOSE (g/day)**
Required dose as scaled from animal antitumor studies	0.12 to 0.28
Required dose as scaled from animal anti-edema studies	0.4 to 3
Required cytotoxic dose as determined from pharmacokinetic calculations	250
Commonly prescribed human dose in noncancerous conditions	0.06 to 0.12
Estimated LOAEL dose	2.2
Tentative dose recommendation for further research	**0.12 to 1.8 grams** *

* *Upper value based on the general linear bioavailability limit of 1.8 grams per day.*

Dose Calculations for Anthocyanins

Even though we are not interested in anthocyanidins for their cytotoxic properties, we include an analysis of the required dose based on cytotoxicity to show that excessive doses would be required. As discussed in Chapter 19, anthocyanins and anthocyanidins are cytotoxic at concentrations between about 5 and 100 μM, with glycosides somewhat less potent than aglycones. This is a rather large range, and possibly anthocyanins and anthocyanidins from some plants are more potent than those from others. Looking at studies where the IC_{50} was below 50 μM (i.e., those on effective anthocyanins and anthocyanidins), the average IC_{50} for aglycones was roughly 6 μM and that for glycosides was about 13 μM, a twofold difference as expected. We use a value of 15 μM for dose calculations for anthocyanins, similar to most other compounds. This may be underestimated, but it does not matter for our purposes because the dose estimate based on this value is already too high even with synergism, and a higher target concentration would only produce a more prohibitive estimate.

Using an oral clearance of 760 L/hr and a target in-vivo concentration of 15 μM (30 μM after adjustment for conjugates), the required anthocyanin dose is about 82 grams every eight hours, or 250 grams per day. This is much larger than the commonly prescribed daily dose of 60 to 120 milligrams used for noncancerous conditions. It is also larger than the range of 400 milligrams to 3 grams that was effective in animal anti-edema studies and the range of 120 to 280 milligrams effective in animal antitumor studies (see Chapter 19).

The LOAEL dose is probably higher than the common dose of 120 milligrams. In one human pharmacokinetic study, a single 1.5-gram dose of anthocyanins was given (in 25 grams of elderberry extract) without ill effects, but the study did not specifically look for adverse reac-

tions.[116] The LOAEL dose for anthocyanidins may be similar to that for proanthocyanidins. No adverse effects were mentioned in animal studies using high proanthocyanidin doses, although again, such reactions were not specifically sought. In one study, oral administration of 400 mg/kg per day prevented acute postoperative edema in rats.[117] The human equivalent is about 6.5 grams. In a second one on rabbits, oral administration of 50 mg/kg per day altered the aortic cholesterol content.[118] The human equivalent is 1.5 grams per day.

The oral LD_{50} of proanthocyanidins in unspecified rodents was 3 g/kg, or the human equivalent of about 29 grams, assuming the study was conducted in mice.[119] If the LOAEL dose is 13- to 75-fold lower than the LD_{50} (see Appendix I), then the LOAEL dose is 390 milligrams to 2.2 grams. Based on the above, we assume the LOAEL dose for both anthocyanidins and proanthocyanidins is 2.2 grams. This value is just below the average LOAEL dose for all flavonoids discussed here, which is 2.9 grams.

Table J.12 summarizes the therapeutic dose estimates for anthocyanins from this appendix and Chapter 19. Based on the available information, it is clear that cytotoxic concentrations of anthocyanins will not be produced in the plasma after oral dosing. Protective effects on the vasculature can be expected at the tentative recommended range, however, and these may inhibit cancer progression through indirect means.

Dose Calculations for Proanthocyanidins

We presume that proanthocyanidins are active against cancer cells in vitro at 15 μM. Although the degree that proanthocyanidins are conjugated in the plasma is unknown, to be conservative we assume they are conjugated like other flavonoids, and we therefore use an in-vivo target of 30 μM after adjustment for conjugates. Using an oral clearance value of 410 L/hr and a 30-μM target, a dose of 29 grams would be required every eight hours, or 87 grams per day, which is prohibitive. This is probably a low estimate, since most in-vitro studies discussed in Chapter 19 reported that concentrations greater than 15 μM are necessary. Because of the high dose requirement, proanthocyanidins are not considered here as cytotoxic compounds.

Proanthocyanidins are available commercially as grape seed or pine bark extract. Doses are normally 50 to 100 milligrams per day for noncancerous conditions, but for stronger effects, up to 300 milligrams daily or more are sometimes prescribed. The estimated LOAEL dose is 2.2 grams per day, as estimated above.

Table J.13 summarizes the therapeutic dose estimates for proanthocyanidins from this appendix and Chapter 19. The same conclusions drawn for anthocyanins above apply for these as well (i.e., they are most useful as indirect-acting compounds).

TABLE J.13 ESTIMATED THERAPEUTIC AND LOAEL DOSES FOR PROANTHOCYANIDINS	
DESCRIPTION	DOSE (g/day)
Required dose as scaled from animal anti-edema studies	0.49 to 6.5
Required cytotoxic dose as determined from pharmacokinetic calculations	87
Commonly prescribed human dose in noncancerous conditions	0.05 to 0.3
Estimated LOAEL dose	2.2
Tentative dose recommendation for further research	**0.49 to 1.8 grams**[*]

[*] *Upper value based on the general linear bioavailability limit of 1.8 grams per day.*

Chapter 20:
Nonflavonoid Phenolic Compounds

CAPE and Propolis

Although CAPE and bee propolis hold promise, as evidenced by their in-vitro effects against cancer cells and in-vivo effects against inflammation, the pharmacokinetic properties of CAPE remain uncertain; they have not been studied in animals or humans. Still, we can estimate a value for the total clearance of CAPE by using the TOC model, which predicted a value of 58 L/hr (see Table I.3). Of all compounds listed in that table, the predictions for CAPE and the related compound caffeic acid are perhaps the most uncertain. This is because of a lack of animal studies. Neither the pharmacokinetic response nor the metabolism of these compounds has been adequately studied.

One pharmacokinetic study was completed on caffeic acid in rabbits, but it was not clear whether it measured free or total caffeic acid. Based on that study, the oral clearance as scaled to humans was 81 L/hr, which is roughly half the value of 140 L/hr predicted by the FOC model.[120] Thus if free clearance was measured, the study suggests that the FOC model overpredicted the value for free oral clearance. On the other hand, if total oral clearance was measured, it suggests that about half the plasma concentration is in the free form (total clearance would be about half the value for free clearance). Although the actual percentage of free caffeic acid (or CAPE) in plasma has not been measured, the value of free ferulic acid, a close relative of caffeic acid and CAPE, has been measured in human urine. One study reported that about half the urinary ferulic acid is in the free form and half is in the conjugate form.[121] Therefore, it is possible that free caffeic acid (and possibly CAPE) accounts for about half the total plasma concentration. This would be a much higher percentage than for all other phenolic compounds discussed, however,

and it would also be much higher than the 0.5-percent value used for curcumin, a compound structurally related to caffeic acid. Lacking additional information, we assume the percentage of free caffeic acid and CAPE in the plasma is about midway between these values, or 24 percent. In addition, we assume the predictions made for free oral clearance by the FOC model are accurate. Thus, using Equation I.2, the predicted total oral clearance values for caffeic acid and CAPE are 34 and 58 L/hr, respectively, as listed in Table I.3. Clearly, additional work remains to determine more trustworthy clearance values.

CAPE is active at roughly 15 μM in vitro. As discussed above, we assume that most of the plasma concentration is in the conjugate form, and therefore our target in-vivo concentration becomes 30 μM. To produce an average total plasma concentration of 30 μM, a CAPE dose of 4 grams would be required every eight hours, or 12 grams per day.

The most common source of CAPE is propolis; its concentration in propolis varies from about 0 to 5 percent.[122, 123] If we assume that propolis contains 2.5 percent CAPE, a CAPE dose of 12 grams would require a propolis dose of 480 grams, which is prohibitive. As discussed in Chapter 20, however, propolis contains additional caffeic acid esters besides CAPE that can contribute to an antitumor effect, although the degree of that contribution is uncertain. One in-vitro study indicated that propolis might be about six times less potent than CAPE, thus we estimate that the required propolis dose would be about 72 grams (12 grams x 6).

A 72-gram propolis dose is much larger than the 1.3-gram dose scaled from a mouse antitumor study in Chapter 20. It is also larger than the range of 1 to 11 grams per day found effective in animal anti-inflammatory experiments (scaled to humans), as discussed in Chapter 20. Clearly, there are uncertainties in the required dose, and additional research is necessary.

TABLE J.14   ESTIMATED THERAPEUTIC AND LOAEL DOSES FOR PROPOLIS

DESCRIPTION	DOSE (g/day)
Required dose as scaled from animal antitumor studies	1.3
Required dose as scaled from animal anti-inflammatory studies	0.96 to 11
Required cytotoxic dose as determined from pharmacokinetic calculations	72
Target dose based on range from animal antitumor studies and pharmacokinetic calculations	1.3 to 72
Minimum required antitumor dose assuming 15-fold synergistic benefits	0.087 to 4.8
Commonly prescribed human dose in noncancerous conditions	0.2 to 3
Estimated LOAEL dose	15
Tentative dose recommendation for further research	**3 to 15**
Minimum degree of synergism required	**uncertain**

contains other active compounds that increase its cytotoxicity about sixfold, we can guess that the LOAEL dose might also be reduced by sixfold. This would suggest that the LOAEL dose for propolis is greater than 14 to 80 grams, the low end of which is roughly similar to that of the mouse studies on propolis. To estimate the LOAEL dose, we use an average of these three values (13, 19, and 14 grams per day), or 15 grams per day.

Table J.14 summarizes the therapeutic dose estimates for propolis from this appendix and Chapter 20. Note that the 15-gram dose of propolis is above the 1.8-gram general bioavailability limit. This dose would contain only about 350 milligrams of CAPE itself, however, and so should not present a bioavailability problem.

Because of the inconsistencies, the required target dose can be estimated only within a large range, 1.3 to 72 grams per day.

As an aside, if the total oral clearance for CAPE were equal to the geometric average value for all other phenolic compounds listed in Tables I.2 and I.3 (excluding caffeic acid), its total clearance would be 16 L/hr. If its free oral clearance were 240 L/hr as predicted by the FOC model, then from Equation I.2 its percentage in the plasma would be 5.8. Using a clearance value of 16 L/hr, the final propolis dose would be 20 grams (3.3 grams x 6), which is still high but more reasonable. If the percentage of free CAPE in the plasma were 0.5 percent, as is used for curcumin, the final propolis dose would be 1.5 grams per day, which is about equal to the doses found effective in animal studies.

In one study, the oral LOAEL dose for propolis in mice was 1.4 g/kg per day.[124] The human equivalent is roughly 13 grams. Similar results were seen in another mouse study, where oral doses of propolis greater than 2 g/kg began to produce signs of toxicity.[125] The human equivalent is about 19 grams per day. The TOPKAT model was not able to predict a LOAEL dose for CAPE itself, but it can be estimated from the LD_{50}. The TOPKAT model predicted a LD_{50} for CAPE greater than 10 g/kg in rats, or the human equivalent of about 160 grams. If the LOAEL dose is 13- to 75-fold lower (see Appendix I), then the CAPE LOAEL dose would be greater than 2.1 to 12 grams, as scaled to humans. Using the assumptions above, this is equal to a propolis dose of greater than 84 to 480 grams. Since propolis

There is some concern that caffeic acid, a metabolite of CAPE, may produce carcinogenic effects. At the propolis doses considered here, however, it does not appear that such effects would occur. Caffeic acid is a common dietary component found in coffee and numerous other foods. People who consume moderately high amounts of coffee ingest about 630 milligrams per day of caffeic acid.[126] Caffeic acid has been reported to be carcinogenic in the forestomach and kidney of rats and mice, apparently by inducing cell proliferation rather than DNA damage.[126, 127] It shares this trait with a number of other antioxidants.[128, 129] On the other hand, because of its antioxidant effects, caffeic acid inhibited chemically induced tumor promotion in some studies, which indicates it can also have anticarcinogenic effects.[130, 131] Indeed, its effects appear to be dose related; low doses may inhibit carcinogenesis and high ones (270 mg/kg in the rat) may promote cellular proliferation that can lead to cancer.[126, 132] The human equivalent of 270 mg/kg is about 4.4 grams per day, which is greater than the total caffeic acid ester content of a 15-gram propolis dose. If propolis contains 19 percent caffeic acid esters, a 15-gram dose would contain 2.9 grams of caffeic acid esters. Moreover, it appears that only caffeic acid and not caffeic acid esters cause carcinogenic effects.[126] At least this is true for chlorogenic acid, the caffeic acid ester that is the primary form of caffeic acid in coffee. CAPE itself and other caffeic acid esters have demonstrated cancer preventive effects in animals and inhibition of mutagenesis in vitro.[133, 134] Although it seems there would be no problem with carcinogenicity, additional study is needed to ensure no carcinogenic potential for propolis exists with the doses calculated here.

Curcumin

Pharmacokinetics studies of curcumin have been performed in mice, rats, dogs, and humans. These reported that after oral administration, only a small concentration of free curcumin exists in the plasma, with the bulk of curcumin being conjugates of it and its primary metabolites. Unfortunately, almost all pharmacokinetic studies have investigated plasma concentrations of the free form, and little is known about pharmacokinetics of the conjugate forms.

In two rat studies, oral administration of 1 and 2 g/kg produced free curcumin plasma concentrations of less than the detection limits (0.05 and 13 µM, respectively).[135, 136] Free curcumin was also below the detection limits in the plasma following oral administration of up to 3.5 g/kg in rats and 1 g/kg in dogs.[137] One rat study with a lower detection limit did measure free curcumin in plasma, however.[138] In this study, the oral clearance based on a dose of 2g/kg was about 7,500 L/hr, as scaled to humans.[a] The equivalent human dose is about 32 grams.

Free curcumin was also measured in one mouse study. The plasma concentration curve of free curcumin after oral administration of 1 g/kg is illustrated in Figure J.6 (based on reference 139). The equivalent human dose is about 9.6 grams. Oral clearance based on this study is 5,600 L/hr, as scaled to humans.

Based on these rat and mouse studies, the human clearance of free curcumin may be about 7,500 to 5,600 L/hr (midrange of 6,500 L/hr). It is uncertain if these values are accurate at doses applicable to humans, since large doses were given in the animal studies. The two rodent pharmacokinetic studies on free curcumin used doses above the general linear bioavailability limit of 600 milligrams per administration (9.6 and 32 grams, scaled to humans). A radiolabeled study on rats indi-

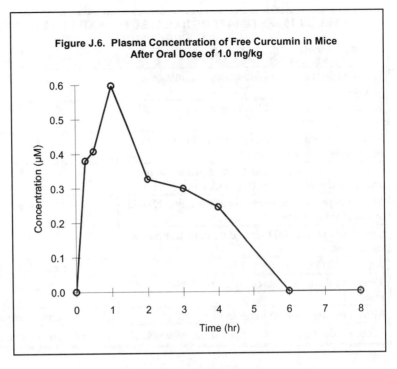

Figure J.6. Plasma Concentration of Free Curcumin in Mice After Oral Dose of 1.0 mg/kg

cated, however, that similar percentages of the administered dose were absorbed when doses ranged from about 1 and 32 grams (as scaled to humans), but it is likely that especially the larger doses would have been metabolized differently than a 600-milligram dose.[140] The FOC model predicted the free oral clearance of curcumin would be 200 L/hr, although this seems underestimated compared to a value of 6,500 L/hr. With no additional data, we use a value of 6,500 L/hr in further calculations.

Due to the low plasma concentrations produced, early researchers concluded that curcumin was not bioavailable, but we now known that it is indeed absorbed but heavily metabolized. For example, one study reported that excretion of conjugated compounds in the urine markedly increased in rats fed curcumin.[135] Furthermore, the radiolabeled study in rats mentioned above suggested that up to 66 percent of a curcumin dose is absorbed but heavily metabolized.

Unfortunately, the oral clearance of total (free plus conjugated) curcumin in plasma has not been studied. Lacking concrete data, we can use the TOC model to predict a value of 33 L/hr (see Table I.3). In Equation I.2, a 0.5 percent value was used as the percent of free compound in plasma. This is relatively low but was used because pharmacokinetic studies suggested that almost all the compound exists as conjugates in plasma.

As seen in Chapter 20, curcumin is active against cancer cells in vitro at a concentration of about 15 µM. Since it occurs in plasma as conjugates, we use a target in-vivo concentration that is twice as large, or 30 µM.

---

[a] In the same study, an oral dose of 2 grams in humans did not significantly increase the plasma concentration of free curcumin. When curcumin was combined with a compound that inhibits conjugation (piperine, from black pepper), a 2-gram dose in humans did raise plasma levels of free curcumin to about 0.5 µM. However, the concentration did not stay high for long (the half-life was only about 15 minutes). Piperine inhibits glucuronide conjugation and has increased the bioavailability of a number of drugs. Given on an empty stomach, it may also increase the bioavailability of free curcumin.

TABLE J.15   ESTIMATED THERAPEUTIC AND LOAEL DOSES FOR CURCUMIN

DESCRIPTION	DOSE (g/day)
Required dose as scaled from animal antitumor studies	0.36 to 3.2
Required dose as scaled from animal anti-inflammatory studies	0.23 to 3.2
Required cytotoxic dose as determined from pharmacokinetic calculations	8.7
Target dose based on range from animal antitumor studies and pharmacokinetic calculations	0.36 to 8.7
Minimum required antitumor dose assuming 15-fold synergistic benefits	0.024 to 0.58
Commonly prescribed human dose in noncancerous conditions	0.75 to 1.5
Estimated LOAEL dose	greater than 43
Tentative dose recommendation for further research	**1.5 to 1.8**[*]
Minimum degree of synergism required	**uncertain**

[*] *Upper value based on the general linear bioavailability limit of 1.8 grams per day.*

TABLE J.16   PHARMACOKINETIC STUDIES OF SILYBIN IN HUMANS

DOSE	MEASURED SUBSTANCE	ORAL CLEARANCE (L/Hr)	REFERENCES
53 mg of silybin in 140 mg of silymarin[*]	free lignan	280	141
53 mg of silybin in 140 mg of silymarin	total lignan	28	141
120 mg of silybin in about 300 mg of silymarin	total lignan	36	142

[*] *Milk thistle contains silymarin, which is a mixture of flavonolignans. The chief active flavonolignan is silybin. The content of silymarin in milk thistle is about 1.5% to 3%.*[143]

To produce a 30 μM average plasma concentration of total curcumin, a dose of 2.9 grams every eight hours would be required, or 8.7 grams per day, which is above the range scaled from animal antitumor studies (0.36 to 3.2 grams) and that scaled from anti-inflammatory studies (0.23 to 3.2 grams). Due to the inconsistencies, the required target dose can be estimated only within a large range, 0.36 to 8.7 grams per day.

The LOAEL dose for curcumin appears to be very high, reportedly greater than 3.5 g/kg in rats and 1 g/kg in dogs.[137] The human equivalents are greater than 58 and 43 grams. Long-term curcumin administration over three generations showed no adverse effects in rats. In some studies, curcumin administration may have increased the incidence of certain cancers in mice, but this has not been confirmed. Oral doses of 2 grams per day for 127 days did not produce adverse effects in HIV-positive individuals.[137] From these findings, we assume the LOAEL dose is more than 43 grams per day. Quite likely, the majority of this dose would be excreted in the feces and not absorbed.

Table J.15 summarizes the therapeutic dose estimates for curcumin in this appendix and Chapter 20.

Arctigenin and Arctium Seed

Unfortunately, the oral clearance of arctigenin has not been studied in humans or animals. However, the clearance for two different lignans—silybin (from milk thistle) and schizandrin (from *Schizandra chinensis*, a plant used in Chinese herbal medicine)—have been studied in humans. Clearance values for silybin and schizandrin can also be predicted by the FOC model. Silybin is actually a hybrid lignan that also has flavonoid aspects, but it is close enough to arctigenin to help verify the accuracy of the FOC model's prediction for arctigenin (see Tables I.2 and I.3).

Table J.16 summarizes data obtained from human pharmacokinetic studies on silybin. Note that the oral clearance for total silybin (free plus conjugates) is about 11-fold lower than for the free form. This suggests that about 11 percent of the total silybin plasma concentration is composed of the free form, a percentage similar to several other compounds discussed here.

The table shows the oral clearance for free silybin is about 280 L/hr, which is nearly identical to the value of 260 L/hr predicted by the FOC model. Furthermore, the FOC model is reasonably accurate for predicting oral clearance of the lignan schizandrin. The clearance of free schizandrin based on a human study (using a dose of 15 milligrams) is 82 L/hr; this is similar to the value of 110 L/hr predicted by the FOC model. The model predicted that the oral clearance for free arctigenin would be lower, at 44 L/hr. Since the model's predictions for silybin and schizandrin appear reasonably accurate, we assume that 44 L/hr for arctigenin is as well.

Clearance for some other lignans is similar to the above-mentioned values. For example, the oral clearance of free sesamin from sesame seeds is about 83 L/hr, as scaled from a rat study (after a dose of 8.4 grams, scaled to humans).[144] Sesamin, like the other lignans, can inhibit proliferation of cancer cells in vitro.[145]

The TOC model discussed in Appendix I can be used to estimate the oral clearance of total arctigenin; in Table I.3 it is predicted to be 5.3 L/hr. As with silybin, we assume that free arctigenin accounts for about 11 percent of the total plasma concentration (a value of 12 percent is used in Equation I.2).

Arctigenin is active in vivo at concentrations of about 15 μM. Since it occurs as conjugates in the plasma, we use a target in-vivo concentration twice as large, or 30 μM. To produce an average plasma concentration of 30 μM, an arctigenin dose of about 470 milligrams every eight hours would be required, or 1.4 grams per day. The average arctigenin content of *Arctium* seed is about 5.6 percent (range 3.2 to 8.4 percent in eight samples), and 95 percent of this is derived from arctiin, the glycoside of arctigenin.[146] Therefore, to produce an arctigenin dose of 1.4 grams, about 27 grams of seed would be needed. This is greater than the commonly prescribed dose of about 9 grams (in decoction) used in Chinese herbal medicine. No animal antitumor studies have been conducted, so we cannot use them to verify the 27-gram estimate.

The LOAEL dose of arctigenin has not been studied in animals. The TOPKAT model predicted a LOAEL dose of only 2.4 mg/kg in rats, or 39 milligrams as scaled to humans. This is likely to be too low, however. For one thing, this dose is unusually low compared to LOAEL doses for other natural compounds (see Table I.5). For another, using the above assumptions, it would be equal to an *Arctium* seed dose of only about 710 milligrams, which is 13-fold lower than the commonly prescribed dose of 9 grams.

The TOPKAT model predicted a rat LD_{50} for arctigenin of 3,000 mg/kg, or about 49 grams, scaled to humans. If this is correct and if the LOAEL dose is 13- to 75-fold lower (see Appendix I), then the LOAEL dose

TABLE J.17 ESTIMATED THERAPEUTIC AND LOAEL DOSES FOR ARCTIGENIN AND *ARCTIUM* SEED		
DESCRIPTION	**ARCTIGENIN DOSE (g/day)**	***ARCTIUM* SEED DOSE (g/day)**
Required cytotoxic dose as determined from pharmacokinetic calculations	1.4	27
Target dose based on pharmacokinetic calculations	1.4	27
Minimum required antitumor dose assuming 15-fold synergistic benefits	0.093	1.7
Commonly prescribed human dose in noncancerous conditions	0.5	9
Estimated LOAEL dose	0.65	12
Tentative dose recommendation for further research	**0.65**	**12**
Minimum degree of synergism required	**2.3-fold potency increase**	

of arctigenin is between 650 milligrams and 3.8 grams per day. The LOAEL dose of *Arctium* seed is then between 12 and 68 grams daily. Conservatively, we take the LOAEL dose to be 650 milligrams of arctigenin, or 12 grams of *Arctium* seed, which is similar to the commonly prescribed dose.

Table J.17 summarizes the therapeutic dose estimates for arctigenin and *Arctium* seed in this appendix and Chapter 20.

Silybin may also have anticancer effects. In vitro, it inhibited proliferation of human ovarian and breast cancer cells at an IC_{50} of 5 to 24 μM. It also effectively competed with estrogen for type II estrogen binding sites, and like other type II-active agents, it acted synergistically with multiple chemotherapy drugs.[147]

Using data in Table J.16, the oral clearance for total silybin is about 28 to 36 L/hr; we can use a midrange value of 32 L/hr in dose calculations. Silybin is active at about 15 μM in vitro, and to account for conjugates we use an in-vivo target concentration of 30 μM. The required silybin dose is then 3.7 grams every eight hours, or 11 grams per day. If milk thistle seeds contain about 2.3 percent silymarin (which is mostly comprised of silybin), a 480-gram daily dose of milk thistle seeds would be needed, which is prohibitive.

Commercial milk thistle extracts contain up to 80 percent silymarin. Therefore, the required dose of this extract may be about 14 grams per day, which is larger than the commonly prescribed one of 250 milligrams to 1 gram for noncancerous conditions. If used in synergistic combinations, the 14-gram extract dose could be reduced to about 930 milligrams, which is within the common dose range but would require the full 15-fold increase in potency we are allowing from synergism.

Flaxseed Lignans

The pharmacokinetic properties of flaxseed lignans have been studied in humans, but dose calculations based on this data are inconsistent with doses scaled from rodent antitumor studies. Those based on the pharmacokinetic and in-vitro data are about 77-fold higher than the 60-gram dose scaled from successful animal experiments. A similar inconsistency has been reported by other authors, who have noted that achievable plasma concentrations of mammalian lignans in humans are far below those required for in-vitro activity.[148]

In one pharmacokinetic study, oral administration of 25 grams per day of flaxseed for eight days produced average total (free plus conjugate) plasma enterodiol and enterolactone concentrations of about 86 nM in healthy women.[148] Assuming that 0.052 percent of flaxseed is converted to mammalian lignans in the human gut, we can use Equation J.3 to estimate that the oral clearance for total mammalian lignans is about 21 L/hr. In contrast, other investigators have measured total plasma lignan values in humans after flaxseed administration that were roughly 8.7 and 14-fold higher, relative to the same dose.[149, 150] The oral clearance based on these studies would then be roughly 1.5 and 2.4 L/hr. The average of all three oral clearance values is 8.3 L/hr, and we use this value in calculations below.

The FOC model predicted a free oral clearance of 57 L/hr for enterolactone, similar to the value of 44 L/hr for arctigenin.[a] The TOC model predicted a total oral clearance of 6.8 L/hr, which is similar to and helps confirm the 8.3-L/hr value estimated above. The 6.8-L/hr value predicted by the TOC model assumes that 12 percent of the enterolactone in the plasma would occur in the free form. This is a reasonable percentage, since it is similar to that for other lignans. Moreover, a human study reported that the free plus sulfate forms accounted for about 21 percent of the total plasma concentration.[55]

Enterolactone is cytotoxic in vitro at concentrations ranging from 10 to 100 µM. Since so few in-vitro studies have been done, we assume that, like most other phenolics, enterolactone will be active at 15 µM. Since enterolactone exists in the plasma primarily as conjugates, the in-vivo target concentration is presumed to be twice as large, or 30 µM. To produce an average plasma concentration of 30 µM, a 590-milligram dose of mammalian lignans would be needed every eight hours, or

1.8 grams per day. Assuming that the yield of enterolactone from flaxseed is 0.052 percent (see Chapter 20), a 1.8-gram dose of enterolactone is supplied by about 3,500 grams of flaxseed per day (or 3.5 grams of SECO, the active flaxseed lignan). This flaxseed dose is excessive and is 58-fold larger than the 60-gram dose scaled from rodent studies cited in Chapter 20.

The reasons for the large difference are not clear. Perhaps the oral clearance value is overestimated. Chronic administration of flaxseed increases tissue levels more effectively than acute exposure, and the human pharmacokinetic studies tested relatively acute exposure (they were conducted over periods of less than two weeks). Alternatively, mammalian lignans possibly are effective at lower concentrations in vivo than the assumed 15-µM concentration, or perhaps the effect of flaxseed in rodents was due to constituents other than SECO. For example, flaxseed contains 35 to 45 percent oil, about half of which is alpha-linolenic acid, an omega-3 fatty acid (see Table 17.1).[151] When scaled to humans, the daily dose of 60 grams of flaxseed would contain about 12 grams of alpha-linolenic acid, which is a considerable amount. Nonetheless, even though alpha-linolenic acid could play a role in flaxseed's antitumor effects, one of the rodent studies administered pure SECO diglycoside (SD), which would not contain alpha-linolenic acid, and the same antitumor effects occurred. This suggests that SECO is capable of producing antitumor effects on its own at the doses used. In summary, questions remain regarding the pharmacokinetics, effective concentrations, and active constituents of flaxseed, and consequently the required dose remains uncertain.

The commonly prescribed flaxseed dose as a bulking agent to treat constipation is 10 to 30 grams daily. The LOAEL dose is uncertain, but it is likely the 60-gram dose scaled from animal experiments would be safe. In two studies, daily doses of 50 grams for four weeks did not produce adverse effects in healthy humans.[152, 153] Thus we assume the LOAEL dose is greater than 60 grams per day.

Table J.18 summarizes the therapeutic dose estimates for flaxseed from this appendix and Chapter 20.

Resveratrol

The pharmacokinetic properties of free resveratrol have been investigated in rats, and the plasma concentration curve after oral administration is shown in Figure J.7 (based on reference 154). Other rat studies have reported similar peak concentrations relative to this dose.[155]

Based on the data in the figure, the estimated human oral clearance of free resveratrol is 45 L/hr. The FOC

---

[a] *The FOC model predicted that the clearance for free enterodiol would be significantly higher, at 770 L/hr. This larger value does not conform with data from the human studies; therefore, we use a clearance value of 57 L/hr for free enterolactone and enterodiol combined.*

model predicted a clearance about sevenfold higher (310 L/hr). It is a judgment call as to which is more accurate, since no human pharmacokinetic studies have been conducted. A value of 310 L/hr is more in keeping with the free oral clearance values for other phenolic compounds discussed (which have a geometric mean free oral clearance of 350 L/hr). It is also in keeping with the free oral clearance values for most flavonoids, which are structurally related to resveratrol. For lack of additional information, we use 310 L/hr, as obtained by the FOC model. It is uncertain why the value based on the rat study is so small in comparison. Perhaps the study inadvertently measured conjugate concentrations in addition to that of the free compound.

The clearance for total resveratrol has not been studied in animals or humans, but we can use the TOC model to estimate a value. As shown in Table I.3, the total oral clearance for resveratrol is predicted to be 4.7 L/hr. This was calculated using a value of 1.5 percent for the percentage of free resveratrol in the plasma. This value is consistent with in-vitro absorption studies using isolated small intestine tissue, as well as values of most flavonoids (for example, genistein).[156]

Resveratrol is active in vitro at concentrations of about 15 µM. Due to the presence of conjugates, we use a target in-vivo concentration of 30 µM. To produce an average concentration of 30 µM in the plasma, 260 milligrams of resveratrol would be required every eight hours, or 770 milligrams per day. A 770-milligram dose is larger than the 68-milligram dose scaled from the rat antitumor study mentioned in Chapter 20. It is also larger than the commonly prescribed dose of 20 milligrams recommended for some resveratrol products. Due to the inconsistencies, the required target dose can be estimated only within a large range, 68 to 770 milligrams per day.

The LOAEL dose of resveratrol is uncertain; animal LOAEL dose studies have not been conducted, and the TOPKAT model was unable to predict a value. It did predict, however, a LD_{50} of 1.9 g/kg in rats, or 31 grams

TABLE J.18 ESTIMATED THERAPEUTIC AND LOAEL DOSES FOR FLAXSEED	
DESCRIPTION	**DOSE (g/day)**
Required dose as scaled from animal antitumor studies	60
Required cytotoxic dose as determined from pharmacokinetic calculations	3,500
Target dose based on range from animal antitumor studies and pharmacokinetic calculations	60 to 3,500
Minimum required antitumor dose assuming 15-fold synergistic benefits	4 to 230
Commonly prescribed human dose in noncancerous conditions	10 to 30
Estimated LOAEL dose	greater than 60
Tentative dose recommendation for further research	**30 to 60**
Minimum degree of synergism required	**uncertain**

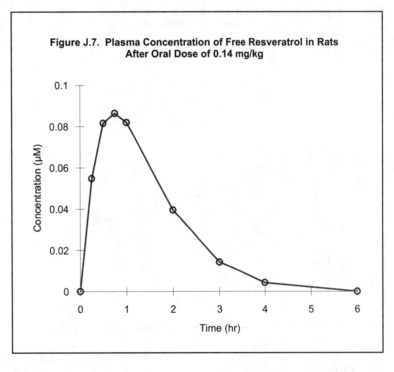

Figure J.7. Plasma Concentration of Free Resveratrol in Rats After Oral Dose of 0.14 mg/kg

as scaled to humans, and this can be used to roughly estimate a LOAEL dose. If we assume that the LOAEL dose is 13- to 75-fold lower than the LD_{50} (see Appendix I), the human LOAEL dose would be 410 milligrams to 2.4 grams per day. Conservatively, we take the LOAEL dose to be 410 milligrams. Obviously, additional toxicity studies are needed to verify this estimate.

Table J.19 summarizes the therapeutic dose estimates for resveratrol in this appendix and Chapter 20.

TABLE J.19 ESTIMATED THERAPEUTIC AND LOAEL DOSES FOR RESVERATROL	
DESCRIPTION	**DOSE (mg/day)**
Required dose as scaled from an animal antitumor study	68
Required cytotoxic dose as determined from pharmacokinetic calculations	770
Target dose based on range from animal antitumor studies and pharmacokinetic calculations	68 to 770
Minimum required antitumor dose assuming 15-fold synergistic benefits	4.5 to 51
Commonly prescribed human dose in noncancerous conditions	20
Estimated LOAEL dose	410
Tentative dose recommendation for further research	**68 to 410**
Minimum degree of synergism required	**uncertain**

In analyzing the mouse data, we supposed that free emodin accounted for 10 percent of the total plasma concentration. This is the approximate percentage suggested by the rat study; it also appears reasonable based on other studies with compounds similar to emodin. Rhein is an anthraquinone closely related to emodin, and diacerein is a drug form of rhein that is better absorbed than rhein itself. In humans, diacerein is excreted in the urine in its free form (20 percent), glucuronide conjugate form (62 percent), and sulfate conjugate form (18 percent).[161]

The oral clearance in humans based on the data in Figure J.8 is 78 L/hr. This is similar to and helps confirm the oral clearance of 110 L/hr predicted by the FOC model, so we use the FOC prediction for dose calculations. Since the clearance of total emodin has not been studied in animals, we can use the TOC model to estimate total oral clearance. As listed in Table I.3, the total oral clearance of emodin is predicted to be 13 L/hr. In using Equation I.2, a value of 12 percent was utilized for the percentage of free emodin in plasma. This is consistent with the rat data mentioned above.

Emodin is active in vitro at a concentration of roughly 15 μM. Since it probably occurs as conjugates, we use a target in-vivo concentration twice that, or 30 μM. To generate an average plasma concentration of 30 μM, 840 milligrams would be needed every eight hours, or 2.5 grams per day. This dose is large and may cause adverse effects, but it is within the range of 330 milligrams to 4.9 grams as scaled from mouse antitumor studies cited in Chapter 20.

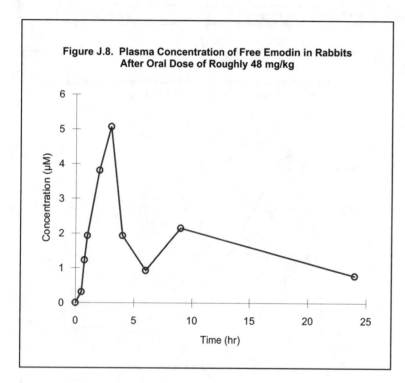

Figure J.8. Plasma Concentration of Free Emodin in Rabbits After Oral Dose of Roughly 48 mg/kg

Emodin

Few studies exist on the pharmacokinetics of emodin after oral administration. One investigated emodin pharmacokinetics in rabbits, but unfortunately, the actual dose given was not clearly specified.[157] The plasma concentration-time curve from this study is shown in Figure J.8. The dose needed to produce this peak concentration can be estimated by using data from three different studies: emodin studies in rabbits and mice and an aloe-emodin one in rats.[158, 159, 160] These suggest that a dose of roughly 48 mg/kg may have produced this peak in rabbits.

The commonly prescribed dose of emodin in noncancerous conditions is about 20 milligrams per day. This is based on the label of some commercial products of *Polygonum cuspidatum* standardized for emodin. A similar dose is obtained when making decoctions from the crude herb, as is done in Chinese herbal medicine. The concentration of emodin in *Polygonum* is approximately 1.1 percent, and the common dose of *Polygonum* is about 15 grams per day (in decoction).[160] Since about 12 percent of the emodin content in plants is extracted by hot water, most decoctions contain about 20 milligrams of emodin.[160] This is lower than the commonly prescribed dose of 100 milligrams per day for the related drug diacerein.[161]

The TOPKAT model predicted a LOAEL dose of 180 mg/kg for emodin in rats. The human equivalent is about 3 grams per day. Like other anthraquinones, emodin may have a purgative effect; the purgative dose in mice is greater than 500 mg/kg for a single administration.[162] The human equivalent is about 4.8 grams. A slight purgative effect was caused by a single dose of 50 mg/kg in rats.[163] The human equivalent is about 810 milligrams. Therefore, we conservatively take the human LOAEL dose to be about 810 milligrams per day.

Table J.20 summarizes the therapeutic dose estimates for emodin from this appendix and Chapter 20.

Hypericin

The pharmacokinetic properties of hypericin have been investigated in humans. In three studies, hypericin doses in the range of 1.5 to 2.2 milligrams in a standardized *Hypericum* extract produced oral clearance values of 3.9, 3.1, and 2.4 L/hr.[164, 165, 166] We use an average of these values, or 3.1 L/hr, in dose calculations. These studies apparently measured free hypericin, even though the resulting oral clearance values are far lower than the geometric mean free oral clearance value for other phenolics (350 L/hr). The next highest free clearance value to 3.1 L/hr is the 44-L/hr value for arctigenin. Since pharmacokinetic studies have not measured the clearance of total hypericin, we can use the TOC model to make a prediction. Using equation I.2 and a value of 12 for the percentage of free hypericin in the plasma, the predicted total oral clearance value is 0.37 L/hr. A 12 percent value is used, since this is in keeping with emodin, the other anthraquinone compound discussed here.

As discussed in Table D.2 (Appendix D), hypericin inhibits proliferation of a variety of cancer cell lines at concentrations of 5 to 25 μM. As with other phenolic compounds, we employ a target concentration of 15 μM and adjust this to 30 μM due to the presence of conjugates. To achieve an average plasma concentration of 30 μM, a dose of 45 milligrams of hypericin would be needed every eight hours, or 130 milligrams per day.

The commonly prescribed daily dose in noncancerous conditions is 900 milligrams of *Hypericum* extract, containing a hypericin dose of about 2.7 milligrams. The LOAEL dose is slightly higher. In one study, a daily total hypericin oral dose of 11 milligrams (containing both hypericin and pseudohypericin) was generally well tolerated, but slight photosensitivity was experienced. Doses as low as 5.6 milligram per day of total hypericin

TABLE J.20 ESTIMATED THERAPEUTIC AND LOAEL DOSES FOR EMODIN	
DESCRIPTION	**DOSE (g/day)**
Required dose as scaled from animal antitumor studies	0.33 to 4.9 (average 2.2)
Required cytotoxic dose as determined from pharmacokinetic calculations	2.5
Target dose based on an average from animal antitumor studies and pharmacokinetic calculations	2.4
Minimum required antitumor dose assuming 15-fold synergistic benefits	0.16
Commonly prescribed human dose in noncancerous conditions	0.02
Estimated LOAEL dose	0.81
Tentative dose recommendation for further research	**0.16 to 0.81**
Minimum degree of synergism required	**3-fold potency increase**

TABLE J.21 ESTIMATED THERAPEUTIC AND LOAEL DOSES FOR HYPERICIN	
DESCRIPTION	**DOSE (mg/day)**
Required dose as scaled from animal antitumor studies (photoactivated)	120 to 920 (average 520)
Required cytotoxic dose as determined from pharmacokinetic calculations (nonphotoactivated)	130
Target dose based on range from animal antitumor studies and pharmacokinetic calculations	130 to 520
Minimum required antitumor dose assuming 15-fold synergistic benefits	9 to 35
Commonly prescribed human dose in noncancerous conditions	2.7
Estimated LOAEL dose	5.6 to 11
Tentative dose recommendation for further research	**5.6 to 11**
Minimum degree of synergism required	**uncertain**

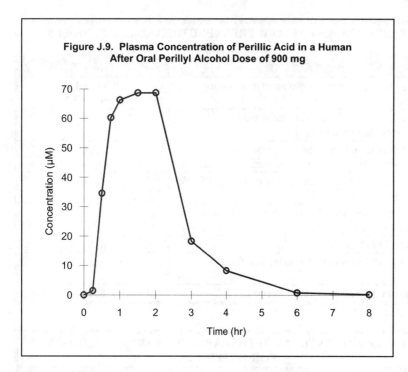

Figure J.9. Plasma Concentration of Perillic Acid in a Human After Oral Perillyl Alcohol Dose of 900 mg

Perillyl alcohol has also been tested in human pharmacokinetic studies. The plasma concentration curve for perillic acid in one human after a 900-milligram dose of perillyl alcohol is shown in Figure J.9 (based on reference 169). The oral clearance derived from this data is about 32 L/hr, a value similar to those from other studies; in a phase I study, the average oral clearance for perillic acid after perillyl alcohol administration was 27 L/hr on day 29. As with the study on limonene, plasma levels were about half as high after repeated administration.[174] On day one, the oral clearance was roughly 11 L/hr, similar to the human oral clearance based on a study in dogs.[170] We use the 27 L/hr value in dose calculations.[b]

Perillic acid inhibits cancer cells in vitro at concentrations of about 520 µM (see Chapter 21). To achieve that average concentration in the plasma, a dose of 124 grams of limonene would be needed every eight hours, or 370 grams per day. The required dose for perillyl alcohol would be 19 grams every eight hours, or 56 grams per day. These doses are prohibitive, but significant amounts of other monoterpenes occur in the plasma after limonene and perillyl alcohol administration, and so lower doses may be effective. When limonene is given orally, the unchanged compound as well as perillyl alcohol and high amounts of dihydroperillic acid and other metabolites are found in the plasma. Indeed, in one study monoterpenes other than perillic acid account for about 71 percent of the total plasma monoterpene concentration after limonene administration.[168] When perillyl alcohol was given, intermediate metabolites such as perillaldehyde occurred in sizable quantities. It is likely that these other monoterpenes and monoterpene metabolites increase the effectiveness of limonene and perillyl alcohol, although to what degree is unknown. One study reported that perillaldehyde is about 2.5-fold more potent than perillyl alcohol, and more than 2.5-fold more potent than perillic acid, in inducing apoptosis in prostate cancer cells.[171]

The doses scaled from animal studies in Chapter 21 suggest that the required limonene dose is about 91 grams per day and the required perillyl alcohol dose is 12 to 24 grams per day. These values are roughly three-

increased photosensitization in sensitive individuals.[166] In a study on HIV-infected patients, a daily oral dose of 35 milligrams was not tolerated.[167] The most common side effect was photosensitivity. Based on all the above, we assume a LOAEL dose of 5.6 to 11 milligrams.[a]

Table J.21 summarizes the therapeutic dose estimates for hypericin from this appendix and Chapter 20.

Chapter 21: Terpenes

Monoterpenes

We first discuss the pharmacokinetics of limonene and perillyl alcohol, then calculate required doses. From these, we estimate the required dose for geraniol.

Based on a phase I trial in which an 18-gram limonene dose was given to humans, the oral clearance for production of perillic acid, the active metabolite of limonene, was 110 L/hr.[168] Plasma concentrations of perillic acid after repeated limonene administrations were about half as high, however, which suggests that treatment induces detoxification enzymes. The oral clearance after repeated administrations was about 220 L/hr, which we use for our calculations.

---

[a] *The TOPKAT model greatly overestimated the LOAEL dose, probably due to the lack of compounds in the model's database that are similar enough to hypericin. The model predicted that the LOAEL dose would be 260 mg/kg in rats. The human equivalent is about 4.2 grams per day.*

[b] *The FOC model predicted an oral clearance of 0.1 L/hr for limonene, 45 L/hr for geraniol, and 51 L/hr for perillyl alcohol, but these values were not based on the production of perillic acid. The prediction for perillic acid itself was 7.7 L/hr, which is lower than the value of 27 L/hr for production of perillic acid from perillyl alcohol, as would be expected.*

to fourfold higher than the doses of 370 and 56 grams per day for limonene and perillyl alcohol calculated above. It is reasonable to assume then that the other monoterpenes in the plasma could account for this three- to fourfold difference.

Doses required for geraniol appear to be lower than those for limonene and perillyl alcohol. As discussed in Chapter 21, geraniol was effective in animal studies at doses of 2.4, 5.8, and 34 grams per day, as scaled to humans. Since the 34-gram dose is much larger than the others, we will assume that the required dose is an average of 2.4 and 5.8 grams, or 4.1 grams.

The maximum tolerated dose of limonene has been investigated in humans; in a phase I study, it was 14 grams per day (8 g/m^2).[168] Dose-limiting toxicities were nausea, vomiting, and diarrhea, all of which were reversible when treatment was discontinued. The LOAEL dose is probably slightly lower than the maximum tolerated dose but greater than 7 grams per day, since one study reported that a limonene dose of 7 grams (100 mg/kg) produced no signs of toxicity in humans.[172]

The maximum tolerated dose of perillyl alcohol has been studied in dogs. In 90- and 28-day studies, it was about 400 and 600 mg/kg per day.[173] The human equivalent of 400 mg/kg is about 18 grams daily. Again, the LOAEL dose is probably slightly lower. In fact, in studies on dogs, the LOAEL dose of perillyl alcohol was about 300 mg/kg per day (about 13 grams per day, scaled to humans).[173] A 13-gram daily dose of perillyl alcohol has been tested in human phase I studies (in three divided doses per day); it was generally well tolerated but did produced mild to moderate gastrointestinal toxicity and fatigue in some patients.[174] (Disease progression was stabilized for six months or more in 4 of the 18 patients who received treatment.) A daily dose of about 9 grams per day was better tolerated. A second phase I study also reported that a dose of 9 to 11 grams was generally well tolerated.[175] Based on these phase I studies, we estimate that the LOAEL dose of perillyl in most patients is about 9 grams per day. At this dose,

only one cancer patient exhibited mild gastrointestinal toxicity.[a]

The animal studies cited in Chapter 21 suggest that geraniol did not cause adverse effects in rodents at a dose equivalent to 34 grams per day in humans; this dose was probably near the maximum tolerated one. Since we do not have actual human or animal LOAEL data for geraniol (or human maximum tolerated dose data), we conservatively estimate that the LOAEL dose is about one-sixth the maximum tolerated rodent dose. (The LOAEL dose for perillyl alcohol was one-third the maximum tolerated rodent dose.) The estimated daily human LOAEL dose for geraniol is then about 5.7 grams.

Table J.22 summarizes the therapeutic dose estimates for monoterpenes from this appendix and Chapter 21.

TABLE J.22 ESTIMATED THERAPEUTIC AND LOAEL DOSES FOR MONOTERPENES			
DESCRIPTION	LIMONENE DOSE (g/day)	PERILLYL ALCOHOL DOSE (g/day)	GERANIOL DOSE (g/day)
Required dose as scaled from animal antitumor studies	91	12 to 24 (average 19)	2.4 to 34 (average 4.1)[*]
Required cytotoxic dose as determined from pharmacokinetic calculations	120[†]	19[†]	uncertain
Target dose based on an average from animal antitumor studies and pharmacokinetic calculations	110	19	4.1
Minimum required antitumor dose assuming 15-fold synergistic benefits	7.3	1.3	0.27
Estimated LOAEL dose	14[‡]	9	5.7
Tentative dose recommendation for further research	**7.3 to 14**	**1.3 to 9**	**0.27 to 5.7**
Minimum degree of synergism required	**7.9-fold potency increase**	**2.1-fold potency increase**	**none**

[*] *The highest of the three available doses was omitted to calculate the average.*
[†] *Assumes that other monoterpenes in the plasma besides perillic acid allow a threefold dose reduction.*
[‡] *Maximum tolerated dose.*

---

[a] *The TOPKAT model predicted a human LOAEL dose of 4.1 grams for perillic acid (as scaled from the rat dose). As mentioned, perillyl alcohol is metabolized to perillic acid in vivo. However, the TOPKAT predictions for limonene and perillyl alcohol itself were greatly underestimated. The model predicted LOAEL doses equivalent to 1.2 grams for limonene and 250 milligrams for perillyl alcohol in humans, respectively. The model was unable to make predictions for geraniol.*

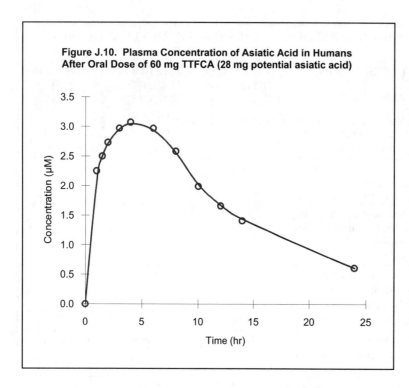

Figure J.10. Plasma Concentration of Asiatic Acid in Humans After Oral Dose of 60 mg TTFCA (28 mg potential asiatic acid)

Centella Triterpenoids

The primary active component of *Centella* triterpenoids is thought to be asiatic acid. (The effects of asiaticoside, a glycoside of asiatic acid, may be mediated through its conversion to asiatic acid in vivo.) The pharmacokinetic parameters of asiatic acid have been studied in humans. The plasma concentration curve after oral administration in one study is shown in Figure J.10 (based on reference 176). Based on data from this study, the oral clearance after a single dose is about 3 L/hr. In another human study, the oral clearance of asiatic acid (and its equivalent dose in asiaticoside) was 20 L/hr.[177] In contrast, the FOC model predicted a higher clearance of 76 L/hr. Because of these differences, we will examine the oral clearance values for other similar compounds.

Asiatic acid is structurally similar to both ursolic acid and boswellic acid. The FOC model predicted clearance values of 29 and 27 L/hr for these compounds. All three compounds are structurally similar to the terpenoid glycyrrhetic acid obtained from licorice. The FOC model predicted an oral clearance of 20 L/hr for this compound, which is reasonably close to the value of 12 L/hr calculated from a human study.[178] In short, we have four similar compounds with more or less similar clearance values predicted by the FOC model and human studies. There are some differences among these values, however, and since few data are available, any attempt to balance these with one another and with their doses

found effective in animal antitumor studies requires a judgment call.

To estimate this balance, we assume that the 76 L/hr value predicted for asiatic acid by the FOC model is overestimated and drop it from further consideration. We can then estimate the oral clearance for asiatic acid as an average of the two human studies discussed above, or 12 L/hr. There are no pharmacokinetic studies for boswellic acid, and the FOC model predicted a clearance of 27 L/hr. Since the FOC model appears to be overestimating the clearance for terpenoid compounds (1.7-fold for glycyrrhetic acid and more for asiatic acid), we take the true clearance to be about half the value predicted. We can estimate then that the oral clearance for boswellic acid is 14 L/hr, which is about equal to our estimate for asiatic acid. Obviously, additional pharmacokinetic studies are needed to determine if these values are accurate, but in the meantime, this method provides a rough estimate.

Assuming that asiatic acid, like the related compound ursolic acid, produces cytotoxic effects in vivo at roughly 15 μM, a dose of 700 milligrams would be needed every eight hours, or 2.1 grams per day. This is similar to and helps confirm the 1.3-gram dose of ursolic and oleanolic acids scaled from mouse antitumor studies in Chapter 21. Human studies suggested that conversion of asiaticoside to asiatic acid is complete.[177] Since TTFCA, the total triterpene fraction of *Centella*, contains about 55 percent asiatic acid (as asiatic acid and asiaticoside), a 2.1 gram dose of asiatic acid would be equal to a TTFCA dose of about 3.8 grams per day. This is about 21-fold higher than the commonly prescribed TTFCA dose of 180 milligrams per day.

Although a 2.1 gram dose of asiatic acid is high and the exact LOAEL dose is uncertain, it is likely to be safe. The TOPKAT model tentatively predicted that the LOAEL dose for asiatic acid would be 460 mg/kg in rats. The human equivalent is about 7.5 grams per day. The TOPKAT model predicted a human LOAEL dose (scaled from rat doses) for boswellic acid of 2.7 grams. Since this is lower, to be conservative we use it as the LOAEL dose for both asiatic and boswellic acid. Therefore, a 2.1-gram dose of asiatic acid is just below the 2.7-gram LOAEL dose.

Table J.23 summarizes the therapeutic dose estimates for asiatic acid in this appendix and Chapter 21.

Boswellic Acid

The pharmacokinetic properties of boswellic acid have not been studied in animals or humans. As discussed above in relation to *Centella* pharmacokinetics, we estimate the oral clearance for boswellic acid is 14 L/hr.

Like asiatic acid, boswellic acid appears to be active in vitro at a concentration of roughly 15 µM. To produce this average plasma concentration, a dose of about 770 milligrams would be needed every eight hours, or 2.3 grams per day. This dose is within the range found effective in animal antitumor studies (0.34 to 2.4 grams daily).

The LOAEL dose predicted by the TOPKAT model is 160 mg/kg in rats. The human equivalent is about 2.7 grams.

Table J.24 summarizes the therapeutic dose estimates for boswellic acid from this appendix and Chapter 21.

Horse Chestnut and Escin

The pharmacokinetics and dose response of escin are perplexing. The bioavailability of escin is low; doses of 50 to 100 milligrams produced a serum concentration of only about 13 nM in healthy subjects. It follows that the oral clearance of escin in humans is high, roughly 300 to 470 L/hr.[179, 180] According to one paper, escin reduces vascular permeability in part by increasing production of prostaglandin F_2, an eicosanoid that causes vessel contraction. This occurs at concentrations of about 4.1 to 9.1 µM in vitro.[181] As discussed in Chapter 21, cytotoxic concentrations are similar (10 µM). Because of the high clearance value and high molecular weight, however, a daily dose of about 100 grams would be required to produce an average plasma concentration of 10 µM. This dose is prohibitive, and it is far higher than the commonly prescribed one of 100 to 150 milligrams per day for treating vascular insufficiency. The high oral clearance value indicates that escin would not be effective in vivo for reducing vascu-

TABLE J.23   ESTIMATED THERAPEUTIC AND LOAEL DOSES FOR ASIATIC ACID

DESCRIPTION	DOSE (g/day)
Required dose as scaled from animal antitumor studies (for oleanolic and ursolic acids)	1.3
Required cytotoxic dose as determined from pharmacokinetic calculations	2.1
Target dose based on an average from animal antitumor studies and pharmacokinetic calculations	1.7
Minimum required antitumor dose assuming 15-fold synergistic benefits	0.11
Commonly prescribed human dose in noncancerous conditions	0.03 to 0.09
Estimated LOAEL dose	2.7
Tentative dose recommendation for further research	**1.7**
Minimum degree of synergism required	**none**

TABLE J.24   ESTIMATED THERAPEUTIC AND LOAEL DOSES FOR BOSWELLIC ACID

DESCRIPTION	DOSE (g/day)
Required dose as scaled from animal antitumor studies	0.34 to 2.4
Required dose as scaled from animal anti-inflammatory studies	0.73 to 3.2
Doses used in human anticancer studies	3.6 to 5.4 as *Boswellia* extract[*]
Required cytotoxic dose as determined from pharmacokinetic calculations	2.3
Target dose based on an average from animal antitumor studies and pharmacokinetic calculations	1.8
Minimum required antitumor dose assuming 15-fold synergistic benefits	0.12
Commonly studied human dose in noncancerous conditions	0.6 (boswellic acid) 0.9 to 1.1 (*Boswellia* extract)
Estimated LOAEL dose	2.7
Tentative dose recommendation for further research	**1.8**
Minimum degree of synergism required	**none**

[*] *The concentration of boswellic acid in the* Boswellia *extracts used is uncertain.*

lar permeability, yet it has been reported effective in placebo-controlled trials (see Chapter 21). The reasons for its effectiveness are uncertain. Perhaps active metabolites of escin are present at higher concentrations than escin itself, or the effect may be due to a very high affinity for vascular tissue or to synergism occurring with other components of horse chestnut extract. To some extent, the latter has been found true. Adding flavonoids that occur naturally in horse chestnut to escin (at a 10:1 ratio) increased escin bioavailability by as

TABLE J.25   ESTIMATED THERAPEUTIC AND LOAEL DOSES FOR ESCIN

DESCRIPTION	DOSE (mg/day)
Required dose as scaled from animal anti-edema studies	150 to 600
Required dose as determined from human anti-inflammatory or anti-edema studies	100 to 150
Required cytotoxic dose as determined from pharmacokinetic calculations	100 grams
Commonly prescribed human dose in noncancerous conditions	100 to 150
Estimated LOAEL dose	150
Tentative dose recommendation for further research	**150**

TABLE J.26   ESTIMATED THERAPEUTIC AND LOAEL DOSES FOR RUSCOGENINS

DESCRIPTION	DOSE (mg/day)
Required cytotoxic dose as determined from pharmacokinetic calculations	1,500[*]
Commonly prescribed human dose in noncancerous conditions	100
Estimated LOAEL dose	130
Tentative dose recommendation for further research	**100 to 130**

[*] *Based on an average clearance value obtained from other simple triterpenoids and saponins.*

much as 50 percent in mice.[182] Still, increased bioavailability alone would not account for the huge difference in dose.

In summary, although issues with pharmacokinetics and dose response are unresolved with respect to vasoprotective concentrations, many animal and human studies have demonstrated that horse chestnut extract is effective in protecting the vascular system and reducing edema. Due to its effects in humans, it is a promising compound for reducing vascular permeability and has the potential to indirectly inhibit cancer progression, but it is unlikely that cytotoxic concentrations could be reached safely in humans after oral administration.

Oral administration of horse chestnut extract is likely to be safe at normal escin doses (100 to 150 milligrams per day), although the risk of adverse effects may increase sharply with larger doses. The oral LD_{50} of sodium beta-escin in mice, rats, and guinea pigs is 134, 400, and 188 mg/kg, respectively (beta-escin is the naturally occurring form).[183] The human equivalents are about 1.3, 6.5, and 3.9 grams, or an average of 3.9 grams. Using the average value and assuming that the LOAEL dose is 13- to 75-fold lower (see Appendix I), the LOAEL dose is likely to be between 52 and 300 mil-

ligrams. The lower portion of this range is well below the normal dose range of 100 to 150 milligrams. Conservatively, we take the LOAEL dose to be 150 milligrams.

Table J.25 summarizes the therapeutic dose estimates for escin in this appendix and Chapter 21.

Butcher's Broom

Ruscogenins, the active saponins in butcher's broom, are considered as indirect-acting compound here, rather than as cytotoxic ones. Nonetheless, there is the possibility that ruscogenins may induce direct cytotoxic effects. Pharmacokinetic studies of ruscogenins in animals or humans are not available, although one source briefly mentions that they are absorbed after oral administration.[184] We can, however, estimate their oral clearance based on that of the other simple triterpenoids and saponins discussed here. The estimated oral clearance values for asiatic acid, boswellic acid, and ginseng metabolites (see below) range from 3.6 to 14 L/hr; we use the average of 9.9 L/hr as an estimate for ruscogenins. (The clearance for escin is not used in making this average, since escin is a more complex saponin.)

As discussed in Chapter 21, ruscogenins may be active in vitro at about 4 μM. This value is from only one study, however, and therefore we assume that ruscogenins, like most other compounds, are active at 15 μM. To produce this average concentration in the plasma would require a dose of about 510 milligrams every eight hours, or 1.5 grams per day, which is about 15-fold higher than the commonly prescribed dose of up to 100 milligrams daily for noncancerous conditions.[185]

It is uncertain whether a dose of 1.5 grams would be safe for long-term use. Although no toxicity studies have been conducted on ruscogenins, the TOPKAT model predicted a LOAEL dose of 7.8 mg/kg in rats. The human equivalent is about 130 milligrams per day. If the maximum safe dose is 130 milligrams, synergistic interactions would need to produce about a 12-fold increase in potency. As discussed in Chapter 21, a 12-fold increase is theoretically possible, but the 1.5-gram target dose is based on very limited pharmacokinetic and in-vitro data; therefore, while direct effects may be possible in synergistic combinations, it is best at this stage to think of ruscogenins as indirect-acting compounds.

Table J.26 summarizes the therapeutic dose estimates for ruscogenins from this appendix and Chapter 21.

Ginseng

Ginseng is characterized in this book as an immune stimulant, but it could also directly inhibit cancer cells. The pharmacokinetic properties of ginseng saponins have been investigated in mice.[186] Since M1 appears to be the active metabolite, we focus on its properties. The plasma concentration curve for M1 in mice after an oral dose of ginsenoside Rb_1 is shown in Figure J.11 (based on reference 187).

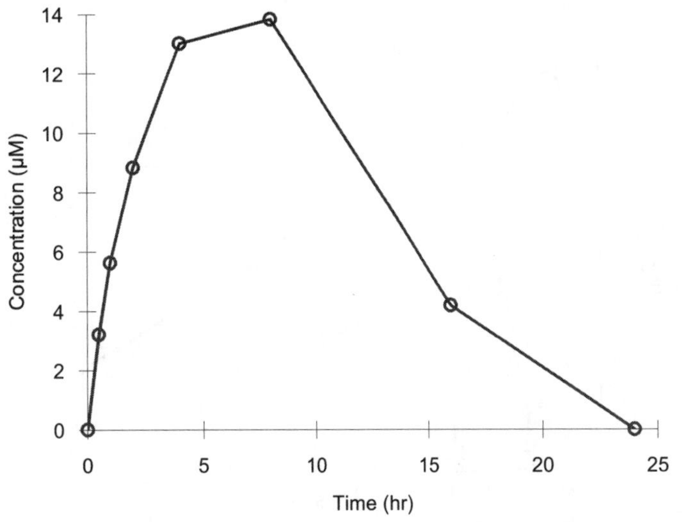

Using the data in this figure, the human oral clearance of M1 after ginseng saponin administration is about 3.6 L/hr. From the discussions in Chapter 21, we estimate M1 is active in vivo at 25 µM and all ginsenosides produce M1 equally. To achieve an average plasma concentration of 25 µM, a ginsenoside dose of 610 milligrams would be required every eight hours, or 1.8 grams per day. This is equal to about 47 grams per day of root, which is greater than the commonly prescribed daily dose of 3 to 9 grams. It is also greater than the human dose of 3.2 to 16 grams of root as scaled from rodent experiments (see Chapter 21). Due to the inconsistencies, the required target dose can be estimated only within a large range, 3.2 to 47 grams per day.

A daily dose of 48 grams would probably cause adverse effects. In Chinese herbal medicine, up to 30 grams per day is sometimes used, but only in acute situations such as hemorrhagic shock.[188] The LOAEL dose of ginseng or its ginsenosides is uncertain. In one study in mice, the intraperitoneal LD_{50} for ginsenosides was 910 mg/kg. The equivalent human oral dose is about 16 grams per day. If we assume the LOAEL dose is 13 to 75-fold lower than the LD_{50} (see Appendix I), then the oral LOAEL dose of ginsenosides in humans would be between 210

Figure J.11. Plasma Concentration of M1 in Mice After Oral Dose of 80 mg/kg Rb1

milligrams and 1.2 grams, or about 5.5 to 32 grams of root. The commonly prescribed dose of 9 grams of root falls within this range. To be conservative, we presume that the LOAEL dose is 9 grams of root per day, or 340 milligrams of ginsenosides.

Table J.27 summarizes the therapeutic dose estimates for ginseng in this appendix and Chapter 21.

TABLE J.27 ESTIMATED THERAPEUTIC AND LOAEL DOSES FOR GINSENG		
DESCRIPTION	**GINSENOSIDE DOSE (mg/day)**	**GINSENG ROOT DOSE (g/day)**
Required dose as scaled from animal antitumor studies	120 to 610	3.2 to 16
Required cytotoxic dose as determined from pharmacokinetic calculations	1,800	47
Target dose based on range from animal antitumor studies and pharmacokinetic calculations	120 to 1,800	3.2 to 47
Minimum required antitumor dose assuming 15-fold synergistic benefits	8 to 120	0.21 to 3.1
Commonly prescribed human dose in noncancerous conditions	110 to 340	3 to 9
Estimated LOAEL dose	340	9
Tentative dose recommendation for further research	**110 to 340**	**3 to 9**
Minimum degree of synergism required for direct inhibition of cancer	**uncertain**	

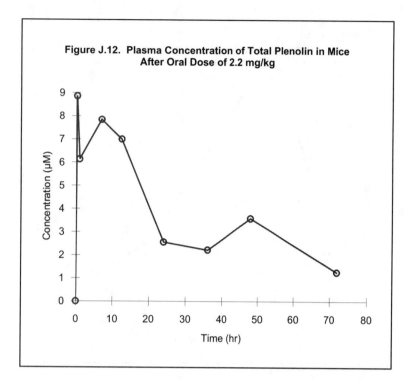

Figure J.12. Plasma Concentration of Total Plenolin in Mice After Oral Dose of 2.2 mg/kg

Parthenolide

The pharmacokinetic properties of parthenolide have not been investigated in rodents or humans, but those for a similar sesquiterpene lactone, plenolin, have been in mice (see Figure J.12).[189, a] Plenolin is a synthetic analog of helenalin, a sesquiterpene lactone isolated from the *Helenium* species. Like the *Tanacetum* species (feverfew, *Tanacetum parthenium*), the *Helenium* species is also a member of the Compositae family. The study in mice was done with radiolabeled plenolin, and therefore it can be expected to generate minimum values for oral clearance. The estimated human oral clearance based on this study is 0.16 L/hr. If the clearance were 7.5-fold higher, as suggested by the average value in Table J.2, it would be 1.2 L/hr.

The FOC model predicted an oral clearance of 1.9 L/h for parthenolide, which would seem reasonable given the data from the radiolabeled study. The model also predicted similar values (5.1 and 6 L/hr) for two other sesquiterpene lactones, helenalin and artemisinin. Helenalin was mentioned above and artemisinin in Chapter 21.

Although the FOC model predicted a clearance for artemisinin of 6 L/hr, the oral clearances calculated from three different human studies on artemisinin were 500, 310, and 430 L/hr (average 410 L/hr).[190, 191, 192] The

meaning of these large differences is unclear, and the implications for estimating parthenolide clearance are uncertain. One might think that the oral clearance for parthenolide and other sesquiterpene lactones could also be as high as 410 L/hr, since their structures are similar to artemisinin. However, based on the small dose of parthenolide that is apparently effective in noncancerous conditions, as well as the radiolabeled data on plenolin and the magnitude of sesquiterpene lactone doses used in rodent antitumor studies, it seems that a clearance value of 1.9 L/hr for parthenolide is more reasonable than one of 410 L/hr. Therefore, we assume the FOC model is accurate for parthenolide and that the oral clearance is 1.9 L/hr.

Parthenolide is active in vitro at concentrations of roughly 5 µM (see Chapter 21). To produce this concentration in plasma, a dose of 19 milligrams every eight hours would be required, or 57 milligrams per day. This is similar to the dose of 96 milligrams per day scaled from the mouse antitumor study mentioned in Chapter 21; however, 57 milligrams per day is about 10-fold greater than the oral doses of up to 5.8 milligrams recommended by some manufacturers for noncancerous conditions. It is also higher than the 0.54-milligram doses used in successful studies on migraine patients.[193]

The LOAEL dose of parthenolide is uncertain. The TOPKAT model predicted that the rat LOAEL dose would be 12 mg/kg per day. The human equivalent would be about 190 milligrams per day. Although this dose may be correct, it is large compared to the commonly prescribed dose of 0.54 to 5.8 milligrams. Because it is so large and there are no animal LOAEL dose studies to back it up, we also estimate a LOAEL dose based on the LD50.

The TOPKAT model predicted that the rat LD50 for parthenolide would be 5 g/kg, or 81 grams as scaled to humans. This estimate is high compared with TOPKAT predictions and animal studies on related compounds. The model predicted that the LD50 for helenalin would be 130 mg/kg, or 2.1 grams as scaled to humans. In addition, the intraperitoneal LD50s of helenalin and plenolin have been reported to be about 43 and 100 mg/kg in mice, respectively.[194] The equivalent human oral doses are about 0.58 and 1.3 grams. The average of these three values (2.1, 0.58, and 1.3 grams per day) is 1.3 grams. If we assume that the human LD50 for parthenolide is 1.3 grams per day, and if the LOAEL dose is 13- to 75-fold lower than the LD50, then the LOAEL dose is

---

[a] *Calculations based on this study assumed a plasma volume of 1.2 milliliters in mice.*

17 to 100 milligrams. Conservatively, we take the LOAEL dose to be 17 milligrams per day.

Table J.28 summarizes the therapeutic dose estimates for parthenolide from this appendix and Chapter 21.

Chapter 22: Lipid-Soluble Vitamins

Vitamin A

Transport and Metabolism of Vitamin A

Because the metabolism, transport, and mode of action of vitamin A differ from most other natural compounds discussed in this book, it is worthwhile to discuss these aspects in more detail.

Most natural compounds affect cancer cells by altering events at the plasma membrane or in the cytoplasm. In contrast, ATRA travels directly to the nucleus and affects gene transcription. The effects of ATRA are mediated through its ability to bind to retinoid receptors in the nucleus. These receptors are the retinoic acid receptor (RAR) and the retinoid X receptor (RXR); both belong to the superfamily of steroid and hormone receptors and function as transcription factors (much like NF-κb) to regulate the expression of various genes.[195]

The transportation and metabolism of retinol in vivo is illustrated in Figure J.13 (adapted from references 196 and 197). Upon absorption, retinyl esters are incorporated, along with other fatty substances such as triglycerides and cholesterol, into a group of fatty substances called chylomicrons. These, in turn, are transported into the general blood circulation via the lymphatic system. Once in the circulation, chylomicron remnants can be absorbed by the liver and by other tissues. In many tissues, the uptake of chylomicron remnants is mediated by the low-density lipoprotein (LDL) receptor.

The liver is the primary metabolism and storage organ for vitamin A. When the need arises, some of the retinyl esters stored there are metabolized to retinol or retinoic acid compounds such as ATRA. Retinol, after binding with retinol-binding protein, enters the circulation, where it can be used by other tissues. ATRA also binds to a transport protein and enters the circulation, but its plasma concentration is generally less than 1 percent of that of retinol.[198] The liver maintains steady plasma concentrations of retinol and ATRA; these concentra-

| TABLE J.28   ESTIMATED THERAPEUTIC AND LOAEL DOSES FOR PARTHENOLIDE ||
DESCRIPTION	DOSE (mg/day)
Required dose as scaled from animal antitumor studies	96
Required cytotoxic dose as determined from pharmacokinetic calculations	57
Target dose based on an average from animal antitumor studies and pharmacokinetic calculations	77
Minimum required antitumor dose assuming 15-fold synergistic benefits	5.1
Commonly prescribed human dose in noncancerous conditions	0.54 to 5.8
Estimated LOAEL dose	17
Tentative dose recommendation for further research	**17**
Minimum degree of synergism required	**4.5-fold potency increase**

tions rise only slightly following ingestion of a meal or supplements containing retinol or retinyl esters.

Under normal circumstances, the circulating levels of retinyl esters (in chylomicrons) and retinol and ATRA (bound to proteins) are adequate to affect gene transcription in appropriate tissues. The word *appropriate* is key here, since tissues vary in their sensitivity to vitamin A. Whether a tissue is influenced depends on the extent of vitamin A uptake by the cell, the extent of vitamin A metabolism within the cell, and the expression of retinoic acid receptors (RAR and RXR) in the cell's nucleus. These three factors form a regulatory system to ensure the correct tissues are affected by vitamin A at the correct time and that its toxic effects do not manifest.

To understand how retinol might be used therapeutically, the uptake and metabolism of vitamin A and the expression of nuclear receptors demand more explanation. Cells can uptake each of the three circulating forms of vitamin A (retinyl esters, retinol, and ATRA or other retinoic acids), but some cells have an affinity for specific forms. For example, chylomicron uptake in some cells is mediated by the LDL receptor, as mentioned above, and cells vary in their expression of this receptor. Regardless of the specific uptake mechanism, about 25 percent of postmeal retinol is cleared from the circulation by tissues other than the liver.[199] Human leukocytes, fat cells, muscle cells, and bone marrow cells are all capable of taking up retinyl esters from chylomicrons.[200–203] Similarly, the uptake of retinol and ATRA from the circulation can also vary. Among other things, retinol and ATRA uptake depends on the expression of certain cellular proteins called cellular retinol-binding proteins (CRBP) and cellular retinoic acid-binding proteins (CRABP).[197] As the names imply,

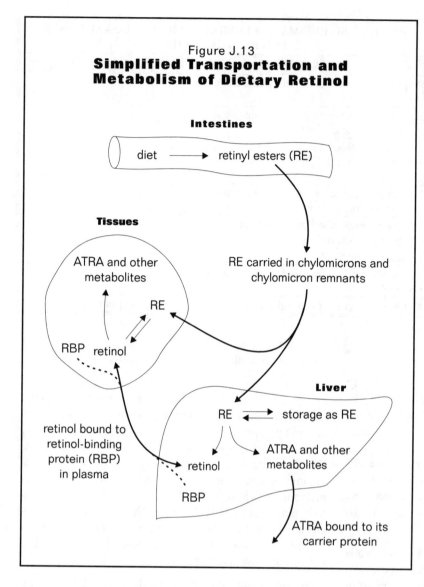

Figure J.13
Simplified Transportation and Metabolism of Dietary Retinol

Intestines

diet ⟶ retinyl esters (RE)

Tissues

ATRA and other metabolites

RE carried in chylomicrons and chylomicron remnants

RE

RBP retinol

retinol bound to retinol-binding protein (RBP) in plasma

Liver

RE ⇌ storage as RE

retinol

ATRA and other metabolites

RBP

ATRA bound to its carrier protein

We can see from the above that the uptake and sensitivity of normal cells to vitamin A can vary depending on a number of factors, such as the presence of LDL receptors, cellular binding proteins, enzymes needed for retinol metabolism, and nuclear receptors.[198, 208, 209] The same is true for cancer cells.[210–214] In fact, it has been postulated that the development of some cancers like breast cancer may be associated with defects in CRBP expression.[215] Such defects would reduce the ability of vitamin A to perform its normal role in controlling cell proliferation. In addition, defects in nuclear receptor expression are associated with the development of promyelocytic leukemia.[216] Thus the effectiveness of retinol or ATRA administration in cancer treatment can be expected to vary depending on the characteristics of the cell line.

Pharmacokinetics of Vitamin A

The pharmacokinetic parameters of retinol, retinyl esters, and ATRA have been investigated in humans, all after retinyl ester administration. Clearance calculations from these studies are summarized in Table J.29. As seen, common clearance values for retinol, retinyl esters, and ATRA are 45, 4.6, and 730 L/hr. In some studies, however, oral administration of retinyl esters did not increase ATRA concentrations. Note that although clearance values for retinol are relatively low, its toxicity is high. Toxic doses (2,700,000 I.U.) of retinyl esters would be required to raise the plasma retinol concentration by even 3 µM, for example. Other human studies indicated that oral administration of 300,000 I.U. of retinyl esters increased average retinol plasma concentrations only by about 20 percent.[217] Thus retinol concentrations are unlikely to change appreciably with retinyl ester (or retinol) administration.

Although we do not discuss ATRA as a treatment agent, we still examine its pharmacokinetics and its commonly used clinical dose. The results allow us to estimate a target in-vivo concentration of ATRA for use with retinyl ester administration.

Clearance of ATRA after its oral administration has been investigated in humans. Studies indicate that its pharmacokinetic properties are highly variable among subjects and change with increasing exposure. As with

these proteins bind retinol and retinoic acid within the cell.

Once in the cell, ATRA is able to directly affect nuclear receptors; however, retinol, the predominant form of vitamin A, must first be metabolized to ATRA. The ability of cells to form ATRA from retinol varies according to a number of factors, which include the amount of CRBP and CRABP within the cell and the presence of needed cellular enzymes.

Once adequate intracellular ATRA concentrations are available, gene transcription can be affected if sufficient amounts of RAR and RXR nuclear receptors are present. Cells vary in their expression of these nuclear factors. In some studies, exposure of normal, precancerous, and cancer cell lines to high concentrations of retinoids upregulated the expression of retinoid nuclear receptors.[204–207] vitamin C, asiatic acid, and possibly many other compounds discussed in this book, prolonged administration induces detoxification enzymes, increases excretion, or both, resulting in lower plasma concentrations. In four studies, the mean oral clearance values for ATRA after its administration were 88, 110, 330, and 750 L/hr (an overall average 320 L/hr).[218–221, a]

In-vitro studies indicate that the IC_{50} of ATRA for inducing differentiation or inhibiting proliferation occurs over a wide range of concentrations, roughly 0.01 to 10 μM depending on the cell line and conditions (see Chapter 22 and Appendix D). The average ATRA dose in clinical studies is roughly 300 to 400 milligrams per day.[218, 219] If the oral clearance is about 320 L/hr as estimated above, from Equation J.3 we can estimate that the average ATRA plasma concentration over a 24-hour period would be about 0.15 μM. Normal plasma levels of ATRA are approximately 4 to 12 nM, or about 19-fold lower than 0.15 μM.[226, 227] An average concentration of 0.15 μM is within the effective range of 0.01 to 10 μM given above and will be used as a target in-vivo concentration. Of course, the selection of this target value is somewhat arbitrary, given the large range of possibilities.

We have determined that the oral clearance of ATRA after oral administration of retinyl esters is about 730 L/hr and that a reasonable in-vivo target concentration is 0.15 μM. Based on these values, a retinal ester dose of 540,000 I.U. would be required every eight hours, or 1,600,000 I.U. per day, to produce cytotoxic concentrations of ATRA in the plasma, but this dose is prohibitive.

We know from in-vitro studies that the IC_{50} of retinyl esters for inhibition of proliferation is about 10 μM (see

TABLE J.29 ORAL CLEARANCE VALUES FOR RETINOIDS AFTER ADMINISTRATION OF RETINYL ESTERS			
DOSE (I.U.)	COMPOUND MEASURED	CLEARANCE (L/Hr)	REFERENCES
Retinol Clearance			
150,000	retinol	24	222
440,000	retinol	65	
Average retinol clearance		45	—
Retinyl Ester Clearance			
150,000	retinyl palmitate	4.8	222
440,000	retinyl palmitate	7.9	
50,000/meter sq.[*]	retinyl esters	1.4	203
100,000	retinyl esters	5.8	223
130,000	retinyl esters	3.2[†]	224
Average retinyl ester clearance		4.6	—
ATRA Clearance			
5,000, 10,000, and 25,000[‡]	ATRA	incalculable[§]	225
150,000	ATRA	580	222
440,000	ATRA	880	
Average ATRA clearance		730[‖]	—

[*] *Dose given to children.*

[†] *Reported as retinol but more likely to be retinyl esters.*

[‡] *Type of ester was not specified. Retinyl palmitate was administered in all other studies.*

[§] *These doses did not produce a change in the area under the curve (AUC).*

[‖] *Omits incalculable values in calculation of average.*

Chapter 22). If the clearance of retinyl esters after their oral administration is 4.6 L/hr (see Table J.29), then a retinyl ester dose of 250,000 I.U. would be required every eight hours, or 740,000 I.U. per day.[b] This is also prohibitive.

We can conclude from the above that orally administered retinyl esters are unlikely to produce cytotoxic concentrations of retinyl esters or ATRA in the plasma, since the doses required would be prohibitive. Thus retinyl esters may be most effective when used in synergistic combinations with other compounds. We can also conclude that after dosing with retinyl esters, the greatest cytotoxic effect is likely to come from elevated retinyl ester plasma concentrations, rather than elevated ATRA ones. However, this conclusion is based on a somewhat arbitrary choice for an effective in-vivo concentration for ATRA (0.15 μM), and it is therefore suspect. Retinol plasma concentrations would likely

---

[a] *The FOC model predicted an oral clearance for ATRA of 2,100 L/hr, which is on average 6.6-fold higher than the values obtained from human studies.*

[b] *One I.U. is equal to 0.3 micrograms of retinol, 0.344 μg of retinyl acetate, and 0.550 μg of retinyl palmitate. Retinyl esters in the plasma and supplements tend to be primarily retinyl palmitate. We use a value of 0.49 μg per I.U. here for mixed retinyl esters.*

TABLE J.30   ESTIMATED THERAPEUTIC AND LOAEL DOSES FOR RETINYL ESTERS

DESCRIPTION	DOSE (I.U./day)
Required dose based on human anticancer studies	16,000 to 270,000 (average of 140,000)
Required cytotoxic dose as determined from pharmacokinetic calculations	740,000
Target dose based on range from human and animal studies and pharmacokinetic calculations	140,000 to 740,000
Minimum required antitumor dose assuming 15-fold synergistic benefits	9,300 to 49,000
Commonly prescribed human dose in noncancerous conditions	2,500 to 5,000
Estimated maximum tolerated dose	50,000 to 600,000
Tentative dose recommendation for further research	**50,000 to 600,000**
Minimum degree of synergism required	**uncertain**

produce the weakest cytotoxic effect. The retinyl ester dose needed to generate a cytotoxic concentration of retinol (about 7 μM, or a change of about 5 μM from baseline) would be about 3,200,000 I.U. per day. This dose is far higher than that for producing cytotoxic concentrations of retinyl esters (740,000 I.U. per day) or ATRA (1,600,000 I.U. per day).

Assuming that cytotoxicity will be caused by retinyl esters in the plasma rather than ATRA or retinol, the target dose for retinyl esters is about 740,000 I.U. per day, as calculated above. This dose, however, is not in close agreement with the average retinyl ester dose of 140,000 I.U. scaled from human studies in Chapter 22. Due to the inconsistencies, the required target dose of retinyl esters can be estimated only within a large range, 140,000 to 740,000 I.U. per day.

Based on a phase I study, the maximum tolerated dose of retinol (apparently as retinol itself) is about 360,000 I.U. per day (200,000 I.U. per square meter).[228] Adverse effects were reversible when it was discontinued. In sensitive patients, the adverse effects included dry skin, increased triglycerides, neuropsychiatric symptoms, headache, hepatomegaly, and lesions on the lips. Other studies indicated that adults can generally tolerate 300,000 to 600,000 I.U. of retinyl esters for several months with no toxicity symptoms.[a] In some studies, 300,000 I.U. of retinyl esters were safe for periods of up to two years, but daily intake as low as 50,000 I.U. was toxic in some individuals if taken for more than 18 months.[195] We assume here that the maximum tolerated

dose of retinyl esters is 50,000 to 600,000 I.U. per day. This wide range reflects the differing sensitivities of patients to vitamin A.

For general health purposes, retinyl ester doses of 5,000 I.U. per day for men and 2,500 I.U. per day for women (excepting pregnant women) are reasonable.[229] In 2,297 healthy subjects, administration of 2,500 I.U. of retinyl esters for periods greater than three years produced no severe adverse effects but may have had a minor impact on the liver.[230] In a study on 146 healthy subjects, no adverse effects were noted at doses of 1,800 I.U. per day for periods up to 12 years.[231]

While oral administration of ATRA itself is generally well tolerated by most patients, serious adverse effects may be encountered in some. Common side effects include dry skin, dry lips, skin rash, headache, and nasal stuffiness. A severe retinoic acid syndrome may be produced in 25 percent of cases at high doses, which can be reversed by corticosteroid administration. An increase in white blood cell count occurs in 30 percent of cases and requires management with chemotherapy or corticosteroids. Based on phase I trials, the maximum tolerated dose of ATRA is about 270 milligrams per day (150 mg/m²). The dose limiting toxicities are usually skin reactions, such as erythema. Other toxicities can include headache, nausea, vomiting, as well as alterations in liver enzyme levels.[232, 233]

Table J.30 summarizes the therapeutic dose estimates for retinyl esters in this appendix and Chapter 22.

Melatonin

The pharmacokinetic properties of melatonin after oral administration have been studied in humans. Figure J.14 illustrates the plasma concentration curve after oral administration of 100 milligrams (based on reference 234). The oral clearance based on this study is 560 L/hr, which is very similar to the values of 530 and 500 L/hr calculated from two other human studies after a single dose of 3 milligrams and multiple administrations of 50 milligrams every four hours, respectively.[235, 236] We use an average value of 530 L/hr in dose calculations. The peak melatonin concentration after the 3-milligram dose was about 16 nM. This dose is equal to the commonly prescribed one in noncancerous conditions.

Melatonin is active against cancer cells at concentrations between about 0.1 to 1 nM, which is within the

---

[a] *It would be expected that retinyl palmitate would be about 1.8-fold less toxic than retinol due to the difference in their molecular weights (i.e., the palmitate group in retinyl palmitate is not toxic, only the retinol group).*

range of normal peak plasma concentrations. Therefore, administration of melatonin may not be needed to produce cancer inhibition. Nonetheless, as discussed in Chapter 22, melatonin administration may increase the chance of producing anticancer effects. Human anticancer studies commonly used melatonin doses of 10 to 20 milligrams per day. Based on the data above, it is likely that a 10-milligram dose would produce a peak concentration of about 53 nM and an average nighttime concentration of about 14 nM. This 14-nM value is reasonably close to the 1-nM concentration found optimally effective in in-vitro studies, which suggests that cytotoxic effects may be occurring in vivo at this dose (concentrations of 100 nM or higher appear to be less effective than concentrations of 1 nM).

The antioxidant effects of melatonin are perplexing. As discussed in Chapter 23, doses of about 20 to 50 milligrams, scaled to humans, produced antioxidant effects in animals. A 50-milligram dose would increase the average nighttime plasma concentration to about 70 nM; however, the antioxidant effects of melatonin are only seen in vitro at very high concentrations, between about 20 and 100 μM.[237] A daily dose of about 15 grams would be needed to produce an average nighttime plasma concentration of 20 μM. Thus the antioxidant effects produced in vivo at small doses are not explained by those seen in vitro. The animal studies suggested that much smaller concentrations (about 28 to 70 nM) may produce antioxidant effects in vivo.

The LOAEL dose for melatonin is uncertain. One recent paper has reported that doses of 10 milligrams per day for 28 to 40 days did not cause adverse effects in healthy subjects.[238] Two reviews of the toxicology of melatonin have also been published, but unfortunately they did not give a LOAEL dose, since the amount of information available is still insufficient.[239, 240] Although no major adverse effects have been reported in any of the literature, even at high doses, minor and transient ones include sleepiness, nightmares, hypotension, sleep disorders, fever, headache, hyperglycemia, dizziness, and other effects. Based on the available information, it appears that doses of 10 milligrams or less are

Figure J.14. Plasma Concentration of Melatonin in Humans After Oral Dose of 100 mg

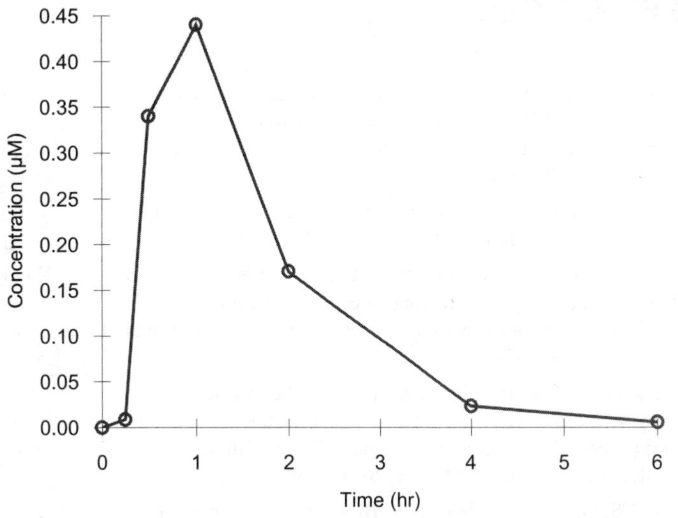

TABLE J.31   ESTIMATED THERAPEUTIC AND LOAEL DOSES FOR MELATONIN

DESCRIPTION	DOSE (mg/day)
Required dose as scaled from animal antitumor studies	commonly 10 to 50
Doses used in human anticancer studies	10 to 50 (commonly 10 to 20)
Required cytotoxic dose as determined from pharmacokinetic calculations	0 to 10
Target dose based on human studies and pharmacokinetic calculations	0 to 20
Minimum required antitumor dose assuming 15-fold synergistic benefits	0.67 to 1.3
Commonly prescribed human dose in noncancerous conditions	3
Estimated LOAEL dose	10 to 50
Tentative dose recommendation for further research	**3 to 20**
Minimum degree of synergism required	**none**

safe in most individuals. The human cancer studies discussed in Chapter 22 suggested that doses of 10 to 50 milligrams were safe. Clearly, more study is required to define the toxicology of melatonin. Lacking additional information, we estimate the LOAEL dose to be between 10 and 50 milligrams per day.

Table J.31 summarizes the therapeutic dose estimates for melatonin in this appendix and Chapter 22. The maximum tentative recommended dose was chosen to be no more than 20 milligrams, since this is the maximum dose used in most human studies.

REFERENCES

1. Fontana RJ, deVries TM, Woolf TF, et al. Caffeine based measures of CYP1A2 activity correlate with oral clearance of tacrine in patients with Alzheimer's disease. Br J Clin Pharmacol 1998 Sep; 46(3):221–8.

2. Berg G, Jonsson KA, Hammar M, et al. Variable bioavailability of papaverine. Pharmacol Toxicol 1988 May; 62(5):308–10.

3. Slevin ML, Joel SP, Whomsley R, et al. The effect of dose on the bioavailability of oral etoposide: Confirmation of a clinically relevant observation. Cancer Chemother Pharmacol 1989; 24(5):329–31.

4. Nakagawa K, Okuda S, Miyazawa T. Dose-dependent incorporation of tea catechins, (-)-epigallocatechin-3-gallate and (-)-epigallocatechin, into human plasma. Biosci Biotechnol Biochem 1997 Dec; 61(12):1981–5.

5. Yang CS, Chen L, Lee MJ, et al. Blood and urine levels of tea catechins after ingestion of different amounts of green tea by human volunteers. Cancer Epidemiol Biomarkers Prev 1998 Apr; 7(4):351–4.

6. Blanchard J, Tozer TN, Rowland M. Pharmacokinetic perspectives on megadoses of ascorbic acid. Am J Clin Nutr 1997 Nov; 66(5):1165–71.

7. Kleine MW, Stauder GM, Gebauer F, et al. Kinetics of proteolytic enzyme activity of serum in a controlled randomized double blind study. 2nd International Congress on Biological Response Modifiers, San Diego, California, USA, Jan 29–31, 1993.

8. Lehmann PV, et al. Beeinflussung der autoimmunen T-cell-antwort durch hydrolytische enzyme. In *Systemisch enzymtherapie. aktueller stand und fortschritte.* Wrba H, Kleine MW, Miehlke K, et al., eds. München, Germany: MMW Medizin Verlag, 1996.

9. Maehder K, Weigelt O. Die Bestimmung der proteolytischen und fibrinolytischen Aktivität auf Blut- und Hämoglobin-Agarplatten. Ar-zneimittel-Forsch 1972; 22:116–117.

10. Biber A, Fischer H, Romer A, Chatterjee SS. Oral bioavailability of hyperforin from hypericum extracts in rats and human volunteers. Pharmacopsychiatry 1998; 31(Suppl 1):36–43.

11. Setchell KD. Absorption and metabolism of soy isoflavones-from food to dietary supplements and adults to infants. J Nutr 2000 Mar; 130(3):654S-5S.

12. Ader P, Wessmann A, Wolffram S. Bioavailability and metabolism of the flavonol quercetin in the pig. Free Radic Biol Med 2000 Apr 1; 28(7):1056–67.

13. Adachi Y, Okazaki M, Ohno N, et al. Enhancement of cytokine production by macrophages stimulated with (1-->3)-beta-D-glucan, grifolan (GRN), isolated from Grifola frondosa. Biol Pharm Bull 1994 Dec; 17(12):1554–60.

14. Xiang DB, Li XY. Effects of Achyranthes bidentata polysaccharides on interleukin-1 and tumor necrosis factor-alpha production from mouse peritoneal macrophages. Chung Kuo Yao Li Hsueh Pao 1993 Jul; 14(4):332–6.

15. Noguchi K, Tanimura H, Yamaue H, et al. Polysaccharide preparation PSK augments the proliferation and cytotoxicity of tumor-infiltrating lymphocytes in vitro. Anticancer Res 1995; 15(2):255–8.

16. Wang SY, Hsu ML, Hsu HC, et al. The anti-tumor effect of Ganoderma lucidum is mediated by cytokines released from activated macrophages and T lymphocytes. Int J Cancer 1997 Mar 17; 70(6):699–705.

17. Sugimachi K, Maehara Y, Kusumoto T, et al. In vitro reactivity to a protein-bound polysaccharide PSK of peripheral blood lymphocytes from patients with gastrointestinal cancer. Anticancer Res 1995 Sep–Oct; 15(5B):2175–9.

18. Conte A, de Bernardi M, Palmieri L, et al. Metabolic fate of exogenous chondroitin sulfate in man. Arzneimittelforschung 1991; 41(7):768–72.

19. Sasaki T, Takasuka N, Chihara G, Maeda YY. Antitumor activity of degraded products of lentinan: Its correlation with molecular weight. Gann 1976 Apr; 67(2):191–5.

20. Yagi A, Nakamori J, Yamada T, et al. In vivo metabolism of aloemannan. Planta Med 1999 Jun; 65(5):417–20.

21. Ikuzawa M, Matsunaga K, Nishiyama S, et al. Fate and distribution of an antitumor protein-bound polysaccharide PSK (Krestin). Int. J Immunopharmac 1988; 10(4):415–423.

22. Lachmann G, Lorenz D, Radeck W, Steiper M. [The pharmacokinetics of the S35 labeled labeled garlic constituents alliin, allicin and vinyldithiine.] Arzneimittelforschung 1994 Jun; 44(6):734–43.

23. Egen-Schwind C, Eckard R, Kemper FH. Metabolism of garlic constituents in the isolated perfused rat liver. Planta Med 1992 Aug; 58(4):301–5.

24. Kleijnen J, Knipschild P, ter Riet G. Garlic, onions and cardiovascular risk factors. A review of the evidence from human experiments with emphasis on commercially available preparations. Br J Clin Pharmacol 1989 Nov; 28(5):535–44.

25. Bensky D, Gamble A. Chinese herbal medicine materia medica. Seattle: Eastland Press, 1993, pp. 441–2.

26. Alnaqeeb MA, Thomson M, Bordia T, Ali M. Histopathological effects of garlic on liver and lung of rats. Toxicology Letters 1996; 85(3):157–164.

27. Fehri B, Aiache JM, Korbi S, et al. Toxic effects induced by repeated administrations of Allium sativm L. aqueous extract. J. Pharm Belg 1991; 46:363–374.

28. Piskula MK, Yamakoshi J, Iwai Y. Daidzein and genistein but not their glucosides are absorbed from the rat stomach. FEBS letters 1999; 447:287–291.

29. Hollman PC, de Vries JH, van Leeuwen SD, et al. Absorption of dietary quercetin glycosides and quercetin in healthy ileostomy volunteers. Am J Clin Nutr 1995; 62:1276–82.

30. Hollman PCH, van Trijp JMP, Mengelers MJB, et al. Bioavailability of the dietary antioxidant quercetin in man. Cancer Letters 1997; 114:139–140.

31. King RA, Broadbent JL, Head RJ. Absorption and excretion of the soy isoflavone genistein in rats. J Nutr 1996 Jan; 126(1):176–82.

32. Bingham SA, Atkinson C, Liggins J, et al. Phyto-oestrogens: Where are we now? Br J Nutrition 1998; 79:393–406.

[33] Pietta PG, Gardana C, Mauri PL. Identification of Gingko biloba flavonol metabolites after oral administration to humans. J Chromatogr B Biomed Appl 1997 May 23; 693(1):249–55.

[34] Griffiths LA, Smith GE. Metabolism of apigenin and related compounds in the rat. Metabolite formation in vivo and by the intestinal microflora in vitro. Biochem J 1972 Jul; 128(4):901–11.

[35] Liebich HM, Forst C. Basic profiles of organic acids in urine. J Chromatogr 1990; 525(1):1–14.

[36] Wojcicki J, Gawronska-Szklarz B, Bieganowski W, et al. Comparative pharmacokinetics and bioavailability of flavonoid glycosides of Ginkgo biloba after a single oral administration of three formulations to healthy volunteers. Mater Med Pol 1995 Oct–Dec; 27(4):141–6.

[37] Da Silva EL, Piskula M, Terao J. Enhancement of antioxidative ability of rat plasma by oral administration of (-)-epicatechin. Free Radic Biol Med 1998 May; 24(7–8):1209–16.

[38] Okushio K, Suzuki M, Matsumoto N, et al. Identification of (-)-epicatechin metabolites and their metabolic fate in the rat. Drug Metab Dispos 1999 Feb; 27(2):309–16.

[39] Piskula MK, Terao J. Accumulation of (-)-epicatechin metabolites in rat plasma after oral administration and distribution of conjugation enzymes in rat tissues. J Nutr 1998 Jul; 128(7):1172–8.

[40] Adlercreutz H, Markkanen H, Watanabe S. Plasma concentrations of phyto-oestrogens in Japanese men. Lancet 1993 Nov 13; 342(8881):1209–10.

[41] Doerge DR, Chang HC, Churchwell MI, Holder CL. Analysis of soy isoflavone conjugation in vitro and in human blood using liquid chromatography-mass spectrometry. Drug Metab Dispos 2000 Mar; 28(3):298–307.

[42] Coldham NG, Sauer MJ. Pharmacokinetics of [(14)C]genistein in the rat: Gender-related differences, potential mechanisms of biological action, and implications for human health. Toxicol Appl Pharmacol 2000 Apr 15; 164(2):206–215.

[43] Hsieh CY, Santell RC, Haslam SZ, Helferich WG. Estrogenic effects of genistein on the growth of estrogen receptor-positive human breast cancer (MCF-7) cells in vitro and in vivo. Cancer Res 1998 Sep 1; 58(17):3833–8.

[44] Crowell JA, Jeffcoat AR, Tyndall LW, Zeisel SH. Clinical phase 1 studies of isoflavones. J Nutr 2000; 130(3):666S.

[45] Shimoi K, Okada H, Furugori M, et al. Intestinal absorption of luteolin and luteolin 7-o-β-glucoside in rats and humans. FEBS Letters 1998; 438:220–224.

[46] da Silva EL, Piskula MK, Yamamoto N, et al. Quercetin metabolites inhibit copper ion-induced lipid peroxidation in rat plasma. FEBS Lett 1998 Jul 3; 430(3):405–8.

[47] Morand C, Crespy V, Manach C, et al. Plasma metabolites of quercetin and their antioxidant properties. Am J Physiol 1998 Jul; 275(1 Pt 2):R212–9.

[48] Manach C, Morand, C, Texier O, et al. Quercetin metabolites in plasma of rats fed diets containing rutin or quercetin. J Nutr 1995; 125:1911–1922.

[49] Noroozi M, Burns J, Crozier A, et al. Prediction of dietary flavonol consumption from fasting plasma concentration or urinary excretion. Eur J Clin Nutr 2000 Feb; 54(2):143–9.

[50] Manach C, Morand C, Crespy V, et al. Quercetin is recovered in human plasma as conjugated derivatives which retain antioxidant properties. FEBS Lett 1998 Apr 24; 426(3):331–6.

[51] Lee MJ, Wang ZY, Li H, et al. Analysis of plasma and urinary tea polyphenols in human subjects. Cancer Epid Biomark Prev 1995; 4:393–399.

[52] Donovan JL, Luthria DL, Stremple P, Waterhouse AL. Analysis of (+)-catechin, (-)-epicatechin and their 3'- and 4'-O-methylated analogs. A comparison of sensitive methods. J Chromatogr B Biomed Sci Appl 1999 Apr 16; 726(1–2):277–83.

[53] Williamson G, Plumb GW, Uda Y, et al. Dietary quercetin glycosides: Antioxidant activity and induction of the anticarcinogenic phase II marker enzyme quinone reductase in Hepalclc7 cells. Carcinogenesis 1996 Nov; 17(11):2385–7.

[54] Manach C, Morand C, Crespy V, et al. Quercetin is recovered in human plasma as conjugated derivatives which retain antioxidant properties. FEBS Letters 1998; 426:331–336.

[55] Adlercreutz H, Fotsis T, Lampe J, et al. Quantitative determination of lignans and isoflavonoids in plasma of omnivorous and vegetarian women by isotope dilution gas chromatography-mass spectrometry. Scand J Clin Lab Invest 1993; 53(Suppl 215):5–18.

[56] Andersson SH, Cronholm T, Sjovall J. Effects of ethanol on conjugated gonadal hormones in plasma of men. Alcohol Alcohol 1987; Suppl 1:529–31.

[57] Myking OL, Digranes O. Conjugated and unconjugated plasma oestrogens in men with chronic alcoholism and in normal men. J Steroid Biochem 1984 Mar; 20(3):799–801.

[58] Townsend PT, Dyer GI, Young O, et al. The absorption and metabolism of oral oestradiol, oestrone, and oestriol. Br J Obst Gyn 1981; 88:846–852.

[59] Barua AB, Duitsman PK, Kostic D, et al. Reduction of serum retinol levels following a single oral dose of all-trans retinoic acid in humans. Int J Vit Nutr Res 1997; 67:423–26.

[60] Barua AB, Batres RO, Olson JA. Characterization of retinyl beta-glucuronide in human blood. Am J Clin Nutr 1989 Aug; 50(2):370–4.

[61] Yamamura Y, Kawakami J, Santa T, et al. Selective high-performance liquid chromatographic method for the determination of glycyrrhizin and glycyrrhetic acid-3-O-glucuronide in biological fluids: Application of ion-pair extraction and fluorescence labelling agent. J Chromatogr 1991 Jun 14; 567(1):151–60.

[62] Yamamura Y, Kawakami J, Santa T, et al. Pharmacokinetic profile of glycyrrhizin in healthy volunteers by a new high-performance liquid chromatographic method. J Pharm Sci 1992 Oct; 81(10):1042–6.

[63] Dalu A, Haskell JF, Coward L, Lamartiniere CA. Genistein, a component of soy, inhibits the expression of the EGF and ErbB2/Neu receptors in the rat dorsolateral prostate. Prostate 1998 Sep 15; 37(1):36–43.

[64] Morand C. Personal communication based on unpublished data. July 2000.

[65] Day AJ, Bao Y, Morgan MR, Williamson G. Conjugation position of quercetin glucuronides and effect on biological activity. Free Radic Biol Med 2000 Dec 15; 29(12):1234–43.

[66] Biesalski HK, Schaffer M. Comparative assessment of the activity of beta-carotene, retinoyl-beta-D-glucuronide, and retinoic acid on growth and differentiation of a human promyelocytic leukemia cell line HL-60. Int J Vitam Nutr Res. 997; 67(5):357–63.

[67] Zile MH, Cullum ME, Simpson RU, et al. Induction of differentiation of human promyelocytic leukemia cell line HL-60 by retinoyl glucuronide, a biologically active metabolite of vitamin A. Proc Natl Acad Sci USA 1987 Apr; 84(8):2208–12.

[68] Janick-Buckner D, Barua AB, Olson JA. Induction of HL-60 cell differentiation by water-soluble and nitrogen-containing conjugates of retinoic acid and retinol. FASEB J 1991 Mar 1; 5(3):320–5.

[69] Yanagihara K, Ito Akihiro, Toge T, et al. Antiproliferative effects of isoflavones on human cancer cell lines established from the gastrointestinal tract. Cancer Res 1993 Dec 1; 53(23):5815–21.

[70] Zhou JR, Mukherjee P, Grugger ET, et al. Inhibition of murine bladder tumorigenesis by soy isoflavones via alterations in the cell cycle, apoptosis, and angiogenesis. Cancer Res 1998 Nov 15; 58(22):5231–8.

[71] Kamei H, Kojima T, Hasegawa M, et al. Suppression of tumor cell growth by anthocyanins in vitro. Cancer Investigation 1995; 13(6):590–594.

[72] Jing Y, Waxman S. Structural requirements for differentiation-induction and growth-inhibition of mouse erythroleukemia cells by isoflavones. Anticancer Res 1995 Jul–Aug; 15(4):1147–52.

[73] Hempstock J, Kavanagh JP, George NJ. Growth inhibition of prostate cell lines in vitro by phytooestrogens. Br J Urol 1998; 82(4):560–3.

[74] Ryu SY, Ahn JW, Kang YH, et al. Antiproliferative effect of arctigenin and arctiin. Arch Pharm Res 1995; 18(6):462–3.

[75] Moritani S, Nomura M, Takeda Y, Miyamoto KI. Cytotoxic components of bardanae fructus (goboshi). Biol Pharm Bull 1996 Nov; 19(11):1515–7.

[76] Kim DH, Kim SY, Park SY, Han MJ. Metabolism of quercitrin by human intestinal bacteria and its relation to some biological activities. Biol Pharm Bull 1999 Jul; 22(7):749–51.

[77] Robinson MJ, Corbett AH, Osheroff N. Effects of topoisomerase II-targeted drugs on enzyme-mediated DNA cleavage and ATP hydrolysis: Evidence for distinct drug interaction domains on topoisomerase II. Biochemistry 1993; 32:3638–3643.

[78] Kim HK, Cheon BS, Kim YH, et al. Effects of naturally occurring flavonoids on nitric oxide production in the macrophage cell line RAW 264.7 and their structure-activity relationships. Biochem Pharmacol 1999 Sep 1; 58(5):759–65.

[79] King RA, Bursill DB. Plasma and urinary kinetics of the isoflavones daidzein and genistein after a single soy meal in humans. Am J Clin Nutr 1998; 67:867–72.

[80] Morton MS, Matos-Ferreira A, Abranches-Monteiro L, et al. Measurement and metabolism of isoflavonoids and lignans in the human male. Cancer Lett 1997 Mar 19; 114(1–2):145–51.

[81] Watanabe S, Yamaguchi M, Sobue T, et al. Pharmacokinetics of soybean isoflavones in plasma, urine and feces of men after ingestion of 60 g baked soybean powder (kinako). J Nutr 1998 Oct; 128(10):1710–5.

[82] Hollman, PC, Gaag MV, Mengelers MJ, et al. Absorption and disposition kinetics of the dietary antioxidant quercetin in man. Free Radical Biology & Medicine 1996; 21(5):703–707.

[83] McAnlis GT, McEneny J, Pearce J, Young IS. Absorption and antioxidant effects of quercetin from onions, in man. European J Clin Nutr 1999; 53:92–96.

[84] Olthof MR, Hollman PC, Vree TB, Katan MB. Bioavailabilities of quercetin-3-glucoside and quercetin-4'-glucoside Do not differ in humans. J Nutr 2000 May; 130(5):1200–3.

[85] Morrice PC, Wood SG, Duthie GG. High-performance liquid chromatographic determination of quercetin and isorhamnetin in rat tissues using beta-glucuronidase and acid hydrolysis. J Chromatogr B Biomed Sci Appl 2000 Feb 11; 738(2):413–7.

[86] Piskula MK. Soy isoflavone conjugation differs in fed and food-deprived rats. J Nutr 2000 Jul; 130(7):1766–1771.

[87] Harada M, Kan Y, Naoki H, et al. Identification of the major antioxidative metabolites in biological fluids of the rat with ingested (+)-catechin and (-)-epicatechin. Biosci Biotechnol Biochem 1999 Jun; 63(6):973–7.

[88] Spencer JP, Chowrimootoo G, Choudhury R, et al. The small intestine can both absorb and glucuronidate luminal flavonoids. FEBS Lett 1999 Sep 17; 458(2):224–30.

[89] Zhang Y, Wang GJ, Song TT, et al. Urinary disposition of the soybean isoflavones daidzein, genistein and glycitein differs among humans with moderate fecal isoflavone degradation activity. J Nutr 1999 May; 129(5):957–62.

[90] Xu X, Wang HJ, Murphy PA, et al. Daidzein is a more bioavailable soymilk isoflavone than is genistein in adult women. J Nutr 1994 Jun; 124(6):825–32.

[91] Xu X, Wang HJ, Murphy PA, Hendrich S. Neither background diet nor type of soy food affects short-term isoflavone bioavailability in women. J Nutr 2000 Apr; 130(4):798–801.

[92] King RA. Daidzein conjugates are more bioavailable than genistein conjugates in rats. Am J Clin Nutr 1998 Dec; 68(6 Suppl):1496S-1499S.

[93] Conquer JA, Maiani G, Azzini E, et al. Supplementation with quercetin markedly increases plasma quercetin concentration without effect on selected risk factors for heart disease in healthy subjects. J Nutr 1998 Mar; 128(3):593–7.

[94] Gerritsen ME, Carley WW, Ranges GE, et al. Flavonoids inhibit cytokine-induced endothelial cell adhesion protein gene expression. Am J Pathology 1995; 147(2):278–292.

[95] Mascolo N, Pinto A, Capasso F. Flavonoids, leukocyte migration and eicosanoids. J Pharm Pharmacol 1988 Apr; 40(4):293–5.

[96] Taguchi K, Hagiwara Y, Kajiyama K, Suzuki Y. [Pharmacological studies of Houttuyniae herba: The anti-inflammatory effect of quercitrin.] Yakugaku Zasshi 1993 Apr; 113(4):327–33.

[97] Romero J, Marak GE Jr, Rao NA. Pharmacologic modulation of acute ocular inflammation with quercetin. Ophthalmic Res 1989; 21(2):112–7.

[98] Wakai K, Egami I, Kato K, et al. Dietary intake and sources of isoflavones among Japanese. Nutr Cancer 1999; 33(2):139–45.

99 Hertog MG, Hollman PC, Katan MB, Kromhout D. Intake of potentially anticarcinogenic flavonoids and their determinants in adults in The Netherlands. Nutr Cancer 1993; 20(1):21–9.

100 Crowell JA, Levine BS, Page JG, et al. Preclinical safety studies of isoflavones. Third International Symposium on the Role of Soy in Preventing and Treating Chronic Disease. October 31-November 3, 1999. Washington, DC. USA.

101 NCI, DCPC. Clinical development plan: Genistein. J Cell Biochem 1996; 26S:114–126.

102 Crowell JA, Jeffcoat AR, Tyndall LW, Zeisel SH. Clinical phase I studies of isoflavones. Third international symposium on the role of soy in preventing and treating chronic disease. October 31-November 3, 1999. Washington, DC. USA.

103 Lee MJ, Wang ZY, Li H, et al. Analysis of plasma and urinary tea polyphenols in human subjects. Cancer Epidemiol Biomarkers Prev 1995 Jun; 4(4):393–9.

104 van het Hof KH, Kivits GA, Weststrate JA, Tijburg LB. Bioavailability of catechins from tea: The effect of milk. Eur J Clin Nutr 1998 May; 52(5):356–9.

105 Unno T, Kondo K, Itakura H, Takeo T. Analysis of (-)-epigallocatechin gallate in human serum obtained after ingesting green tea. Biosci Biotechnol Biochem 1996 Dec; 60(12):2066–8.

106 Maiani G, Serafini M, Salucci M, et al. Application of a new high-performance liquid chromatographic method for measuring selected polyphenols in human plasma. J Chromatography B 1997; 692:311–317.

107 van het Hof KH, Kivits GAA, Weststrate JA, Tijburg LBM. Bioavailability of catechins from tea: The effect of milk. Eur J Clin Nutr 1998 May; 52(5):356–9.

108 NCI/DCPC. Clinical development plan: Tea extracts. Green tea polyphenols. Epigallocatechin gallate. J Cell Biochem Suppl 1996; 26:236–57.

109 Yamane T, Nakatani H, Kikuoka N, et al. Inhibitory effects and toxicity of green tea polyphenols for gastrointestinal carcinogenesis. Cancer 1996 Apr 15; 77(8 Suppl):1662–7.

110 Pietta P, Simonetti P, Gardana C, et al. Relationship between rate and extent of catechin absorption and plasma antioxidant status. Biochem Mol Biol Int 1998 Dec; 46(5):895–903.

111 Chen L, Lee MJ, Li H, Yang CS. Absorption, distribution, elimination of tea polyphenols in rats. Drug Metab Dispos 1997 Sep; 25(9):1045–50.

112 Nakagawa K, Miyazawa T. Chemiluminescence-high-performance liquid chromatographic determination of tea catechin, (-)-epigallocatechin 3-gallate, at picomole levels in rat and human plasma. Anal Biochem 1997 May 15; 248(1):41–9.

113 Morazzoni P, Livio S, Scilingo A, et al. Vaccinium myrtillus anthocyanosides pharmacokinetics in rats. Arzneimittelforschung 1991 Feb; 41(2):128–31.

114 Lapara J, Michaud J, Masquelier J. Etude pharmacocinetique des oligomeres flavanoliques. Plantes Medicinales et Phytotherapie 1977; 11:133–142.

115 Schwitters B, Masquelier J. OPC in practice; bioflavinoids and their application. Rome, Italy: Alfa Omega Publishers, 1993, pp. 57–8.

116 Cao G, Prior R. Anthocyanins are detected in human plasma after oral administration of an elderberry extract. Clin Chem 1999 Apr; 45(4):574–6.

117 Doutremepuich JD, Barbier A, Lacheretz F. Effect of Endotelon (procyanidolic oligomers) on experimental acute lymphedema of the rat hindlimb. Lymphology 1991 Sep; 24(3):135–9.

118 Wegrowski J, Robert AM, Moczar M. The effect of procyanidolic oligomers on the composition of normal and hypercholesterolemic rabbit aortas. Biochem Pharmacol 1984 Nov 1; 33(21):3491–7.

119 Huynh HT, Teel RW. Selective induction of apoptosis in human mammary cancer cells (MCF-7) by pycnogenol. Anticancer Res 2000 Jul–Aug; 20(4):2417–20.

120 Uang YS, Kang FL, Hsu KY. Determination of caffeic acid in rabbit plasma by high-performance liquid chromatography. J Chromatogr B Biomed Appl 1995 Nov 3; 673(1):43–9.

121 Bourne LC, Rice-Evans C. Bioavailability of ferulic acid. Biochem Biophys Res Commun 1998 Dec 18; 253(2):222–7.

122 Grunberger, D. Personal communication. Sept 1997.

123 Bailey D, Boik J. Unpublished observations. 1999.

124 Burdock GA. Review of the biological properties and toxicity of bee propolis (propolis). Food and Chemical Toxicology 1998; 36(4):347–63.

125 Park EH, Kim SH, Park SS. Anti-inflammatory activity of propolis. Arch Pharm Res 1996; 19(5):337–341.

126 Lutz U, Lugli S, Bitsch A, et al. Dose response for the stimulation of cell division by caffeic acid in forestomach and kidney of the male F344 rat. Fundam Appl Toxicol 1997 Oct; 39(2):131–7.

127 Ito N, Hirose M, Takahashi S. Cell proliferation and forestomach carcinogenesis. Environ Health Perspect 1993 Dec; 101 Suppl 5:107–10.

128 Ito N, Imaida K, Hirose M, Shirai T. Medium-term bioassays for carcinogenicity of chemical mixtures. Environ Health Perspect 1998 Dec; 106 Suppl 6:1331–6.

129 Hirose M, Takesada Y, Tanaka H, et al. Carcinogenicity of antioxidants BHA, caffeic acid, sesamol, 4-methoxyphenol and catechol at low doses, either alone or in combination, and modulation of their effects in a rat medium-term multi-organ carcinogenesis model. Carcinogenesis 1998 Jan; 19(1):207–12.

130 Kaul A, Khanduja KL. Polyphenols inhibit promotional phase of tumorigenesis: Relevance of superoxide radicals. Nutr Cancer 1998; 32(2):81–5.

131 Tanaka T, Kojima T, Kawamori T, et al. Inhibition of 4-nitroquinoline-1-oxide-induced rat tongue carcinogenesis by the naturally occurring plant phenolics caffeic, ellagic, chlorogenic and ferulic acids. Carcinogenesis 1993 Jul; 14(7):1321–5.

132 Lutz WK. Dose-response relationships in chemical carcinogenesis: Superposition of different mechanisms of action, resulting in linear-nonlinear curves, practical thresholds, J-shapes. Mutat Res 1998 Sep 20; 405(2):117–24.

133 Rao CV, Desai D, Kaul B, et al. Effect of caffeic acid esters on carcinogen-induced mutagenicity and human colon adenocarcinoma cell growth. Chem Biol Interact 1992 Nov 16; 84(3):277–90.

[134] Huang MT, Ma W, Yen P, et al. Inhibitory effects of caffeic acid phenethyl ester (CAPE) on 12-O-tetradecanoylphorbol-13-acetate-induced tumor promotion in mouse skin and the synthesis of DNA, RNA and protein in HeLa cells. Carcinogenesis 1996 Apr; 17(4):761–5.

[135] Ravindranath V, Chandrasekhara N. Absorption and tissue distribution of curcumin in rats. Toxicology 1980; 16:259–265.

[136] Wahlstrom B, Blennow G. A study on the fate of curcumin in the rat. Acta Pharmacol et Toxicol 1978; 43:86–92.

[137] NCI, DCPC. Clinical development plan: Curcumin. J Cell Biochem 1996; 26S:72–85.

[138] Shoba G, Joy D, Joseph T, et al. Influence of piperine on the pharmacokinetics of curcumin in animals and human volunteers. Planta Medica 1998; 64:353–356.

[139] Pan MH, Huang TM, Lin JK. Biotransformation of curcumin through reduction and glucuronidation in mice. Drug Metab Dispos 1999 Apr; 27(4):486–94.

[140] Ravindranath V, Chandrasekhara N. Metabolism of curcumin—studies with [3H]curcumin. Toxicology. 1981–82; 22(4):337–44.

[141] Rickling B, Hans B, Kramarczyk R, et al. Two high-performance liquid chromatographic assays for the determination of free and total silibinin diastereomers in plasma using column switching with electrochemical detection and reversed-phase chromatography with ultraviolet detection. J Chromatogr B Biomed Appl 1995 Aug 18; 670(2):267–77.

[142] Schulz HU, Schurer M, Krumbiegel G, et al. [The solubility and bioequivalence of silymarin preparations.] Arzneimittelforschung 1995 Jan; 45(1):61–4.

[143] Bruneton J. Pharmacognosy, phytochemistry, and medicinal plants. Secaucus, NY: Lavoisier Publishing, 1995, p. 250.

[144] Umeda-Sawada R, Ogawa M, Igarashi O. The metabolism and distribution of sesame lignans (sesamin and episesamin) in rats. Lipids 1999 Jun; 34(6):633–7.

[145] Miyahara Y, Komiya T, Katsuzaki H, et al. Sesamin and episesamin induce apoptosis in human lymphoid leukemia molt 4B cells. Int J Mol Med 2000 Jul; 6(1):43–6.

[146] Sun WJ, Sha ZF, Gao H. Determination of arctiin and arctigenin in Fructus Arctii by reverse-phase HPLC. Yao Hsueh Hsueh Pao 1992; 27(7):549–51.

[147] Scambia G, De Vincenzo R, Ranelletti FO, et al. Antiproliferative effect of silybin on gynaecological malignancies: Synergism with cisplatin and doxorubicin. Eur J Cancer 1996 May; 32A(5):877–82.

[148] Nesbitt PD, Lam Y, Thompson LU. Human metabolism of mammalian lignan precursors in raw and processed flaxseed. Am J Clin Nutr 1999 Mar; 69(3):549–55.

[149] Morton MS, Wilcox G, Wahlqvist ML, Griffiths K. Determination of lignans and isoflavonoids in human female plasma following dietary supplementation. J Endocrinol 1994 Aug; 142(2):251–9.

[150] Atkinson DA, Hill HH, Shultz TD. Quantification of mammalian lignans in biological fluids using gas chromatography with ion mobility detection. J Chromatogr 1993 Aug 11; 617(2):173–9.

[151] Bruneton J. Pharmacognosy, phytochemistry, and medicinal plants. Secaucus, NY: Lavoisier Publishing, 1995, p. 106.

[152] Cunnane SC, Hamadeh MJ, Liede AC, et al. Nutritional attributes of traditional flaxseed in healthy young adults. Am J Clin Nutr 1995 Jan; 61(1):62–8.

[153] Cunnane SC, Ganguli S, Menard C, et al. High alpha-linolenic acid flaxseed (Linum usitatissimum): Some nutritional properties in humans. Br J Nutr 1993 Mar; 69(2):443–53.

[154] Bertelli AA, Giovannini L, Stradi R, et al. Kinetics of trans- and cis-resveratrol (3,4',5-trihydroxystilbene) after red wine oral administration in rats. Int J Clin Pharmacol Res 1996; 16(4–5):77–81.

[155] Bertelli A, Bertelli AAE, Gozzini A, Giovannini L. Plasma and tissue resveratrol concentrations and pharmacological activity. Drugs Exp Clin Res 1998; 24(3):133–8.

[156] Kuhnle G, Spencer JP, Chowrimootoo G, et al. Resveratrol is absorbed in the small intestine as resveratrol glucuronide. Biochem Biophys Res Commun 2000 May 27; 272(1):212–7.

[157] Pang Z, Wang B, Li S. Study on the pharmacokinetics of emodin and chrysophanol in rabbits. J of Xi'an Medical University 1993; 14(4):346–249.

[158] Lang W. Pharmacokinetic-metabolic studies with ^{14}C-aloe emodin after oral administration to male and female rats. Pharmacology 1993; 47(suppl 1):110–119.

[159] Mengs U, Krumbiegel G, Volkner W. Lack of emodin genotoxicity in the mouse micronucleus assay. Mutat Res 1997; 393(3):289–293.

[160] Liang JW, Hsiu SL, Wu PP, Chao PDL. Emodin pharmacokinetics in rabbits. Planta Medica 1995; 61:406–408.

[161] Nicolas P, Tod M, Padoin C, Petitjean O. Clinical pharmacokinetics of diacerein. Clin Pharmacokinet 1998 Nov; 35(5):347–59.

[162] Natori S, Ikekawa N, Suzuki M, eds. Advances in natural products chemistry; extraction and isolation of active compounds. New York: John Wiley & Sons, 1981.

[163] Bachman M, Schlatter C. Metabolism of [14C]emodin in rat. Xenobiotica 1981; 11(3):217–25.

[164] Staffeldt B, Kerb R, Brockmoller J, et al. Pharmacokinetics of hypericin and pseudohypericin after oral intake of the Hypericum perforatum extract LI 160 in healthy volunteers. J Geriatr Psychiatry Neurol 1994 Oct; 7 Suppl 1:S47–53.

[165] Kerb R, Brockmoller J, Staffeldt B, et al. Single-dose and steady-state pharmacokinetics of hypericin and pseudohypericin. Antimicrobial Agents and Chemotherapy 1996; 40(9):2087–2093.

[166] Brockmoller J, Reum T, Bauer S, et al. Hypericin and pseudohypericin: Pharmacokinetics and effects on photosensitivity in humans. Pharmacopsychiatry 1997 Sep; 30 Suppl 2:94–101.

[167] Gulick RM, McAuliffe V, Holden-Wiltse J, et al. Phase I studies of hypericin, the active compound in St. John's Wort, as an antiretroviral agent in HIV-infected adults. Ann Intern Med 1999 Mar 16; 130(6):510–4.

[168] Vigushin DM, Poon GK, Boddy A, et al. Phase I and pharmacokinetic study of d-limonene in patients with advanced cancer. Cancer Chemother Pharmacol 1998; 42(2):111–7.

[169] Zhang Z, Chen H, Chan KK, et al. Gas chromatographic-mass spectrometric analysis of perillyl alcohol and metabolites in

plasma. J Chromatogr B Biomed Sci App 1999 May 14; 728(1):85–95.

170 Phillips LR, Malspeis L, Supko JG. Pharmacokinetics of active drug metabolites after oral administration of perillyl alcohol, an investigational antineoplastic agent, to the dog. Drug Metab Dispos 1995 Jul; 23(7):676–80.

171 Boon PJ, van der Boon D, Mulder GJ. Cytotoxicity and biotransformation of the anticancer drug perillyl alcohol in PC12 cells and in the rat. Toxicol Appl Pharmacol 2000 Aug 15; 167(1):55–62.

172 Crowell PL, Elson CE, Bailey HH, et al. Human metabolism of the experimental cancer therapeutic agent d-limonene. Cancer Chemother Pharmacol 1994; 35:31–37.

173 NCI, DCPC. Clinical development plan: L-perillyl alcohol. J Cell Biochem 1996; 26S:137–148.

174 Ripple GH, Gould MN, Stewart JA, et al. Phase I clinical trial of perillyl alcohol administered daily. Clinical Cancer Res 1998; 4:1159–1164.

175 Hudes GR, Szarka CE, Adams A, et al. Phase I pharmacokinetic trial of perillyl alcohol (NSC 641066) in patients with refractory solid malignancies. Clin Cancer Res 2000 Aug; 6(8):3071–80.

176 Grimaldi R, De Ponti F, D'Angelo L, et al. Pharmacokinetics of the total triterpenic fraction of Centella asiatica after single and multiple administrations to healthy volunteers. A new assay for asiatic acid. J Ethnopharmacol 1990 Feb; 28(2):235–41.

177 Rush WR, Murray GR, Grahm DJM. The comparative steady-state bioavailability of the active ingredients of Madecassol. Eur J Drug Metab Pharmacokinet 1993 Oct–Dec; 18(4):323–6.

178 Cantelli-Forti G, Maffei F, Hrelia P, et al. Interaction of licorice on glycyrrhizin pharmacokinetics. Environ Health Perspectives 1994; 102(suppl 9):65–68.

179 Oschmann R, Biber A, Lang F, et al. [Pharmaokinetics of beta-escin after administration of various Aesculus extract containing formulations.] Pharmazie 1996 Aug; 51(8):577–81.

180 Kunz K, Lorkowski G, Petersen G, et al. Bioavailability of escin after administration of two oral formulations containing aesculus extract. Arzneimittelforschung 1998 Aug; 48(8):822–5.

181 Longiave D, Omini C, Nicosia S, Berti F. The mode of action of aescin on isolated veins: Relationship with PGF2 alpha. Pharmacol Res Commun 1978 Feb; 10(2):145–52.

182 Obolentseva GV, Khadzhai Ya I. Effect of escin and a flavonoid complex prepared from horse chestnut on inflammatory edema. Farmakol Toksikol 1969; 32(2):174–7.

183 Hampel H, Hofrichter G, Liehn H, et al. Pharmacology of escin isomers, especially alpha-escin. Forschungslab 1970; 20(2):209–15.

184 Bruneton J. Pharmacognosy, phytochemistry, medicinal plants. Secaucus, NY: Lavoisier Publishing, 1995, p. 557.

185 Murray MT. The healing power of herbs. 2nd ed. Rocklin, CA: Prima Publishing, 1992, pp. 385–6.

186 Hasegawa H, Sung JH, Benno Y. Role of human intestinal Prevotella oris in hydrolyzing ginseng saponins. Planta Medica 197; 63:436–440.

187 Wakabayashi C, Hasegawa H, Murata J, Saiki I. In vivo antimetastatic action of ginseng protopanaxadiol saponins is based on their intestinal bacterial metabolites after oral administration. Oncol Res 1997; 9(8):411–7.

188 Bensky D, Gamble A. Chinese herbal medicine materia medica. Seattle: Eastland Press, 1993, p. 315.

189 Grippo AA, Wyrick SD, Lee KH, et al. Disposition of an antineoplastic sesquiterpene lactone, [3H]-plenolin, in BDF1 mice. Planta Medica 1991; 57:309–14.

190 Chan KL, Yuen KH, Jinadasa S, et al. A high-performance liquid chromatography analysis of plasma artemisinin using a glassy carbon electrode for reductive electrochemical detection. Planta Med 1997 Feb; 63(1):66–9.

191 Benakis A, Paris M, Loutan L, et al. Pharmacokinetics of artemisinin and artesunate after oral administration in healthy volunteers. Am J Trop Med Hyg 1997 Jan; 56(1):17–23.

192 De Vries PJ, Dien TK, Khanh NX, et al. The pharmacokinetics of a single dose of artemisinin in patients with uncomplicated falciparum malaria. Am J Trop Med Hyg 1997 May; 56(5):503–7.

193 Heptinstall S, Awang DV, Dawson BA, et al. Parthenolide content and bioactivity of feverfew (Tanacetum parthenium (L.) Schultz-Bip.). Estimation of commercial and authenticated feverfew products. J Pharm Pharmacol 1992 May; 44(5):391–5.

194 Chapman DE, Roberts GB, Reynolds DJ, et al. Acute toxicity of helenalin in BDF1 mice. Fundam Appl Toxicol 1988 Feb; 10(2):302–12.

195 NCI, DCPC. Clinical development plan: Vitamin A. J Cellular Biochem 1996; 26S:269–307.

196 Blomhoff R, Skrede B, Norum KR. Uptake of chylomicron remnant retinyl ester via the low density lipoprotein receptor: Implications for the role of vitamin A as a possible preventive for some forms of cancer. J Intern Med 1990 Sep; 228(3):207–10.

197 Napoli JL. Biochemical pathways of retinoid transport, metabolism, and signal transduction. Clin Immunol Immunopathol 1996 Sep; 80(3 Pt 2):S52–62.

198 Kurlandsky SB, Gamble MV, Ramakrishnan R, Blaner WS. Plasma delivery of retinoic acid to tissues in the rat. J Biol Chem 1995 Jul 28; 270(30):17850–7.

199 van Bennekum AM, Kako Y, Weinstock PH, et al. Lipoprotein lipase expression level influences tissue clearance of chylomicron retinyl ester. J Lipid Res 1999 Mar; 40(3):565–74.

200 Skrede B, Blomhoff R, Maelandsmo GM, et al. Uptake of chylomicron remnant retinyl esters in human leukocytes in vivo. Eur J Clin Invest 1992 Apr; 22(4):229–34.

201 Karpe F, Humphreys SM, Samra JS, et al. Clearance of lipoprotein remnant particles in adipose tissue and muscle in humans. J Lipid Res 1997 Nov; 38(11):2335–43.

202 Wolf G. Uptake of retinoids by adipose tissue. Nutr Rev 1994 Oct; 52(10):356–8.

203 Skrede B, Lie SO, Blomhoff R, Norum KR. Uptake and storage of retinol and retinyl esters in bone marrow of children with acute myeloid leukemia treated with high-dose retinyl palmitate. Eur J Haematol 1994 Mar; 52(3):140–4.

204 Takeyama K, Kojima R, Ohashi R, et al. Retinoic acid differentially up-regulates the gene expression of retinoic acid receptor alpha and gamma isoforms in embryo and adult rats. Biochem Biophys Res Commun 1996 May 15; 222(2):395–400.

205 Lovat PE, Annicchiarico-Petruzzelli M, Corazzari M, et al. Differential effects of retinoic acid isomers on the expression of nuclear receptor co-regulators in neuroblastoma. FEBS Lett 1999 Feb 26; 445(2–3):415–9.

206 Dahiya R, Boyle B, Park HD, et al. 13-cis-retinoic acid-mediated growth inhibition of DU-145 human prostate cancer cells. Biochem Mol Biol Int 1994 Jan; 32(1):1–12.

207 Spinella MJ, Dmitrovsky E. Aberrant retinoid signaling and breast cancer: The view from outside the nucleus. J Natl Cancer Inst 2000 Mar 15; 92(6):438–40.

208 Smeland S, Bjerknes T, Malaba L, et al. Tissue distribution of the receptor for plasma retinol-binding protein. Biochem J 1995 Jan 15; 305 (Pt 2):419–24.

209 Bhat PV. Tissue concentrations of retinol, retinyl esters, and retinoic acid in vitamin A deficient rats administered a single dose of radioactive retinol. Can J Physiol Pharmacol 1997 Jan; 75(1):74–7.

210 Rundhaug J, Gubler ML, Sherman MI, et al. Differential uptake, binding, and metabolism of retinol and retinoic acid by 10T1/2 cells. Cancer Res 1987 Nov 1; 47(21):5637–43.

211 Jurukovski V, Simon M. Reduced lecithin:retinol acyl transferase activity in cultured squamous cell carcinoma lines results in increased substrate-driven retinoic acid synthesis. Biochim Biophys Acta 1999 Jan 4; 1436(3):479–90.

212 Shao Z, Yu L, Shen Z, Fontana JA. Retinoic acid nuclear receptor alpha(RAR alpha) plays a major role in retinoid-mediated inhibition of growth in human breast carcinoma cells. Chin Med Sci J 1996 Sep; 11(3):142–6.

213 Shyu RY, Jiang SY, Huang SL, et al. Growth regulation by all-*trans* retinoic acid and retinoic acid receptor messenger ribonucleic acids expression in gastric cancer cells. Eur J Cancer 1995; 31A(2):237–43.

214 Moasser MM, DeBlasio A, Dmitrovsky E. Response and resistance to retinoic acid are mediated through the retinoic acid nuclear receptor gamma in human teratocarcinomas. Oncogene 1994 Mar; 9(3):833–40.

215 Kuppumbatti YS, Bleiweiss IJ, Mandeli JP, et al. Cellular retinol-binding protein expression and breast cancer. J Natl Cancer Inst 2000 Mar 15; 92(6):475–80.

216 Tallman MS, Wiernik PH. Retinoids in cancer treatment. J Clin Pharmacol 1992 Oct; 32(10):868–88.

217 Copper MP, Klaassen I, Teerlink T, et al. Plasma retinoid levels in head and neck cancer patients: A comparison with healthy controls and the effect of retinyl palmitate treatment. Oral Oncol 1999 Jan; 35(1):40–4.

218 Conley BA, Egorin MJ, Sridhara R, et al. Phase I clinical trial of all-*trans* retinoic acid with correlation of its pharmacokinetics and pharmacodynamics. Cancer Chemother Pharmacol 1997; 39(4):291–9.

219 Trump DL, Smith DC, Stiff D, et al. A phase II trial of all-*trans* retinoic acid in hormone-refractory prostate cancer: A clinical trial with detailed pharmacokinetic analysis. Cancer Chemother Pharmacol 1997; 39(4):349–56.

220 Adamson PC, Pitot HC, Balis FM. Variability in the oral bioavailability of all-*trans* retinoic acid. J Natl Cancer Inst 1993 Jun 16; 85(12):993–6.

221 Guiso G, Rambaldi A, Dimitrova B, et al. Determination of orally administered all-*trans* retinoic acid in human plasma by high-performance liquid chromatography. J Chromatogr B Biomed Appl 1994 Jun 3; 656(1):239–44.

222 Buss NE, Tembe EA, Prendergast BD, et al. The teratogenic metabolites of vitamin A in women following supplements and liver. Hum Exp Toxicol 1994 Jan; 13(1):33–43.

223 Reinersdorff DV, Bush E, Liberato DJ. Plasma kinetics of vitamin A in humans after a single oral dose of [8,9,19–13C]retinyl palmitate. J Lipid Res 1996 Sep; 37(9):1875–85.

224 Tsutani H, Ueda T, Uchida M, Nakamura T. Pharmacological studies of retinol palmitate and its clinical effect in patients with acute non-lymphocytic leukemia. Leuk Res 1991; 15(6):463–71.

225 Chen C, Mistry G, Jensen B, et al. Pharmacokinetics of retinoids in women after meal consumption or vitamin A supplementation. J Clin Pharmacol 1996 Sep; 36(9):799–808.

226 Meyer E, Lambert WE, De Leenheer AP. Simultaneous determination of endogenous retinoic acid isomers and retinol in human plasma by isocratic normal-phase HPLC with ultraviolet detection. Clin Chem 1994 Jan; 40(1):48–57.

227 Napoli JL. Quantification of physiological levels of retinoic acid. Methods Enzymol 1986; 123:112–24.

228 Goodman GE, Alberts DS, Earnst DL, Meyskens FL. Phase I trial of retinol in cancer patients. J Clin Oncol 1983 Jun; 1(6):394–9.

229 Murray MT. Encyclopedia of nutritional supplements. Rocklin, CA: Prima Publishing, 1996, p. 36.

230 Cartmel B, Moon TE, Levine N. Effects of long-term intake of retinol on selected clinical and laboratory indexes. Am J Clin Nutr 1999 May; 69(5):937–43.

231 Sibulesky L, Hayes KC, Pronczuk A, et al. Safety of <7500 RE (<25000 IU) vitamin A daily in adults with retinitis pigmentosa. Am J Clin Nutr 1999 Apr; 69(4):656–63.

232 Lee JS, Newman RA, Lippman SM, et al. Phase I evaluation of all-*trans* retinoic acid in adults with solid tumors. J Clin Oncol 1993 May; 11(5):959–66.

233 Budd GT, Adamson PC, Gupta M, et al. Phase I/II trial of all-*trans* retinoic acid and tamoxifen in patients with advanced breast cancer. Clin Cancer Res 1998 Mar; 4(3):635–42.

234 Vakkuri O, Leppaluto J, Kauppila A. Oral administration and distribution of melatonin in human serum, saliva and urine. Life Sci 1985 Aug 5; 37(5):489–95.

235 Shirakawa S, Tsuchiya S, Tsutsumi Y, et al. Time course of saliva and serum melatonin levels after ingestion of melatonin. Psychiatry Clin Neurosci 1998 Apr; 52(2):266–7.

236 Kane MA, Johnson A, Nash AE, et al. Serum melatonin levels in melanoma patients after repeated oral administration. Melanoma Res 1994 Feb; 4(1):59–65.

237 Rapozzi V, Comelli M, Mavelli I, et al. Melatonin and oxidative damage in mice liver induced by the prooxidant antitumor drug, adriamycin. In Vivo 1999 Jan–Feb; 13(1):45–50.

[238] de Lourdes M, Seabra V, Bignotto M, et al. Randomized, double-blind clinical trial, controlled with placebo, of the toxicology of chronic melatonin treatment. J Pineal Res 2000 Nov; 29(4):193–200.

[239] Arendt J. Safety of melatonin in long-term use. J Biol Rhythms 1997 Dec; 12(6):673–81.

[240] Guardiola-Lemaitre B. Toxicology of melatonin. J Biol Rhythms 1997 Dec; 12(6):697–706.

SUPPLEMENTAL MATERIAL FOR CHAPTER 19

Supplemental material for Chapter 19, "Flavonoids," contains of Table K.1, which summarizes studies on the cytotoxic effects of flavonoids against cancer cells. See also Tables D.1 and D.2 which review studies on the ability of flavonoids and other compounds to induce differentiation and apoptosis.

TABLE K.1 SELECTED STUDIES ON THE IN-VITRO CYTOTOXIC EFFECTS OF FLAVONOIDS	
CELL LINE	**EFFECTS**
Apigenin	
Human breast cancer	For estrogen-dependent cells, the IC_{50}s for genistein and apigenin were about 15 and 7 μM, respectively. For estrogen-independent cells, the IC_{50}s were about 520 and 7 μM, respectively.[1]
Human breast cancer	IC_{50} = 13 μM.[2]
Nasopharynx carcinoma (KB line)	IC_{50} = 27 μM. Apigenin was inactive in three in-vivo NCI standard test systems.[3]
Mouse leukemia	IC_{50} = about 15 μM. The effect may have been due to topoisomerase inhibition.[4]
Four human thyroid cancer cell lines	IC_{50} from 22 to 32 μM.[5]
Five human cancer cell lines	IC_{50} = 16 to 29 μM.[6]
Luteolin	
Human leukemia	Complete ATP depletion and inhibition of glucose uptake at 30 μM.[7]
Four human thyroid cancer cell lines	IC_{50} from 22 to 32 μM.[5]
Five human cancer cell lines	IC_{50} = 7 to 15 μM.[6]
Four human cancer cell lines	IC_{50} = 1.3 to 3.1 μM. Luteolin was the most effective of 27 flavonoids tested.[8]
Androgen-independent rat prostate cancer	70% to 80% inhibition at 10 μM.[9]
Genistein	
Estrogen-dependent and estrogen-independent human breast cancer cells	IC_{50} = 24 to 44 μM. The effects were not reduced by overexpression of the multidrug-resistance gene.[10]
	IC_{50} = 21 to 31 μM.[11]
	Cell inhibition at 40 to 50 μM. The effect appeared to be due to PTK inhibition.[12]
Estrogen-dependent human breast cancer	IC_{50} = 19 μM. Inhibition was reversed by the addition of excess estrogen. Inhibition by other flavonoids was not affected by estrogen.[13]
	At low concentrations (1 nM to 1 μM) genistein stimulated cell proliferation. At concentrations greater than 10 μM, however, cell proliferation was strongly inhibited.[14, 15]
Three human breast cancer cell lines	Cell inhibition at 7 to 37 μM. Genistein acted synergistically with doxorubicin.[16]
	IC_{50} = 10 μM. Normal fibroblasts were not affected. Genistein counteracted the growth-stimulatory effects of estrogen and growth factors.[17]
Human breast cancer	In 1:1 combinations with other flavonoids, the IC_{50} was 7 to 11 μM.[18]
Human breast cancer	Inhibited DNA synthesis by 49% at 37 μM. The effect appeared to be due to PTK and *ras* inhibition.[19]
Human breast cancer	IC_{50} = 8.8 μM.[20]
Rat prostate cancer	70% to 80% inhibition at 0.1 to 10 μM in an androgen-independent cell line.[9]

TABLE K.1   SELECTED STUDIES ON THE IN-VITRO CYTOTOXIC EFFECTS OF FLAVONOIDS *(continued)*

CELL LINE	EFFECTS
Human prostate cancer cells obtained from patients	Dose-dependent inhibition at 5 to 37 μM.[21]
Human prostate cancer	$IC_{50} = 40$ μM. The expression of PSA was also reduced.[22]
Two human prostate cancer cell lines	$IC_{50} = 16$ to 100 μM.[23]
Six human prostate cancer cell lines	$IC_{50} = 35$ to 110 μM. The average IC_{50} was 75 μM.[24]
Human prostate cancer	$IC_{50} =$ about 38 μM.[25]
Human and rat prostate cancer	$IC_{50} =$ about 22 to 73 μM.[26]
Three human testicular cancer cell lines	$IC_{50} =$ about 130 to 185 μM.[27]
Human brain cancer	$IC_{50} = 5$ to 10 μM.[28]
Three human brain cancer cell lines	$IC_{50} = 8$ μM. The effect appeared to be due to PKC inhibition. Although genistein is a weak inhibitor of PKC, in this study it inhibited PKC secondary to PTK inhibition. Growth factors in the culture stimulated PTK, which in the absence of genistein led to downstream stimulation of PKC.[29]
Human stomach cancer	$IC_{50} = 10$ to 23 μM.[30]
	$IC_{50} = 20$ μM (after 4 days).[31]
Human myelogenous and human T lymphocytic leukemia	Caused 100% cell death in HML cells at 37 μM. IC_{50} in HLL cells was 11 μM. Genistein was not cytotoxic to normal lymphocytes.[32]
Rat lymphoma	$IC_{50} = 15$ to 25 μM.[30]
Human colon cancer	$IC_{50} =$ about 45 μM.[33]
Six neuroblastoma cell lines	Inhibited five of six cell lines. $IC_{50} =$ about 19 μM.[34]
Four human bladder cancer cell lines	$IC_{50} =$ about 37 to 74 μM. The motility of cell lines that express EGF was also inhibited at 37 μM.[35]
ras-dependent human bladder cancer	$IC_{50} =$ about 37 μM. Cell migration was also reduced, possibly due to an inhibition of kinases.[36]
Twelve different human cell lines	IC_{50} from 24 to 185 μM. The average was 65 μM.[37]
Quercetin	
Skin cancer	Of eight flavonoids tested, quercetin and luteolin were the most potent at inhibiting proliferation of skin cancer cells. Their IC_{50}s were 19 and 21 μM, respectively.[38]
Human leukemia	$IC_{50} =$ about 10 μM.[39]
Human leukemia	$IC_{50} = 43$ μM.[40]
Human ovarian cancer	$IC_{50} = 66$ μM. Synergistic inhibition occurred when genistein was added to the culture.[41]
Human ovarian cancer	Dose-dependent inhibition between 10 nM and 10 μM.[42]
Human non-small-cell lung cancer	Dose-dependent inhibition between 10 nM and 1 μM.[43]
Squamous cell carcinoma	Proliferation was inhibited at 26 μM.[44]
Human breast cancer	Dose-dependent inhibition between 17 μM and 33 μM.[45]
Human stomach cancer	$IC_{50} = 32$ to 55 μM.[46]
Human meningioma	Inhibition at 10 μM.[47]
Human lymphoblastoid	Dose-dependent inhibition between 10 nM and 10 μM.[48]
Human melanoma	Dose-dependent inhibition between 1 nM and 1 μM.[49]

REFERENCES

1 Guthrie N, Carroll KK. Inhibition of mammary cancer by citrus flavonoids. Adv Exp Med Biol 1998; 439:227–236.

2 Hirano T, Oka K, Akiba M. Antiproliferative effects of synthetic and naturally occurring flavonoids on tumor cells of the human breast carcinoma cell line, ZR-75-1. Res Commun Chem Pathol Pharmacol 1989 Apr; 64(1):69–78.

3 Edwards JM. Antineoplastic activity and cytotoxicity of flavones, isoflavones, and flavanones. J Natural Products 1979; 42:85–91.

4 Jing Y, Waxman S. Structural requirements for differentiation-induction and growth-inhibition of mouse erythroleukemia cells by isoflavones. Anticancer Res 1995 Jul–Aug; 15(4):1147–52.

5 Yin F, Giuliano AE, Van Herle AJ. Growth inhibitory effects of flavonoids in human thyroid cancer cell lines. Thyroid 1999 Apr; 9(4):369–76.

6 Ryu SR, Choi SU, Lee CO, et al. Antitumor activity of some phenolic compounds in plants. Arch Pharm Res 1994; 17(1):42–44.

7 Post JF, Varma RS. Growth inhibitory effects of bioflavonoids and related compounds on human leukemic CEM-C1 and CEM-C7 cells. Cancer Lett 1992 Dec 24; 67(2–3):207–13.

8 Kawaii S, Tomono Y, Katase E, et al. Antiproliferative activity of flavonoids on several cancer cell lines. Biosci Biotechnol Biochem 1999 May; 63(5):896–9.

9 Ho SM, Chun J. Inhibition of cell growth in an androgen-independent rat prostatic cell line (AIT) by phytochemicals. Adv Exp Med Biol 1996; 401:319.

10 Peterson G, Barnes S. Genistein inhibition of the growth of human breast cancer cells: Independence from estrogen receptors and the multi-drug resistance gene. Biochem Biophys Res Commun 1991; 179(1):661–7.

11 Constantinou AI, Krygier AE, Mehta RR. Genistein induces maturation of cultured human breast cancer cells and prevents tumor growth in nude mice. Am J Clin Nutr 1998 Dec; 68(6 Suppl):1426S-1430S.

12 Tetsuka T, Srivastava SK, Morrison AR. Tyrosine kinase inhibitors, genistein and herbimycin A, do not block interleukin-1 beta-induced activation of NF-kappa B in rat mesangial cells. Biochem Biophys Res Commun 1996 Jan 26; 218(3):808–12.

13 So FV, Guthrie N, Chambers AF, Carroll KK. Inhibition of proliferation of estrogen receptor-positive MCF-7 human breast cancer cells by flavonoids in the presence and absence of excess estrogen. Cancer Lett 1997 Jan 30; 112(2):127–33.

14 Zava DT, Duwe G. Estrogenic and antiproliferative properties of genistein and other flavonoids in human breast cancer cells in vitro. Nutr Cancer 1997; 27(1):31–40.

15 Wang TTY, Sathyamoorthy N, Phang JM. Molecular effects of genistein on estrogen receptor mediated pathways. Carcinogenesis 1996; 17(2):271–275.

16 Monti E, Sinha BK. Antiproliferative effect of genistein and adriamycin against estrogen-dependent and -independent human breast carcinoma cell lines. Anticancer Res 1994 May–Jun; 14(3A):1221–6.

17 Fioravanti L, Cappelletti V, Miodini P, et al. Genistein in the control of breast cancer cell growth: Insights into the mechanism of action in vitro. Cancer Lett 1998 Aug 14; 130(1–2):143–52.

18 So FV, Guthrie N, Chambers AF, et al. Inhibition of human breast cancer cell proliferation and delay of mammary tumorigenesis by flavonoids and citrus juices. Nutr Cancer 1996; 26(2):167–81.

19 Clark JW, Santos-Moore A, Stevenson LE, Frackelton AR. Effects of tyrosine kinase inhibitors on the proliferation of human breast cancer cell lines and proteins important in the ras signaling pathway. Int J Cancer 1996; 65:186–191.

20 Balabhadrapathruni S, Thomas TJ, Yurkow EJ, et al. Effects of genistein and structurally related phytoestrogens on cell cycle kinetics and apoptosis in MDA-MB-468 human breast cancer cells. Oncol Rep 2000 Jan; 7(1):3–12.

21 Geller J, Sionit L, Partido C, et al. Genistein inhibits the growth of human-patient BPH and prostate cancer in histoculture. Prostate 1998; 34(2):75–79.

22 Onozawa M, Fukuda K, Ohtani M, et al. Effects of soybean isoflavones on cell growth and apoptosis of the human prostatic cancer cell line LNCaP. Jpn J Clin Oncol 1998 Jun; 28(6):360–3.

23 Peterson G, Barnes S. Genistein and biochanin A inhibit the growth of human prostate cancer cells but not epidermal growth factor receptor tyrosine autophosphylation. Prostate 1993; 22(4):335–45.

24 Rokhlin OW, Cohen MB. Differential sensitivity of human prostatic cancer cell lines to the effects of protein kinase and phosphatase inhibitors. Cancer Letters 1995; 98:103–110.

25 Hempstock J, Kavanagh JP, George NJ. Growth inhibition of prostate cell lines in vitro by phyto-oestrogens. Br J Urol 1998 Oct; 82(4):560–3.

26 Naik HR, Lehr JE, Pienta KJ. An in vitro and in vivo study of antitumor effects of genistein on hormone refractory prostate cancer. Anticancer Res 1994 Nov–Dec; 14(6B):2617–9.

27 Kumi-Diaka J, Rodriguez R, Goudaze G. Influence of genistein (4',5,7-trihydroxyisoflavone) on the growth and proliferation of testicular cell lines. Biol Cell 1998 Jul; 90(4):349–54.

28 Schweigerer L, Christeleit K, Fleischmann G, Adlercreutz H, et al. Identification in human urine of a natural growth inhibitor for cells derived from solid paediatric tumours. Eur J Clin Invest 1992; 22(4):260–4.

29 Baltuch GH, Yong VW. Signal transduction for proliferation of glioma cells in vitro occurs predominantly through a protein kinase C-mediated pathway. Brain Res 1996 Feb 26; 710(1–2):143–9.

30 Buckley AR, Buckley DJ, Gout PW, Liang H, et al. Inhibition by genistein of prolactin-induced Nb2 lymphoma cell mitogenisis. Mol Cell Endocrinol 1993 Dec; 98(1):17–25.

31 Matsukawa Y, Marui N, Sakai T, Satomi Y, et al. Genistein arrests cell cycle progression at G2-M. Cancer Res 1993; 53(6):1328–31.

32 Hirano T, Gotoh M, Oka K. Natural flavanoids and lignans are potent cytostatic agents against human leukemic HL60 cells. Life Sciences 1994; 55(13):1061–9.

[33] Kuo SM. Antiproliferative potency of structurally distinct dietary flavonoids on human colon cancer cells. Cancer Letters 1996; 110:41–48.

[34] Brown A, Jolly P, Wei H. Genistein modulates neuroblastoma cell proliferation and differentiation through induction of apoptosis and regulation of tyrosine kinase activity and N-myc expression. Carcinogenesis 1998 Jun; 19(6):991–7.

[35] Theodorescu D, Laderoute KR, Calaoagan JM, Gulding KM. Inhibition of human bladder cancer cell motility by genistein is dependent on epidermal growth factor receptor but not p21ras gene expression. Int J Cancer 1998 Dec 9; 78(6):775–82.

[36] Lu HQ, Niggemann B, Zanker KS. Suppression of the proliferation and migration of oncogenic ras-dependent cell lines, cultured in a three-dimensional collagen matrix, by flavonoid-structured molecules. J Cancer Res Clin Oncol 1996; 122(6):335–42.

[37] Fajardo I, Quesada AR, Nunez de Castro I, et al. A comparative study of the effects of genistein and 2-methoxyestradiol on the proteolytic balance and tumour cell proliferation. Br J Cancer 1999 Apr; 80(1–2):17–24.

[38] Huang YT, Hwang JJ, Lee PP, et al. Effects of luteolin and quercetin, inhibitors of tyrosine kinase, on cell growth and metastasis-associated properties in A431 cells overexpressing epidermal growth factor receptor. Br J Pharmacol 1999 Nov; 128(5):999–1010.

[39] Uddin S, Choudhry MA. Quercetin, a bioflavonoid, inhibits the DNA synthesis of human leukemia cells. Biochem Mol Biol Int 1995 Jul; 36(3):545–50.

[40] Xiao D, Zhu SP, Gu ZL. Quercetin induced apoptosis in human leukemia HL-60 cells. Chung Kuo Yao Li Hsueh Pao 1997 May; 18(3):280–3.

[41] Shen F, Weber G. Synergistic action of quercetin and genistein in human ovarian carcinoma cells. Oncol Res 1997; 9(11–12):597–602.

[42] Scambia G, Ranelletti FO, Panici PB, et al. Inhibitory effect of quercetin on OVCA 433 cells and presence of type II oestrogen binding sites in primary ovarian tumours and cultured cells. Br J Cancer 1990 Dec; 62(6):942–6.

[43] Caltagirone S, Ranelletti FO, Rinelli A, et al. Interaction with type II estrogen binding sites and antiproliferative activity of tamoxifen and quercetin in human non-small-cell lung cancer. Am J Respir Cell Mol Biol 1997 Jul; 17(1):51–9.

[44] Kandaswami C, Perkins E, Drzewiecki G, et al. Differential inhibition of proliferation of human squamous cell carcinoma, gliosarcoma and embryonic fibroblast-like lung cells in culture by plant flavonoids. Anticancer Drugs 1992 Oct; 3(5):525–30.

[45] Markaverich BM, Roberts RR, Alejandro MA, et al. Bioflavonoid interaction with rat uterine type II binding sites and cell growth inhibition. J Steroid Biochem 1988; 30(1–6):71–8.

[46] Yoshida M, Sakai T, Hosokawa N, et al. The effect of quercetin on cell cycle progression and growth of human gastric cancer cells. FEBS Lett 1990 Jan 15; 260(1):10–3.

[47] Piantelli M, Rinelli A, Macri E, et al. Type II estrogen binding sites and antiproliferative activity of quercetin in human meningiomas. Cancer 1993 Jan 1; 71(1):193–8.

[48] Scambia G, Ranelletti FO, Benedetti Panici P, et al. Type-II estrogen binding sites in a lymphoblastoid cell line and growth-inhibitory effect of estrogen, anti-estrogen and bioflavonoids. Int J Cancer 1990 Dec 15; 46(6):1112–6.

[49] Piantelli M, Maggiano N, Ricci R, et al. Tamoxifen and quercetin interact with type II estrogen binding sites and inhibit the growth of human melanoma cells. J Invest Dermatol 1995 Aug; 105(2):248–3.

SOFTWARE AND SERVICES

This appendix lists the software and services generously provided to help in preparing this book.

MATHCAD AND AXUM

Mathcad is a robust advanced calculation software package for the technical community. This application tool is designed to solve complex mathematical problems (i.e., linear, nonlinear, quadratic, and mixed-integer programming), create graphs and sketches, and share results via the Internet. Axum is a technical publication-quality graphing and data analysis package used for exploring, customizing, and presenting data. Several of the figures shown in this book were created in Axum, and it was used to perform linear regression analysis for the models discussed in Appendix I.

Contacts:

MathSoft, Inc.
101 Main Street
Cambridge, MA 02142-1521
E-mail: info@mathsoft.com
Web: www.mathsoft.com
Phone: 617-577-1017
Sales: 1-800-628-4223

MOLECULAR MODELING PRO™

Molecular Modeling Pro™ is a 3-D chemical modeling program that allows estimation of over 70 physical descriptors based on chemical structure and also allows structure minimization, structural modeling, and graphical display in several formats. Molecular Modeling Pro™ was used along with the Topix program to generate descriptors for use in the Free Oral Clearance (FOC) model described in Appendix I.

Contacts:

ChemSW, Inc.
420 F Executive Court North
Fairfield, CA 94585-4019
Web: www.chemsw.com
Phone: 707-864-0845

NEUROGENETIC OPTIMIZER

Neurogenetic Optimizer is a neural network development program that uses genetic algorithms to simultaneously optimize the inputs and structure of a neural network. The program can automatically test hundreds of combinations of input variables and neural designs to evolve optimum solutions. Neurogenetic Optimizer was tested as an alternative to standard linear regression analysis for the models discussed in Appendix I.

Contacts:

BioComp Systems, Inc.
4018 148th Ave. NE
Redmond, WA 98052
E-mail: info@biocompsystems.com
Web: www.biocompsystems.com
Phone: (425) 869-6770
Sales: (800) 716-6770

TOPIX

Topix is a program that calculates structural descriptors based on 2-D chemical structures. It calculates both simple descriptors such as ring counts, as well as various substructure and topological descriptors. Topix was used along with Molecular Modeling Pro™ to generate descriptors for the Free Oral Clearance (FOC) model described in Appendix I.

Contacts:

E-mail: helpdesk@lohninger.com
Web: www.lohninger.com

TOPKAT TOXICITY ASSESSMENT

TOPKAT is a software package that computes and automatically validates assessments of toxic and environmental effects of chemicals solely from molecular structure. TOPKAT employs Quantitative Structure Toxicity Relationship (QSTR) models for assessing various measures of toxicity. In addition to selling the TOPKAT program, Oxford Molecular also provides a toxicity assessment service for those who would like to submit individual compounds for analysis. This service provided LD_{50} and LOAEL dose estimates for most of the natural compounds discussed in this book (see Appendix I).

Contacts:

Oxford Molecular Group, Inc.
11350 McCormick Road, Executive Plaza III,
Suite 1100
Hunt Valley, MD 21030
Web: www.oxmol.com
Phone: (410) 527-4500
Sales: (800) 876-9994

WINNONLIN®

WinNonlin® is comprehensive pharmacokinetic, pharmacodynamic, and PK/PD link modeling program that supports both compartmental and noncompartmental analysis. It allows simultaneous fitting of functions and differential equations, complex statistical analysis, analysis and simulation based on predefined and user defined libraries, and complex graphical output. WinNonlin® was used to conduct all pharmacokinetic modeling and produce all pharmacokinetic graphics that appear in this book. WinNonlin® is a registered trademark of Pharsight Corporation.

Contacts:

Pharsight Corporation
800 W. El Camino Real, Suite 200
Mountain View, CA 94040
E-mail: info@pharsight.com
Web: www.pharsight.com
Phone: 650-314-3800

NATURAL COMPOUNDS RESEARCH FUND

This book presents many reasons to believe that natural compounds hold promise in cancer treatment. The field is in its infancy, however, and many new studies are needed. The anticancer effects of natural compounds, both alone and in combination, must be better characterized, and their potential to cause adverse effects must be more fully investigated. Completion of these tasks will require adequate funding, but such funding is not easily obtained through traditional sources. If the ideas and material presented here inspire you, and if you have the ability to help, we need your assistance.

M. D. Anderson Cancer Center at the University of Texas in Houston has agreed to create a fund expressly for donations to further research on natural compounds in cancer treatment. My colleague, Robert A. Newman, Ph.D., Pharmacology Section Chief, will directly oversee this fund. M. D. Anderson Cancer Center is one of the world's leading cancer research institutions; information about it can be found at www.mdanderson.org.

All donations will be deeply appreciated and will help further scientific investigation of nontoxic natural compounds in cancer therapy. For additional information on this fund, please visit the Oregon Medical Press web site at www.ompress.com. Tax-deductible donations can be sent to:

M. D. Anderson Cancer Center
P.O. Box 297153
Houston, Texas 77297
Attention: Natural Compounds Research Fund

1,25-D$_3$	active form of Vitamin D$_3$	m^2	square meters of body surface area
AFR	ascorbate free radical	MAPK	mitogen-activated protein kinase
AP-1	activator protein-1	mg, mM	milligrams, millimoles
ATP	adenosine triphosphate	MHC	major histocompatibility complex
ATRA	all-*trans* retinoic acid	MMP	matrix metalloproteinase
AUC	area under the curve	MRD	maximum recommended dose
bFGF	basic fibroblast growth factor	MTD	maximum tolerated dose
CAM	cell adhesion molecule	NAC	*N*-acetylcysteine
CAPE	caffeic acid phenethyl ester	NADH	reduced nicotinamide adenine dinucleotide
CD	cluster of differentiation (e.g., CD44)	NF-κB	nuclear factor-kappa B
Cdk	cyclin-dependent kinase	ng, nM	nanograms, nanomoles
CL	clearance	NK cell	natural killer cell
COX-1 and -2	cyclooxygenase 1 and 2	NO$^•$	nitric oxide
DADS	diallyl disulfide	NOAEL	no-observable-adverse-effects level
DHA	docosahexaenoic acid	O$_2$	molecular oxygen
DHAsc	dehydroascorbate	O$_2^{•-}$	superoxide radical
DNA	deoxyribonucleic acid	OH$^•$	hydroxyl radical
ECM	extracellular matrix	PDGF	platelet-derived growth factor
EGCG	epigallocatechin gallate	PG	prostaglandin (e.g., PGE$_2$)
EGF	epidermal growth factor	PhK	phosphorylase kinase
EPA	eicosapentaenoic acid	PI kinase	phosphatidylinositol kinase
FGF	fibroblast growth factor	PKC	protein kinase C
FOC	free oral clearance	PSK	polysaccharide K
g	grams	PSP	polysaccharide peptide
GAG	glycosaminoglycan	PTK	protein tyrosine kinase
GGT	gamma-glutamyl transpeptidase	RNA	ribonucleic acid
GM-CSF	granulocyte-macrophage colony stimulating factor	ROS	reactive oxygen species
GTE	green tea extract	SAM	*S*-adenosylmethionine
H$_2$O$_2$	hydrogen peroxide	SECO	secoisolariciresinol
HMGR	hydroxymethylglutaryl-coenzyme A reductase	SHBG	sex hormone binding globulin
I.U.	international units	SOD	superoxide dismutase
IC$_{50}$	50% inhibitory concentration	TGF	transforming growth factor
ICAM	intercellular adhesion molecule	TIMP	tissue inhibitors of metalloproteinase
IFN	interferon	TNF	tumor necrosis factor
IGF	insulin-like growth factor	TOC	total oral clearance
IL	interleukin (e.g., IL-2)	TTFCA	total triterpenic fraction of *Centella asiatica*
kg	kilograms	μg, μM	micrograms, micromoles
LAK	lymphokine-activated killer cell	uPA	urokinase plasminogen activator
LD$_{50}$	lethal dose (in 50% of animals)	VCAM	vascular cell adhesion molecule
LOAEL	lowest-observable-adverse-effects level	VEGF	vascular endothelial growth factor
LT	leukotriene (e.g., LTB$_4$)	VES	vitamin E succinate

INDEX

Page numbers in bold refer to the location of the topic's primary discussion. Page numbers in italics refer to information contained in tables. Please refer to the acronym list for all abbreviations.

ABOUT THE AUTHOR

John Boik received his Masters degree in Acupuncture and Oriental Medicine (MAcOM) from the Oregon College of Oriental Medicine in Portland and his Bachelors degree in civil engineering from the University of Colorado in Boulder. He has been national board certified in both acupuncture and Chinese herbology by the National Commission for the Certification of Acupuncturists (NCCA) and now devotes his full time to writing and research. He currently serves on the Editorial Review Board for the journal *Alternative Medicine Review*. This is his second book, his first being *Cancer and Natural Medicine: A Textbook of Basic Science and Clinical Research*.